Lippincott's
Textbook for
PERSONAL SUPPORT WORKERS

BRIEF CONTENTS

Unit 1   **Introduction to Health Care**   1

Chapter 1   The Canadian Health Care System   3
Chapter 2   The Personal Support Worker   14
Chapter 3   Professionalism and Job-Seeking Skills   25
Chapter 4   Legal and Ethical Issues   45
Chapter 5   Communication Skills   57
Chapter 6   Those We Care For   80

Unit 2   **Safety**   101

Chapter 7   Communicable Disease and Infection Control   103
Chapter 8   Bloodborne and Airborne Pathogens   130
Chapter 9   Workplace Safety   140
Chapter 10   Patient and Resident Safety and Restraints   160
Chapter 11   Positioning, Lifting, and Transferring Patients and Residents   179
Chapter 12   Basic First Aid and Emergency Care   213

Unit 3   **Basic Patient and Resident Care**   233

Chapter 13   The Patient or Resident Environment   235
Chapter 14   Admissions, Transfers, and Discharges   250
Chapter 15   Bedmaking   262
Chapter 16   Vital Signs, Height, and Weight   278
Chapter 17   Cleanliness and Hygiene   313
Chapter 18   Grooming   348
Chapter 19   Basic Nutrition   371
Chapter 20   Assisting With Urinary and Bowel Elimination   396

Unit 4   **Death and Dying**   433

Chapter 21   Caring for People Who Are Terminally Ill   435
Chapter 22   Caring for People Who Are Dying   445

Unit 5   **Structure and Function of the Human Body**   463

Chapter 23   Basic Body Structure and Function   465
Chapter 24   The Integumentary System   481

Chapter 25   The Musculoskeletal System   505
Chapter 26   The Respiratory System   540
Chapter 27   The Cardiovascular System   564
Chapter 28   The Nervous System   582
Chapter 29   The Sensory System   597
Chapter 30   The Endocrine System   619
Chapter 31   The Digestive System   632
Chapter 32   The Urinary System   647
Chapter 33   The Reproductive System   660

Unit 6   **Special Care Concerns**   677

Chapter 34   Caring for People With Developmental Disabilities   679
Chapter 35   Caring for People With Mental Illness   690
Chapter 36   Caring for People With Dementia   703
Chapter 37   Caring for People With Cancer   720
Chapter 38   Caring for People With HIV/AIDS   730

Unit 7   **Acute Care**   739

Chapter 39   Caring for Surgical Patients   741
Chapter 40   Caring for Mothers and Newborns   759
Chapter 41   Caring for Pediatric Patients   775

Unit 8   **Home Health Care**   789

Chapter 42   Introduction to Home Health Care   791
Chapter 43   Safety and Infection Control in the Home Health Care Setting   803

Glossary   815
Appendix A   Answers to the What Did You Learn? Exercises   835

Appendix B   Introduction to the Language of Health Care   837

Index   849

Lippincott's

Textbook for PERSONAL SUPPORT WORKERS

A Humanistic Approach to Caregiving

CANADIAN EDITOR

Marilyn A. McGreer, BSc, LPN
Career Coach
Bredin Institute Health Career Program for the Internationally Educated Health Professionals
Former (2004–2009) Coordinator of the Health Care Aide Program, Instructor, and Instructional
  Assistant in the Practical Nurse Program
NorQuest College
Edmonton, Alberta, Canada

Pamela J. Carter, RN, BSN, MeD, CNOR
Program Coordinator/Instructor
School of Health Professions
Davis Applied Technology College
Kaysville, Utah

Wolters Kluwer | Lippincott Williams & Wilkins
Health
Philadelphia • Baltimore • New York • London
Buenos Aires • Hong Kong • Sydney • Tokyo

Executive Acquisitions Editor: Elizabeth Nieginski
Development Editor: Melanie Cann
Product Manager: Laura Scott
Design Coordinator: Holly McLaughlin
Illustration Coordinator: Brett MacNaughton
Manufacturing Coordinator: Karin Duffield
Prepress Vendor: Aptara, Inc.

10 9 8 7 6 5 4 3 2

Printed in USA.

Library of Congress Cataloging-in-Publication Data

Carter, Pamela J.
 Lippincott's textbook for personal support workers : a humanistic
approach to caregiving / Pamela J. Carter ; Marilyn A. McGreer, Canadian editor.
   p. ; cm.
 Other title: Textbook for personal support workers
 Canadian adaptation of: Lippincott's textbook for nursing assistants.
2nd ed. c2008.
 Includes index.
 ISBN 978-1-60831-170-5
 1. Nurses' aides—Canada. I. McGreer, Marilyn A. II. Carter, Pamela J. Lippincott's
textbook for nursing assistants. III. Title. IV. Title: Textbook for personal support workers.
 [DNLM: 1. Nurses' Aides—Canada. 2. Caregivers—Canada. 3. Nursing
Care—Canada. WY 193 L324LT 2011]
 RT84.C3685 2011
 610.7306'98—dc22

                                                                    2010018490

Care has been taken to confirm the accuracy of the information presented and to describe generally accepted practices. However, the author(s), editors, and publisher are not responsible for errors or omissions or for any consequences from application of the information in this book and make no warranty, expressed or implied, with respect to the currency, completeness, or accuracy of the contents of the publication. Application of this information in a particular situation remains the professional responsibility of the practitioner; the clinical treatments described and recommended may not be considered absolute and universal recommendations.

The author(s), editors, and publisher have exerted every effort to ensure that drug selection and dosage set forth in this text are in accordance with the current recommendations and practice at the time of publication. However, in view of ongoing research, changes in government regulations, and the constant flow of information relating to drug therapy and drug reactions, the reader is urged to check the package insert for each drug for any change in indications and dosage and for added warnings and precautions. This is particularly important when the recommended agent is a new or infrequently employed drug.

Some drugs and medical devices presented in this publication have Food and Drug Administration (FDA) clearance for limited use in restricted research settings. It is the responsibility of the health care provider to ascertain the FDA status of each drug or device planned for use in his or her clinical practice.

LWW.com

ABOUT THE AUTHORS

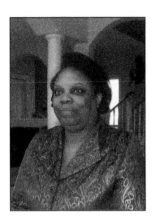

Marilyn McGreer is a home economist and licensed practical nurse. She holds a bachelor of science degree in home economics—specialization family studies—from the University of Alberta, and a licensed practical nurse certificate with a specialty in immunization, from NorQuest College. She also holds certificates in prenatal training and early childhood education.

She recently worked as the coordinator for NorQuest College in Edmonton, Alberta, where she managed and supervised the delivery of the Health Care Aide Program, which won the 2007 award for team excellence. In this role she supervised personal support worker instructors and represented the college working with external stakeholders on various committees, including a curriculum committee of the Association of Canadian Community Colleges. While at NorQuest, she helped to develop an admission test and personal support worker program for students in the English-as-a-second-language program. Her health care experience includes work as a medication nurse, complex care in an adult day program, geriatric care, and acute care. She has also taught courses for a private vocational college in medical administration, anatomy and physiology, and early childhood, and has worked as an instructional assistant in the practical nurse program at NorQuest College.

She holds a professional membership in the Alberta Human Ecology and Home Economics Association and is currently chair of the Fredrickson-McGregor Education Foundation for Licensed Practical Nurses in Alberta. She is a career coach at Bredin Institute in Edmonton, Alberta, where she guides internationally educated health professionals through their registration and licensure process, to obtain credentials for employment in the Canadian health care system.

She is passionate about lifelong learning and enjoys working with culturally diverse populations.

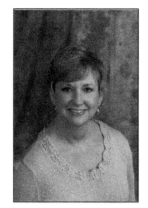

Pamela Carter is a registered nurse and an award-winning teacher. After receiving her bachelor's degree in nursing from the University of Alabama in Huntsville, she immediately began a career as a perioperative nurse. Over the course of her nursing career, she also worked in a physician's office and as a staff nurse in an intensive care unit.

She started teaching informally while serving as an officer in the U.S. Air Force Nurse Corps. She formally entered the field of health care education by accepting a position at the Athens Area Technical Institute in Athens, Georgia, where she taught surgical technology. After obtaining a master's degree in adult vocational education from the University of Georgia, she moved to Florida and took a position teaching nursing assisting students. She continued teaching nursing assisting after accepting a position at Davis Applied Technology College in Kaysville, Utah. During her first year at Davis Applied Technology College, she piloted a new "open-entry/open-exit" method of curriculum delivery for the nursing assistant program at the college and was awarded the superintendent's Award for Outstanding Faculty for her work. She then opened a surgical technology program at the college and has obtained national accreditation from the Commission on Accreditation of Allied Health Education Programs (CAAHEP) for delivery of this program using the "open-entry/open-exit" method. In 2002, she received a National Merit Award for having her program rank in the top 10% in the nation for students passing their national certification exam.

In addition to writing *Lippincott's Textbook for Nursing Assistants*, the original U.S. edition from which this textbook was adapted, she has also authored *Lippincott's Essentials for Nursing Assistants*, *Lippincott's Advanced Skills for Nursing Assistants*, and *Lippincott's Textbook for Long-Term Care Nursing Assistants*. Pamela's writing style reflects her love of teaching, and of nursing. She is grateful for the opportunity that teaching and writing have afforded her to share her experience and knowledge with those just entering the health care profession, and to help those who are new to the profession to see how they can have a profound effect on the lives of others.

A very special thanks to my family. My husband, Ted, for his ongoing support and belief in my abilities. My beautiful daughters, Priscilla, for the stimulating discussions and emotional support, and Sarah, for her bright spirit and wonderful cooking. My son, Sebastian, for his logical mind and warm heart. To my own dear mother and my sisters Janet, Norma, and Sharon, thank you for your prayers, kind words, and unceasing encouragement. I love you all! To all the many students who have taught me so much over the years—thank you, you are all very dear to me.

M.A.M.

To all of the instructors who teach personal support workers—you give so much of yourselves to your students. Not only do you introduce them to the health care profession, you also mentor them, guide them, and inspire them to become the future of humanistic care.

P.J.C.

LETTER FROM THE CANADIAN EDITOR

I am proud to be the Canadian Editor of *Lippincott's Textbook for Personal Support Workers: A Humanistic Approach to Caregiving.* This book has been adapted for the personal support worker who is employed in Canada in private or public health care facilities or in a client's home. The purpose is to provide the instructor and the student a reference book that reflects our Canadian health care system and its health care practices. The health care language of the textbook is consistent with the values and principles enshrined in the Canadian Charter of Rights and Freedoms. It addresses the uniqueness of each health care jurisdiction provincially and territorially and outlines legislation applicable to those regions, including the code of ethics for persons in care. Each chapter is carefully designed to allow the student an opportunity to apply reflective practice thinking.

Across the country the personal support worker is recognized as an important contributor to the health care system. In some jurisdictions a special event is set aside to celebrate and recognize the contribution that the personal support worker provides as a member of the care team. It is my intention that this textbook supports and endorses the contribution of the personal support worker across the country. This Canadian adaptation is written to address the personal support worker's educational needs, including knowledge of the historical origin of the Canadian health care system, the early developments of the Canada Health Act, Canada's Privacy Law, and Canada's First Nation's traditional medicinal practices.

My sincere desire is that this textbook will be embraced and used in classrooms across the country where personal support worker education and training is delivered with the same enthusiasm and excitement that I had adapting this textbook for the Canadian market.

Marilyn McGreer

PREFACE

Personal support worker education is changing. Indeed, it must change if we are to keep pace with the needs of the health care industry. Today, the number of personal support workers employed by hospitals, acute and extended care facilities, hospice agencies, and home health care agencies is growing rapidly. In addition, the composition of the long-term care population (the population most frequently cared for by personal support workers) is changing. Shorter hospital stays and advances in medicine and technology mean that today's long-term care resident tends to be older, sicker, and in need of more assistance with activities of daily living than the resident of 15 years ago. As educators, we must seek to provide our students with the skills and knowledge that they will need to meet the changing needs of their patients, residents, and clients and to advance in their own careers.

In the past, the focus of personal support worker education was on skill competency. However, that focus is shifting now toward graduating personal support workers who not only possess the technical skills they need to provide competent care, but also the compassion and the communication and critical thinking skills they need to function effectively in the health care setting. It is no longer enough for personal support workers to be competent at changing bed linens and measuring vital signs. Today's personal support worker must also be able to recognize the person within the patient, resident, or client and to understand that each person they are responsible for providing care for is unique and special, with individual needs that are very different from those of the person in the next bed. This textbook, *Lippincott's Textbook for Personal Support Workers*, has been written not only to help students develop the skills they need to become personal support workers, but also to introduce them to a very humanistic approach to caregiving.

THEMES AND FEATURES

Three key beliefs informed the writing of this textbook:

1. Students need a textbook that captures their interest and increases their desire to learn.
2. Graduates of personal support worker training programs must be able to provide competent, skilled care in a compassionate way.
3. The personal support worker is a vital member of the health care team.

These beliefs form the basis for the textbook you hold in your hands.

WRITTEN WITH THE STUDENT IN MIND

One of the primary goals in writing this textbook was to make the information it contains interesting and accessible to the student. Great care has been taken to present the student with a textbook that is easy and enjoyable to read, with a well-developed art program and proven learning aids.

A Student-Focused Writing Style

Educators know that a student can easily understand complex information if it is explained in a way that the student can understand. *Lippincott's Textbook for Personal Support Workers* uses a conversational, yet professional, writing style that respects the student's intelligence. Concepts are presented in a straightforward, accessible way, and the text is enlivened through the frequent use of examples and anecdotes from the author's own experience with patients and residents. Recognizing that many students entering personal support worker training programs speak English as a second language or are resource students, each chapter has been thoroughly reviewed by a special needs consultant to ensure an appropriate reading level.

An Art Program Developed Alongside the Text

The purpose of an art program is to reinforce and expand on concepts discussed in the text. To do this effectively, the art must be planned and developed alongside the manuscript. Numerous photographs, both alone and in combination with line art that has been created specifically for this textbook, help students to visualize and remember important concepts.

Proven Learning Aids in Every Chapter

Learning and remembering new information is challenging for many students. To help them meet the challenge of mastering the information in the textbook, we have developed features to assist students with studying and internalizing information:

- **What Will You Learn?** Each chapter begins with a "What Will You Learn?" section, which previews the chapter and helps to focus the student's reading. Each "What Will You Learn?" section begins with a paragraph that introduces the topic of the chapter to the student and explains why the topic is important. This introductory paragraph is then followed by a list of learning objectives and vocabulary words.
- **Summary.** Each chapter ends with a summary in a unique narrative outline format. This summary helps students to review the key, "take home" concepts of the chapter.
- **What Did You Learn?** Multiple-choice and matching exercises at the end of each chapter provide students with the opportunity to evaluate their understanding of the material they have just studied. Answers to these exercises are given in Appendix A.
- **Highlighted figure, table, and box call-outs.** The references to figures, tables, and boxes are highlighted with colour in the narrative, helping students to quickly find their place in the text after stopping to look at a figure, table, or box.

DESIGNED TO PREPARE STUDENTS FOR CLINICAL PRACTICE

It is the author's desire to help prepare students to enter the health care profession with the knowledge, skills, and confidence that education and training can provide. Several of the textbook's features were designed specifically to help prepare the student for clinical practice:

- **Procedures.** Certainly, a major objective of any personal support worker training course is to ensure that graduates are able to provide care in a safe and correct manner. Seventy-eight core procedures are presented in this text. The procedures for each chapter are grouped at the end of the chapter to avoid breaking up the text with lengthy boxes. Each procedure box begins with a "Why You Do It" statement, to help students understand the "why behind the what," an understanding that is the foundation for the development of critical thinking skills. The concepts of privacy, safety, infection control, comfort, and communication are emphasized consistently in every procedure. "Getting Ready" and "Finishing Up" steps are included in every procedure box to help students remember these very important pre- and post-procedure actions. The steps of the procedure are given using clear and concise language, and photographs and illustrations are provided as necessary. An icon identifies procedures that are demonstrated on *Lippincott's Video Series for Nursing Assistants.*
- **Guidelines Boxes.** These boxes summarize general guidelines for various aspects of the personal support worker's job. The unique "What You Do/Why You Do It" format helps students to understand why things are done a certain way. Rather than just presenting students with an endless list of guidelines to memorize, these boxes help them to remember why these guidelines are important to follow.
- **Tell the Nurse! Notes.** A recurrent theme throughout the book is the important role the personal support worker plays in making observations about a patient's or resident's condition and reporting these observations to the nurse. The "Tell the Nurse!" notes highlight and summarize signs and symptoms that a personal support worker may observe that should be reported to the nurse.
- **Stop and Think! Scenarios.** Each chapter concludes with one or more "Stop and Think!" scenarios. These scenarios, which are excellent tools for initiating classroom discussion, encourage students to think critically to solve problems and help them to see

that many situations they will encounter in the workplace do not have cut-and-dried answers.

- **Helping Hands and a Caring Heart: Focus on Humanistic Health Care Boxes.** These boxes, found throughout the text, encourage students to empathize with those in their care, and emphasize the importance of meeting patients' and residents' emotional and spiritual needs, as well as their physical needs.

INSTILLS IN STUDENTS PRIDE IN THEMSELVES AND THEIR CHOSEN PROFESSION

It is important to impress upon students entering the health care profession that no one is "just" a personal support worker. Personal support workers are often the members of the health care team with the most day-to-day contact with patients, residents, and clients. As such, they bear a large part of the responsibility for the well-being of those in their care. To highlight the contributions that personal support workers make, each unit in the textbook concludes with a patient's, resident's, client's, or family member's first-person account of how a personal support worker had a positive impact on their lives or the lives of their loved ones. The goal of these "Personal Support Workers Make a Difference!" stories is to help students to see that personal support workers are vital members of the health care team. Personal support workers who feel that they can and do make a difference in the lives of others will go the "extra mile" to ensure that the care they provide is humanistic.

AN OVERVIEW OF *LIPPINCOTT'S TEXTBOOK FOR PERSONAL SUPPORT WORKERS*

Lippincott's Textbook for Personal Support Workers is a comprehensive textbook, designed to prepare students to work as personal support workers in any health care setting, as well as to open their eyes to the many career opportunities that exist within the health care field and to entice them to further their learning. Canada is in the midst of a health care crisis—profound demographic changes have led to an ever-widening

gap between the number of people who need care and the number of people who are qualified to provide that care. Educators of future health care professionals are charged with providing the community with competent, dedicated, compassionate caregivers. In recognition of this need, this textbook has been designed to be in accordance with standards for curriculum development established by each provincial and territorial government legislation responsible for the oversight of health care practices and education in Canada.

A lifelong interest in learning new information is an important quality for any health care professional to have, as the body of information related to medicine and health care is constantly evolving. A lifelong interest in learning benefits the recipients of care as well as the caregivers themselves. Awareness of career pathways allows those just entering the health care profession to set goals for career advancement and reach them, over time receiving higher levels of compensation for higher levels of experience, skills, and responsibilities.

This textbook consists of eight units. The following is a brief survey of these units and the information they contain.

UNIT 1: INTRODUCTION TO HEALTH CARE

The six chapters that make up Unit 1 provide the student with basic background knowledge. Chapter 1 begins with an overview of how health care has evolved, and continues to evolve, in Canada. It then provides the student with a basic understanding of how the governmental regulations that control health care standards and payment came into existence. Chapter 1 also provides an overview of the many different types of health care facilities, and introduces the idea of holistic, humanistic health care and the "health care team." Chapter 2 focuses on the personal support worker's roles and responsibilities as a member of the health care team, and on the concept of delegation. Professionalism, the concept of work ethic, and job-seeking skills are thoroughly discussed in Chapter 3, introducing students to the idea that a professional attitude promotes respect and is necessary for career advancement. Legal and ethical issues, including patient and resident rights, are covered in Chapter 4. Communication, one of the most essential responsibilities of the personal support worker, is discussed in Chapter 5. This unit concludes with

Chapter 6, which focuses on the central member of the health care team—the patient, resident, or client. This final chapter introduces the concept of human needs and explains how the person being cared for in a health care setting has many needs other than those specifically associated with illness or disability.

UNIT 2: SAFETY

The six chapters that compose Unit 2 are concerned with the measures taken to ensure safety. Chapters 7 and 8 cover communicable disease, and how the spread of communicable disease is prevented in the health care setting. Chapter 9 deals with workplace safety, and includes an extensive discussion about the importance of using proper body mechanics to prevent work-related injuries. Also in Chapter 9, the student is introduced to the "Getting Ready" and "Finishing Up" steps that are taken before and after each procedure. Chapter 10 explores some of the conditions that put patients, residents, or clients at risk for injury, followed by a discussion about methods used to prevent accidents from occurring. In Chapter 11, the techniques used to safely assist patients, residents, and clients with repositioning and transferring are covered. This unit concludes with Chapter 12, which contains information related to recognizing emergencies and responding to them.

UNIT 3: BASIC PATIENT AND RESIDENT CARE

The eight chapters in this unit focus on the skills and equipment used to provide basic daily care to patients, residents, and clients. Chapters 13 and 14 introduce the student to the health care environment and explain the processes for admitting, transferring, or discharging patients, residents, and clients. Chapter 15 covers bedmaking. Chapter 16 covers vital signs, with an emphasis on exactly what function of the body is being measured and situations that may alter these measurements. Also included are practical tips to take the mystery out of taking vital sign measurements, procedures that many students find intimidating and difficult to master at first. Chapters 17 and 18 cover bathing and grooming, with a focus on empathizing with the person receiving the care. In Chapter 19, the Canada Food Guide is reviewed, along with basic information about nutrition and the personal support worker's role in assisting patients or residents

with meeting their nutritional needs. We conclude Unit 3 with Chapter 20, a discussion about assisting with elimination. Again, much emphasis is placed on empathizing with the patient, resident, or client who requires assistance with this most intimate of activities.

UNIT 4: DEATH AND DYING

This unit has been written as two separate chapters to emphasize that a person may cope with a terminal illness and the stages of grief for a long period of time before the actual physical process of dying takes place. Chapter 21 introduces the student to the stages of grief within the context of a discussion about terminal illness. Important concepts such as advance directives, wills, and palliative care are also introduced in this chapter. Chapter 22 focuses on the care a personal support worker provides to the dying person and his or her family members in the hours immediately leading up to, and following, death. Both chapters in this unit include discussions about the grief a personal support worker can expect to feel when a patient, resident, or client dies or receives a diagnosis of a terminal illness.

UNIT 5: STRUCTURE AND FUNCTION OF THE HUMAN BODY

Having a basic understanding of how each of the body's organ systems functions in health is essential to understanding how failure of an organ system to work properly leads to disease and disability. This unit begins with Chapter 23, which provides an overview of the body's organization and introduces the student to rehabilitation and restorative care as methods used to restore function when function has been changed or lost. The next 10 chapters (Chapters 24 through 33) each cover one of the organ systems. A basic explanation of the normal structure and function of the organ system is given, with an emphasis on homeostasis. Next, the normal effects of aging are discussed and differentiated from the effects of disease and disability. Key disorders specific to that particular body system are then discussed. Diagnostic tests and treatments are covered next, along with rehabilitation and restorative care measures specific to the organ system under discussion. Throughout these chapters, the personal support worker's role in recognizing problems and providing care is emphasized.

UNIT 6: SPECIAL CARE CONCERNS

This unit, which consists of five chapters, introduces the student to the special needs of certain groups of people. In Chapter 34, some of the major types of developmental disabilities are reviewed. Chapter 35 is dedicated to a discussion about mental illness, including the importance of recognizing depression in elderly patients, residents, and clients. In Chapter 36, the student is introduced to the idea of dementia, and provided with specific information about how to communicate with, and care for, people who have this devastating condition. Chapter 37 discusses the diagnosis and treatment of cancer, as well as the special needs of people with cancer. The final chapter in this unit, Chapter 38, discusses the special needs of the person who is HIV-positive or has AIDS.

UNIT 7: ACUTE CARE

Personal support workers provide care in many different types of health care settings. Many work in hospitals and clinics and assist nurses in caring for patients with acute conditions. The focus of the three chapters in Unit 7 is on special populations of patients that the personal support worker may encounter in the acute care setting. Chapter 39 is dedicated to the surgical patient, Chapter 40 to obstetrical patients and newborns, and Chapter 41 to the pediatric patient.

UNIT 8: HOME HEALTH CARE

The two chapters in this final unit introduce the student to the home health care setting. Building on the basic knowledge and skills presented in previous units, this unit explores some of the concerns and issues that are unique to the home health care setting. Chapter 42 provides the student with an overview of what home health care is, who might require it, and how it is paid for, and explores some of the qualities that a person must have to succeed as a home support worker. Chapter 43 covers specific issues related to safety and infection control within the home.

GLOSSARY AND APPENDICES

The textbook concludes with two appendices and a comprehensive glossary. Appendix A contains the answers to the "What Did You Learn?" exercises that appear at the end of each chapter.

Appendix B introduces the student to the language of health care. We chose to include this discussion about medical terminology as an appendix so that it could be introduced at any point during the training course and referred to frequently. The tables containing common roots, prefixes, suffixes, and abbreviations are in close physical proximity to the glossary for easy and quick reference.

The glossary is the most comprehensive found in any personal support worker textbook. A precise definition of each vocabulary word is given. The number in parentheses at the end of each entry indicates the chapter where the term is introduced as a vocabulary word. Extensive cross-references remind students of synonyms and antonyms and help them to differentiate related words.

A COMPREHENSIVE PACKAGE FOR TEACHING AND LEARNING

To further facilitate teaching and learning, a carefully designed ancillary package is available. In addition to the usual print resources, we are pleased to present multimedia tools that have been developed in conjunction with the text.

RESOURCES FOR STUDENTS

- **Student Resource CD-ROM and thePoint.** Interactive learning resources are provided on the CD-ROM packaged with the textbook at no additional charge. Students can also access these resources on thePoint at http://thePoint.lww.com/McGreer1e using the codes printed in the front of their textbooks. Features include:
  - *Watch and Learn!* —A series of video clips that support information given in the text.
  - *Personal Support Workers Make a Difference!*—A feature that allows the student to listen to first-person accounts of how personal support workers have made a difference in the lives of patients, residents, clients, and family members.
- ***Workbook for Lippincott's Textbook for Personal Support Workers.*** This workbook provides the student with a fun and engaging way of reviewing important

concepts and vocabulary. Multiple-choice questions, matching exercises, true-false exercises, word finds, crossword puzzles, colouring and labelling exercises, and other types of active-learning tools are provided to appeal to many different learning styles. The workbook also contains procedure checklists for each procedure in the textbook.

RESOURCES FOR INSTRUCTORS

Tools to assist you with teaching your course are available upon adoption of this text on thePoint, at http://thePoint.lww.com/McGreer1e and on the Instructor's Resource DVD-ROM:

- The **Test Generator** lets you put together exclusive new tests from a bank containing nearly 1,000 multiple-choice questions to help you assess your students' understanding of the material.
- An extensive collection of materials is provided for each book chapter:
  - **Pre-Lecture Quizzes** (and answers) are quick, knowledge-based assessments that allow you to check students' reading.
  - **PowerPoint Presentations** provide an easy way for you to integrate the textbook with your students' classroom experience, via either slide shows or handouts.
  - **Guided Lecture Notes** walk you through the chapters, objective by objective, and provide you with corresponding PowerPoint slide numbers.
  - **Discussion Topics** (and suggested answers) can be used as conversation starters or in online discussion boards.
  - **Assignments** (and suggested answers) include group, written, clinical, and web assignments.
- An **Image Bank** lets you use the photographs and illustrations from this textbook in your PowerPoint slides or as you see fit in your course.
- **Discussion Points for the Stop and Think! Scenarios** in the book are provided to guide discussion.
- **Answers to the exercises in the Workbook for Lippincott's Textbook**

for Personal Support Workers are provided.
- Information about classroom management, including a **sample syllabus,** is available.

ADDITIONAL RESOURCES

- *Lippincott's Video Series for Nursing Assistants.* Procedure-based modules provide step-by-step demonstrations of the core skills that form the basis of the daily care the personal support worker provides. "Getting Ready" and "Finishing Up" actions are reviewed on every procedure-based module, and the concepts of privacy, safety, infection control, comfort, and communication are emphasized throughout. Four non-procedure–based modules, on the topics of preparing for entry into the workforce, caring for people with dementia, death and dying, and communication and patient and resident rights, are also available.
- **Copper Ridge *Dementia Care Modules.*** Developed by the esteemed Copper Ridge Institute in affiliation with Johns Hopkins University School of Medicine, this two CD set consists of nine interactive modules designed to teach students how to care for people with dementia. The causes and types of dementia are reviewed, along with dementia-related behaviours and the best way to manage them. Communication and compassion are emphasized throughout. Learning is enhanced through video clips, interactive exercises, and short multiple-choice quizzes at the conclusion of each module.

It is with great pleasure that the authors and publisher introduce these resources—the textbook, the ancillary package, the videos, and the Copper Ridge modules—to you. One of our primary goals in creating these resources has been to share with those just entering the health care field our sense of excitement about the health care profession, and our commitment to the idea that being a personal support worker involves much more than just "bedpans and blood pressures." We hope we have succeeded in that goal, and we welcome your feedback.

TO THE STUDENT

Welcome! By enrolling in this personal support worker training course, you have taken a big first step. You may be taking this course for any number of different reasons. For example, you may be taking this course to "test the waters"—to see if working in health care is something you really want to do. Or, you may already know that you want to work in health care, and you are taking this course because it is the first step toward reaching your goal.

Health care is an exciting, yet demanding, field. During your training course, you will be expected to learn and apply a lot of new information. You will even have to learn a new language, the language of health care! I am Pam Carter, and I am the author of the U.S. textbook from which this Canadian textbook was adapted. It is my pleasure and honor to assist you on your journey toward becoming a health care professional.

HOW TO USE THE BOOK TO PREPARE FOR CLASS AND STUDY

Learning is an active process. You need to read, take notes, and ask questions about anything you are having trouble understanding. Most students who are successful learners take a three-step approach to learning:

PREVIEW

During the *preview* stage of learning, you focus on preparing yourself for class. Most likely, your instructor will give you reading assignments that must be completed before each class. The course *syllabus* that you will receive at the beginning of the course will tell you when each reading assignment must be completed. The reading assignments give you the chance to get a general idea of what is going to be discussed in the next class.

To prepare for class, just read the assignment as if you were reading a novel or a newspaper for enjoyment. As you read the chapter, look for the "Watch and Learn!" icon too. This symbol lets you know that you can use the CD-ROM in the front of your book to watch a video clip that supports the information you are reading about. During the preview, you do not need to take notes or try to memorize facts—just read through the material to get the "big picture" of the information you are about to learn. Some people find it helpful to read the chapter out loud to themselves (or into a tape recorder, so that they can listen to the chapter again later). Others like to highlight parts of the chapter using a highlighting pen, or make notes in the margin. Learning becomes much easier when you discover what methods work best for you.

To assist you with previewing, each chapter in the book begins with a "What Will You Learn?" section. This section contains a list of specific goals for the chapter, called *learning objectives*. Learning objectives tell you what you will be expected to know or be able to do to demonstrate complete understanding of the material in the chapter. During the preview stage, the learning objectives are useful for giving you an overview of the key goals of the chapter.

The "What Will You Learn?" section also contains a list of the new vocabulary words you will need to learn. The vocabulary words, which appear in **bold type** throughout the chapter, are listed in the order that they appear. You can look each word up in the glossary at the back of the book to find a complete definition. Familiarizing yourself with the chapter's vocabulary words before class puts you one step ahead, because when you hear those words in class, they will not sound strange to you, and you may already know what they mean.

VIEW

The *viewing* stage is when you get down to business and really work to understand the material. During the classroom lecture or discussion, highlight important points and take notes as you need to. Ask questions about any of the material that you do not fully understand. Remember, there are no "stupid" questions! If you do not fully understand something, you need to speak up so that the instructor can help you. This is your instructor's job.

REVIEW

After class, go back over the notes you took in class, and re-read the chapter in your book. Some students like to read the entire chapter over again. Others just skim the chapter, paying close attention to the topics they still have questions about. Read the chapter summary, which reviews the key concepts of the chapter. If you are using the student workbook in your class, complete the exercises by looking the answers up in the textbook chapter. Looking for the answers is another way of reviewing the information in the chapter, and many students find that the act of writing the answers down helps them to remember the information.

When you feel comfortable with your understanding of the material, test yourself! Go back to the learning objectives in the "What Will You Learn?" section at the beginning of the chapter and pretend they are questions. Try to answer them. If you have trouble answering them, then you know you need to review certain parts of the chapter again. You can also test yourself using the "What Did You Learn?" section, at the end of each chapter. The answers to the questions in the "What Did You Learn?" section are in Appendix A in the back of the book so that you can see how well you understood the material you just studied. Again, if you have trouble answering these questions, then you will know that your studying is not quite finished! You may need to read certain parts of the chapter again, or ask your instructor for help.

Try to set aside short periods of time for studying each day. For example, you might study for 30 to 45 minutes, take a break to attend to other activities or chores, and then come back and study for another 30 to 45 minutes. After 30 to 45 minutes of studying, most people become tired and lose their ability to concentrate. Studying in short bursts will help keep you focused on the material you are trying to learn.

HOW TO PREPARE FOR TESTS

Did you learn the material or not? This is what instructors want to know when they give tests, quizzes, and exams. Not doing well on a test does not mean that you are a failure. It just means that you need to figure out what went wrong, and make an effort to improve the next time. Perhaps you did not study as well as you could have for the test. Or maybe you got so nervous, you forgot everything you learned when it came time to take the test!

The course syllabus will tell you when a test is scheduled to be given, and what material it will cover. Mark these dates on your calendar, so you are not surprised! Preparing for a test should not be a major event. If you use the preview–view–review approach and study each day, when it comes time to prepare for the test, you will be very well prepared. In the days leading up to the test, all you will need to do is review the material that will be covered on the test one more time, by skimming the chapters in the book and reviewing the notes you took in class.

When it comes time to actually take the test, remember the following tips:

- Relax! You have prepared for this test, and you know the answers to these questions!
- Take a deep breath and make sure you read the directions carefully. The directions will tell you whether there is only one correct answer for each question, or whether it is possible for a question to have more than one correct answer.
- Read each question completely and carefully. Many students answer questions incorrectly simply because they are in a hurry and miss important words, like "except" or "not."
- If the question is a multiple-choice question, try to state the answer in your head before looking at the answer choices. Then read each answer choice before choosing the one that best matches the answer you have in your head. This will increase your confidence that the answer you have selected is the correct one.
- After selecting an answer, avoid second-guessing yourself. Research has shown that

your first choice is most likely to be correct, if you studied the material well. Sometimes, however, you will come across a question later in the test that makes you realize that you answered an earlier question incorrectly. In this case, when you are sure that you have made a mistake, it is all right to go back and change your answer. But if you do not have a clear idea of what the correct answer is, doubting your first choice will most likely result in changing a correct answer to an incorrect one!

• If you cannot answer a question, go on to the next. Often, another question on the test will jog your memory and help you to remember the answer to the question you skipped earlier. Just remember to go back over your answer sheet before you hand in your test to make sure you have answered all of the questions.

Many people think that the goal of studying is to pass a test. It is true that as you work through your training course, you will have to pass many tests. And some provinces and territories require people who want to be personal support workers to pass a certification exam at the end of the training course. But passing the test is a short-term goal. It is more important for you to be able to remember and use the information that you learned during your training course long after you complete the course and pass the certification exam. The people you will be caring for are depending on you to be knowledgeable and good at what you do. They are trusting you with their health and well-being. Study hard, ask questions, and remember that each and every person you care for throughout your career deserves the same type of competent, compassionate care that you would expect to be given to your own mother, father, spouse, sibling, or child. As a personal support worker, you will have the chance to have a positive effect on the lives of many people.

Caring for those in need is very important work. As a personal support worker, your role is an emotionally supportive one that will expose you to the best and worst of people and situations. But with the proper basic nursing skills, knowledge, and experience, your career will be very rewarding. The more you learn, the more effective you will be in your career. Remember, learning is a lifelong process. I wish you every success as you begin your journey as a personal support worker.

Pam Carter

REVIEWERS OF THIS EDITION

Many thanks to the Canadian instructors who read the manuscript during its various stages of development and provided us with valuable suggestions for improving it:

DEBRA BELL, RNA
Teacher Assistance in Health Care Facilities
Lennoxville Vocational Training Centre
Lennoxville, Quebec, Canada

Mary C. BOIVIN, RN, BA
Clinical Coordinator
Personal Support Worker Program
Cambrian College of Applied Arts & Technology
Sudbury, Ontario, Canada

VALERIE BROWN
Personal Support Worker Program
Georgian College
Ontario, Canada

KELLY BUTLER, RN, BScN, BEd, MScN
Professor, Nursing
Lambton College
Sarnia, Ontario, Canada

JENNIFER LAW, RPN, RN, BScN
Professor of Nursing
Hunter Institute of Technology & Advanced
  Learning
Toronto, Ontario, Canada

LINDA POIRIER, RN, BScN, MHS
Nursing Professor
Sir Sandford Fleming College
Peterborough, Ontario

MARY POWER, RN
Coordinator, Personal Support Worker Program
St. Clair College
Windsor, Ontario, Canada

TRACI PREISTLY, RN
Instructor, Healthcare Programs
Robertson College
Red River Community College
Winnipeg, Manitoba, Canada

LEANNE ROBB, RN, BSN, MaED
Instructor/Program Leader
Camosun College
Victoria, British Columbia, Canada

DEBORAH SCHUH, RN
Faculty, School of Health & Community Services
Coordinator, Personal Support Worker Program
Durham College
Oshawa, Ontario, Canada

BRENDA WASYLIK, RN, BScN
Program Coordinator
University College of the North
Swan River, Manitoba, Canada

REVIEWERS OF THE U.S. 2nd EDITION

NAOMI ADAMS *Northern Virginia Community College–Woodbridge, Woodbridge, Virginia*

CHRISTINE ALGER *The State University of New York–Stony Brook, Stony Brook, New York*

ROBERTA BARTEE *Delgado Community College–Charity, New Orleans, Louisiana*

JUDITH BATEMAN *Black Hawk College–Quad-Cities Campus, Moline, Illinois*

TAMMY BRYANT *Southwest Georgia Technical College, Thomasville, Georgia*

DIANE CARDAMONE *Wake Technical Community College, Raleigh, North Carolina*

SALLY CHRISTIANSEN *Waukesha County Technical College, Pewaukee, Wisconsin*

DEREK COPPLE *Palo Verde College, Blythe, California*

DEBRA CUMMINGS *Monroe Community College, Rochester, New York*

DENISE FORD *Chattanooga State Technical Community College, Chattanooga, Tennessee*

KATHY GIRARD *Lake Technical Center, Eustis, Florida*

LORI RAE HAMILTON *Otero Junior College, La Junta, Colorado*

MARIE HERMARY-MUNRO *Red Deer College, Red Deer, Alberta, Canada*

ANN HESS *Johnson County Community College Area Vocational School, Overland Park, Kansas*

KARRIE JO HOLMES *Uintah Basin Applied Technology College, Vernal, Utah*

KIMBERLEY JOHNSTON *Sir Sanford Fleming College, Peterborough, Ontario, Canada*

GAIL JOSEPH *Madison Area Technical College, Prairie du Sac, Wisconsin*

LAURIE LIVINGOOD *Tulsa Technology Center, Tulsa, Oklahoma*

JOAN MATSUKAWA *Kapiolani Community, College, Honolulu, Hawaii*

ANJENETTE MILLIGAN *Florence-Darlington Technical College, Florence, North Carolina*

JOANNE MOATS *Seminole Community College, Sanford, Florida*

LINDA PARRY *Indian River Community College, Ft. Pierce, Florida*

ELIZABETH PELHAM *Our Lady of the Lake College, Baton Rouge, Louisiana*

TOMMIE PNIEWSKI *Hopkinsville Community College, Hopkinsville, Kentucky*

PAT REINHART *Minneapolis Community and Technical College, Minneapolis, Minnesota*

JUDITH RYAN *College of Dupage, Glen Ellyn, Illinois*

PAMELA SMITH *Front Range Community College–Larimer, Fort Collins, Colorado*

MICHELLE SNOW *CNA Educational Services, Inc. Kaysville, Utah*

MARSHA STERNARD *Northeast Wisconsin Technical College–Sturgeon Bay Campus, Sturgeon Bay, Wisconsin*

JUDITH SWAN *Northcentral Technical College, Wausau, Wisconsin*

PATRICIA TARGETT *Naugatuck Valley Community College, Waterbury, Connecticut*

SUE TREITZ *Arapahoe Community College, Littleton, Colorado*

SUSAN WORTH *Madison Area Technical College, Madison, Wisconsin*

PEGGY YOUNG *Central Maine Medical Center School of Nursing, Lewiston, Maine*

ACKNOWLEDGEMENTS

This textbook was written and published through the combined efforts of many people. The planning, manuscript development, editing, design, and production processes involved the contributions of many dedicated individuals. We would like to especially thank Corey Wolfe, Instructional Services Consultant; Elizabeth Nieginski, Executive Acquisitions Editor; Melanie Cann, Senior Development Editor; and Laura Scott, Associate Product Manager, for their ongoing support throughout this project. Special thanks to Sharon Lauman for the many hours of typing and to Marilyn's daughter, Priscilla, for her editorial comments and review.

CONTENTS

UNIT 1

INTRODUCTION TO HEALTH CARE   1

CHAPTER 1
THE CANADIAN HEALTH CARE SYSTEM   3

Health Care Delivery, Past and Present   4
The Role of the Government in Health Care   6
   Roles and Responsibilities of the
     Federal Government   6
   Roles and Responsibilities of the Provincial
     or Territorial Government   6
Paying for Health Care   6
Health Care Organizations   7
   Types of Health Care Organizations   7
   Structure of Health Care Organizations   10
The Health Care Team   10

CHAPTER 2
THE PERSONAL SUPPORT WORKER   14

Nursing, Past and Present   15
Regulated Versus Non-regulated Health
   Care Professions   15
Education of the Personal Support Worker   16
Responsibilities of the Personal Support
   Worker   17
The Nursing Team   17
Delegation   20

CHAPTER 3
PROFESSIONALISM AND
JOB-SEEKING SKILLS   25

What is a Professional?   26
What is a Work Ethic?   27
   Punctuality   27
   Reliability   28
   Accountability   28
   Conscientiousness   28

   Courtesy and Respectfulness   28
   Honesty   29
   Cooperativeness   29
   Empathy   29
   A Desire to Learn   29
Personal Health and Hygiene   29
   Maintaining your Physical Health   29
   Maintaining your Emotional Health   31
   Personal Hygiene and Appearance   31
Job-Seeking Skills   32
   Defining the Ideal Job   32
   Finding Job Openings   35
   Preparing Résumés, Cover Letters,
     and Reference Lists   35
   Putting in Applications   36
   Going on Interviews   40
   Leaving a Job   42

CHAPTER 4
LEGAL AND ETHICAL ISSUES   45

Basic Human Rights   46
Basic Rights of People Who are
   Receiving Health Care   47
   Patients' Rights   47
   Residents' Rights   47
Laws: A Way of Preserving Patients'
   and Residents' Rights   48
   Violations of Civil Law   48
   Violations of Criminal Law: Abuse   51
Ethics: Guidelines for Behavior   52
   Professional Ethics   53
   Personal Ethics   53
Protecting Yourself from Legal and Ethical
   Difficulties   53

CHAPTER 5
COMMUNICATION SKILLS   57

What is Communication?   58

Communicating Effectively 59
  Tactics that Enhance Communication 61
  Blocks to Effective Communication 64
  Conflict Resolution 64
Telephone Communication 66
Communication Among Members of
  the Health Care Team 67
  Reporting 68
  Recording 69
  The Nursing Process 75

CHAPTER 6
THOSE WE CARE FOR 80

Patients, Residents, and Clients 81
Growth and Development 83
  Infancy (Birth to 1 Year) 85
  Toddlerhood (1 to 3 Years) 85
  Preschool (3 to 5 Years) 86
  School-age (5 to 12 Years) 87
  Adolescence (12 to 20 Years) 87
  Young Adulthood (20 to 40 Years) 88
  Middle Adulthood (40 to 65 Years) 88
  Later Adulthood (65 to 75 Years) 89
  Older Adulthood (75 Years and Beyond) 89
Basic Human Needs 89
  Maslow's Hierarchy of Human Needs 89
  Human Sexuality and Intimacy 92
Culture and Religion 94
Quality of Life 96

UNIT 2

SAFETY 101

CHAPTER 7
COMMUNICABLE DISEASE AND
INFECTION CONTROL 103

What is a Microbe? 104
  Bacteria 105
  Viruses 105
  Fungi 107
  Parasites 107
Defenses against Communicable
  Disease 107
  The Immune System 107
  Antibiotics 109
Communicable Disease and the
  Chain of Infection 109

Infection Control in the Health Care Setting 112
  Medical Asepsis 112
  Surgical Asepsis 116
  Barrier Methods 116
  Isolation Precautions 118

Procedure 7-1: Handwashing 122
Procedure 7-2: Removing Gloves 123
Procedure 7-3: Putting on a Gown 124
Procedure 7-4: Removing a Gown 125
Procedure 7-5: Putting on and Removing a
  Mask 126
Procedure 7-6: Removing More Than One Article of
  Personal Protective Equipment (PPE) 127
Procedure 7-7: Double-Bagging (Two Workers) 127

CHAPTER 8
BLOODBORNE AND
AIRBORNE PATHOGENS 130

Bloodborne Diseases 131
  Bloodborne Transmission 131
  Hepatitis and Hiv/Aids 131
  Protecting Yourself from Bloodborne
    Diseases 134
Airborne Diseases 136
  Airborne Transmittal 136
  Tuberculosis 137
  Protecting Yourself from Airborne
    Diseases 138

CHAPTER 9
WORKPLACE SAFETY 140

Protecting your Body 141
  The "ABCs" of Good Body Mechanics 141
  Lifting and Back Safety 142
Following Procedures 144
Preventing Falls 148
Preventing Chemical Injuries 149
Preventing Electrical Shocks 150
Fire Safety 150
  Preventing Fires 150
  Reacting to a Fire Emergency 154
Disaster Preparedness 156

CHAPTER 10
PATIENT AND RESIDENT
SAFETY AND RESTRAINTS 160

Accidents 161
  Risk Factors 161
  Avoiding Accidents 163
  Reporting Accidents 166

Restraints   166
   Use of Restraints   166
   Complications Associated with Restraint Use   169
   Restraint Alternatives   171
   Applying Restraints   173

Procedure 10-1: Applying a Vest Restraint   175
Procedure 10-2: Applying Wrist or Ankle Restraints   176
Procedure 10-3: Applying Lap or
   Waist (Belt) Restraints   177

CHAPTER 11
POSITIONING, LIFTING, AND TRANSFERRING
PATIENTS AND RESIDENTS   179

Positioning Patients and Residents   180
   Basic Positions   182
   Repositioning a Person   185
Transferring Patients and Residents   187
   Transferring a Person to and from a Wheelchair
     or Chair   188
   Transferring a Person to and from a Stretcher   188
   Transferring a Person Using a Mechanical Lift   188
   Assisting a Person with Walking (Ambulating)   189

Procedure 11-1: Moving a Person to the Side
   of the Bed (One Worker)   193
Procedure 11-2: Moving a Person to the Side
   of the Bed (Two Workers)   193
Procedure 11-3: Moving a Person up in Bed
   (One Worker)   195
Procedure 11-4: Moving a Person Up in
   Bed (Two Workers)   196
Procedure 11-5: Raising a Person's Head and
   Shoulders   196
Procedure 11-6: Turning a Person
   Onto his or her Side   197
Procedure 11-7: Logrolling a Person
   (Two Workers)   198
Procedure 11-8: Applying a Transfer (Gait) Belt   199
Procedure 11-9: Transferring a Person from
   a Bed to a Wheelchair (One Worker)   200
Procedure 11-10: Transferring a Person From a
   Bed to a Wheelchair (Two Workers)   202
Procedure 11-11: Transferring a Person From a
   Wheelchair to a Bed   203
Procedure 11-12: Transferring a Person From a
   Bed to a Stretcher (Four Workers)   204
Procedure 11-13: Transferring a Person From a
   Stretcher to a Bed (Four Workers)   205
Procedure 11-14: Transferring a Person Using a
   Mechanical Lift (Two Workers)   206
Procedure 11-15: Assisting a Person With Sitting
   on the Edge of the Bed ("Dangling")   208
Procedure 11-16: Assisting a Person With Walking
   (Ambulating)   209

CHAPTER 12
BASIC FIRST AID AND
EMERGENCY CARE   213

Responding to an Emergency   214
Basic Life Support Measures   216
Emergency Situations   217
   "Heart Attacks" and Strokes   217
   Fainting (Syncope)   218
   Seizures   219
   Hemorrhage   220
   Shock   220
   Airway Obstructions ("Choking")   220
The Chain of Survival   222

Procedure 12-1: Performing Abdominal Thrusts in
   Conscious Adults and Children
   Older Than 1 Year   224
Procedure 12-2: Relieving a Foreign-body Airway
   Obstruction in Unconscious Adults and Children Older
   Than 1 Year   225
Procedure 12-3: Performing Chest Thrusts in Conscious
   Adults and Children Older Than 1 Year   226
Procedure 12-4: Clearing the Airway in
   a Conscious Infant   227
Procedure 12-5: Clearing the Airway in an Unconscious
   Infant   228

UNIT 3

BASIC PATIENT AND
RESIDENT CARE   233

CHAPTER 13
THE PATIENT OR RESIDENT
ENVIRONMENT   235

The Patient or Resident Unit   236
   Hospitals   236
   Long-term Care Facilities   237
   Assisted-living Facilities   238
   Home Health Care   238
Ensuring Comfort   238
   Cleanliness   239
   Odour Control   239
   Ventilation   240
   Room Temperature   240
   Lighting   240
   Noise Control   241
Furniture and Equipment   241
   Beds   241

Chairs   244
Over-Bed Tables   244
Storage Units   244
Call Light and Intercom Systems   245
Privacy Curtains and Room Dividers   246
Other Equipment   246
Personal Items   246

CHAPTER 14
ADMISSIONS, TRANSFERS,
AND DISCHARGES   250

Admissions   251
The Admissions Process   252
Tactics for Making a New Patient or Resident
     Feel Welcome   253
Transfers   257
Discharges   258

CHAPTER 15
BEDMAKING   262

Linens and other Supplies for Bedmaking   263
Linens   263
Other Bedmaking Supplies   265
Handling of Linens   265
Standard Bedmaking Techniques   268
Closed (Unoccupied) Beds   269
Occupied Beds   271

Procedure 15-1: Making an Unoccupied (Closed)
     Bed   272
Procedure 15-2: Making an Occupied Bed   274

CHAPTER 16
VITAL SIGNS, HEIGHT, AND WEIGHT   278

What Do Vital Signs Tell Us?   280
Measuring and Recording Vital Signs   280
Body Temperature   281
Factors Affecting the Body Temperature   281
Measuring the Body Temperature   281
Normal and Abnormal Findings   284
Pulse   285
Factors Affecting the Pulse   286
Measuring the Pulse   286
Normal and Abnormal Findings   287
Respiration   287
Factors Affecting Respiration   288
Measuring Respiration   288
Normal and Abnormal Findings   288
Blood Pressure   289
Factors Affecting Blood Pressure   289

Measuring Blood Pressure   290
Normal and Abnormal Findings   293
Height and Weight   294
Measuring Height and Weight   294
Measuring Vital Signs in Children   296

Procedure 16-1: Measuring an Oral Temperature
     (Glass or Electronic Thermometer)   298
Procedure 16-2: Measuring a Rectal Temperature
     (Glass or Electronic Thermometer)   299
Procedure 16-3: Measuring an Axillary Temperature
     (Glass or Electronic Thermometer)   301
Procedure 16-4: Measuring a Tympanic Temperature
     (Tympanic Thermometer)   302
Procedure 16-5: Taking a Radial Pulse   303
Procedure 16-6: Taking an Apical Pulse   304
Procedure 16-7: Counting Respirations   305
Procedure 16-8: Measuring Blood Pressure   305
Procedure 16-9: Measuring Height and Weight Using an
     Upright Scale   307
Procedure 16-10: Measuring Weight Using a Chair
     Scale   308
Procedure 16-11: Measuring Height and Weight Using a
     Tape Measure and a Sling Scale   309

CHAPTER 17
CLEANLINESS AND HYGIENE   313

The Benefits of Personal Hygiene   314
Scheduling of Routine Care   315
Assisting with Oral Care   316
Providing Oral Care for a Person with Natural
     Teeth   316
Providing Oral Care for a Person with Dentures   317
Providing Oral Care for an Unconscious Person   318
Assisting with Perineal Care   318
Providing Perineal Care for Female Patients
     and Residents   322
Providing Perineal Care for Male Patients
     and Residents   322
Assisting with Skin Care   322
Bathing   322
Massage   328

Procedure 17-1: Brushing and
     Flossing the Teeth   330
Procedure 17-2: Providing Oral Care for a
     Person with Dentures   332
Procedure 17-3: Providing Oral Care for an
     Unconscious Person   333
Procedure 17-4: Providing Female Perineal Care   334
Procedure 17-5: Providing Male Perineal Care   336
Procedure 17-6: Assisting with a Tub
     Bath or Shower   338
Procedure 17-7: Giving a Complete Bed Bath   340

Procedure 17-8: Giving a Partial Bed Bath   342
Procedure 17-9: Giving a Back Massage   344

CHAPTER 18
GROOMING   348

Assisting with Hand and Foot Care   350
   Care of the Hands   350
   Care of the Feet   351
Assisting with Dressing and Undressing   352
Assisting with Hair Care   354
   Shampooing the Hair   356
   Styling the Hair   356
   Preventing Tangles   357
Assisting with Shaving   357
   Assisting Men   357
   Assisting Women   358
Assisting with the Application of
   Make-up   358

Procedure 18-1: Assisting With Hand Care   360
Procedure 18-2: Assisting With Foot Care   361
Procedure 18-3: Assisting a Person
   With Dressing   362
Procedure 18-4: Changing a Hospital Gown   364
Procedure 18-5: Shampooing a
   Person's Hair in Bed   365
Procedure 18-6: Combing a Person's Hair   366
Procedure 18-7: Shaving a Person's Face   367

CHAPTER 19
BASIC NUTRITION   371

Food and How our Bodies use it   372
   Types of Nutrients   374
   A Balanced Diet   375
Factors that Affect Food Choices and
   Eating Habits   375
Special Diets   379
Meal Time   380
   Preparing for Meal Time   381
   Assisting the Person to Eat   382
   Feeding Dependent Patients and Residents   383
   Measuring and Recording Food Intake   384
Other Ways of Providing Fluids and Nutrition   385
   Intravenous (Iv) Therapy   385
   Enteral Nutrition   386
   Total Parenteral Nutrition (Hyperalimentation)   388
Fluids and Hydration   388
   Fluid Balance   388
   Offering Fluids   389
   Measuring and Recording Intake and Output   389

Procedure 19-1: Feeding a Dependent Person   392

CHAPTER 20
ASSISTING WITH URINARY AND BOWEL ELIMINATION   396

Assisting with Elimination   397
   Elimination Equipment   397
   Promoting Normal Elimination   399
   Obtaining Urine and Stool Specimens   402
Urinary Elimination   403
   Measuring Urine Output   404
   Urinary Catheterization   405
   Urinary Incontinence   411
Bowel Elimination   414
   Problems With Bowel Elimination   414
   Enemas   416
   Rectal Suppositories   418

Procedure 20-1: Assisting a Person
   With Using a Bedpan   420
Procedure 20-2: Assisting a Man
   With Using a Urinal   421
Procedure 20-3: Collecting a Routine Urine
   Specimen   422
Procedure 20-4: Collecting a Midstream
   ("Clean Catch") Urine Specimen   423
Procedure 20-5: Collecting a Stool Specimen   425
Procedure 20-6: Providing Catheter Care   426
Procedure 20-7: Emptying a Urine Drainage Bag   427
Procedure 20-8: Administering a Soapsuds Enema   428

UNIT 4

DEATH AND DYING   433

CHAPTER 21
CARING FOR PEOPLE WHO ARE TERMINALLY ILL   435

Stages of Grief   437
Wills   440
Dying with Dignity   440
   Advance Directives   440
   Hospice Care   441
Effects of Caring for the Terminally Ill
   on the Caregiver   442

CHAPTER 22
CARING FOR PEOPLE WHO ARE DYING   445

Caring for a Dying Person   447
Meeting the Dying Person's Physical Needs   448
   Meeting the Dying Person's Emotional Needs   450

Care of the Family   451
Postmortem Care   454

Procedure 22-1: Providing Postmortem Care   457

UNIT 5

STRUCTURE AND FUNCTION OF THE HUMAN BODY   463

CHAPTER 23
BASIC BODY STRUCTURE AND
FUNCTION   465

How is the Body Organized?   466
   Cells   466
   Tissues   467
   Organs   468
   Organ Systems   469
Health and Disease   469
   Categories of Disease   471
   Risk Factors for Disease   471
Rehabilitation and Restorative Care   472
   The Role of the Personal Support Worker   473
   Types of Rehabilitation   475

CHAPTER 24
THE INTEGUMENTARY SYSTEM   481

Structure of the Integumentary System   483
   Skin   483
   Accessory Structures (Appendages)   483
Function of the Integumentary System   484
   Protection   484
   Maintenance of Fluid Balance   484
   Regulation of Body Temperature   484
   Sensation   485
   Vitamin D Production   485
   Elimination and Absorption   485
The Effects of Aging on the Integumentary
   System   485
   Changes in Physical Appearance   486
   Fragile, Dry Skin   486
   Thickening of the Nails   487
   Less Efficient Temperature Regulation   487
Disorders of the Integumentary System   487
   pressure Ulcers   487
   Wounds   494
   Burns   497
   Lesions   498

Procedure 24-1: Assisting the Nurse With a
   Dressing Change   501

CHAPTER 25
THE MUSCULOSKELETAL SYSTEM   505

Structure of the Musculoskeletal System   506
   The Skeletal System   506
   The Muscular System   508
Function of the Musculoskeletal System   509
   Protection   509
   Support   509
   Movement   509
   Heat Production   511
   Calcium Storage   511
   Production of Blood Cells   512
The Effects of Aging on the
   Musculoskeletal System   512
   Loss of Bone Tissue   513
   Loss of Muscle Mass   513
   Wear and tear on the Joints   514
Disorders of the Musculoskeletal System   514
   Osteoporosis   514
   Arthritis   515
   Muscular Dystrophy   517
   Fractures   518
   Amputations   521
General Care Measures   523
   Range-of-motion Exercises   523
   Heat and Cold Applications   524
   Rehabilitation   527

Procedure 25-1: Assisting a Person With Passive
   Range-of-Motion Exercises   530
Procedure 25-2: Giving a Moist Cold Application   535
Procedure 25-3: Giving a Dry Cold Application   536
Procedure 25-4: Giving a Dry Heat Application With an
   Aquamatic Pad   537

CHAPTER 26
THE RESPIRATORY SYSTEM   540

Structure of the Respiratory System   541
   Airway   541
   Lungs   542
Function of the Respiratory System   543
   Ventilation   543
   Gas Exchange   543
The Effects of Aging on the Respiratory
   System   544
   Less Efficient Ventilation   545
   Increased Risk of Respiratory Infections   545
Disorders of the Respiratory System   546

Infections   546

Asthma   547

Chronic Obstructive Pulmonary Disease   548

Cancer   549

Pneumothorax and Hemothorax   550

Respiratory Therapy   551

Oxygen Therapy   551

Mechanical Ventilation   556

Suctioning   559

General Care Measures   559

Observation   560

Promoting Comfort   561

CHAPTER 27
THE CARDIOVASCULAR SYSTEM   564

Structure of the Cardiovascular System   565

Blood   565

Blood Vessels   567

Lymphatic System   567

Heart   569

Function of the Cardiovascular System   571

Transport   571

Regulation   573

Protection   573

The Effects of Aging on the Cardiovascular System   573

Less Efficient Contraction   574

Decreased Elasticity of the Arteries and Veins   574

Decreased Numbers of Blood Cells   574

Disorders of the Cardiovascular System   574

Disorders of the Blood   574

Disorders of the Blood Vessels   575

Disorders of the Heart   576

Diagnosis of Cardiovascular Disorders   578

Cardiac Rehabilitation   579

CHAPTER 28
THE NERVOUS SYSTEM   582

Structure of the Nervous System   583

The Central Nervous System   584

The Peripheral Nervous System   585

Function of the Nervous System   586

Regulation of the Internal Environment   586

Interaction with the External Environment   586

The Effects of Aging on the Nervous System   586

Slowed Conduction Times   586

Memory Changes   587

Disorders of the Nervous System   587

Transient Ischemic Attacks   587

Stroke   588

Parkinson's Disease   589

Epilepsy   590

Multiple Sclerosis   591

*Amyotrophic Lateral Sclerosis
(Lou Gehrig's Disease)   591*

Head Injuries   591

Spinal Cord Injuries   591

Diagnosis of Neurologic Disorders   592

Rehabilitation   592

CHAPTER 29
THE SENSORY SYSTEM   597

Structure of the Sensory System   598

General Sense   598

Touch   598

Position   599

Pain   599

Taste and Smell   601

Sight   601

Structure of the Eye   602

Function of the Eye   602

The Effects of Aging on the Eye   603

Disorders of the Eye   604

*Caring for Eyeglasses, Contact Lenses,
and Prosthetic Eyes   606*

Hearing and Balance   609

Structure of the Ear   609

Function of the Ear   610

The Effects of Aging on the Ear   610

Disorders of the Ear   611

Procedure 29-1: Assisting a Person With
an In-the-Ear Hearing Aid   616

CHAPTER 30
THE ENDOCRINE SYSTEM   619

Structure of the Endocrine System   620

Function of the Endocrine System   620

Pituitary Gland   621

Pineal Gland   622

Thyroid Gland   622

Parathyroid Glands   623

Thymus Gland   623

Adrenal Glands   624

Pancreas   624

Sex Glands   625

The Effects of Aging on
the Endocrine System   625

Disorders of the Endocrine System   625

Pituitary Gland Disorders   625
Thyroid Gland Disorders   626
Adrenal Gland Disorders   626
Diabetes   627

CHAPTER 31
THE DIGESTIVE SYSTEM   632

Structure of the Digestive System   633
The Digestive Tract   633
The Accessory Organs   636
Function of the Digestive System   636
Digestion   636
Absorption   636
Excretion   637
Effects of Aging on the Digestive System   637
Less Efficient Chewing and Swallowing   637
Less Efficient Digestion   637
Increased Risk for Constipation   637
Disorders of the Digestive System   637
Ulcers   638
Hernias   638
Gallbladder Disorders   638
Cancer   639
Diagnosis of Digestive Disorders   639
Caring for a Person with an Ostomy   639

Procedure 31-1: Providing Routine Ostomy Care   643

CHAPTER 32
THE URINARY SYSTEM   647

Structure of the Urinary System   648
The Kidneys   648
The Ureters   649
The Bladder   649
The Urethra   649
Function of the Urinary System   650
Removal of Liquid Wastes   650
Maintenance of Homeostasis   650
The Effects of Aging on the Urinary System   651
Disorders of the Urinary System   651
Infections   652
Kidney Stones (Renal Calculi)   652
Kidney (Renal) Failure   653
Tumours   655
Diagnosis of Urinary Disorders   657

CHAPTER 33
THE REPRODUCTIVE SYSTEM   660

The Female Reproductive System   662
Structure of the Female Reproductive System   662
Function of the Female Reproductive System   664
The Effects of Aging on the Female Reproductive System   664
Disorders of the Female Reproductive System   665
Common Diagnostic Procedures   667
Common Surgical Procedures   668
The Male Reproductive System   668
Structure of the Male Reproductive System   668
Function of the Male Reproductive System   669
The Effects of Aging on the Male Reproductive System   670
Disorders of the Male Reproductive System   670
Common Diagnostic Procedures   671
Sexually Transmitted Infections   671
Types of Sexually Transmitted Infections   672
Prevention of Sexually Transmitted Infections   673

UNIT 6

SPECIAL CARE CONCERNS   677

CHAPTER 34
CARING FOR PEOPLE WITH DEVELOPMENTAL DISABILITIES   679

What is a Developmental Disability?   680
Special Needs of People with Developmental Disabilities   680
Special Education   680
Protection of Rights   681
Emotional and Social Needs   681
Types of Developmental Disabilities   682
Mental Retardation   682
Down Syndrome   683
Autism   683
Cerebral Palsy   683
Fragile X Syndrome   684
Fetal Alcohol Syndrome   684
Spina Bifida   684
Hydrocephalus   684
Caring for a Person with a Developmental Disability   685
Communicating with a Person with a Developmental Disability   686
Meeting the Physical Needs of a Person with a Developmental Disability   687

CHAPTER 35
CARING FOR PEOPLE WITH
MENTAL ILLNESS   690

Mental Health   691
    Coping Mechanisms   692
    Defense Mechanisms   693
Causes and Treatment of Mental Illness   694
Types of Mental Illness   695
    Anxiety Disorders   695
    Depression   696
    Bipolar Disorder (Manic Depression)   697
    Schizophrenia   697
    Eating Disorders   697
Caring for a Person with Mental Illness   698
    Listening and Observing   698
    Assisting with Activities of Daily Living   700

CHAPTER 36
CARING FOR PEOPLE WITH
DEMENTIA   703

What is Dementia?   704
Types of Dementia   705
    Alzheimer's Disease   705
    Vascular (Multi-infarct) Dementia   706
Behaviours Associated with Dementia   707
    Types of Behaviours   708
    Managing Difficult Behaviours   710
Caring for a Person with Dementia   711
    Meeting the Physical Needs of a Person
        with Dementia   711
    Meeting the Emotional Needs of a Person
        with Dementia   715
Effects on the Caregiver of Caring for the Person
    with Dementia   717

CHAPTER 37
CARING FOR PEOPLE WITH CANCER   720

What is Cancer?   721
    Types of Cancer   722
    Causes of Cancer   722
Detection of Cancer   723
    Warning Signs of Cancer   723
    Routine Physical Examinations and Screening Tests   724
Treatment of Cancer   725
Caring for a Person with Cancer   726
    Meeting the Physical Needs of a
        Person with Cancer   726
    Meeting the Emotional Needs of a Person
        with Cancer   727

CHAPTER 38
CARING FOR PEOPLE WITH HIV/AIDS
730

What is Aids?   731
    Who is at Risk for Hiv/Aids?   732
    A Global Health Crisis   732
Protection of Rights   733
Caring for a Person with Aids   734
    Meeting the Physical Needs of a Person with Aids   734
    Meeting the Emotional Needs of a Person with Aids   735

UNIT 7

ACUTE CARE   739

CHAPTER 39
CARING FOR SURGICAL PATIENTS   741

Care of the Pre-operative Patient   743
    Emotional Preparation   743
    Physical Preparation   746
Care of the Post-operative Patient   749
    Preventing Complications   750
    Assisting with Positioning   752
    Assisting with Nutrition   753
    Assisting with Elimination   753
    Assisting with Hygiene   753
    Assisting with Walking (Ambulation)   753

Procedure 39-1: Applying Anti-embolism (TED)
    Stockings   755

CHAPTER 40
CARING FOR MOTHERS AND
NEWBORNS   759

The Antepartum (Prenatal) Period   760
    Physical Changes in Pregnancy   760
    Routine Prenatal Care   760
    Complications During Pregnancy   762
    Meeting the Pregnant Woman's Physical Needs   762
    Meeting the Pregnant Woman's Emotional
        Needs   762
Labour and Delivery   763
    Labour   763
    Delivery   763
    Immediately Following Delivery   764
The Postpartum Period   764
    Care of the Mother   764
    Care of the Baby   766

CHAPTER 41
CARING FOR PEDIATRIC PATIENTS   775

Caring for Infants   777
  Meeting the Infant's Physical Needs   777
  Meeting the Infant's Emotional Needs   777
  Meeting the Infant's Need for Safety   777
Caring for Toddlers   778
  Meeting the Toddler's Physical Needs   779
  Meeting the Toddler's Emotional Needs   779
  Meeting the Toddler's Need for Safety   780
Caring for Preschoolers   780
  Meeting the Preschooler's Physical Needs   780
  Meeting the Preschooler's Emotional Needs   780
  Meeting the Preschooler's Needs for Safety   781
Caring for School-age Children   781
  Meeting the School-age Child's Physical Needs   781
  Meeting the School-age Child's Emotional Needs   782
  Meeting the School-age Child's Need for Safety   782
Caring for Adolescents   782
  Meeting the Adolescent's Physical Needs   782
  Meeting the Adolescent's Emotional Needs   783
  Meeting the Adolescent's Need for Safety   783
Child Abuse   783
  Forms of Abuse   784
  Risk Factors for Child Abuse   784
  Role of the Personal Support Worker in
    Reporting Abuse   785

UNIT 8

HOME HEALTH CARE   789

CHAPTER 42
INTRODUCTION TO HOME HEALTH
CARE   791

What is Home Health Care?   792

Paying for Home Health Care   792
  The Health Care Team   793
Responsibilities of the Home Support Worker   794
  Personal Care   795
  Homemaking   796
Qualities of the Successful Home Support
  Worker   797
  Ability to Work Independently   797
  Ability to be Organized and Manage Time   797
  Reliability   798
  Ability to Set Professional Boundaries   799

CHAPTER 43
SAFETY AND INFECTION CONTROL IN THE
HOME HEALTH CARE SETTING   803

Workplace Safety   804
  Accidents and Medical Emergencies   804
  Abusive Situations   806
Infection Control   806
  Maintaining a Sanitary Environment   807
  Using Standard Precautions   809
Personal Safety   810

GLOSSARY   815

APPENDIX A
ANSWERS TO THE WHAT DID YOU LEARN?
EXERCISES   835

APPENDIX B
INTRODUCTION TO THE LANGUAGE OF
HEALTH CARE   837

INDEX   849

INTRODUCTION TO HEALTH CARE

1 The Canadian Health Care System
2 The Personal Support Worker
3 Professionalism and Job-Seeking Skills
4 Legal and Ethical Issues
5 Communication Skills
6 Those We Care For

Welcome to the health care field! Today in Canada, the health care field is one of the largest fields, producing jobs for more than 1.5 million people across the country. Unit 1 introduces you to the health care field, and to your role as a personal support worker. Basic concepts and skills that you will use everyday in your work as a personal support worker are also reviewed in Unit 1.

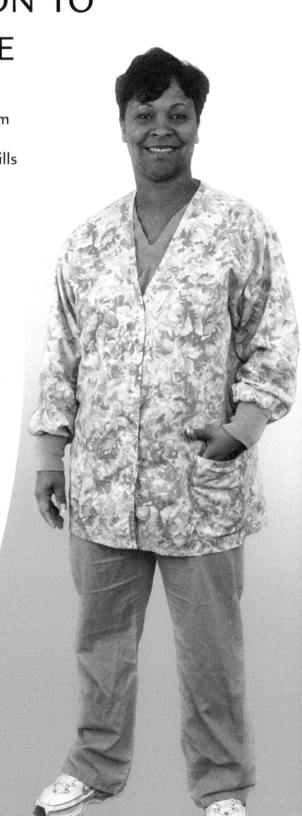

Photo: Welcome to the health care field! Personal support workers are key members of the health care team.

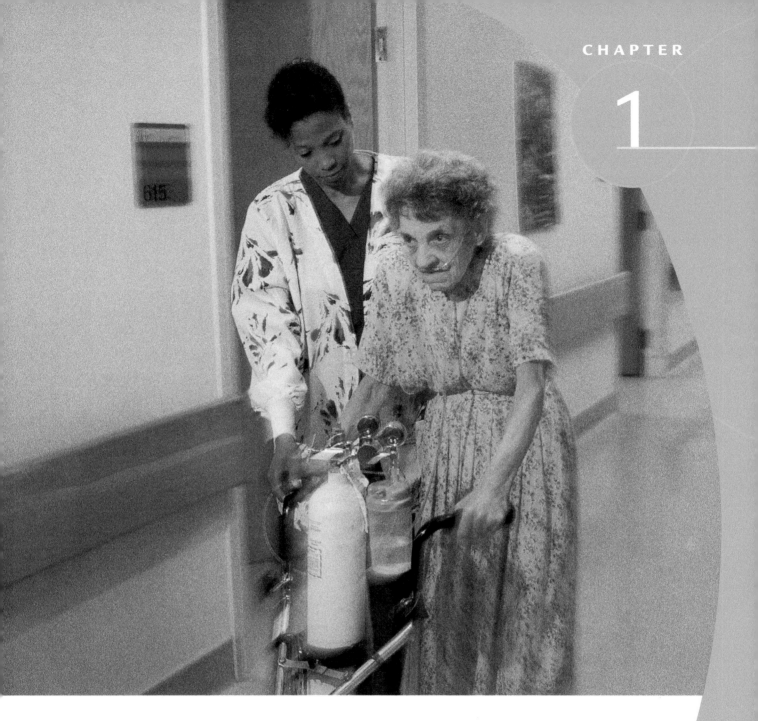

The Canadian Health Care System

WHAT WILL YOU LEARN?

As a health care professional, you will be part of the health care system. In this chapter, you will learn about the history of our health care system, the role that government plays in our health care system, and how health care is paid for in Canada. We will also discuss the many different types of organizations that make up the health care system. Finally, we

Photo: Health care is a people-oriented business.

will discuss the health care team, and the importance of taking a holistic, humanistic approach to health care. When you are finished with this chapter, you will be able to:

1. Identify changes that have occurred in how health care is delivered.
2. Describe the roles and responsibilities of the federal government and the provincial/territorial governments with regard to health care.
3. Discuss how health care is paid for in Canada.
4. Describe the different types of health care organizations.
5. Briefly explain the structure of a health care organization.
6. Describe how the members of the health care team work together to provide care, and explain what a holistic, humanistic approach to health care means.

Vocabulary

Canada Health Act (1984)	Patient	Resident	Hospice organization
Health Canada	Sub-acute care unit (skilled nursing unit, skilled nursing facility)	Assisted-living facility	Health care team
Medicare		Home health care agency	Holistic care
Mission	Long-term care facility (nursing home)	Client	
Hospital			

HEALTH CARE DELIVERY, PAST AND PRESENT

The history of medicine in Canada can be traced back to Canada's First Nations people. Each tribe had its own healer, or medicine man. The medicine man treated illness with spiritual cures, plant remedies, and other traditional practices. Caring for the sick and delivering babies were primarily the responsibility of the women of a tribe.

When the English and French early settlers arrived in Canada in the 1600s, they brought Western medical practices with them. Until the early 1800s, the quality of health care in Canada was variable. Health care delivery focused mainly around the home and family. The health care provider was trained in general health care skills. He or she would deliver the babies, attend to wounds and broken bones, and provide comfort to both the dying person and the family (Fig. 1-1). Patients were at the mercy of the health care provider, and there was little the family could do if the care they received was poor. Hospitals were not-for-profit charitable organizations that usually had religious affiliations and provided care primarily for the poor. Unfortunately, early hospitals typically caused more illness than they helped (Fig. 1-2).

During the 1800s and 1900s, there were many advancements in health care in Canada. The first medical schools were established in Eastern Canada in the 1820s. During the mid-1800s, a number of advances were made in public sanitation and hygiene, leading to improvements such as the provision of safe drinking water and the establishment of garbage services to remove waste from the cities. In the early 1900s, the construction of government-run hospitals began. These hospitals cared primarily for patients suffering from mental illnesses and tuberculosis.

Throughout the 1920s and 1930s, public demand for more government involvement in providing improved health care for all Canadians increased. Many Canadians wanted the government to establish a national health insurance system. However, the Great Depression made putting such an idea into action financially difficult for the government. In addition, doctors throughout the country did not readily embrace the idea of a national health insurance system. Doctors set their own fees. People who could not afford the fees had to rely on assistance from charitable institutions, such as the Victorian Order of Nurses, or religious institutions, such as the Catholic and Protestant churches.

In 1947, the province of Saskatchewan, under the leadership of Premier Tommy Douglas, introduced government-funded health insurance for its residents. This early form of government-funded health insurance came about due to a constant

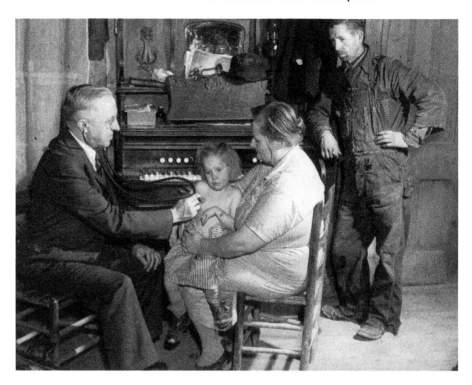

Figure 1-1
In the past, health care was delivered in the home, usually by a "family doctor." (*Hafton/Archive by Getty Images.*)

shortage of doctors in the province. To attract doctors to their towns, the municipal governments offered to subsidize (pay for) the doctors' practices. By the 1960s, similar subsidy models had been adopted by other levels of government throughout the country. In 1961, Tommy Douglas introduced the universal medicare legislation in Saskatchewan, and became known as the father of medicare. This began the groundbreaking work for the federal government's plan. In 1968, the federal government of Lester B. Pearson introduced a universal health care plan, the Medical Care Act. This act was revised and updated in 1984 and renamed the **Canada Health Act.** The

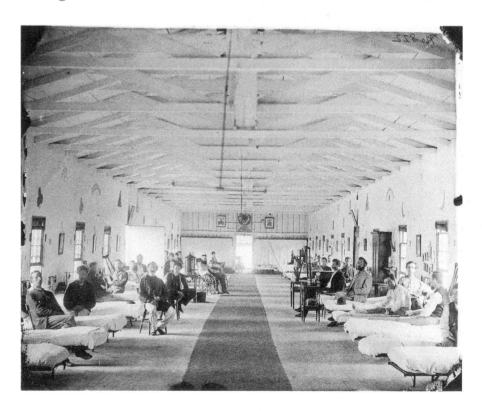

Figure 1-2
Modern ideas about hospital cleanliness and patient care did not exist in the 1800s.

Canada Health Act of 1984 established publically funded health care insurance in Canada.

THE ROLE OF THE GOVERNMENT IN HEALTH CARE

The federal government and the provincial/territorial governments share the responsibility for health care in Canada.

ROLES AND RESPONSIBILITIES OF THE FEDERAL GOVERNMENT

The federal government is responsible for:

- Developing and administering government policies and programs that promote health and wellness and prevent disease. The goal of these policies and programs is to ensure the health and wellness of the Canadian population. **Health Canada** is the federal department responsible for the development of these programs and policies.
- Providing financial support to the provinces and territories. The Canada Health Act outlines the five criteria that the provinces and territories must meet in order to qualify for federal financial support (Box 1-1).
- Delivering health care services to First Nations and Inuit people living on reserves, members of the Royal Canadian Mounted Police, veterans, inmates in federal penitentiaries, and refugee protection claimants.
- Transferring health-related tax benefits for medically insured health services to provincial/territorial governments.

ROLES AND RESPONSIBILITIES OF THE PROVINCIAL OR TERRITORIAL GOVERNMENT

The provincial/territorial government is responsible for:

- Meeting the criteria outlined in the Canada Health Act (see Box 1-1).
- Covering, free of charge, all medically necessary hospital and doctor services provided to permanent residents.
- Developing and administering the health care insurance plan.
- Deciding where hospitals will be located; how many doctors, nurses, and other health care professionals are needed; and how much money will be spent on health care services.
- Deciding how much coverage will be provided to permanent residents for health care services that are not medically necessary, such as ambulance services, prescription plans, optometry, dentistry, and home care services.

PAYING FOR HEALTH CARE

Canada has a national health insurance program that is legislated by the Canada Health Act. This program is often referred to unofficially as **"Medicare."** Medicare was created to ensure that all Canadians have access to medically necessary hospital and doctor services on a prepaid basis through the health insurance legislation of each province or territory. The Canadian health care system is mostly publicly funded. Approximately 30% of Canadian health care is paid for privately.

Most of the health care services that are paid for privately are either not covered by

BOX 1-1	The Five Criteria for Federal Financial Support as Specified in the Canada Health Act (1984)

Public administration. The insurance plan must be managed on a non-profit basis by a public authority accountable to the provincial/territorial government.

Comprehensiveness. The insurance plan must cover all medically necessary services in a hospital setting.

Universality. All permanent residents of a province or territory must be covered by the

public insurance plan on the same terms and conditions.

Portability. All permanent residents of a province or territory must be covered by the public insurance plan wherever they are treated in Canada.

Accessibility. All permanent residents of a province or territory must have access to medically necessary services regardless of their income, age, health, status, or financial circumstances.

Medicare or only partially covered. Approximately 65% of Canadians have some form of supplementary private health insurance plan. Many of these plans are through their employers, or through private companies such as the Worker's Compensation Board in British Columbia.

Medicare today faces many challenges across the country. The rising cost of health care is making it difficult for the program to sustain itself. In addition, wait times for medical services are often long. In an effort to address the challenge of long wait times, the federal government has charged the provinces and territories with guaranteeing timely access to health care in at least one of the following priority areas: cancer care, hip and knee replacement, cardiac care, diagnostic imaging, cataract surgeries, and primary care.

HEALTH CARE ORGANIZATIONS

As a personal support worker, you will be employed by a health care organization. All health care organizations have a purpose, or **mission.** Some health care organizations, such as university hospitals, are associated directly with a school. The primary mission of a university hospital may be to train people in the field of health care. Other health care organizations are associated with a religious group. Some health care organizations are owned by corporations and use the health care industry as a financial investment in order to turn a profit. Although some health care organizations have very specific missions, others combine many of the following:

- To prevent disease by providing immunizations, teaching people how to control chronic health problems, and identifying factors that could place a person at risk for a disease
- To detect and treat disease
- To promote health by teaching people about ways to achieve and maintain both physical and mental fitness
- To offer rehabilitation (restorative care) services in order to help people return to their highest possible level of physical or emotional function
- To provide emergency care to people with life-threatening illnesses or injuries

- To educate health care professionals by providing work-based training for medical students, student nurses, and many other types of students training for a career in the health care field

TYPES OF HEALTH CARE ORGANIZATIONS

There are many different types of health care organizations. Depending on where you live, you may be able to work as a personal support worker in all of these organizations, or just some. For example, in some provinces or territories, personal support workers are only employed in long-term care facilities (nursing homes), but in others, personal support workers can work in hospitals.

Hospitals

Probably the best-known type of health care organization is the **hospital.** The services provided by a hospital differ according to the hospital's mission and location. Some hospitals, such as children's hospitals, women's centers, cancer centers, or orthopedic hospitals, have very specific missions, either in terms of the type of people they serve or the services that they offer. Other hospitals, sometimes called "general hospitals," provide a variety of services, such as:

- Delivering babies
- Diagnosing diseases
- Treating diseases with medications, surgery, or both
- Providing emergency and intensive care services
- Providing mental health services
- Providing rehabilitation and physical therapy

People who receive the services of a hospital are typically referred to as **patients.** A hospital may admit a patient for care (have the patient stay for one or more nights). This is called inpatient care. Or a hospital may provide its services on an outpatient basis (the patient goes home the same day). For example, a patient with cancer who returns to the hospital every day for a period of time to receive radiation therapy would be receiving outpatient care.

Sub-acute Care Units (Skilled Nursing Units)

The care provided in a hospital is costly, and the number of beds in the hospital is limited.

Therefore, once a patient has recovered enough to be out of danger, he or she is usually moved from the medical–surgical unit. Often, these patients still need some care from a skilled health care professional. This care may be provided in a **sub-acute care unit** (also called a **skilled nursing unit** or a **skilled nursing facility).** A sub-acute care unit may be a unit within a hospital or a long-term care facility, or it may be a separate facility.

Patients in sub-acute care units may require intravenous medications, physical therapy, respiratory care or ventilator services, or wound management. The care given in these units focuses on rehabilitation and helping the patient to move from hospital care to home care (Fig. 1-3). Some patients in sub-acute care units recover fully, but others may need to move to a long-term care facility or arrange for continued care from home health care services after they return home.

Long-Term Care Facilities (Nursing Homes)

A **long-term care facility (nursing home)** is for people who are unable to care for themselves at home, yet do not need to be hospitalized (Fig. 1-4). Because the long-term care facility becomes the person's home, either temporarily or permanently, people being cared for in long-term care facilities are referred to as **residents,** rather than patients. Some residents will stay in the facility for a short period of time, until they are well enough to return home. Others will remain in the long-term care facility for the rest of their lives.

There are many reasons why a person would need to move to a long-term care facility. Many residents are elderly, but younger adults and children with conditions resulting from accidents or birth defects may also live in long-term care facilities. As with hospitals, long-term care facilities may provide care to residents with a wide variety of needs, or they may specialize. For example, some long-term care facilities provide skilled nursing care for residents who are unable to provide any of their own daily care. Others specialize in caring for residents with Alzheimer's disease. Still others help residents who have had a stroke or suffered a head injury to regain function.

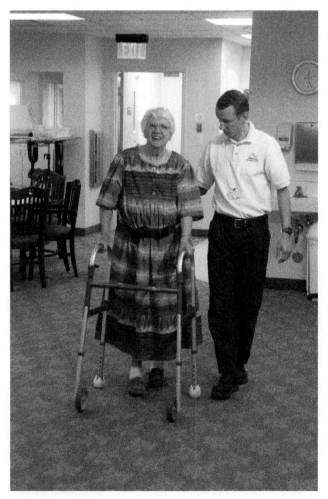

Figure 1-3
The care provided in sub-acute care units, also called skilled nursing units or skilled nursing facilities, often focuses on rehabilitation. Here, a physical therapist teaches a patient how to use a walker.

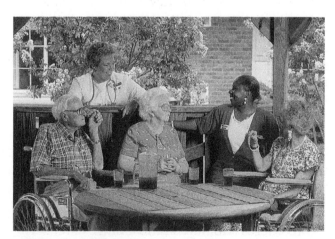

Figure 1-4
Residents of long-term care facilities (nursing homes) are unable to care for themselves at home, yet do not need to be hospitalized. (© *Will & Deni McIntyre/Photo Researchers, Inc.*)

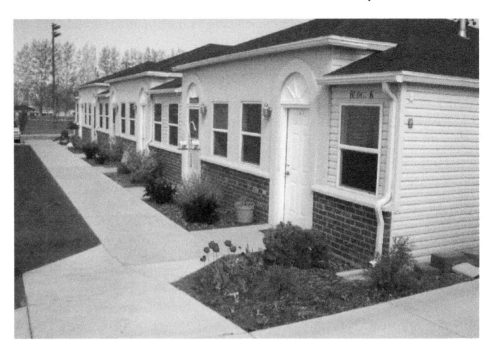

Figure 1-5
Residents of assisted-living communities often live in individual apartments. These residents are able to provide most of their own care but need help with certain things, such as medications, transportation, meals, or housekeeping. (*Courtesy of Country Pines Retirement Community, Clinton, UT.*)

Assisted-Living Facilities (Group Homes)

An **assisted-living facility** is a type of long-term care facility. People who live in an assisted-living facility are able to provide most of their own care, but they may need some limited help with medications, transportation, meals, and housekeeping. The residents of an assisted-living facility usually live in private apartments or a group home (a small home-like facility located in a residential neighborhood) and can feel safe and secure knowing that if they need help, someone is nearby to provide it, 24 hours a day (Fig. 1-5). Many retirement communities offer both assisted-living services and long-term care services. If the resident's needs change, he or she can move to the long-term care facility to receive more advanced care.

Home Health Care Agencies

Home health care agencies provide skilled care in a person's home (Fig. 1-6). In the home health care setting, people who receive care are typically called **clients,** rather than patients or residents. Home health care services are available for people of all ages with any number of different medical needs. For example, a new mother and her baby may need home care, especially if the baby was born too early. A person recovering from an accident, a stroke, or surgery may also need home care.

Hospice Organizations

Hospice organizations provide care for people who are dying and their families. People are able to receive the services of a hospice organization when they know that they have only 3 to

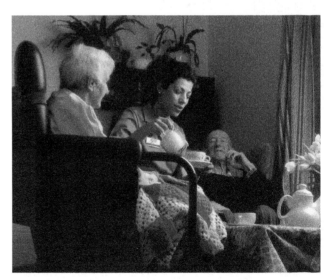

Figure 1-6
Personal support workers who work for home health care agencies provide health care to people in their homes. A home health care aide's responsibilities might also include preparing and serving light meals and light housekeeping, depending on the client's needs and agency policy. (*SPL/CL Photo Researchers, Inc.*)

6 months to live. The focus of hospice care is on relieving pain and providing emotional and spiritual support for both the dying person and the family. Hospice care can be provided in the home, hospital, or long-term care facility, or in a facility devoted exclusively to providing care to the dying.

STRUCTURE OF HEALTH CARE ORGANIZATIONS

Most health care organizations are set up in a way similar to that shown in Figure 1-7. Most are governed by a board of trustees (also called a board of directors), and most have divisions (groups in charge of certain aspects of the organization's function). An administrator or chief executive officer (CEO) usually manages the organization and is the link between the board and the organization.

The board is made up of community members. The board sets policies to ensure that the care offered by the organization is safe and of good quality. The board also makes sure that the organ-

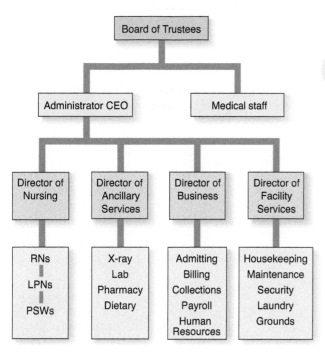

Figure 1-7
Most health care organizations are organized in similar ways. Each division within a health care organization is responsible for one key aspect of the organization's function.

ization meets the needs of the community. For example, think about a rural community where there is only one hospital. This hospital does not provide obstetric services, which means that pregnant women must travel out of the area to deliver their babies. The hospital's board surveys the people in the town and determines that the hospital needs to offer obstetric services in order to meet the community's needs. The board then develops a plan to get funding to build a maternity ward, and to find qualified people to staff it.

Each division within a health care organization is responsible for one key aspect of the organization's function. Each division is managed by a division director or division manager. The medical services division is led by a medical director, and is responsible for the doctors on staff. Nursing services is headed by a director of nursing (DON) or chief nursing officer (CNO), and is responsible for all aspects of the organization that have to do with patient or resident care. Business services is led by a business director, and usually oversees admissions, billing, and payroll. The business division may also oversee maintenance and housekeeping. The ancillary services division typically contains the departments in the organization that provide patient or resident services, such as social services and dietary services.

THE HEALTH CARE TEAM

Within each facility, care of patients or residents is provided by a **health care team,** made up of many people with different types of knowledge and skill levels (Fig. 1-8). The patient or resident is always the focus of the health care team's efforts. The goal of the health care team is to provide **holistic care** (care of the whole person, physically and emotionally). Each member of the health care team's job is as important as any other member's. Think of the members of the health care team as links in the chain of care provided for the patient or resident. Because a chain is only as strong as its weakest link, each member of the health care team must provide care to the best of his or her ability. For example, the maintenance staff keeps the facility running smoothly by keeping equipment in good working order. The housekeeping staff keeps the facility clean. The people who work in the lab must be precise when performing laboratory studies and writing reports. In

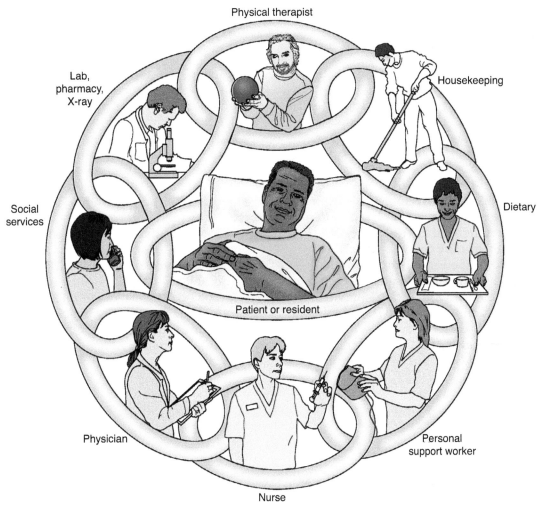

Physical therapist

Lab, pharmacy, X-ray

Housekeeping

Social services

Dietary

Patient or resident

Physician

Personal support worker

Nurse

Figure 1-8
Care is provided by the health care team. The patient or resident is the primary focus of the health care team's efforts. Because a chain is only as strong as its weakest link, each member of the health care team must provide care to the best of his or her ability.

short, everyone must provide competent care in order for the health care team to function properly.

In addition to taking a holistic approach to health care, the health care team takes a humanistic approach to health care. A humanistic approach to health care is one that focuses on the person receiving care. When we take a humanistic approach to health care, we:

- Consider the qualities that make the person unique, and use that knowledge to guide the care that we provide
- Imagine how it would feel to be in the person's situation, and act with empathy and compassion

- Consider the person's emotional, social, and spiritual needs, as well as his or her physical needs

To practice a humanistic approach to health care, spend time with your patients or residents and get to know them as individuals. Using that knowledge, think about things you can do that will help them to feel more comfortable, both physically and emotionally. Act with compassion. Everyone will benefit! You will have the satisfaction of knowing that you are providing the best care possible, and your patients or residents will feel well cared for and valued as individuals. That is what a humanistic approach to health care is all about.

SUMMARY

- Society has always sought to care for the sick and injured.
  - In Canada during the 1700s, 1800s, and early part of the 1900s, most people who needed health care received it in their homes. Most care was provided by family members and a "family doctor."
  - Throughout the 1920s and 1930s, public demand for more government involvement in providing improved health care for all Canadians increased. The Medical Care Act (1968) and the Canada Health Act (1984) led to the establishment of the present-day Canadian health care system.
- The federal government and the provincial/ territorial governments share the responsibility for health care in Canada.
- The Canada Health Act (1984) established publically funded health care insurance in Canada, and ensured that all Canadians have access to medically necessary hospital and doctor services on a prepaid basis.
- There are many different types of health care organizations, including hospitals, sub-acute care units (skilled nursing units), long-term care facilities (nursing homes), assisted-living facilities, home health care agencies, and hospice organizations.
- Health care is provided by a team of people, each with different areas of expertise and job responsibilities.
  - As a personal support worker, you are a critical part of the health care team.
  - The health care team takes a humanistic (person-focused), holistic (taking into account the person's physical needs, as well as emotional ones) approach to health care.

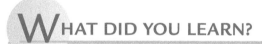

WHAT DID YOU LEARN?

Multiple Choice

Select the single best answer for each of the following questions.

1. The Canada Health Act was passed in:
   a. 1968
   b. 1900
   c. 1984
   d. 1930
2. In Canada, health care is the responsibility of the:
   a. Federal government
   b. Provincial/territorial government
   c. Consumer
   d. Federal and provincial/territorial governments
3. Health Canada is:
   a. A provincial health department
   b. A federal health department

   c. A provincial tax program
   d. A federal tax program
4. The first province in Canada to practice universal health coverage in 1947 was:
   a. Manitoba
   b. Alberta
   c. Saskatchewan
   d. Ontario
5. The Medical Care Act was passed in:
   a. 1968
   b. 1900
   c. 1984
   d. 1930

Matching

Match each type of health care facility with its appropriate description.

_____ 1. Assisted-living facility

_____ 2. Long-term care facility (nursing home)

_____ 3. Hospice

_____ 4. Home health care agency

_____ 5. Sub-acute care unit (skilled nursing unit, skilled nursing facility)

a. Place where people who can provide for most of their own care but who need limited assistance can live

b. Provides skilled care in a person's home

c. Provides care for people who cannot care for themselves, yet are not ill enough to be hospitalized

d. Care devoted exclusively to the dying

e. Provides care that is focused on rehabilitation; assists patients in making the transition from hospital care to home care

STOP and Think!

Think about what health care was like in Canada 100 years ago. How has health care delivery changed in Canada since the early 1900s? What aspects of the "old-fashioned" way of delivering health care were good? Not so good? What aspects of modern health care delivery are good? Not so good?

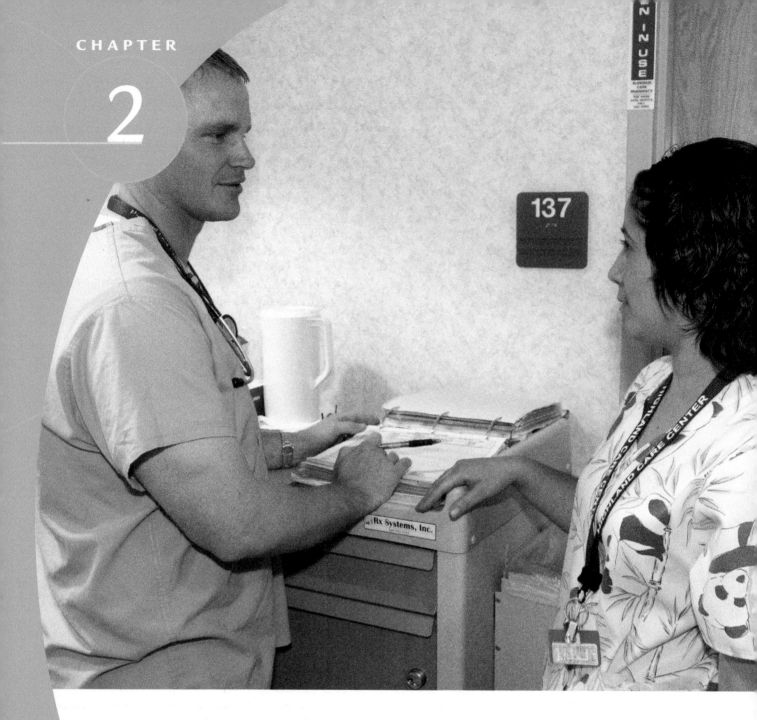

The Personal Support Worker

WHAT WILL YOU LEARN?

In the previous chapter, you were introduced to the idea of a "health care team," a group of employees with varying types of knowledge and skill levels who provide holistic care to a patient or resident. If you think of the members of the health care team as "links" in the chain of care, then as a personal support worker, you are a very critical "link." What contributions does the personal support worker make to the health care team, and

Photo: Nurses and personal support workers work together to provide patient or resident care.

what education is needed to become a personal support worker? In this chapter we will answer those questions, as well as describe the various ways in which nursing care can be delivered. We will also discuss how the personal support worker and nurse interact to achieve the goal of safe, efficient patient or resident care. When you are finished with this chapter, you will be able to:

1. Discuss requirements for personal support worker training.
2. Discuss the responsibilities of the personal support worker.
3. List the members of the nursing team, and describe the role of each team member.
4. Discuss the delegation process as it relates to the personal support worker.
5. List the five rights of delegation.

Vocabulary

Regulated health care profession	Licensed practical nurse (LPN) or registered nurse's assistant (RNA)	Charge nurse	Functional (modular) nursing
Non-regulated health care profession		Head nurse	Team nursing
Competency evaluation	Registered nurse (RN) or registered psychiatric	Director of nursing (DON)	Delegate
Reciprocity	nurse (RPN)	Primary nursing	Five rights of delegation
			Scope of practice

NURSING, PAST AND PRESENT

Very simply stated, the field of nursing involves caring for others. People who enter the field of nursing, such as nurses and personal support workers, provide physical and emotional care for people who are sick, disabled, or injured. Many nurses also work to keep people healthy, by teaching them about ways to maintain health and prevent illness.

Perhaps you have heard of Florence Nightingale. Florence Nightingale (1820–1910) was a British nurse who is credited with making nursing into the profession that it is today (Fig. 2-1). Ms. Nightingale started training programs for nurses and set up practices for hospital cleanliness and patient care that are followed to this day. By establishing educational standards for nursing professionals, Ms. Nightingale improved conditions for both the people receiving health care and those providing it. For the first time, those in the nursing field were regarded as professionals in their own right, with specialized knowledge, skills, and responsibilities.

The knowledge, skills, and responsibilities of the personal support worker have grown over the years too. Early personal support workers were employed in long-term care facilities and hospitals to help the nurses care for residents and patients. These personal support workers usually did not have training in the health care field, which led to poor care in many cases. Today's personal support workers, however, are well-trained members of the health care team with many important responsibilities.

REGULATED VERSUS NON-REGULATED HEALTH CARE PROFESSIONS

Health care professions are either regulated or non-regulated. A **regulated health care profession** is self-governed and associated with a professional organization called a college.

The college sets educational and licensing requirements for its members. The college establishes a scope of practice, a code of ethics, and standards of conduct that its members must adhere to. The college has a legislated responsibility to its members and to the public to ensure that the roles and responsibilities of its profession are clearly defined and followed by members of the profession. Nursing is a regulated profession, and in each province and territory across Canada there is a professional licensing body of nurses.

In contrast, a **non-regulated health care profession** does not have a professional self-governing

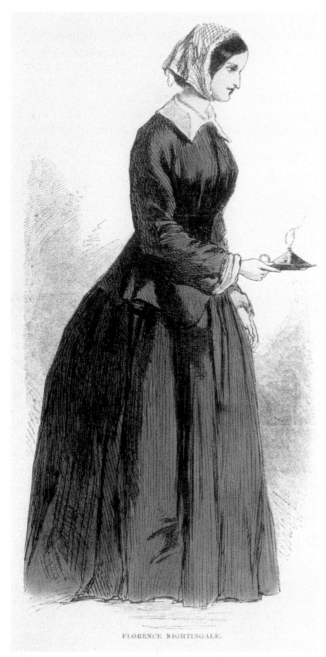

Figure 2-1
Florence Nightingale was a British nurse who established educational standards for nursing professionals. (© *National Library of Medicine/Photo Researchers, Inc.*)

health care professionals. For example, if you are employed to work in a recreation department of a long-term care facility, you may report directly to a recreational therapist. If you work in a group home (a small facility located in a residential neighborhood), then your supervisor could be a social worker. Some clients prefer to employ personal support workers directly. When you work directly for a client, the client is your supervisor.

EDUCATION OF THE PERSONAL SUPPORT WORKER

Requirements for personal support worker training vary across the country. In some provinces, the training program is provincially legislated. Training is offered in both public and private community colleges, as well as on the job (for example, some long-term care facilities offer on-the-job training). Most training programs are 20 to 32 weeks in length. Training programs may be offered on a full-time or part-time basis. The training program includes classroom lectures, hands-on practice of skills (usually in a laboratory setting), and supervised experience in a health care setting (Fig. 2-2).

As you complete your personal support worker training, you will study communication skills, infection control, safety and emergency

college. At present, the profession of personal support worker is non-regulated. Even though personal support workers do not have a self-governing college that governs their role, personal support workers are accountable to their employers, their supervisors, and to their patients, residents, or clients. In most settings, personal support workers are supervised by nurses. However, depending on where you work, you could be supervised by other

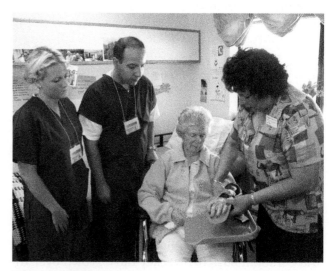

Figure 2-2
Part of a personal support worker's training involves working with patients or residents in an actual health care setting.

procedures, residents' rights, basic nursing skills, personal care skills, feeding techniques, and skin care. You will also learn how to help patients and residents move from place to place, change positions, dress, and perform range-of-motion exercises. In addition, you will learn the signs and symptoms of common diseases and how to care for people who have problems with thinking and memory. During the practical experience portion of the program you will practice performing nursing care procedures on real people.

At the conclusion of your training program, you may need to take a **competency evaluation.** The competency evaluation may include a written test and a skills test (during which you will be asked to perform selected nursing skills learned in the training program). The actual number of test questions that you must answer and skills that you must demonstrate is determined by your training program. Some training programs do not require a written test at the end of the program. Instead, an experienced personal support worker may be assigned to evaluate your work performance.

Upon successfully completing the training program, you will receive the appropriate documentation for certification. Remember that requirements for training (that is, the program length and required hours of actual supervised experience in a health care setting) vary across the country. You may be required to complete additional hours of training as you move from one province or territory to another. The principle of **reciprocity** means, however, that in many cases, your certificate will be valid in another province or territory once you have obtained the necessary additional hours of training.

RESPONSIBILITIES OF THE PERSONAL SUPPORT WORKER

As a personal support worker, most of your responsibilities will relate to meeting the basic physical needs of patients and residents, which include hygiene, safety, comfort, nutrition, exercise, and elimination. You may also be responsible for helping to keep your patients' or residents' environment clean and neat. In addition to taking care of patients' or residents' physical needs, you will play an important role in meeting patients' or residents' emotional needs. Talking with patients or residents to see how they are responding to

their treatments and care and providing encouragement are important parts of your job. Because you will have many opportunities to interact with your patients or residents, you will be in a unique position to observe changes in a patient's or resident's physical or mental status, and to report these observations to the nurse. You may be responsible for documenting your observations. Finally, you may be responsible for helping your patients or residents and their family members to understand and follow medical instructions. A typical job description for a personal support worker is shown in Figure 2-3.

THE NURSING TEAM

The nursing team, a subset of the health care team, is responsible for providing care to the patient or resident (Table 2-1). At minimum, the nursing team consists of a nurse and a personal support worker. The nurse is either a **licensed practical nurse (LPN) or a registered nurse's assistant (RNA)**, or a **registered nurse (RN), or a registered psychiatric nurse (RPN).** The nurse carries out the doctor's orders, and the personal support worker helps the nurse. Other members of the nursing team may include a **charge nurse,** an RN/RPN or LPN/RNA who supervises the other nurses for a particular shift, and a **head nurse,** an RN/RPN who is in charge of a department or section. Each health care organization has an RN/RPN who directs all of the nursing care within that facility. This person is the **director of nursing (DON).**

The way in which the members of the nursing team work together varies, depending on the setting. For example, in the home health care setting, the case manager (an RN/RPN) develops a care plan along with the client and his or her family, and the personal support worker follows this plan when she visits the client. Often, in this situation, the personal support worker is the only health care provider who sees the client daily. The nurse may see the client only when she visits the home in a supervisory capacity (for example, every few weeks).

In the hospital or other settings where all of the members of the nursing team are "on-site," several different models for organizing the team's efforts have been developed.

- In **primary nursing,** one nurse (an RN/RPN or an LPN/RNA) is assigned several patients or residents, and is responsible for planning and carrying out

---

JOB DESCRIPTION

Job Title: Health Care Aide (HCA) Personal Support Worker (PSW)	Department: Nursing	Division: Bonnechere Manor	Reports to: Resident Care Coordinator(s)
Revision Date: March 2008	Salary Grid:		

Position Summary:
Under the direction and supervision of the Resident Care Coordinator(s), the Health Care Aide/Personal Support Worker provides resident-focused personal care within an interdisciplinary team consistent with the Mission and Philosophy of Care at Bonnechere Manor.

Qualifications:
- Personal Support Worker Certificate, Health Care Aide Certificate or equivalent formal education from an approved school
- Certificate – Food Safety Awareness Program recognized by a Public Health Unit
- Experience in long term care setting an asset
- Therapeutic verbal and written communication skills in English
- Ability to work well with others in a team approach and to adapt to changing situations
- Physically capable of performing assigned duties within a flexible work schedule inside a 24-hour-a-day, 7-day-a-week operation
- Demonstrates regular attendance standards in keeping with the County Attendance Support Program
- Ability to meet and maintain health requirement as per Long Term Care Legislation
- Current WHMIS certification, an asset
- Computer skills, an asset

Position Responsibilities:
Delivers resident-focused care within full scope of practice of a PSW/HCA, in a home-like environment, respecting the individuality and dignity of each resident/family and co-workers, including the completion of the following duties:

1. Performs the responsibilities of the position within the legislative and regulatory standards set out in the applicable Provincial and Municipal Acts. Performs the responsibilities of the position consistent with the Operational policies of the County of Renfrew.

2. Participates in all aspects of personal resident care to ensure the physical, psychological, social and spiritual needs of each resident/family are met under the direction of the Registered Staff and/or Resident Care Coordinator(s).

3. Utilizes therapeutic communication by establishing a working relationship with resident/families and co-workers for the purpose of meeting resident needs; ensures respect, dignity, individuality of each resident and staff member.

4. Participates with other team members in formulating, delivering and reporting daily resident care needs and personal preferences by:
   - Attending and gathering pertinent data from report
   - Seeking direction from Registered Staff
   - Observing residents for any changes and reporting immediately to the Registered Staff
   - Assessing behaviours and activities of daily living and reporting in oral and/or written form at designated times
   - Reporting unusual events promptly and directly to Registered Staff

Figure 2-3
It is always a good idea to be very familiar with your formal job description at each facility where you work. Here is an example of a typical job description for a personal support worker. (*Courtesy of County of Renfrew, Ontario, Canada.*)

5. Delivers effective and efficient care under the direction of the Registered Staff that promotes resident/family choice and acknowledges resident strengths and limitations, as well as the need for safety and the safety of other resident/family and staff.

6. Consistent with resident-focused care approach to meet resident needs and demonstrates initiative to:
   • Assist with serving meals, feeding, providing nourishment supplements
   • Assist with transporting and transferring resident as needed
   • Respond to any resident in need and assists any employee in need of help
   • Under the direction of Registered Staff, applies treatment creams to residents

7. Ensures daily, the neatness of residents' rooms, furniture, clothes closets, mobility devices, tub/washrooms, utility rooms and kitchen/serveries.

8. Participates in multidisciplinary committee work as required:
   • Care conferences as directed
   • Unit meetings, general staff meetings, and PSW/HCA meetings

9. Participates in continuing education, relevant to LTC, to ensure skills and abilities are maintained and enhanced.

10. Participates in continuous quality improvement of the care unit and associated care services by:
    • Ongoing collection and documentation of CMI data
    • Using supplies in a cost-efficient manner as per product guidelines
    • Offering suggestions to Resident Care Coordinator(s) regarding resource allocation
    • Participating in continuing education, relevant to LTC, to ensure skills and abilities are maintained and enhanced

11. Creates a facility environment that protects confidentiality of residents, staff, and activities of Bonnechere Manor.

12. Protects own health and health of others by adopting safe work practices, reporting unsafe conditions immediately, and attending all relevant in-services regarding occupational health and safety. Follows all Guidelines for employees and employers as legislated under the Ontario Occupational Health and Safety Act.

> The foregoing description reflects the general duties necessary to describe the principal functions of the job identified and shall not be construed to be all of the work requirements that may be inherent in this classification.

Figure 2-3 (*Continued*)

all aspects of care for those people. The nurse performs all of the nursing duties for his or her patients, from feeding and bathing to giving medications and other treatments. Other nurses and personal support workers are responsible for the primary nurse's patients or residents when the primary nurse is not on duty, but all nursing efforts on behalf of those patients or residents are directed and coordinated by the primary nurse.

• In **functional (modular) nursing,** each member of the nursing team carries out the same assigned task for all patients or residents. For example, for a particular group or unit of patients or residents, one nurse may administer all medications while another nurse does assessments and special treatments. One personal support worker may be assigned to take vital signs and assist with meals, while another is assigned bathing and bedmaking.

• In **team nursing,** a team leader (an RN/RPN) determines all of the nursing needs for the patients or residents assigned to the team, and assigns tasks according to each team member's skills and level of responsibility. For example, the nurse may assist the personal support worker with bathing a patient or resident, and then give that person his or her medication. Or two

Table 2-1	The Nursing Team	
TEAM MEMBER	**REQUIREMENTS TO PRACTICE**	**CONTRIBUTION TO TEAM**
Registered nurse (RN) OR Registered psychiatric nurse (RPN)	A baccalaureate degree from a liberal arts college or university OR A 2-year diploma from an accredited community college PLUS A license obtained by passing a provincial/territorial examination	Develops care plans and coordinates all aspects of patient or resident care Provides nursing care to patients or residents Delegates selected aspects of patient or resident care to other team members, and supervises these team members as they carry out the delegated tasks
Licensed practical nurse (LPN) OR Registered nurse's assistant (RNA)	A certificate or a diploma from a 12- to 18-month training program offered by accredited community college PLUS A license obtained by passing a provincial/territorial examination	Provides nursing care to patients or residents Delegates selected aspects of patient or resident care to other team members, and supervises these team members as they carry out the delegated tasks
Personal support worker OR Health care support worker Health care aide Continuing care aide Nursing home attendant Home support worker	A certificate from an approved school OR equivalent formal education from an approved school OR A willingness to be trained by the employer	Assists the RN/RPN or LPN/RNA with providing nursing care to patients or residents; responsibilities include basic nursing tasks related to meeting hygiene, safety, comfort, nutrition, exercise, and elimination needs

personal support workers may work together to complete the tasks usually handled by personal support workers, such as bathing and bedmaking.

No matter which nursing care model is used in the health care facility where you work, you will be the team member responsible for providing most of the personal care for your patients or residents. One of your most important duties while you are providing this care will be to notice changes in a patient's or resident's condition and to report these changes to the nurse.

DELEGATION

To **delegate** a task means to give another person permission to perform that task on your behalf. The nurse is responsible for providing safe nursing care to the public. This means that the nurse is responsible for planning and coordinating the care plan for patients or residents. In order to ensure that the nursing team functions efficiently, a nurse has the authority to delegate selected tasks to a personal support worker.

Typically, the nurse will delegate nursing tasks related to routine care (hygiene, comfort, exercise) to personal support workers. An RN/RPN can also delegate certain nursing tasks, such as data collection and documentation, to a personal support worker. However, nursing tasks that require professional judgment, such as assessment, planning, or evaluating, cannot be delegated to a personal support worker. For example, a personal support worker can take a person's vital signs and record this information on the person's chart, but the personal support worker is not qualified to interpret the data.

Understanding how a nurse decides which tasks to delegate will help you to understand why you may be asked to do certain tasks but not others. When delegating a task, the nurse must know the abilities and qualifications of the personal support worker, and she or another licensed nurse must be available to provide supervision. In addition, the nurse must consider the patient's or resident's individual needs. To enable nurses to make good decisions about which tasks to delegate and to whom, the National Council of State Boards of Nursing (NCSBN) (an American organization) has developed guidelines called the **five rights of delegation** (Table 2-2).

Table 2-2 Five Rights of Delegation

	QUESTIONS THE PERSONAL SUPPORT WORKER MUST CONSIDER	QUESTIONS THE NURSE MUST CONSIDER
The right task	Is this a task that can be delegated? Does the nurse practice act allow me to delegate the task? Is the task in the job description for the personal support worker?	Does the state allow me to perform this task? Have I been trained to do this task? Do I have experience performing this task? Is this task in my job description?
The right circumstance	What is the patient's or resident's condition? Is he or she stable? What are the needs of the patient or resident at this time?	Can I perform this task safely, given the patient's or resident's condition?
The right person	Does the personal support worker have the right training and experience to safely complete the task?	Am I confident that I can perform this task safely? Do I have any reservations about performing this task, and if so, what are they?
The right direction	Am I able to give the personal support worker clear direction regarding how to perform this task? Am I able to explain to the personal support worker what is expected?	Did the nurse give me clear instructions? Do I understand what the nurse expects?
The right supervision	Will I be available to supervise and answer questions?	Will the nurse be available to supervise and answer questions?

You and the nurse share the responsibility for making sure that delegated tasks are carried out without causing harm to the patient or resident. The nurse is responsible for making good decisions about which tasks to delegate, and for providing adequate supervision. You are responsible for recognizing which delegated tasks are within your **scope of practice** (the range of tasks that you are legally permitted to do as a personal support worker) and range of abilities, and using this knowledge as the basis for either accepting or refusing the assignment. Your scope of practice will be determined by provincial or territorial legislation, as well as by your facility.

Just as a nurse uses the five rights of delegation to decide which tasks to delegate and to whom, you can use the five rights of delegation to help you decide whether to accept or decline a delegated task (see Table 2-2). When you agree to perform a task, you accept responsibility for your actions. You must ask for help when you have questions or are unsure about how to proceed, and you must communicate with the nurse by reporting what you have done and what you observed.

You should never refuse an assignment simply because you do not want to do it. You must have a good reason for refusing to carry out an assign-

ment, or you could lose your job. Valid reasons for refusing an assignment include the following:

- The task is not in your job description. Box 2-1 summarizes tasks that are generally outside the scope of practice of a personal support worker.
- Carrying out the task could result in harm to the patient or resident.
- The task is illegal or unethical.
- The nurse is not available to supervise your efforts.
- You do not have the proper equipment.
- The directions are not clear.
- You are not able to perform the task safely.
- You have not received adequate training about the task or the equipment used.

If you do make the decision to decline a task that you have been assigned to do, it is your responsibility to state clearly that you are not going to do the task and your reason why. Failure to communicate your refusal to complete a task to the person requesting your help can jeopardize the care or safety of the patient or resident. The person requesting your help assumes that you are doing the task, unless he or she hears otherwise. Declining a task is a discussion that you should have privately with the person requesting the task of you. Do not discuss the issue in front of the resident, patient, or visitors.

BOX 2-1	Tasks That Are Generally Beyond the Personal Support Worker's Scope of Practice

Administering medications (including oxygen). Some states allow personal support workers to administer medications to residents in assisted-living facilities, if the personal support worker has undergone specialized training to do so. Generally, only a licensed nurse (an RN/RPN or LPN/RNA) or doctor is allowed to give medications. Personal support workers may assist patients in taking medication by bringing water or helping to open the medicine bottle.

Receiving verbal orders (in person or over the telephone) from doctors. Licensed nurses (RN/RPNs or LPN/RNAs) are the only personnel authorized to receive doctors' orders.

Diagnosing illnesses and prescribing medications. Only doctors can diagnose illnesses and prescribe medical or surgical treatment.

Supervising other personal support workers. Licensed nurses (RN/RPNs or LPN/RNAs) are responsible for supervising personal support workers.

Performing procedures that require sterile technique. Personal support workers are permitted to assist a nurse in performing a sterile procedure, but they are not trained to do these procedures themselves.

Inserting or removing tubes from a person's body (bladder, esophagus, trachea, nose, ears). Personal support workers generally are not trained in procedures that involve inserting or removing tubes from a patient's or resident's body. Exceptions may be made if the personal support worker has had the opportunity to practice a procedure under an instructor's supervision.

General guidelines for accepting or declining an assignment are given in Guidelines Box 2-1. A good general rule to keep in mind is that you should not perform any task that is not listed in your job description. Because a personal support worker's duties can vary from province to province, and also from facility to facility, you must be familiar with your formal job description. Ask your supervisor about anything you do not understand. This is important to protect yourself, as well as your patients or residents.

Guidelines Box 2-1	Guidelines for Accepting or Declining an Assignment

WHAT YOU DO	WHY YOU DO IT
Always ask the nurse for clarification if there is something you do not understand.	It is your responsibility to make sure you know what is to be done and how it is to be done before going to the patient or resident.
Never perform a task that you have not been taught to do, or that you feel uncomfortable doing, unless you are supervised by a nurse.	The nurse is ultimately responsible for ensuring the patient's or resident's safety. This means that it is the nurse's responsibility to ensure that whoever is performing the task on his or her behalf is qualified to do so, and capable. It is irresponsible for you to misrepresent your abilities, or to proceed unsupervised with a task that you are not fully capable of doing well.
Never ignore an assignment because you do not know how to perform the task or the task is beyond your scope of practice.	The patient's or resident's needs must be attended to, either by you or by someone else. If you feel that you cannot perform the task that you are being asked to do, explain your concerns to the nurse so that she can either help you with the task or reassign it.

SUMMARY

- No matter what the setting, personal support workers are an integral part of the nursing team, a subset of the health care team.
  - Like all of the members of the nursing team, personal support workers undergo training that authorizes them to perform certain tasks.
  - Personal support workers assist the nurse by performing basic nursing functions, such as those related to hygiene, safety, comfort, nutrition, exercise, and elimination.
- In order to ensure that the nursing team operates smoothly and efficiently, a "chain of command" exists. This means that licensed nurses (RN/RPNs or LPN/RNAs) are able to assign (delegate) certain tasks to personal support workers.
  - The delegation of tasks cannot be taken lightly by either the delegator (the licensed nurse) or the delegatee (the personal support worker). Both share the responsibility of ensuring that the procedure is carried out without harm to the patient or resident.
  - The personal support worker must know which tasks are within his or her scope of practice, and which tasks are not.

WHAT DID YOU LEARN?

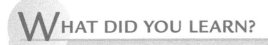

Multiple Choice

Select the single best answer for each of the following questions.

1. Personal support workers are:
   a. Licensed health care workers
   b. Non-regulated health care workers
   c. Members of the regulatory nursing body
   d. Members of a professional organization
2. As a personal support worker, it is your responsibility to:
   a. Plan the patient's or resident's care
   b. Perform the tasks your supervisor assigns to you
   c. Do the best you can without asking for help
   d. Compare assignments with your co-workers
3. If you do not know how to do an assigned task, you should:
   a. Call another personal support worker for help
   b. Ask the patient or resident how he prefers to have it done
   c. Ask the nurse for help
   d. Follow the instructions in the procedure manual

4. Personal support workers work under the supervision of:
   a. A doctor
   b. A registered nurse/registered psychiatric nurse (RN/RPN) or licensed practical nurse/registered nurse's assistant (LPN/RNA)
   c. Other personal support workers
   d. The long-term care facility administrator
5. To "delegate" means to:
   a. Do what you are told to do
   b. Give another person permission to perform a task on your behalf
   c. Transfer your duties to another personal support worker
   d. Have the charge nurse take your assignment

6. The term "scope of practice" refers to:
   a. The tasks a patient or resident asks you to perform
   b. The tasks your co-workers ask you to help them with
   c. The range of tasks that you are legally permitted to do
   d. The tasks that your supervisor has assigned to you

STOP and Think!

The nurse you are working with has asked you to remove Mrs. Thompson's urinary catheter. Your facility trains personal support workers to perform this task, and you have just completed that training. Removing Mrs. Thompson's urinary catheter will be the first time you will have a chance to perform this new skill on a "real" person, and you are uncomfortable. What should you do?

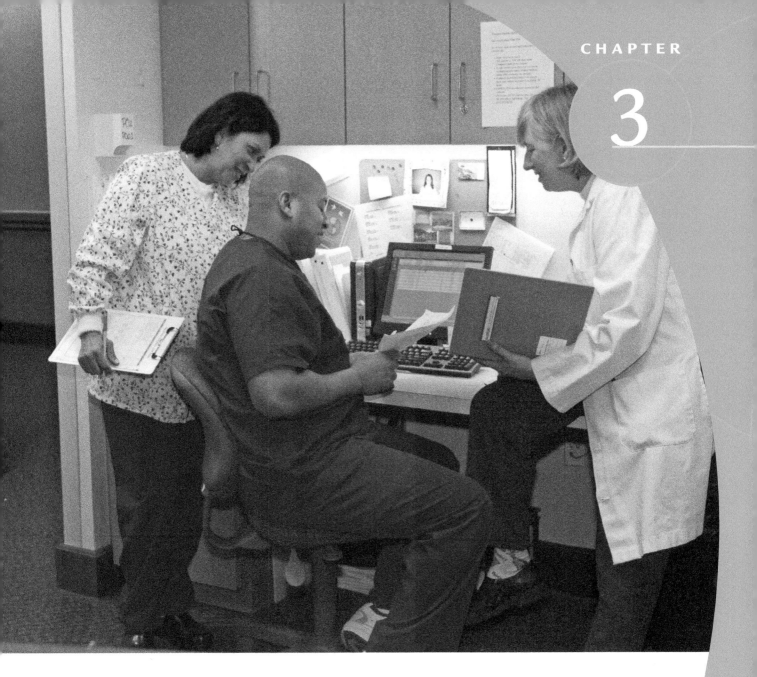

Professionalism and Job-Seeking Skills

WHAT WILL YOU LEARN?

While having the knowledge and ability to perform your duties well is essential, showing professionalism and a strong work ethic are important too. In this chapter, we will explore the qualities of professionalism and a strong work ethic, and how possessing these qualities can help you to get a job, and excel at it. In addition, we will provide

Photo: The health care industry relies on all types of professionals to provide quality care to patients and residents.

an overview of the process of applying and interviewing for a job. It may seem odd to be talking about how to get a job at the beginning of the book, but knowing what is expected of a good employee helps you to make a great impression while you are still a student. When you are finished with this chapter, you will be able to:

1. Define the terms *professional* and *professionalism*.
2. Discuss characteristics that health care workers demonstrate that promote professionalism and explain the importance of each characteristic.
3. Define the term *work ethic* and describe how good work habits promote professionalism.
4. Understand the importance of personal health and hygiene for the health care worker.
5. Describe considerations one must explore when seeking employment.
6. List several sources of employment information for jobs in the health care industry.
7. Discuss the application process necessary for obtaining employment.
8. Describe how to make a good impression during a job interview.
9. Describe the proper way to resign from a job.

Vocabulary

Professional	Hygiene	Reference list	Interview
Professionalism	Résumé	Human resources (HR)	
Attitude	Canadian Human Rights	department	
Work ethic	Law	(personnel)	
Empathy			

WHAT IS A PROFESSIONAL?

What exactly is a professional? And how is professionalism measured? One definition of a professional is "a person with much experience and great skill in a specified role" who is "engaged in a specific occupation for pay or as a means of livelihood." Another definition relates the word "professional" to a "profession," or a sacred vow. The relationship between the word "profession" (in the sense of a sacred vow) and the word "professional" (in the sense of one who takes a sacred vow) is especially applicable to those of us who consider ourselves "health care professionals," for we do practice that "sacred vow" of providing care for those in need.

The health care industry gives the title of **professional** to those who have credentials, obtained through education and training, that enable them to become licensed or certified to practice a certain profession. This industry certainly relies on all types of professionals, such as physicians, nurses, and personal support workers, to provide quality care to patients and residents. However, many people who are considered professionals do not need a license or a certificate to perform their

jobs, and they may not even need a specific educational background. Being a professional also means having a professional attitude, or exhibiting **professionalism.**

An **attitude** is the side of ourselves that we display to the world, communicating outwardly how we feel about things. A person's attitude is apparent from things he says (and the way he says them), the way he behaves, and the way he looks. You may have heard it said about a person that he or she "has an attitude," meaning that the person's outward behaviour is unpleasant. Well, an attitude is something we all possess and it can be positive instead of negative.

Possessing a positive attitude in the workplace means that you are caring and compassionate toward your patients or residents, and that you demonstrate a commitment to doing your job to the best of your ability at all times. This commitment to doing your best is the attitude that defines professionalism, the attitude of being a professional. While your job as a personal support worker will allow you to earn a paycheck, a true professional views her work as a reflection of the role she plays in society. Income is important, but so is the sense of pride you will feel as a result of setting high standards for your performance and obtaining satisfaction from the work you do, and in knowing that you are helping others. Regardless of the level of education, certification, or experience a health care professional has, professionalism is all about exhibiting the right attitude, to co-workers, patients or residents, and visitors. Professionalism is a choice you make and requires effort. What attitude will you choose to show?

WHAT IS A WORK ETHIC?

A **work ethic** can be described in many ways and measured by any number of standards, but simply put, it relates specifically to your attitude toward your work. Professionalism and a strong work ethic go hand in hand.

A strong work ethic is what separates an average employee from a great employee (Fig. 3-1). Two personal support workers can have solid skills and be very good at getting their work done on time, but the personal support worker with the strongest work ethic will be the one who enjoys the greatest professional success. A good work ethic not only allows a person to grow in her career (because her employer will be satisfied with the quality of her work), it allows her to experience the emotional rewards of knowing that she has made her best effort.

There are many qualities that are associated with a strong work ethic, such as cheerfulness and enthusiasm, a willingness to volunteer for new assignments, and a desire to learn new skills. A personal support worker with a strong work ethic is someone you can depend on and trust, someone who treats others with kindness, respect, and compassion. People with strong work ethics know how to do their jobs well, they like their jobs, and they continue to learn and improve. Let's discuss some specific qualities that define a good work ethic.

PUNCTUALITY

Being punctual means that you are on time, or a little bit early. Arriving to work on time prepared to start your duties is vital in the health care industry (Fig. 3-2). Many people are relying on you! The staff working the shift before yours is anxious for you to relieve them so that they can go home to their families and other responsibilities. If

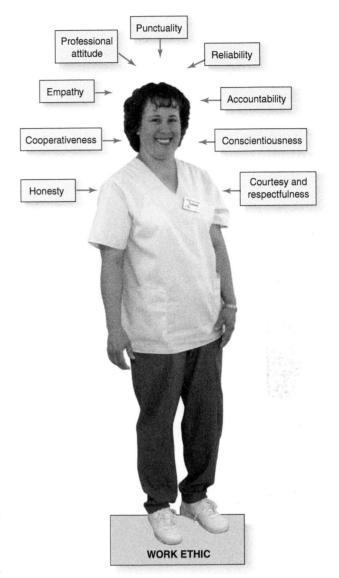

Figure 3-1
Professionalism and a strong work ethic go hand in hand. Many qualities contribute to a strong work ethic.

you work a morning shift, patients and residents will need your assistance in getting out of bed and preparing for breakfast, diagnostic tests, or surgery.

Organization is necessary to achieve punctuality. If you work a morning shift, plan ahead the evening before by packing your lunch and making sure your uniform is clean and pressed. If you have children, pack their lunches, lay out their clothes for the next day, and make sure any papers they need for school are completed. Setting the alarm 15 minutes earlier will not significantly affect the

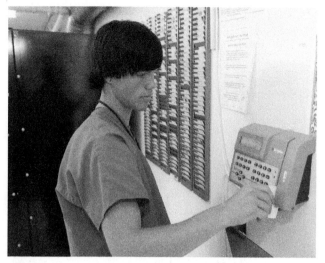

Figure 3-2
Being punctual means that you are on time or a little early. It is important to come to work on time because many people are relying on you!

amount of sleep you get, but it will allow you that extra time you need to have breakfast before work, or tend to any small last-minute crises.

RELIABILITY

Reliability is an essential characteristic for a personal support worker. Reliability means that others can count on you to come to work every day, as scheduled, and to remain there during your entire shift (in other words, that your attendance is consistent). Everyone certainly has to miss a day of work occasionally for sickness or emergencies, but frequent absences are a very poor reflection on your work ethic. Have alternative plans for transportation and childcare in place before the need arises, and try to keep yourself healthy to decrease your need to take sick days. Poor attendance and chronic lateness are primary reasons employers take corrective action against personal support workers.

Reliability also means that others can count on you to do your job conscientiously and well, with minimal supervision. Your supervisor should not feel the need to look over your shoulder or "check up" on you to make sure your work has been finished.

ACCOUNTABILITY

Accountability is also an essential characteristic for a personal support worker. An accountable person accepts responsibility for his or her actions, and the results of those actions. Being accountable means that you can accept criticism that is intended to help you improve, admit a mistake, and work to correct the situation. Although it can be difficult to admit that you have made a mistake, trying to conceal a mistake or blame it on someone else will only make matters worse. By acknowledging a mistake and taking measures to correct it, you are not only acting in the best interest of your patient or resident, you are letting your supervisors and co-workers know that you can be trusted to do your job to the best of your ability at all times, and that you are interested in learning how to prevent similar mistakes from happening in the future.

CONSCIENTIOUSNESS

Conscientious personal support workers take their assignments seriously and make sure they follow directions carefully. They demonstrate responsibility by asking for additional explanation or clarification when necessary, seeking help with difficult tasks, and admitting that they may not know how to perform a particular task. If you have not been shown how to do a procedure that you have been asked to do, show that you are interested in learning how. A conscientious personal support worker attends to details and goes the extra mile to complete a task with care. When you act conscientiously, you leave your patients or residents feeling like they are special and have received the "royal treatment."

COURTESY AND RESPECTFULNESS

Always treat other people with respect, both your patients or residents and your co-workers. The phrases *please, thank you,* and *excuse me* can improve the quality of almost any interaction. Avoid using "baby talk" or "talking down" to patients or residents. Address people as they prefer to be addressed. If in doubt, err on the side of formality ("Dr. Smith," "Mrs. Jones," "Mr. Davis," "Ms. Thomson"). Being polite and having good manners are correct in any situation. Considering another person's feelings and beliefs shows that you truly care about the person.

Show respect for your co-workers and supervisors by not saying anything negative about them to your patients or residents, or other co-workers. Do not speak poorly about your place of employment to others, even if there are things that you are not happy with. People who hear you say negative things about your place of employment will begin to wonder about you and why you continue to work there if the situation is so bad. If the person you are speaking to is a patient or resident (or a family member of a patient or resident), he or she may begin to question the quality of care that is being given.

HONESTY

Honesty is a critical quality for health care workers to have. You are expected to accurately record vital signs and other information about the condition of the people you care for. You will have access to people's valuables, especially in the long-term care and home health care settings. You will be trusted with information of a very private nature regarding people's care and medical condition. Patients and residents will come to trust you and confide in you. If you act in a way that gives your patients or residents reason to lose confidence in their ability to trust you, it will be very difficult to reestablish your relationship.

COOPERATIVENESS

Being able to cooperate, or work as part of a team, is essential in the health care industry. Professionals with many different levels of education and areas of training work together to benefit the people they care for. Remember how important your part of the chain of care is and what an essential role you play in providing for the care and comfort of your patients or residents, and use this as a driving force. Making an effort to get along with your co-workers will make your work easier and will ease the burden on your co-workers as well. A good personal support worker does not wait for a co-worker to ask for help; he or she sees a need and offers a helping hand. You will undoubtedly have to work with people you may not especially like, but a professional is able to put his or her personal feelings aside for the benefit of the patient or resident.

EMPATHY

Empathy means that you are able to try and imagine what it would feel like to be in another person's situation. There are times when co-workers, patients or residents, or the family members of patients or residents will really try your patience, but if you think of how you would feel if you were in a similar situation, you may

find that you are able to understand the offending behaviour better. Empathy gives us another perspective and helps us to be kinder and more tolerant. Treating people with kindness is a better reflection of professionalism than, for example, displaying superior intellect.

A DESIRE TO LEARN

Although you may have completed your training as a personal support worker, you will never stop needing to learn new things. The field of health care is constantly changing, and new techniques and treatments are developed daily. To provide the best possible care to your patients or residents, you must continue to learn new ways of caring for them. It is not the responsibility of your supervisor or your place of employment to keep you up to date on new health care issues. It is your responsibility. There are many professional journals, some specifically for personal support workers, that cover new information that is important for you to know. Learn about the illnesses or conditions that the people you are caring for have. Ask questions about new techniques or treatments you see being used. This way, you become more involved as a member of the health care team because you have a better understanding of the care being given.

PERSONAL HEALTH AND HYGIENE

To care for your patients or residents to the best of your ability, you must first care for yourself. By taking proper care of yourself, you demonstrate that you are a professional who takes her responsibilities seriously.

MAINTAINING YOUR PHYSICAL HEALTH

The duties of a personal support worker require much physical effort. You will be constantly lifting, bending, walking, and reaching as you perform your daily tasks at work. As you will learn in later chapters, there are many risks to your health and physical condition in the health care profession. Your employer, your co-workers, your family, and especially your patients or residents rely on you to be able to do your duties. In addition to giving you more energy, staying physically fit keeps your body strong and allows you to

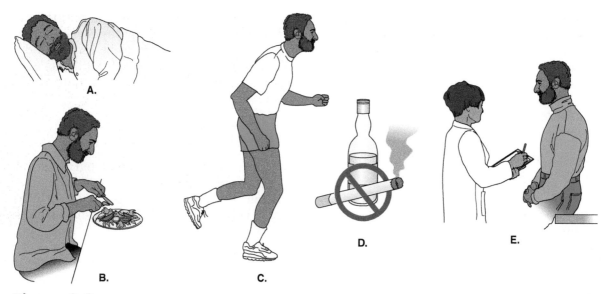

Figure 3-3

There are many things you can do to keep your body in good physical condition. **(A)** Get enough sleep. **(B)** Eat well-balanced meals. **(C)** Exercise regularly. **(D)** Avoid smoking, excessive alcohol consumption, and the use of recreational drugs. **(E)** Get routine physical examinations to detect health problems early.

avoid many types of job-related injuries (Fig. 3-3). To keep your body in good physical condition:

- **Get enough sleep.** Most people need an average of 6 to 8 hours of sleep to function properly. Not only does rest relax the muscles, it also relaxes the mind and allows you to think clearly. Too little rest can weaken your immune system, making you more likely to get infections, such as cold and flu viruses.

- **Eat well-balanced meals.** A working body needs good nutrition, a subject you will learn more about in Chapter 19. You need fuel for your muscles and for your brain. Avoid fad diets because they often are responsible for the loss of muscle mass and strength.

- **Exercise regularly.** Regular physical exercise gives you more strength and energy, and keeps your heart and lungs healthy. In addition, regular exercise helps reduce the mental stress that sometimes goes along with intensely emotional jobs, such as those in the health care field.

- **Do not smoke.** Smoking causes the blood vessels in the body to narrow, reducing the flow of oxygen-carrying blood to the body's cells. It is well known that smoking is associated with lung cancer, emphysema, and heart disease. Infertility, impotence, and an

increased risk of miscarriage are other negative effects of smoking. In addition to being a health risk, smoking makes your clothes and breath smell bad.

- **Do not take recreational drugs and limit your alcohol intake.** Recreational drugs are associated with many health problems. Many employers now perform drug screening of potential employees. Although many people feel that there is nothing wrong with occasionally having a drink if this is something you enjoy, drinking too much or too frequently can negatively impact your health and leave you unable to perform your job to the best of your ability. The health care profession needs workers who are clear-headed and able to make good decisions on behalf of others. Do not report to work while under the influence of recreational drugs or alcohol, or use these substances while on duty—doing so is dangerous for you, as well as for your patients or residents.

- **Have a routine physical examination.** Many chronic illnesses, such as high blood pressure and diabetes, go undetected until they have caused permanent damage to your body. Many types of cancers can be cured if detected early enough. Uncorrected vision and hearing problems can lead to errors when taking vital signs or reading medication labels. Routine physical examinations can help you to detect problems early, so that actions can be taken to correct them.

MAINTAINING YOUR EMOTIONAL HEALTH

Caring for others is an emotionally demanding job, as well as a physically demanding one, for many reasons:

- Due to the shortage of health care workers, as well as a need to cut costs, many facilities are understaffed, which means that employees are often overworked.
- Not all patients or residents are happy or grateful for the care they are receiving. Many people in need of care do not feel well and, as a result, may be difficult or hard to manage. Sometimes a person who is ill or worried will become angry or very critical and he or she will take these feelings out on you, even though you have done nothing wrong.
- As a health care worker, you will have to face the death of some of your patients or residents. This can be difficult, especially in situations where you have had a chance to develop a relationship with the patient or resident and his or her family members.

Fortunately, there are actions you can take to help keep your emotions in check while you are on the job, and prevent emotional "burn-out":

- **Maintain your physical health.** It is proven that physical activity relieves mental and emotional stress.
- **Be sure to schedule time for yourself.** Most of us are not just caregivers in the workplace; we are caregivers at home as well. It is important to make time for yourself, to do what you like to do, in order to avoid feeling overwhelmed by your responsibilities at home and at work.
- **Take advantage of counselling services offered by your employer, or confide in a clergy member.** Talking to a professional can help you to manage work-related stress and define your feelings and beliefs about difficult subjects, such as death and dying (Fig. 3-4).
- **When a situation becomes particularly "heated" at work, take a physical and emotional break.** Have someone relieve you (or make sure your patients are safe), and take a walk outside to calm down.

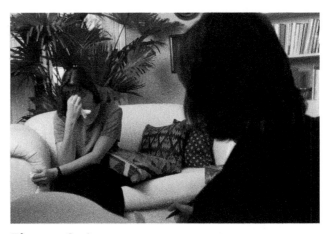

Figure 3-4
Talking with a counsellor can help you to manage work-related stress.

- **Ask to be assigned to different work areas, or to different patients or residents, occasionally.**

PERSONAL HYGIENE AND APPEARANCE

Personal **hygiene,** or cleanliness, addresses several issues. First, it promotes a professional image. If you care enough about yourself to keep yourself clean and neat, the people you care for will feel that you will do the same for them. Would you want to be cared for by someone with breath or body odors, or dirty hair? Second, good personal hygiene helps to prevent the spread of infection, both to your patients or residents and to you and your family. In a health care setting, the potential to come into contact with all types of "germs" is increased, and practicing good personal hygiene is necessary. To practice good personal hygiene:

- Bathe daily and use a deodorant.
- Shampoo your hair regularly and treat dandruff or other scalp conditions.
- Keep your nails short and clean.
- Brush and floss your teeth, and use mouthwash. Visit a dentist regularly. Poor dental health can cause breath odors and gum infections.
- Men should shave daily, or keep facial hair neatly groomed and trimmed.
- Wear a clean, pressed uniform each day.
- Wash your hands often.

Practicing good personal hygiene is essential to presenting a professional image. When you

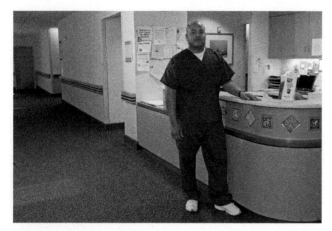

Figure 3-5
In the health care field, many of the traits we have come to associate with a professional image are related to maintaining safety and health.

picture a health care professional, what does she look like? Is she wearing a wrinkled, stained uniform? Is her hair unkempt? Are her shoes dirty? Of course not! The health care worker you picture in your mind is clean and neat, with an unwrinkled uniform and clean shoes (Fig. 3-5). Her hair is neatly styled and held back off the face. She wears few accessories. A watch with a second hand is an essential part of a personal support worker's uniform, but bracelets, necklaces, rings, and dangling earrings are not. In the health care field, many of the traits we have come to associate with a professional image are related to maintaining safety and health. Guidelines for a professional appearance are given in Guidelines Box 3-1.

JOB-SEEKING SKILLS

You are currently in the process of training to become a personal support worker. You may have chosen to take this training for any number of reasons. You may have an interest in the health care profession and are taking this course to explore that interest. You may be entering the workforce after spending years raising a family, or you may find yourself in need of work due to a change in your financial situation. You may be applying to nursing school and require the personal support worker training to meet admission criteria. Regardless of your reason or reasons for entering the health care field, you will find many opportunities to put your training to use. The health care field is one of the most rapidly grow-

ing areas, and the trend is expected to continue. Long-term care facilities, home health care agencies, hospice organizations, hospitals, doctor's offices, dialysis centers, rehabilitation centers, and many other types of health care organizations employ personal support workers. Perhaps you already know what type of health care organization you would like to work in, or perhaps you will have to try a few different things before you find your special place.

DEFINING THE IDEAL JOB

So, you're ready to get a job. Before you begin the process of responding to notices about job opportunities, completing applications, and going on interviews, it is important that you take time to explore what you really want from your employment and what you will be able to offer to your employer (Fig. 3-6). Some questions to consider are:

- **What type of facility do you want to work at?** Do you like working with elderly people? If so, you might like working in a long-term care facility. Maybe you have always wanted to work with disabled children, or find the idea of caring for people in their homes appealing. Maybe you would thrive as part of the team working in the fast-paced environment of an acute care setting. Focusing on your interests, likes, and dislikes will help you to narrow the search, increasing the chance that you will find a job you will enjoy.
- **Are there limitations on the hours or shifts you are available to work?** If you are a parent with small children, you may be limited to working certain shifts depending on your childcare arrangements. Do not lead an employer to believe that you are available for any shift if you can realistically only work evenings.
- **Do you have reliable transportation to get to work?** Your employer will rely on you to come to work as scheduled and on time. If you rely on public transportation, apply for work at facilities serviced by that particular transportation method.
- **What are some of your personality strengths?** Are you self-motivated and independent, or do you like more supervision and guidance? A personal support worker who works well independently would be an asset for a home health care agency, while one who prefers more supervision would

Guidelines Box 3-1 Guidelines for a Professional Appearance

WHAT YOU DO	WHY YOU DO IT
Style your hair neatly and away from your face.	Securing your hair away from your face keeps it away from equipment, out of your eyes, and out of your work. If your hair is not secured back, when you move your hair out of your eyes, any dirt on your hands will be transferred to your hair and face.
Keep your nails short and clean, with smoothly filed edges.	Germs can hide under the tips of long nails. Long nails can also scratch a person's skin. Frequent handwashing can cause acrylic and false nails to lift, allowing water to become trapped underneath and lead to a fungal infection in the nailbed.
Leave bracelets, necklaces, rings, and dangling earrings at home.	A child or confused person might pull dangling earrings through your earlobes. Necklaces and bracelets get in the way, and can get caught in equipment and broken. If you wear rings, germs can become trapped underneath them, which makes handwashing less effective. Rings can also scratch a person's skin when you are providing care.
If you wear makeup, apply it lightly and tastefully.	Wearing too much makeup, or makeup that is too bright or too dark, does not contribute to a professional appearance.
If you wear cologne or perfume, it should be of a light fragrance and lightly applied.	Many people are sensitive to fragrances and may find perfume or cologne that is of a strong scent or heavily applied offensive.
Wear a clean, pressed uniform each day. Make sure that your shoes are polished.	Attention to details, such as making sure that your uniform is wrinkle-free and your shoes are polished, says to others that you care about your appearance. A clean uniform is also essential for limiting the spread of infection.
If you have a tattoo or body piercing, try to select a uniform style that will conceal it. If you are thinking about getting a tattoo or body piercing, consider its location carefully.	Many people feel that tattoos and body piercings make a person look less professional.
Practice good personal hygiene and grooming daily.	Good personal hygiene helps to prevent breath and body odors and limits the spread of infection. In addition, if you care enough about yourself to keep yourself clean and neat, the people in your care will feel that you will do the same for them.

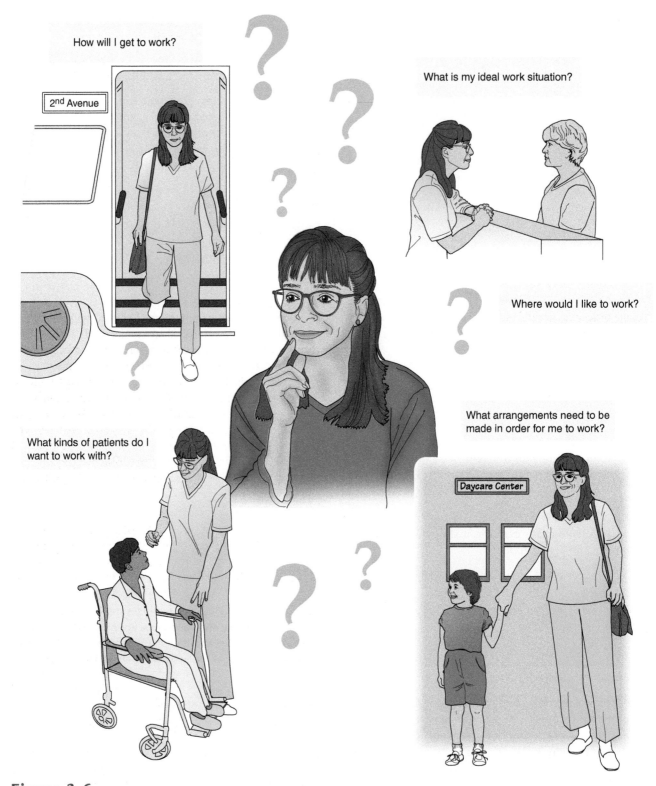

Figure 3-6
The first step to finding a job is thinking about what sort of situation best fits your personality, lifestyle, and interests.

probably be better suited for working in a facility.

FINDING JOB OPENINGS

Once you have some specific goals in mind, where do you start your search? There are many places to search for job openings. Certainly the classified ads in the local newspaper is a great place to start. Telephone directories list facilities and agencies that hire personal support workers. You could try calling these organizations directly, or checking the Internet to see if the organizations you are interested in post job openings on their websites. In addition, you can use the Internet to check sites dedicated to helping people find jobs. The school that you are attending may offer a job placement service, where you can check job listings and obtain help with writing a résumé. You could also check for job postings on the bulletin board in the facility where you are receiving clinical training. Last but not least, friends and co-workers may know of openings. Start a list of positions that you hear of that interest you, so that you will have the information readily available.

PREPARING RÉSUMÉS, COVER LETTERS, AND REFERENCE LISTS

Résumé

Before actually making application for a particular job, you must prepare a **résumé,** a brief document that gives a possible employer general information about you and your education and work experience. Résumés should be typed or printed using a computer on white or off-white paper. With résumés, "plain" is best—no fancy lettering or designs are necessary! A résumé contains only facts and should be kept to one page, if at all possible (Fig. 3-7). Your résumé should include:

- Your full name, address, telephone number, and, if you have one, your e-mail address
- A short objective, or career goal
- A history of your education (list the schools you attended most recently first, and for each school, include the dates you attended the school and the degree you graduated with)
- An employment history (list each of your previous employers, and for each employer,

include the dates that you worked there, your job title, and your primary job duties)

Listing volunteer work on your résumé is appropriate, but only if it relates to the job you are applying for. There is some information that should never be included on a résumé, including your age, marital status, weight, religion, sexual preference, and whether or not you have children (or are planning to have them). This information should not matter to an employer who is considering you as an employee. In fact, according to the **Canadian Human Rights Law,** it is against the law for an employer to ask a candidate questions related to these subjects at any time during the hiring process.

Cover Letter

You may also want to prepare a cover letter to send out with your résumé. A cover letter is written as a way of introducing yourself to a potential employer. Your résumé contains information about your education, training, and experience, but a cover letter goes beyond the straight facts. A cover letter says, "Hello, this is why I want to work for your organization, and this is why I am the best person for the job" (Fig. 3-8). Your cover letter should be fairly short and typed or printed using a computer on white or off-white paper. Pay special attention to your grammar and spelling.

Reference List

The last document you should prepare before applying for a job is a reference list. A **reference list** is a list of three or four people who would be willing to talk to a potential employer about your abilities. When considering people to include on your reference list, think about people who know you well and have worked with you in a professional capacity, such as your teachers, co-workers, or previous supervisors. Before listing a person as a reference, make sure you have his or her permission to do so. Some people may hesitate to act as a reference. For example, they may not want their contact information given out, they may be too busy, or they may not think you did as good a job for them as you thought you did. After a person has agreed to be your reference, make sure you have accurate contact information for that person, including his or her full name and title (if any), a current and complete address, and a telephone number. Type your reference list on a sheet of paper that matches your résumé. Some employers will ask for a list of references at the time you turn in an application; others will want you to write your references on

---

SUZIE SMITH
123 NORTH AVENUE
ANYWHERE, CANADA
(123) 456-7890

Career Objective:

To obtain a position as a Personal Support Worker in a rehabilitation-centered healthcare facility that will allow me to use my skills to assist those in need.

Education:

Anywhere Vocational Center	May–July 2006
Anywhere, Canada	Personal Support Worker Course
	Certification: August 2006
State Jr. College	August–December 2005
Anywhere, Canada	General Studies
Anywhere High School	Graduated: June 2005
Anywhere, Canada	High School Diploma

Certifications:

Personal Support Worker	August 2006 (Current)
CPR Certification	July 2006 (Current)

Employment History:

Sunshine Assisted Living	August 2006–Present
Anywhere, Canada	

Rehabilitation Unit. Provided assistance with activities of daily living for residents, with an emphasis on rehabilitation. Worked closely with physical therapists to carry out therapy plan with meals and ambulation.

Quality Printing	July 2005–July 2006
Anywhere, Canada	

Cashier/Customer Service. Worked part-time while attending college. Responsible for assisting customers with print orders and making end-of-day bank deposits.

Volunteer History:

Hospice	June 2004–July 2006
Anywhere, Canada	

Respite Volunteer. Provided respite relief for families receiving hospice care. Sat with patients and read to them.

Figure 3-7
A résumé is a short, precise document with information about you, your work experience, and your education.

the actual application form. Either way, you will be prepared with correct and current information. How efficient and organized you will appear at that first meeting!

PUTTING IN APPLICATIONS

Now that you have thought about your ideal work situation, prepared a list of job opportunities to pursue, written your résumé and cover letter, and gathered your references, you are ready to place applications. Although it is acceptable and common practice to just stop by organizations where you are interested in working and ask to complete an application, you may want to call ahead to ask if there are any positions open for personal support workers. Even if there are not any immediate openings, most facilities will keep applications on file for approximately 6 months, so ask if you may place an application to be kept on file.

Suzie Smith
123 North Avenue
Anywhere, Canada
February 1, 2008

Sandra Jones, Director of Human Resources
Sunny Hills Rehabilitation Center
1234 South Avenue
Anywhere, Canada

Dear Ms. Jones,

I would like to express my interest in the Personal Support Worker (PSW) position at Sunny Hills Rehabilitation Center that was listed in the local want ads. In July, 2006, I completed my PSW training at Anywhere Vocational Center. Since that time, I have been employed at Sunshine Assisted Living as a PSW in their rehabilitation unit.

I am a hard worker and I learn new skills easily. I love working with the elderly and have heard that your facility is a very enjoyable place to work.

Thank you for taking the time to review and consider my application. I am available for an interview at your convenience and look forward to meeting with you soon.

Sincerely,

Suzie Smith

Suzie Smith, PSW

Figure 3-8
A cover letter is a letter that you write to go along with your résumé. Your cover letter allows you to explain more fully why you want to work for a particular organization, and what qualities you have that make you the ideal person for the job opening in question.

In some facilities, the director of nursing (DON) handles the hiring of personal support workers. In others, hiring is handled through the **human resources (HR) department (personnel).** Usually, when you go to an organization to complete a job application, the receptionist at the main desk will give you the application to complete (Fig. 3-9).

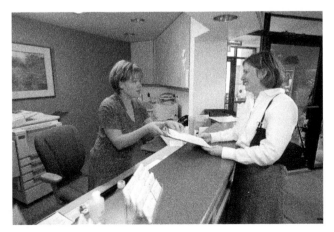

Figure 3-9
When you go to complete your application form, take your résumé, cover letter, and references with you, and dress neatly.

When you go to complete your application, take your résumé and references with you and dress appropriately, even though you expect only to complete the application and leave. Some facilities may choose to interview you at that time, especially if there is an opening. Appropriate dress means "clean and neat." Make sure your clothes are pressed and clean and your shoes are polished. Hair should be neatly arranged and out of your face. Jewelry should be simple and minimal, and if you wear perfume or cologne, the fragrance should be light. Women should make sure that their makeup is tastefully applied. Even if you do not interview, this will be the first impression you make on a possible employer. You can be sure that the people who do the hiring for the organization will do some preliminary screening by asking the receptionist whether you appeared neat and well organized, and what your attitude was like.

A job application is a standardized form used to obtain basic pertinent information, such as which position you are applying for, how you can be reached, and what shifts you can work (Fig. 3-10). Remember the time you spent earlier thinking about practical factors

(*Text continued on page 40*)

HIGHLAND CARE CENTER
APPLICATION FOR EMPLOYMENT

Highland Care Center is an equal opportunity employer, dedicated to a policy of non-discrimination in employment on any basis, including race, color, age, sex, religion, national origin or disability. Highland supports hiring people who have disabilities and meets all Human Resources and Skill Development Canada requirements to provide reasonable accommodations for people with disabilities who are qualified to do the job. A mandatory drug test will be performed within 90 days of hire. Criminal background checks will be made on all new employees.

PERSONAL INFORMATION

Name: _____ Date: _____

Please list any other names you have been known by or employed under: _____

Phone Number: _____ Social Insurance Number: _____

Position Desired: _____ Salary Desired: _____

Present Address: _____

| Street | City | Province | Area Code |

Permanent Address (if different from above): _____

| Street | City | Province | Area Code |

Have you ever applied for employment with Highland before? Yes _____ No _____ If yes, when? _____

Have you ever worked for Highland before? Yes _____ No _____ If yes, when? _____

Available for: Full Time _____ Part Time _____ On Call _____ Shifts available for: Morning _____ Afternoon _____ Night _____

If hired, when would you be available to begin work? _____

Are you eligible for employment in Canada? Yes _____ No _____

How did you learn about Highland Care Center? _____

Have you ever been convicted of a felony or misdeamor? Yes _____ No _____ Do you smoke? Yes _____ No _____

Upon hire a criminal background check will be conducted.

EDUCATION	Name and Location of School	Graduate?
High School		
College		
Business/Trade/Tech.		

List Other Job-Related Skills: _____
_____

Special Skills or Qualifications: _____
_____

Figure 3-10

A job application is a standardized form used to obtain basic information about each person who applies for a job with the organization. It is a legal document, and your signature at the bottom states that all of the information you have provided is true and accurate.

Please list your previous work experience below beginning with your present or most recent employer for the past five years or your last three employers, whichever you feel will provide us with the most helpful information about you.

Dates of Employment Must list month and year	Name, Address, Phone Number of Employer Name of Supervisor	Ending Wage	Ending Position	Reason for Leaving
Begin Date _____ End Date _____				
Begin Date _____ End Date _____				
Begin Date _____ End Date _____				

If a previous employer is not to be contacted, designate which

one: _____

Are there any comments you would like to share ? _____
_____

The information provided in this Application for Employment is true, correct and complete. If employed, any misstatement or omission of fact on this application may result in my dismissal. I understand that acceptance of an offer of employment does not create a contractual obligation upon Highland Care Center to continue to employ me in the future. Daywest HealthCare Services, Inc. Is a drug & alcohol free workplace. As a condition of employment all employees must successfully pass a drug test which will be administered some time during their orientation period. Criminal background checks will be made on all new employees.

Signature:_____ Date:_____

FOR HIGHLAND USE ONLY

Interviewed by: _____ Date:_____

References:

Person Contacted, Place and Date: _____

Person Contacted, Place and Date: _____

Person Contacted, Place and Date: _____

Remarks: _____
_____
_____

HIGHLAND CARE CENTER
RELEASE OF INFORMATION

Applicant Name: _____

Social Insurance #: _____ Date:_____

I authorize Highland Care Center to seek and obtain information from employers, supervisors and colleagues regarding the following as well as any other job-related information which will enable the facility to evaluate my suitability for employment.

____ work habits ____ technical skills

____ performance record ____ vaccination records

____ ability to form effective working relationships with co-workers

____ other: _____

I authorize those contacted to release this information to Highland Care Center.

By initialing below, I authorize Highland Care Center to obtain information from:

____ All former employers and current employer

____ Former employers only

Signature:_____ Date:_____

Figure 3-10 (*Continued*)

that needed to be taken into consideration, such as childcare arrangements and transportation? Now you will be able to easily answer the questions on the application about your availability for work. The application form will also require you to provide information about your education, your work history, and the reasons you left your previous job. There are many legitimate reasons why a person would leave a place of employment:

- "I left to take a position that is closer to home."
- "I left because I was offered better hours/a pay increase."
- "I left to have children."
- "I left to go to school."
- "I left because we moved to a new city or town."
- "I left because I was laid off."

The reason for leaving a job could be that you were fired. If so, be honest. Your chances of finding new employment are much better if a potential employer hears the truth from you, instead of finding it out by calling your references. When giving a reason for leaving a job, avoid speaking negatively about your previous employer, even if the situation was not ideal. Doing so reflects poorly on you as a potential employee.

Some facilities will allow you to take the application home to be filled out and returned at a later date. Others will require you to complete the application while you are there. Most facilities will also request a copy of your résumé and reference list, along with the completed application. Be prepared to complete the application form in the facility. Have notes available with details that you will need to complete the application. Use blue or black ink and write clearly. The application form is a legal document, and your signature at the bottom states that all the information is true and accurate. An employer who finds out that you lied about any information on the application form has grounds to fire you without notice.

Ask for an appointment for an interview when you submit your cover letter, résumé, reference list, and completed application. Some facilities will make the appointment at this time. Others may want to review your résumé and application and call you for an appointment at a later date. If you have not heard from a potential employer in 1 week's time, it is appropriate to call and ask about the status of your application. A follow-up call shows a potential employer that you have initiative and are interested in the job.

GOING ON INTERVIEWS

You have an appointment for that interview! An **interview** is the chance for a potential employer to meet you personally and learn more about you in an effort to determine if you are the right person for the job. Equally as important, the interview is a chance for *you* to learn more about the employer and the position, in an effort to determine if they are right for you. Being properly prepared for the interview will allow you to gather as much information about the organization and the job as possible during the interview, so that you can make an informed decision about the job if it is offered to you. In addition, being properly prepared can make all the difference in how a potential employer views your potential! Your résumé and application contain all of the "hard" facts about your education and experience, but you are the one responsible for persuading the interviewer of your interest in the job, dedication to your profession, and abilities.

Before going to the interview, make a list of questions you would like answers to, and refer to this list during the interview. This shows that you are interested in the position and are taking the opportunity to interview seriously. Some questions you might want to ask include:

- "What are the major responsibilities or duties of the position? May I have a copy of the job description?"
- "Do you have to replace personal support workers often, here? If so, why?"
- "May I see the unit where I will be working and meet the person who will be supervising me?"
- "What do you think personal support workers like best about working here? Least?"
- "How many personal support workers staff each unit?"
- "When would I be eligible for a performance evaluation, and what are the standards I will be evaluated against?"
- "What qualities are you looking for in a personal support worker?"
- "What opportunities exist for career growth and furthering my education?"

You are interviewing for a job in the health care setting, so help the interviewer see you as a part of his or her staff. Present yourself as a

Figure 3-11

Dress like the professional that you are when you go for your interview! Clean, neat hair and nails and polished shoes are appropriate for both men and women. **(A)** An appropriate outfit for a man would be slacks, a button-down shirt or a polo shirt, and a belt. A tie is optional. **(B)** For a woman, an appropriate outfit would be a skirt and a blouse, with stockings. Make-up and jewelry should be kept to a minimum.

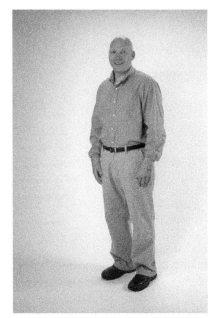
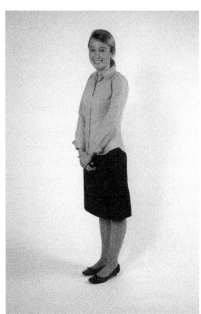

A

B

well-groomed professional (see Guidelines Box 3-1 and Fig. 3-11). Make sure your clothing is pressed and all repairs, such as missing buttons or loose seams, have been taken care of before the interview. Your shoes should be clean and polished. If you are a man, wear slacks (not jeans), a button-down shirt or a polo shirt, and a belt, and possibly a sport jacket if the weather is cool. A tie is optional. If you are a woman, wear a skirt (or dress slacks) and a blouse or a simple dress. Wear stockings, and make sure that the hem length of your skirt or dress is modest.

Carrying a small notebook containing the questions you want to ask during the interview and a copy of your résumé, reference list, and your certificate and transcript looks very professional. Do not chew gum during the interview, and make sure your cellular phone is turned off. You only have one chance to make a first impression, so make it a good one!

Give yourself adequate time to get to the interview. Ideally, you will arrive a few minutes early. After being introduced to the interviewer, shake his or her hand and take a seat when you are invited to do so. Do not address the interviewer by his or her first name, unless the interviewer specifically asks you to. Thank the person for the opportunity to interview at the beginning of the interview.

During the interview process, sit up straight and try not to fidget. You might be nervous and that is certainly understandable, but try to appear as confident and comfortable as you can under the circumstances. Maintain good eye contact during the interview and speak clearly. Common questions an interviewer might ask a candidate are listed in Box 3-1. Most interviewers will ask a potential employee about his or her strengths and weaknesses. Think about this ahead of time, and be honest. We all have some terrific strengths and we also have our weaknesses. Remember that a person who is aware of a weakness is capable of working to improve it. Try to answer questions concisely yet completely; it is best if you can strike a balance between listening and talking. If you do not know the answer to a question, simply say that you do not know—most interviewers are quick to recognize bluffing.

At the end of the interview, the interviewer will usually give you an opportunity to ask any questions that you may have. Now is the time to refer to your list! Asking questions of your own indicates that you have an active interest in making sure that you are a good fit for the job and the organization. The interviewer may have discussed salary and benefits (medical benefits, dental benefits, retirement plans, holiday and sick time, schedule for pay increases) during the

Common Interview Questions

"Tell me about yourself. Why did you become a personal support worker?"

"What part of your last job did you like the most? The least?"

"Why are you leaving your current job?" (or, "Why did you leave your last job?")

"What are you looking for in a manager?"

"How do you describe your work habits?"

"How do you set priorities?"

"How do you handle yourself under stress?"

"How do you handle problems with patients or co-workers?"

"Tell me about a specific situation that interfered with your ability to do your job, and how you handled it."

"What is the most satisfying workday you have had this year? Why?"

"Do you have a mentor? What have you learned from this person?"

"Who in your life would you consider to be 'successful'? Why?"

"What do you consider to be your greatest strength? Your greatest weakness?"

"Where do you want to go with your career? What steps have you taken to achieve your goal?"

"What is it about our organization that appeals to you?"

February 6, 2008

Dear Ms. Jones,

I would like to thank you for the opportunity to interview for the personal support worker position at Sunny Hills Rehabilitation Center. I was impressed by the quality of your facility and the competence of your staff and would like very much to become a member of your health care team. I look forward to hearing from you in the near future.

Thank you,

Suzie Smith

Figure 3-12
After your interview, send a thank-you note to the person who interviewed you, thanking her for her time and restating your interest in the position and the organization.

course of the interview, but if he or she did not, it is best not to ask about these things now. The proper time to discuss pay and benefits is when a job offer is made. When the interview is over, thank the interviewer again for his or her time, and for considering you for the position. If the interviewer did not mention when you can expect to hear from him or her regarding the position, ask. Then leave! The interview is over, and there is nothing left to do but write a thank-you note.

You should write a short thank-you note within 1 day of interviewing for the position, thanking the interviewer for considering you for the position and briefly explaining why you are excited about the possibility of working for his or her organization (Fig. 3-12). Everyone wants to be complimented on his or her organization, and your interest in being a part of that organization is a compliment. You may hand-write your thank-you note on a plain notecard, or type it.

As with dropping off the application, if you do not hear from the organization you interviewed with within the amount of time specified at the close of the interview, it is appropriate to follow-up with a telephone call. When a representative

of the organization calls to offer you a job, you can take this opportunity to ask any questions that may have occurred to you since the interview, or that were not appropriate to ask during the interview. If you need time to think about the offer, it is acceptable to ask the person who has offered you the job if you can call him or her back with an answer within the next day or so.

Applying and interviewing for jobs can be a time-consuming process that requires a lot of effort. By taking the time to prepare, you increase your chances of finding a situation where you will be happy and satisfied with your work.

LEAVING A JOB

Chances are, you will accept many different jobs over the course of your career. When leaving a job, give your employer at least 2 weeks' notice so that arrangements can be made to cover your shifts. Write a letter stating your desire to leave the job and the date of your last day on the job. Even if you were not happy at that particular place of employment, the professional thing to do is to thank your employer for the opportunity to work there. Leave on a positive note because you may need a reference from your present place of employment for a future job opportunity. You may even wish to work for your present employer again sometime in the future.

SUMMARY

- The health care industry relies on all types of professionals to provide quality care to patients and residents.
  - Professionals, such as doctors, nurses, and personal support workers, have certain credentials that are obtained through education and training.
  - Being a professional also means having a professional attitude.
- You must exhibit a strong work ethic in order to be successful and grow professionally.
  - A personal support worker with a strong work ethic possesses qualities that make her both pleasant to work with and dependable.
  - A personal support worker with a strong work ethic demonstrates compassion and respect for his patients or residents.
  - A personal support worker with a strong work ethic continues to learn so that his or her patients or residents receive the best possible care.
- In order to care for your patients or residents to the best of your ability, you must first care for yourself.

- Taking care of the body's physical needs helps keep your body strong, healthy, and able to handle the physical demands of being a personal support worker.
- Taking steps to maintain your emotional health helps to prevent emotional "burnout" and helps you to keep your emotions in check, both at work and at home.
- Good personal hygiene helps to prevent the spread of infection and promotes a professional appearance.
- Job-seeking skills are useful for finding an employment situation that matches your individual needs.
  - Advance planning about the type of employment you want helps to give your job search direction.
  - Résumés provide potential employers with information about your education and skills. Job applications are legal documents that provide pertinent information about your employment history.
  - A job interview is an opportunity for the potential employer to evaluate you, and for you to evaluate the potential employer.

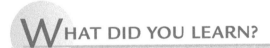

WHAT DID YOU LEARN?

Multiple Choice

Select the single best answer for each of the following questions.

1. A person with much experience and great skill in a specified role is referred to as a(n):
   a. Apprentice
   b. Professional
   c. Graduate
   d. Novice
2. In Canada, personal support workers can be employed at all of the following except:
   a. Hospitals
   b. Long-term care facilities
   c. Research centers
   d. Rehabilitation centers
3. A short, precise document with information about you, your work experience, and your education is called a:
   a. Minimum Data Set (MDS)
   b. Résumé

   c. Reference
   d. Cover letter
4. All of the following information should be included on your résumé, except for your:
   a. Name
   b. Address
   c. Employment history
   d. Religion
5. An organization's human resources (HR) department is also known as:
   a. Personnel
   b. Dietary
   c. Administration
   d. Education

6. Which one of the following is a standardized form that is also a legal document used when applying for a job?
   a. Résumé
   b. Cover letter
   c. Reference list
   d. Application

7. The chance for a potential employer to meet you personally occurs during the:
   a. Application process
   b. Interview process
   c. Job posting process
   d. Reference checking process

8. A personal support worker can promote his or her own physical health by doing all of the following except:
   a. Eating well-balanced meals
   b. Getting plenty of rest
   c. Smoking and drinking socially
   d. Attending aerobics classes

9. A personal support worker's personal cleanliness is referred to as:
   a. Grooming
   b. Neatness
   c. Hygiene
   d. Fashion

10. Qualities that characterize a good work ethic include all of the following except:
    a. Reliability
    b. Punctuality
    c. Honesty
    d. Tardiness

11. What type of a personal support worker accepts responsibility for his or her actions?
    a. An accountable personal support worker
    b. A respectful personal support worker
    c. A courteous personal support worker
    d. A punctual personal support worker

12. What type of a personal support worker is able to imagine what it would feel like to be in another person's situation?
    a. A creative personal support worker
    b. An empathetic personal support worker
    c. An experienced personal support worker
    d. An honest personal support worker

13. What type of a personal support worker can be counted on to come to work every day?
    a. A punctual personal support worker
    b. A personal support worker with access to public transportation
    c. A reliable personal support worker
    d. An ethical personal support worker

STOP and Think!

Imagine that you have just completed your personal support worker training and taken the state test. While you are waiting for your test results, you decide to begin reading job postings to see what opportunities are available. At this point, you are considering several options. You are excited about beginning your career in the health care field, and you are anxious to get into the workforce and put your new skills to use. However, you think that you might also want to continue your education, and become either a licensed practical nurse (LPN) or a registered nurse (RN) someday. What sorts of organizations may be looking for personal support workers in your community? How could working as a personal support worker now help you to further define your career goals?

You are a personal support worker student completing your training in a local health care facility. Do you think that the nurses and personal support workers view you as a potential employee? What actions can you take as a student to make a good impression?

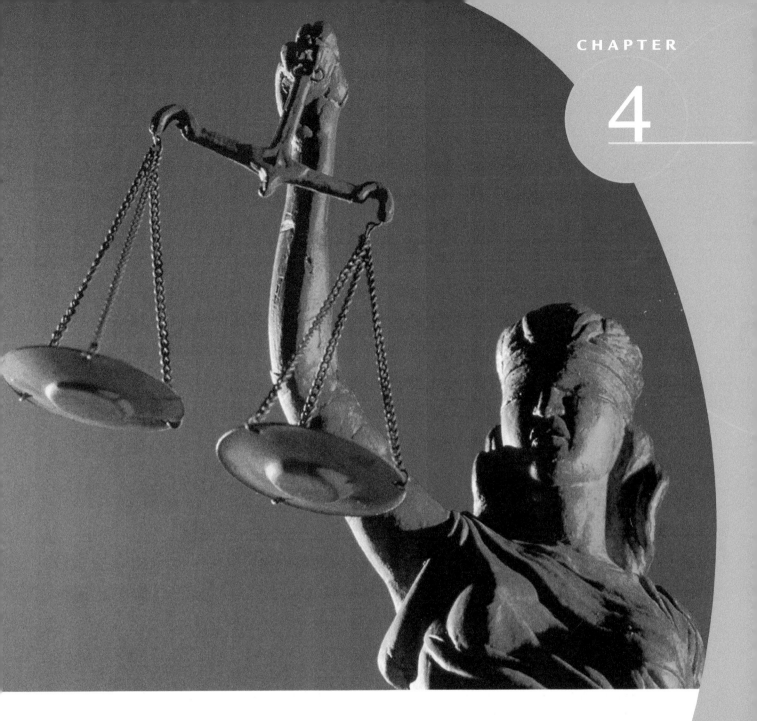

Legal and Ethical Issues

WHAT WILL YOU LEARN?

As members of society, we make decisions every day about how to behave. Some of these decisions are dictated by society's laws, or rules established by the governing authority, and we act a certain way because we know that failing to obey these rules can result in punishment. Other decisions are dictated by our own personal ethical code, or moral sense of what is right and wrong. Many factors influence an individual's ethical code,

Photo: Lady Justice symbolizes the fair and equal administration of the law. (© Jupiter Images.)

including spiritual beliefs and values instilled by the person's family. Generally, when we act according to our ethical code, we act a certain way because we believe it is the right way to act, not because we risk punishment if we do not behave in that way. Obeying society's laws and upholding our own personal ethical standards allow us to function as members of society. Just as laws and ethics guide our behavior in society, laws and ethics guide our behavior in the workplace, as health care providers. (Recall the discussion in Chapter 3 about the importance of having a "work ethic.") This chapter explores some of the legal issues that can affect you, as a personal support worker, and describes general ethical principles that should guide your behavior in the workplace. When you are finished with this chapter, you will be able to:

1. Discuss basic human rights that all Canadians are entitled to, as outlined in the Canadian Charter of Rights and Freedoms.
2. Discuss the basic rights of people who are receiving health care.
3. Discuss the legal aspects of health care delivery.
4. List common legal violations that are related to the provision of health care.
5. Display the awareness that health care workers must have in order to avoid legal dilemmas.
6. Define the types of abuse and describe signs that indicate abuse.
7. Discuss the health care worker's obligations in the reporting of suspected abuse.
8. Explain the difference between legal and ethical issues.
9. Describe the ethical standards that govern the nursing profession in particular, and the health care profession in general.

Vocabulary

Right	Malpractice	False imprisonment	Sexual abuse
Laws	Intentional tort	Invasion of privacy	Elder abuse
Civil laws	Defamation	Confidentiality	Ethics
Criminal laws	Slander	Canada Privacy Act	Beneficence
Litigation	Libel	Larceny	Nonmaleficence
Liability	Assault	Abuse	Justice
Tort	Battery	Physical abuse	Fidelity
Unintentional tort	Informed consent	Psychological	Autonomy
Negligent	Fraud	(emotional) abuse	Value

BASIC HUMAN RIGHTS

A **right** is something a person is entitled to receive. All Canadians are entitled to basic human rights, as outlined in the Canadian Charter of Rights and Freedoms. The Charter is part of the Canadian Constitution. As such, federal and provincial/territorial laws must uphold its principles. Each province and territory has a human rights code that is consistent with the basic human rights outlined in the Charter. These basic human rights include:

- Freedom of religion
- Freedom of conscience (thought), belief, and expression (including freedom of press and other forms of media communication)
- Freedom of peaceful assembly and association (that is, the right to gather with others to support a common cause)
- The right to vote, and the right to participate in political activities
- The right to enter Canada, remain in Canada, and leave Canada
- The right to life, liberty, and security of person
- The right to equal treatment for all under the law (that is, protection from discrimination)

One way the government works to preserve its citizens' basic human rights is by making and enforcing laws. **Laws** are rules that are made by a controlling authority, such as the provincial/territorial or federal government. By formally establishing principles to guide behavior, laws give society a way of settling disputes in a civilized, orderly way. Laws enacted by the federal and provincial/territorial governments serve to protect basic human rights for all people, regardless of race, religion, gender, or income.

BASIC RIGHTS OF PEOPLE WHO ARE RECEIVING HEALTH CARE

In Canada, health care legislation (laws) help to ensure that all patients, residents, and clients receive safe, skillful medical care. These laws uphold the Canadian values of freedom, equality, and dignity for all. Each province or territory has its own set of laws that protect the rights of people who are receiving health care. Some provinces or territories have created "bills of rights" for people receiving health care, based on these laws.

PATIENTS' RIGHTS

In general, patients have the right to:

1. Receive considerate and respectful care
2. Receive information about their diagnosis, treatment, and prognosis
3. Make decisions about their plan of care, and to refuse a recommended treatment
4. Specify their wishes regarding health care in advance in case the time comes when they can no longer make those wishes known themselves (see Chapter 21 for more details)
5. Have privacy
6. Expect that all communication (written and oral) pertaining to their care will be treated with confidentiality
7. Review the records related to their medical care, and to have the information they contain explained or interpreted as necessary
8. Suggest alternatives to their planned care, or to transfer to another facility if they so desire
9. Be informed of any business relationships between parties that influence the care they receive (for example, the hospital and an insurance provider; the hospital and a university)
10. Participate in, or decline to participate in, experimental studies

11. Be informed of their options for care when they are discharged from the hospital
12. Know how the hospital settles disputes, what the hospital charges for its services, and what options for payment are available

Patients are responsible for:

1. Cooperating with health care providers
2. Respecting the property, comfort, environment, and privacy of other patients
3. Making an effort to understand, and follow, instructions concerning treatment
4. Providing accurate and complete information about their health status by answering questions as truthfully and completely as possible
5. Ensuring payment for services received (including providing insurance information in a cooperative and timely manner)
6. Informing the health care staff of any medications brought from home
7. Accepting responsibility for the consequences of refused treatment or disregarded instructions

RESIDENTS' RIGHTS

Each province and territory in Canada has laws that protect the rights of residents of long-term care facilities and community care facilities. Examples include the Nursing Homes Act in Alberta and the Long-Term Care Act in Ontario. All residential facilities within the province or territory must comply with these laws. Failure to comply could result in facility closure, severe fines, or both.

Although the specific laws vary depending on the province or territory, all of the laws have the common purpose of maintaining the health, safety, and well-being of residents. In all provinces and territories, residents have the following general rights:

1. Residents have the right to make decisions regarding their care, including choosing their own physician, participating in planning and implementing their own care, having their individual needs and preferences accommodated, and voicing grievances about care.
2. Residents have the right to privacy, including privacy while receiving treatments and nursing care, making and receiving telephone calls, sending and receiving mail, and receiving visitors. Residents have the right to confidentiality of personal and medical records.
3. Residents have the right to be free from physical or psychological abuse, including the improper use of restraints.

4. Residents have the right to receive visitors, and to share a room with a spouse if both partners are residents in the same facility.
5. Residents have the right to use personal possessions.
6. Residents have the right to control their own finances.
7. Residents have the right to information about eligibility for Medicare, and to be protected against discrimination.
8. Residents have the right to information about the facility's compliance with regulations, planned changes in living arrangements, and available services (and the fees for these services).
9. Residents have the right to remain in the facility unless transfer or discharge is required by a change in health or ability to pay, or the facility is closed.
10. Residents have the right to organize and participate in groups organized by other residents, or the families of residents. For example, residents or their families may organize groups dedicated to improving life for residents, by suggesting changes that could be made at the facility or by planning group outings and activities. Residents also have the right to participate in social, religious, and community activities of their choosing.
11. Residents have the right to information about advocacy groups.
12. Residents have the right to choose to work at the facility, either as volunteers or as paid employees. For many people, working or helping others gives them a sense of purpose. However, under no circumstances is a resident obligated to work (for example, in exchange for services).

In respecting the rights of patients and residents, health care workers behave according to legal standards; they also behave according to ethical standards.

LAWS: A WAY OF PRESERVING PATIENTS' AND RESIDENTS' RIGHTS

There are two types of laws: civil laws and criminal laws. **Civil laws** are concerned with the relationships among individuals. **Criminal laws** are concerned with the relationship between the individual and society as a whole. People found guilty of violating civil laws usually must pay a fine or make a financial settlement to the party that was wronged. Those who violate criminal laws are often sentenced to prison. **Litigation** is the lawsuit, or legal action, taken against a person who is accused of breaking a law. The responsibility of an individual to act within the confines of the law is called **liability.** Each individual is considered responsible, and held accountable, for his or her own actions in accordance with the law.

VIOLATIONS OF CIVIL LAW

When a patient or resident is admitted to a health care facility, he signs a form giving the facility permission to provide medical care. A health care worker employed by that facility likewise agrees to provide that care to the patient or resident. This arrangement is a contractual agreement. Contracts, such as the contract that exists between a personal support worker and the person she cares for, fall under the jurisdiction of civil law. When this civil law is violated, a **tort,** or wrong, is committed. An **unintentional tort** occurs when someone causes harm or injury to another person or that person's property without the intent to cause harm. A person who commits an unintentional tort is considered **negligent** for failing to do what a "careful and reasonable" person would do (Fig. 4-1). For example, in each of the following scenarios, the personal support worker would be considered negligent:

- A personal support worker becomes distracted by another resident's needs and forgets to lock the wheels on the wheelchair she has just placed by the resident's bed. As the resident moves from the bed to the wheelchair, the wheelchair rolls, causing the resident to fall.
- While changing a patient's bed linens, a personal support worker forgets to check the linens for personal objects. As a result, the patient's dentures are sent to the laundry with the soiled linens, and the dentures are damaged when they go through the washing machine.
- A personal support worker who is caring for a resident with a reputation for complaining fails to report the resident's complaints of pain to the nurse. It turns out that this time the resident's complaints were valid.

Negligence committed by people who hold licenses to practice their profession, such as doctors, nurses, lawyers, dentists, and pharmacists,

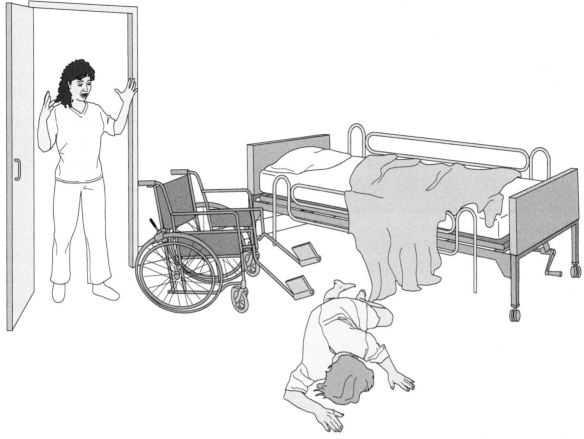

Figure 4-1
The personal support worker who was responsible for this patient has committed an unintentional tort and would be considered negligent for failing to lock the wheels on the wheelchair, an action that could have prevented the patient from falling.

is considered **malpractice.** Personal support workers (who receive certification, but not licensure) cannot be charged with neligence.

A violation of civil law committed by a person with the intent to do harm is considered an **intentional tort.** Intentional torts that personal support workers are particularly at risk for committing in the workplace include defamation, assault, battery, fraud, false imprisonment, invasion of privacy, and larceny.

Defamation

Defamation is making untrue statements that hurt another person's reputation. Statements in oral form are called **slander,** while statements in written form are called **libel.** It is best to avoid saying negative things or spreading rumors about a co-worker, supervisor, doctor, patient, or resident (Fig. 4-2). Although it is easy to become hurt, angry, or defensive when you feel that someone has treated you unfairly, making untrue remarks

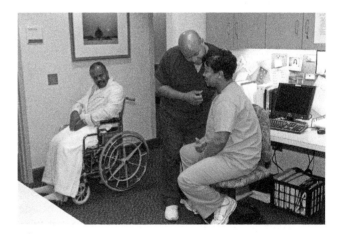

Figure 4-2
Never say negative things or spread rumors about co-workers, patients, or residents. Doing so is unprofessional, and it could get you in trouble with the law!

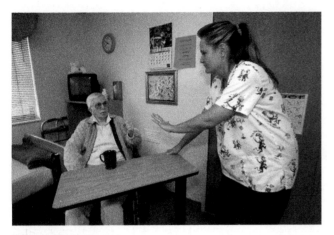

Figure 4-3
Try to avoid letting your emotions get out of check. Making angry gestures toward another is considered assault.

about that person is not the professional way to handle these feelings.

Assault

Assault is threatening or attempting to touch a person without his or her consent, causing that person to fear bodily harm (Fig. 4-3). A person can be found guilty of committing assault on the basis of an angry statement ("If you get up out of that wheelchair once more without calling for help, I'll tie you down!") or an angry gesture (shaking a fist in someone's face or acting as if you are going to slap her). Even very patient people can become frustrated occasionally. To avoid doing something you will regret later, "take a break" (physically and emotionally) when you feel your emotions get on edge.

Battery

Battery is touching a person without his or her consent. For example, a health care worker could be accused of battery for physically restraining a person who is trying to leave the room, or for performing a procedure for which the person or the person's family has not given consent. To avoid being charged with battery, health care providers must obtain **informed consent** from patients and residents before starting a treatment or procedure. Informed consent, which is discussed in detail in Chapter 39, implies that the person has been informed of the need for a procedure or treatment, and that he has given his permission to the health care provider to perform the procedure or administer the treatment. Even if a person initially consents to a treatment or procedure, he is able to

withdraw that consent and refuse the treatment or procedure at any time.

Fraud

Fraud is deception that could cause harm to another person. A health care worker who misrepresents her professional qualifications (for example, by telling a patient or resident that she is a nurse when she is not, or lying about previous training or employment on a job application) is committing fraud.

False Imprisonment

False imprisonment is confining another person against his or her will. In the health care setting, it is sometimes necessary to confine a person to a chair, a bed, or a room to maintain that person's safety (or the safety of others). However, the use of restraints can be considered false imprisonment if the restraints are not justified for the safety of the patient, the resident, or the staff (see Chapter 10).

Invasion of Privacy

Invasion of privacy is violating another person's right to keep certain information and aspects of himself away from the examination of others. In the health care setting, discussing a patient's or resident's physical condition, diagnosis, prognosis, or behavior in a public area (such as an elevator, hallway, or cafeteria) violates that person's right to confidentiality, and can be considered an invasion of privacy if someone overhears your discussion (Fig. 4-4). **Confidentiality** means keeping personal

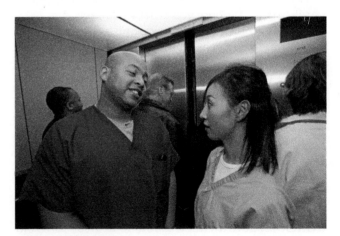

Figure 4-4
It is fine to chat with co-workers in public areas about topics that are not related to work, but never discuss your patients or residents, or their care, in a place where you could be overheard by others.

information that someone shares with you to yourself. Confidentiality applies not only to spoken and observed information, but also to written information. Always make sure that charts, medical records, or computer screens with patient or resident information are not left where others can read them. The only time it is acceptable to discuss a patient or resident is when it is necessary to exchange information about that person's care with someone else who is directly involved in caring for that person. Failure to maintain a person's physical privacy (for example, by leaving a door or curtain open during a procedure, or exposing a person's entire body when it is only necessary to expose a certain part) is also considered an invasion of privacy. In most facilities a confidentiality agreement is signed as a condition of employment. The personal support worker could be terminated for violation of this agreement.

The **Canada Privacy Act** took effect in 1983. There are two federal privacy laws, the Privacy Act and the Personal Information Protection and Electronic Documents Act (PIPEDA). Both of these laws protect the privacy rights of Canadians by establishing ground rules for how organizations may use, collect, or disclose personal information. The Privacy Commissioner of Canada is the federal authority that deals with privacy complaints and conducts investigations. In addition to the federal laws, every province and territory in Canada has privacy legislation that outlines specific rules on how to use, collect, and disclose patients' or residents' personal health information to health care providers and other health care organizations. Provincial/territorial privacy legislation:

- Regulates who has the right to view a person's medical records, data, or other private information
- Sets standards on how a person's medical information is to be stored and transmitted from one place to another
- Requires that health care organizations set policies that allow a patient or resident to have access to his or her medical records

Larceny

Larceny is stealing. In the health care setting, especially in the long-term care and home health care settings, but also in the hospital setting, health care workers have access to patients' or residents' personal belongings. It is never acceptable to take something belonging to another person, even if the item is not of great monetary value or if the person does not seem to "need" it. People who are elderly or ill are particularly vulnerable to theft, and not just at the hands of health care workers—family members, neighbors, or fellow residents may also commit larceny. As a personal support worker, it is important for you to be aware of others who may steal from one of your patients or residents, and to report any suspicions according to your facility's or agency's policy.

VIOLATIONS OF CRIMINAL LAW: ABUSE

Abuse, the repetitive and deliberate infliction of injury on another person, is a criminal act, and is punishable by a court of law. A person can commit abuse by *actively doing something to* another person, or by *failing to do something for* another person, such as provide adequate care or attention. Abuse takes many forms. The injury that results from the abuse may be physical or emotional.

Forms of Abuse

Physical abuse results in injury to the abused person's body. Striking, biting, slapping, shaking, and handling another person roughly are all forms of physical abuse. In a situation where one person depends on another for care, the caregiver can commit physical abuse by failing to provide for the basic physical human needs (adequate food and drink and physical cleanliness) of the person in his or her care. In the health care setting, failure to reposition a person frequently can lead to pressure ulcers and is also considered a form of physical abuse.

Psychological (emotional) abuse can be inflicted in many ways. Making another person fearful by threatening him with physical harm or abandonment is one form of psychological abuse, as is teasing a person in a cruel way. Isolating a person by preventing him from interacting with others (an act called *involuntary seclusion*) is another form of psychological abuse. Involuntary seclusion can involve keeping a person in a room alone with the door closed. In extreme cases, it may involve locking a person in a closet or attic for years.

Sexual abuse is forcing another person to engage in sexual activity. Making inappropriate, sexually aggressive comments or threats is also a form of sexual abuse.

Risk Factors for Abuse

Anyone can become the victim of abuse, but those who depend on others for their care (the very young, the disabled, and the elderly) are particularly at risk. The greater the disability, the more at risk the person is for abuse or neglect.

Elder abuse is the abuse of an older person. Elder abuse takes many forms:

- Infliction of physical pain or injury
- Failure to provide food, water, care, and medications
- Involuntary confinement or seclusion
- Withholding of Canada Pension checks and other sources of income (or intentional mismanagement of funds)
- Sexual abuse

Perpetrators of Abuse

There are many reasons why a person may become abusive toward another. Sometimes, abuse is rooted in the desire of one person to overpower and dominate another. Many abusers were victims of abuse themselves. Other times, in a situation where a person requires a great deal of care, the primary caregiver may become overly tired, frustrated, and overwhelmed by the responsibility of providing care, leading to abuse and neglect. This is often the case with an adult child who finds herself in the situation of caring for an ill and demanding elderly parent, without the proper training or support system.

Even people who are trained to administer care may become overwhelmed by their responsibilities or a particular situation. A health care worker is particularly at risk for becoming abusive when the patient or resident is "difficult" or hard to manage, and the relationship is long term, rather than short term. As described in Chapter 3, many facilities have counselling services to help employees deal with the emotional stress that caring for others can create.

Regardless of the reason abuse occurs, abuse is never an acceptable form of behavior! Be very careful not to place yourself in the position of potentially abusing a patient or resident. Being found guilty of abuse could destroy your potential for future employment in the health care field.

Role of the Personal Support Worker in Reporting Abuse

As a personal support worker, you may find yourself in a situation where you suspect that one of your patients or residents is being abused (Box 4-1). Laws require that any health care worker who suspects the abuse of a child or elderly person must report his or her suspicions to the proper

---

BOX 4-1 Signs of Abuse

- Poor personal hygiene, as evidenced by an unclean body, clothes, or both; an unshaven face or uncombed hair; skin irritation (from wearing urine-soaked undergarments for long periods of time); dried stool on buttocks; or a lack of oral hygiene
- Loss of weight or dehydration (see Chapter 19 for signs and symptoms of dehydration)
- Unexplained bruises or bruises in various stages of healing; explanations of injuries that are not consistent with the location of the injury
- Patches of missing hair
- Burn marks from cigarettes or abrasions from ropes or other bindings
- Unclean or unsafe living conditions, as evidenced by rotting food, unchanged sheets, or a lack of heat or water services
- An anxious, fearful, or withdrawn demeanor, especially in the presence of the abuser
- Uncontrolled medical conditions (possibly the result of a lack of prescribed medication or treatment)
- Bruising, chafing, or discharge from the genital area

---

authorities. Your facility or agency will have specific policies regarding the chain of reporting. Some organizations will require that you report to your supervisor or nurse, while others require reporting to a risk management representative. It is not your responsibility to investigate whether or not abuse has actually occurred, or who has caused it. The provincial/territorial agency that handles abuse reports will proceed through the proper channels. Your responsibility is to simply report your suspicions.

ETHICS: GUIDELINES FOR BEHAVIOR

As you have learned, laws serve to preserve basic human rights. As such, laws generally deal with issues that are either "black" or "white": an action is either within the law, or outside of it. But what about situations that are not so easily defined? The dramatic changes in health care that have been brought about by advances in technology and research have greatly impacted legal and ethical issues surrounding the medical profession, and have created some unique moral dilemmas. Consider the following questions:

- What should be done with human embryos that have been frozen for future use, if the parents decide they do not want to have any more children?
- How does one decide who receives a donor organ, when there are so many people in need but few organs available?
- When does human life begin?
- Should doctors be allowed to end a person's life, at that person's request?

Clearly, these are difficult questions to answer because the answers depend on the individual's values and beliefs. When definitive answers to questions are not available, we rely on ethical standards to decide what to do. **Ethics** are moral principles or standards that govern conduct. The word "ethics" comes from the Greek word *ethos*, which means "beliefs that guide life." Ethical standards, which are less rigid than laws, help us to determine the difference between right and wrong in areas where the law fears to tread.

PROFESSIONAL ETHICS

Each profession has a code of ethics, or guidelines pertaining to standards of conduct and practice, for that profession. The code of ethics for personal support workers falls within the Canadian Nurses Association (CNA) code of ethics for nursing (Box 4-2). In addition, there are some general ethical principles that guide all health care workers:

- **Beneficence.** Do good for those in your care by preventing harm and promoting the health and welfare of the person above all else.

BOX 4-2	Code of Ethics for Personal Support Workers

- Treat patients and residents with respect for their individual needs and values.
- Respect the patient's or resident's right to choice in regard to the individual's right to control his or her own care.
- Hold confidential all information about patients and residents learned in the health care setting.
- Be guided by consideration for the dignity of patients and residents.
- Fulfill the obligation to provide competent care to patients and residents.

- **Nonmaleficence.** Avoid harming those in your care. Use kindness and gentleness when administering care.
- **Justice.** Treat people fairly and equally, regardless of race, religion, culture, disability, or ability to pay.
- **Fidelity.** Act with integrity to earn others' trust.
- **Autonomy.** Respect a person's rights and personal preferences.
- **Confidentiality.** Maintain a person's privacy by allowing the person to discuss sensitive issues with the knowledge that the information will be kept secret.

PERSONAL ETHICS

Many factors influence a person's ethics, which are derived from a person's values. A **value** is a cherished belief or principle. Factors that influence a person's values include his or her religious or spiritual beliefs, level and type of education, culture and heritage, and life experiences. Each person's value system is unique, and as a personal support worker, you need to think about how you feel about certain moral and ethical issues. Only then will you be able to understand that although another person's values may differ from yours, that person's values are as important to her as yours are to you. Respect for the individual is one of the principles that forms the basis of the code of ethics for nursing (Fig. 4-5).

Ethical dilemmas arise when we attempt to judge other people by our own ethical standards. Satisfactory resolutions to ethical dilemmas in the health care field can be obtained only by allowing the patient or resident to become an informed, active participant in his or her care, and by following ethical standards when administering care.

PROTECTING YOURSELF FROM LEGAL AND ETHICAL DIFFICULTIES

During your career, you will be exposed to a variety of circumstances and situations. Always bear in mind the legal and ethical responsibilities and obligations that you have as a caregiver. Make sure that you are familiar with your employer's policies, and with your duties and obligations as listed in your job description. Be aware of the scope of practice for personal support worker in your province or territory. Do not make decisions or perform duties that are not within your scope

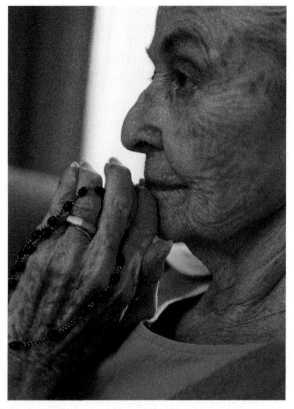

Figure 4-5
Values, which are derived from religious and spiritual beliefs, culture and heritage, and a person's family, are the basis of ethics. Not everyone has the same values. It is important to recognize and respect your patients' or residents' values, even if they are not the same as yours.

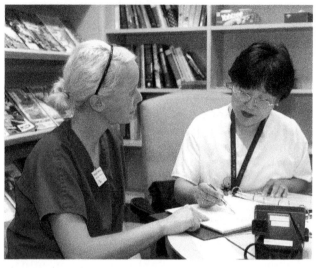

Figure 4-6
In order to stay within the legal limits of your job, know your scope of practice (as defined by the province or territory and your job description), familiarize yourself with your employer's "policies and procedures" manual, and always seek clarification from your supervisor if there is something you do not understand.

of practice, as defined by facility policy, your job description, and your province's or territory's regulations. Keeping yourself informed is critical to ensure that the care you give is within the legal limits of your job (Fig. 4-6). Finally, if you find yourself in a situation that may pose legal liability issues for you or your employer, or you are facing an ethical dilemma that you are not sure how to resolve, be sure to share your concerns with your supervisor.

SUMMARY

- A professional acts in a way that is legally and ethically appropriate.
- Each province and territory has legislation that protects the people who receive our care.
- Laws are rules that are made by a controlling authority, such as the provincial/territorial or federal government, that serve to protect basic human rights.
  - Civil laws are concerned with relationships between individuals. Criminal laws are concerned with the relationship between an individual and society as a whole.
  - An unintentional tort occurs when someone causes harm or injury to another person or that person's property without the intent to cause harm. A person who commits an unintentional tort is considered negligent for failing to do what a careful and reasonable person would do.
  - A violation of civil law committed by a person with the intent to do harm is called an intentional tort. Examples of intentional torts that may be committed by personal support workers in the workplace are defamation, assault, battery, fraud, false imprisonment, invasion of privacy, and larceny.
- Abuse, the repetitive and deliberate infliction of injury on another person, is a criminal act and is punishable by a court of law.
  - Abuse can be committed by either actively doing something to another

person, or by failing to do something for another person.

- Abuse can be physical or emotional.
- People who depend on others for their care, such as the very young, the disabled, and the elderly, are particularly at risk for abuse.
- Laws require that any health care worker who suspects the abuse of a child or elderly person must report his or her suspicions to the proper authorities.

- Ethics are moral principles or standards that govern conduct. Ethical dilemmas in the health care field can be solved only by allowing the patient or resident to become an informed, active participant in his or her care, and by following ethical standards when providing care.

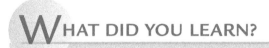

WHAT DID YOU LEARN?

Multiple Choice

Select the single best answer for each of the following questions.

1. All of the following are legal terms that relate to making false statements that injure another person's reputation except:
   a. Defamation
   b. Battery
   c. Slander
   d. Libel

2. If a personal support worker fails to raise the side rails on the bed of a confused patient, and the patient falls out of bed and is injured, the personal support worker may be charged with:
   a. Malpractice
   b. Negligence
   c. An intentional tort
   d. Assault

3. Which legislation protects the rights of residents of long-term or community care facilities?
   a. Canada Health Act
   b. Canadian Charter of Rights and Freedom
   c. Health Canada
   d. Provincial/territorial long-term care and community care legislation

4. Which ethical principle relates to the concepts of informed consent and a person's right to refuse treatment?
   a. Beneficence
   b. Autonomy
   c. Fidelity
   d. Justice

5. Confidentiality means:
   a. Only sharing information with those directly involved in a patient's or resident's care
   b. Respecting a patient's or resident's right to privacy

   c. Never sharing information with anyone
   d. Both "a" and "b"

6. All residents have basic rights. Which of the following is a basic right of residents?
   a. Right to choice
   b. Right to privacy and confidentiality
   c. Right to be free from verbal abuse, or any other abuse
   d. All of the above

7. You are a personal support worker working in a home health care setting. You suspect that one of your clients is being emotionally and physically abused by her husband. What should you do first?
   a. Call the police
   b. Keep your suspicions to yourself but continue to observe the situation
   c. Immediately report your suspicions to the case manager
   d. Tell another personal support worker at the agency

8. One of your fellow personal support workers has been having a very hard time with one of her residents. The resident is confused and, as a result, is being uncooperative. In a moment of complete frustration, your co-worker says to the resident, "If you don't shut up and behave yourself right now, I'm going to slap you!" What kind of an intentional tort has this personal support worker committed?
   a. Assault
   b. Battery
   c. Negligence
   d. Malpractice

9. A personal support worker answers the telephone at the nursing station. The doctor who is calling wants to give a verbal order, and the personal support worker tells the doctor that she is a nurse and can take the order. What intentional tort has the personal support worker committed?
   a. Slander
   b. Fraud
   c. Libel
   d. Informed consent

10. What does the provincial privacy legislation protect?
    a. The patient's or resident's right to privacy
    b. The patient's or resident's right to sue negligent health care workers
    c. The patient's or resident's right to be free from abuse
    d. The patient's or resident's right to choose who will provide his or her care

Matching

Match each numbered item with its appropriate lettered description.

E 1. Civil laws

A 2. Liability

D 3. Fraud

B 4. Ethics

C 5. Beneficence

a. The responsibility of an individual to act within the confines of the law
b. A system of moral principles or standards used to govern conduct
c. Protecting a patient or resident from harm
d. Deception that could cause harm to another person
e. Laws that deal with relationships between individuals

STOP and Think!

A licensed practical nurse (LPN) who works with you in a long-term care facility stops in Mrs. Taylor's room to give Mrs. Taylor her daily medications. Mrs. Taylor is in the bathroom and you are changing the linens on her bed. The nurse hands you the medication cup, which contains three pills, and asks you to have Mrs. Taylor take the pills as soon as she comes out of the bathroom. You are aware that in your province, personal support workers who work in long-term care facilities are not allowed to give medications. When you mention your concern about giving Mrs. Taylor her medication to the nurse, she says, "It's okay; the other personal support workers do this for me all of the time." What should you do?

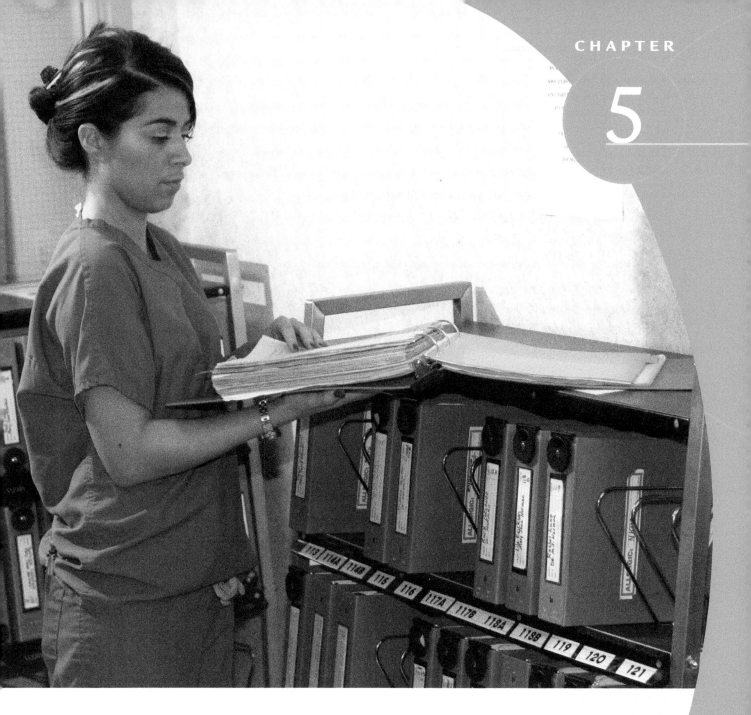

Communication Skills

WHAT WILL YOU LEARN?

Being able to effectively communicate, or participate in the exchange of information, is a critical skill for all people in the health care field to possess. Every day, you will need to communicate with your patients or residents, and with other members of the health care team. If just one link in the chain of communication is broken, the quality of care given

Photo: A personal support worker checks a resident's medical record. The medical record is one way members of the health care team share information with one another.

to the patient or resident can suffer. In this chapter, we will describe techniques for, as well as obstacles to, effective communication. In addition, we will review some of the tools that are commonly used by members of the health care team to ensure that information is readily available to all who are involved with the care of a patient or resident. When you are finished with this chapter, you will be able to:

1. Define communication.
2. Describe the two major forms of communication, and give examples of each.
3. Discuss techniques that promote effective communication.
4. Describe blocks to effective communication and discuss methods used to avoid them.
5. Identify causes of conflict, and discuss ways of resolving conflicts.
6. Demonstrate proper telephone communication skills.
7. Discuss the methods of reporting and recording information in a health care setting.
8. Explain how the patient's or resident's medical record makes communication easier among members of the health care team.
9. Describe communication technologies that are being used in the health care field today.
10. Explain why the personal support worker is a vital link in the communication chain, and describe how the personal support worker communicates information to other members of the health care team.
11. List the steps of the nursing process, and describe how the nursing team uses the nursing process to plan the patient's or resident's care.
12. Understand the role of effective communication in the provision of quality health care.

Vocabulary

Communication	Observation	Reporting	Care plan
Verbal communication	Objective data	Recording	Nursing process
Nonverbal communication	Signs	Medical record (chart)	Nursing diagnosis
Conflict	Subjective data	Kardex	Interventions
	Symptoms		Goals

WHAT IS COMMUNICATION?

Communication is the exchange of information. The key to understanding what communication truly is lies within the word "exchange." If you exchange gifts with another person, you give that person a gift, and in return, you receive one back. In the exchange of information that defines communication, there is a constant back-and-forth flow of information. Communicating is not just about telling someone something (giving information). It is also about listening and observing (receiving information).

For effective communication to occur, all of the people who are involved must actively participate in the exchange of information. Communication involves at least two people, a *sender* and a *receiver.* The sender is the person with information to share, and the receiver is the person for whom the information is intended. The sender delivers the information in the form of a *message,* which the receiver may or may not understand. Through *feedback,* or a return message, the receiver lets the sender know whether the message was received and understood (Fig. 5-1). Note that as information is transmitted back and forth, the sender and the receiver switch roles.

There are two major forms of communication, verbal and nonverbal. **Verbal communication** involves the use of language, either spoken or written. Sign language, a system of hand gestures used to make letters of the alphabet and words, is also considered a form of verbal communication. Verbal communication tends to be deliberate—when we use language to express a thought, it is usually with the intent of giving specific information to another person.

Nonverbal communication, on the other hand, tends to be more subtle. In nonverbal

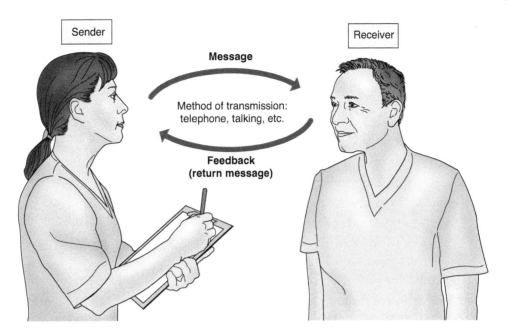

Figure 5-1
Communication involves the back-and-forth flow of information between a sender and a receiver.

communication, a person gives information through the use of facial expressions, gestures, body language, and tone of voice. For example, consider a resident with disabling arthritis. Not wanting to seem a "burden" to the health care staff, the resident may tell you that she feels fine when you ask. However, you note that she makes a face when she tries to get out of her chair and her voice seems strained. These observations suggest that the resident is not being entirely truthful with you about how she is feeling. Of the two forms of communication, nonverbal communication is perhaps the most reliable method of "reading" another person, especially in the health care field. For various reasons, such as embarrassment, shyness, or a fear of being perceived as foolish, people may not say what they really mean. Being observant and aware of others' nonverbal cues will give you a greater understanding of what your patients or residents are feeling and thinking.

COMMUNICATING EFFECTIVELY

As a personal support worker, you must be a successful communicator, both as a sender and a receiver of information, with both those you care for and your co-workers. For example, you will use communication skills to comfort, reassure, and teach your patients or residents.

Because personal support workers typically spend more time with patients and residents, and get to know them better than any other member of the health care team, you will become one of the strongest links between the patient or resident and the other health care team members. As you form relationships with your patients or residents, they will talk to you, confide in you, listen to you, and trust you. In addition, by carefully watching your patients or residents for nonverbal communication cues, you may be the first member of the health care team to notice that Mr. Jones' colour is not quite right, or that Mrs. Smith is having abdominal pain after eating, even though she is not complaining verbally.

In addition to communicating well with patients or residents, communicating well with your co-workers is also essential. Supervisors will delegate tasks to you, and you must be sure that you understand what they are asking you to do and how you are to go about doing it. Additionally, you will be the "eyes and ears" of the nurses, physical therapists, dietitians, social workers, and other members of the health care team. Relaying vital information about your patient's or resident's condition to the nurse is an essential part of your duties. As a personal support worker, you are not trained to diagnose and treat medical problems. However, your knowledge of your patient or resident will allow you to gather important information that, when communicated to the nurse, will alert the health care

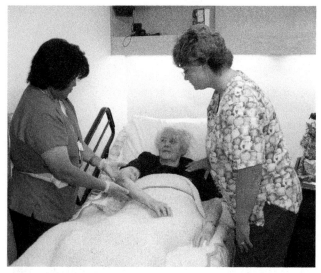

Figure 5-2
As a personal support worker, you are an important link between the patient or resident and the other members of the health care team.

team members to changes in that person's condition and influence the care he or she receives. Your responsibility as a communication link between the patient or resident and the rest of the health care team is very important (Fig. 5-2)!

Clearly, it is important for a personal support worker to learn good communication skills. There are many ways that communication can fail. Remember that good communication is a "two-way street" and involves the *exchange* of information. To see where problems in communication can occur, let's look at each part of the process of exchanging information:

1. **The sender creates a message.** Information needs to be organized and relevant to the person who will be receiving it. Your message, whether it is spoken or written, should convey the relevant facts, organized in an easily accessible manner. Use language that the receiver understands—this could mean getting help from an interpreter, if the receiver does not speak the same language you do, or using simple, common words in place of more complex, medical words. Speak clearly and loudly enough for the receiver to hear you without straining. Written messages should be legible and organized so that the information is complete and concise.

2. **The sender delivers the message.** Information can be transmitted from one person to another in many different ways. Speaking directly to another person, or "face-to-face," permits nonverbal communication to take place. Other methods of transmission, such as letters, memos, e-mails, telephone calls, and intercom conversations, are primarily methods of verbal communication. Nonverbal communication is impossible with these methods of transmission because the sender and the receiver are physically separated. When relying on a written form of transmission, be sure your handwriting is neat and your spelling is accurate. With oral methods of transmission, such as telephone calls and intercom conversations, it is important to ensure that background noise or static does not interfere with the receiver's ability to hear your message.

3. **The receiver receives the message.** For successful communication to occur, the receiver must be physically able to receive the message and mentally engaged in the communication exchange. For example, a person with a hearing loss could not physically receive a spoken message. A person who cannot read would not be able to understand a message sent in written form. A person who has had a stroke may be able to hear your words perfectly, but may not be able to understand their meaning. Sign language or communicating through nonverbal means (for example, nodding your head "yes" to a person's question) would not be effective if the person is blind. These are all examples of physical problems that can interfere with a person's ability to receive a message. Communication can also fail when a receiver is mentally distracted, or not really paying attention to the sender.

4. **The receiver provides feedback.** Have you ever spoken to someone and had him ignore you? Did you wonder whether or not the person even heard you? You did not receive feedback from that person. Feedback, like the other parts of communication, can be verbal (spoken or written) or nonverbal. During an exchange of information, it is important for the receiver to provide feedback to the sender, and it is important for the sender to listen and watch for this feedback. If the receiver does not provide feedback, the sender should make an effort to get a response of some sort. When feedback does not occur, or indicates that the message the sender sent was not interpreted correctly, other methods of enhancing communication may be necessary.

TACTICS THAT ENHANCE COMMUNICATION

Good communication skills will serve you well, both in your professional life and your personal life. There are many ways you can enhance communication with others.

When You Are the Receiver, Be a Good Listener

Listening is perhaps the most useful communication skill, especially in the health care setting. Active listening requires focusing your attention on the speaker. Sit down or assume a relaxed posture so you do not appear rushed or in a hurry to move on, and make eye contact with the person (Fig. 5-3). Do not interrupt or try to finish the person's sentence for her. Interrupting a person may make her forget what she was trying to tell you in the first place. Let the person finish what she was saying before you ask another question or make a comment, and focus on the person and the information she is trying to give you—try not to think about what *you* intend to do or say next. After the person has finished speaking, you should ask questions to help clarify any information that you do not understand. Your comments and questions will let the speaker know whether you understood her message, or whether she needs to provide additional information.

When You Are the Sender, Make Sure Your Message Is Clear

Speak clearly and use words that the person you are speaking to understands. A nurse or a fellow personal support worker will understand medical

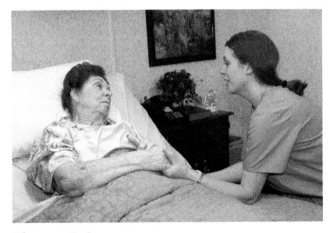

Figure 5-3
Being a good listener is essential to being a good communicator.

terminology, and using medical terminology is appropriate when you are communicating with one of your co-workers. However, a patient, resident, or family member may not be familiar with medical terminology. To make sure the patient or family member understands your message, try to use common words instead of technical words whenever it is appropriate to do so. For example, you could say, "Miss Lewis, we're going to go for a walk down the hall now, to get you up and moving" instead of "Miss Lewis, I'm going to ambulate you now."

Sometimes, it is necessary to communicate with someone who does not speak the same language you do, or who has a physical problem that makes certain forms of communication less effective than others. To meet the regulation that requires patients and residents to give informed consent for treatments and procedures, health care facilities must provide interpreters for patients or residents who speak languages other than English. By definition, a person cannot give informed consent unless he understands what he is consenting to! A hearing-impaired person may need a sign language interpreter to assist with communication, or you could try writing out important questions for the person to read and respond to. A picture board, a tool that allows a person to point to a picture of what he or she is trying to say, is often useful when trying to communicate on a basic level with someone who speaks a different language or is hearing impaired (Fig. 5-4). More information about communicating with patients and residents with special needs can be found in Chapters 34 and 35.

If a patient or resident seems to have difficulty understanding you when you are talking to him, make sure that there is not too much background noise. If the person usually wears glasses or a hearing aid, check to make sure that these aids are in place and the hearing aid is turned on.

Learn Techniques for Encouraging People to Talk

When you need to get information from someone, try asking the person an open-ended question. Questions that can be answered with a simple "yes" or "no" usually get just that response, and the conversation ends. In contrast, open-ended questions encourage the person to talk. Another question that can cause a conversation to end is "Why?" If a patient complains that he does not like his dinner or choice of snack, instead of asking "Why?" (which can be intimidating), you could ask the person to tell you what his favorite

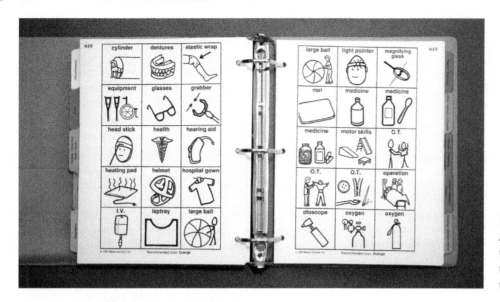

Figure 5-4
A picture board can be used to communicate when illustrations are more effective than words.

food or snack is. For example, consider the following two conversations:

Conversation 1

> **Personal support worker:** "Good morning, Mr. Hopkins. Did you have breakfast this morning?"
> **Mr. Hopkins:** "No."
> **Personal support worker:** "Why not?"
> **Mr. Hopkins:** "I don't know . . . I just wasn't hungry, I guess."

Conversation 2

> **Personal support worker:** "Good morning, Mr. Hopkins. What did you have for breakfast this morning?"
> **Mr. Hopkins:** "Not much. They sent up scrambled eggs. I don't care for scrambled eggs, so I just had some buttered toast and coffee."
> **Personal support worker:** "I didn't know you didn't like scrambled eggs! Let me see what I can do about that. Do you dislike eggs in general, or just scrambled eggs? In the meantime, are you hungry?"

In the second conversation, the personal support worker achieved two key goals: She engaged Mr. Hopkins in the conversation, and in the process, she made him feel as though she really cared about him as an individual.

Rephrasing what someone says to you is another way to encourage someone to talk. For example, if one of your residents tells you that she feels sad and lonely, instead of asking "Why?" try repeating the person's statement back to her as a question: "You are feeling sad and lonely?" By rephrasing and asking an open-ended question, you will invite the person to say more. In addition, encouraging the person to talk more about what she is feeling shows the person that you are actively listening to what she is saying to you.

Usually, asking open-ended questions is better than asking questions that can be answered with a simple "yes" or "no." But in some situations, a "yes or no" question may be better. For example, asking questions that can be answered with a short "yes" or "no" (or a nod or shake of the head) is appropriate when you are caring for a patient or resident who is having trouble breathing or who finds it very difficult to speak.

Provide and Seek Feedback

Providing and seeking feedback is a critical communication skill that will come into play with both your co-workers and your patients or residents. Consider two conversations, one between you and the nurse, and the other between you and one of your patients or residents. In the first, you are the "receiver"—the nurse is asking you to do a task. After the nurse has finished speaking, you could say, "Let me make sure I understand this correctly," and repeat the information back to her. What awesome feedback! The nurse now knows that you were listening, and that you understand what is being asked of you (Fig. 5-5). The *exchange* of information has occurred. You are communicating effectively.

In the second conversation, you are the "sender" and one of your residents is the "receiver"—you are trying to give instructions to the resident about

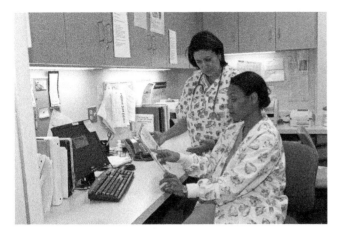

Figure 5-5
By indicating to the nurse that she understands what she is being asked to do, this personal support worker is providing good feedback.

how to use the call light control system in the room, and you want to make sure that he understands how the system works. You might say, "Now repeat that information back to me so I can make sure you've got it," but asking for feedback in this way could be intimidating to the resident. A more gracious way of finding out whether the resident understood your message would be to say, "Now, if you could just repeat these instructions back to me so I can make sure I didn't leave anything out." This approach makes the resident feel that he is helping you by repeating the information, and in the process, you are able to tell whether or not he understands your instructions clearly.

Be Mindful of Your Body Language and Tone of Voice

Use appropriate body language when listening or talking to other people. Negative body language, such as crossing your arms across your chest, tapping your feet or fingers, rolling your eyes, or constantly looking at your watch or toward the door, sends the very clear message that you are bored or uninterested (Fig. 5-6). In contrast, displaying positive body language, such as facing the person, nodding as he speaks, smiling or looking serious as appropriate, and making occasional vocal sounds, such as "uh huh" or "hmm," indicates to the person that you are interested in what he is saying. Positioning your body so you are at eye level with the speaker also shows interest (Fig. 5-7). Children are especially responsive to the adult who comes "down to their level" to listen to what they have to say.

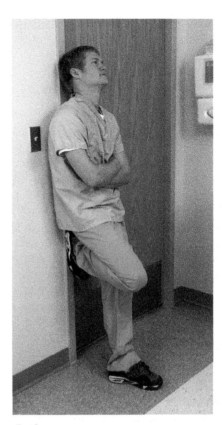

Figure 5-6
If you were a patient or resident, what message would this personal support worker be sending to you?

Tone of voice is important too. A sharp or hurried tone of voice suggests to the person that you are impatient or angry. In contrast, speaking slowly in a soothing tone of voice suggests that you are calm, competent, and kind.

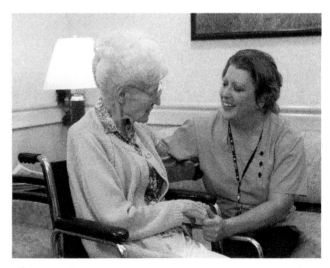

Figure 5-7
Putting yourself at eye level with a patient or resident indicates to the person that you are interested in what he or she has to say, and that you have time to listen.

This relaxes the other person and is a useful technique for calming a person who is frightened or upset.

Remember the Value of Silence and a Comforting Touch

There will be many times throughout your career as a personal support worker when words will not be enough to communicate your care and concern to a patient or resident, or to a family member of one of your patients or residents. Silence and a comforting touch will say more than words can (Fig. 5-8). Touch is perhaps the most universal of all languages, but remember to be sensitive to the individual's comfort level. Many patients and residents appreciate affection and will enjoy a hug or sitting and holding your hands as you talk. Other people may not be as comfortable with affection, and will be satisfied with a light pat on the shoulder or top of the hand as you greet them or say good-bye.

In addition to allowing us to communicate when words are not enough, touch is comforting and establishes a bond. So much has been written about the "healing powers of touch"—for example, consider the role of therapeutic massage in the treatment of physical ailments. Research has also shown that babies, even when given adequate food and physical care, fail to grow and thrive without human touch and attention.

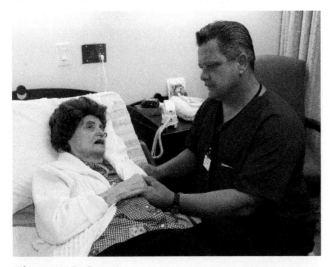

Figure 5-8
Of the many techniques for enhancing communication, nothing says "I care about you and I want to help you" more effectively than a simple touch on a person's hand or shoulder.

BLOCKS TO EFFECTIVE COMMUNICATION

Some behaviors and attitudes can block effective communication. Perhaps the most common obstacle to effective communication is not listening carefully to what another person is saying. You must be especially careful not to "tune out" your patients or residents, despite the fact that you will be busy, and many of the people you will care for could be easily labeled "complainers." Imagine the consequences if you ignore a patient's or resident's complaint, and it turns out to be valid.

Being judgmental of others will also block communication. If a person feels that you do not believe or respect what he is trying to tell you, he will most likely stop talking and will probably refuse to answer any questions you may ask later. A judgmental attitude, indicating that you do not really care to hear what the person is trying to tell you, can be revealed through negative body language or comments you may make. Communication blocks can occur when you assume that someone else knows what you are thinking. Your patient should know that she should not adjust the flow rate on her intravenous (IV) line, shouldn't she? Your co-workers should know without bothering you that Mrs. Jones has already been up to the bathroom, shouldn't they? Your husband should know why you are mad at him, shouldn't he? The assumption that other people know what you know, think the way you think, and feel the way you feel presents a major block to effective communication and can lead to conflict and confusion. To avoid this communication pitfall, be proactive in your interactions with others, and keep them informed. For example, give instructions and gentle reminders to patients or residents, tell your co-workers what has already been accomplished and what still needs to be done before you go on break, and ask your husband to take out the trash instead of getting angry because he did not think of it himself!

CONFLICT RESOLUTION

Conflict, or discord resulting from differences between people, can occur when one person is unable to understand or accept another's ideas or beliefs. Conflict can also arise when one person's expectations for another differ from that person's expectations for himself. Other times, conflict arises because one person misunderstands another person's words or intentions. How many times have you been angry with a friend because you thought she said or meant one thing, only to find out after talking with her that what you thought she said or meant is not what she said or meant at all? Conflict can occur when another person's needs or wants conflict with our own needs and wants.

Some degree of conflict in our lives is inevitable because we are individuals with unique personalities, feelings, and beliefs. Conflict is a fairly common occurrence in the health care field, because health care is a people-oriented business. It is also a very emotional business. Patients and residents are sick, hurting, confused, and frightened. Family members feel helpless and sad. Personal support workers and other health care workers are often stressed by the emotional and physical demands of their work. As a result, conflicts may arise between a member of the health care team and a patient or resident, between two patients or residents, or between two members of the health care team (Fig. 5-9). Getting along with other people, while a very important part of your job, can sometimes be the hardest part of your job.

Conflict makes the people directly involved, as well as those around them, uncomfortable. This discomfort can affect a patient's or resident's ability to recover or a staff member's quality of work.

Good communication is essential to preventing conflict, as well as helping to resolve it. If you find yourself involved in a conflict, remember what it means to be a professional, and take the time to talk calmly with the person with whom you are upset. It is important to address areas of conflict early, before they have time to get worse and involve more people. Approaches for resolving conflict include the following:

- Ask to speak privately with the person you have a conflict with. Because the two of you may be able to resolve your disagreement on your own, try this approach before asking a supervisor to mediate, if at all possible. Remain polite and professional and thank the person for her time.
- During your conversation, focus on the specific area of conflict. Do not focus on how you feel about the other person, or how you think she should have acted under the circumstances.
- Be specific about what you understand the problem to be, and express why you are upset in terms of "I," rather than the more accusatory "you." For example, instead of saying, "You really hurt my feelings by what you said the other day," say, "I am bothered by what you said the other day." In this manner, you take responsibility for the emotion and allow the other person to explain her side of the story.
- Be prepared to hear how the other person may feel toward you or the problem, even if it is not pleasant. Perhaps you were the one who was initially misunderstood.
- Be gracious enough to apologize for misunderstanding the other person, or for being the one who was misunderstood.
- Ask the other person for insight into solutions for resolving the conflict. Her suggestions may surprise you!
- Sometimes it is necessary to "agree to disagree." People with differing opinions and beliefs can focus on the things they have in common, such as caring about the patient's or resident's well-being, and still disagree on certain issues (Fig. 5-10). Learning to respect others' beliefs is an important part of being professional.
- If you are unable to resolve a conflict with a co-worker, a patient or resident, or a patient's or resident's family member on your own, seek the advice of your supervisor. A conflict that affects the quality of the care you provide must not be allowed to continue!

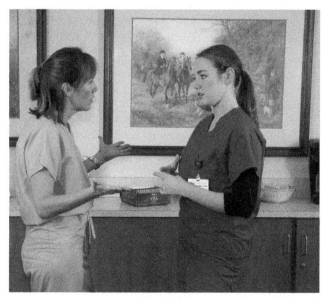

Figure 5-9
Conflict can occur between two members of the health care team or between a member of the health care team and a patient, resident, or visitor. Poor communication is one of the most common reasons conflict occurs!

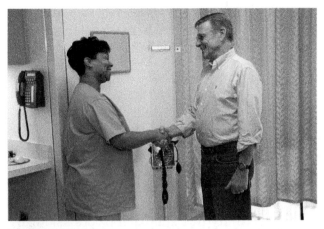

Figure 5-10
Sometimes, the best solution to a conflict is to simply "agree to disagree." Instead of focusing on your differences, focus on your similarities. In the professional setting, for example, even if you and a resident's family member cannot agree about what is "best" for the resident, you can certainly respect the fact that both of you care deeply about the resident and want to do what is best for him.

TELEPHONE COMMUNICATION

The telephone is a primary tool of communication in the health care field. Other departments will call to verify an order or request, doctors will call to ask about a patient or resident or to give orders, and family members will call to get an update on the condition of a loved one. The telephone at the

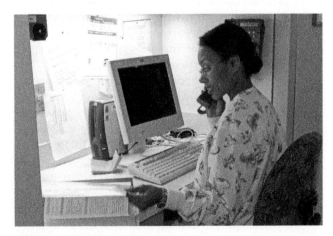

Figure 5-11
Developing a good phone manner is important, because you will find yourself frequently using the telephone to communicate!

BOX 5-1 Telephone Etiquette

- Answer the telephone promptly, within the first three rings.
- Answer with a pleasant greeting, such as "Good morning" or "Good afternoon."
- Identify yourself by name and title and by your unit or floor according to facility policy: "3 West; Mary Smith, PSW, speaking."
- Because the caller obviously needs something (otherwise, he would not be calling), ask "How may I help you?"
- Know how to perform basic functions using your facility's telephone system, such as how to transfer a call or place a caller on hold.
- If you must place a caller on hold, ask her permission first ("May I put you on hold for a minute?"). Be aware of the length of time a caller has been on hold; if the time becomes excessive (more than 5 minutes), ask the caller if she wants to continue to hold, leave a message, or call back later.
- If the person the caller wants to speak to is unavailable, offer to take a message. When taking a telephone message, be sure to write down the date and time of the call, the name of the caller, a telephone number where the caller can be reached, and your name. Write clearly, and ask the caller to spell his or her name if you are not sure how to spell it. Be sure to deliver the message to the person for whom it was intended.
- A personal support worker is not to take doctor's orders, receive or give results of diagnostic tests, or release patient or resident information to anyone, even family members. Calls of this nature should be handled by a nurse.
- Do not use the telephone at the nurse's station to make or receive personal calls. Personal calls should be made from a pay phone or your own cellular phone, while you are on break or at lunch. Never tie up a telephone used for health care communication by using it for personal business.

nursing station is in use constantly—it is almost as if a teenager lives there! As a personal support worker, you will usually be required to answer the telephone, either at the nursing station or in a patient's or resident's room (Fig. 5-11). Proper telephone etiquette is reviewed in Box 5-1.

When you answer the telephone, make sure your voice is pleasant and unhurried. Believe it or not, a caller can "hear a smile" in your voice. This can be very comforting to an anxious family member who is calling to check on a sick loved one. You must remember to be as professional on the telephone as you are in person. There will be times when a caller may be impatient or angry; resist the urge to respond in a similar manner. You do not know the cause of the caller's impatience or anger, and you certainly do not want to add to it. The way you handle yourself on the telephone reflects directly on your facility. If callers perceive you as kind and professional when they speak to you on the phone, they will feel that the people you are caring for are receiving the same kind, professional care.

Confidentiality is of concern when the telephone is used as a means of communication. When you are discussing a person's care over the telephone, be sure that other patients, residents, or visitors cannot overhear your conversation. Know your facility's policy regarding what information can be provided over the telephone. For example, some facilities, such as those that provide mental health care or substance abuse rehabilitation, protect their patients' and residents' right to privacy through policies that prohibit staff from confirming or denying that a person is even receiving treatment at the facility. To give out such information could result in litigation against the facility, and ultimately cost you your job. The Canada Privacy Act of 1983 discussed in Chapter 4, specifically regulates who may be given information about a person in a health care facility.

COMMUNICATION AMONG MEMBERS OF THE HEALTH CARE TEAM

As you have already learned, the personal support worker plays a very important role in gathering and sharing information about patients and residents with other members of the health care team. As you interact with your patients or residents, you will have the opportunity to make observations. An **observation** is something that you notice about the patient or resident, typically related to a change in the person's physical or mental condition. The amount of time you will spend with your patients or residents, combined with the type of duties you are responsible for performing daily (for example, bathing, feeding, ambulating, toileting), will give you a chance to observe things that other health care team members may overlook.

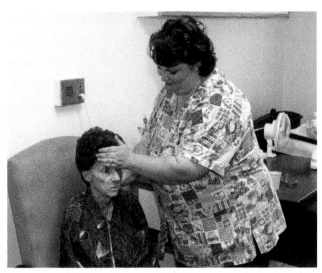

Figure 5-12
When you make an objective observation, you obtain information using one of your five senses. Here, the personal support worker is feeling the resident's forehead to assess whether or not the skin is hot and dry or cool and clammy.

Two types of data can lead to observations: objective data and subjective data. **Objective data** are information that you obtain directly, through measurements or by using one of your five senses. In the professional setting, the senses you will use most often are sight, hearing, touch, and smell. For example, certain indicators of a person's health, called vital signs, can be objectively measured. (The vital signs are temperature, pulse, respiratory rate, and blood pressure.) You can see the colour of a person's skin, and feel that it is cool and clammy (Fig. 5-12). You can see the colour of a person's urine, smell any foul odour, and measure the amount. You can hear wheezing or gurgling as a person breathes. You can see bruises, swelling, or rashes on the skin when you help a person bathe. You can see how much breakfast the person ate and measure how much juice she drank. These are all objective observations. Objective observations, such as an elevated temperature, a rash, or a low urine output, are called **signs.** **Subjective data,** on the other hand, are information that cannot be objectively measured or assessed. The basis for a subjective observation is usually a person's complaint, or **symptom.** For example, a patient or resident may tell you that he has a headache or stomachache. You cannot see, feel, measure, or hear his pain, but he can describe it to you (Fig. 5-13).

When you are communicating subjective observations to the other health care team members, it

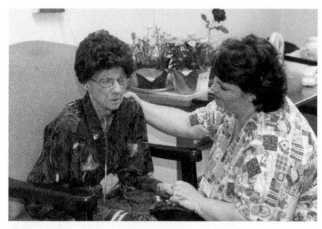

Figure 5-13
A subjective observation is information that is derived "second-hand." This personal support worker knows that her resident is experiencing stomach pain because the resident is describing it to her, not because she detected the resident's pain using one of her five senses.

is useful to quote the person directly, whether you are relaying the complaint verbally (reporting) or writing the information in the person's medical record (recording). It is also useful to support subjective observations with objective ones. For instance, Mrs. White tells you that she feels dizzy when she stands up (a subjective observation). To gather more information, you ask Mrs. White if she has gotten dizzy before, and whether or not her dizziness is accompanied by a headache or nausea. Her answers to these questions would also be subjective observations. Next, you observe Mrs. White's skin for paleness or redness; touch her skin to see if it is warm, or cool and clammy; measure her blood pressure; and take her pulse. All of these objective observations give you still more information. By gathering objective facts to add to Mrs. White's subjective statements, and then organizing this information in a logical way and relaying it to the nurse, you are truly communicating! Not only have you told the nurse about Mrs. White's symptoms, you have given her objective data that may help determine what is causing those symptoms.

Once you have made an observation, you must decide on the most effective method of communicating that observation to the nurse. Personal support workers use two methods of communicating observations about their patients or residents and documenting the care provided so that other health care team members are kept "in-the-know." These methods are reporting and recording. Some observations need to be reported to the nurse immediately, such as a patient's or

resident's complaint of pain or a change in her vital signs. Other observations only need to be recorded in the person's medical record. Throughout this text, observations that need to be reported to the nurse immediately are highlighted as "Tell the Nurse!" notes.

REPORTING

Reporting is the spoken exchange of information between health care team members. Reporting is used throughout the shift to communicate changes about a patient's or resident's status to other health care team members (Fig. 5-14). Personal support workers use reporting to communicate the following information to the nurse:

- Observations that suggest a change in the patient's or resident's condition
- Observations regarding the patient's or resident's response to a new treatment or therapy
- A patient's or resident's complaints of pain or discomfort
- A patient's or resident's refusal of treatment
- A patient's or resident's request for clergy

When reporting information, follow the guidelines that help promote effective communication. Make sure the information you are reporting is accurate—refer to the patient or resident by name and room number, and if you are reporting measurements, such as vital signs, write the numbers down so you do not forget them or report them incorrectly. Report your observations in an orderly, concise manner. Avoid adding information that is not relevant to what you are trying to communicate. Use correct terminology

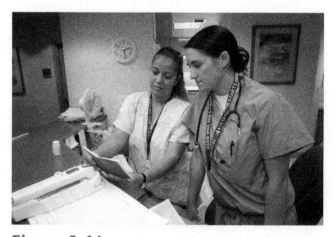

Figure 5-14
This personal support worker is reporting a change in one of her resident's vital signs to the nurse.

when reporting, and make sure the person you are reporting to gives you feedback so that you know he received the information and will act on it.

Reporting is also routinely used when shifts change to keep the staff members who are coming to work aware of all the information that is necessary to ensure a smooth continuation of care for the patient or resident. For example, the end-of-shift report is when oncoming staff members would be informed of new patients or residents and their care requirements, changes in the care plan for established patients or residents (such as new orders or treatments), and changes in a patient's or resident's status (such as rest or appetite changes).

RECORDING

Recording, sometimes referred to as "charting," is communicating information about a patient or resident to other health care team members in written form. Tools associated with recording include the medical record (chart) and the Kardex.

Medical Record (Chart)

A person's **medical record (chart)** is a legal document where information about the person's current condition, the measures that have been taken by the medical and nursing staff to diagnose and treat the condition, and the person's response to the treatment and care provided are recorded. Because the medical record, a legal document, is a formal accounting of the care the person received from the health care facility, it can be retrieved at any time and used in a court of law as evidence in a litigation claim.

The medical record is usually organized in sections with specific forms contained in each section. Some of these forms provide general information about the patient or resident. Others are specific to a particular health care department. The forms used may vary depending on the type of facility or health care agency. Typically, however, a medical record contains the following forms:

- **Admission sheet.** The admission sheet provides standard information about the person, including the person's name, address, date of birth and age, Social Insurance number, gender, insurance and employment information, emergency notification information, and advance directive information.

- **Medical history.** Usually, the medical record contains a dictated and typed medical history from the person's doctor. The medical history contains information about the person's previous surgeries and medical conditions, current medications, allergies, and current medical diagnosis.

- **Nursing history.** The nursing history is completed by the nurse at the time of the person's admission to the facility. The nursing history provides information related to the person's care needs, such as information about physical disabilities or limitations, bowel and bladder habits, dietary preferences, and use of ambulation aids. An example of a nursing history is given in Chapter 14.

- **Physician's order sheet.** The physician's order sheet is used by the doctor to communicate to the other members of the health care team what should be done for the patient or resident. For example, the doctor may use the physician's order sheet to order treatments (such as medications), specify dietary orders or activity status, or order diagnostic tests.

- **Medication administration record (MAR).** The medications ordered for the patient or resident are listed here, along with the dosage and the time at which they are to be administered. This form is also used to record when medications are given, and by whom. Some long-term care and assisted-living facilities provide additional training to allow personal support workers to give medications. If giving medications is within your scope of practice, then you will record your activities on the MAR.

- **Physician's progress notes.** The doctor uses this form to record his notes and observations about the person's progress and response to treatment.

- **Narrative nurse's notes.** The nurse uses this form to document the person's complaints (symptoms) and the actions taken by the nursing staff in response to them (Fig. 5-15). Some facilities allow personal support workers to make notations in the narrative nurse's notes, and some do not.

- **Graphic sheet.** This is where information that is gathered routinely—such as vital signs, the frequency of urination and bowel movements, and food and fluid intake—is documented (Fig. 5-16). Some long-term care facilities use a type of graphic sheet to record a resident's activities of daily living

Date	Time	Department (Nursing, P. T., etc.)	Prob. No.	◄ Progress Note	◄ Signature/Title
12/02	1410	n		P. Abdish,CNA	Resident c/o pain in Rt. arm. BP 142/86,
					P. 92, R. 18, T. 99.2(o). RN notified.
12/02	1415	n		S. Carter, RN	Demeral 50mg, p.o. administered. Rt. arm elevated on
					pillow. Fingers warm and pink.
12/02	1500	n		S. Carter, RN	Resident states "My arm feels much
					better now."

Patient's Name (Last, First, MI)	Attending Physician	Room Number	Patient Number
Hayes, Ethel J	Sanders	302	1301

Figure 5-15
The care provided by the nursing staff, and the patient's or resident's response to this care, is documented in the narrative nurse's notes.

(ADLs) and exercise therapy. The graphic sheet is the form used by personal support workers most often to document the care they provide.

- **Miscellaneous documents.** Laboratory reports, radiology reports, and reports related to other diagnostic tests or therapeutic treatments are usually included in specific sections of the person's medical record.

The information recorded on these various forms allows the members of the health care team to communicate with each other efficiently. For example, consider the following scenario:

Three days ago, Mrs. Wilson was admitted to 2 North for abdominal pain. Yesterday, when Mrs. Wilson's doctor reviewed the graphic sheet in Mrs. Wilson's chart, she saw that Mrs. Wilson had developed a fever. The doctor recorded her observations and impressions on the physician's progress notes form, and then ordered an antibiotic for Mrs. Wilson using the physician's order sheet. The unit clerk read the physician's order sheet and notified the pharmacy about the antibiotic. After giving the antibiotic to Mrs. Wilson, the nurse recorded when the antibiotic was given on the MAR. Throughout the rest of that day and night, the personal support workers who were caring for Mrs. Wilson measured and recorded Mrs. Wilson's temperature at regular intervals on the graphic sheet. When the doctor made her rounds the next day, she was able to see that the antibiotic had been given as ordered

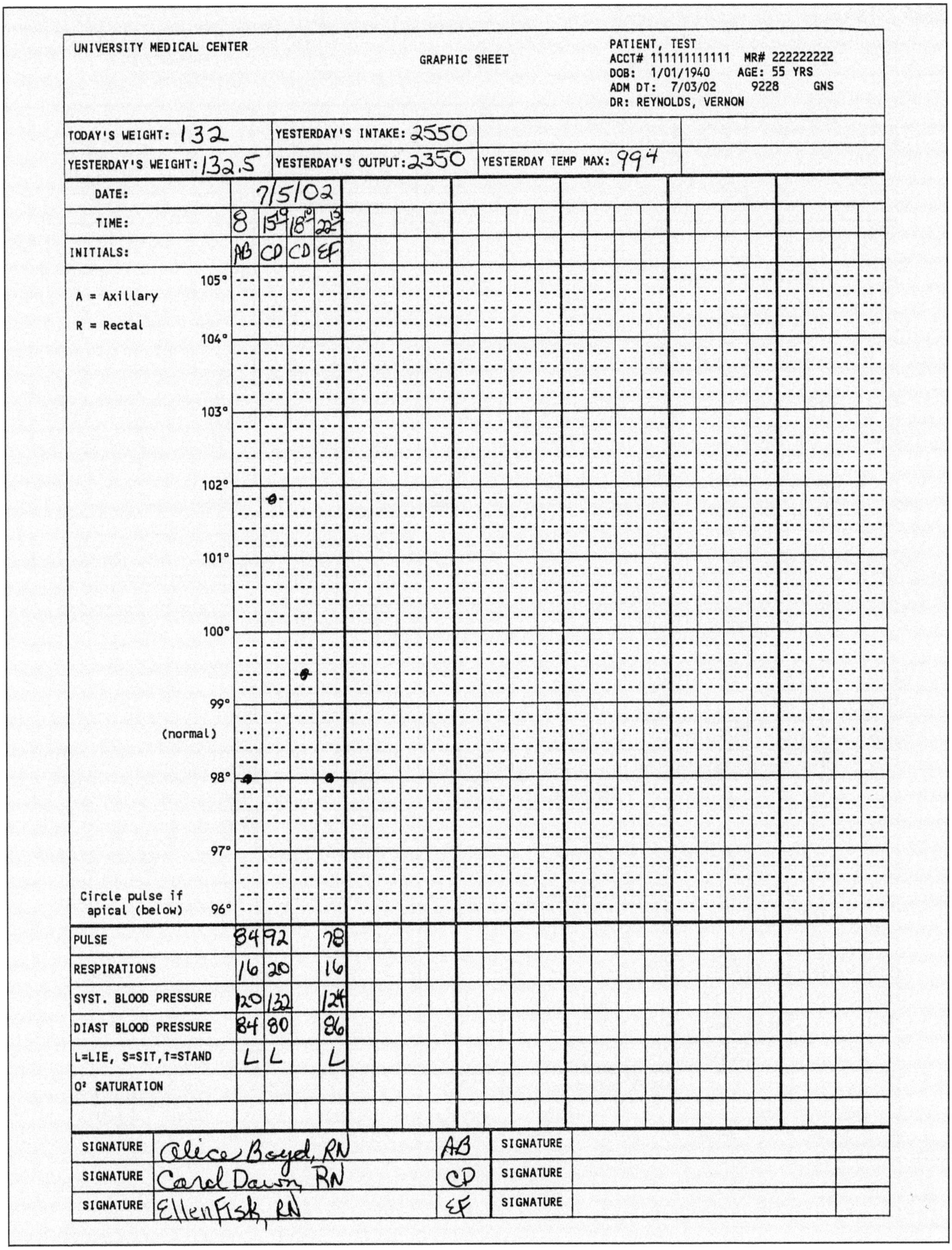

UNIVERSITY MEDICAL CENTER	GRAPHIC SHEET	PATIENT, TEST ACCT# 111111111111 MR# 222222222 DOB: 1/01/1940 AGE: 55 YRS ADM DT: 7/03/02 9228 GNS DR: REYNOLDS, VERNON

TODAY'S WEIGHT: 132	YESTERDAY'S INTAKE: 2550		
YESTERDAY'S WEIGHT: 132.5	YESTERDAY'S OUTPUT: 2350	YESTERDAY TEMP MAX: 99⁴	

DATE:	7/5/02
TIME:	8 15¹⁵ 18¹⁰ 22¹⁵
INITIALS:	AB CD CD EF

A = Axillary
R = Rectal

(temperature graph, 105° down to 96°, normal at 99°)

Circle pulse if apical (below)

PULSE	84 92	78
RESPIRATIONS	16 20	16
SYST. BLOOD PRESSURE	120 132	124
DIAST BLOOD PRESSURE	84 80	86
L=LIE, S=SIT, T=STAND	L L	L
O² SATURATION		

SIGNATURE	Alice Boyd, RN	AB	SIGNATURE	
SIGNATURE	Carol Dawn, RN	CD	SIGNATURE	
SIGNATURE	Ellen Fisk, RN	EF	SIGNATURE	

Figure 5-16
The graphic sheet is used to record information that is more easily and accurately expressed visually, as opposed to verbally. For example, here you can see how the patient's temperature has changed throughout the day.

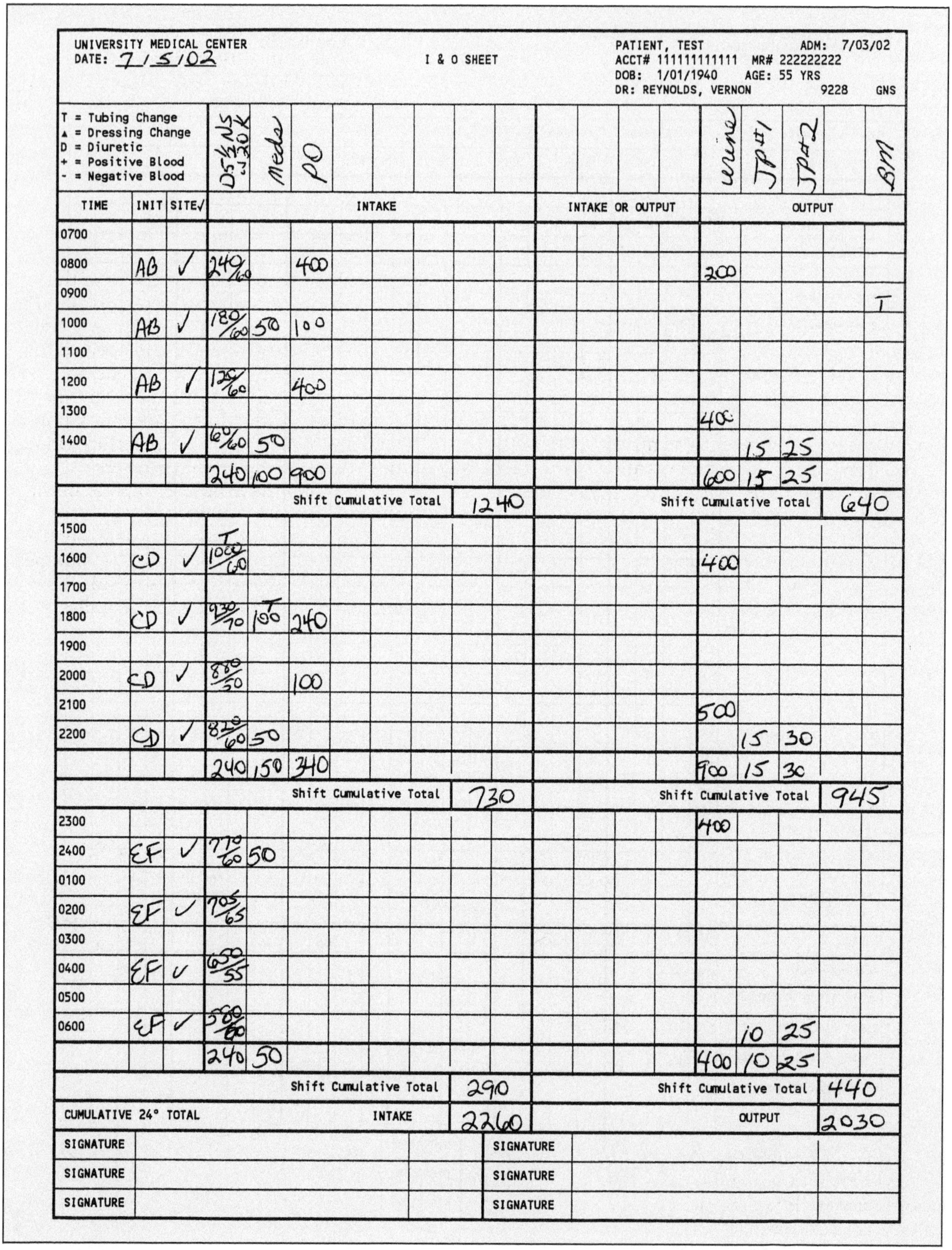

UNIVERSITY MEDICAL CENTER
DATE: 7/5/02

I & O SHEET

PATIENT, TEST ADM: 7/03/02
ACCT# 111111111111 MR# 222222222
DOB: 1/01/1940 AGE: 55 YRS
DR: REYNOLDS, VERNON 9228 GNS

Legend:
- T = Tubing Change
- ▲ = Dressing Change
- D = Diuretic
- + = Positive Blood
- − = Negative Blood

Intake columns: D5½NS w30K | Meds | PO
Output columns: urine | JP#1 | JP#2 | BM

TIME	INIT	SITE✓	D5½NS w30K	Meds	PO	INTAKE OR OUTPUT	urine	JP#1	JP#2	BM
0700										
0800	AB	✓	240/60		400		200			
0900										T
1000	AB	✓	180/60	50	100					
1100										
1200	AB	✓	125/60		400					
1300							400			
1400	AB	✓	60/60	50				15	25	
			240	100	900		600	15	25	
Shift Cumulative Total						1240	Shift Cumulative Total			640
1500			T							
1600	CD	✓	1000/60				400			
1700										
1800	CD	✓	930/70 (T)	100	240					
1900										
2000	CD	✓	880/50		100					
2100							500			
2200	CD	✓	820/60	50				15	30	
			240	150	340		900	15	30	
Shift Cumulative Total						730	Shift Cumulative Total			945
2300							400			
2400	EF	✓	770/60	50						
0100										
0200	EF	✓	705/65							
0300										
0400	EF	✓	650/55							
0500										
0600	EF	✓	580/60					10	25	
			240	50			400	10	25	
Shift Cumulative Total						290	Shift Cumulative Total			440
CUMULATIVE 24° TOTAL					INTAKE	2260			OUTPUT	2030

SIGNATURE
SIGNATURE
SIGNATURE

SIGNATURE
SIGNATURE
SIGNATURE

Figure 5-16 (Continued)

and could tell by the temperature recordings that Mrs. Wilson was responding to the medication.

By using the medical chart properly, the health care team members were able to communicate with each other in an organized, efficient way. The doctor did not need to find the nurse or personal support worker to ask whether Mrs. Wilson was receiving the antibiotic, or to find out whether her fever had gone away.

Each facility or agency has specific policies about whether or not a personal support worker is allowed to record information in the medical record. In some agencies or facilities, you may be able to record information on the graphic sheet, but not on the narrative nurse's notes. In others, you will be required to make entries in the narrative nurse's notes as documentation of the care you provide and the observations you make. Whenever you enter information on a person's medical record, date and time your entry correctly. Most medical facilities and agencies use the 24-hour time clock, also called "military time," for recording the time in a patient's med-

ical record (Fig. 5-17). Guidelines for recording are given in Guidelines Box 5-1.

The way information is organized and entered into a medical record, and the policies dictating who is permitted to enter information into the record, differ from facility to facility. However, two policies regarding the handling of medical records are always the same, no matter where you work:

- The information contained in a person's medical record is considered confidential and is only to be read by members of the health care team who are directly involved in the care of that person and need access to the information in the record to provide that care. For example, although a custodial worker is part of the health care team, he does not need access to the information in the medical record in order to perform his duties. Therefore, custodial workers generally do not have access to patients' or residents' charts.
- To keep patients and residents safe, each form in the medical record must be stamped or printed with the patient's or resident's identification information. Accidentally

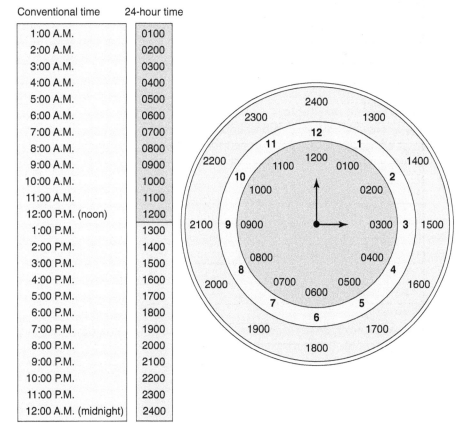

Figure 5-17
Most medical facilities and agencies use the 24-hour time clock, also referred to as "military time," for recording the time in a patient's medical record. The 24-hour time clock eliminates the need to differentiate between morning (A.M.) and night (P.M.), thus reducing errors in recording. On the 24-hour time clock, the morning hours are the same as on the conventional clock. To indicate a time in the afternoon, add "12" to the time on the conventional clock. When time is stated according to the 24-hour time clock, the first two numbers indicate the hour and the last two numbers indicate the minute (for example, 8:24 P.M. conventional time = 2024 military time). Conventional time = *grey*; morning hours = *beige*; afternoon hours = *blue*.

Conventional time	24-hour time
1:00 A.M.	0100
2:00 A.M.	0200
3:00 A.M.	0300
4:00 A.M.	0400
5:00 A.M.	0500
6:00 A.M.	0600
7:00 A.M.	0700
8:00 A.M.	0800
9:00 A.M.	0900
10:00 A.M.	1000
11:00 A.M.	1100
12:00 P.M. (noon)	1200
1:00 P.M.	1300
2:00 P.M.	1400
3:00 P.M.	1500
4:00 P.M.	1600
5:00 P.M.	1700
6:00 P.M.	1800
7:00 P.M.	1900
8:00 P.M.	2000
9:00 P.M.	2100
10:00 P.M.	2200
11:00 P.M.	2300
12:00 A.M. (midnight)	2400

WHAT YOU DO	WHY YOU DO IT
Write legibly, using blue or black ink. Your facility may have specific policies regarding the colour of ink used.	It is important to write legibly to avoid miscommunication. A pen is used instead of a pencil because pencil can be erased, enabling someone to change the person's medical record. Blue and black ink reproduce best when a document is photocopied.
Always sign or initial your entry, according to facility policy.	By signing or initialing your entry, you indicate that you are the person who needs to be consulted if further clarification of the information you have entered is necessary. Additionally, signing or initialing your entry indicates that you accept legal responsibility for what you have written.
Only record observations that you have made, or care that you have given. Do not make entries for another person.	By making an entry in a medical record, you accept legal responsibility for that entry. Therefore, it is best to record only information that you, personally, can vouch for.
Date and time your entries correctly (see Fig. 5-17).	The date and time that actions occurred or observations were made are extremely important elements of the medical record, which is a legal account of care provided.
Check the patient's or resident's name on the medical record and on the form where you are recording.	By verifying the patient's or resident's identification information, you will ensure that you are recording the person's information in the correct medical record.
Use appropriate medical terminology and facility-approved abbreviations when recording.	Using correct terminology and abbreviations will prevent others from having to second-guess your meaning.
Do not record care as given or procedures as performed before you have provided the care or performed the procedure. Only document after the fact.	You may become distracted or involved in another situation that prevents you from carrying out the duties you have already charted. If you record duties as "completed" in the medical record, but then do not actually complete these duties, you will have committed fraud.
Record information in a timely manner. If you must wait to record something, keep notes about your observations and care so that the information you record in the medical record will be accurate.	If you wait until the end of your shift to record, you may forget important information.
If you make an error, do not erase, use correction fluid to cover, or scribble through the mistaken entry. Simply draw a line through the mistake and initial it according to facility policy.	Striking through an error is the only legal way to indicate a change in the medical record. Erasing or using correction fluid to correct an error could be seen as an attempt to hide or change existing information.
Remember that in a liability situation, care not recorded was care not provided.	Proper and conscientious recording of patient or resident information protects the patient or resident, your employer, and you.

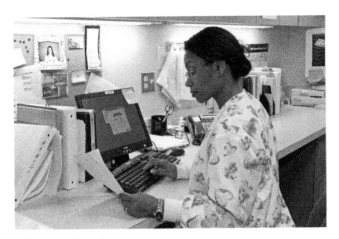

Figure 5-18
Computerized charting is becoming more widespread.

placing a physician's order sheet meant for one person in another person's medical record could cause someone to receive a treatment or medication in error. A miscommunication of this nature could have serious, possibly even fatal, consequences.

As the use of computers becomes more widespread, computerized charting is replacing paper charting in some facilities and agencies (Fig. 5-18). In computerized charting, the person's medical record is maintained by entering data into a computer in response to the computer's prompts, rather than by filling in a paper form. Medical records created in this way tend to be more accurate and legible because they are typed rather than handwritten. Using a computer to maintain and access a patient's or resident's medical record does not require advanced computer training. If your facility or agency uses computerized charting, your employer will provide training in the use of the computer as part of your new employee orientation. During this training, you will learn how to enter data about your patients or residents, as well as how to quickly retrieve information you need about a patient or resident in order to provide his or her care.

Although computerized charting offers many advantages over paper charting, patient and resident confidentiality is a primary concern when the computer is used to store patient data. To promote patient or resident confidentiality, each user of the computer is assigned a password, which permits the user to have access to certain patients' or residents' medical records. Never give anyone else your password or leave the computer active after you have used it. If you fail to log off after using the computer, the information on the screen may be visible or accessible to people who are not authorized to have access to it. Additionally, if you fail to log off when you are finished with the computer, someone else could enter information under your password, and it will appear as if you have entered it. Computer monitors should be positioned so that the screen is not visible to the public when you are working. Your facility or agency will have specific policies (mandated by HIPAA) regarding computer use and confidentiality. Make sure you are familiar with these policies, and follow them carefully.

Kardex

The **Kardex** is a card file containing condensed versions of each patient's or resident's medical record. The Kardex card contains a summary of the person's current diagnosis, the diagnostic tests and treatments ordered by the doctor, and information about routine care measures, such as the person's diet, level of ambulation, and bathing schedule (Fig. 5-19). The Kardex card is updated as the person's condition or doctor's orders change. By providing a one-page summary of the patient's or resident's medical record, the Kardex card keeps health care team members from having to search through the entire record every time they need information about the person's status and care plan.

THE NURSING PROCESS

Although the doctor is responsible for diagnosing a person's medical problems and ordering medication or other therapies to correct those problems, the nursing team is responsible for carrying out the doctor's orders and providing holistic care to the patient or resident. To achieve its goals, the nursing team develops a specific plan of care, called the **care plan,** for each patient or resident. The communication method that is used to develop the care plan is called the **nursing process.** The nursing process allows members of the nursing team to communicate with one another regarding the patient's or resident's specific needs (in regard to nursing care), what steps will be taken to meet those needs, and whether or not the steps were effective in meeting the person's needs. The care plan, which comes from the nursing process, makes sure that all members of the nursing team are "on the same page." The nurse who is acting as the nursing team leader is responsible for developing the care plan. She does this with the help of other health care team members, including the patient or

ADVANCED DIRECTIVES

_X_ Living will   ____ Autopsy request
____ Do not resuscitate ____ Feeding restrictions
____ Do not hospitalize ____ Medication restrictions
_X_ Organ donation   ____ Other treatment restrictions
____   ____ NONE OF THE ABOVE

Allergies: **Sulfa**

(Write in red or highlight)

Nutritional/Oral

Diet _Regular_

Supplements: _n/a_

Meal Location: Breakfast _Dining room_
                 Lunch _Dining room_
                 Dinner _Dining room_

____ Swallowing Difficulty   ____ Thicken Liquids
____ Tube Feeding   ____ NPO
____ I-O   ____ Fluid Restriction
____ TPN

Elimination   QOL program(s) _n/a_
Bladder:
_X_ Continent ____ Incontinent ____ Catheter

Bowel:
_X_ Continent ____ Incontinent ____ Ostomy

Cognition
____ Short term memory problem
____ Decision-making difficulty
____ Difficulty expressing self

Oriented to:
_X_ Person   _X_ Place
_X_ Time   _X_ Situation

Behavior   QOL program _n/a_
____ Verbally Abusive
____ Physically Abusive
____ Socially Inappropriate
____ Resistant to Care
____ Wandering/Exit Seeking   QOL program _n/a_

Communication
Primary Language:
_X_ English _____ Other: _____
____ Alternative methods used:
____ Communication board   ____ Writing
____ Sign language   ____ Gestures
____ Other _____

Appliances
____ Hearing Aide ____ R ____ L
_X_ Glasses ____ Contacts
_X_ Dentures ____ Upper ____ Lower _X_ Partial
____ Anti-embolism hose
_X_ Prosthesis/Splint/Brace (description) _Cast-Rt_
     Forearm

Respiratory
                        ____ Pulse Oximetry
____ Tracheostomy   ____ Oxygen
____ Ventilator   ____ Suctioning
Skin Management   QOL program _____
____ Turn & Position   ____ Other _____
____ Mattress

Additional Quality of Life Program(s) or Medical
Specialty Treatment Program(s)
Physical Therapy rt. arm

ADL's		Self-Performance				Support (# of Persons)	
Bathing _____	I	S	Ⓛ	E	T	①	2
Dressing_____	I	S	Ⓛ	E	T	①	2
Toileting_____	Ⓘ	S	L	E	T	1	2
Eating_____	I	S	Ⓛ	E	T	①	2
Transferring_____	Ⓘ	S	L	E	T	1	2
Walking_____	I	S	Ⓛ	E	T	①	2

I - Independent   E - Extensive
S - Supervised   T - Total
L - Limited

Mobility: Weight bearing status _good_
____ Mechanical lift   ____ W/chair
____ ROM   ____ Walker
     _X_ AROM   _X_ Cane
     ____ PROM   ____ Other: ____
____ Bedfast/chairbound
Weight schedule _X_ mo ____ why ____ other
     QOL program _____
Restraint: Type: _____ When: _____
     QOL Program

Resident Preferences:	Bathing type:	Bathing Day/time:
	____ Shower	
Name: _Miss (Ethel)_	_X_ Tub	M Ⓣ W Ⓣⱨ
Time to arise _7 am_	____ Other:	F Sⓐ Su
Time to rest: _1 pm_		
Time to retire _10 pm_		AM Ⓟⓜ
Likes/dislikes: ____		

Special Precautions:
Please assist at mealtime by opening milk and cutting food into
small pieces

Diagnoses:
Primary: _____
Secondary: _FX Rt. radius & ulna_

RESIDENT NAME	ADMISSION DATE	PHYSICIAN	DOB	AGE	Medical Record Number
Ethel Hayes	12/01/06	_Sanders_	03/06/1929	77	1301

Figure 5-19

The Kardex card, kept in a Kardex file, summarizes the most up-to-date information about a patient's or resident's condition and care needs.

resident, the personal support worker, and members of specific departments, such as dietitians, social workers, and physical therapists.

The nursing process is organized into a series of steps:

1. **Assessment.** During this step, information specific to the patient or resident is gathered. Sources of this information are the person's medical history, the nursing history, family members, and most importantly, the person himself. As part of the assessment process, the nurse examines the patient or resident and asks questions about his abilities, level of discomfort, eating and toileting habits, and specific needs.

2. **Diagnosis.** Using the information gathered during the assessment step, the nurse then develops a **nursing diagnosis,** or a statement that describes a problem the person is having, as well as the cause of the problem. Unlike a medical diagnosis, which states a medical problem that must be identified and managed by a doctor, a nursing diagnosis states a problem that the nursing staff can identify and treat independently. For example, consider a person who has a broken arm. The medical diagnosis for this person might be "fractured radius and ulna." The nursing diagnosis might be "impaired nutritional status due to inability to feed self because of dominant hand being in a cast."

3. **Planning.** The next step in the nursing process involves making a plan for the person's care. Using information obtained from the nursing diagnosis, the nurse develops **interventions** (actions that will be taken to help the person) and **goals** (descriptions of what the interventions are meant to achieve). For example, in order to achieve the goal of

improved nutritional status for the person with the cast on his arm, the intervention may be to cut the person's food into bite-sized pieces to make it easier for him to eat. The interventions and goals that have been set for the patient or resident are written down in a formal way. This document (the care plan) becomes part of the patient's or resident's medical record and may be included on the Kardex.

4. **Implementation.** During the implementation step, the interventions that were detailed in the care plan are carried out. (The care plan specifies the team members who are responsible for doing each intervention.)

5. **Evaluation.** During the evaluation step, the nursing team checks the effectiveness of the care plan and revises it as necessary. Is the care plan working? Are the goals being met? What needs to be improved or changed to meet the goals? Has the patient's or resi-dent's status changed? Is the existing care plan still appropriate for the patient or resident? If certain interventions are not working, or if the goals have been met, the care plan will change.

The nursing process is ongoing. The nursing staff continually assesses the patient or resident and adjusts the care plan as the person's needs change. As a personal support worker, you will participate in the nursing process by carrying out interventions and communicating observations to the nurse. When you communicate observations to the nurse, you help him or her with the assessment and evaluation steps of the nursing process. Your observations and communications to the nurse and other health care team members will ensure that the patient or resident remains the focus of quality, compassionate care that is carefully planned, implemented, and evaluated.

SUMMARY

- Communication is the exchange of information.
  - For good communication to occur, a sender must send a clear message directly to a receiver who can understand the message. The receiver must provide feedback that lets the sender know that the message was heard "loud and clear."
  - Effective communication among health care team members is essential to ensure that patients or residents receive top-quality, safe care. It is important for personal support workers to have good communication skills because the exchange of information with patients, residents, and co-workers is a key part of the personal support worker's job.
  - Personal support workers are an important link between the patient or resident and other members of the health care team. The personal support worker is often the first member of the health care team to become aware of a change in a patient's or resident's condition that could be a sign of something serious.
- There are many ways to improve communication with others.
  - Listening is one of the most important communication skills, especially in the health care field.
  - Speaking clearly, asking open-ended questions, and using appropriate body language when talking with other people are other ways to improve communication.
- Reporting and recording are two methods of communication used by the health care team to make sure that everyone involved in the care of a patient or resident has current, reliable information about that person. Observations about a patient's or resident's condition are reported, recorded, or both. Observations may be subjective or objective.
  - Reporting is the spoken exchange of information between members of the health care team. Observations about a change in a patient's or resident's condition must be reported to the nurse immediately.
  - Recording is the written exchange of information between members of the health care team. Recording is done in the person's medical record or chart.
- The nursing process is a communication method that allows members of the nursing team to meet a patient's or resident's specific care needs. The personal support worker plays a role in the nursing process by carrying out interventions and communicating observations to the nurse.

WHAT DID YOU LEARN?

Multiple Choice

Select the single best answer for each of the following questions.

1. Which one of the following is an open-ended question?
   a. "Are you Mrs. Brown?"
   b. "Mr. Jones, when you were growing up, what was your favorite meal?"
   c. "Are you feeling okay, Mrs. Smith?"
   d. "It's beautiful outside today, Mrs. Murphy! Do you want to go for a walk?"

2. Which one of the following is an example of positive body language?
   a. Nodding encouragingly as someone speaks
   b. Crossing your arms across your chest
   c. Tapping your feet or fingers
   d. Rolling your eyes

3. An example of an action that blocks effective communication is:
   a. Interrupting
   b. Not listening carefully
   c. Being judgmental
   d. All of the above

4. Which one of the following is an objective observation?
   a. "Mr. Wohl says that his back hurts when he coughs."
   b. "Ms. O'Connell's urine is cloudy, and has a strong odour."
   c. "Mr. McAndrews is complaining of a headache."
   d. "The resident in room 201B is complaining of a stomachache."

5. Which one of the following is an example of nonverbal communication?
   a. Using sign language to communicate with a deaf person
   b. Recording vital sign measurements in a patient's or resident's chart
   c. Gently touching a patient or resident on the shoulder to reassure her
   d. Making a telephone call

6. What usually forms the basis for a subjective observation?
   a. A symptom, or patient complaint
   b. A measurement
   c. A doctor's order
   d. All of the above

7. Which step of the nursing process involves gathering information about a patient or resident?
   a. Implementation
   b. Assessment
   c. Planning
   d. Evaluation

8. With regard to telephone communication, personal support workers are responsible for all of the following except:
   a. Writing down the caller's name and telephone number if the person the caller wants to speak to is not available, and delivering this message to the intended recipient
   b. Answering the telephone promptly, with a pleasant greeting
   c. Taking down doctor's orders if the nurse is not available and a doctor calls
   d. Identifying themselves to the caller by name and title, per facility policy

9. When recording information in a person's medical chart, what should you remember to do?
   a. Use pencil so that errors can be corrected neatly
   b. Sign or initial and date and time your entry, per facility policy
   c. Update all of your patients' or residents' charts at one time at the end of each shift
   d. All of the above

10. What is it called when people have differences and they are unable to come to an agreement?
    a. Communication
    b. Conflict
    c. Culture
    d. Personality difference

Matching

Match each numbered item with its appropriate lettered description.

_____ **1.** Admission sheet

_____ **2.** Narrative nurse's notes

_____ **3.** Medical history

_____ **4.** Physician's order sheet

_____ **5.** Graphic sheet

a. Used to record patient complaints and the actions that were taken by the nursing team to provide relief

b. Used to record routine data, such as vital signs, frequency of urination and bowel movements, and food and fluid intake

c. Used to order diagnostic tests and treatments, and to specify dietary orders or activity status

d. Typed or dictated document that lists a patient's previous surgeries and medical conditions, current medications, allergies, and current medical diagnosis

f. Document that contains essential information about the patient, including his or her name and address, birth date, insurance information, advance directives information, and emergency contact information

STOP and Think!

You are caring for Mr. Thompson today and notice that he seems distracted and is having difficulty speaking clearly. You know that you should report this to the nurse immediately.

What other subjective and objective data should you gather to report to the nurse? How can you make sure that the nurse receives the information from you?

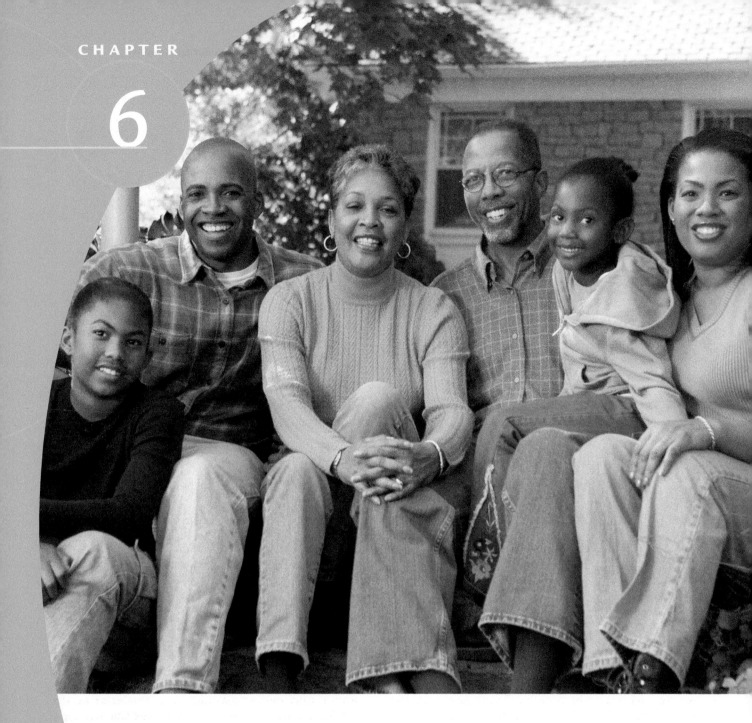

Those We Care For

As we start on the final chapter in this introductory unit, you are probably beginning to realize that there is much more to being a personal support worker than blood pressures and bedpans. A health care worker can go to the most well-known schools, receive the most

Photo: Throughout the course of our lives, we pass through a series of stages. Here, members from the same family represent the stages of school age, adolescence, young adulthood, and middle adulthood. (© Jupiter Images.)

intense training, and graduate at the top of his class, but if he is not able to connect on a human level with his patients or residents, he will fail. In this chapter, we will explore the qualities that we, as humans, share, as well as the ones that make us unique individuals. When you are finished with this chapter, you will be able to:

1. Recognize that health care is a people-focused service.
2. Discuss why people need health care intervention.
3. Differentiate between acute, chronic, and terminal conditions, and give an example of each.
4. Describe how the health care industry classifies people, and list the types of people you might have the opportunity to work with.
5. List and briefly describe the stages of human growth and development.
6. Understand that developmental changes are common throughout the life span of a person.
7. Draw Maslow's hierarchy of basic human needs, and explain each level.
8. Describe ways that a personal support worker helps patients and residents to meet their needs.
9. Understand the difference between sex and sexuality and discuss how a person's sexuality can be affected by illness.
10. Explain the concept of diversity, and why it is important for health care workers to recognize their patients' and residents' diversity.

Vocabulary

Acute illness	Puberty	Sex	Masturbation
Chronic illness	Menarche	Heterosexual	Culture
Terminal illness	Nocturnal emissions	Homosexual	Race
Growth	Menopause	Bisexual	Religion
Development	Need	Transsexual	
Tasks	Sexuality	Transvestite	
Neonate	Intimacy	Coitus	

PATIENTS, RESIDENTS, AND CLIENTS

If someone asked you "As a personal support worker, who do you care for?" you might answer (depending on where you work) "I care for patients," or "I care for residents," or "I care for clients." (As you will recall from Chapter 1, a patient is a person who is receiving health care in a hospital, clinic, or extended-care facility. A resident is a person who is living in a long-term care facility or an assisted-living facility, and a client is a person who is receiving care in his or her own home, from a home health care agency.) These are all terms for people who, because they are sick, injured, or unable to care for themselves, need the services that the health care industry offers. At the most basic level, patients, residents, and clients are "those we care for."

There are three general types of illnesses or conditions that can cause a person to need health care services. An **acute illness** is a condition characterized by a rapid onset and a relatively short recovery time. Because the onset is rapid, acute illnesses are usually unexpected. Conditions such as pneumonia, appendicitis, a broken bone, or labour and delivery would be considered acute conditions. In contrast, a **chronic illness** is a condition that is ongoing. A person with a chronic illness generally needs continuous medication or treatment to control the condition. Occasionally, acute flare-ups of the chronic condition lead to hospitalization. Examples of chronic illnesses include diabetes, asthma, arthritis, and high blood pressure (hypertension). Finally, a **terminal illness** is an illness or condition from which recovery is not expected. People who have a terminal illness will die as a result of their illness, usually within a short period of time. Examples of terminal illnesses include some types of cancer, end-stage emphysema, and some heart conditions.

To make providing care more efficient, the health care industry groups people according to

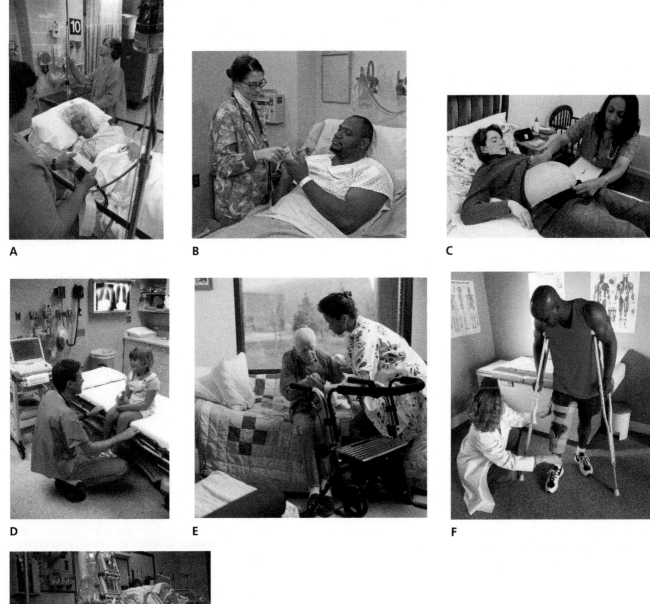

Figure 6-1
Examples of the many ways in which people are grouped by the health care industry. **(A)** Surgical patient. **(B)** Medical patient. **(C)** Obstetrical patient. **(D)** Pediatric patient. **(E)** Geriatric patient. **(F)** Rehabilitation patient. **(G)** Intensive care patient. (*F,* © *LWA-Stephen Welstead/CORBIS; **G,** © Grafton Marshall Smith/CORBIS.*)

their ages, illnesses or medical conditions, or special health care needs (Fig. 6-1). For example, it would not make sense to have adults and small children on the same ward, or a critically ill person rooming with a woman who is recovering from delivering a baby. In some cases, specialized training is needed to care for a certain type of patient, so it would make sense to group all of the patients requiring that type of specialized care

together. Examples of terms that are often used to describe people, based on the person's age, illness, or special health care needs, include the following:

• **Surgical patients** have illnesses or conditions that are treated by surgery, such as appendicitis or certain types of tumors. Surgical patients are admitted to the hospital for surgery and the recovery period afterward. Many surgical procedures are performed on an outpatient basis, which means that the patient is admitted to the hospital for surgery, but then sent home to recover. The care of surgical patients is discussed in Chapter 39.

- **Medical patients** have an illness or condition that is treated with interventions other than surgery, such as medication, physical therapy, or radiation. Examples of medical conditions include pneumonia, myocardial infarction ("heart attack"), stroke, and some stomach disorders (such as ulcers).
- **Obstetrical patients** are those who are pregnant or have just given birth. Obstetrical care extends throughout the pregnancy and labour and delivery, and then continues for about 8 weeks after delivery. Although most obstetrical patients are admitted to the hospital for the actual labour and delivery, and remain hospitalized for a brief time afterward, most of the care before and after the delivery is provided on an outpatient basis (unless the mother or baby experiences complications). The care of obstetrical patients is discussed in Chapter 40.
- **Pediatric patients** are children and adolescents. Pediatrics has become a specialty because children and teenagers are at risk for some diseases that adults are not. In addition, sometimes special considerations must be taken into account when providing treatments and care for younger patients because a child's body does not function in exactly the same way an adult's does. Sometimes an entire facility is dedicated to the care of the pediatric patient. Other times, a special unit within the hospital or long-term care facility is designated as the pediatrics unit. The care of pediatric patients is discussed in Chapter 41.
- **Geriatric patients** are elderly people. Health care workers who specialize in geriatrics are trained to recognize the physical and mental effects of the normal aging process and help older people adjust to these changes. They are also trained to care for people with diseases that are particularly common among this age group.
- **Psychiatric patients** are people with impaired mental health. Psychiatric patients are often treated on an outpatient basis, using a combination of counselling and medication. However, mentally ill people who are a danger to themselves or others may be admitted to a health care facility for treatment.
- **Rehabilitation patients** are those who are undergoing therapy to restore their highest level of physical, emotional or mental, or vocational functioning. People born with physical disabilities or deformities may require physical rehabilitation. So might people who have had a stroke or are recovering from surgery or an injury. Emotional or mental rehabilitation may be necessary for people with substance abuse problems. Vocational rehabilitation focuses on providing the person with special training after an injury or surgery so that he or she can return to a particular type of work. Rehabilitation facilities or units provide services both on an inpatient and outpatient basis.
- **Sub-acute or extended-care patients** are usually recovering from an acute illness or condition. They do not need the total care provided by a hospital, but are not quite ready to return home. They may continue to have a need for intravenously administered medications, physical therapy, or other treatments that cannot be provided by untrained caretakers.
- **Intensive care patients** need very specialized, or intensive, care and are usually admitted to an intensive care unit or a special care unit. After heart or brain surgery, or after a heart attack or stroke, a patient will stay in the special care unit until her condition improves. She will then be moved to a regular hospital unit.

As you can see, the people we care for can be classified in many different ways. However, those in need of health care services are not merely defined by their illnesses and disabilities. First and foremost, patients, residents, and clients are human beings. In the rest of this chapter, we will take a closer look at some of the things that all people have in common, as well as some of the things that make us different.

GROWTH AND DEVELOPMENT

Throughout the course of our lives, we all pass through a series of stages. We are constantly changing, from conception until the time of death.

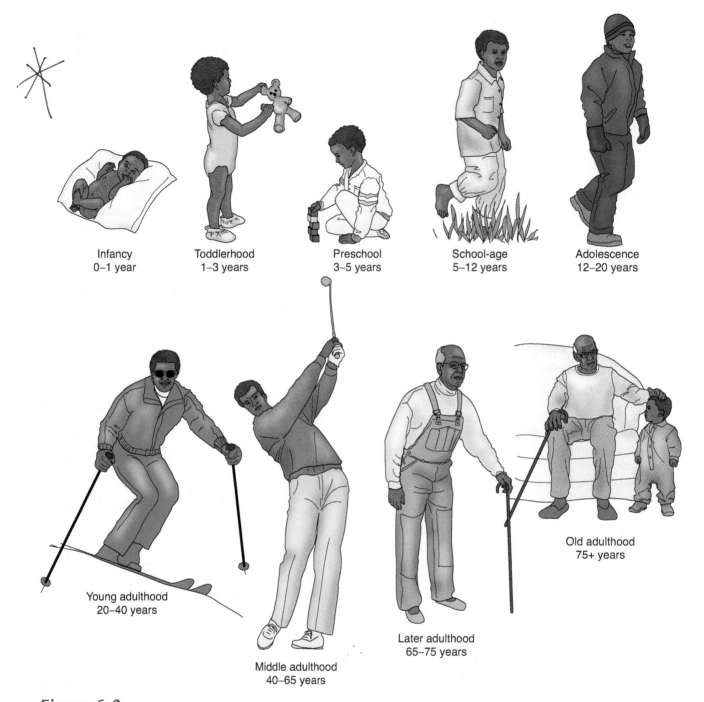

Infancy
0–1 year

Toddlerhood
1–3 years

Preschool
3–5 years

School-age
5–12 years

Adolescence
12–20 years

Young adulthood
20–40 years

Middle adulthood
40–65 years

Later adulthood
65–75 years

Old adulthood
75+ years

Figure 6-2
Everyone passes through the same stages of growth and development.

Changes that occur physically are known as **growth.** Changes that occur psychologically or socially are known as **development.** Growth is demonstrated by changes in height and weight and by physical maturation of the body's organ systems. Development is evidenced by changes in a person's behaviour and way of thinking. Both growth and development occur in an orderly fashion and progress from the simple to the com-

plex. Physically, a baby must develop the muscle strength and coordination that will enable him to sit, then stand, and finally to walk. Developmentally, that baby will smile at his mother, then coo, say his first word, and soon speak in complete sentences.

The process of growth and development is divided into stages of normal progression (Fig. 6-2). Although all people progress through the stages of growth and development in a series of expected steps, they do not progress through the stages at the same rate. For example, one child may walk at 8 months and speak his first word at 10 months. His sister, on the other hand, may talk relatively early at 7 months, but not walk until the age of 14 months. Although the stages of growth and development can be generalized by age, it is important to note that each person, like the brother and sister described here, progresses through the stages at his or her own pace. A person cannot progress to the next stage without successfully completing the **tasks,** or growth and development milestones, associated with the stage she is currently in. With young children and teenagers, it is quite common to see some overlap in the stages. This is because growth and development occur unevenly, or in spurts, with one part occurring faster than the other. A 5-year-old may have quickly matured emotionally and prefers the company of older children, but lacks certain motor skills that would allow him to ride a bike or play baseball. This can be quite frustrating for the child until he has physically grown enough to keep up. Another child may reach physical maturity quickly, but will then need to "catch up" emotionally. The basic principles of growth and development are highlighted in Box 6-1.

Psychologists are people who study the mind and behaviour. Many psychologists have developed theories about human development throughout the life span. Depending on which psychologist's work you study, you may find that the growth and development stages are defined slightly differently, in terms of age ranges and tasks. Additionally, the age at which a person begins or ends a certain stage of development varies slightly according to the individual. Figure 6-2 and the descriptions of the various stages in the sections that follow are generalizations, obtained from the large amount of research that has been done on the subject of human growth and development. Throughout your career as a personal support worker, you may have the opportunity to care for people of all different ages, from premature newborns to those who have lived for more than a century. As a person grows and ages, the physical and psychological changes that occur affect the type of care the person needs, and the way in which we communicate with him or her. Becoming familiar with the various stages of growth and development, and the tasks commonly associated with these stages, will help you become a more able caregiver.

INFANCY (BIRTH TO 1 YEAR)

Infancy is the stage during which physical and psychological changes occur most rapidly. By his first birthday, an infant will typically weigh three times what he did when he was born, and he will have progressed from a totally helpless **neonate** (a newborn infant, 28 days or younger) to a child learning how to walk (Fig. 6-3). During this stage, new tasks are accomplished on a weekly and monthly basis. The infant begins to smile and laugh, recognize parents and siblings, play peek-a-boo, and say simple words. He progresses from drinking only mother's milk or formula to feeding himself solid foods. What a year!

TODDLERHOOD (1 TO 3 YEARS)

Physical growth slows down during toddlerhood, but development of the muscular and nervous systems allows the toddler to become quite active. The toddler can walk, run, climb, jump, and peddle a tricycle easily (Fig. 6-4). Suddenly, parents and caretakers must work hard to remove unsafe objects and curb the natural curiosity of the toddler! In addition to allowing increased mobility, development of the muscular and nervous systems permits greater control of the bladder and bowels, so this is when toilet training begins.

Developmentally, the toddler learns the words to express emotions, such as "sad" or "scared,"

BOX 6-1	Principles of Growth and Development

- Growth and development occur continuously throughout a person's life span, from conception until death.
- Growth and development occur step by step and in an orderly progression. Each stage has specific characteristics and tasks that must be accomplished before the person can progress to the next stage.
- Growth and development tasks progress from the simple to the complex.
- Growth and development tasks progress from head to toe, and from the center of the body outward.
- Growth and development occur at variable rates for each individual, and may occur unevenly or in spurts.

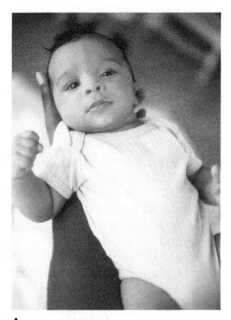

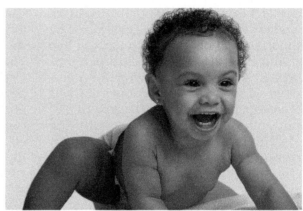

A   B

Figure 6-3
During the infancy stage, growth and development tasks are accomplished in leaps and bounds. Within the space of a year, an infant goes from being totally helpless **(A)** to being able to move around independently **(B)**.

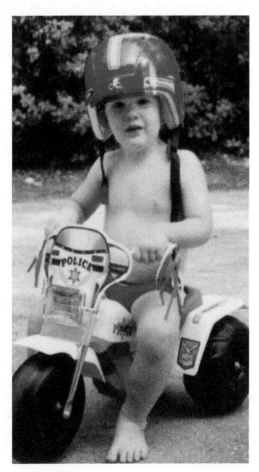

Figure 6-4
During the toddler stage, development of the nervous and muscular systems leads to increased mobility.

and is able to express herself in short, complete sentences. Toddlers become quite independent and sometimes have trouble following rules of behaviour. The toddler's world revolves around the toddler! Toddlers will engage actively in play, but usually play alone or alongside another child without many interactions. Toddlers do not separate from a parent or familiar caregiver easily. Therefore, medical procedures that require separation of the child and the caregiver can be very frightening for a toddler.

PRESCHOOL (3 TO 5 YEARS)

The preschooler is an adventure waiting to happen! The preschooler's physical coordination improves a great deal, and he learns to dress himself and tie his own shoes. Toileting becomes more independent. Preschoolers become involved in playing with other children, and will use their active imaginations to create detailed play stories and scenes (Fig. 6-5). During this stage, children become aware of gender differences and roles and are very curious about the differences between boys and girls. They ask questions all the time and love to have stories told or read to them. As the preschooler begins to know the difference between right and wrong behaviour, he begins to develop a conscience and is able to more easily follow rules.

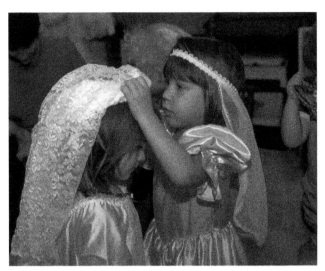

Figure 6-5
Preschoolers enjoy interacting with others and playing "make-believe." (© *Joseph Sohm; Chromo Sohm, Inc./CORBIS.*)

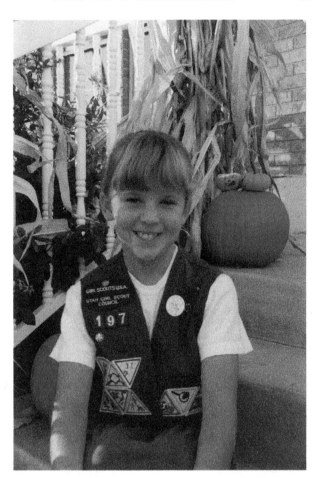

Figure 6-6
School-aged children like activities that allow them to interact with members of the same sex.

SCHOOL-AGE (5 TO 12 YEARS)

The school-aged child experiences several major physical growth spurts, which lead to increases in both height and weight. As her fine motor skills develop, the child's ability to write and draw improves. Play usually involves groups of same-sex friends. Popular activities, such as belonging to a scout troop, help with developing gender identity (Fig. 6-6). With school attendance comes an ability to follow society's rules. Children in this age group actively seek approval from authority figures and peers. They develop logical thinking patterns and learn to incorporate other people's perspectives into their own thinking. Morals develop and school-aged children may feel very strongly about issues being either right or wrong, with no grey area. Spirituality and religious beliefs, as well as a concern for other living things, also take root during this developmental stage.

ADOLESCENCE (12 TO 20 YEARS)

The ages of children in this developmental stage vary considerably. Adolescence begins at the onset of **puberty,** when the secondary sex characteristics appear and the reproductive organs begin to function. In girls, the onset of puberty usually occurs between the ages of 10 and 14 years, and in boys, it occurs between the ages of 12 and 16 years.

Physical growth and development during adolescence is considerable. In girls, the development of breasts and the growth of hair in the pubic and armpit (axillary) regions occur before the onset of menstruation, or **menarche.** Throughout adolescence, a girl's breasts continue to develop and her hips broaden, leading to the curves that characterize the female shape. In boys, the genitals increase in size. Pubic, axillary, and facial hair develops, and the voice deepens. Ejaculation, or the release of semen, signals the onset of puberty; adolescent boys often experience **nocturnal emissions** (commonly known as "wet dreams") while sleeping. A growth spurt occurs, and the adolescent boy may gain more than a foot in height over the course of a few months. His shoulders broaden and his muscles become more developed.

Psychologically, the period of adolescence is stormy. Adolescents may be self-conscious about their changing bodies and increased awareness of their own sexuality (Fig. 6-7). They are torn between wanting to be treated as grown-ups and

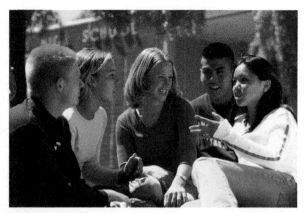

Figure 6-7
Adolescence can be a difficult yet exciting time.

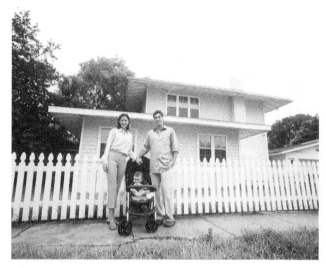

Figure 6-8
Many young adults choose to get married and begin families of their own.

being afraid to make their own decisions. Adolescents experiment with new styles of dress and hair, and follow very closely with their friends. They begin to date and to question the moral teachings of authority figures and parents. As a result, experimentation with alcohol, drugs, and sex may occur during this stage. As a reflection of their increasing emotional maturity, adolescents take jobs to make extra cash, learn to drive, and begin to make plans for their future education or the beginning of a career.

YOUNG ADULTHOOD (20 TO 40 YEARS)

After the turmoil of adolescence, young adulthood comes as a relief. Young adults typically enjoy stable, supporting friendships and good health. The primary tasks of this stage include completing one's education, starting a career, and, possibly, finding a partner and marrying. The young adult learns to be successful on her own, and if she marries, adjusts to living with a partner. Many young adults choose to start families (Fig. 6-8). For many women, the most significant physical change that will occur during young adulthood is pregnancy. Otherwise, the physical changes that occur in young adults are generally minor. The adult height is achieved during adolescence.

MIDDLE ADULTHOOD (40 TO 65 YEARS)

Middle adulthood frequently finds people at the height of their careers and productivity. Many middle adults find themselves in the role of

caretaker to their children as well as to their aging parents. As the children grow up and become less reliant, many middle adults find that they have more time to travel or participate in leisure activities (Fig. 6-9). During middle adulthood, many people become grandparents. Physically, the middle adult begins to show signs of aging, such as wrinkles or a few grey hairs. Women typically experience **menopause** (cessation of menstruation and fertility) in their early 50s. Although good health is usually still enjoyed, some chronic illnesses, such as hypertension and diabetes, become apparent during this stage.

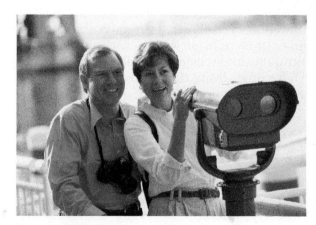

Figure 6-9
Many middle adults have raised their families and now have more time to reconnect as a couple and pursue their own interests and hobbies.

LATER ADULTHOOD (65 TO 75 YEARS)

During this stage, the physical signs of aging and the development of chronic illnesses become more prevalent. Strength diminishes, as do many senses, such as hearing and sight. Retirement may place the older adult on a fixed income, but those who have planned wisely are able to travel and pursue hobbies that they did not have time for when they were employed (Fig. 6-10). During this stage, many people must cope with the loss of friends or a spouse due to death.

OLDER ADULTHOOD (75 YEARS AND BEYOND)

During this stage, a primary task is preparing for one's own death. Although some older adults continue to be relatively healthy and independent, many must adjust to failing health and a

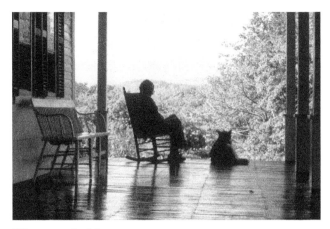

Figure 6-11
Many older adults feel that they have lived a good life. (© Bill Binzen/CORBIS.)

growing dependency on others. Even if their health or physical abilities prevent them from being totally independent, many older adults continue to feel fulfilled and needed until death, and enjoy sharing the wisdom of their years with younger people (Fig. 6-11).

BASIC HUMAN NEEDS

Clearly, all patients and residents are not alike. The people you will care for will be in different growth and development stages, and as such, they will have different needs. The primary mission of health care is to tend to the physical and emotional needs of those we care for. But what exactly are these needs?

MASLOW'S HIERARCHY OF HUMAN NEEDS

A **need** is something that is essential for a person's physical and mental health. Abraham Maslow (1908–1970), a famous American psychologist, defined what he thought to be the basic human needs, and then arranged them in a pyramid to show that certain needs are more basic than other needs (Fig. 6-12). Maslow's pyramid, called *Maslow's hierarchy of human needs*, reflects Maslow's belief that the more basic, lower-level needs must be met, at least to some degree, before the higher-level needs can be met. Many people can meet their needs with little or no outside help. But people who are ill, injured, or disabled must rely on the help of the health care team to make sure that their needs are met.

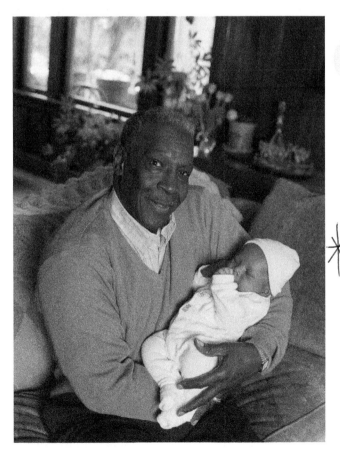

Figure 6-10
During late adulthood, many people retire from their careers and begin to enjoy the results of a lifetime of hard work, such as grandchildren and travel.

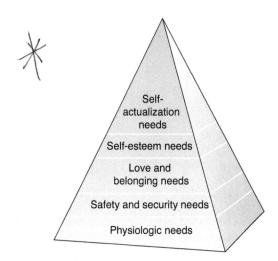

Figure 6-12
Maslow's hierarchy of human needs. A "hierarchy" shows the relationship of one idea to another. By arranging the basic human needs in a pyramid shape, Maslow created a visual representation of the idea that basic needs must be fulfilled before more complex ones.

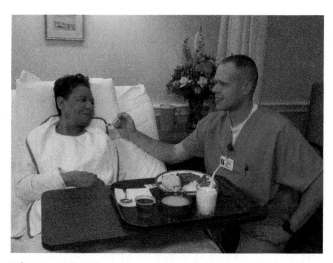

Figure 6-13
The personal support worker shown here is helping his resident to meet her need for nutrition, one of the most basic human needs.

Physiologic Needs

The most basic level in Maslow's hierarchy of needs is physiologic (physical) needs, such as oxygen, water, food, shelter, elimination, rest and sleep, physical activity, and sexuality. Meeting the physiologic needs is essential for survival. Therefore, meeting these needs is of the highest priority. A person must have enough oxygen or he will die within minutes. Water and food are essential for life, as is the ability of the body to eliminate waste products, such as carbon dioxide, urine, and feces. Shelter protects a person from the elements and extremes in temperature. Rest and sleep are essential for preventing physical exhaustion, which can lead to disability and illness. Physical activity keeps the nervous, skeletal, and muscular systems functioning and prevents wasting. Sexuality involves both the individual's need to have a sexual identity, as well as the need to engage in sexual activity, which allows for a species to reproduce and avoid extinction. Personal support workers perform many duties that assist patients in meeting their physiologic needs: Assisting with meals, toileting, ambulating, and providing a relaxing environment in which to sleep are just some of the many ways you will help people to meet their most basic needs (Fig. 6-13).

Safety and Security Needs

Safety and security needs are both physical and emotional. Not only must we *be* safe, we must also *feel* safe. For example, parents of young children take measures, such as covering electrical outlets, padding sharp surfaces, and keeping household cleaners and medications in a locked cabinet, to make sure that their children remain physically safe from harm. Personal support workers follow policies and procedures that are designed to ensure their own safety, as well as that of their patients or residents. For example, to prevent the spread of infection, a personal support worker follows the procedure for handwashing. To protect a resident who is at risk for falling, the personal support worker always makes sure that the resident has his walker close at hand. In the next unit, Unit 2, you will learn about the many ways in which personal support workers work to ensure their own safety, as well as that of the people they care for.

The emotional part of safety and security involves trusting others and being free of fear of harm. For example, parents help their children feel safe and secure by tucking them into bed at night, establishing routines, and letting them know that "mommy and daddy will always be there." A personal support worker can help a patient or resident feel safe by remembering that the entire experience of being in an unfamiliar place and having unfamiliar tests and treatments done is very frightening for many people. By explaining procedures and having questions answered promptly, the personal support worker can help to relieve much of this anxiety (Fig. 6-14).

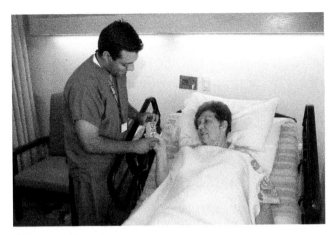

Figure 6-14
Understanding how the bed-positioning controls work can make a nervous patient or resident feel more secure in her unfamiliar environment.

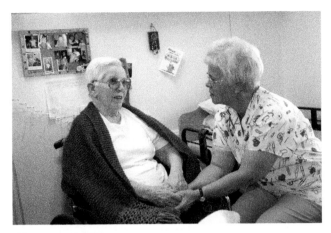

Figure 6-15
All human beings need to feel that they are loved and needed by others.

Love and Belonging Needs

All people need to feel loved, accepted, and appreciated by others. People meet this need for one another by showing affection and forming close (intimate) relationships. Family life helps us to meet our love and belonging needs. We need to feel that we are part of an accepting group. When this need is unmet, feelings of loneliness and isolation develop. Babies and children fail to grow, and older people can actually "die of loneliness." Being a patient or a resident in a health care facility can cause a person to feel isolated, unlovable, and unappreciated. Patients and residents often feel that they have become a medical condition, instead of a person. By taking an interest in the person and showing respect for the person's specific likes and dislikes, personal support workers can help to meet that person's need to feel loved, accepted, and appreciated by others. A smile, a kind word, or a gentle touch can go a long way toward making someone feel loved, appreciated, and like she "belongs" (Fig. 6-15).

Self-Esteem Needs

Self-esteem is influenced by how a person perceives herself, and how she thinks others perceive her. Everyone wants to be respected and thought well of by others. Being hospitalized or moving to a long-term care facility can affect a person's self-esteem in many ways. Many things can affect the self-esteem of a person who is receiving health care, such as:

- Having to wear a hospital gown
- Having surgery that might cause the person's physical appearance to change

- Having to depend on others for something one used to be able to do for oneself

Personal support workers help to preserve their patients' and residents' self-esteem by providing for privacy when it is necessary to expose someone's body, by allowing people to wear their own clothing (as opposed to a hospital gown) whenever possible, and by assisting people with basic grooming (Fig. 6-16).

Self-Actualization Needs

The highest level on the hierarchy of needs is self-actualization. To achieve self-actualization, a person must reach his or her fullest potential. Most of us try throughout life to meet this need,

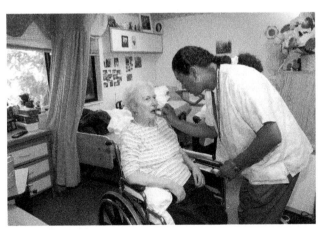

Figure 6-16
By helping this resident to look her best, this personal support worker is helping to foster the resident's self-esteem.

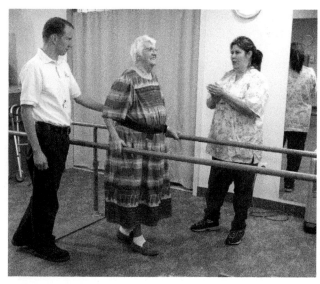

Figure 6-17
Helping patients and residents to set small, realistic goals helps them to meet their need for self-actualization.

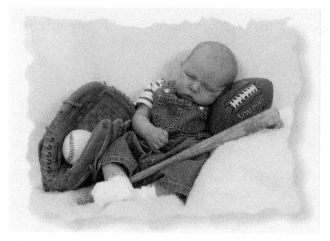

Figure 6-18
Society influences our ideas about our sexuality from an early age.

because we are constantly setting new goals for ourselves. As a health care worker, you will have the unique opportunity to help the people you care for achieve self-actualization, by helping them to set small, realistic goals for a positive outcome (Fig. 6-17). Examples of goals that patients or residents may have include taking one step (for a person who has had a stroke), delivering a healthy baby (for a pregnant woman), or returning home (for a person who has broken a hip).

The needs of the people you care for will change as their conditions improve or decline. By helping people to meet their most essential needs first, you will enable them to meet their higher-level needs. For example, it is difficult to work on a person's self-esteem if he is struggling to breathe! Recognizing needs that people have difficulty meeting on their own, and helping them to meet these needs, is one of the most valuable contributions you will make as a personal support worker.

HUMAN SEXUALITY AND INTIMACY

All human beings are sexual beings. **Sexuality** is an integral part of our personalities; it is how a person perceives his or her maleness or femaleness. Sexuality differs from **intimacy,** which is a feeling of emotional closeness to another, and **sex,** which is the physical activity one engages in to obtain sexual pleasure and reproduce. A

person's sexuality can be influenced by many factors, including the person's culture and religious beliefs. From birth, we are surrounded by symbols of our sexuality—little boys receive baseball mitts and miniature toolboxes "just like Dad's"; little girls receive dolls and tea sets (Fig. 6-18). We grow up being taught by our parents and peers what is appropriate behaviour for a "little girl" or for a "big boy."

As we progress through the developmental stages of life, we develop personal ideas and beliefs about our own sexuality. Many women like to express their sexuality by dressing in a feminine manner and wearing makeup, while others may prefer a more casual, natural look. Men also have preferences in their dress. For example, some feel most masculine in suits and ties, others in jeans and boots. People also develop preferences for the types of people they are sexually attracted to. For example, **heterosexuals** are attracted to members of the opposite sex, while **homosexuals** are attracted to members of the same sex. **Bisexuals** are attracted to members of both sexes.

Sometimes, a person's feelings about his or her sexuality do not correspond with the person's physical body. These people, called **transsexuals,** believe that they should be members of the opposite sex. Some transsexuals have a surgical procedure (a "sex change operation") to physically become a member of the opposite sex, after receiving psychiatric counselling to ensure that they are good candidates for the surgery. In other cases, the way a person chooses to express his or her sexuality does not match what society has defined as typically "male" or "female." For example, a **transvestite** is a person who becomes sexually excited by dressing as a member of the opposite sex. Most transvestites are men who prefer to dress like women. A person with transvestite tendencies is not necessarily a transsexual or a homosexual—in fact, most transvestites are heterosexual men.

As a personal support worker, you will meet people whose feelings about their sexuality, and the ways in which they express these feelings, might be very different from your feelings about your sexuality and the way you express those feelings. You must avoid being judgmental or critical of how another person chooses to express his or her sexuality. Acceptance of another person's views does not mean that you approve of that person's beliefs and practices. It only means that you respect that person's right to make his or her own decisions.

Because society so often associates youth and beauty with sexuality, we often do not consider the sexual needs of aging people. Sexuality (or the need to think of oneself as a sexual being) and intimacy (the need to share emotional closeness with another) are basic human needs, common to all people, young and old (Fig. 6-19). Many elderly people in long-term care facilities have lost their sexual partners, either as a result of death or divorce. Quite often, they have the chance to find happiness again in their golden years with someone they meet in a nursing facility.

Although sexual activity is a part of some intimate relationships, it is not necessarily a part of all. Many people share intimacy by just cuddling or caressing. Sometimes illness or physical disabilities make **coitus** (sexual intercourse) difficult or impossible, but there are other ways in which two people can love each other.

There are many ways that, as a personal support worker, you can help patients and residents to fulfill their need to be thought of as sexual beings, and to engage in intimate relationships with others:

- Avoid being judgmental.
- Help your patients and residents with rituals that make them feel either feminine or masculine, such as dressing and applying make-up, perfume, or aftershave lotion.
- Allow for privacy. If the person is in a private room, close the door and use a "do not disturb" sign as the person requests. If the person has a roommate, suggest to the roommate that the two of you take a walk or participate in another activity, outside of the room. Privacy is necessary for people in intimate relationships, whether or not they involve coitus (sexual intercourse). It is also necessary for people who want to engage in **masturbation** (stimulation of the genitals for sexual pleasure or release, by a means other than sexual intercourse).
- If a person is masturbating in a public room (some confused patients or residents will do this), take the person to his or her room and provide for safety and privacy.
- Always knock before entering a person's room. If you do interrupt a sexual encounter, excuse yourself quietly and say you will return later.

Some people become sexually aggressive and will behave in an unpleasant or unwelcome way toward you or another patient or resident. It is important for you to be able to recognize situations that could be considered sexual abuse or assault. However, before you get upset and report the person's inappropriate behaviour to a supervisor, stop and think about a few things. Although a patient or resident, especially if he or she is elderly, may seem unattractive to you, think about what that person sees when he or she looks at you. You may be young and very attractive. You

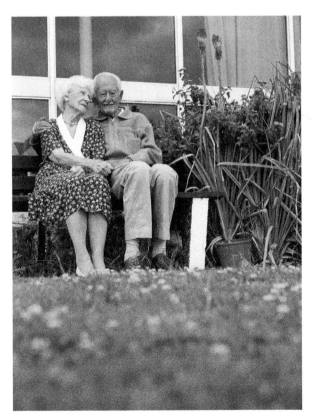

Figure 6-19
Sexuality and intimacy are basic human needs for everyone, young and old.

may remind the patient or resident of his or her spouse, when that person was young. The patient or resident may have poor eyesight and mistake you for someone else, or he or she may be confused or disoriented as a result of a disease process. Although it is totally inappropriate for you to attend to the sexual needs of your patients or residents, it is important to avoid being unkind or hateful in your response. Depending on the situation, tell the patient or resident kindly, yet firmly, that you are not going to do what he or she is asking you to do, or that he or she must not touch you in that manner. Avoid giggling or teasing the patient or resident in a flirtatious manner. This will only serve to reinforce the inappropriate behaviour. If the behaviour does not stop, or if the behaviour is directed at another patient or resident, you should discuss the matter with your supervisor.

CULTURE AND RELIGION

You can see that there are many things that, as human beings, we all have in common. For example, everyone has the same basic needs, although some needs may be more pressing than others at any given time for any one individual. Similarly, we all pass through the same stages of growth and development, although not at the same time or at the same rate. Culture, the subject of this section, is another thing that makes human beings human. All people have a culture, although everyone's culture is not the same. **Culture** is made up of the beliefs (including religious or spiritual beliefs), values, and traditions that are customary to a group of people. It is a view of the world that is handed down from generation to generation. A culture can be shared by people of the same race or ethnicity, by people who live within the same geographic area or speak the same language, or by a combination of these two (Fig. 6-20). While racial identity is often mixed with a person's culture, **race** is a general characterization that describes skin color, body stature, facial features, and hair texture.

One of the most unique things about the Canada is the diversity of cultures that are represented here (Box 6-2). Diversity has enriched this country, yet problems can arise when people are not sensitive to, or respectful of, the cultural uniqueness of each individual. As a health care worker, it is important for you to learn as much as possible about the characteristics of other cultural or ethnic groups of people, because your

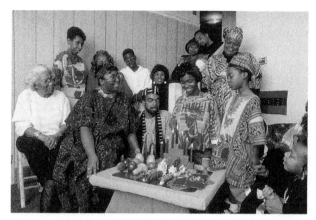

Figure 6-20
This African American family is celebrating Kwanzaa, a holiday celebrated by Africans and people of African descent throughout the world. Kwanzaa, a celebration of African history and culture, with a special emphasis on family life, occurs from December 26 through January 1. Kwanzaa is a cultural holiday, not a religious one. Celebrants are united by their African heritage, not their religion. (© *Lawrence Migdale*.)

patients or residents will have cultural differences that may affect their preferences regarding health care. Additionally, a primary goal of the nursing team is to provide for the comfort of those we care for. A person who feels that his culture is not understood or respected by the people who are caring for him will feel uncomfortable.

There are many ways in which a health care worker can accidentally be disrespectful of a patient's or resident's culture, which can lead to

BOX 6-2	Canada's Ethnic Groups

According to Statistics Canada 2006 Census, there are more than 200 ethnic groups living in Canada. The Ethnic Origin Classifications are:

Aboriginals, which includes First Nations, Metis, and Inuit
British Isles, which includes English, Irish, Scottish, and Welsh
Caribbean Origin
Latin, Central, and South American Origin
European Origin
African Origin
Asian Origin
Arab Origin

conflict. Sometimes, misunderstandings occur simply because a health care worker is not aware of how a certain person's culture influences her behaviour. Although it is difficult to make generalizations about culture—not everyone from the same geographic region, or with the same skin tone, necessarily has the same beliefs or value system—being aware of what a patient or resident is telling you can help you to know when cultural differences need to be taken into account. Areas where culture and health care often intersect include beliefs and practices associated with food and meals; religious beliefs and practices; and attitudes toward health, sickness, and death.

Liking certain types of food, or food prepared a specific way, is very cultural. For example, a person from the Asian community may prefer rice to potatoes. Sometimes, a patient or resident may request or refuse a certain food or combination of foods in order to follow religious beliefs or practices. For example, a person of the Catholic faith may not want to eat meat on Fridays during Lent, and a person of the Jewish faith may follow the practice of not drinking milk with a meal that contains meat. In some cultures, it is believed that certain combinations of foods can aid or inhibit healing. For example, according to Taoism (a philosophy that originated in Asia), illness occurs when the body is out of balance. To restore balance, certain foods may be chosen over others. If one of your patients or residents requests or denies a certain food or combination of foods for religious or other reasons, be sure to tell the nurse. The nurse will work with the dietary department to meet the person's request.

A person's spiritual beliefs, or **religion,** are often very closely linked with his or her culture. Members of some cultural groups have certain rituals that they feel will bring them good luck or aid in healing. For example, you may encounter a person from Turkey who believes hanging an "evil eye" talisman will ward off bad spirits, or a person from Panama who believes that wearing strings on the wrist will relieve pain. A person might want to light candles while praying to a specific saint. Many people are very spiritual and find comfort and solace in prayer, reading scriptures or spiritual books, singing, and praying. If a patient or resident asks to see a spiritual leader or clergy member, communicate the request promptly and according to your facility's policy, and allow for privacy during the visit. Other persons' religious beliefs may be very different from yours, but you can be certain

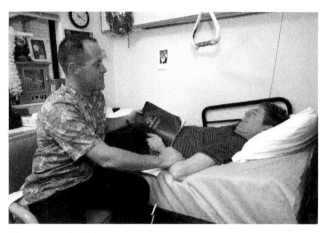

Figure 6-21
A personal support worker can help people to obtain comfort from their religious beliefs, even if he or she does not share those same beliefs.

that their beliefs are as important to them as yours are to you. You do not have to believe in a person's religion to offer the kind of care that reading their scriptures to them when they cannot will show (Fig. 6-21).

There are other examples of cultural practices that we must be respectful of, even if we think they are wrong. Remember, your culture gave you your value system, and your patient's or resident's culture gave her her value system. Respecting another person's values does not mean that you have to agree with that person, or her values. For example, some cultures do not allow women certain freedoms that we take for granted in this country. Imagine that you are a male personal support worker, caring for a Middle Eastern woman. In some Middle Eastern cultures, a woman is not allowed to be questioned or examined by a male health care provider unless her husband is present. Your patient's husband has not yet arrived at the hospital, and you need to perform a procedure for this patient. Although it would be tempting to go ahead with the procedure without the husband present, you know that your patient would not be comfortable if you were to put her in a difficult situation. You would be devaluing her belief system by trying to overrule it.

Throughout your career, you may be lucky enough to care for people from many different cultural and religious backgrounds. You will most likely encounter situations, practices, and beliefs that no book could have prepared you for! Take time to listen to your patients or residents, and to learn from them. Exposure to cultures other than your own is enriching, both professionally and personally.

QUALITY OF LIFE

As a health care professional, you are trained to care for a person's physical needs. Treating illness and promoting good health are two primary goals of all health care providers. However, sometimes we are so focused on treating a patient's or resident's problems, we forget to consider the desires of the individual. A humanistic approach to health care, as you have learned, takes into account a person's emotional, social, and spiritual needs as well as his or her physical ones. Making an effort to accommodate a person's cultural beliefs and practices is one way that health care workers provide humanistic care. Another way is by allowing patients and residents to make decisions related to their own quality of life.

As a personal support worker, you will learn that a person who has diabetes must control her diet carefully. You will learn that a person with heart disease should eat fewer foods high in cholesterol and stop smoking. But, what if your patient or resident does not comply with the recommendations of the health care team? Is the woman with diabetes a bad person if she truly loves sweets and does not want to give them up? Is the man with heart disease a bad person if he cannot bear to give up his daily breakfast of eggs and bacon at the diner? What if a person refuses a treatment or surgery that may prolong his or her life? Should the health care worker simply write that person off and focus only on those willing to follow medical advice?

Helping Hands and a Caring Heart

FOCUS ON HUMANISTIC HEALTH CARE

Focus for a moment on why people need health care and what it is like to be a patient or resident. Being sick, injured, or unable to care for oneself creates a state where a person will need the services the health care industry offers. People do not choose illness or infirmity, and most very desperately want to "get better" quickly.

What is it like to be a patient? Patients feel scared and lonely. They feel sick. They are unsure about their health, now and in the future. Some patients worry about whether they will be able to return to work, and they are concerned about how their illness will affect the financial future of their families. Others worry about how they will look after

surgery (for example, a woman who has had a mastectomy to treat breast cancer may worry that her husband will no longer find her attractive). Some medical treatments can also cause a change in a person's physical appearance (for example, loss of hair as a result of chemotherapy). Patients worry about spouses, children, and pets at home, and whether they are being cared for properly. They worry about the emotional effects of their illness on their family members. The hospital environment itself can be frightening and uncomfortable, full of strange noises and smells. If you were in this situation how would you feel and how might this affect your behaviour?

Similarly, what is it like to be a resident? Imagine what it would be like to have to move from a home you loved to a long-term care facility. You have lived a long, full life. You have worked hard and raised a family. You really liked your little house with your cat and the shady back porch where you could sit on hot summer evenings. Now, you are not managing as well as you once did—you have fallen twice, and left the teakettle on numerous times and forgotten about it. Even though, logically, you know it makes sense to move to a place where there is always someone around to "take care of you," when you gave up your home, you gave up a certain amount of your independence along with it. You cannot take all of your furniture, and you must find a new home for your pet cat. You have a roommate (at your age!) and you have to eat the meals that are prepared for you, when they are served to you. Gone are the lazy summer evenings eating peaches on the porch for dinner and relaxing in the bathtub with a glass of wine. How would you feel about this loss of independence, and how might this affect your behaviour? People who find themselves as patients and residents often feel that they are at the mercy of the health care industry. While some patients and residents are cheerful, compliant, and grateful, others may be depressed, angry, anxious, or just downright mean. When you must care for a patient or resident who makes you wish you had never chosen to be a personal support worker (and you can be certain you *will* encounter patients or residents like this), stop and think for a moment about the reasons that person may be acting out of sorts. When you look beyond the illness or condition, past the technical duties and procedures, and into that person's eyes, you will find your reason for choosing to be a personal support worker . . . a person who needs you very much.

If a health care worker gives a person the proper information about his illness or condition, and educates him about the steps that can be taken to treat or resolve the condition, then the health care worker has provided the person with the information he needs to make a conscientious decision concerning his own health. The person must make these decisions according to his own personal values and sense of what is best for himself, as an individual. This is where the idea of *quality of life* comes into play. Quality of life has to do with getting satisfaction and comfort from the way we are living. The idea of what quality of life means differs for each person and may vary as a person's situation changes. For example, during your career as a health care worker, you will care for terminally ill people who want every treatment available to help them fight for life, even if the procedures are dangerous or painful. You will also care for terminally ill people who decline painful or risky treatments because they feel that their ability to enjoy life and derive pleasure from living will be too compromised by the treatments. Each of your patients and residents must be allowed to make decisions concerning his or her quality of life. In order to provide holistic care for your patients or residents, you must respect their decisions related to maintaining their quality of life.

SUMMARY

- Patients, residents, and clients are people who need the services of the health care industry because they are sick, injured, or unable to care for themselves.
  - Acute, chronic, or terminal illnesses can cause a person to need health care services.
  - People in health care settings are grouped according to their ages, illnesses or medical conditions, or special health care needs.
- People in health care settings have many different physical and emotional needs.
  - Basic needs must be met before higher-level needs can be met.
  - Maslow's hierarchy of human needs includes physiologic needs, safety and security needs, love and belonging needs, self-esteem needs, and self-actualization needs.
  - Sexuality is how a person perceives his or her maleness or femaleness. Sexuality differs from intimacy (the need to feel emotionally close to another person) and from sex (a physical act engaged in for pleasure and reproduction). Sexuality and intimacy are basic human needs.
  - Patients and residents who are not able to meet their needs on their own rely on the health care team to recognize and help meet these needs for them.
- The people you will care for are individuals, with unique feelings, memories, goals, and personalities.
  - You will care for people in varying stages of growth and development.
  - You will care for people from different cultural and religious backgrounds.
  - Recognizing and respecting the differences in the people you care for will allow you to provide humanistic care. When you provide humanistic care, you make a difference in the lives of your patients or residents and their family members.

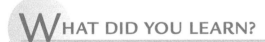HAT DID YOU LEARN?

Multiple Choice

Select the single best answer for each of the following questions.

1. Sally is caring for Mrs. Norville, who lives in a long-term care facility. Sally encourages Mrs. Norville to make her own decisions about what to do each day. She helps her with dressing and grooming, but lets her do as much as she can for herself. These activities help fulfill Mrs. Norville's need for:
   a. Security
   b. Shelter
   c. Spirituality
   d. Self-esteem

2. When caring for people from different cultures, you should try to:
   a. Understand and respect their special needs
   b. Encourage them to change their beliefs while in your facility
   c. Pretend that the cultural differences do not exist
   d. Avoid talking to them

3. Which one of the following is an example of an acute condition?
   a. Appendicitis
   b. Emphysema
   c. Diabetes
   d. High blood pressure (hypertension)

4. A resident's religion forbids him from eating pork. Pork chops are being served for dinner. What should you do?
   a. Tell the resident that religious restrictions on diet do not count in times of illness
   b. Ask the nurse to call the dietary department
   c. Insist that the resident eat the pork, because it contains protein, an essential nutrient
   d. Reassure the resident by telling him that the doctor ordered this diet

5. A resident in a long-term care facility may show her sexuality by doing all of the following except:
   a. Desiring sexual intercourse
   b. Engaging in public fondling
   c. Giving her granddaughter a doll for her birthday
   d. Applying makeup and scented powder before receiving a male visitor

6. Which one of the following is not a basic human need?
   a. Fear
   b. Self-actualization
   c. Self-esteem
   d. Water

7. Which one of the following is a basic social need?
   a. Food
   b. Water
   c. Air
   d. Love

8. What is a person who becomes sexually excited by dressing as a member of the opposite sex called?
   a. A transsexual
   b. A transvestite
   c. A bisexual
   d. A homosexual

Matching

Match each numbered item with its appropriate lettered description.

_D_ 1. Infancy
_C_ 2. Toddlerhood
_F_ 3. Preschool
_G_ 4. School-aged
_A_ 5. Adolescence
_B_ 6. Middle adulthood
_E_ 7. Older adulthood

a. A 16-year-old girl going to the junior prom
b. A 42-year-old executive running his own company
c. A 2-year-old boy starting toilet training
d. A 6-month-old girl learning to sit up
e. A 92-year-old great-grandmother moving to a long-term care facility
f. A 4-year-old boy learning to tie his shoes
g. An 11-year-old Boy Scout participating in his troop's annual canned food drive

STOP and Think!

You are caring for Mr. Spencer, who was admitted to your long-term care facility yesterday. Yesterday, he was quiet and polite. Today, however, he is hostile and mean. He refused to go to the dining room for lunch and knocked the tray you brought him to the floor. He keeps yelling at you, saying, "This feels like a prison!" Why do you think Mr. Spencer is acting this way? What could you do to help him?

Personal Support Workers Make a Difference!

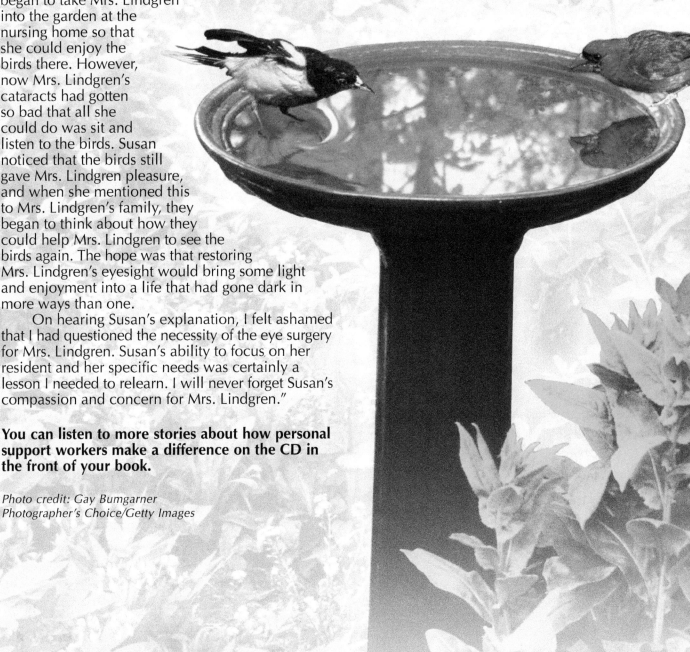

"I am an operating room nurse, and I care for many elderly patients who are having cataract surgery. Many of my elderly patients are very healthy, and excited about having surgery to restore their vision.

Not too long ago, we were scheduled to perform cataract surgery on a resident from a local nursing home, Mrs. Lindgren. I was somewhat surprised to meet my patient! Mrs. Lindgren had Alzheimer's disease and was quite confused. Susan, a personal support worker who had cared for Mrs. Lindgren regularly for about 3 years, came with her to the surgery. Needless to say, I pondered the wisdom of putting Mrs. Lindgren through surgery, which would most certainly be a frightening experience for her. What was the surgeon thinking?

When I expressed my concerns to Susan, she told me a little bit about Mrs. Lindgren. Susan told me that before Mrs. Lindgren's Alzheimer's disease had progressed to the point where she was no longer able to care for herself, she had loved to sit in her garden and watch the birds gather around the many bird baths that she kept filled. Knowing this, Susan began to take Mrs. Lindgren into the garden at the nursing home so that she could enjoy the birds there. However, now Mrs. Lindgren's cataracts had gotten so bad that all she could do was sit and listen to the birds. Susan noticed that the birds still gave Mrs. Lindgren pleasure, and when she mentioned this to Mrs. Lindgren's family, they began to think about how they could help Mrs. Lindgren to see the birds again. The hope was that restoring Mrs. Lindgren's eyesight would bring some light and enjoyment into a life that had gone dark in more ways than one.

On hearing Susan's explanation, I felt ashamed that I had questioned the necessity of the eye surgery for Mrs. Lindgren. Susan's ability to focus on her resident and her specific needs was certainly a lesson I needed to relearn. I will never forget Susan's compassion and concern for Mrs. Lindgren."

You can listen to more stories about how personal support workers make a difference on the CD in the front of your book.

Photo credit: Gay Bumgarner
Photographer's Choice/Getty Images

2

SAFETY

7 Communicable Disease and Infection Control
8 Bloodborne and Airborne Pathogens
9 Workplace Safety
10 Patient and Resident Safety and Restraints
11 Positioning, Lifting, and Transferring Patients and Residents
12 Basic First Aid and Emergency Care

As you have learned, being a personal support worker is physically demanding work that places you in close contact with people. Many of the people you will care for will be ill, injured, frail, or a combination of the three. Not only must you know how to protect yourself in the workplace (from communicable disease and from physical injury), but you must also know how to protect those entrusted to your care. Maintaining safety is the focus of Unit 2.

Photo: A personal support worker helps a resident to walk safely.

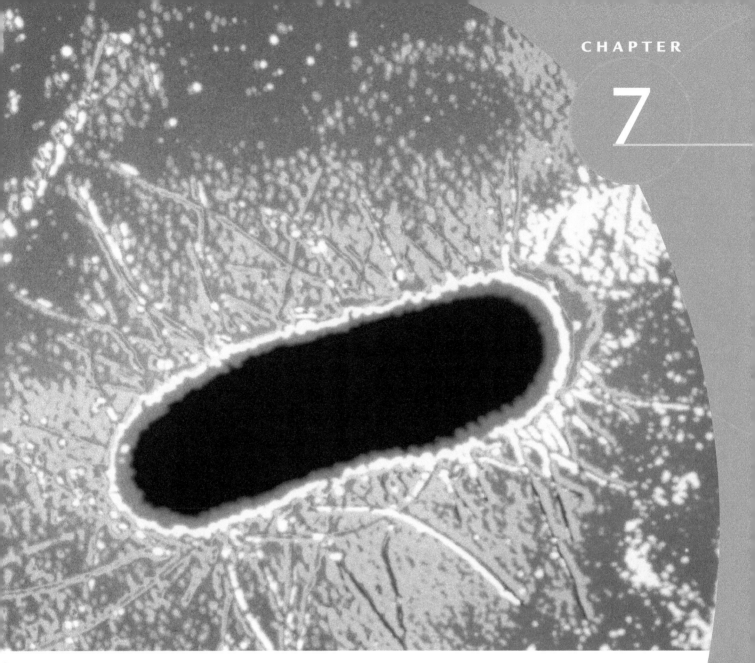

Communicable Disease and Infection Control

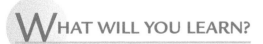HAT WILL YOU LEARN?

Communicable diseases are diseases that can be spread from one person to another. There are many factors that come together in the health care setting to make it easy for communicable diseases to spread. In this chapter, you will learn how to minimize these factors, so that

Photo: Escherichia coli, a microbe that can cause disease. Colour was added to this photograph, which was taken with a special microscope (a tool that is used to see things that are not visible to the naked eye). (© Howard Sochurek/CORBIS.)

you can protect yourself, your family members, and your patients or residents from catching a communicable disease. You will also learn about the causes of communicable disease, and the ways communicable diseases are spread from one person to another. After all, it is hard to protect yourself and others from communicable disease if you do not know what causes it or how it is spread! When you are finished with this chapter, you will be able to:

1. List the different types of "germs" (microbes) that cause disease and discuss the conditions that are essential for their survival and growth.
2. Define the terms *normal flora* and *pathogen*.
3. Explain the defense mechanisms the body uses to keep us from getting sick.
4. Define the term *infection* and describe the chain of events required for infection to occur.
5. List factors that can make a person more likely to get an infection.
6. Define the term *health care–associated infection* and discuss ways a person could get an infection within the health care system.
7. List the four major methods of infection control.
8. List the four techniques of medical asepsis.
9. State how personal protective equipment is used in infection control.
10. List the standard precautions that are taken with every patient or resident.
11. Describe the three types of transmission-based precautions and explain when they are used.
12. Demonstrate proper handwashing, gloving, masking, gowning, and double-bagging technique.

Vocabulary

Communicable disease	Methicillin-resistant	Virulence	Transient flora
Microbe	*Staphylococcus aureus*	Health care–associated	Personal protective
(microorganism)	(MRSA)	infections (HAIs)	equipment (PPE)
Normal (resident) flora	Vancomycin-resistant	Nosocomial infections	Isolation precautions
Pathogens	enterococcus (VRE)	Infection control	Standard precautions
Opportunistic microbes	Infection	Medical asepsis	Transmission-based
Colonies	Chain of infection	Sanitization	precautions
Aerobic	Contaminated	Antisepsis	Airborne precautions
Anaerobic	Fomite	Disinfection	Droplet precautions
Antibodies	Vector	Sterilization	Contact precautions

WHAT IS A MICROBE?

A **microbe,** also called a **microorganism,** is a living thing that cannot be seen with the naked eye. Many (but not all) microbes consist of just one cell. (To give you an idea of how small a cell is, consider that it is estimated that the adult human body is composed of approximately 50 million *million* cells!) Microbes are found in the air, in the soil, in water, in food, and in and on the bodies of plants and animals, including humans.

Most microbes cause no harm and are actually essential for healthy living. For example, some of the microbes that live in the human digestive tract help us to get certain vitamins from the foods that we eat. Others help to maintain an environment that is unfriendly to harmful microbes. The harmless microbes that help the human body to function properly are called **normal (resident) flora.**

Some microbes, however, can cause illness and are known as **pathogens.** Sometimes microbes can be considered normal flora in one part of the body and pathogens in another. For example, *Escherichia coli* is a microbe that normally lives in our large intestines, where it is harmless. However, when *E. coli* finds its way out of the intestine and into another part of the body where it is not normal flora, such as the bladder, it can cause an infection. These types of microbes are called **opportunistic microbes.** Given the chance, opportunistic microbes can change from harmless to pathogenic.

There are many different types of microbes that live and prosper among us. Microbes can generally be classified as bacteria, viruses, fungi, or parasites (Table 7-1).

BACTERIA

Bacteria cause many of the infections you will encounter in the health care setting. Many scientists believe that bacteria lived on Earth long before any other life forms. Bacteria have been found in polar ice caps, as well as in deep cracks in the ocean floor. The ability of bacteria to adapt to all sorts of environments is proof of this life form's ability to survive.

Most bacteria consist of only one cell, and reproduce by dividing in half. Although bacteria usually consist of only one cell, they often group together to form **colonies.** Scientists classify and name bacteria in many different ways:

- By their shape
- By the way they arrange themselves in a colony
- By the way they stain (how they react to the dye scientists use to make microbes more visible under a microscope)

For example, round bacteria are called *cocci,* rod-shaped bacteria are called *bacilli,* and spiral-shaped or curved bacteria are called *spirilla* (Fig. 7-1). Bacterial colonies may consist of pairs of bacteria (indicated by the prefix *diplo-*), chains of bacteria (indicated by the prefix *strepto-*), or grape-like clusters of bacteria (indicated by the prefix *staphylo-*). So, what would you know if you saw the word *Staphylococcus aureus* on a person's medical record? You would know that

this person had an infection caused by a round bacterium (*-coccus*) that arranges itself in clusters (*Staphylo-*)! There are thousands of types of bacteria and not all of them are named using this method. However, this example illustrates how you can learn the meaning of a word that might be unfamiliar to you by taking it apart. In Appendix B, "Introduction to the Language of Health Care," you can learn about many more prefixes, suffixes, and roots that are used to form words commonly used in the health care setting.

Bacteria, like all other living things, have certain basic requirements for survival. These requirements vary, according to the type of bacteria. For example, some bacteria, called **aerobic** bacteria, need oxygen to live. Others, called **anaerobic** bacteria, die if oxygen is present. Most bacteria that can cause illness need a warm, moist, dark environment and a source of nutrition in order to grow—requirements the inside of the human body meets perfectly! Some types of bacteria can surround themselves with a hard shell, called an *endospore,* and enter a state of inactivity. If the inactive bacterium's best growing conditions become available, the bacterium will become active again. Because of their protective endospores, these types of bacteria are very difficult to kill using the standard techniques described later in this chapter. Examples of illnesses caused by bacteria that form endospores include tetanus (lockjaw) and botulism (food poisoning).

Bacteria are the most common cause of infection in the health care setting. Some common illnesses caused by bacteria include "strep throat" (caused by *Streptococcus pyogenes*), some bladder infections (such as those caused by *E. coli*), and some skin infections (such as those caused by *S. aureus*). Several types of small, rod-shaped bacteria are transmitted by ticks and fleas and cause diseases such as Rocky Mountain spotted fever and typhus. Bacteria are also responsible for some types of pneumonia and some infections of the reproductive and urinary systems.

VIRUSES

Viruses, the smallest of all microbes, can only be seen using a special kind of microscope, called an electron microscope. Viruses are not even complete cells—they are just small bundles of protein. Because viruses are not complete cells, they cannot carry out normal cellular activities, such as reproduction, by themselves. Instead, they must take over a host cell, usually a plant or animal cell. Once inside the host cell, the virus

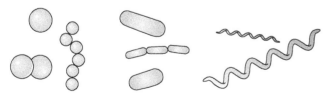

A. Cocci (spheres)   **B.** Bacilli (rods)   **C.** Spirilla (spirals)

Figure 7-1

Bacteria can be **(A)** spherical, **(B)** rod-shaped, or **(C)** spiral-shaped.

Table 7-1   Types of Microbes

	TYPE	EXAMPLES OF COMMONLY CAUSED INFECTIONS
	Bacteria	"Strep throat," urinary tract infections, abscesses, tuberculosis (TB), bacterial meningitis, Lyme disease, Rocky Mountain spotted fever, syphilis
	Viruses	HIV/AIDS, hepatitis, fever blisters, common cold
	Fungi	Ringworm, "athlete's foot," vaginal yeast infections (candidiasis), oral yeast infections (thrush)
	Parasites Insects	Scabies, pediculosis (lice)
	Helminths (worms)	Pinworm infestation
	Protozoa	Malaria, amebic dysentery

Top to bottom: *Lester V. Bergman/CORBIS.* © *Ron Boardman; Frank Lane Picture Agency/CORBIS.* © *Lester V. Bergman/CORBIS.* © *Mike Buxton; Papilio/CORBIS.* © *Lloyd Birmingham/Custom Medical Stock Photo.* © *Lester V. Bergman/CORBIS.*

uses the host cell's "machinery" to make copies of itself. Eventually, the virus and all of its copies (called *progeny*) break through the host cell's wall, killing the host cell and freeing the viruses to infect other, neighboring host cells. Many illnesses are caused by viruses, including the common cold, fever blisters (caused by herpes simplex virus), chickenpox (caused by varicella zoster virus), hepatitis, and acquired immunodeficiency syndrome (AIDS, caused by human immunodeficiency virus, or HIV).

FUNGI

Fungi are a group of plant-like organisms that scientists have classified together because of certain characteristics, including the makeup of their cell walls. Not all fungi are microscopic—for example, mushrooms are a type of fungus! Other types of fungi you may be familiar with include yeasts (such as the yeast that is used to make bread rise and beer foamy) and molds (such as the mildew that grows inside a shower stall or the growths that appear on bread and cheese if left too long). Many fungi help us (or, at least, do not harm us). However, some fungi are capable of causing illness. If you have ever had ringworm (caused by *Tinea corporis*), athlete's foot (caused by *Tinea pedis*), thrush (a yeast infection in the mouth), or candidiasis (a vaginal yeast infection), then you have been the victim of a fungus!

PARASITES

Parasites live in or on a host, such as a plant or animal, and use that host for food and protection. Some parasites can be transmitted from one person to another through physical contact. For example, scabies, an itchy skin condition, is caused by a mite that burrows under the skin. Pediculosis (lice) is caused by wingless insects that live on the scalp or body and feed on the host's blood. Both scabies and lice are often seen in the health care setting. Other parasites are transferred from one person to another through feces or blood.

Helminths, a type of parasite, are worm-like organisms that live in the human body (as well as the bodies of other animals). Examples of helminths include pinworms, tapeworms, and roundworms. Although the way these organisms are transmitted from one host to another varies, transmission usually involves eating or inhaling the worm eggs, which then grow in the host's digestive tract. The mature worms produce eggs or larvae of their own, which are then passed out of the host's body with the feces. Once the eggs reach the outside world again, they are free to be eaten or inhaled by another host, and the life cycle of the helminth continues.

Protozoa, another type of parasite, are said to be "animal-like" because they can take in food. Protozoa cause illnesses such as malaria (transmitted by the bite of a mosquito) and amebic dysentery (a type of diarrhea caused by drinking water contaminated with protozoa).

DEFENSES AGAINST COMMUNICABLE DISEASE

THE IMMUNE SYSTEM

Many, many microbes share the Earth with us. If microbes are everywhere, and some of them can make us sick, then why aren't we all always sick? The answer to this question lies in the body's immune system, the wonderful defense system that protects us from infection. Some of the body's defenses are nonspecific, which means that they help to protect us from all pathogens. Other defenses are specific, which means that they help to protect us only from certain pathogens.

Nonspecific Defense Mechanisms

Our main nonspecific defense mechanism is healthy, intact skin and mucous membranes. Skin that is without cuts, scrapes, or wounds physically prevents pathogens from entering the body. In addition, the natural lubricants on our skin contain substances that help to prevent the growth of pathogens. Mucous membranes line all of the organ systems that come in contact with the outside world (the respiratory, digestive, urinary, and reproductive systems). The special cells of the mucous membranes secrete mucus, a sticky substance that creates a physical barrier by trapping and destroying pathogens. Keeping the skin clean helps to reduce the number of pathogens on the skin. Good oral hygiene and drinking plenty of fluids helps to keep mucous membranes functioning properly. These are important measures to take for yourself, as well as for your patients or residents. Stomach acid (which kills many of the microbes contained in the food we eat), tears (which contain a substance that kills microbes), and the acts of coughing and sneezing (which remove inhaled microbes) are also nonspecific defense mechanisms that prevent microbes from "setting up shop" in our bodies.

If a pathogen manages to get past these first lines of defense and an infection results, the body activates a general immune response that helps to fight off the infection. Blood vessels around the site of the infection dilate (widen), allowing more blood flow to the area. The increased blood flow brings more oxygen and nutrients to the tissues, along with large numbers of white blood cells (leukocytes). White blood cells destroy pathogens that invade the body, either by eating them (Fig. 7-2) or by secreting substances that cause them to die. The increased blood flow causes the infected area to become red, warm, swollen, and painful (Fig. 7-3). A person who is fighting off an infection may have a high body temperature (fever). If you remember, most pathogens prefer a nice, normal body temperature. The fever helps to destroy the pathogens and is a normal response for many infections.

As a personal support worker, it is important for you to watch for signs of infection in your patients or residents. Many patients or residents may not be able to communicate that they do not feel well or that they have pain. Some infections, if not treated at an early stage, can be very dangerous for people. If one of your patients or

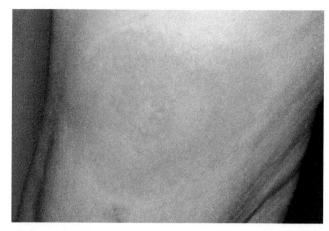

Figure 7-3
The site of infection is typically hot, red, swollen, and painful. This means the body's general immune response is at work! (*Custom Medical Stock Photo.*)

residents has signs or symptoms of an infection, the doctor may order a diagnostic test, called a *culture and sensitivity*, to find out which microbe is causing the infection and which medication is best suited to fight it. The culture and sensitivity may be performed on urine, wound drainage, or other body fluids or substances.

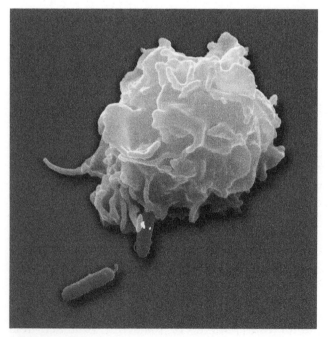

Figure 7-2
In this photograph, a white blood cell (*white*) is killing a pathogen (*red*) by eating it. This is a process called phagocytosis (*phago-* means "eat" and *cyt-* means "cell"). (*SPL/Photo Researchers, Inc.*)

TELL THE NURSE

Possible signs of infection that should be reported to the nurse immediately include:

- An increase in body temperature
- A rapid pulse, a rapid respiratory rate, or changes in blood pressure
- Pain or difficulty breathing
- Redness, swelling, or pain
- Foul-smelling or cloudy urine
- Pain or difficulty urinating
- Diarrhea or foul-smelling feces
- Nausea or vomiting
- Lack of appetite
- Skin rashes
- Fatigue
- Increased confusion or disorientation
- Any unusual discharge or drainage from the body

Specific Defense Mechanisms

The body's nonspecific defense mechanisms, including physical barriers and the general immune response, are one way our immune systems help us to prevent and fight off infections. The immune system also has the ability to develop specialized proteins called **antibodies,** which help our bodies to fight off specific microbes. A person develops antibodies following exposure to the microbe. This exposure may come from a previous infection with the microbe, or through a vaccination (shot). For example, the antibodies that build up in the body following a case of measles or chickenpox are the reason most of us only get these "childhood diseases" once. Similarly, when you get your annual "flu shot," what you are getting is a dose of the virus strains that cause the flu. The viruses have been killed, so that you do not actually get sick, but the exposure is enough to cause your immune system to begin producing antibodies against those particular strains of the virus. That way, if you are exposed later, you will be immune.

ANTIBIOTICS

Many times, our immune systems can fight off invading pathogens on their own. Other times, however, some outside help is required. An *antibiotic* is a drug that is able to kill bacteria or make it difficult for them to reproduce and grow. The first antibiotic, penicillin, came into widespread use during World War II, and completely changed how we treat infectious disease. Today, there are many types of antibiotics, used to treat many different types of bacterial infections. Antimicrobial agents (used to treat fungal and parasitic infections) and antiviral agents (used to treat some viral infections) are other drugs that we use to treat infection.

Antibiotics and other medications used to treat infection are not always effective against all infections. Bacteria, as you will recall, are very adaptable organisms that have been around since the beginning of time. As such, some bacteria have used their ability to change to develop resistance to the antibiotics used to fight them. This means that the antibiotics that used to work against these bacteria no longer work. Two types of bacteria, **methicillin-resistant Staphylococcus aureus (MRSA)** and **vancomycin-resistant enterococcus (VRE),** have become resistant to two of the most powerful antibiotics we have invented to date (methicillin and vancomycin).

S. aureus and enterococci are common microbes. *S. aureus* is often found on a person's skin and is transmitted easily through person-to-person contact. Enterococci are commonly found in a person's digestive tract and are transmitted through contact with feces. In a health care setting, these pathogens can be very dangerous because many patients and residents do not have healthy immune systems and, therefore, are less able to fight off infection. If infection occurs, it is difficult to treat because these microbes have become resistant to the drugs used to treat them in the past. MRSA and VRE are well-known examples of bacteria that have developed resistance to antibiotics. It is reasonable to expect that in the future, other bacteria will become resistant to antibiotics as well.

Although antibiotics have given us more options for treating infectious disease than we had in the past, they do not work against all pathogens all of the time. The best policy is to avoid infection in the first place. You can keep your immune system strong and healthy through proper nutrition, adequate rest, and regular exercise. You can also take steps to limit your exposure to pathogens. In the next few sections, we will look at how pathogens are spread from one person to another, and what you can do to help control their spread.

COMMUNICABLE DISEASE AND THE CHAIN OF INFECTION

An **infection** is an illness caused by a pathogen (a microbe that can cause illness). Infections can be local (affecting a small, defined area of the body), generalized (affecting a general area or an organ), or systemic (affecting the entire body). Many, but not all, infections are communicable, which means that they can be transmitted from one person to another, either directly or indirectly. Sometimes the terms *communicable* and *contagious* are used to mean the same thing, but the two terms are not truly synonymous. *Contagious* is more accurately used to describe an infection that can be easily transmitted from one person to another through casual contact, such as a common cold. For example, you can get a cold just by touching a button in an elevator after someone who has a cold has touched it, or by sitting next to someone with a cold on a crowded bus. Therefore, a common cold is not only communicable, it is contagious. On the other hand, infections such as AIDS and hepatitis, while still

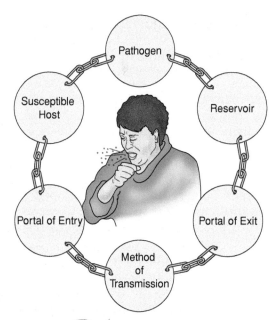

Figure 7-4 Watch & Learn

The chain of infection. For a person to get an infection, all six links in the chain must be present.

communicable, are not considered contagious because they are not transmitted through casual contact.

For a person to get a communicable infection, six key conditions must be met. These six key elements are known as the **chain of infection** (Fig. 7-4).

1. A *pathogen* must be present.
2. A *reservoir* must be present. A reservoir is a place where something is stored. In this case, a reservoir is a place that is suitable for the pathogen's survival. Pathogens collect in the reservoir, and sometimes, they multiply there as well. Possible reservoirs of pathogens include humans and other animals, food, water, milk, and objects that come in contact with an infected person's secretions or body fluids.
3. A *portal of exit* must be available. The portal of exit is the way the pathogen leaves the reservoir. (The word *portal* means "door.") The way a pathogen leaves its reservoir varies, depending on the type of pathogen and the reservoir. For example, when the reservoir is a human being, common portals of exit for pathogens include the digestive tract (through feces, saliva, or vomitus), the respiratory tract (through mucus), the genitourinary tract (through urine, semen, or vaginal secretions), and the skin (through blood, pus, or other drainage from wounds).

4. A *method of transmission* must be available. After the pathogen leaves its reservoir via the portal of exit, it must have a way of physically getting from one person to another. This is called the pathogen's method of transmission, and it may be direct or indirect. Direct transmission requires close contact between an infected and a noninfected person. Pathogens can be directly transmitted when a noninfected person makes physical contact with an infected person, or inhales or ingests droplets exhaled by the infected person (for example, when that person coughs, talks, or sneezes). Indirect transmission occurs when a noninfected person comes into contact with a non-living object that has been **contaminated** (soiled) by pathogens. These objects are called **fomites.** For example, a water glass or a bed sheet can become a fomite if it becomes contaminated by pathogens from a person with an infection, because if a noninfected person uses the contaminated water glass or sleeps on the contaminated bed linens, he could become infected (Fig. 7-5). Other pathogens, such as the protozoan that causes malaria, are transmitted by way of a **vector,** or a living creature (in the case of malaria, a mosquito). Some pathogens can be transmitted by more than just one method.

5. A *portal of entry* must be available. Now that the pathogen has left its reservoir and been successfully transmitted to another person, it must have a way of entering the new person's body. The respiratory, urinary, digestive, and reproductive systems are common portals of entry. So are breaks in the skin. A pathogen can leave one person's body and be transmitted to another person, but if the

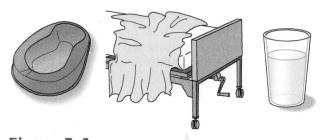

Figure 7-5

Pathogens can live on objects such as linens, bedpans, and drinking glasses. When an uninfected person touches or uses these items, he might pick up some of the pathogens on them and become sick. Non-living objects that are capable of transmitting disease are called fomites.

pathogen is not able to enter the new person's body, infection will not occur.

6. A *susceptible host* must be available. Microbes that can cause infection enter the human body continuously. The defense systems of the body, both those we are born with and those we acquire (such as vaccines), can fight off most of these pathogens. However, many factors can place us at risk for infection. This is when the pathogen "makes its move." Risk factors that make a person more likely to get an infection include:

- **Very young or very old age.** The very young and the very old are more likely to get an infection. The young have not had time to develop an effective defense mechanism for fighting infections, and the elderly lose their defenses as they age.
- **Poor general health.** A person who is sick or debilitated ("worn down") is more at risk for infection because the body's defenses are already weakened by illness. Therefore, the person is not able to fight off the pathogen as easily. Additionally, certain medical treatments, such as chemotherapy or radiation therapy, can affect the functioning of the body's immune system and put a person more at risk for infection.

- **Stress and fatigue.** Lack of rest and emotional stress can affect the body's ability to defend itself from pathogens.
- **Indwelling medical devices.** Medical devices, such as catheters, feeding tubes, and intravenous (IV) lines, increase a person's risk of infection by providing a portal of entry for pathogens.

Many of the people you will care for as a personal support worker have risk factors for infection. Your patients or residents will be sick, recovering from surgery, elderly, or have a chronic illness or conditions that will increase their risk of getting an infectious disease. A major part of your responsibility in caring for other people involves protecting them from infection.

The chain of infection can be broken by taking away just one of the six required elements (Fig. 7-6). For example, taking the right antibiotic for a bacterial infection quickly turns a person's body into an unfriendly reservoir for bacteria. Covering an infected wound with a dressing eliminates a pathogen's portal of exit by containing the pathogen within the dressing. Washing your hands and making sure that linens, utensils, glassware, and other possible fomites are properly cleansed eliminate a method of transmission. Wearing gloves and keeping your skin healthy and intact remove one potential portal of

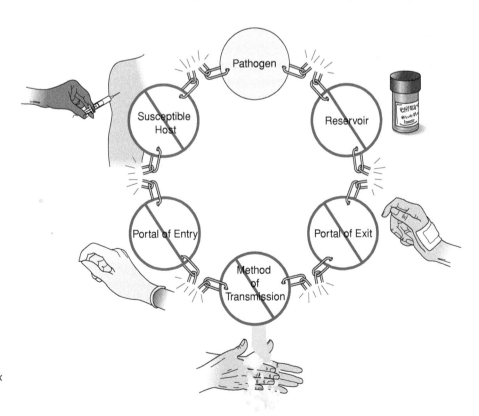

Figure 7-6
The chain of infection can be broken by removing just one of the six elements that must be present for infection to occur.

entry available to pathogens. Receiving required immunizations and maintaining general good health make you a less susceptible host. All of these actions break a link in the chain of infection, stopping the infection from being transmitted. Other factors that determine whether or not an infection will be transmitted are the **virulence** (strength or disease-producing potential) of the pathogen and the actual number of pathogens that enter the body.

INFECTION CONTROL IN THE HEALTH CARE SETTING

What do you picture when you think of a health care facility? Health care professionals in clean, fresh uniforms, a smell of antiseptic in the air, and miles of shiny tile floors? Most of us think of health care facilities as clean, possibly even sterile, environments. Maintaining cleanliness in health care facilities is essential, because exposure to pathogens is increased in these settings. Additionally, most of the people in health care facilities are there because they are not in good overall health. Therefore, their potential to become infected is increased.

Health care–associated infections (HAIs) are infections that people get while they are in the hospital or other health care setting. A patient or resident can get an HAI while he or she is receiving care. Or a health care worker can get an HAI while providing care. Infections acquired by patients or residents while they are in a health care facility are also called **nosocomial infections.** The most common method of transmission for HAIs, including the very dangerous VRE, is on the hands of health care workers.

All health care facilities follow basic practices that are designed to decrease the chance that an infection will be spread from one person to another. These practices are called **infection control.** There are four major methods of infection control—medical asepsis, surgical asepsis, barrier methods, and isolation precautions.

MEDICAL ASEPSIS

Medical asepsis involves physically removing or killing pathogens, and is primarily achieved through processes involving soap, water, antiseptics, disinfectants, or heat. The goal of medical asepsis is to remove pathogenic microbes from surfaces, equipment, and the hands of health care workers. There are four techniques that make up the practice of medical asepsis: sanitization, antisepsis, disinfection, and sterilization (Fig. 7-7):

- **Sanitization** is the word we use to describe practices associated with basic cleanliness, such as handwashing, cleansing of eating utensils and other surfaces with soap and water, and providing clean linens and clothing. Sanitization practices physically remove pathogens, thereby preventing their spread. General guidelines for maintaining a sanitary environment in a health care setting or home are given in Guidelines Box 7-1.
- **Antisepsis** takes sanitization one step further, by actually killing microbes or stopping them from growing. An antiseptic is a chemical that is capable of killing a pathogen, or preventing it from growing. Antiseptics can be used on the skin or other surfaces to kill pathogens. Rubbing alcohol and iodine are common antiseptics used on the skin to prevent infection. Many soaps used in the health care setting now contain an antiseptic agent as well.
- **Disinfection** involves the use of stronger chemicals to kill pathogens. The chemicals used for disinfection are too strong to be used on the skin. Instead, disinfectants are used to clean non-living objects that come in contact with body fluids or substances, such as bedpans, urinals, and tray tables.
- **Sterilization** is the most thorough method of killing microbes. Sterilization is used on objects that must be completely free of any microbes, such as surgical instruments, hypodermic needles, or IV catheters. These objects must be sterilized because they are placed in the patient's or resident's body. Therefore, they can act as portals of entry for microbes. Many disposable items used in health care settings, such as hypodermic needles, IV catheters, and urinary catheters, are sterilized and packaged by the manufacturer. Reusable items, such as surgical instruments, are usually cleaned and sterilized in the health care facility. Items are sterilized either by placing them in an autoclave (a machine that uses pressurized steam heat to kill microbes) or by soaking them in chemicals that destroy all microbes. Although covering items in boiling water will kill most microbes, boiling is not an effective method of sterilization.

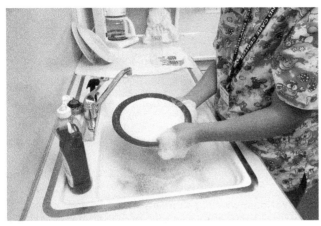

A. Sanitization

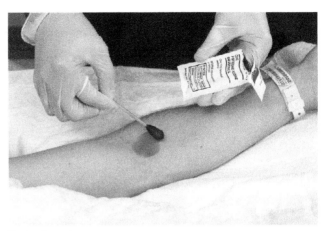

B. Antisepsis

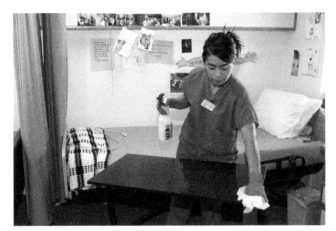

C. Disinfection

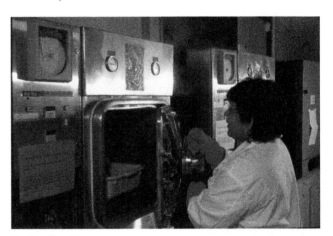

D. Sterilization

Figure 7-7
There are many approaches to medical asepsis, a general term used to describe techniques used to remove or kill microbes. **(A)** Sanitization is physically removing microbes from surfaces. Here, a home support worker washes dishes. **(B)** Antisepsis involves the use of agents that kill microbes or slow down their growth, such as iodine (Betadine) or rubbing alcohol. Here, a nurse cleans a patient's skin with a Betadine swab. **(C)** Disinfection also involves the use of agents that kill microbes. Because disinfectants are strong chemicals, disinfection is used only to clean non-living objects. This personal support worker is using a disinfectant to clean an over-bed table.
(D) Sterilization involves the use of pressurized steam heat or very strong chemicals to kill microbes. This technician is opening a steam autoclave, a device used to sterilize instruments and equipment. (**D,** © *Wedgwood/Custom Medical Stock Photo.*)

Before disinfecting or sterilizing an object, the object must be cleaned first using basic sanitization methods. The chemicals used to disinfect or sterilize an object cannot work properly unless the surface to be disinfected or sterilized is clean and free of any organic material (material from a living organism, such as blood, urine, or feces). Organic materials contain fats and proteins that coat the surface of the object, much like an egg yolk coats the surface of a plate. If the plate is not washed with detergent and warm water before the egg yolk dries, the hardened yolk becomes very difficult to remove. The same principle applies to dirty bedpans, urinals, and other pieces of equipment—if the piece of equipment is not washed first using soap and water, any organic material that is present can harden, making it difficult for the disinfectant or sterilization agent to kill the microbes underneath the dried material. Therefore, equipment must be properly cleaned using basic sanitization methods before moving on to disinfection or sterilization.

Guidelines Box 7-1   Guidelines for Maintaining a Sanitary Environment

WHAT YOU DO	WHY YOU DO IT
Wash your hands after contact with any body fluid or substance, whether it is your own or another person's. Examples of body fluids and substances include blood, saliva, vomitus, urine, feces, vaginal discharge, semen, wound drainage, pus, mucus, and respiratory secretions.	Pathogens often leave the body through the gastrointestinal tract, genitourinary tract, respiratory tract, or breaks in the skin. In addition, some pathogens are transmitted in blood and other body secretions, such as breast milk.
Wash your hands frequently, especially after using the bathroom; before handling food, drink, or eating utensils; and before and after any contact with a patient or resident.	Frequent handwashing eliminates a method of transmission for microbes.
Cover your mouth or nose with a tissue when you cough or sneeze, and teach your patients and residents to do the same. Dispose of tissues properly by placing them in a waste container.	Some microbes are transmitted in particles of saliva or sputum. Covering your nose or mouth with a tissue contains these particles and helps to prevent the spread of infection.
Provide each patient or resident with individual personal care items, such as toothbrushes, drinking glasses, towels, washcloths, and soap.	If not properly cleaned after use, these items can act as fomites. Therefore, it is better to limit their use to one person.
Keep contaminated or dirty items, such as soiled linens, away from your uniform.	Microbes can be transferred from the dirty item to your uniform, which can then act as a fomite.
When cleaning, take care not to stir up dust. For example, wiping dusty surfaces with a damp cloth or mop helps prevent the movement of dust and lint into the air. Do not shake linens when making beds.	Dust can act as a fomite and carry microbes from one area to another.
Dispose of garbage properly.	If not disposed of properly, garbage can provide an ideal environment for microbial growth, especially if the garbage contains food or other materials susceptible to rotting.
Follow established procedures for preparing dirty linens and clothing for the laundry.	Soiled linens and clothing act as fomites and must be handled in a way that will lessen the chance of someone else coming in contact with the contaminated item.
Maintain good personal hygiene, and help your patients or residents to do the same. Bathing, washing hair, brushing teeth, and wearing clean clothing are all grooming practices that help prevent the spread of infection.	Personal grooming practices help to reduce the number of microbes present on the skin.

Handwashing

As a personal support worker, the technique of medical asepsis that you will use most frequently is handwashing. According to the Canadian Center for Occupational Health and Safety (CCOHS), *handwashing is the single most important method of preventing the spread of infection.* This is true in the "real world," as well as in the health care setting. However, in the health care setting, handwashing takes on a special importance because the chance of picking up a pathogen and passing it on to someone else is greater than in normal, everyday life. In addition, many of the people who are in health care facilities are less able to handle an infection, should they get one. The easiest way to protect yourself and your patients or residents is to be conscientious about washing your hands!

Before you move from one person's room to another in a health care facility, you must always wash your hands. In the process of taking care of your patients or residents, you will collect microbes on your hands. These microbes could then be easily transferred to the next patient or resident you care for, yourself, or one of your family members. Failing to wash your hands before giving care to a patient or resident could even be considered abuse.

There are two main types of microbes found on a person's hands. Earlier in this chapter, you learned about the first type, normal (resident) flora. These are the microbes that normally live on a person's skin and usually do not cause infections. Normal flora lives deep in the pores of the skin and cannot be totally removed. The other type of microbe typically found on a person's hands is called **transient flora.** Transient flora is picked up from touching contaminated objects or people who have an infectious disease. Most nosocomial infections are caused by transient flora—the hands of the health care worker serve as the method of transmission from one person to another. Transient flora lives on the surface of the skin and is easily removed by proper handwashing.

There are differences in opinion about handwashing techniques, such as the time required, the type of cleaning agents that should be used, and the frequency with which handwashing should occur. Certain situations may require specific handwashing techniques. For example, health care workers who work in the operating room, intensive care unit, neonatal unit, or labour and delivery units may be required to use an antiseptic cleaning agent, a scrub brush, or both because patients in these settings have higher

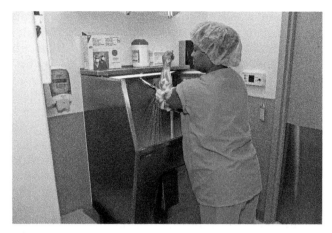

Figure 7-8
This person is performing a surgical scrub in preparation for entering an operating room.

infection risks (Fig. 7-8). Antiseptic cleaning agents remove the transient flora from the surface of the skin. They also slow down the growth of the normal flora, which can be helpful in certain areas of health care. Procedure 7-1 describes the basic handwashing procedure. Although the specifics of how handwashing is performed vary from setting to setting, one aspect of handwashing always remains the same—it must be performed thoroughly, properly, and consistently. At the minimum, wash your hands:

- When you first arrive at your facility
- Before entering a patient's or resident's room
- Before entering a "clean" supply room
- Before obtaining clean linen from a linen cart
- Before handling a patient's or resident's meal tray
- Before you go on break and before you leave your shift
- Before and after drinking, eating, or smoking
- Before and after inserting contact lenses
- After using the bathroom
- After coughing, sneezing, or blowing your nose
- After touching anything that may be considered dirty—especially objects contaminated with blood or other body fluids or substances
- After picking an object up from the floor
- After removing disposable gloves, including those times when you are replacing a torn glove
- After handling your hair or applying makeup or lip gloss

When washing your hands, make sure you clean those areas where microbes love to hide, under and around the fingernails and between the fingers. As you learned in Chapter 3, long fingernails do not really have a place in the personal support worker's professional life. Long fingernails trap microbes underneath them and therefore are harder to clean. Nail polish cracks and peels, providing many places for transient microbes to hide. False nails, acrylics, and wraps often lift, creating an excellent breeding ground for microbes. Many health care facilities ban the use of these types of nail treatments by anyone involved in providing hands-on care for patients or residents.

It is also not a good idea to wear rings and bracelets while on the job. Many health care workers think that by removing their jewelry before washing their hands, they can remove any microbes trapped underneath the jewelry. But, think about this: even if you remove your jewelry before you wash your hands, the jewelry itself is still dirty, so you will be putting dirty jewelry back on to your clean hands. For the sake of efficiency and cleanliness, it is best to keep your fingernails short and unpolished, and to leave your jewelry at home when performing your duties as a personal support worker.

A good lather of soap and the physical motion of rubbing your hands together remove skin oils and lotions, which can harbor microbes. Rinsing thoroughly removes microbes, along with the dirt and lather. Because frequent handwashing can cause the skin to become excessively dry, leading to cracking, applying a lotion or hand cream after washing is recommended. Remember, your own intact skin is important to help protect you from infection too.

While nothing can replace the effectiveness of good handwashing to remove visible dirt, blood, or other body fluids or substances, the CCOHS has issued guidelines recommending the use of alcohol-based hand rubs for routine hand decontamination. Alcohol-based hand rubs have several advantages:

- Using an alcohol-based hand rub is quicker than washing your hands at the sink, which means that during duties that require frequent handwashing, using an alcohol-based hand rub can save time.
- Alcohol-based hand rubs are gentler on the skin than soap and water.
- Alcohol-based hand rubs are used without water, so they can be used anywhere. In many facilities, alcohol-based hand rubs can be dispensed at the patient's or resident's bedside, saving many trips back and forth to the sink. Many even come in containers small enough to be carried in your uniform pocket.

It is very simple to use an alcohol-based hand rub. The label on the product will tell you how much product to use. Apply this amount to one of your palms and rub your hands together, covering your hands and fingers (front and back) with the product. Continue rubbing your hands together until your skin is dry. That's all there is to it!

Remember, if your hands are visibly soiled with dirt, blood, or other body fluids or substances, you must wash them at the sink, using soap and water. However, if your hands are not visibly soiled, then it is acceptable to use an alcohol-based hand rub to decontaminate your hands, instead of handwashing.

SURGICAL ASEPSIS

Surgical asepsis is used for procedures that involve entering a person's body. Examples of procedures that require surgical asepsis include surgical procedures, injections, the insertion of IV catheters, and the insertion of urinary catheters. Because these procedures disrupt the body's natural protective barriers, all instruments and equipment used must be sterile, or totally free from microbes. In most provinces and territories, performing procedures that require surgical asepsis is not within a personal support worker's scope of practice. However, some facilities will provide extra training in this area if performing procedures that require surgical asepsis is part of your job description.

BARRIER METHODS

In addition to medical asepsis and surgical asepsis, barrier methods are used to control infection in the health care setting. A *barrier* is an object that physically prevents microbes from reaching a health care provider's skin or mucous membranes. Examples of barriers used in infection control, called **personal protective equipment (PPE),** include disposable gloves, gowns, masks, and protective eyewear. While in use, the barrier becomes contaminated with microbes and must be removed in a way that prevents transmission of the microbes onto the skin of the health care worker.

Gloves

Gloves are the most commonly used barrier method. Gloves are worn in the following situations:

- When there is a possibility that you will come in contact with body fluids or substances
- When you are performing or assisting with perineal care (cleaning of the area between the legs)
- When you are performing or assisting with mouth care
- When you have a cut or abrasion on your hands
- When you are shaving a patient or resident
- When you are performing care on a patient or resident who has an open wound or other break in the skin

To effectively prevent contamination of your hands, gloves must be intact (without holes or tears), and they must fit properly. Gloves that are too tight are uncomfortable. Gloves that are too loose will not stay on your hands. Many people are allergic or sensitive to latex, the material that is most commonly used to make disposable gloves. If you or someone you are caring for is sensitive to latex, then you should use gloves made from another synthetic material, such as vinyl. Health care facilities must provide non-latex barrier methods for people who are sensitive to latex.

The most common error made by people who wear gloves for barrier protection is becoming too comfortable with the fact that they are protecting themselves, and forgetting to protect others! If you are wearing gloves and you touch a surface that is contaminated, then your gloves become contaminated. If you then touch another surface, such as the side rail, light switch, or doorknob, with your contaminated gloves, the pathogens will be transferred from your gloves to that surface. The next person who touches the surface could then pick up the microbes you deposited there with your dirty gloves (Fig. 7-9). Gloves that become contaminated with material that may contain pathogens should be removed before touching any other surface. You may need to change gloves several times during one procedure to prevent the transfer of microbes from dirty areas to clean areas (for example, when cleaning feces from a person who has soiled himself, or changing soiled sheets). And always wash your hands after removing your gloves. Procedure 7-2 describes the proper way to remove gloves.

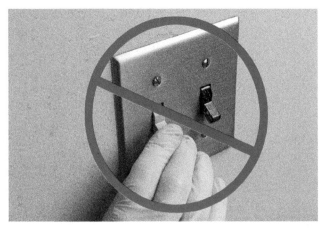

Figure 7-9
Do not make this mistake! By touching the light switch with her gloved hands, this personal support worker has transferred whatever microbes were on her gloves onto the light switch, where they could be easily transferred onto the hands of the next person who turns on the light.

Gowns

A gown (fabric or paper) should be used when it is likely that your uniform will be soiled with body fluids or substances. Many gowns that are used for PPE are fluid-resistant. The use of the gown prevents contamination of your uniform. Each gown is worn only once. Any gown, fabric or paper, is considered contaminated if it becomes wet. Procedures 7-3 and 7-4 describe how to put on and take off a gown, respectively.

Masks

Masks prevent you from breathing in microbes through your nose or mouth, and are worn when there is a chance that you will be exposed to pathogens that are transmitted through the air or in droplets of saliva. For example, the pathogens that cause measles and tuberculosis (TB) are airborne pathogens, and the pathogens that cause pneumonia, strep throat, and meningitis are transmitted in droplets of saliva. You could be exposed to these pathogens when a person with one of these diseases talks, coughs, or sneezes.

Surgical masks are most commonly used, but if you are caring for a person with TB, you may be required to wear a special high-filtration mask (Fig. 7-10). Surgical masks are "one size fits all," but high-filtration masks are available in various sizes and you must be fitted for them in advance. All masks are used only once. You must discard and replace your mask if it becomes wet or

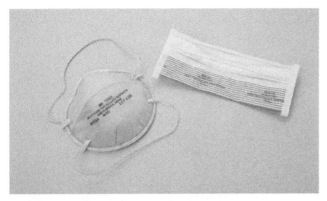

Figure 7-10
Masks cover your nose and mouth and protect you from inhaling pathogens that are transmitted in the air or in saliva. (*Left*) A high-filtration respirator mask, worn when caring for people with tuberculosis (TB). (*Right*) A surgical mask.

soiled. Procedure 7-5 explains how to put on and take off a mask.

Protective Eyewear

Goggles, face shields, and other types of protective eyewear are used to protect your eyes from substances that may splash (Fig. 7-11). Blood and other body fluids, as well as the fluid used to clean wounds, may contain pathogens, which can enter your body through your eyes. Goggles fit close to your face and can be worn over prescription eyeglasses. Face shields may be attached to a mask, or to an elastic band that fits around the head. Your employer is required to provide you with appropriate protective eyewear.

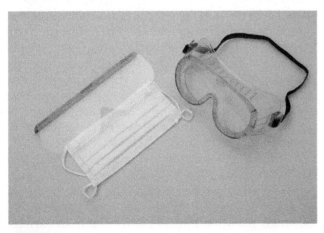

Figure 7-11
Face shields (*left*) and goggles (*right*) are used to protect your eyes from substances that may splash.

In many situations, you may need to wear more than one article of PPE. The best sequence for putting these items on is as follows: gown, mask, protective eyewear, gloves. The order of removal is: gloves, protective eyewear, gown, mask. Procedure 7-6 describes how to remove PPE when more than one article is being used. After use, PPE is considered contaminated. Removal of PPE in the correct sequence helps to protect you from infection. For instance, you would not want to remove your mask first, because this would mean that you would have to touch your face with your contaminated gloves.

ISOLATION PRECAUTIONS

The last major method of controlling the spread of infection throughout a health care facility is by using isolation precautions. **Isolation precautions** are guidelines, based on a pathogen's method of transmission, that we follow to contain the pathogen and limit others' exposure to it as much as possible.

Standard Precautions

Standard precautions are precautions that health care workers take with every patient or resident to protect themselves from pathogens that are transmitted in blood. Standard precautions involve the use of barrier methods, as well as certain environmental control methods, to protect the health care worker (Box 7-1). *For these methods to be effective, they must be used consistently.*

Transmission-Based Precautions

Transmission-based precautions are used when a person is known to have a disease that is transmitted a certain way, for example, via the air, in droplets, or by direct contact.

- **Airborne precautions** are used when caring for people infected with pathogens that can be transmitted through the air. Airborne pathogens enter the respiratory tract of people breathing the same air as the infected person. Therefore, airborne precautions include placing the person in a private room with the door closed, wearing a mask when caring for the person, and minimizing the amount of time the person spends out of his private room. When it is necessary for the infected person to leave his room, he wears a mask. Diseases caused by pathogens that can be transmitted in the air include TB,

BOX
7-1 Standard Precautions

1. Gloves must be worn if the *possibility* exists that the hands could come in contact with blood or other body fluids. Gloves must also be worn when touching any surface or linen that could be contaminated with infected materials. Remember that you cannot see a virus with the naked eye.

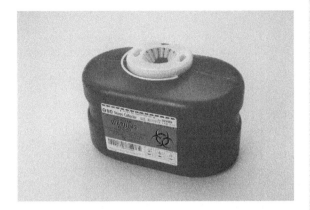

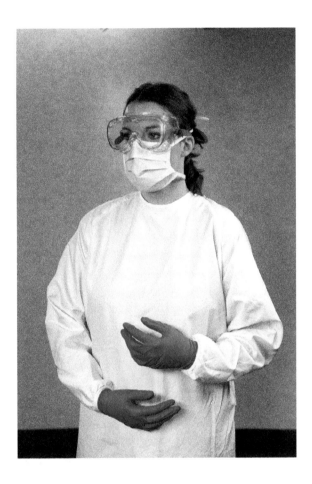

4. Sharps, such as used needles, razors, or broken glass, must be disposed of properly in labeled, approved containers. Contaminated, broken glass items should not be handled, even with gloved hands. They should be swept or vacuumed up for disposal.
5. Spills of blood or other body fluids must be cleaned up promptly with an approved viricidal cleaning agent or a solution of 1 part household bleach to 10 parts water. Personal protective equipment (PPE), such as gloves and a gown, should be worn while cleaning up spills.

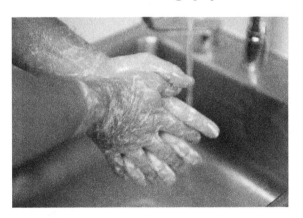

2. A waterproof (impervious) gown must be worn if the *possibility* exists that your clothes could become soiled with blood or other body fluids.
3. A mask, face shield, and eye goggles must be worn if the *possibility* exists that blood or other body fluids could splash or spray.

6. **Handwashing is the single most important method of preventing the spread of infection!** Hands must be washed when you remove your gloves. If accidental exposure to blood or other body substances occurs, hands must be washed thoroughly and immediately.

chickenpox, and measles. Airborne precautions are listed in Box 7-2.

- **Droplet precautions** are used when caring for people with diseases caused by pathogens that are transmitted by direct exposure to droplets released from the

mouth or nose (for example, when the person coughs, sneezes, or talks). Droplet precautions must also be taken when performing procedures that involve contact with an infected person's mouth or nose. Diseases caused by pathogens that can be

BOX 7-2   Airborne Precautions

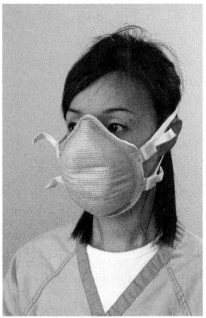

1. Patients or residents known or suspected to be infected with an airborne pathogen are to be placed in private rooms with special ventilation systems.
2. Health care workers should wear masks when caring for patients or residents with known or suspected tuberculosis (TB). If the health care worker has not been exposed to measles or chickenpox (and is therefore not immune), then he is at risk for these diseases, and a mask should be worn when caring for patients or residents with measles or chickenpox. If the health care worker is immune to measles or chickenpox, a mask is not necessary.
3. A surgical mask should be placed over the patient's or resident's face if she must be transported from one location to another. Transport of the patient or resident should be kept to a minimum.
4. All precautions for preventing transmission of TB should be implemented if the patient or resident is known or suspected to have TB.

transmitted in droplets include mumps, influenza, whooping cough, strep throat, scarlet fever, rubella, meningitis, pneumonia, diphtheria, and epiglottitis. Droplet precautions are the same as airborne precautions, except that it is usually only necessary to wear a mask when you are within 91.44 cm of the infected person.

- **Contact precautions** are used when caring for people with diseases caused by pathogens that are transmitted directly (by touching the person) or indirectly (by touching fomites). Diseases that can be transmitted by contact include skin and wound infections, digestive tract infections, and some respiratory tract infections. Contact precautions involve using barrier methods whenever you must touch the infected person or items contaminated with wound drainage or body substances. Contaminated linen and waste materials must be contained and disposed of properly. Procedure 7-7 describes how to transfer contaminated items out of a person's room when contact precautions are being followed.

Helping Hands and a Caring Heart

FOCUS ON HUMANISTIC HEALTH CARE

When caring for a person with a communicable disease, it is very important to remember the person. We work hard to follow all of the procedures that help to prevent the spread of infection, and this is a very important part of providing care. However, sometimes it is easy to forget about how the person with the infection might feel. A person with a communicable disease often feels dirty or unwanted. Think about it—how would you feel if a health care worker had to wear gloves or a mask every time he or she came near you? When airborne or droplet precautions are in effect, the person with the communicable disease may feel isolated and lonely, and desperately miss the company of other people. Friends and family members may avoid visiting the person. When you are caring for a patient or resident with a communicable disease, checking on the person frequently and taking the time to talk with the person when you are providing care can help to make the person feel better.

SUMMARY

- A huge variety of microbes share our planet.
  - Major types of microbes include bacteria, viruses, fungi, and parasites.
  - Some cause disease, and are called pathogens, while others are harmless. Harmless microbes that live in and on our bodies are called normal flora.
- Our immune systems help us to fight off infections.
  - The human immune system's nonspecific defense mechanisms include the physical barriers provided by the skin and mucous membranes, and the general immune response.
  - The human immune system's specific defense mechanisms include antibodies.
- Health care facilities provide the perfect environment for the spread of infection.
  - The chain of infection describes the elements that must be present in order for infection to occur. The six elements of the chain of infection are pathogen, reservoir, portal of exit, method of transmission, portal of entry, and susceptible host.
  - Breaking just one link in the chain of infection stops the spread of infection from one person to another.
- Some of the people you will care for will be receiving health care because they have a serious communicable disease. Others may have a serious communicable disease and not even know it. In addition, many of the people you will care for will be more at risk for catching a communicable disease because they are not entirely healthy to begin with. Therefore, infection control is very important in the health care setting.
- Health care workers take many approaches to infection control. As a personal support worker, it is your ethical and legal responsibility to protect your patients or residents from infectious disease. You must also protect yourself and your family members. The techniques used to help control the spread of infection are effective only if performed properly and consistently.
- Medical asepsis involves physically removing or killing pathogens.
  - Methods of medical asepsis include sanitization, antisepsis, disinfection, and sterilization.
  - Handwashing, a form of medical asepsis, is the single most important method of controlling the spread of infection.
- Surgical asepsis is required for procedures that involve entering a person's body.
- Barrier methods prevent a pathogen from gaining access to a health care worker's body. Commonly used barrier methods include gloves, gowns, masks, and protective eyewear.
- Isolation precautions are based on a pathogen's mode of transmission (blood, air, droplet, direct contact).

Handwashing

WHY YOU DO IT   Handwashing is the most important method of preventing the spread of infection.

1. Gather needed supplies, if not present at the handwashing area: *soap or the cleansing agent specified by your facility, hand lotion* (optional), *paper towels, a nailbrush* (optional), *an orange stick* (optional).

2. Stand away from the sink, so that your uniform does not touch the sink. Push your sleeves up your arms 4 to 5 inches; if you are wearing a watch, push it up too.

3. Use a clean paper towel to turn on the faucet, adjusting the water temperature until it is warm. Dispose of the paper towel in a facility-approved waste container.

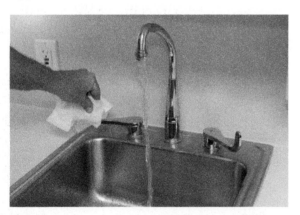

Step 3 Use a clean paper towel to turn on the faucet.

4. Wet your hands, keeping your fingers pointed down. This will cause the water to run off your fingertips and into the sink. Do not allow water to run up your forearms.

5. Press the hand pump or step on the foot pedal to dispense the cleaning agent into one cupped hand.

6. Lather well, keeping your fingers pointed down at all times. Make sure the lather extends at least 1 inch past your wrists.

7. Rub your hands together in a circular motion, washing the palms and backs of your hands. Interlace your fingers to clean the spaces between your fingers. Continue for at least 15 seconds.

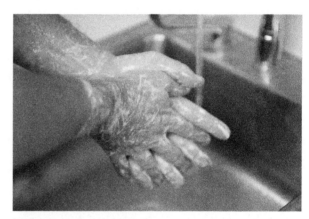

Step 7 Interlace your fingers.

8. Rub the fingernails of one hand against the palm of the opposite hand to force soap underneath the tips of the fingernails, *or* clean underneath the tips of the fingernails with the blunt edge of an orange stick or a nailbrush.

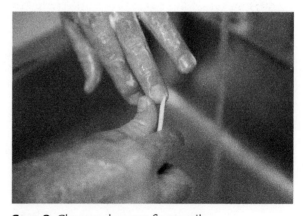

Step 8 Clean under your fingernails.

9. Rinse your hands, keeping your fingers pointed down at all times.

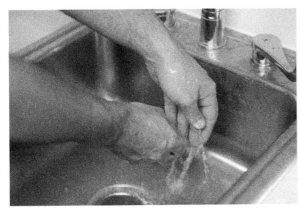

Step 9 Always point your fingertips down.

10. Dry your hands thoroughly with a clean paper towel. Dispose of the paper towel in a facility-approved waste container, being careful not to touch the container.

11. With a new paper towel, turn off the faucet. Carefully dispose of the paper towel.

12. As you leave the handwashing area, if there is a doorknob, open the door by covering the doorknob with a clean paper towel. If there is no doorknob, push the door open with your hip and shoulder to avoid contaminating your clean hands.

13. After leaving the handwashing area, apply a small amount of hand lotion to keep your skin supple and moist.

PROCEDURE 7-2

Removing Gloves

WHY YOU DO IT Removing your gloves properly prevents you from contaminating your skin or uniform.

1. With one gloved hand, grasp the other glove at the palm and pull the glove off your hand. Keep the glove you have removed in your gloved hand. (Think, "glove to glove.")

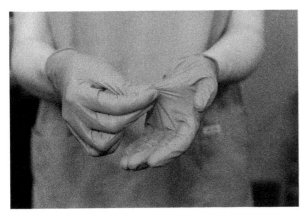

Step 1 "Glove to glove."

2. Slip two fingers from the ungloved hand underneath the cuff of the remaining glove, at the wrist. Remove that glove from your hand, turning it inside-out as you pull it off. (Think, "skin to skin.")

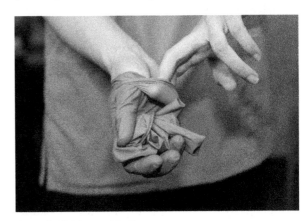

Step 2 "Skin to skin."

3. Dispose of the soiled gloves in a facility-approved waste container.

4. Wash your hands.

PROCEDURE / 7-3

Putting on a Gown

WHY YOU DO IT   Putting on a gown properly prevents your uniform from becoming soiled with body fluids.

1. Gather needed supplies: *a gown, gloves.*
2. Remove your watch and place it on a clean paper towel or in your pocket. (If you are wearing jewelry, remove that as well.) Roll up the sleeves of your uniform so that they are about 10–15 cm above your wrists.
3. Wash your hands.
4. Put on the gown by slipping your arms into the sleeves.

5. Secure the gown around your neck by tying the ties in a simple bow or by fastening the Velcro™ strips.
6. Reach behind yourself and overlap the edges of the gown so that your uniform is completely covered. Secure the gown at your waist by tying the ties in a simple bow or by fastening the Velcro™ strips.

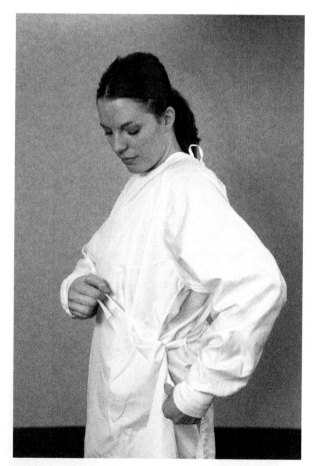

Step 6 Overlap and tie.

7. Put on the gloves. The cuffs of the gloves should extend over the cuffs of the gown.

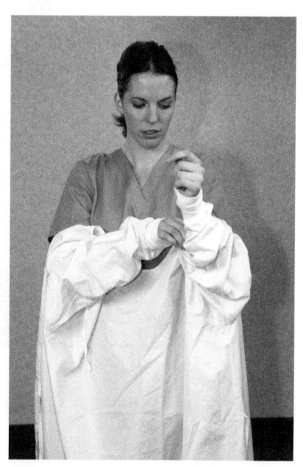

Step 4 Slip your arms into the sleeves.

PROCEDURE 7-4

Removing a Gown

WHY YOU DO IT Removing a gown properly prevents you from contaminating your skin or uniform.

---

1. Untie the waist ties (or undo the Velcro™ strips at the waist).

2. Remove and dispose of your gloves as described in Procedure 7-2.

3. Untie the neck ties (or undo the Velcro™ strips at the neck). Be careful not to touch your neck or the outside of the gown.

4. Grasping the gown at the neck ties, loosen it at the neck.

5. Slip the fingers of your dominant hand under the cuff of the gown on the opposite sleeve, and pull the sleeve over your hand. Be careful not to touch the outside of the gown with either hand.

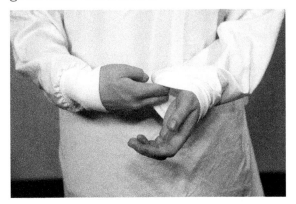

Step 5 Be careful not to touch the outside of the gown.

6. Use your gown-covered hand to pull the sleeve over your other hand, and then pull the gown off both arms.

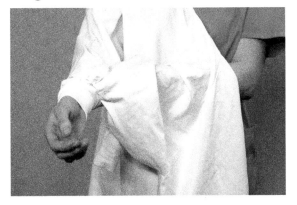

Step 6 Use your gown-covered hand to pull the sleeve over your other hand.

7. Holding the gown away from your body, roll it downward, turning it inside out as you go. Take care to touch only the noncontaminated side of the gown.

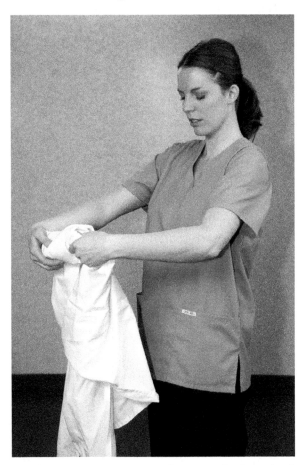

Step 7 Hold the gown away from your body and roll it downward, turning it inside out.

8. After the gown is rolled up, contaminated side inward, dispose of it in a facility-approved container.

9. Wash your hands.

PROCEDURE 7-5

Putting on and Removing a Mask

WHY YOU DO IT   Putting on a mask properly prevents pathogens that are transmitted through the air or in droplets from entering your nose and mouth. Removing a mask properly prevents you from contaminating your skin or uniform.

Putting on a Mask

1. Gather needed supplies: *a mask.*
2. Wash your hands.
3. Place the mask over your nose and mouth, being careful not to touch your face with your hands.

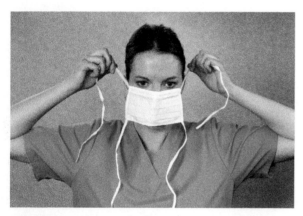

Step 3 Be careful not to touch your face with your hands.

4. Tie the top strings of the mask securely behind your head.

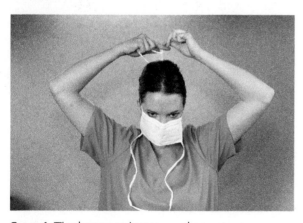

Step 4 Tie the top strings securely.

5. Tie the bottom strings of the mask securely behind your neck. Make sure that the mask fits snugly around your face. You want to breathe through the mask, not around it.

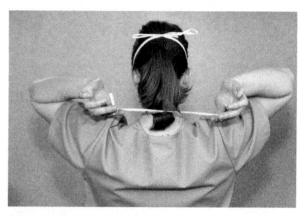

Step 5 Tie the bottom strings securely.

Removing a Mask

1. Wash your hands. (You do not want to touch your face with dirty hands.)
2. Untie the bottom strings first, and then untie the top strings.
3. Remove the mask by holding the top strings. Dispose of the mask, holding it by its ties only, in the facility-approved container located inside the patient's or resident's room.
4. Wash your hands.

PROCEDURE 7-6

Removing More Than One Article of Personal Protective Equipment (PPE)

WHY YOU DO IT   Removing PPE in the proper order helps to prevent you from contaminating your skin or uniform.

1. Untie the gown's waist ties (or undo the Velcro™ strips at the waist).
2. Remove and dispose of your gloves as described in Procedure 7-2.
3. Remove your protective eyewear.
4. Untie the gown's neck ties (or undo the Velcro™ strips at the neck), and loosen the gown at the neck. Remove and dispose of the gown as described in Procedure 7-4.
5. Remove and dispose of the mask as described in Procedure 7-5.
6. Wash your hands.

PROCEDURE 7-7

Double-Bagging (Two Workers)

WHY YOU DO IT   Double-bagging helps to keep any pathogens that may be on the outside of the bag from spreading to other places.

1. The personal support worker inside the person's room places the contaminated items into an isolation bag (usually a colour-coded plastic bag) and secures the bag with a tie.
2. Another personal support worker, referred to as the "clean" personal support worker, stands outside of the person's room, holding a plastic bag cuffed over her hands. The cuff at the top of the bag protects the "clean" personal support worker's hands.
3. The personal support worker inside the isolation unit deposits the bag of contaminated items into the bag held by the "clean" personal support worker.
4. The "clean" personal support worker secures the top of the plastic bag tightly and disposes of the double-bagged items according to facility policy.

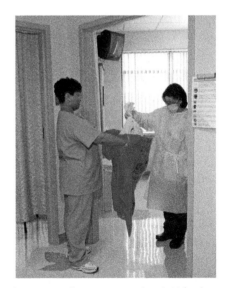

Step 3 The personal support worker inside the room places the bag of contaminated items in the bag held by the personal support worker outside of the room.

WHAT DID YOU LEARN?

Multiple Choice

Select the single best answer for each of the following questions.

1. When you wash your hands, you should:
   a. Use the hottest water possible
   b. Scrub with a brush for 3 minutes
   c. Rinse with your fingers pointed up
   d. Rinse with your fingers pointed down

2. When should you wash your hands?
   a. When you wake up in the morning and before you go to bed at night
   b. Before and after contact with a patient or resident
   c. When the charge nurse tells you to
   d. When you notice that they look or feel dirty

3. You have been told to follow contact precautions with one of your residents. Therefore, this resident's soiled linen should be:
   a. Thrown away
   b. Bagged prior to removing it from the room
   c. Taken directly to the laundry
   d. Placed in the linen hamper

4. Which of the following procedures best destroys all bacteria?
   a. Sterilizing
   b. Washing with bleach
   c. Soaking in alcohol
   d. All of the above

5. Bacteria may enter the body through:
   a. The mouth
   b. The nose
   c. Cuts in the skin
   d. All of the above

6. Which statement about the handwashing procedure is correct?
   a. As long as soap is used, the temperature of the water does not matter
   b. The faucet is clean and may be touched during handwashing
   c. Wash at least 2.54 cm above the wrist
   d. All of the above

7. Microbes can be spread by:
   a. Looking at a person with a communicable disease
   b. Coughing or sneezing
   c. Touching a person with a communicable disease
   d. Both "b" and "c"

8. Which one of the following statements about protective gowns is true?
   a. The outside is considered the "clean" side
   b. The gown opens in the front
   c. A gown may be used more than once
   d. A gown is considered contaminated when wet

9. Which one of the following could be a fomite?
   a. A water glass that has been used
   b. A mosquito
   c. Linens that have just come back from the laundry
   d. A cut in the skin

10. Which one of the following must be present in order for infection to spread?
    a. A personal support worker
    b. An indwelling medical device
    c. A susceptible host
    d. A patient or resident who looks ill

11. When are goggles a necessary part of personal protective equipment (PPE)?
    a. Whenever blood is present
    b. Whenever blood may splash or spray
    c. Whenever you are taking care of a person with tuberculosis (TB)
    d. Goggles are not really a necessary part of PPE

12. For health care workers, which of the following is the most important method of preventing the spread of infection?
    a. Standard precautions
    b. Handwashing
    c. Wearing gloves
    d. Wearing gowns and goggles

13. Personal protective equipment (PPE) refers to:
    a. Sterilization and disinfection
    b. Security personnel
    c. Disposable gloves, face masks, and gowns
    d. Isolation precautions

Matching

Match each numbered item with its appropriate lettered description.

_____ 1. Communicable disease

_____ 2. Pathogen

_____ 3. Leukocyte

_____ 4. Opportunistic microbe

_____ 5. Fomite

_____ 6. Aerobic

_____ 7. Health care–associated infection (HAI)

_____ 8. Vector

_____ 9. Anaerobic

_____10. Antibody

a. Describes bacteria that need oxygen to survive

b. Special proteins that help fight specific pathogens

c. Can be transferred from one person to another

d. Microbe that can cause illness

e. Non-living object that is contaminated

f. White blood cell

g. Can change from harmless to pathogenic, given a chance

h. Infection gotten in the health care setting

i. A living creature that transmits disease

j. Describes bacteria that die if oxygen is present

STOP and Think!

Several residents in your care have come down with a nasty intestinal virus that causes diarrhea. One resident, Mrs. Grande, is so weak that she was unable to get out of bed in time and soiled her clothing and bedding. Where is the most likely portal of exit for this pathogen? What steps should you take when cleaning up Mrs. Grande that will help to keep this virus from being spread to other residents, your co-workers, and you?

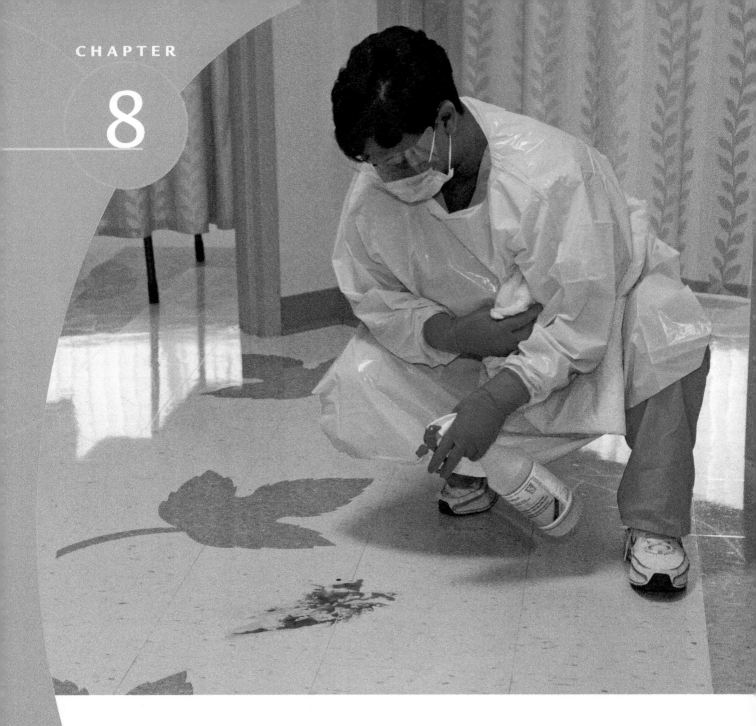

Bloodborne and Airborne Pathogens

WHAT WILL YOU LEARN?

As a personal support worker, you will have close contact with patients and residents, some of whom will have life-threatening communicable diseases. Although your risk of getting these diseases is real, there are things you can do to minimize that risk. In this chapter, you will learn about some of the communicable diseases that pose the most risk to health care

Photo: Following standard precautions, such as wearing personal protective equipment (PPE) whenever contact with blood or other body fluids is likely, helps to protect you from bloodborne pathogens.

workers, and how these diseases are transmitted. You will learn what you can do to minimize your risk of getting one of these infections. And you will also learn about the standards that have been developed by the Canadian Center for Occupational Health and Safety (CCOHS) with the goal of protecting you at work while you provide quality care for your patients or residents. When you are finished with this chapter, you will be able to:

1. Describe how bloodborne pathogens are transmitted.
2. Describe two major bloodborne diseases that pose a threat to the health care worker.
3. Describe measures a health care worker can take to protect himself or herself from exposure to bloodborne pathogens.
4. List the CCOHS standards for bloodborne pathogens.
5. Identify the requirements for an exposure control plan.
6. Describe how airborne pathogens are transmitted.
7. Describe a major airborne disease that poses a threat to the health care worker.
8. Describe measures a health care worker can take to prevent the spread of airborne pathogens.

Vocabulary

Bloodborne pathogen	Canadian Center for	Human	T cell
Body fluids	Occupational Health	immunodeficiency	CCOHS Bloodborne
Hepatitis	and Safety (CCOHS)	virus (HIV)	Pathogens Standard
Hepatitis A virus (HAV)	Hepatitis C virus (HCV)	Acquired	Exposure control plan
Oral–fecal route	Hepatitis D virus (HDV)	immunodeficiency	Airborne pathogen
Hepatitis B virus (HBV)	Hepatitis E virus (HEV)	syndrome (AIDS)	Tuberculosis (TB)
Carrier			

BLOODBORNE DISEASES

BLOODBORNE TRANSMISSION

A **bloodborne pathogen** is a disease-producing microbe that is transmitted to another person through blood or other body fluids. **Body fluids** are liquid or semi-liquid substances produced by the body, such as blood, urine, feces, vomitus, saliva, drainage from wounds, sweat, semen, vaginal secretions, tears, cerebrospinal fluid, amniotic fluid, and breast milk. For a bloodborne pathogen to be transmitted from one person to another, blood or body fluids from an infected person must enter the bloodstream of a person who is not infected. There are several ways this could occur in the workplace:

- Needlesticks (puncture wounds caused by dirty hypodermic needles)
- Cuts from contaminated, broken glass (such as that from a broken blood tube)
- Direct contact between infected blood and broken skin, mucous membranes, or the eyes

Additionally, bloodborne pathogens can be transmitted via sexual intercourse, or through blood transfusions.

Several diseases are caused by bloodborne pathogens. The most common are:

- Hepatitis B, C, and D
- Human immunodeficiency virus (HIV), which causes acquired immunodeficiency syndrome (AIDS)
- Malaria
- Syphilis
- Ebola

Of these, hepatitis and HIV pose the greatest occupational risk to the health care worker.

HEPATITIS AND HIV/AIDS

Hepatitis

Hepatitis is inflammation of the liver, the organ that removes toxic substances from the bloodstream (Fig. 8-1). Hepatitis is most commonly caused by a viral infection, but it may also be caused by chemicals, drugs, or drinking alcohol.

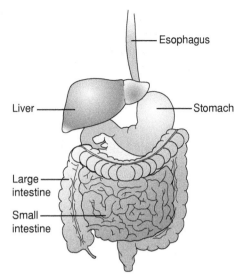

Figure 8-1
Hepatitis is inflammation of the liver, the organ that removes toxic substances from the blood.

Some infections with a hepatitis virus are mild, producing no lasting effects on the liver. Others are chronic and affect the liver's ability to function over time. If the liver failure is severe, the person will die unless she receives a liver transplant. Currently, five types of hepatitis virus have

been identified: the hepatitis A, B, C, D, and E viruses.

Hepatitis A virus

Hepatitis A virus (HAV) is not a bloodborne pathogen. This virus is transmitted through the **oral–fecal route,** which means that the virus lives in the digestive tract of an infected person and leaves the person's body through the feces. The feces can contaminate food or water. Then, when a person eats or drinks the contaminated food or water, he becomes infected. (*Oral* means mouth. In this case, the infection is transmitted by taking contaminated food or water into the mouth.) For example, HAV can be passed on when a food service worker who has the virus uses the restroom but fails to wash her hands properly before returning to work and handling a customer's food (Fig. 8-2). Hepatitis A outbreaks are also found in areas where raw sewage comes in contact with bodies of water where shellfish, such as oysters, live. The virus infects the shellfish and is then passed on to unsuspecting people who eat the contaminated shellfish raw. Fortunately, the illness caused by HAV (commonly referred to as *infectious hepatitis*) is usually acute and the person usually recovers fully. An effective vaccine against this virus is available and recommended for the general public.

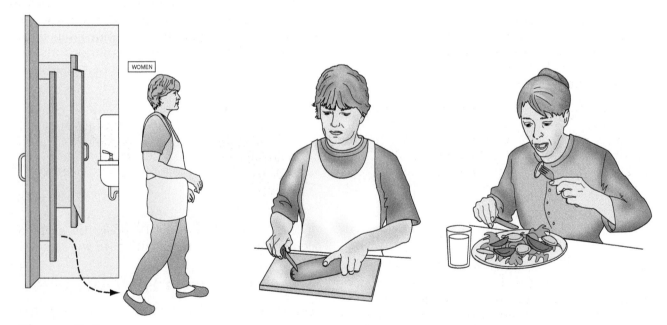

Figure 8-2
Hepatitis A virus (HAV) is transmitted via the oral–fecal route. The virus lives in an infected person's digestive tract and leaves the body in the feces. If the person's hands become contaminated with feces and then the person handles food, the infection could be passed on to the person who eats the contaminated food.

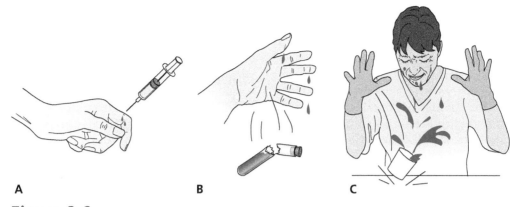

A   B   C

Figure 8-3

In the workplace, hepatitis B virus (HBV) can be transmitted by **(A)** a needlestick injury, **(B)** cuts from contaminated glass, or **(C)** direct contact with blood, for example, through a blood splash to the face.

Hepatitis B virus

Hepatitis B virus (HBV), a bloodborne pathogen, is a serious threat for the health care worker. The virus is found in blood, as well as in other body fluids, such as semen and vaginal secretions. This means that HBV can be transmitted through transfusion of infected blood or blood products, across the placenta from mother to infant, and through unprotected sexual intercourse (both heterosexual and homosexual). Health care workers are at risk for getting HBV through:

- Needlestick injuries
- Cuts from contaminated objects
- Exposure of broken skin or mucous membranes to contaminated blood or other body fluids (Fig. 8-3).

In addition to blood, semen, and vaginal secretions, body fluids known to carry high amounts of HBV include wound drainage and cultures, cerebrospinal fluid, amniotic fluid, and breast milk. Other body secretions do not typically have high viral counts unless there is visible blood present.

Infection with HBV causes an acute illness in most people, but some people can be infected by the virus and never develop symptoms. These people are considered **carriers.** Carriers do not have symptoms of the disease and therefore may be unaware that they have it. However, the virus lives in their bodies and can be transmitted to another person. Between 5% and 10% of HBV infections become chronic. People with chronic infections may never have symptoms and become carriers. Or, they may have flare-ups of symptoms every so often, resulting in months of

disability. An effective vaccination against HBV is available and is recommended by the Canadian Center for Occupational Health and Safety (CCOHS) for health care workers, as well as the general public (Fig. 8-4).

Health care workers who have any direct contact with patients or residents can be exposed to body fluids that contain HBV. Although the virus is not known to be transmitted in saliva, the gums of people with periodontal (gum) disease may bleed during oral care and tooth brushing, exposing the health care worker to potentially contaminated blood. There is always the risk of nicking a patient or resident with the razor during shaving, and patients or residents may fall and injure themselves, resulting in wounds that

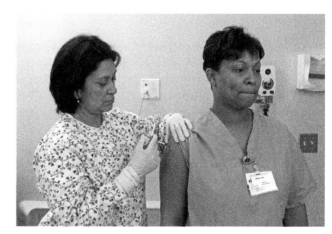

Figure 8-4

A vaccine against hepatitis B virus (HBV) is available. The Canadian Center for Occupational Health and Safety (CCOHS) requires employers to make the vaccine available to personal support workers free of charge.

bleed. A used hypodermic needle could be lost in the bed linens or accidentally tossed in the trash, placing an unsuspecting health care worker at risk for a puncture injury. Because of these occupational risks, the CCOHS recommends that all health care workers who have even the slightest potential for being exposed to blood or contaminated body fluids should receive the hepatitis B vaccination, which provides immunity to the virus. The CCOHS requires employers to offer this vaccine to employees free of charge.

Hepatitis C virus

Hepatitis C virus (HCV) is also a bloodborne pathogen. The most common mode of transmission is through contaminated blood transfusions, although some needlestick exposures have caused infection. Although the mode of HCV transmission is mainly bloodborne, in more than 40% of people who are diagnosed with HCV, no obvious route of transmission is found. The illness that results from infection with HCV tends to be more chronic and serious than that resulting from infection with HBV. As many as 85% of people with hepatitis C develop chronic disease, and of these, 20% go on to develop end-stage cirrhosis (a fatal liver disease), liver failure, or liver cancer. Hepatitis C is the leading cause for liver transplantation in Canada and the United States. Currently, no vaccine against HCV is available.

Hepatitis D virus

Hepatitis D virus (HDV), also a bloodborne pathogen, is found only in people who are already infected with HBV. Vaccination against HBV protects against HDV.

Hepatitis E virus

Hepatitis E virus (HEV) is not a bloodborne type of hepatitis. Like HAV, HEV is spread through the oral–fecal route of transmission. HEV infection is most common in countries with poor sanitation controls. There is no vaccination to protect against this virus.

HIV/AIDS

Human immunodeficiency virus (HIV) is the virus that causes **acquired immunodeficiency syndrome (AIDS).** HIV is a bloodborne pathogen, and is transmitted in the same way as HBV. Its effect on the body, however, is very different.

As described in Chapter 7, the human immune system recognizes and destroys pathogens (microbes that can enter the body and cause illness). One way the immune system does its job is

through **T cells,** special white blood cells (leukocytes) that play a role in the immune response to invading pathogens. There are two main types of T cells. One type of T cell recognizes cells that are foreign to the body, such as those infected by viruses, and kills them by producing substances that cause the foreign cells to burst. The other type of T cell produces substances that help other cells in the immune system to defend the body against pathogens.

T cells are the main target of HIV (Fig. 8-5). The virus invades the T cell. But, instead of killing the T cell immediately, it uses the T cell to make copies of itself and increase its numbers. Eventually, the virus kills the T cell, and then the virus (and all of its copies) moves on to repeat the process in other T cells. This process, over time, results in an increase in the virus count and a decrease in the T cell count.

In addition to invading and killing T cells, HIV invades the cells that form new T cells. This causes the body to produce T cells that cannot recognize pathogens. The body then becomes unable to recognize and fight off infections, leading to the condition known as AIDS. People with AIDS do not die from the virus itself. They die from infections that the body is no longer able to fight. To date, there is no cure for AIDS and no vaccine to prevent HIV.

PROTECTING YOURSELF FROM BLOODBORNE DISEASES

Standard Precautions

Bloodborne pathogens, such as HIV and HBV, pose an occupational risk to the health care worker (Table 8-1). Because of the type of work you do, you will come in contact with substances that carry these viruses. Additionally, in many cases, you will not be able to easily identify patients or residents who have these diseases. For example, HIV can be present in the blood of an infected person for a long time without causing symptoms or being detected using the diagnostic tests that are currently available. Similarly, the viruses that cause hepatitis B and hepatitis C can live in a person's body without causing signs or symptoms. For these reasons, we in the health care field *must* treat each patient or resident we have contact with as if he or she *may* be infected with a bloodborne pathogen. This is why standard precautions (see Chapter 7, Box 7-1) are taken with each patient or resident.

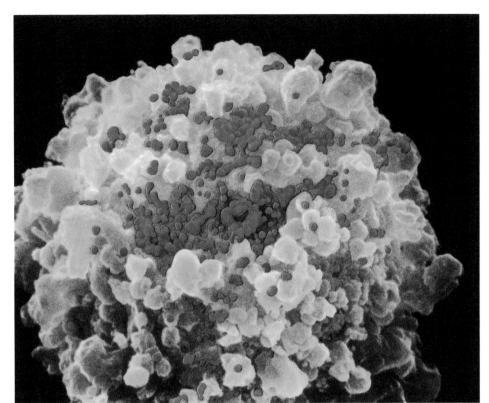

Figure 8-5

This photograph was taken by a special microscope, and color was added to enhance it. It shows a T cell (*green*) that is infected with the human immunodeficiency virus (HIV), shown in *red*. Infection with HIV can lead to the development of acquired immunodeficiency syndrome (AIDS), a fatal disease. (*NIBSC/Photo Researchers, Inc.*)

Table 8-1	Comparison of Hepatitis B Virus (HBV) and Human Immunodeficiency Virus (HIV)	
	HEPATITIS B VIRUS (HBV)	**HUMAN IMMUNODEFICIENCY VIRUS (HIV)**
Virus's ability to live outside of the body	HBV can live on a dry surface in the form of dried blood or body fluid for as long as **7 days.**	HIV can live for up to **24 hours** on a dry surface.
Virus content per cc/mL of blood*	**1,000,000,000 (1 billion)** virus particles per cc/mL of blood	**1,000 (1 thousand)** virus particles per cc/mL of blood
Risk of getting virus from a needlestick injury	**6%–30%**	**Less than 0.1%**[†]
Modes of transmission	Not transmitted by casual contact. Outside of the health care profession, HBV can be transmitted by having unprotected sexual intercourse or sharing needles used to inject drugs. It can also be transmitted to a fetus across the placenta or following exposure to the mother's blood during birth.	Not transmitted by casual contact. Outside of the health care profession, HIV can be transmitted by having unprotected sexual intercourse or sharing needles used to inject drugs. It can also be transmitted to a fetus across the placenta or following exposure to the mother's blood during birth.
Associated annual death rate among health care workers	Approximately 250 health care workers die each year from HBV	Statistic not available

*One cc/mL of blood is equal to approximately one large drop of blood. Therefore, even minor cuts can be significant in terms of their ability to expose the health care worker to bloodborne pathogens.
[†]97.7% of occupational exposures do not result in HIV infection.

BOX 8-1   CCOHS Bloodborne Pathogens Standard

- People working in an area where exposure to bloodborne pathogens is possible must receive training on the risks associated with bloodborne pathogens and on the methods they can use to safeguard themselves. Proof of initial training (at orientation) is to be on file in the employee's records, and training must be updated annually.
- Employers must make the hepatitis B vaccine available to workers who are at risk, free of charge. If an employee refuses the vaccination, a disclaimer signed by the employee must be kept on file. If the employee decides to accept the vaccine at a later date, the employer must provide it.
- The employer must provide adequate personal protective equipment (PPE), as required by the employee's duties. This includes gloves (non-latex, if the employee has allergies), face and eye protection, gowns and aprons, and scrub attire. It is the employee's responsibility to use the PPE consistently and conscientiously.

- Environmental control methods must be used to protect both the employees and the patients or residents. Environmental control methods include special ventilation systems to keep the air clean, procedures for the disposal of liquid waste, the availability of sharps disposal containers, and procedures for handling contaminated linen and trash. Housekeeping and cleaning methods must also meet CCOHS's standards.
- Each health care facility must have an **exposure control plan** in place in case an employee is exposed to blood or other body fluids from a patient or resident. The exposure control plan states what actions must be taken if an employee is exposed to blood or other body fluids while on the job. This plan must be up to date, available in written form, and available to all employees. It is the employee's responsibility to report any exposure incidents so that the employer can arrange for appropriate medical tests and treatment.

For standard precautions to be effective, they must be used consistently with every patient or resident.

It is important to remember that although those who choose to work in the health care field place themselves at risk for exposure to substances that can cause disease, the risk of encountering these substances outside of the workplace also exists. In fact, your behaviour outside the workplace could put you at much higher risk for getting one of these diseases. For example, having unprotected sexual intercourse is the most common way of getting HBV and HIV, and the rate of new hepatitis B and AIDS cases is growing fastest among young, heterosexual men and women. Your job exposes you to risks, such as needlesticks, that people in other professions do not need to worry about. But, if you follow the standard precautions, your risk of getting a bloodborne disease in the workplace will probably be lower than your risk of getting a bloodborne disease outside of it!

CCOHS Bloodborne Pathogens Standard

Your safety in the workplace is a shared responsibility. You are responsible for following the standard precautions. Your employer is responsible for making sure that you have the equipment and training you need to maintain your safety in

the workplace. To help employers to meet their responsibilities toward their employees, the CCOHS has created certain standards that all employers must follow, called the **CCOHS Bloodborne Pathogens Standard** (Box 8-1).

Any health care facility that does not follow the CCOHS standards for bloodborne pathogens may risk heavy fines and serious penalties, such as closure of the facility. For health care workers who do not follow standard precautions, the penalty can be even greater—a deadly illness. Additionally, if you have an exposure accident and were not following the recommended precautions, you may not be covered by worker's compensation if you become sick as a result of the exposure. The consequences of not following proper procedures in the workplace are not worth the risk.

AIRBORNE DISEASES

AIRBORNE TRANSMITTAL

Airborne pathogens are disease-producing microbes that are transmitted through the air. When an infected person coughs or sneezes, the pathogens leave the body through particles of saliva or sputum (Fig. 8-6). As these particles spray through the air, they dry out and remain in

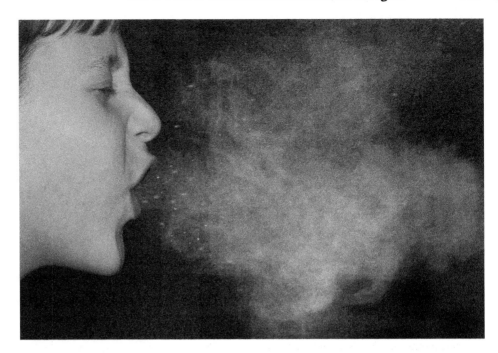

Figure 8-6
A typical sneeze sends several thousand droplets of microbe-containing mucus and saliva into the air. (*Getty Images/William Radcliffe.*)

the air for a long time (much like particles of dust caught in a shaft of sunlight). Like dust, the dried-out droplets containing pathogens are in the air we breathe and on the surfaces we touch. Infection spreads when a person breathes the air containing the suspended pathogens. Infections that are transmitted in this way include measles, chickenpox, and tuberculosis (TB). Although vaccines are available to prevent measles and chickenpox, there is currently no vaccine against TB.

TUBERCULOSIS

Tuberculosis (TB) is an infection caused by a bacterium that usually infects the lungs, but may also infect the kidneys or bones. The bacteria are present in the sputum of an infected person and are spread by airborne droplets when the person coughs, sneezes, speaks, or sings. People who have close, frequent contact with a person who has TB are most likely to get the disease. A person infected with TB may have the disease for years before she shows any symptoms.

In the early 1900s, TB caused many deaths. It was often called "consumption" because the disease progressed slowly and caused a wasting effect on the person. (In other words, the person grew very thin, and appeared to be eaten, or "consumed," by the disease.) During this time, people with TB were usually sent to special hospitals called *sanatoriums*, which offered treatment and also served as a way of limiting the spread of the disease, by keeping people with TB

away from others. In the early 1950s, the development of antibiotics that worked against the bacterium that causes TB resulted in a decrease in the number of people with the disease. However, since the mid-1980s, there has been an increase in the number of new cases of TB. Many factors seem responsible for these new cases:

- Strains of the bacterium that cause TB have become resistant to the antibiotics used to treat the infection, making the antibiotics less effective.
- People with immunodeficiency syndromes, such as AIDS, are more at risk for infections such as TB, and the number of people with immunodeficiency syndromes has increased.
- More people are traveling to developing nations, where TB is still common.
- People who are poor or who live in crowded urban areas (for example, homeless people, illegal immigrants) are at increased risk for TB.

People who get TB need to be treated for a long time, with many different antibiotics. Unfortunately, the people who are most likely to get the disease are least likely to complete the course of treatment for it because they lack money, a stable home, or both.

Because the number of new TB cases is increasing, and because the disease may go undiagnosed, a very real potential for exposure to TB in the workplace exists. Because health care workers are at risk for getting TB from patients or residents, health care facilities regularly screen

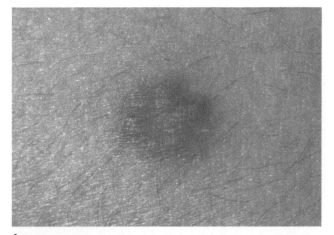

A

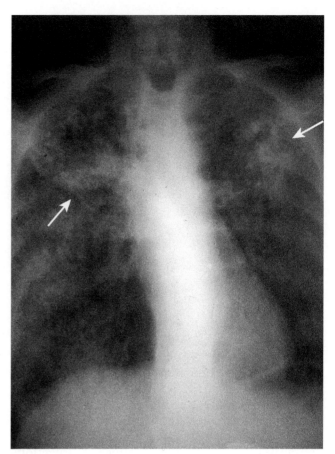

B

Figure 8-7

Health care facilities and agencies routinely screen employees for tuberculosis (TB). **(A)** A simple skin test is used to screen for exposure to TB. A person who has been exposed to the bacterium that causes TB will develop redness and swelling in the area (*shown here*). A person who has not been exposed will not have any reaction to the tuberculin. **(B)** TB causes changes in the lungs that can be seen on a chest x-ray (*arrows*). The chest x-ray of a person with a TB infection in the upper part of the lungs is shown here. (**A,** *Dr. P. Marazzi, Photo Researchers, Inc.;* **B,** *B. Bates M.D./Custom Medical Stock Photo.*)

employees for TB using a simple skin test. A small amount of test material, called tuberculin, is placed under the skin on the arm using a needle or tines. In a few days, the area is checked. A person who has been exposed to the bacterium that causes TB will develop redness and swelling in the area (Fig. 8-7A). A person who has not been exposed will not have any reaction to the tuberculin. Testing positive on a skin test does not mean that you have TB, just that you have been exposed to it. Additional tests, such as a chest x-ray, are necessary to determine if a person actually has TB (see Fig. 8-7B).

PROTECTING YOURSELF FROM AIRBORNE DISEASES

If a patient or resident is known or suspected to have an airborne disease, such as TB, airborne precautions (see Chapter 7, Box 7-2) are taken.

SUMMARY

- Hepatitis B virus (HBV), hepatitis C virus (HCV), hepatitis D virus (HDV), and human immunodeficiency virus (HIV) are bloodborne pathogens that a health care worker may be exposed to. These viruses cause serious, possibly even life-threatening, diseases.
  - For a bloodborne pathogen to be transmitted from one person to another, blood or body fluids from an infected person must enter the bloodstream of a noninfected person.
    - Needlesticks, cuts from contaminated glass, and splashes and sprays of contaminated blood can put a health care worker at risk for a bloodborne disease.

- Bloodborne diseases can also be transmitted through sexual intercourse and through blood transfusions.
- A person who is infected with a bloodborne pathogen may not appear to be ill.
- You and your employer share the responsibility for maintaining your safety in the workplace.
  - Employers must follow the standards outlined by the Canadian Center for Occupational Health and Safety (CCOHS) to ensure that the work environment is safe (the CCOHS Bloodborne Pathogens Standard).
  - Employees must follow the recommended precautions for preventing the spread of disease (standard precautions). Following the recommended standard precautions, at all times, is the single most important thing you can do to ensure your own safety.

- A vaccine against HBV is available, and offers protection against HDV as well. Currently, there is no vaccine available for HCV or HIV.
- Tuberculosis (TB) is caused by an airborne pathogen. The pathogen that causes TB is spread when an infected person coughs, sneezes, speaks, or sings.
  - The number of TB cases is on the rise. A person with TB may not appear to be ill.
  - Although antibiotics are available to treat TB, treatment is difficult, time-consuming, and expensive. There is currently no vaccine available for TB.
- You will face exposure to many infections, some life-threatening, while caring for others. Learning about these infections and how they are transmitted, as well as staying well informed about new developments and treatments for these diseases, will allow you to provide quality care to those you are responsible for.

WHAT DID YOU LEARN?

Multiple Choice

Select the single best answer for each of the following questions.

1. Hepatitis B virus (HBV), a bloodborne pathogen, can be found in all of the following body fluids except:
   a. Blood
   b. Semen
   c. Wound drainage
   d. Sweat
2. Human immunodeficiency virus (HIV) can be transmitted through all of the following means except:
   a. Blood splash to mucous membrane
   b. Sexual intercourse
   c. Sharing needles
   d. A mosquito bite

3. A vaccination against which one of the following bloodborne diseases is available?
   a. Lyme disease
   b. AIDS
   c. Hepatitis C
   d. Hepatitis B
4. Hepatitis B is a viral disease of the:
   a. Spleen
   b. Liver
   c. Blood
   d. Heart

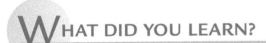 **and Think!**

You are walking past the TV room of the nursing facility where you work. You hear a call for help. As you enter the room, you see that Mr. Torres has a pretty bad nosebleed. There is blood on his hands and clothes, and some has puddled on the floor. What should you do as you rush to help Mr. Torres? How will you clean up the blood afterward?

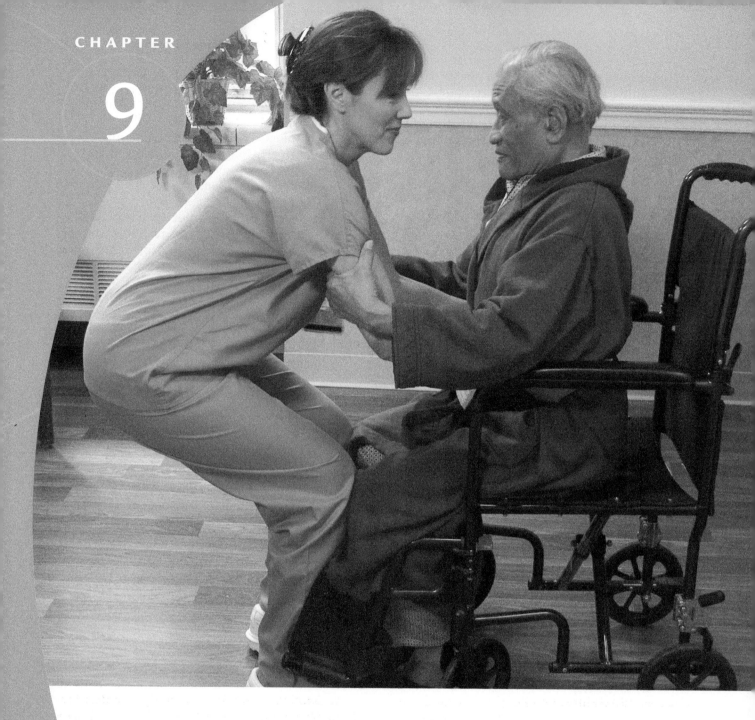

Workplace Safety

WHAT WILL YOU LEARN?

As you have learned in Chapters 7 and 8, the risk of infectious disease is a work-related hazard faced by all people in the health care system—patients and residents, family members and visitors, and health care workers. Although minimizing the spread of infectious disease is a major safety concern for health care workers, it is not the only one. In this chapter, we

Photo: A personal support worker uses good body mechanics to protect herself from injury while assisting a resident to stand.

will explore other threats to the safety of people who work or live in a health care facility, and the measures you can take to minimize these threats. When you are finished with this chapter, you will be able to:

1. Define the term *body mechanics* and demonstrate actions that make the body more effective when working.
2. Demonstrate the use of good body mechanics when lifting.
3. Describe ways to prevent back injury.
4. Explain why personal support workers follow procedures when providing patient or resident care.
5. List the steps that are taken before and after every patient or resident care procedure, and explain why these steps are taken.
6. Describe hazards that increase the risk of falls in the health care setting.
7. Demonstrate how to assist a person who is falling.
8. Describe chemical hazards found in the health care setting.
9. Discuss electrical hazards found in the health care setting and ways to avoid them.
10. List the elements necessary for a fire to start and continue to burn.
11. Describe the RACE fire response plan.
12. Demonstrate how to use a fire extinguisher.
13. List disaster situations that may affect a health care facility, and describe the focus of a disaster preparedness plan in a hospital versus in a long-term care facility.

Vocabulary

Body mechanics	Procedure	Materials Safety Data	RACE fire response
Alignment	Pre-procedure actions	Sheet (MSDS)	plan
Balance	Post-procedure	Grounded	Disaster
Coordinated body	actions		
movement			

PROTECTING YOUR BODY

Performing the same action over and over places stress on the body—for example, think of the stress on a baseball catcher's knees as he squats, then stands, then squats again hundreds of times throughout a single game. In addition, moving a large, awkward, or heavy object also places strain on the body and can lead to injury. As a personal support worker, you will place stress on your body as you lift, push, pull, stoop, and bend repeatedly on a daily basis. In addition, in many cases, you will need to move a person or piece of equipment that is larger and heavier than you are. There is no doubt about it—being a personal support worker is extremely physically demanding! Fortunately, by practicing good body mechanics and learning proper lifting techniques, you can minimize your risk for physical injury.

THE "ABCs" OF GOOD BODY MECHANICS

The efficient movement and use of the body is accomplished through good **body mechanics.** The basic components (the "ABCs") of good body mechanics are **A**lignment, **B**alance, and **C**oordinated movement.

Alignment is simply good posture. For the body to work most efficiently, proper alignment is necessary to ensure that no excess strain is placed on the joints and muscles. The back is held in a "neutral" position, with the natural curvature of the lower back intact. Imagine that you are looking at a person who is holding her body in proper alignment (Fig. 9-1). On the side view, you would be able to draw a straight line connecting the person's ear, shoulder, hip, knee, and ankle. From the front view, you would be able to draw a straight line connecting the nose, the

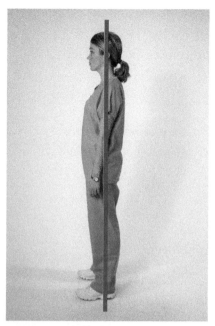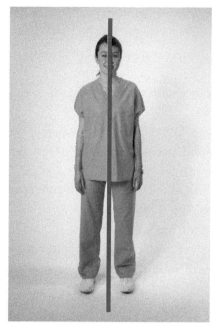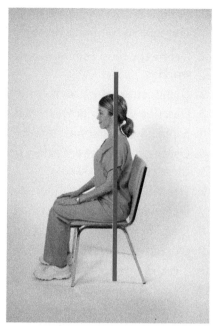

Figure 9-1
When the body is held in proper alignment, the back is in a "neutral" position, with the curve of the lower spine intact. Holding the body in proper alignment prevents strain on the joints and muscles.

sternum (breastbone), and the navel, and then continuing between the legs, dividing that space equally in half.

Balance is stability produced by the even distribution of weight. Balance involves holding your center of gravity, or area of largest mass, close to your base of support. For example, when you are standing, your base of support is your feet (which are placed squarely on the floor), and your centre of gravity is your torso, the heaviest part of your body. The larger your base of support, and the closer the heaviest part of your body is to that base of support, the more balanced you will be. How, then, can you stabilize your body and maximize your ability to remain balanced? There are two ways:

- You can increase your base of support by spreading your feet further apart.
- You can bring your centre of gravity closer to your base of support by bending at the knees and hips, so that your torso is closer to your feet.

Imagine that you are standing with your legs together and your ankles touching. If someone pushed you, you might lose your balance and fall. Now imagine that you are standing with your feet about shoulder-width apart. The same shove might not cause you to lose your balance. And if you were then to lower your body into a squat, it would be even harder to push you over! Increasing your base of support by standing with your feet apart, and positioning yourself so that your centre of gravity (your torso) is close to your base of support (your feet), improves your balance and is a very important part of practicing good body mechanics (Fig. 9-2).

Coordinated body movement involves using the weight of your body to help with movement. For example, when moving a person up in bed, you stand facing the bed, with your feet apart. As you step sideways to move the person's head and shoulders up, you transfer your weight from one foot to the other and the momentum helps you to move the person (Fig. 9-3).

LIFTING AND BACK SAFETY

Practicing good body mechanics is important, especially when you must lift heavy equipment or move people who have trouble moving on their own. Lifting is a required task for personal support workers who provide direct care to patients or residents. Therefore, it is important to learn proper technique. Failure to use good body mechanics when lifting something or someone can result in back injuries. Back injuries are the most common work-related injury in the nursing field. Injuries of the back range from muscle strains and soreness to ruptured vertebral discs

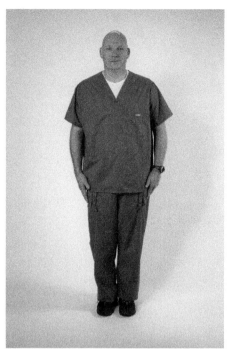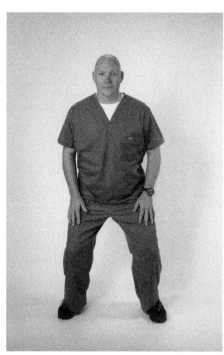

Figure 9-2
Maintaining balance. Spreading your feet apart and bending at the hips and knees improves your ability to stay balanced.

(a condition that may require surgery and a long recovery period). Back injuries are painful and costly (in terms of medical care and missed work), and can be serious enough to end your career and prevent you from participating in other activities that you enjoy. If you do not take precautions to prevent back injuries, you could find yourself in the position of being the patient instead of the care provider!

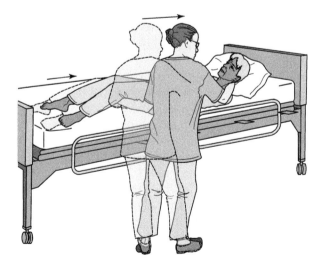

Figure 9-3
Coordinated body movement involves using the weight of your body to help with movement. When the personal support worker steps sideways, shifting her weight from her left foot to her right, the momentum of her body helps to move the person up in bed.

If you have ever watched the weightlifting event in the Olympics, you know that competitive weightlifters can lift more than 500 pounds. The weightlifter's lifting technique is an excellent example of good body mechanics being used. The athlete squats low to the ground, using his arms and shoulders to pull the weight close to his body at chest level. He then uses his hips and legs to stand up with the weight. After becoming upright, he widens his base of support by moving one foot ahead of the other. These manoeuvres allow the large, strong muscles of the body to do the work of lifting and also protect the back from injury.

The muscles of the arms and legs are attached to the long bones in our limbs. The muscle contracts by pulling against the bone it is attached to. This allows us to move and to lift weight. In contrast, the muscles of the back are flat and fan-like, and are not designed to lift weight. When the competitive weightlifter lifts his weights, he uses his leg muscles, not his back muscles. As he raises himself out of the squat, he uses the powerful muscles in his buttocks, hips, and thighs to move himself, and the weight, upward. Although you will not be required to practice competitive weightlifting at work, you should try to imitate the professionals with your technique! For example, if you had to move a patient or resident from the bed to a chair, you would bend your knees and hold the person close to the center of your body. Then,

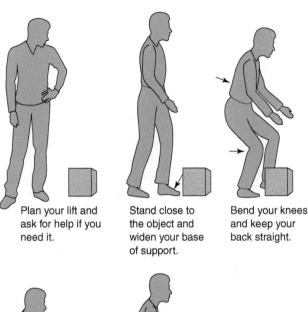

Plan your lift and ask for help if you need it.

Stand close to the object and widen your base of support.

Bend your knees and keep your back straight.

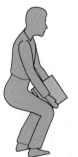 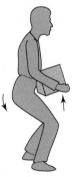

Tighten your stomach muscles.

Lift with your leg muscles.

Figure 9-4
Proper lifting technique.

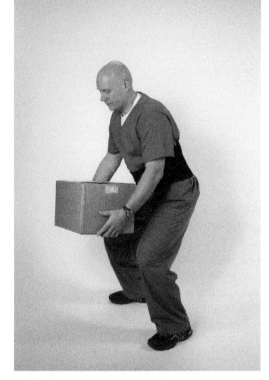

Figure 9-5
A back support can help to hold your body in proper alignment when lifting.

you would use the muscles in your thighs and hips to lift and move the person from the bed to the chair. Proper lifting technique is summarized in Figure 9-4.

Many health care facilities and agencies require employees who must lift to wear back supports. If your facility requires you to wear a back support when lifting, make sure you have been properly trained in its correct use. Use the support correctly. Improper or prolonged use of a back support can actually weaken the back muscles. But, when used correctly, the back support will remind you to hold your body in proper alignment when lifting. Bending at the waist with a tight back support around you is very uncomfortable (Fig. 9-5).

Guidelines for protecting yourself from injury as a result of the physical nature of your job are summarized in Guidelines Box 9-1. To protect your health, remember the principles of good body mechanics and apply them consistently, both at work and at home.

FOLLOWING PROCEDURES

To ensure that the care you provide is safe and correct, you will follow specific procedures. A **procedure** is a series of steps followed in a particular order. Following the recommended steps of a procedure helps to protect the person you are caring for, and it protects you.

Certain steps, called **pre-procedure actions,** are followed before performing any procedure on a patient or resident. In this book, we call these actions "Getting Ready" steps (Guidelines Box 9-2). The "Getting Ready" steps promote efficiency, safety, courtesy, and respect of the patient's or resident's rights. Similarly, there is a group of actions that are routinely performed at the end of each procedure, called **post-procedure actions.** In this book, we call these actions "Finishing Up" steps (Guidelines Box 9-3). The "Finishing Up" steps promote comfort, safety, and communication among members of the health care team. As you review the procedure boxes throughout this book, you will see references to these "Getting Ready" and "Finishing Up" steps in each of them.

(*Text continued on page 148*)

Guidelines Box 9-1	Guidelines for Protecting Yourself From Physical Injury
WHAT YOU DO	*WHY YOU DO IT*
Make a habit of practicing good posture.	Keeping the body in proper alignment, regardless of the activity, reduces stress and fatigue to the muscles and joints.
Create a solid base of support by moving your feet apart, either by widening your stance or by placing one foot in front of the other.	A solid base of support improves your balance, reducing the chance that you will injure yourself during the manoeuvre.
Allow the weight of your own body to assist in pulling or pushing heavy objects.	Using coordinated body movement to move something minimizes the stress on your body while making the task you are trying to accomplish easier.
When moving or lifting people or objects, place your body as close as possible to the object being moved.	Bringing your body's center of gravity closer to the object improves your balance and allows the strong muscles of the shoulders and upper arms to assist in the move.
Squat, do not lean over, to lower your center of gravity when lifting.	Lowering your center of gravity improves your balance. However, this lowering should be accomplished by squatting, rather than leaning over. Squatting allows you to use the strong muscles of your lower body to move yourself, and the weight, upward. Leaning over while lifting weight strains the back joints and muscles.
Use the large, strong muscles of the hips, buttocks, and thighs to do the lifting.	Using the strong muscles of the legs to move yourself upward is preferable to placing strain on the muscles of the back, which are not meant to be used to lift substantial amounts of weight.
Do not lift heavy objects from a position higher than your head. Use a step stool or a short safety ladder to raise your entire body closer to the desired level.	Attempting to lift a heavy object from an awkward position (for example, with your arms raised above your head) interferes with your ability to balance and places you at risk for injury.
If an object is very heavy, do not attempt to lift it. Instead, pull, push, or roll the object.	Pushing, pulling, or rolling a heavy object places less strain on your body because you can use your body weight to help you accomplish the task. In other words, you can use the principle of coordinated movement.
Use assistive devices whenever possible to make the job easier.	Hand carts and dollies permit the easy movement of objects by placing them on wheels. Gait belts, draw sheets, and mechanical lifts (discussed in detail in Chapter 11) help make moving people easier.

(continued)

Guidelines Box 9-1 Guidelines for Protecting Yourself From Physical Injury (continued)

WHAT YOU DO	WHY YOU DO IT
Ask for help when lifting or moving heavy people or objects. You should also get help when you need to move a person who cannot offer any assistance, or is combative.	Heavy or awkward loads increase your risk of injury (and, if you are attempting to lift a person, increase that person's risk of injury as well). A person who is "dead weight" or uncooperative is both heavy and awkward.
Keep your body in good physical condition by exercising regularly, eating nutritious foods, and getting enough rest.	Your body can be compared to an automobile. It must be properly maintained in order to provide you with years of solid performance.

Guidelines Box 9-2 Guidelines for Getting Ready (Pre-procedure Actions)

WHAT YOU DO	WHY YOU DO IT
WASH your hands. Apply gloves and follow standard precautions if contact with blood or body fluids is possible.	Washing your hands and taking standard precautions prevents the spread of infection.
GATHER needed supplies.	Having everything you need before you start promotes efficiency.
KNOCK on the door and identify yourself by name and title to the person.	Knocking before you enter protects the person's right to privacy. Identifying yourself respects the person's right to know who is providing care.
IDENTIFY the person, and greet him or her by name. Methods of identifying patients and residents will vary depending on where you work. Common methods of identifying people in health care facilities include wrist bands and photographs.	Identifying the person ensures that the procedure is being done on the correct patient or resident. Greeting the person by name is courteous.
EXPLAIN the procedure and encourage the person to participate as appropriate.	Explaining the procedure lets the person know what to expect and helps him to understand how he can help.

Guidelines Box 9-2 Guidelines for Getting Ready (Pre-procedure Actions) (continued)

WHAT YOU DO	WHY YOU DO IT
PROVIDE PRIVACY by showing any visitors where they may wait, if necessary, until you have completed the procedure. Close the door and the curtain. Drape the person for modesty as appropriate.	Asking visitors to leave the room, closing the door and curtain, and draping the person for modesty protects the person's right to privacy.
SEE TO SAFETY. Take safety precautions by following standards of body mechanics, equipment use, and infection control. In procedures that involve getting a person out of bed, lower the bed to its lowest position. This decreases the distance between the bed and the floor, should the person fall. In procedures that involve providing care while the person remains in bed, raise the bed to a comfortable working height. This protects your back.	Following standards of body mechanics, equipment use, and infection control keeps you and your patients or residents safe.

Guidelines Box 9-3 Guidelines for Finishing Up (Post-procedure Actions)

WHAT YOU DO	WHY YOU DO IT
CONFIRM that the person is comfortable and in good body alignment.	Proper body alignment is most comfortable for the person. It relieves strain on the muscles and joints, promotes good heart and lung function, and helps prevent contractures and pressure ulcers.
LEAVE the call light control, telephone, and fresh water within easy reach of the person.	Having necessary items nearby promotes independence and helps to prevent falls.
SEE TO SAFETY. Return the bed to the lowest position, lock the wheels, and raise the side rails (if side rails are in use).	Lowering the bed, locking the wheels, and raising the side rails (if side rails are in use) helps to prevent falls.
OPEN the curtain and door if desired by the patient or resident, and inform visitors that they may return to the room.	Opening the curtain and door and letting visitors know that they can return helps to prevent feelings of isolation.

(continued)

Guidelines Box 9-3   Guidelines for Finishing Up (Post-procedure Actions) (continued)

WHAT YOU DO	WHY YOU DO IT
WASH your hands. If gloved, remove and discard the gloves following facility policy, and then wash your hands.	Washing your hands prevents the spread of infection.
REPORT AND RECORD actions as required by your facility.	Reporting lets the nurse know that you have completed the task and allows you to update the nurse about any changes in the patient's or resident's status. Recording formally documents the care that was provided and ensures that all members of the health care team have the same information about the patient's or resident's status and care.

You must learn these steps and perform them before and after every procedure.

PREVENTING FALLS

In Chapter 10, you will learn about situations that increase a patient's or resident's risk for falling, such as poor vision, a limited ability to move, or confusion. But what about factors that increase a personal support worker's chances of falling?

Personal support workers work hard and have many duties that must be completed during a shift. Being in too much of a hurry can increase your risk of falling. Even in an emergency situation, when you need to move quickly, be aware of your surroundings and move only as fast as you are safely able. You are not a help in an emergency if you fall and hurt yourself!

Wet floors also increase your risk of falling. Helping patients and residents with showers and baths often results in water on the floor. A resident who is incontinent (unable to control her bladder) can leave a puddle of urine in the hallway that you could slip in, especially if you are in a hurry. If you see water or other fluids or substances on the floor, you should immediately stop what you are doing and dry the area (Fig. 9-6). Failure to do so puts you, your patients or residents, visitors, and co-workers at risk for falling.

Be aware of objects in your path that could cause you to trip. Electrical cords can also pose a tripping hazard. Try to position furniture so that the electrical cords for lamps and other appliances are close to the outlet.

Make sure that you can see clearly. Night lights positioned near the floor are useful in a health care setting. They allow you to see where you are going without disturbing the patient or resident by turning on the overhead light.

Helping a very weak, unsteady, or uncooperative person to walk or transfer from one place to another without help can cause both of you to

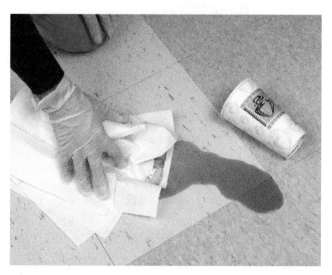

Figure 9-6
Mopping up spills is an important safety measure. Failing to do so can lead to falls.

BOX
9-1 Minimizing the Risk of Injury as a Result of a Fall

1. If the person complains of dizziness or seems unsteady, help him to sit in a chair. If a chair is not close by, help the person to sit on the floor. Stay with the person and call for assistance. This action can prevent a fall completely.

2. If a fall cannot be avoided, place your body behind the person and place your arms around his torso, pulling him close to your body. Do not grab the person's arm in an attempt to prevent the fall, because doing so may actually cause more extensive injuries in some people (such as elderly people, who may have brittle bones, and people with weaknesses on one side of the body).

3. With the person's body pulled close to yours, widen your base of support by placing one foot behind the other, and allow the person to slide down your body toward the floor.

4. As the person slides down, squat while still supporting his body and gently lower him to the floor. Lower yourself to the floor and assume a sitting position with the person's head in your lap.

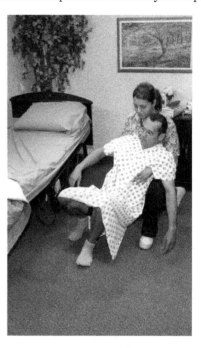

5. Stay with the person and call for assistance.

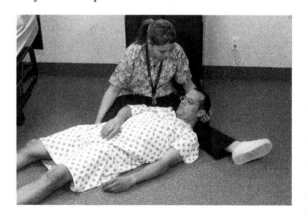

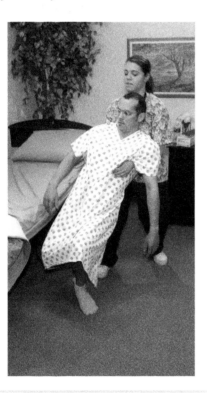

fall. You may not want to ask a busy co-worker for help, but resist the temptation to "go it alone." If the patient or resident you are attempting to help falls, she will take you with her, potentially resulting in serious injury to you both. Attempting to prevent a patient or resident from falling can also result in a back injury for you. Please ask for help whenever you feel you need it in order to safely continue. If you are assisting a person who begins to fall, follow the steps in Box 9-1 to minimize the risk of injury for everyone involved.

PREVENTING CHEMICAL INJURIES

Health care facilities use many chemicals on a daily basis—for example, cleaning solutions and disinfectants, sterilizing agents, and chemotherapeutic drugs. Many of these chemicals can be harmful if they are inhaled, swallowed, absorbed through the skin, or splashed in the eyes. Some chemicals are relatively harmless alone but can become dangerous if accidentally mixed with another product.

The Canadian Centre for Occupational Health and Safety (CCOHS) requires all employers to maintain a list of the chemicals that are used in the facility, from household cleaners to highly toxic solutions, and to inform and educate all workers about the chemicals that are in use in their workplace. One way of communicating information about chemicals to employees is through a **Materials Safety Data Sheet (MSDS),** which the manufacturer of the chemical is required to supply (Fig. 9-7). The MSDS for each chemical in use must be kept on file and be readily available in each unit of the health care facility. The manufacturer must renew the MSDS every 3 years (or sooner, if there is a change in the product). The MSDS summarizes key information about the chemical, such as what it is made from, which exposures may be dangerous, what to do if an exposure occurs, and how to clean up spills. Container labels also provide information about the chemicals in the container, and all containers must be clearly labeled. As a personal support worker, it is your responsibility to be familiar with the chemicals that you may come in contact with in your facility, and to know the proper, safe way to handle each chemical in use.

PREVENTING ELECTRICAL SHOCKS

There are many electrical appliances used in the health care setting, from complex monitoring devices to the common hair dryer. Knowing how to safely operate and maintain electrical equipment in the workplace will help create a safe working environment for you and a safe living environment for your patients or residents.

Precautions, such as using grounded appliances and power strips, help to minimize the risk of electrical shock. Most electrical equipment used in the health care setting is **grounded.** This means that it has a way of returning stray electrical current to the outlet so that the risk of electrical shock is reduced. Grounding may be achieved through a three-prong plug (Fig. 9-8A) or a safety outlet with a ground-fault breaker (Fig. 9-8B). The use of extension cords is not recommended and outlets should not be overloaded. If more than two items must be plugged into an outlet, a facility-approved power strip should be used (Fig. 9-8C).

As a personal support worker, you must be alert for electrical items that pose potential shock or fire hazards. Residents of long-term care facilities often bring small electrical items with them to furnish their rooms, such as radios, televisions, and table lamps. Most facilities require items like these to be inspected by the maintenance department before the resident can use them. However, if you should notice anything unsafe about an electrical appliance that is being used, such as frayed wires or loose plugs, you should remove the appliance from use immediately. This is true of facility-owned equipment as well, such as electrically controlled hospital beds and call light controls. Most health care facilities have a system for tagging a defective item and sending it for repair (Fig. 9-9). Follow your facility's policy. Failure to properly tag a defective electrical device could result in injury or even death to the next person who uses it.

When using electrical equipment, be aware of the safety hazard posed by operating an electrical appliance around water. Do not operate hair dryers, electric razors, curling irons, radios, or other electrical appliances around showers and bathtubs. The risk of electrical shock or electrocution must be taken seriously.

FIRE SAFETY

In a health care facility, a fire that gets out of control can have tragic consequences. Not only does the facility house hundreds of people, many of these people are relatively unable to help themselves in the event of an emergency. As a health care worker, you must know how to prevent fires in the workplace, and what to do in the event that a fire does occur.

PREVENTING FIRES

For a fire to occur, three elements must be present: fuel (something that burns), heat (something to ignite the fuel), and oxygen (Fig. 9-10).

Common sources of fuel in the health care setting include:

- Cloth, such as bed linens, mattresses, and clothing
- Paper
- Substances that easily catch fire and burn quickly, such as cooking oil, gasoline, and nail polish remover
- The building itself

Heat can be provided by:

- An electrical spark (such as may occur with a frayed electrical cord, a "short" in a piece

MSDS: 3M BRAND DISINFECTANT CLEANER
March 08, 2006

```
------------------------------------------------------------------
   5. ENVIRONMENTAL INFORMATION      (continued)
------------------------------------------------------------------
```

RECOMMENDED DISPOSAL:
  Discharge spent solutions and small quantities (less than 5 gal.(19
  L)) to a wastewater treatment system. Flush spent solutions and
  small quantities (less than 5 gal.(19 L)) to a wastewater treatment
  system. Reduce discharge rate if foaming occurs. Incinerate in a
  permitted hazardous waste incinerator in the presence of a
  combustible material.

  Empty container may be sanitary landfilled.

ENVIRONMENTAL DATA:
  Not determined.
        6
REGULATORY INFORMATION:
  Volatile Organic Compounds: ca. 4.00 gms/liter.
  VOC Less H2O & Exempt Solvents: N/D.

  Since regulations vary, consult applicable regulations or authorities
  before disposal. U.S. EPA Hazardous Waste Number = D002 (Corrosive)

EPCRA HAZARD CLASS:
  FIRE HAZARD: Yes PRESSURE: No REACTIVITY: No ACUTE: Yes CHRONIC: Yes

```
------------------------------------------------------------------
   6. SUGGESTED FIRST AID
------------------------------------------------------------------
```

EYE CONTACT:
  Immediately flush eyes with large amounts of water for at least 15
  minutes. Get immediate medical attention.

SKIN CONTACT:
  Immediately flush skin with large amounts of water for at least 15
  minutes in a chemical safety shower while removing contaminated
  clothing and shoes. Get immediate medical attention. Wash
  contaminated clothing before reuse.

INHALATION:
  If signs/symptoms occur, remove person to fresh air. If
  signs/symptoms continue, call a physician.

IF SWALLOWED:
  If swallowed, do NOT induce vomiting. Give victim two glasses of
  water. Call a physician immediately. Never give anything by mouth to
  an unconscious person.

  Note to physician: Probable mucosal damage may contraindicate the use
  of gastric lavage.

```
------------------------------------------------------------------
```
Abbreviations: N/D - Not Determined N/A - Not Applicable CA - Approximately

Figure 9-7
Part of a Materials Safety Data Sheet (MSDS). The MSDS provides important information about
each chemical in use in the workplace.

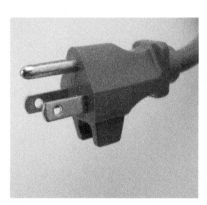
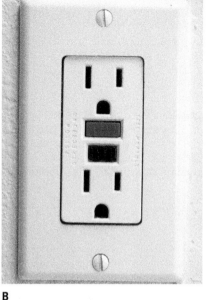
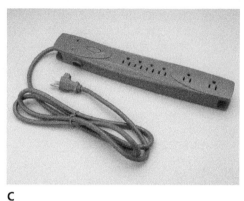

A   B   C

Figure 9-8
(A) Three-prong plugs, **(B)** outlets with ground-fault breakers, and **(C)** power strips help to reduce the risk of electrical shock and fire.

of electrical equipment, or even a lightning strike)
- Lighted smoking materials (such as cigarettes, cigars, or matches)
- Lighted candles
- Heating elements (such as radiators or furnaces)
- Stoves

Oxygen is found in the air around us, and generally the better the air supply, the better a fire will burn. Remember that in a health care facility, many patients and residents receive oxygen therapy, which increases the content of the oxygen in the air in the immediate area. Safety precautions that are used to prevent fires (Guidelines Box 9-4) are extremely important when oxygen therapy is in use. The patient or

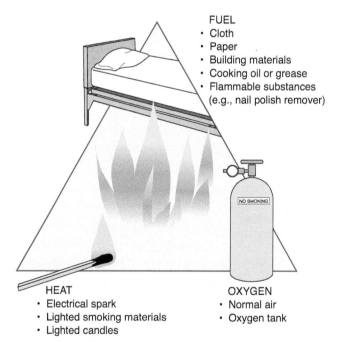

FUEL
- Cloth
- Paper
- Building materials
- Cooking oil or grease
- Flammable substances (e.g., nail polish remover)

HEAT
- Electrical spark
- Lighted smoking materials
- Lighted candles

OXYGEN
- Normal air
- Oxygen tank

Figure 9-9
If you notice that a piece of electrical equipment is malfunctioning or presents a safety hazard, follow your facility's policy for removing it from use and getting it repaired.

Figure 9-10
Three things must be present for a fire to occur: fuel, heat, and oxygen.

Guidelines Box 9-4	Guidelines for Preventing Fires
WHAT YOU DO	*WHY YOU DO IT*
Supervise patients or residents who are disoriented or who may fall asleep while smoking, any time that they smoke.	A sleepy or disoriented person is not paying close attention to the lighted smoking material, which increases the chance that a fire will start.
Do not allow any patient or resident to smoke in bed, especially if the person is receiving oxygen therapy.*	A person who smokes in bed is bringing all three elements necessary for a fire together (fuel = bed linens; heat = lighted smoking material; oxygen = surrounding air). Smoking in bed is especially dangerous because the person is more likely to fall asleep and forget about the lighted smoking material. In addition, the use of oxygen therapy increases the oxygen content of linens and bedding in the immediate area. If burning ashes from a cigarette should happen to drop on the bed, a fire would be more likely to start and would burn much faster as a result of the added oxygen.
Do not provide patients or residents who are receiving oxygen therapy with wool or mohair blankets.	These materials can produce sparks of static electricity, which could lead to a fire.
If smoking is permitted in the facility, make sure that all smoking occurs only in designated smoking areas.	Designated smoking areas have ashtrays for properly extinguishing lit smoking materials. They are also located in a part of the building where oxygen therapy is not in use.
Keep smoking materials, lighters, and matches in a place where children and confused patients or residents cannot reach them.	Children do not understand that playing with these materials can be dangerous. A confused person is not able to use these materials responsibly on his or her own, and should be supervised.
Keep all electrical equipment in good working order.	A spark from a frayed wire, an improperly grounded plug, or an electrical "short" can start an electrical fire.
Handle flammable substances safely and clean up any spills immediately. Do not use flammable substances near a heat source such as a hair dryer or heater, or while smoking.	Flammable substances ignite easily and burn quickly. Therefore, if they come in contact with a heat source, a fire is likely to start.
Report any malfunctioning smoke detectors immediately.	A smoke detector is the best early fire detection device available, but only if it is functioning properly.
Investigate smoke or smells of anything burning promptly. Be aware of the location of fire alarms and fire extinguishers and know how to activate and use them.	Early investigation and quick action can help to contain a fire before it gets out of control.
Be familiar with your facility's fire safety policies and know the location of all exits.	If a fire does occur, you may need to evacuate patients or residents. You will be much more effective in your duties if you are able to remain calm, and your calmness will also help to calm others.

*Although health care facilities prohibit smoking in patient or resident rooms, some people may forget or disregard the rules.

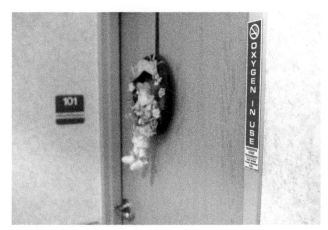

Figure 9-11
Oxygen therapy is common in health care facilities. "Oxygen In Use" signs are posted to warn patients or residents and their visitors that extra precautions are needed when oxygen therapy is in use.

resident and any visitors should be made aware of the added risks (Fig. 9-11).

REACTING TO A FIRE EMERGENCY

Sometimes, despite taking precautions, a fire will occur. In some cases, the fire will be small and can be dealt with rather easily if the situation is addressed promptly and correctly. For example, imagine a fire that begins in a resident's room because a visitor drops a half-lit cigarette in a wastebasket full of paper, or a stovetop fire that begins in the hospital kitchen. In both of these situations, an alert person who knew what to do could control the fire, and it is possible that others outside of the immediate area would not even be aware of the disturbance. However, sometimes a fire can begin on a much larger scale, for example, as a result of faulty electrical wiring in the walls of the building, a gas leak, or even a terrorist attack. In situations like these, a large-scale evacuation (removal) of those in the facility will most likely be necessary.

The general actions that are taken in the event of a fire emergency are known as the **RACE fire response plan** (Fig. 9-12):

Remove any patients or residents who are in immediate danger to safety. Escort people who can walk. Use wheelchairs for unsteady people. To prevent a confused or disoriented person from accidentally wandering back into the fire area, assign

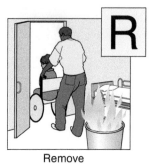
Remove

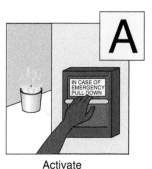
Activate

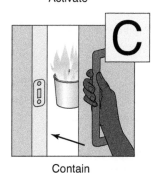
Contain

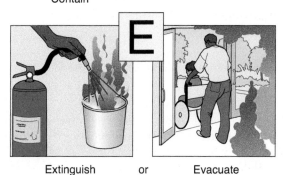
Extinguish   or   Evacuate

Figure 9-12
The RACE fire response plan.

another, alert patient or resident or a visitor to attend to the person. People who cannot get out of bed should be moved in their beds, if possible. If the bed cannot be moved out of the room, or if stairs must be used, the patient or resident can be pulled to safety using the linens from the bed (Box 9-2). Some facilities will train you in

---

BOX 9-2 | **Using Bed Linens to Evacuate a Bedridden Person**

1. Loosen the bottom sheet from the foot of the person's bed.
2. Make sure that the bed is lowered to its lowest position and that the wheels are locked.
3. Grasp the top of the bottom sheet near the person's head and shoulders. Have a co-worker grasp the bottom sheet at the foot of the bed. Using the sheet, gently lower the person to the floor, feet first.
4. Pull the sheet, with the person cradled in it, toward the nearest exit.
5. If it is necessary to move the person down stairs, support the person's upper body by pulling up on the sheet and proceed down the steps backward. Do not allow the person's body to bump against the steps.

---

special techniques that are used to carry a person to safety.

Activate the alarm, if the alarm has not been sounded. Follow your facility's policy for reporting a fire. For example, you may be required to pull the fire alarm, or use the intercom or telephone system.

Contain the fire by closing doors and windows. This action helps to slow the spread of the fire.

Extinguish the fire if possible, or, if the fire is large or spreading quickly,

Evacuate the building.

Extinguishing Fires

As you know, there are three elements that must be present for a fire to continue burning—fuel, heat, and oxygen. If you remove just one of these elements, you can put out (extinguish) the fire. Not all fires are alike. Fires are classified as either "A" type, "B" type, or "C" type fires (Table 9-1). This classification determines the best way to put them out.

A commonly used tool for putting out fires is a fire extinguisher (Fig. 9-13). There are fire extinguishers that are specific for each type of fire, but the most common type of fire extinguisher, an ABC extinguisher, can be used for all types of fires. ABC fire extinguishers use carbon dioxide to remove the oxygen from the fire. This smothers the fire, putting it out. All health care facilities must have easily accessible fire extinguishers, in case a fire should occur. You are responsible for knowing where fire extinguishers

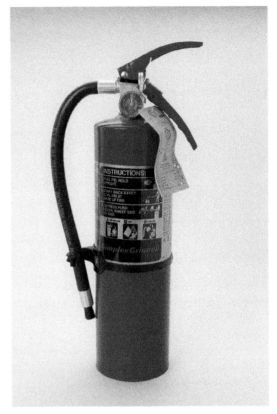

Figure 9-13
An ABC fire extinguisher is effective against all types of fires.

are kept in your facility. During your orientation, you will be trained in the use of your facility's fire extinguishers, and these instructions will be reviewed with you each year. In the event of a small fire, you should be able to use a fire extinguisher to put the fire out safely and effectively. When using a fire extinguisher, remember the word **PASS:**

Pull the safety pin out.
Aim the hose toward the base of the fire.
Squeeze the handle.
Spray the contents of the fire extinguisher at the base of the fire, sweeping from side to side.

Evacuating the Building

If a large, uncontrollable fire breaks out, you will need to know how to get your patients or residents and yourself to safety. Health care facilities must regularly practice and evaluate fire safety plans. You should take these fire drill exercises seriously so that if a fire emergency should occur,

Table 9-1   Types of Fires

TYPE	DESCRIPTION	METHOD OF EXTINGUISHING
A	Fueled by ordinary material such as wood, paper, cloth, leaves, and grass	Water effectively extinguishes a Type A fire by removing the heat.
B	Fueled by a petroleum product (e.g., gasoline, automotive oil), cooking oil, or grease	Do not try to put these fires out with water! Instead, smother the fire by sprinkling powder (such as baking soda) on it or by using a fire extinguisher made for a Type B fire. A stovetop fire that starts in a pan can be extinguished by covering the pan and removing it from the heat source.
C	An electrical fire	Attempting to put an electrical fire out with water can result in shock or electrocution. Use a fire extinguisher that is specific to an electrical fire instead.

your actions will be almost second nature. By knowing what to do and acting calmly, you will increase the efficiency of the evacuation and help to calm those around you.

DISASTER PREPAREDNESS

A **disaster** is a sudden, unexpected event that causes injury to many people, major damage to property, or both. Disasters can be caused by acts of nature (such as tornadoes, earthquakes, hurricanes, floods, blizzards, or ice storms), or they may be the result of explosions, accidents, or acts of war or terrorism. Acts of terrorism can easily be targeted at vulnerable areas such as health care facilities and schools. These acts could include the use of explosives, the release of chemicals (for example, nerve gas agents), or the release of biological agents (such as anthrax).

Your facility or agency will have a disaster preparedness plan that will direct the actions of the health care team in the event of such an occurrence. If you work for a hospital, your facility's disaster plan may focus on preparing staff to handle the simultaneous admission and treatment of multiple people with injuries. If you work in a nursing facility, the focus of your facility's disaster plan may be more on how to provide safe care for your residents in the event of a power failure. In the event of a disaster, you may have to help evacuate residents and patients to safer quarters. Know the particular duties that will be required of you in the event of a disaster and remain calm.

SUMMARY

- There are many factors that contribute to workplace safety and there are many people that the safety of the workplace affects.
  - It is your responsibility to help make your workplace safe, both for yourself and others, by following the guidelines for safety and by reporting any unsafe conditions to the appropriate person.
  - The Canadian Center for Occupational Health and Safety (CCOHS) oversees safety regulations in all types of workplaces and addresses everything from safe lifting techniques to the control of hazardous materials.
    - CCOHS mandates that employers inform workers of all safety risks that are present in their workplace.
    - CCOHS requires employers to provide regular training about the safety risks in the work environment, and how injury is to be avoided. Your employer must keep records of any training you have received that meets CCOHS regulations.
- Practicing good body mechanics allows you to use your body effectively when lifting and moving patients and equipment, and helps to protect you from injury as you perform your daily duties.
  - The "ABCs" of good body mechanics are alignment, balance, and coordinated movement.
  - Learning proper lifting technique is especially critical to preventing back injuries.
- Following procedures when providing patient or resident care helps to ensure that the care you provide is safe and correct.
  - Pre-procedure actions ("Getting Ready" steps) are taken before every patient or resident care procedure. These actions promote efficiency, safety, and respect of the patient's or resident's rights.
  - Post-procedure actions ("Finishing Up" steps) are taken after every patient or resident care procedure. These actions promote comfort, safety, and communication among members of the health care team.
- Falling poses a risk to both the health care worker and the patient or resident. Asking for assistance and knowing how to properly assist a person who is falling can help to prevent injuries to everyone involved.
- Most health care facilities use many chemicals in their daily operation. Information about how to respond to a chemical exposure is found on the Materials Safety Data Sheet (MSDS), which each chemical manufacturer must supply, and on the labeled container.
- Malfunctioning electrical appliances, or electrical appliances that are used improperly, can lead to electric shock, electrocution, and electrical fires.
- A fire in a health care facility can have tragic consequences because many of the people who are housed in health care facilities are unable to move independently or quickly in the event of a fire.
  - Three elements are necessary to start a fire and keep it burning: fuel, heat, and oxygen.
  - The RACE fire response plan describes the general actions that are to be taken in the event of a fire emergency: **R**emove people in the immediate area, **A**ctivate the alarm, **C**ontain the fire, and **E**xtinguish or **E**vacuate as indicated by the situation.
  - In the event of a disaster, follow your facility's disaster preparedness plan.

WHAT DID YOU LEARN?

Multiple Choice

Select the single best answer for each of the following questions.

1. In the event of a fire in a resident's room, your first action should be to:
   a. Remove the resident to a safe place
   b. Get the fire extinguisher
   c. Sound the fire alarm
   d. Notify the head nurse

2. When lifting, remember to use the large muscles of your:
   a. Chest
   b. Hips, buttocks, and thighs
   c. Back
   d. Shoulders

3. You accidentally knock over a water pitcher, spilling water on the floor of a patient's room. What should you do?
   a. Call housekeeping
   b. Continue with your assignment and make a mental note to wipe up the spill later
   c. Throw a towel over the spill to absorb the liquid and alert others to be careful
   d. Wipe the spill up immediately

4. While you are walking with Mrs. Davis in the hallway, she complains of dizziness. Your first response should be to:
   a. Assist her into a nearby chair and call for help
   b. Assist her to the floor and go get help
   c. Ask Mrs. Davis to breathe deeply and reassure her that everything will be fine
   d. Encourage Mrs. Davis to continue walking because she needs the exercise

5. As you come around the corner on your unit, you hear Mrs. Petersen shouting in alarm, and you see smoke and flames coming from the wastebasket in her room. You should:
   a. Run to the telephone and call the fire department
   b. Take Mrs. Petersen's cigarettes away
   c. Assist Mrs. Petersen out of the room and close the door
   d. Throw water on the flames

6. Using good body mechanics to lift an object off the floor means that you would:
   a. Use a mechanical lift
   b. Kneel down to get the broadest base of support and lift up

   c. Squat and lift with your legs
   d. Lean over at the waist, keeping your back flat

7. Unsafe conditions in a health care facility can be caused by:
   a. Health care workers who allow patients or residents to get out of bed
   b. Health care workers who stop doing an assigned task to clean up a spill
   c. Overloaded outlets and extension cords
   d. Patients and residents who smoke in "smoking only" areas

8. All of the following actions could cause a fire except:
   a. Using a three-prong plug
   b. Emptying an ashtray into a wastebasket
   c. Smoking in a room where a person is receiving oxygen therapy
   d. Placing a stack of linens on a heating unit to warm them

9. Where should you direct the foam when using a fire extinguisher to put out a fire?
   a. At the base of the fire
   b. In a circle around the fire, to prevent the fire from spreading
   c. At the top of the fire
   d. Anywhere in the general area of the fire

10. What are the "ABCs" of good body mechanics?
    a. Assess, Balance, Complete
    b. Assign, Begin, Complete
    c. Alignment, Balance, Coordinated movement
    d. Attempt, Brace, Change

11. You are a new personal support worker and have been assigned to clean the room of a resident who has just been discharged. The nurse shows you the cleaning closet, which contains towels, rags, and containers holding liquids and powders of various colors and odours. How can you find out what cleaning products are appropriate for your assigned task?
    a. Read the care plan
    b. Read the Material Safety Data Sheet (MSDS)
    c. Use your senses—smell the contents of each container and use whichever has the most pleasant smell

d. There is no need to find out which product is most appropriate—the cleaning closet contains only products used for cleaning

12. Following pre-procedure and post-procedure actions before and after each procedure is important to:
    a. Prevent the patient or resident from becoming confused
    b. Ensure that the care you give is safe and correct
    c. Make the nurse happy
    d. Pass the certification exam

13. Which one of the following is a pre-procedure ("Getting Ready") step?
    a. Report and record
    b. Identify the person
    c. Confirm that the person is comfortable and in good body alignment
    d. Open the curtain or door

14. How do you "see to safety" before and after performing a procedure?
    a. Use good body mechanics
    b. Use equipment properly
    c. Practice infection control
    d. All of the above

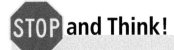

STOP and Think!

You work on the second floor of a long-term care facility. As you are walking down the hall toward the nursing station, you hear one of your residents, Miss Verna, call for help. When you look into her room, you see that her wastebasket is on fire. What should you do? Is it possible to accomplish more than one step of the RACE plan at once?

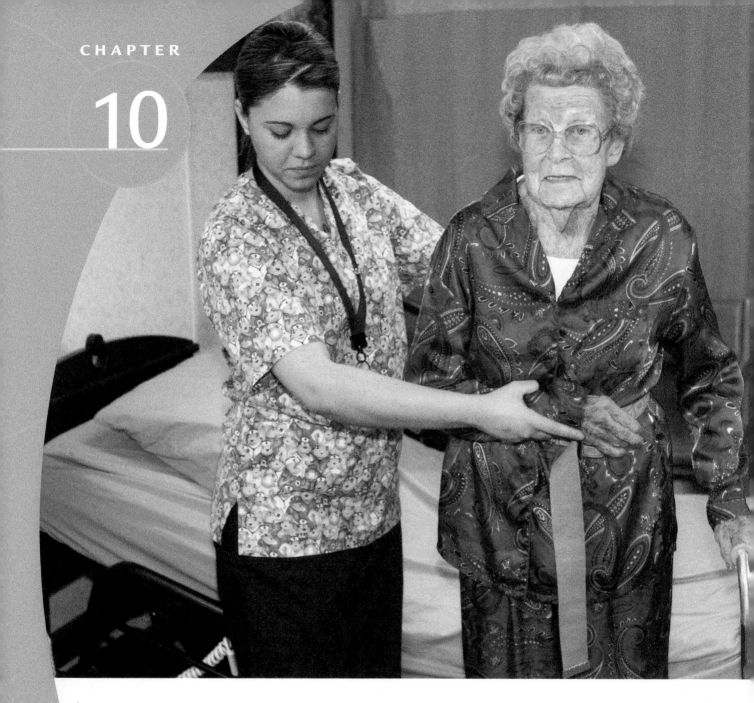

Patient and Resident Safety and Restraints

WHAT WILL YOU LEARN?

Life has taught us many lessons in safety. When you were a child, your parents reminded you to look both ways before crossing the street. As a teen learning to drive, you were cautioned to wear your seatbelt and to observe the rules of the road. As an adult, you

Photo: As a personal support worker, you will play an important role in keeping your patients or residents safe. Here, a personal support worker helps a resident to get out of bed safely.

remember to lock the door at night and turn off the coffeepot before you leave home. As you remember from Chapter 6, safety is a basic human need. If we feel safe, we can relax and rest and we feel secure and comfortable. The previous chapters have explained principles and procedures designed to help keep you safe while you perform your duties as a personal support worker. In this chapter, we will focus on principles and procedures that help to keep those you care for safe. When you are finished with this chapter, you will be able to:

1. Identify risk factors that may put people in a health care facility at higher risk for accidents and injury.
2. Describe basic safety methods designed to prevent accidents in a health care facility.
3. Understand the importance of reporting and recording accidents.
4. List the different types of restraints.
5. Identify safety concerns of restraint use.
6. Describe methods used to reduce the need for restraints.
7. Demonstrate the proper application of a vest restraint, a wrist or ankle restraint, and a lap or waist (belt) restraint.

Vocabulary

Paraplegia	Comatose	Physical restraint	Restraint alternatives
Quadriplegia	Incident (occurrence)	Chemical restraint	
Hemiplegia	report		

ACCIDENTS

RISK FACTORS

For many reasons, certain groups of people are more at risk than others to have an accident (Fig. 10-1). Recognizing the factors that can increase a person's chances of having an accident will help you minimize the chance that an accident will occur.

Age

Infants and young children are at high risk for accidents. Infants are helpless. As a result, they are prone to accidental suffocation and falls. Young children are not helpless, but they lack knowledge about things that are dangerous. As a result, young children are at risk for injuries such as falls, burns, poisoning, and drowning. You can find out more about safety issues related to children in Chapter 41.

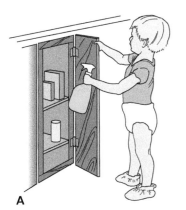
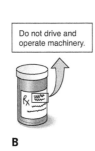
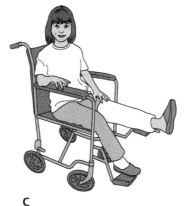
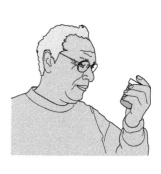

A   B   C   D

Figure 10-1
Some factors that place people at risk for accidents: **(A)** very young or very old age; **(B)** medication effects; **(C)** impaired mobility (an inability to move easily); **(D)** sensory impairment (an inability to see, hear, smell, taste, or detect pain or changes in temperature).

The elderly are at high risk for accidents also. Although an elderly person can recognize a dangerous situation, some of the physical and mental effects of the aging process can affect his or her ability to be safe.

Medication

The effects of medications, especially pain medications, can affect the ability of a person to be safe, regardless of age or other factors. For example, under the influence of a pain medication (which has a sedative effect), a person who normally smokes a cigarette while watching the evening news could fall asleep in front of the television while smoking, causing a fire. Driving and operating machinery are dangerous under the influence of some medications. Medications that affect blood pressure can cause a person to become dizzy if he or she stands up quickly, leading to a fall. Some medications cause confusion in the elderly, especially if they are not taken properly.

Paralysis

Paralysis (an inability to move or to feel) can be caused by a spinal cord injury or a stroke ("brain attack"). Depending on where a spinal cord injury occurs, a person can be paralyzed from the waist down, or from the neck down. Paralysis from the waist down is known as **paraplegia.** Paralysis from the neck down is known as **quadriplegia.** A quadriplegic or paraplegic person's abilities vary, according to the exact level of the spinal injury. A stroke can cause **hemiplegia,** or paralysis on one side of the body. Not only is a person with paraplegia, quadriplegia, or hemiplegia unable to move the affected areas of his body, he is usually unable to sense pain, heat, or cold in these areas. The inability to move properly increases the person's risk for falling. The lack of sensation increases the person's risk for other injuries, such as burns.

Poor Mobility

An inability to move easily can put a person at risk for falling. Pain and stiffness from arthritis can make it difficult for a person to get around easily. A stroke can sometimes cause a person to shuffle his feet when he walks. This can make a person more likely to trip over carpeted areas and uneven outside surfaces. Although elderly people tend to have more trouble with mobility than younger people, this is a risk factor that can affect all age groups. For example, a person recovering from knee surgery or a broken leg will be more likely to fall because of difficulty with mobility.

Sensory Impairment

We rely on our five senses (vision, hearing, touch, smell, and taste) to give us information about our environment and to keep us safe. Perhaps the sense we rely on the most is sight—not being able to see clearly can put anyone at risk for accidents. Poor vision increases the risk of falls, especially on stairs or over objects left on the floor. A person who wears bifocals may misjudge distance when stepping on or off curbs and steps, leading to falls. Additionally, poor vision can increase the chances of accidental poisoning from medications, if the person is not able to clearly read the directions on the medication label.

Our sense of hearing also plays a large role in keeping us safe. A person with hearing difficulties may not be able to hear signs of danger approaching, such as the sound of an oncoming car. She may also miss warning alarms, such as the sound made by a smoke or carbon monoxide detector. When receiving instructions or directions (for example, regarding how to take a medication), a hearing-impaired person may be able to hear part of what is being said, but not enough to understand completely.

Touch and smell play a role in informing us about our environment as well. Certain conditions, such as diabetes, can decrease a person's sense of touch. People with an impaired sense of touch may not be able to tell that their bath water is too hot, leading to increased risk for burns. Because their ability to feel pain is lessened, they may be unaware that a favorite pair of shoes is causing blisters, leading to infection. Similarly, a decreased ability to smell (such as often occurs as part of the normal aging process) can leave a person unable to detect spoiled food, a natural gas leak in the home, or smoke.

Limited Awareness of Surroundings

There are many reasons a person may not be aware of his surroundings. Confusion and disorientation can be caused by reactions to medication, head injuries, dementia, and other medical conditions. It can also be caused by something as simple as a change in environment or forgetting to put one's glasses on. Confusion can cause a person in a health care facility to forget to call for help when he needs to get up. A person who is unconscious or **comatose** is totally unable to respond to his environment and will also need your assistance to remain safe.

As you can see, there are many factors that can affect a person's ability to avoid accidents. When several of these factors are combined, complex safety issues can result. As a personal support worker, you must evaluate each person and situation individually so that you can provide a safe environment for those you care for.

AVOIDING ACCIDENTS

Many accidents that occur in health care facilities could have been prevented. Most safety measures do require an extra step or two, meaning more work for already overworked staff members. However, remember your obligation to provide the same quality of care for your patients or residents that you would want for a member of your own family. Take that extra step to help ensure the safety of those you care for.

Preventing Falls

Falls are the leading cause of accidental death among elderly people. Falls are also the most common type of accident that occurs in the health care setting. In Chapter 9, you learned how to assist a person who is falling. However, preventing a fall is always the best policy.

Many health care facilities, especially hospitals and long-term care facilities, evaluate each new patient or resident for factors that increase the person's risk for falls (Fig. 10-2). Measures that can be taken to prevent falls are then included in the person's care plan. Guidelines for preventing falls are given in Guidelines Box 10-1.

PATIENT FALL RISK SCORES					Patient Score			
					TIME			
PARAMETERS	4	3	2	1				
Age	–	80+	70 to 79	–				
Mental status	Intermittent confusion or impulsiveness (or both)	–	Confused (baseline)	–				
Elimination	Can't wait or won't wait	Independent and incontinent	Needs assistance	Indwelling catheter				
History of falling	History of multiple falls (3 or more)	–	Has fallen 1 or 2 times	–				
Gait and balance	Unsteady or poor balance standing or walking	Orthostatic hypotension	–	Needs supervision or assistance with equipment				
Medications (By drug class below)	3 or more drug classes	2 drug classes	1 drug class	–				

TOTAL RISK SCORES

Drug classes:
1. **Cardiovascular** (antihypertensives, vasodilators, antiarrhythmics, nitrates)
2. **Psychoactive** (sedatives, hypnotics, barbiturates, anxiolytics, antihistamines, anticonvulsants, antidepressants)
3. **Pain** (narcotics, patient-controlled analgesia, epidural)
4. **Diuretics and cathartics**
5. **Anesthetics** (first 24 hours post-op)

Total risk scores:
9 to 20 = extremely high risk
5 to 8 = high risk
0 to 4 = low risk
If score is > 4, falls prevention protocol should be implemented.

DATE	TIME	NAME

Figure 10-2
Many health care facilities use a form like this one to assess a new patient's or resident's risk of falling. Once the risk factors are known, precautions can be taken to decrease the person's risk of falling. (*Adapted with permission from Abington Memorial Hospital Department of Nursing, Abington, PA.*)

Guidelines Box 10-1 Guidelines for Preventing Falls

WHAT YOU DO	WHY YOU DO IT
Check the person's clothing and shoes. Clothing should fit properly. Shoes should provide good foot support and have nonskid soles.	Long or loose clothing (such as a robe) or shoes that provide inadequate foot support or have slippery soles could lead to tripping.
Encourage the person to use rails along hallways and stairways while walking.	The additional support offered by rails may be all that is needed to allow a person to move about safely and independently.
Observe the person for signs of unsteadiness and offer physical assistance as needed.	Offering assistance as needed allows the person to remain as independent as possible, while minimizing the risk of falls.
Observe the person's ability to use walking aids, such as canes and walkers, and correct incorrect use.	Using a piece of equipment improperly can be just as hazardous as not using it at all.
Check equipment, such as walkers and wheelchairs, to ensure that it is in good condition. Nonskid tips should be intact on walkers. Wheelchair wheel locks should function properly.	Malfunctioning or broken equipment increases a person's risk for accidents.
Make sure a patient or resident who needs glasses is wearing them when he or she is out of bed.	A person who cannot see clearly is more at risk for falls.
Remove any clutter or obstacles from walkways and provide adequate lighting.	Proper lighting enhances the ability to see. Removal of obstructions is an easy way to minimize falls.
Keep beds in the lowest position. Keep bed wheels locked.	Keeping the bed in the lowest position minimizes the distance from the bed to the floor, should the person fall out of bed. Keeping the wheels on the bed locked prevents the bed from rolling. A rolling bed could result in injury to the personal support worker, the patient or resident, or both.
Keep side rails up or down, according to the care plan for that particular person.	Side rails can prevent a person from falling out of bed. Because side rails are considered a form of restraint, they should always be lowered, unless the person's medical condition is such that he or she needs the protection that is offered by having the side rails raised.
Always make sure the call light control is within easy reach of the person. Answer call lights promptly, and offer to help the person with toileting frequently.	Many falls are the result of a person trying to make it to the bathroom without assistance.

Guidelines Box 10-1	Guidelines for Preventing Falls (continued)
WHAT YOU DO	*WHY YOU DO IT*
Wipe up any spills immediately.	Wet surfaces may not be obvious (especially to people with some degree of visual impairment) and greatly increase the risk of slipping.
Keep people who are at risk for falling and disoriented close to the nurses' station. Offer frequent assistance with walking.	Keeping a person who is disoriented and at risk for falling close to the nurses' station allows staff to "keep an eye" on the person, and also minimizes the chance that a person who feels lonely will try to get up to look for company. A person who is offered help with walking on a regular basis is less likely to try to get up on his or her own, thereby minimizing the chance of a fall.
Orient a newly admitted patient or resident to the unit and his or her room.	Falls and other accidents often occur when a person is unfamiliar with his or her surroundings.

Preventing Burns

As you learned earlier, people who have a reduced sense of touch (reduced sensation) may be at risk for burns. A burn can be life-threatening to a patient or resident. Measures for preventing burns include the following:

- If a person will be taking a tub bath or shower, always check the water temperature first using a bath thermometer. The water temperature should be between 40.5°C (105°F) and 46°C (115°F). If the person is elderly, the water temperature should be at the lower end of this range. Many long-term care facilities have whirlpool tubs that allow you to set the water temperature before filling the tub.
- If you will be giving a person a bed bath, you should measure the temperature of the water in the basin. The water in the basin can be hotter than the water in a bathtub or shower because it cools off quickly and the person will not be immersed in it. The temperature range for a bed bath is between 43.3°C (110°F) and 46°C (115°F).
- Teach patients or residents who will be bathing themselves to check the water temperature with a thermometer or a hand or wrist before getting into the bathtub or shower.
- Use extreme care with heat applications (discussed in detail in Chapter 25).
- Warn people that a food or beverage is hot before giving it to them. Many burns occur

when hot liquids (such as soup, coffee, or tea) spill. Some people may need a cup with a lid for their coffee or tea if weakness or unsteadiness puts them at risk for spilling.
- Follow the guidelines for using electrical appliances that are given in Chapter 9. Electrical burns can occur if an appliance malfunctions or is used near water.

Preventing Accidental Poisonings

Many people think of accidental poisonings as a problem that affects only children, but elderly people are at risk for accidental poisonings too. Poor eyesight, confusion, or a decreased sense of taste or smell can cause an elderly person to eat or drink something that will cause her harm. Accidental poisonings can also occur if a person takes too much, or the wrong, medication. An elderly person might not be able to read the medication label, or he might forget that he has already taken his medication that day, and take it again. To minimize the risk of accidental poisonings:

- Never store household cleaners or other chemicals in containers meant for food or beverages.
- Keep household cleaners and chemicals in a locked cabinet.
- Make sure the contents of all containers are clearly marked on the outside.
- Provide help with reading labels as necessary.

REPORTING ACCIDENTS

Accidents will happen despite the precautions taken by even the most conscientious of health care workers. Some accidents occur as a result of faulty equipment or from unfamiliarity with new equipment. Other accidents are the result of carelessness on the part of a health care worker or family member of the patient or resident involved. When accidents do occur, you must know exactly how to report the accident at your particular facility or organization.

All accidents are to be verbally reported immediately to the nurse. In addition, most facilities require the accident to be reported in written form as well. This written report is called an **incident (occurrence) report.** It generally takes the form of a preprinted document that must be completed (Fig. 10-3). Information about the accident should be provided in a straightforward and factual manner, without opinion or blame.

The completed incident (occurrence) report is used by the quality assurance department and is very important for follow-up. For example, consider a situation where an accident has occurred because a wheelchair's brakes did not hold properly. Following the completion of the proper forms by the personal support worker, the quality assurance department might find that several similar accidents have occurred with wheelchairs of the same type, or after repairs from the same shop, or on the same shift of work scheduling. This would show a trend that could help prevent accidents like this from happening in the future.

Some health care workers hesitate to report an accident because they feel responsible for the accident or are afraid they will be blamed for the accident. Other times, they know that a co-worker will be blamed for carelessness and do not want to report the co-worker's error to a supervisor. As described in Chapter 3, the personal support worker must be honest and dependable in carrying out her duties. Reporting accidents promptly helps to protect your patients, your facility, and yourself.

RESTRAINTS

Restraints, referred to as "reminder devices" in some facilities, are sometimes necessary to help keep a person safe. Restraints are used to restrict a person's freedom of movement, or to prevent a person from reaching parts of his body. For example, a restraint might be used for an agitated, disoriented patient who continually tries to remove an intravenous (IV) line from her arm.

Restraints can be either physical or chemical. A **physical restraint** is a device that is attached to or near a person's body to limit a person's freedom of movement or access to her body (Fig. 10-4). Physical restraints confine a person to a bed or a chair or prevent movement of a specific body part and cannot be easily removed by the restrained person. Physical restraints can be applied to parts of the body, such as the wrists, ankles, chest, waist, or elbows. Additionally, some types of chairs or attachments to chairs can act as restraints. So can the side rails of beds or tightly tucked sheets. Not permitting a person free access to other rooms or parts of the facility is also considered a form of physical restraint.

A **chemical restraint** is any medication that alters a person's mood or behaviour, such as a sedative or tranquilizer. There is a fine line between using medications to help calm an anxious, combative (physically aggressive), or agitated (very upset) person and using medications for staff convenience. These medications should assist in the control of anxiety, combative behaviour, or agitation. They should not be used in so high a dose as to make the person sleepy or unable to function in a normal fashion.

USE OF RESTRAINTS

Restraints are never used as punishment or for the staff's convenience. They are used to provide postural support, to protect the patient or resident from harm, or to protect the staff from harm (in the case of a combative or violent patient). Restraints are to be used only if all other methods have failed (see the section below "Restraint Alternatives") and the person is considered to be a danger to herself or others if restraints are not applied. Examples of situations where the use of restraints may be appropriate (Fig. 10-5) include, but are not limited to:

- A person who is at risk for falling but cannot remember to call for help before attempting to get up
- A person who is at risk for wandering away from a facility, because of dementia
- A person who attempts to remove or pull out tubing necessary for medical treatment (this is particularly common among small children, confused patients or residents, and patients or residents who are intubated and uncomfortable)

COMMUNITY NURSING SERVICE
INCIDENT REPORT

EMPLOYEE INVOLVED:

Name: _____

Address: _____

Phone: _____

Employee: _____
(RN, PT, Aide, etc.)

PATIENT INVOLVED:

Name: _____

Address: _____

Phone: _____

FID #: _____

OTHERS INVOLVED: Name: _____ Phone: _____

Address: _____ Relationship: _____

- -

Date of Incident: _____ Time of Incident: _____

Location of Incident: _____

Incident Reported to: _____ Time: _____ Date: _____

DESCRIPTION OF INCIDENT: (Complete Workers Comp. form if on-job injury)

_____
Employee Signature

FOLLOW-UP

Family aware of incident: _____

Physician aware of incident: _____

Action Taken:

Follow-up / Supervisor's Comments:

Figure 10-3

An incident (occurrence) report like this one must be completed if an accident occurs. The report provides information that might help to prevent a similar accident from happening again.

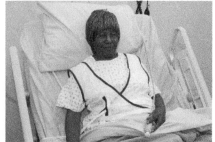

A. Vest restraint

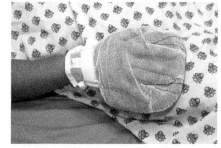

D. Mitt restraint

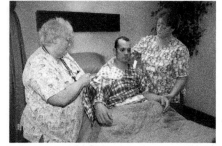

B. Jacket restraint

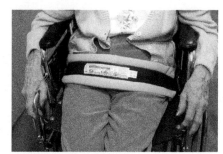

E. Lap restraint

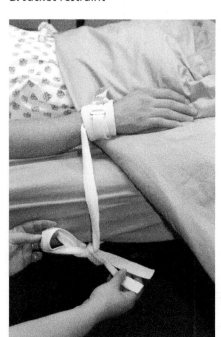

C. Wrist restraint

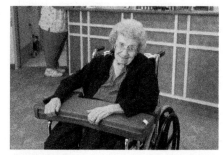

F. Lap buddy

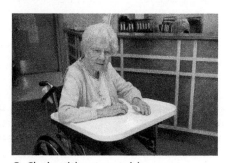

G. Chair with a tray table

Figure 10-4
Physical restraints are attached on or near a person's body. They limit freedom of movement. Some examples of physical restraints are shown here. **(A)** A vest restraint. **(B)** A jacket restraint. **(C)** A wrist restraint. **(D)** A mitt restraint. **(E)** A lap restraint. **(F)** A lap buddy and **(G)** a chair with a tray table are considered restraints if the person cannot remove the lap buddy or tray table independently.

- A person who has overdosed on alcohol or medications and is demonstrating combative behaviour (due to withdrawal symptoms) or is on suicide precautions

The use of restraints is clearly defined in legal guidelines and standards issued by health care facilities. The improper use of restraints can be considered holding a person against his or her will, or false imprisonment. Current standards of care set forth by Canadian hospitals and long-term care facilities require that health care facilities minimize their use of restraints, or follow a policy of "least restraint." Each health care facility has policies and procedures detailing the use of restraints for patients and residents. As a personal support worker, you must understand your facility's policies, and your responsibilities, regarding the use of restraints. Failure to follow these policies can result in a situation that is dangerous for your patient or resident.

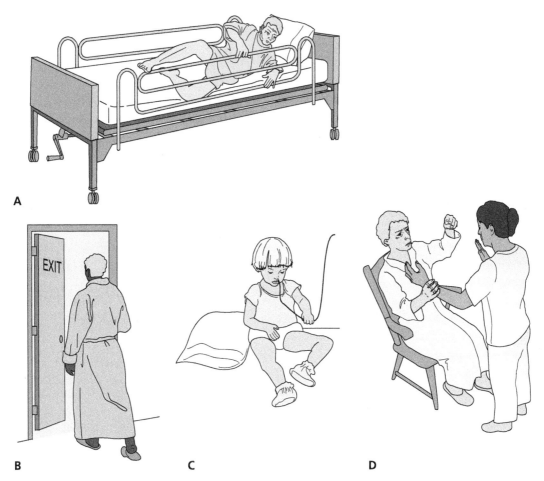

Figure 10-5
Restraints are to be used only with a doctor's order and only if the person is considered to be a danger to himself or others if restraints are not applied. The use of restraints is a last resort. However, in some situations, the use of a restraint may be appropriate. **(A)** A person who is at risk for falling but will not stay in his bed or a chair and will not call for help may need to be restrained. **(B)** A person who may wander away from the facility may need to be restrained. **(C)** A person who tries to remove tubing needed for medical treatment may need to be restrained. **(D)** A person who is combative (physically aggressive) may need to be restrained.

Additionally, failure to follow these policies can leave you and your facility open for litigation. Guidelines for the use of restraints are given in Guidelines Box 10-2.

COMPLICATIONS ASSOCIATED WITH RESTRAINT USE

Many complications can result from the use of restraints. Restraints are dangerous even when used properly, but doubly so if they are not. A person who is restrained is eight times more likely to die than a person who is not restrained. Consider the following:

- Strangulation (cutting off the person's air supply) can occur if a vest restraint is

improperly applied or if the restraint gets tangled in a piece of furniture.
- Bruises, nerve damage, and skin abrasions can result if a restrained person pulls at the restraint.
- Permanent tissue damage as a result of impaired blood flow can occur if a restraint is placed incorrectly or too tightly. All of the tissues of the body require oxygen to live, and oxygen is carried to the tissues in the blood. If something stops blood from flowing to a certain part of the body, the affected tissues can be permanently damaged from lack of oxygen. In some cases, amputation (removal of a limb) may even be necessary.
- Broken bones and other serious injuries can occur if a restrained person tries to get out

Guidelines Box 10-2 Guidelines for Using Restraints

WHAT YOU DO	WHY YOU DO IT
Do not use a restraint without a written doctor's order that states the reason for the restraint.	Canadian hospitals and long-term care facilities protect patients and residents from being unnecessarily restrained through policy and procedure—the philosophy of "least restraint."
Never use a restraint to "punish" a patient or resident, or for your own convenience.	Physically and emotionally, the use of restraints has a very negative impact on the person's quality of life. Therefore, restraints are only used when absolutely necessary, after all other methods of ensuring the person's safety have failed.
Use the least restrictive restraint for the least amount of time.	Minimizing the use of restraints is important to preserve the person's quality of life.
Follow the manufacturer's instructions, nurse's direction, and facility policy for applying restraints.	Improper application of restraints can lead to serious medical complications, injury, or even death.
Use a restraint that is the correct size and in good condition.	If the restraint is too large, the person may be able to remove it, either completely or partially. This puts the person at risk for falling and strangulation. If the restraint is too small, complications such as restriction of blood supply to areas beyond the restraint can result. If the restraint is in poor condition, it may not properly restrain the person, or the person may be injured when the restraint is applied.
Use commercial restraints. Do not use makeshift restraints, such as bed sheets or locks.	Using anything other than a commercial restraint to restrain a person is unprofessional and dangerous.
Restraints are always applied over clothing, pajamas, or a gown.	Clothing offers a layer of protection between the restraint and the person's skin.
Restraints are tied in simple, quick-release knots placed out of reach of the patient's or resident's hands.	Quick-release knots must be used in case a person needs to be released from the restraint quickly due to an emergency (for example, choking).
Ensure that you have enough help when applying a restraint.	Attempting to apply a restraint to an uncooperative, combative person can lead to injury of the person, you, or both.
Check on the restrained person every 15 minutes to make sure that feeling and blood flow are normal in any restrained extremity (arm or leg).	A restraint that is applied too tightly can lead to poor blood flow, which in turn can lead to permanent tissue or nerve damage. In addition, checking on the person regularly helps to prevent him or her from feeling abandoned.

(continued)

Guidelines Box 10-2 Guidelines for Using Restraints (continued)

WHAT YOU DO	WHY YOU DO IT
Completely remove the restraint every 2 hours, for a total of 10 minutes.	Releasing the restraint allows you to reposition the person. All patients and residents should be repositioned at least every 2 hours, whether they are restrained or not.
Record any care given to a restrained person promptly and according to your facility's policy.	In a litigation situation, any action not recorded is considered not done. You can provide the best care possible, but if you do not record it, your effort will not protect you or your facility if legal action is taken.
Use restraints only if you have been properly trained in their use.	**Incorrect use of restraints can result in death!**

of the restraints. For example, a person restrained in a chair may still try to get up, which could result in injury if the chair overturns. Similarly, a person who is improperly restrained in a bed could slide between the bed and the side rails, or attempt to climb over the side rails, actions that could lead to injury or death if the restraint gets caught in the side rails.

- Pneumonia, pressure ulcers, and blood clots (complications of immobility) can occur if a person is left in a restraint for too long.
- Incontinence (an inability to control one's bowel, bladder, or both) can occur if a person is not taken to the bathroom regularly.
- The mental effects associated with the use of restraints can be serious and include agitation, increased confusion, humiliation, and embarrassment.

Helping Hands and a Caring Heart

FOCUS ON HUMANISTIC HEALTH CARE

Physically and emotionally, restraints have a very negative impact on a person's quality of life. Imagine how you would feel if you had to be "tied down." You might feel embarrassed, frightened, or humiliated. As a personal support worker, there are many things you can do that may eliminate or reduce the need for restraints. These things require planning and effort, but the effort is considered part of the quality, individualized care that should be given to each person.

RESTRAINT ALTERNATIVES

Although the use of physical or chemical restraints is not forbidden by any regulating agency, measures must be taken to avoid their use. In other words, **restraint alternatives** must be sought and used. The measures taken to avoid the use of restraints on a person must be documented before resorting to the use of restraints to protect that person's safety.

Some alternatives to using chemical or physical restraints are shown in Figure 10-6. For example, a personal support worker can:

- Provide an environment in which the person feels safe and secure. Placing a confused person close to the nurses' station, where he can be observed and the person can, in turn, watch others and not feel left alone, is often helpful. Taking time to speak to the person often or sitting beside him while you complete paperwork offers the person company and companionship. Soft music, television, or other methods of entertainment can be calming.

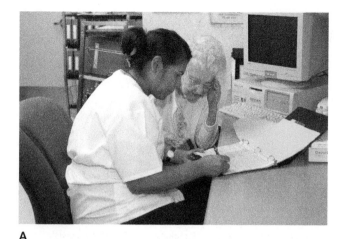

A

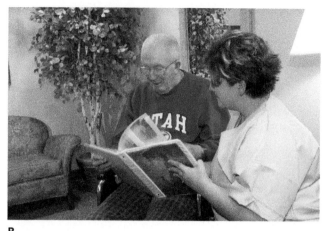

B

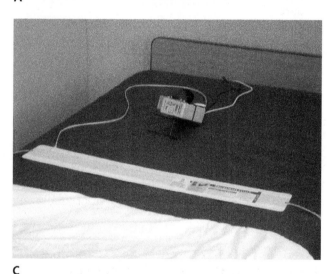

C

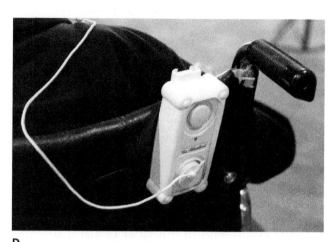

D

Figure 10-6

Alternatives to physical and chemical restraints should always be tried first. **(A)** Moving the person to a place, such as near the nurses' station, can help ease feelings of loneliness. Sometimes all people want is company or to be where the action is. **(B)** Volunteers, other residents, or family members can be called on to provide company to a person too. **(C)** A pressure-sensitive bed monitoring system is shown here. The pressure-sensing mat is secured across the mattress (under the sheet), located where the person's buttocks will be. The monitor, shown here next to the mat, is then usually hung from the headboard, out of the person's reach and sight. If the person tries to get out of bed, an alarm will sound, alerting the staff that the person needs help. Systems like this are helpful for patients or residents who are likely to fall if they try to get up unassisted. Similar systems are available for chair or wheelchair seats as well. **(D)** A wanderer monitoring system is a sensor that is attached to the person's wheelchair or worn around the wrist or ankle. If the person tries to leave the facility through a doorway that leads to an unsafe area, an alarm will sound, alerting the staff so that someone can guide the person back to safety. Systems like this are useful for patients or residents who are likely to stray away from the facility, such as those with dementia. (*C, courtesy of Bed-Check® Corp., Tulsa, OK.*)

- Provide frequent attention to the person's physical needs. Take the person to the bathroom and offer a drink or snack regularly, per facility policy or more frequently if necessary. Assist the person with walking or change her position frequently, to help maintain comfort.

Answer call lights promptly and make sure that the call light control is within easy reach of the person.
- Explain procedures and reassure the person. Being in a situation or having a condition that requires the use of restraints can be confusing and embarrassing.

- Get help from family members, volunteers, or other residents of the facility. Providing companionship can be an effective alternative to the use of restraints. Additionally, this approach improves the quality of a person's life.
- Use restraint methods that are less restrictive. For example, pressure-sensitive alarm systems are placed on a person's wheelchair seat or bed. If the person tries to get up without help, the alarm will sound, alerting the staff. Sometimes the alarm will remind the person to call for help when he needs to get up. Another type of alarm system, called a wanderer monitoring system, involves a small sensor that is worn around the wrist or ankle, or placed on the person's wheelchair. If the person tries to leave the facility, an alarm will sound, alerting the staff so that the person can be gently and safely led back inside. These sensors work the same way as anti-shoplifting devices in shopping malls.

APPLYING RESTRAINTS

In some situations, restraint alternatives will not be enough to keep the patient or resident safe, and it will be necessary to apply a physical restraint. Only a doctor can order a restraint for a patient or resident. If a doctor orders a restraint for one of your patients or residents, always follow your facility's policies regarding the application and use of restraints in order to protect yourself, your facility, and, most important, your patient or resident.

Most facilities require either a registered nurse (RN)/registered psychiatric nurse (RPN) or a licensed practical nurse (LPN)/registered nursing assistant (RNA) to apply the restraint, but as a personal support worker, you will be responsible for providing care for the person while he is restrained. For example, you must check on the person every 15 minutes and help him with repositioning, range-of-motion exercises, and meeting nutritional and toileting needs. The restraint must be removed every 2 hours. Be sure to consider how frightening and humiliating it can be for a person to be restrained. Do not forget to provide the care necessary to meet the person's emotional, as well as his physical, needs. All care that you give to a restrained person must be recorded promptly.

In addition to providing and recording care, you will also be responsible for observing the person's response to the restraint and reporting any signs of trouble to the nurse immediately.

TELL THE NURSE

Each time you attend to a person who is wearing a restraint, you should be alert to signs and symptoms related to the use of the restraint. Tell the nurse immediately if:

- The restrained person complains of, or shows any signs of, shortness of breath or difficulty breathing
- The hand or foot beyond the restraint is pale, blue, or cold
- The restrained person complains of pain, numbness, or tingling at or below a restrained body part
- The restrained person has become more confused, disoriented, or agitated

Any restraint that is tied should be tied with a "quick-release" knot (Fig. 10-7). A quick-release knot, or slip knot, will hold tightly if the restrained person pulls against it, but can be undone quickly by pulling on its "tails." The use of a quick-release knot will allow you to free a person from a restraint quickly in the event of an emergency.

Applying a Vest Restraint

A vest restraint is applied to a person's chest to protect the person from falling out of bed or a chair. The person's arms are placed through the armholes of the vest, and the flaps of the vest are crossed over each other, across the person's chest. A vest restraint should never be put on backward (that is, with the back of the vest on the person's chest and the flaps crossed across her back). Putting the vest on backward can cause the person to strangle if she slides down against the improperly placed restraint, because the back of the restraint is higher than the front. The procedure for applying a vest restraint is given in Procedure 10-1.

A jacket restraint is similar to a vest restraint, in that it is applied to the chest, but a jacket restraint has sleeves and closes in the back.

Applying Wrist or Ankle Restraints

In some cases, wrist or ankle restraints are applied to keep a person from moving his arms, legs, or both. When keeping a person in bed is the goal, the doctor may specify the number of extremities that are to be restrained. For example, a two-point restraint would involve two extremities (for example, both wrists), a three-point restraint

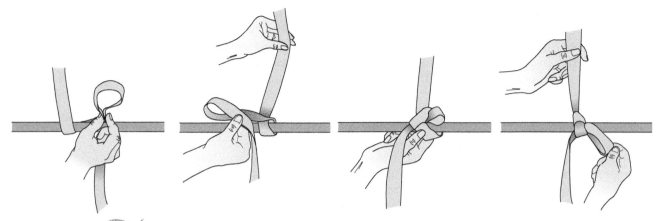

Figure 10-7 Watch & Learn

To make a quick-release knot, make a regular overhand knot, but slip a loop (instead of the end of the strap) through the first loop.

would involve three extremities, and a four-point restraint would involve all four extremities.

Although wrist restraints are sometimes used to confine a person to bed, a more common use is to prevent a person from removing tubes and catheters. When preventing a person from removing a tube or catheter is the purpose of the wrist restraint, a mitt restraint may be used instead. This mitten-like variation of a wrist restraint restricts finger movement. A mitt restraint prevents the person from grasping tubes or catheters, but allows for more freedom of arm movement.

The procedure for applying wrist or ankle restraints is given in Procedure 10-2.

Applying Lap or Waist (Belt) Restraints

Lap restraints are used to prevent a person from sliding out of a chair. Waist (belt) restraints can be used to secure a person in a chair or in a bed. The procedure for applying a lap or waist (belt) restraint is given in Procedure 10-3.

SUMMARY

- Safety is a basic human need.
  - If we feel safe, we can relax and rest because we feel secure and comfortable.
  - Personal support workers are responsible for helping to ensure the safety of those they care for.
- There are many factors that can put a person at increased risk for an accident, including age, impaired mobility, use of certain medications, and sensory impairment.
- Most accidents that occur in a health care facility are avoidable.
  - Providing for the safety of those we care for is a never-ending process.
  - A personal support worker must be continuously aware, observing patients and residents and their environment for safety risks. Personal support workers must also perform their duties in accordance with specified policies and procedures that have been established for safety.

- If an accident does occur, it should be reported immediately and an incident (occurrence) report should be completed promptly. Proper reporting and recording of accidents helps to protect your patients and residents, your facility, and yourself.
- Restraints are sometimes necessary to help ensure a person's safety. Because the use of restraints can be associated with complications (and possibly even death), restraints are used only when all other measures to ensure a person's safety have failed.
  - Restraints are never used to punish a person, or for the convenience of the staff.
  - Physically and emotionally, restraints have a very negative impact on a person's quality of life. The use of restraints requires extra care on the part of the personal support worker to protect the patient's or resident's safety and dignity.

Applying a Vest Restraint

WHY YOU DO IT   A vest restraint is applied to a person's chest to prevent the person from falling out of bed or a chair.

Getting Ready WORKTEPS

1. Complete the "Getting Ready" steps.

Supplies

- vest restraint in proper size

Procedure

2. Get help from a nurse or another personal support worker, if necessary.

3. Assist the person to a sitting position by locking arms with him or her.

4. Support the person's back and shoulders with one arm while slipping the person's arms through the armholes of the vest using your other hand. Apply the restraint according to the manufacturer's instructions. The vest should cross in the front, across the person's chest.

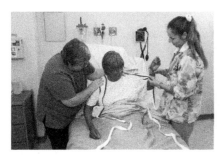

Step 4 Support the person's back and shoulders while slipping her arms through the armholes of the vest.

5. Make sure there are no wrinkles across the front or back of the restraint.

6. Bring the ties through the slots.

7. Help the person to lie or sit down.

8. Make sure the person is comfortable and in good body alignment.

9. If the person is in a chair, thread the straps *between* the seat and the armrest or *between* the back of the seat and the back of the chair, according to the manufacturer's directions. If the person is in bed, attach the straps to the bed frame, never the side rails. Always use the quick-release knot approved by your facility.

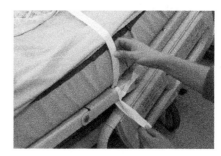

Step 9 Attach the straps to the bed frame, never the side rails.

10. Make sure the restraint is not too tight. You should be able to slide a flat hand between the restraint and the person. Adjust the straps if necessary.

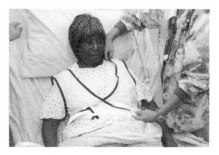

Step 10 Check to make sure the restraint is not too tight.

(continued)

Finishing Up CLSOWR

11. Complete the "Finishing Up" steps.

12. Check on the restrained person every 15 minutes.

13. Release the restraint every 2 hours and:

   a. Reposition the person.

   b. Meet the person's needs for food, fluids, and elimination.

   c. Give skin care and perform range-of-motion exercises.

14. Reapply the restraint.

15. Report and record the procedure, noting the type of restraint used, the time the restraint was applied, and the person's response to the restraint. Include any other relevant observations and sign the chart. Be sure to include your title as well as your name.

PROCEDURE 10-2

Applying Wrist or Ankle Restraints

WHY YOU DO IT   Wrist or ankle restraints are applied to keep a person from moving his arms, legs, or both.

Getting Ready WGKIEPS

1. Complete the "Getting Ready" steps.

Supplies

- appropriate number of wrist restraints, ankle restraints, or both

Procedure

2. Get help from a nurse or another personal support worker, if necessary.

3. Apply the wrist or ankle restraint following the manufacturer's instructions. Place the soft part of the restraint against the skin.

4. Secure the restraint so that it is snug, but not tight. You should be able to slide two fingers under the restraint.

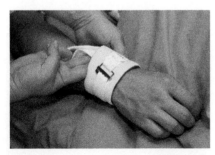

Step 4 You should be able to slip two fingers between the person's wrist and the restraint.

5. Attach the straps to the bed frame. Always use the quick-release knot approved by your facility.

6. If applying more than one restraint, repeat steps 3 through 5.

Finishing Up CLSOWR

7. Complete the "Finishing Up" steps.

8. Check on the restrained person every 15 minutes.

9. Release the restraint every 2 hours and:

   a. Reposition the person.

   b. Meet the person's needs for food, fluids, and elimination.

   c. Give skin care and perform range-of-motion exercises.

10. Reapply the restraint.

11. Report and record the procedure, noting the type of restraint used, the time the restraint was applied, and the person's response to the restraint. Include any other relevant observations and sign the chart. Be sure to include your title as well as your name.

PROCEDURE 10-3

Applying Lap or Waist (Belt) Restraints

WHY YOU DO IT Lap restraints are used to prevent a person from sliding out of a chair. Waist (belt) restraints can be used to secure a person in a chair or in a bed.

Getting Ready WCKIEpS

1. Complete the "Getting Ready" steps.

Supplies

- lap or waist restraint in proper size

Procedure

2. Get help from a nurse or another personal support worker, if necessary.

3. If the person is in a chair, assist him or her to a proper sitting position, making sure that the person's hips are as far back against the back of the chair as possible. (If the person is in a wheelchair, make sure the brakes are locked first, and position the footrests to support the person's feet.)

4. Wrap the restraint around the person's abdomen, crossing the straps behind the person's back.

5. Bring the ties through the loops at the sides of the restraint, according to the manufacturer's directions.

6. Make sure the person is comfortable and in good body alignment.

7. Thread the straps between the chair arm and the chair back before securing the straps out of the person's reach, at the back of the chair. Always use the quick-release knot approved by your facility.

8. Secure the restraint, making sure it is not too tight. You should be able to slide a flat hand between the restraint and the person.

Finishing Up CLSowR

9. Complete the "Finishing Up" steps.

10. Check on the restrained person every 15 minutes.

11. Release the restraint every 2 hours and:
    a. Reposition the person.
    b. Meet the person's needs for food, fluids, and elimination.
    c. Give skin care and perform range-of-motion exercises.

12. Reapply the restraint.

13. Report and record the procedure, noting the type of restraint used, the time the restraint was applied, and the person's response to the restraint. Include any other relevant observations and sign the chart. Be sure to include your title as well as your name.

WHAT DID YOU LEARN?

Multiple Choice

Select the single best answer for each of the following questions.

1. After applying a restraint to a patient or resident:
   a. Try to ignore the person's complaints; he or she just wants attention
   b. Check the restraint every 6 hours
   c. Change the restraint once a day
   d. Remove the restraint at least every 2 hours

2. Vest restraints are applied so that the flaps:
   a. Cross in the back
   b. Cross in the front
   c. Are left open
   d. Are wrapped tightly around the person's chest

3. Which one of the following should not be done when applying a restraint to a patient or resident?
   a. Explain the procedure to the patient or resident
   b. Introduce yourself by name and title
   c. Make sure the patient or resident is asleep
   d. Make sure you have a written doctor's order for the restraint

4. A person with quadriplegia is paralyzed:
   a. From the waist down
   b. From the neck down
   c. On the left side
   d. On the right side

5. What is the leading cause of accidental death among elderly people?
   a. Burns
   b. Falls
   c. Poisonings
   d. Drowning

6. Mary is helping Mr. Watkins to get out of bed when he becomes dizzy, loses his balance, and falls. How should Mary report this accident?
   a. She should tell the nurse about it
   b. She should fill out an incident (occurrence) report
   c. She should tell the nurse about it and fill out an incident (occurrence) report
   d. She should tell the doctor about it

7. Why is a restraint used?
   a. To make caregiving easier for the staff
   b. To punish residents or patients who refuse to follow the rules
   c. To protect a person from harming himself or others, when all other methods of keeping the person safe have failed
   d. All of the above

8. You work in the pediatrics unit of a hospital. One of your small patients has a nasogastric feeding tube that is causing her discomfort, and she keeps trying to pull it out. What should you do to prevent the child from removing the feeding tube?
   a. Apply a mitt restraint
   b. Report your observations to the nurse
   c. Explain to the child that she has to leave the tube alone
   d. Use a sensor alarm

STOP and Think!

Mr. Lovell, one of the residents with dementia at the long-term care facility where you work, has become very agitated. He is prone to falling, and should not get up without help. However, today he is refusing to stay in his bed or his wheelchair. You get him settled, and then as soon as you leave the room, he tries to get up again. This has happened twice, and you are only in the first hour of your shift. You are very concerned that Mr. Lovell will fall and hurt himself, but you cannot stay with him all day because you have other residents to attend to. Describe some things that you could do to help protect Mr. Lovell.

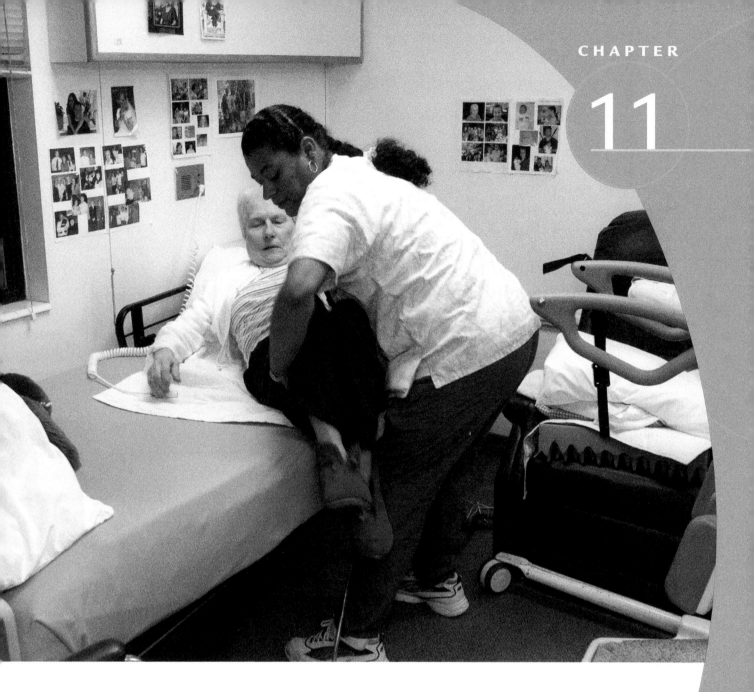

Positioning, Lifting, and Transferring Patients and Residents

WHAT WILL YOU LEARN?

Have you ever been awakened from sleep because the position you were in was uncomfortable? If so, you probably rolled over, found a more comfortable position, and went back to sleep. Can you imagine what it would be like to be unable to change positions, especially if the position you were in was uncomfortable? Most of the people you will care for as a

Photo: A personal support worker helps a resident to transfer out of bed.

personal support worker will be able to move with little or no help. But others will need help to reposition themselves or get out of their bed or chair.

Repositioning, lifting, and transferring people is a major part of the personal support worker's daily routine. You will do this many times a day. By following the guidelines for body mechanics and back safety that you learned in Chapter 9, you can protect yourself from fatigue and injury. In this chapter, you will learn how to keep your patients or residents safe while assisting them with movement. When you are finished with this chapter, you will be able to:

1. Explain the complications of immobility.
2. Describe proper body alignment, and explain why it is important.
3. Identify the different body positions and explain the purpose of regular, frequent repositioning.
4. Discuss safety measures related to lifting and transferring people.
5. Demonstrate techniques of safe lifting and transfer.

Vocabulary

Pressure ulcers	Fowler's position	Prone position	Transfer
Contractures	Semi-Fowler's (low	Sims' position	Weight bearing
Body alignment	Fowler's) position	Shearing	Transfer belt (gait belt)
Supportive devices	High Fowler's position	Friction	Ambulate
Supine (dorsal	Lateral position	Logrolling	
recumbent) position			

POSITIONING PATIENTS AND RESIDENTS

Changing position frequently helps us to stay comfortable while we are sitting or lying down. It also prevents complications that can result from spending long periods of time in the same position. Additionally, in a health care setting, a person may need to get into a certain position to have a procedure done, or to recover from one. Although many of your patients or residents will be able to reposition themselves, some will need your help. For these reasons, helping people who must stay in bed or a wheelchair to reposition themselves is an important responsibility of the personal support worker.

There are many reasons why a person may not be able to shift positions without help. For example, the person could be recovering from surgery, wearing a body cast, or in traction. He or she may be totally or partially paralyzed, unconscious or in a coma, or very weak from a disease or illness. For these people, the inability to change positions regularly can lead to discomfort and, potentially, serious complications. For example, consider a person with limited mobility who has been positioned in a sitting position in bed. With time, this person will

begin to slide down in the bed, leading to discomfort and an inability to breathe easily (Fig. 11-1).

In addition to discomfort, a person who cannot reposition herself is at risk for developing complications (Fig. 11-2). Some of the most serious complications affect the skin, bones and muscles, lungs, and heart:

- **Integumentary system (skin).** The most common complication of immobility is pressure ulcers. **Pressure ulcers,** also known as *decubitus ulcers* or *bed sores,* form when bony areas press against the mattress. The pressure slows down blood flow to the tissues that are pressed between the bone and the mattress. This results in a sore, which can be very difficult to heal and might even be fatal. Pressure ulcers are discussed in detail in Chapter 24.
- **Musculoskeletal system (bones and muscles). Contractures,** discussed in detail in Chapter 25, occur when a joint is held in the same position for too long a time. Contractures cause stiffness and shortening of the tendons, leading to loss of motion of the joint that may be permanent. Long-term immobility can also cause loss of muscle

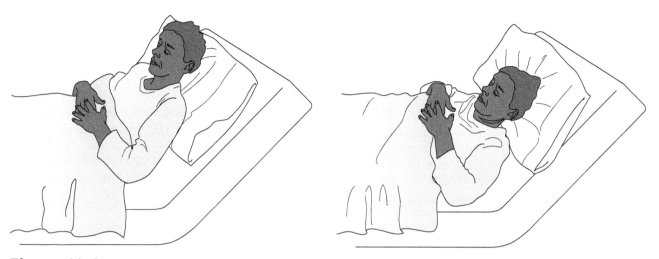

Figure 11-1
Gravity causes a person who is sitting in bed to slide down over time, leading to discomfort and interfering with the person's ability to breathe.

mass and strength. Finally, immobility can cause the loss of calcium from the bones, making the bones brittle and more likely to break.

- **Respiratory system (lungs).** Lying in one position for a long period of time can prevent the lungs from completely filling with air when the person breathes. This causes the small air sacs in the lungs, called *alveoli*, to close. As a result, the person's ability to get oxygen into his or her bloodstream is decreased. In addition, decreased filling of

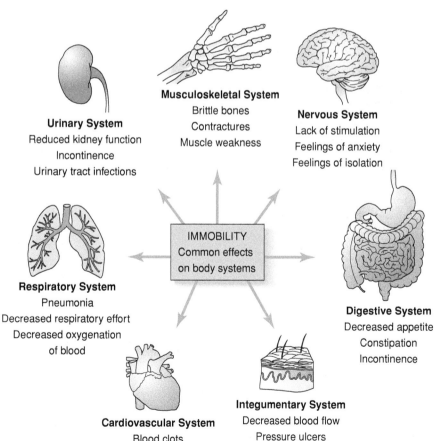

Urinary System
Reduced kidney function
Incontinence
Urinary tract infections

Musculoskeletal System
Brittle bones
Contractures
Muscle weakness

Nervous System
Lack of stimulation
Feelings of anxiety
Feelings of isolation

IMMOBILITY
Common effects
on body systems

Respiratory System
Pneumonia
Decreased respiratory effort
Decreased oxygenation
of blood

Digestive System
Decreased appetite
Constipation
Incontinence

Cardiovascular System
Blood clots
Reduced blood flow

Integumentary System
Decreased blood flow
Pressure ulcers

Figure 11-2
Immobility can cause complications in almost every body system.

the lungs with air allows fluids and mucus to collect in the lungs. This fluid and mucus creates an environment that is favourable for the types of bacteria that cause pneumonia.

- **Cardiovascular system (heart).** When we walk, the large muscles in our legs contract. Contraction of the leg muscles squeezes the veins, helping to move blood from the legs back up to the heart. People who must stay in bed are not using their leg muscles. Therefore, the blood flow from the legs back up to the heart becomes slow. This situation can lead to the formation of blood clots in the lower legs.

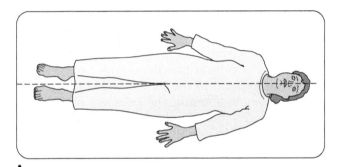

A

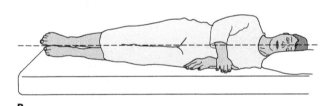

B

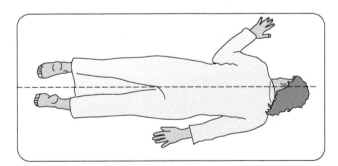

C

Figure 11-3

When a person is in proper body alignment, an imaginary straight line can be drawn connecting the person's nose, breastbone (sternum), and pubic bone. **(A)** Proper body alignment for a person who is lying on her back in bed (supine). **(B)** Proper body alignment for a person who is lying on her side in bed (lateral). **(C)** Proper body alignment for a person who is lying on her stomach in bed (prone).

BASIC POSITIONS

Proper positioning is necessary for good **body alignment** and may help relieve some of the discomfort associated with a person's medical condition. A person in proper body alignment is positioned so that his spine is not twisted or crooked. To check for alignment, imagine a line that connects the person's nose, breastbone (sternum), and pubic bone, and then continues between the person's knees and ankles. This imaginary line should be straight whether the person is lying on his back, side, or abdomen (Fig. 11-3). If the person's legs are spread apart, each leg should be the same distance from the imaginary line. When helping to position one of your patients or residents, imagine yourself in that particular position and remember how your body is most comfortable.

Proper body alignment is most comfortable for the patient or resident. It relieves strain on muscles and joints, promotes good heart and lung function, and helps prevent contractures and pressure ulcers. Sometimes **supportive devices,** such as pillows; rolled sheets, towels, or blankets; and devices designed specifically for the purpose of offering support (Fig. 11-4), are needed to keep the person in proper body alignment. Learning to position these supports correctly is essential. Proper use of supportive devices helps to keep your patients or residents both safe and comfortable. Make sure you ask the nurse or physical therapist about the proper use of any supportive devices for your patients or residents.

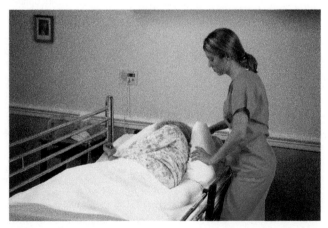

Figure 11-4

Some people require extra support to maintain proper body alignment. This support can be achieved by using pillows; a rolled-up towel, sheet, or blanket; or a supportive device made especially for this purpose.

There are several basic positions that are used when a person must stay in bed or seated for long periods of time (Fig. 11-5). As a personal support worker, you may see variations on these positions for reasons specific for your patient or resident. A doctor may order restrictions on positions for a person after some surgeries or diagnostic procedures. Refer to the care plan or ask the nurse if there are any limitations or special positioning needs the person may have.

Supine (Dorsal Recumbent) Position

When a person is in the **supine (dorsal recumbent) position,** she is lying on her back. The bed is flat and the person's head is supported by a pillow. Sometimes, pillows are placed to support the arms and hands as well. Some people may be more comfortable with a pillow under their knees and lower legs to take strain off the lower back. Others may ask for a small pillow under their lower back.

Fowler's Position

A variation of the supine position is **Fowler's position,** in which the head of the bed is elevated to between 45 and 60 degrees. In **semi-Fowler's (low Fowler's) position,** the head of the bed is elevated approximately 30 to 45 degrees. In **high Fowler's position,** the head of the bed is elevated approximately 60 to 90 degrees (Fig. 11-6). The knee-gatch area of the bed may be bent or a pillow may be placed under the person's knees and calves. Pillows may also support the arms and hands.

The semi-Fowler's position is comfortable for people who are resting in bed and want to read, watch television, or talk with visitors. It is also the most comfortable position for a person who has trouble breathing when lying flat. Some medical conditions, such as hiatal hernia with reflux, and some treatments, such as tube feedings, require the person to be positioned in the semi-Fowler's position. High Fowler's position is useful when a person is eating a meal in bed, and during grooming procedures.

Lateral Position

A person who is in the **lateral position** is lying on his side. When documenting the lateral position, the side of the person that is on the bed is used as the descriptor. For example, a person lying with his left side down on the mattress is in "left lateral position." The person's lower leg is straight and his upper leg is slightly bent at the knee, so that the knees are not pressed together.

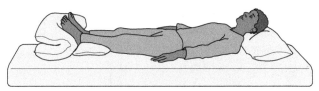

A Supine (dorsal recumbent) position

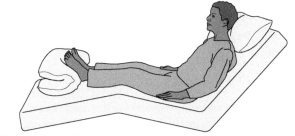

B Fowler's position

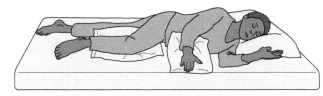

C Lateral position

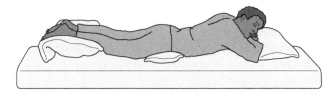

D Prone position

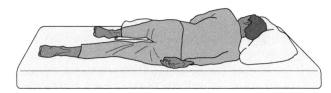

E Sims' position

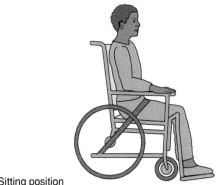

F Sitting position

Figure 11-5

There are several basic positions that are used when a person must remain in bed or seated for a long period of time. **(A)** Supine position. **(B)** Fowler's position. **(C)** Lateral position. **(D)** Prone position. **(E)** Sims' position. **(F)** Sitting position.

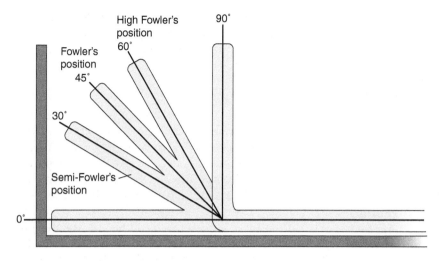

Figure 11-6
In Fowler's position, the head of the bed is elevated. Variations of Fowler's position include semi-Fowler's (low Fowler's) position and high Fowler's position.

Pillows are placed under the person's head and neck, between the legs, and under the upper arm to keep the spine in alignment. A small pillow or rolled sheet may be placed close against the back to keep the person from rolling backward.

A variation of the lateral position may be used to keep pressure off the side of the hip. In the semi–side-lying position, pillows are placed either against the person's back and hip or along the front of her body. The pillows cause the person to lie either a little more forward or a little more toward the back. When the pillows are placed along the person's back and hip, she will lie a little more on her back, leaning toward the pillows. When the pillows are placed along the person's front, she will lie a little more on her abdomen.

The lateral position is often used for people with back pain, to relieve pressure on the spine, and for those in a body cast. Also, the lateral position is part of the cycle of positions for people who are unable to reposition themselves—the person is moved from the supine position to the lateral position, then back to the supine position, and then to the lateral position on the other side every 2 hours, routinely.

Prone Position

A person who is in the **prone position** is lying on his abdomen with his head turned to one side. A small pillow is placed under the person's head. Another small pillow is placed under the lower abdomen and pelvis to allow room for the chest to expand when the person breathes. (Alternatively, a rolled towel can be placed under each of the person's shoulders to reduce pressure on the chest.) A pillow is also placed under the person's shins to keep the feet in proper position. The per-

son's arms are bent at the elbows and his hands are placed on either side of the head, palms facing down. Many people, especially elderly people, are not comfortable in the prone position. Make sure you check with the nurse before placing a person in this position.

Sims' Position

Sims' position is an extreme side-lying position that is almost prone. The person's head is turned to one side and her knee on that side is bent sharply and supported by a pillow. The corresponding arm is bent at the elbow with the hand in front of the face, palm down, resting on a pillow. The lower leg is straight and the lower arm extends out from the side with the hand down near the hips and the palm turned upward. Sims' position is used for people who are receiving enemas, and to relieve pressure on areas that may be prone to developing pressure ulcers, such as the coccyx (the "tailbone") and the greater trochanter of the femur (the "hip bone").

Sitting Position

Positioning and body alignment are important for everyone, not just people who must stay in bed. Proper sitting position holds a person's body in correct alignment while she is sitting in a chair. The person's feet should rest flat on the floor or on the footrests of the wheelchair. Her knees are bent at approximately 90 degrees and the calves of her legs do not touch the chair. The person's buttocks and back rest against the back of the chair. Paralyzed arms should be supported on pillows. A person who cannot hold her body upright for long periods of time may need postural supports to assist in good body alignment.

REPOSITIONING A PERSON

Some people will have conditions that require repositioning as frequently as every hour, but most people will require repositioning every 2 hours. Each time you reposition a person, you should be alert to signs and symptoms of complications related to immobility.

TELL THE NURSE

Possible signs and symptoms of complications related to immobility that should be reported to the nurse immediately include:

- Reddened skin, especially over bony areas, that does not return to its normal color after gentle massage of the surrounding tissue

- Pale, white, or shiny skin over a bony area

- Tears, scrapes, or skin that looks burned

- Hot, reddened, painful areas in the lower legs (do not rub these areas because doing this could dislodge a blood clot, which could then move to a vital organ such as the heart, lungs, or brain)

- New occurrence of urinary or bowel incontinence

- New complaints of pain on movement

- Any disconnected or heavily draining tubes or drains

To assist a person who is in bed into a new position, you will need to know how to lift and turn the person without causing injury to yourself or the person you are trying to move. People who are being moved in bed are particularly at risk for shearing and friction injuries if they are not moved properly. Perhaps you remember sliding across a vinyl car seat or down a metal sliding board while wearing shorts, and feeling pain as you moved and your skin "stuck to" the vinyl or metal. That pain is similar to the pain caused by shearing and friction. **Shearing** is caused by pulling a person across a sheet or other surface that offers resistance. When a person is pulled against a surface that offers resistance, the skin is dragged in a direction opposite that of the underlying tissues and muscles, injuring the blood vessels and connective tissue under the skin and starting the process of skin breakdown. **Friction** occurs when two surfaces, such as a sheet and the person's skin, rub against each other. The rubbing action can injure the skin and contribute to skin breakdown. The risk of shearing and friction can be minimized by rolling or lifting, instead of pulling or dragging, a person who needs to be moved. Guidelines for repositioning a person are given in Guidelines Box 11-1.

Moving a Person to the Side of the Bed

There are many reasons why you may need to reposition a person so that he is lying on one side of the bed or the other. For example, if you want to turn a person, you would first want to move the person to the side of the bed so that when the turn is completed, he is in the middle of the bed (not on one side). You might also need to move a person to the side of the bed before performing a personal care procedure, so that the person is closer to you during the procedure. Depending on the situation, you may be able to move the person to the side of the bed by yourself (Procedure 11-1), or you may need help (Procedure 11-2). Generally speaking, you should get help from a co-worker if the patient or resident is large, seriously ill or injured, or uncooperative.

Helping a Person to Move Up in Bed

As mentioned earlier, people who are sitting up in bed tend to slide down, toward the foot of the bed, over time. To keep a person who is sitting in bed comfortable and in proper body alignment, you must help him with moving up in the bed periodically. Again, depending on the situation, you may be able to do this by yourself (Procedure 11-3), or you may need assistance (Procedure 11-4).

Raising a Person's Head and Shoulders

Often, you will need to lift a person's head and shoulders away from the bed. For example, you may need to do this to help a person with drinking or to rearrange the pillow. Procedure 11-5 explains how to lift a person's head and shoulders away from the bed safely.

Turning a Person On to His or Her Side

Helping a person to roll over in bed helps to keep the person comfortable. It also helps to prevent many of the complications associated with remaining in a single position for a long period of time. The person may be turned away from you (Procedure 11-6) or toward you, depending on the situation. Make sure that the side rail on the opposite side of the bed is raised whenever you are turning a person away from you.

Logrolling a Person

Logrolling is performed whenever it is necessary to move a person who has had back surgery or an

Guidelines Box 11-1 Guidelines for Repositioning a Person

WHAT YOU DO	WHY YOU DO IT
Plan how you will reposition the person and get help from others if necessary.	Depending on the person's medical condition or size, extra equipment or people may be necessary. Planning ahead helps to ensure that the procedure will be carried out efficiently, and with the most consideration for the person's safety and comfort.
Know the specific positioning guidelines for each person in your care. Refer to the care plan or ask the nurse as necessary.	Depending on the person's medical condition, some positions may be required and others may not be allowed. Failure to follow your patient's or resident's specific positioning guidelines can cause the person injury or discomfort.
Reposition the person at least every 2 hours, or according to the care plan.	Regular repositioning is necessary to prevent complications of immobility, such as pressure ulcers.
Explain the procedure to the person, even if he is unconscious.	Understanding how the procedure is done builds trust and helps the person feel like an active participant. Although an unconscious person will not be able to assist in the procedure, the person may still be aware that he is being moved. Telling the person what you are doing as you are doing it helps to reassure the person.
Make sure that you allow the person to assist in the repositioning to the full extent of her ability.	Being able to assist with one's own repositioning promotes feelings of independence and lessens the embarrassment some people may feel over having to rely on someone else for assistance.
Provide for the person's modesty by keeping his body covered.	Keeping the person's body covered preserves his dignity.
Take care to protect any tubes or drains from being pulled out while the person is being moved.	Dislodging tubes or drains is painful for the person. In addition, if tubes or drains become dislodged, it is necessary to reinsert them, which can cause additional discomfort.
Use good body mechanics when helping to reposition a person.	Using good body mechanics will protect you, as well as the patient or resident, from injury.
Use a gentle touch to avoid injury to delicate skin and fragile bones. Use a lift sheet to reposition the person whenever possible. (A lift sheet, also called a draw sheet, is a small sheet that is placed over the bottom sheet so that it extends from the person's shoulders to below her buttocks. Lift sheets are discussed in detail in Chapter 15.)	A lift sheet allows you to lift the person (instead of dragging her across the sheets). This helps to prevent shearing and friction injuries.

Guidelines Box **11-1** Guidelines for Repositioning a Person (continued)	
WHAT YOU DO	*WHY YOU DO IT*
Avoid moving or lifting someone by holding on to his arm or leg.	You could pull the arm or leg out of its socket, or stretch the joint beyond its range of motion.
After repositioning a person, make sure that the bed linens are free of wrinkles, and that the person's clothing is not twisted or wrinkled up underneath the person.	Lying on wrinkled bed linens or clothing can lead to skin breakdown. Skin breakdown increases the person's risk of getting a pressure ulcer.
Gently move the person's clothing aside to check the person's skin, especially on the part of the body the person was just lying on.	Reddened or pale skin can be a sign that a pressure ulcer is starting.

injury to the spine. In turning, the person's body is moved in segments (first the upper body is turned and then the lower body, or vice versa). In logrolling, the person is rolled in one fluid motion so that the head, torso, and legs move as one unit and the body (the "log") is kept in alignment. Two or three workers, plus a lift sheet, are usually necessary to logroll a person. Procedure 11-7 explains how to logroll a person safely.

TRANSFERRING PATIENTS AND RESIDENTS

To **transfer** means to move from one place to another. As a personal support worker, you will help people with transfers many times each day. For example, people transfer from the bed to a chair and back again, or from a wheelchair to a dining chair or commode and back again. Many people are able to transfer from one place to another with little or no help, while others require a lot of help. The assistance you offer will vary from just providing a steadying hand to totally lifting a person from one place to another.

A person's ability to assist with her own transfers may be affected by the person's ability to bear weight. **Weight bearing** refers to a person's ability to stand on one or both legs. A limited ability to bear weight could be caused by surgery that affects the legs, injury to one or both

legs, or paralysis. Some people with paraplegia have learned to transfer themselves by using their arms to support the weight of their body as they move from one surface to another.

A **transfer belt** is a webbed or woven belt with a buckle that is used to assist a weak or unsteady person with standing, walking, or transferring. (When used to help a person walk, a transfer belt is called a **gait belt.**) The belt is approximately 3 to 5 centimetres wide, and it is 137 to 152 centimetres long. Many health care facilities require personal support workers to use a transfer belt when helping people to stand, walk, or transfer. The transfer belt is applied around the person's waist (Procedure 11-8), giving the personal support worker a place to grasp and support the person (other than by the person's arms or ribcage). When using a transfer belt, remember:

- Some patients or residents may have medical conditions that make it dangerous to use a transfer belt on them. For example, a transfer belt should not be applied to a person who is recovering from abdominal surgery. Transfer belts are also not used with people with certain heart disorders. If you are in doubt about using a transfer belt on a patient or resident, check the care plan or ask the nurse for specific directions.
- A transfer belt is only an assist device and should never be used to "lift" a person who is unable to bear weight. A person who is unable to bear weight should be moved with a mechanical lift device.

Before beginning a transfer, advance planning is always necessary. Ask the nurse or physical therapist about any specific limitations the patient or resident has and what the recommended method of transfer is. Many care plans will also have this information. Gather any needed equipment (for example, a mechanical lift or wheelchair) and make sure the equipment is in good working condition. If necessary, move the furniture in the room to make space for a safe transfer. Finally, ask others for help as necessary.

It is important that you learn safe transfer techniques to protect yourself and your patients or residents. Accidents are common during the act of transferring, for both the personal support worker and the person being transferred. Regardless of the particular type of transfer, the safety measures summarized in Guidelines Box 11-2 should always be followed. Specific procedures for various types of transfers are described in the sections that follow.

Helping Hands and a Caring Heart

FOCUS ON HUMANISTIC HEALTH CARE

Remember that a person who needs your assistance during a transfer may feel weak and shaky. The person may be frightened, or embarrassed about having to rely on others to help her do something that always seemed so easy before. Always explain the transfer procedure to the person, and make certain she understands how she is expected to help. Allow the person to assist as much as possible. Encouragement and reassurance from you, along with firm, steady assistance, will help your patient or resident gain confidence in her own abilities and learn to trust that you will be there to offer help as necessary. Promoting a person's independence is an important part of providing humanistic care.

TRANSFERRING A PERSON TO AND FROM A WHEELCHAIR OR CHAIR

Wheelchair use, although a common practice, presents some specific safety issues. Wheelchairs, like any other piece of equipment, need to be checked before use to ensure safety. Check to make sure that there are no broken or missing parts, that the wheels turn smoothly, that any safety straps are secure, and that the brakes hold well. Trying to transfer a person into or out of a wheelchair with unlocked or poorly locked wheels is a common cause of accidents. Procedure 11-9

describes how to transfer a person into a wheelchair or chair by yourself. Procedure 11-10 describes how to transfer a person into a wheelchair or chair with assistance. Procedure 11-11 explains how to transfer a person from a wheelchair or chair to a bed.

TRANSFERRING A PERSON TO AND FROM A STRETCHER

Stretchers are used to transport people to other parts of the facility for surgery or diagnostic testing. Critically ill and comatose people are also transported on stretchers. Procedure 11-12 describes how to transfer a person from a bed to a stretcher. Procedure 11-13 describes how to transfer a person from a stretcher to bed.

TRANSFERRING A PERSON USING A MECHANICAL LIFT

A mechanical lift is used to move people who are very heavy or who are unable to assist in the transfer (Fig. 11-7). Because using a mechanical lift is safer for both the patient or resident and the staff, many facilities encourage the use of these devices. Before using a mechanical lift, always make sure the person you need to transfer weighs less than the weight limit specified on the lift. Some facilities require two staff members to

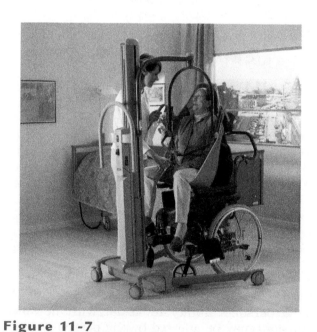

Figure 11-7
A mechanical lift is used to move a person who is very heavy, completely unable to assist with the move, or both. There are many different types of mechanical lifts in use. You should be trained how to operate the lift at the facility where you work before using it. (*Photo courtesy of ARJO.*)

Guidelines Box 11-2 Guidelines for Assisting a Person With Transferring

WHAT YOU DO	WHY YOU DO IT
Plan how you will transfer the person and get help from others if necessary.	Depending on the person's medical condition or size, extra equipment or people may be necessary. Planning ahead helps to ensure that the procedure will be carried out efficiently, and with the most consideration for the person's safety and comfort.
Explain the procedure to the person, even if he is unconscious.	Understanding how the procedure is done builds trust and helps the person feel like an active participant. Although an unconscious person will not be able to assist in the procedure, the person may still be aware that he is being moved. Telling the person what you are doing as you are doing it helps to reassure the person.
Use correct body mechanics. Keep your body close to the person and bend at the knees. Use a transfer belt.	Using good body mechanics will protect you, as well as the patient or resident, from injury.
Make sure that beds are lowered to their lowest position and wheels are locked on beds, stretchers, and wheelchairs.	Lowering the bed to the lowest position makes it easier and safer for the person to transfer, because the lowest position allows the person to put his feet on the floor. Locking the wheels on equipment prevents the equipment from moving out from under the person as he transfers.
Check the person's clothing and shoes. Clothing should fit. Shoes should provide good foot support and have nonskid soles.	Long or loose clothing and shoes that do not provide enough support or have slippery soles could lead to tripping.
Plan the transfer so that the person is leading with her strongest side, if possible.	Doing so allows the person to bear weight in the direction she is going.
Do not allow a person to hold on to you around your neck. Instead, have an unsteady person grasp the arm of the chair or your arm for support.	If the person stumbles or falls while grasping you around the neck, you could be injured.
Do not place your hands under a person's arms to help support him.	If the person stumbles or falls, he may be injured when you lift up as he is falling down.

operate the mechanical lift. Make sure you know your facility's policy. Procedure 11-14 describes one method of transferring a person using a mechanical lift. Because lifts from different manufacturers may vary greatly in their procedures for use, do not use a mechanical lift until you have been taught specifically how to use that lift.

ASSISTING A PERSON WITH WALKING (AMBULATING)

Some patients and residents may be able to transfer without using a wheelchair or stretcher, if they are offered assistance with ambulating. To **ambulate** means to walk. It is important to

Table 11-1   Assistive Devices for Walking (Ambulating)

DEVICE	WHO USES IT	HOW IT IS USED
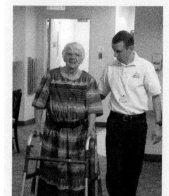 Walker	People who can bear weight but may be weak or unsteady	**Proper fit:** Handgrips level with the person's hips **Proper technique:** The person grasps the top of the frame, lifts the walker up, and places it squarely on the ground 25 to 45 centimetres in front of his or her body. The tips of the walker are placed flat on the floor. Using the top of the frame for support, the person moves one leg forward and then the other, stepping into the frame of the walker. The process is then repeated. The person can use the top of the frame for support between steps if necessary.
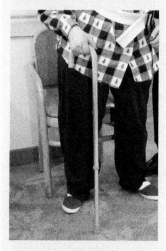 Cane (may have one tip, three tips, or four tips)	People who can bear weight but are weak on one side	**Proper fit:** Handle level with the person's hip **Proper technique:** The person holds the cane on his or her strong side, placing it in front of the body and using it to support his or her weight while moving. The tip of the cane is placed flat on the floor. If the person is using a three- or four-tipped cane, all of the tips are placed flat on the floor at the same time. The weaker leg is moved forward first, followed by the stronger leg. The personal support worker stands slightly behind and to the side of the person, on the person's weak side.
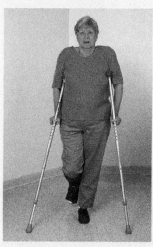 Crutches	People who cannot bear full weight on one leg	**Proper fit:** Top of the crutches rest against the person's sides, not underneath the arms **Proper technique:** The person supports his or her weight with hands on the handgrips (not under the arms). The tips of the crutches are placed flat on the floor. The nurse or physical therapist will teach the person how to move using the crutches.

encourage people who are able to walk (either with or without assistance) to do it on a regular basis. Walking helps to preserve mobility, improves heart and lung function, and promotes digestion. In addition, walking helps the person to remain as independent as possible for as long as possible. A person who feels weak or unsteady benefits, both physically and emotionally, from being encouraged to walk with assistance.

Sitting on the edge of the bed, also called "dangling," is the first step for someone who is going to get out of bed and walk. Procedure 11-15 explains how to help a person to sit on the edge of the bed. When a person has been resting in bed, especially for a long time, sitting up and then standing causes blood to flow to the legs and away from the head. This can lead to dizziness and fainting. Dangling allows time for the heart and blood vessels to make up for the change in position. Blood flow is sent to the head. This reduces the person's risk of falling due to dizziness or loss of consciousness.

There are many different devices people use to help them walk (Table 11-1). These devices are specially fitted to the individual and, therefore, should not be shared.

Procedure 11-16 describes how to assist a person with walking. Be alert to potential problems and be sure to report these to the nurse. Safety guidelines for assisting a person with walking are summarized in Guidelines Box 11-3.

Guidelines Box 11-3	Guidelines for Assisting a Person With Walking (Ambulating)
WHAT YOU DO	**WHY YOU DO IT**
Use correct body mechanics.	Using good body mechanics will protect you, as well as the patient or resident, from injury.
Use a transfer belt on the person according to your facility policy and the care plan.	The transfer belt gives you a safe place to grasp and support the person.
Watch the person for fatigue or discomfort.	A person who is tired or uncomfortable is at greater risk for tripping or fainting.
Check the person's clothing and shoes. Clothing should fit. Shoes should provide good foot support and have nonskid soles.	Long or loose clothing and shoes that do not provide enough support or have slippery soles could lead to tripping.
Check ambulation devices to ensure that they are in good condition. Tips on canes and walkers should not be cracked, worn, or missing.	The tips on canes and walkers provide traction. If they are cracked or worn, they can slip, causing the person to fall.
Request help from a co-worker as necessary when you must assist a weak, unsteady, or uncooperative person with walking.	A person who is weak, unsteady, or uncooperative is likely to fall, injuring both of you. Having help from a co-worker makes a fall less likely.
Allow the person to "dangle" for the specified amount of time before assisting the person to stand up.	Allowing a person time to "dangle" before getting out of bed reduces the person's risk of falling due to dizziness or loss of consciousness.
Ensure that the person is using ambulation devices correctly.	Using an ambulation device correctly reduces the person's risk of slipping and falling.

TELL THE NURSE ⓘ

Each time you assist a person with a transfer, tell the nurse immediately if:

- The person complains of dizziness, shortness of breath, chest pain, a rapid heartbeat (palpitations), or sudden head pain

- The person complains of pain when he tries to bear weight, and this is new

- You observe any changes in the person's usual grip, strength, or ability

- A usually cooperative person refuses to participate ("I just don't feel like it today")

- The equipment is not working properly or is broken

SUMMARY

- For many different reasons, people in a health care setting may be unable to reposition themselves without assistance.
  - The resulting immobility can cause serious complications, including pressure ulcers, contractures, pneumonia, and the formation of blood clots in the legs.
  - Preventing the complications of immobility, through frequent repositioning and transferring, is a major responsibility of the personal support worker.
    - Some people will have conditions that require frequent, regular repositioning, as often as every hour, but at least every 2 hours.
    - There are several basic positions that are used when a person must remain in bed for extended periods of time: the supine (dorsal recumbent), Fowler's, lateral, prone, and Sims' positions. Proper positioning helps to ensure proper body alignment, which relieves strain on the muscles and joints, promotes good heart and lung function, and helps to prevent contractures and pressure ulcers. It is essential for comfort.
    - When repositioning a person, it is important to take care to prevent shearing and friction injuries to the skin.
- Personal support workers also help people to transfer from one place to another many times throughout the day.
  - Advance planning and proper technique help to ensure a safe transfer.
  - Some patients and residents may be able to walk on their own, with help. Encouraging and assisting patients and residents to walk enhances their quality of life by providing both physical and emotional benefits.

11 PROCEDURES

PROCEDURE **11-1**

Moving a Person to the Side of the Bed (One Worker)

WHY YOU DO IT Moving a person to the side of the bed is a necessary first step in many procedures, such as the procedures for turning a person onto his or her side, assisting a person to sit on the edge of the bed, or assisting a person to get out of bed.

Getting Ready WCKIEpS

1. Complete the "Getting Ready" steps.

Procedure

2. Make sure that the bed is positioned at a comfortable working height (to promote good body mechanics) and that the wheels are locked.

3. Place the pillow at the head of the bed, on its edge against the headboard. This gets the pillow out of the way.

4. If the side rails are in use, lower the side rail on the working side of the bed. The side rail on the opposite side of the bed should remain up. Lower the head of the bed so that the bed is flat (as tolerated). Fanfold the top linens to the foot of the bed.

5. Stand at the side of the bed with your feet spread about 30.5 cm apart and with your knees slightly bent to protect your back.

6. Gently slide your hands under the person's head and shoulders and move the person's upper body toward you.

7. Gently slide your hands under the person's torso and move the person's torso toward you.

8. Gently slide your hands under the person's hips and legs and move the person's lower body toward you.

9. Now, position the person as planned (for example, in the prone or lateral position).

10. Reposition the pillow under the person's head and straighten the bottom linens. Draw the top linens over the person. Raise the head of the bed as the person requests.

11. Make sure that the bed is lowered to its lowest position and that the wheels are locked. If the side rails are in use, return them to the raised position.

Finishing Up CLSOWR

12. Complete the "Finishing Up" steps.

PROCEDURE **11-2**

Moving a Person to the Side of the Bed (Two Workers)

WHY YOU DO IT This method of moving a person to the side of the bed is safer for both you and the person if the person is large, very ill or injured, or uncooperative. Using a lift sheet also helps to prevent shearing and friction injuries.

Getting Ready WCKIEpS

1. Complete the "Getting Ready" steps.

Supplies

● lift sheet (if one is not already on the bed)

(continued)

Procedure

2. Make sure that the bed is positioned at a comfortable working height (to promote good body mechanics) and that the wheels are locked.

3. Place the pillow at the head of the bed, on its edge against the headboard. This gets the pillow out of the way.

4. If the side rails are in use, lower the side rails. Lower the head of the bed so that the bed is flat (as tolerated). Fanfold the top linens to the foot of the bed.

5. If the lift sheet is already on the bed, make sure that it is positioned so that it is under the person's shoulders and hips. (If a lift sheet is not already on the bed, position one under the person's shoulders and hips.)

6. Stand at the side of the bed, opposite your co-worker, with your feet spread about 30.5 cm apart and with your knees slightly bent to protect your back.

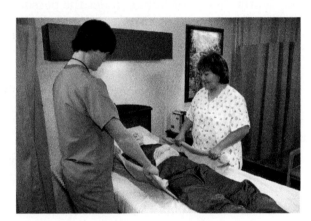

Step 6 Stand opposite your co-worker.

7. Grasp the edge of the lift sheet and roll it over as close to the person's body as possible. This will provide for a better grip. (Your co-worker does the same.)

8. Grasp the rolled edge of the lift sheet with both hands, palms and fingers facing down. One hand should be level with the person's shoulders and the other should be level with his or her hips.

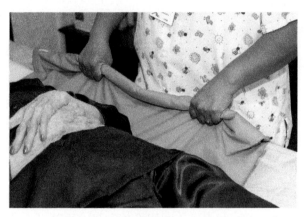

Step 8 Grasp the rolled lift sheet with both hands, palms and fingers facing down.

9. On the count of "three," slowly and carefully lift up on the lift sheet in unison and move the person to the side of the bed.

10. Now, position the person as planned (for example, in the prone or lateral position).

11. Reposition the pillow under the person's head and straighten the bottom linens. Draw the top linens over the person.

12. Make sure that the bed is lowered to its lowest position and that the wheels are locked. If the side rails are in use, return them to the raised position.

Finishing Up   CLSOWR

13. Complete the "Finishing Up" steps.

PROCEDURE 11-3

Moving a Person up in Bed (One Worker)

WHY YOU DO IT Gravity causes a person who is sitting in bed to slide down over time, leading to discomfort and interfering with the person's ability to breathe. Helping the person to move up in bed promotes comfort and makes it easier for the person to breathe.

Getting Ready WGKIEpS

1. Complete the "Getting Ready" steps.

Procedure

2. Make sure that the bed is positioned at a comfortable working height (to promote good body mechanics) and that the wheels are locked.

3. If the side rails are in use, lower the side rail on the working side of the bed. The side rail on the opposite side of the bed should remain up. Fanfold the top linens to the foot of the bed.

4. Place the pillow at the head of the bed, on its edge against the headboard. This gets the pillow out of the way. It also pads the headboard in case you move the person up a little too much or too fast!

5. **Method "A":**

   a. Face the head of the bed. Position your outside foot (that is, the foot that is farthest away from the edge of the bed) 30.5 cm in front of the other foot and bend your knees slightly to protect your back.

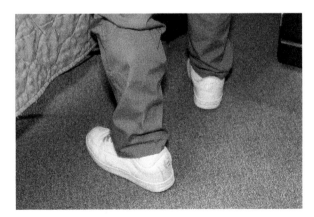

Step 5 Position your outside foot 30.5 cm in front of your inside foot.

   b. Place your arm that is nearest the head of the bed under the person's head and shoulders. Lock your other arm with the person's arm that is closest to you.

   c. Have the person bend her knees.

   d. Tell the person that on the count of "three," she is to lift her buttocks and press her heels into the mattress as you lift her shoulders. On the count of "three," help the person to move smoothly toward the head of the bed.

6. **Method "B":**

   a. Have the person grasp the head of the bed or a trapeze, if there is one.

   b. Face the head of the bed. Position your outside foot (that is, the foot that is farthest away from the edge of the bed) 30.5 cm in front of the other foot and bend your knees slightly to protect your back.

   c. Place your hands under the person's back and buttocks.

   d. Have the person bend his knees.

   e. Tell the person that on the count of "three," he is to lift his buttocks and press his heels into the mattress. On the count of "three," help the person to move smoothly toward the head of the bed.

7. Reposition the pillow under the person's head and straighten the bottom linens. Draw the top linens over the person. Raise the head of the bed as the person requests.

8. Make sure that the bed is lowered to its lowest position and that the wheels are locked. If the side rails are in use, return them to the raised position.

Finishing Up CLSOWR

9. Complete the "Finishing Up" steps.

PROCEDURE 11-4

Moving a Person Up in Bed (Two Workers)

WHY YOU DO IT   This method of moving a person up in bed is safer for both you and the person if the person is large, very ill or injured, or uncooperative. Using a lift sheet also helps to prevent shearing and friction injuries.

Getting Ready   WGKIEPS

1. Complete the "Getting Ready" steps.

Supplies

● lift sheet (if one is not already on the bed)

Procedure

2. Make sure that the bed is positioned at a comfortable working height (to promote good body mechanics) and that the wheels are locked.

3. Place the pillow at the head of the bed, on its edge against the headboard. This gets the pillow out of the way. It also pads the headboard in case you move the person up a little too much or too fast!

4. If the side rails are in use, lower the side rails. Lower the head of the bed so that the bed is flat (as tolerated). Fanfold the top linens to the foot of the bed.

5. If the lift sheet is already on the bed, make sure that it is positioned so that it is under the person's shoulders and hips. (If a lift sheet is not already on the bed, position one under the person's shoulders and hips.)

6. Stand at the side of the bed, opposite your co-worker, with your feet spread about 30.5 cm apart and with your knees slightly bent to protect your back.

7. Grasp the edge of the lift sheet and roll it over as close to the person's body as possible. This will provide for a better grip. (Your co-worker does the same.)

8. Grasp the rolled edge of the lift sheet with both hands, palms and fingers facing down. One hand should be level with the person's shoulders and the other should be level with his or her hips.

9. On the count of "three," slowly and carefully lift up on the lift sheet in unison and move the person toward the head of the bed. Avoid dragging the person across the bottom linens.

10. Reposition the pillow under the person's head and straighten the bottom linens. Draw the top linens over the person. Raise the head of the bed as the person requests.

11. Make sure that the bed is lowered to its lowest position and that the wheels are locked. If the side rails are in use, return them to the raised position.

Finishing Up   CLSOWR

12. Complete the "Finishing Up" steps.

PROCEDURE 11-5

Raising a Person's Head and Shoulders

WHY YOU DO IT   Raising the person's head and shoulders away from the bed is necessary when you need to adjust the pillow and during some care procedures, such as dressing. Knowing how to perform this procedure safely prevents injury to you and your patient or resident.

Getting Ready   WGKIEPS

1. Complete the "Getting Ready" steps.

Procedure

2. Make sure that the bed is positioned at a comfortable working height (to promote good body mechanics) and that the wheels are locked.

3. Place the pillow at the head of the bed, on its edge against the headboard. This gets the pillow out of the way.

4. If the side rails are in use, lower the side rail on the working side of the bed. The side rail on

the opposite side of the bed should remain up. Fanfold the top linens to the foot of the bed.

5. Face the head of the bed. Position your outside foot (that is, the foot that is farthest away from the edge of the bed) 30.5 cm in front of the other foot, and bend your knees slightly to protect your back.

6. Slide one hand under the person's shoulder that is nearest to you.

7. Slide the other hand under the person's upper back.

8. On the count of "three," slowly and carefully lift the person's head and shoulders.

9. Reposition the pillow under the person's head and straighten the bottom linens. Draw the top linens over the person. Raise the head of the bed as the person requests.

10. Make sure that the bed is lowered to its lowest position and that the wheels are locked. If the side rails are in use, return them to the raised position.

Finishing Up CLSOWR

11. Complete the "Finishing Up" steps.

PROCEDURE 11-6

Turning a Person Onto His or Her Side

WHY YOU DO IT   The lateral position is part of the cycle of positions for people who are unable to reposition themselves. The person is moved from the supine position to the lateral position, then back to the supine position, and then to the lateral position on the other side.

Getting Ready WCKIEpS

1. Complete the "Getting Ready" steps.

Supplies

● additional pillows (if not already in the room)

Procedure

2. Make sure that the bed is positioned at a comfortable working height (to promote good body mechanics) and that the wheels are locked.

3. Place the pillow at the head of the bed, on its edge against the headboard. This gets the pillow out of the way.

4. If the side rails are in use, lower the side rail on the working side of the bed. The side rail on the opposite side of the bed should remain up. Lower the head of the bed so that the bed is flat (as tolerated). Fanfold the top linens to the foot of the bed.

5. Stand at the side of the bed with your feet spread about 30.5 cm apart and with your knees slightly bent to protect your back.

6. Move the person to the side of the bed nearest you.

7. Cross the person's arm that is nearest you over the person's chest.

8. Bend the person's leg that is nearest you, placing the foot on the bed. (Or, cross the person's leg that is nearest to you over his or her other leg.)

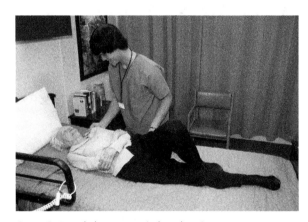

Step 8 Bend the person's leg that is nearest you, placing the foot on the bed.

9. Roll the person onto his or her side:

   a. To roll the person away from you: Place one of your hands on the person's shoulder that is nearest you, and place your other hand on the person's hip that is nearest you. Gently roll the person away from you, toward the opposite side of the bed.

(continued)

b. To roll the person toward you: Raise the side rail and move to the other side of the bed. Lower that side rail. Place one hand on the person's shoulder that is farthest away from you, and place your other hand on the person's hip that is farthest away from you. Gently roll the person toward you.

10. Reposition the pillow under the person's head and straighten the bottom linens. Support the person by placing a pillow lengthwise between the person's legs. The person's lower leg should be straight, and the upper leg should be slightly bent at the knee. Place additional pillows under the person's upper arm, and behind his or her back. Draw the top linens over the person.

11. Make sure that the bed is lowered to its lowest position and that the wheels are locked. If the side rails are in use, return them to the raised position.

Finishing Up CLSoWR

12. Complete the "Finishing Up" steps.

PROCEDURE 11-7

Logrolling a Person (Two Workers)

WHY YOU DO IT Logrolling is done whenever it is necessary to move a person who has had back surgery or an injury to the spine. The person is rolled in one fluid motion so that the head, torso, and legs move as one unit and the body is kept in alignment.

Getting Ready WCKIEpS

1. Complete the "Getting Ready" steps.

Supplies

- lift sheet (if one is not already on the bed)

Procedure

2. Make sure that the bed is positioned at a comfortable working height (to promote good body mechanics) and that the wheels are locked.

3. Place the pillow at the head of the bed, on its edge against the headboard. This gets the pillow out of the way.

4. If the side rails are in use, lower the side rail on the working side of the bed. The side rail on the opposite side of the bed should remain up. Lower the head of the bed so that the bed is flat (as tolerated). Fanfold the top linens to the foot of the bed.

5. Stand with the other worker on the side of the bed with the lowered side rail. Stand facing the bed with your feet spread about 30.5 cm apart and with your knees slightly bent to protect your back. One worker is aligned with the person's head and shoulders; the other is aligned with the person's hips.

6. Place your hands under the person's head and shoulders while your co-worker places his or her hands under the person's hips and legs (or vice versa). Lifting in unison, gently move the person toward the side of the bed closest to you.

7. Place a pillow lengthwise between the person's legs and fold the person's arm so that it will be on top of his chest when he is turned.

8. Raise the side rail and make sure that it is secure.

9. Go to the opposite side of the bed and lower the side rail.

10. Working with the other worker, turn the person onto his side.

   a. If a lift sheet is being used, turn the person by reaching over him and grasping the lift sheet. One worker should place one hand on the lift sheet at the level of the person's shoulder and the other hand at the level of the person's hip; the other worker should place one hand on the lift-sheet at the level of the person's hip and the other at the level of the person's calves.

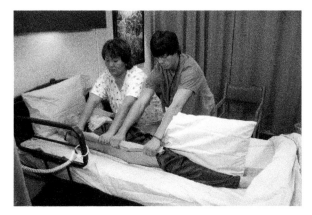

Step 10a Reach over the person and grasp the lift sheet.

b. If a lift sheet is not being used, one worker should position his or her hands on the person's shoulders and hips and the other worker should place his or her hands on the person's thigh and calves.

11. On the count of "three," roll the person toward the side on which you are standing in a single movement, being sure to keep the person's head, spine, and legs aligned.

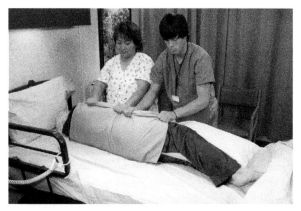

Step 11 On the count of "three," roll the person in one fluid movement.

12. Reposition the pillow under the person's head and straighten the bottom linens. Support the person by bolstering his back with pillows. The pillow between the person's legs should remain in place, and additional pillows or folded towels should be used to support the person's arms. Draw the top linens over the person.

13. Make sure that the bed is lowered to its lowest position and that the wheels are locked. If the side rails are in use, return them to the raised position.

Finishing Up CLSOWR
14. Complete the "Finishing Up" steps.

PROCEDURE 11-8

Applying a Transfer (Gait) Belt

WHY YOU DO IT The transfer belt gives you a safe place to grasp and support the person when assisting the person with standing, transferring, or walking.

Getting Ready WGKIEP5
1. Complete the "Getting Ready" steps.

Supplies
● transfer belt

Procedure
2. If the person is in bed, make sure that the bed is lowered to its lowest position and that the wheels are locked. If the side rails are in use, lower the side rail on the working side of the bed. The side rail on the opposite side of the bed should remain up. Fanfold the top linens to the foot of the bed. Assist the person to sit on the edge of the bed.

3. Apply the belt around the person's waist, over his or her clothing. Buckle the belt in the front by threading the tongue of the belt

(continued)

through the side of the buckle that has "teeth" first, and then placing the tongue of the belt through the other side of the buckle.

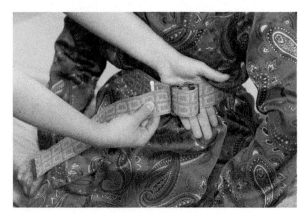

Step 3 Thread the tongue of the belt through the side of the buckle that has "teeth" first.

4. Before tightening the belt, turn it so that the buckle is off-center in the front or to the side.
5. Tighten the belt and check for fit. The belt should be snug, but you should be able to slip your fingers between the belt and the person's waist. When applying a transfer belt

to a woman, make sure that her breasts are not trapped underneath the belt.
6. Use an underhand grasp when holding the belt to provide greater safety.

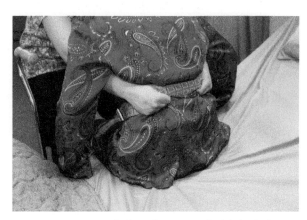

Step 6 Use an underhand grasp to hold the belt.

Finishing Up CLSOWR

7. When the person has finished transferring and is ready to return to bed, reverse the procedure.
8. Complete the "Finishing Up" steps.

PROCEDURE 11-9

Transferring a Person From a Bed to a Wheelchair (One Worker)

WHY YOU DO IT   Wheelchairs are used to transport people who have trouble walking. Using proper technique helps to keep both you and the person safe during the transfer from bed to wheelchair.

Getting Ready WGKIEDS
1. Complete the "Getting Ready" steps.

Supplies
- wheelchair
- lap blanket (optional)
- person's robe
- person's slippers or shoes
- transfer belt

Procedure
2. Determine the person's strongest side, and then place the wheelchair alongside the bed.

Position the wheelchair so that the person will move toward the chair "strong side first." Whenever possible, position the wheelchair so that it is against a wall or a solid piece of furniture so that it will not slide backward during the transfer.
3. Lock the wheelchair wheels, and either remove the footrests or swing them to the side.
4. Fanfold the top linens to the foot of the bed.
5. Make sure that the bed is lowered to its lowest position and that the wheels are locked. Raise the head of the bed as tolerated.

6. Help the person to move toward the side of the bed where the wheelchair is located.

7. Assist the person to dangle.

8. Allow the person to rest on the edge of the bed. The person should be sitting squarely on both buttocks, with her knees apart and both feet flat on the floor (to offer a broad base of support). The person's arms should rest alongside her thighs. Watch for signs of dizziness or fainting. Position yourself in front of the person so that you can offer assistance in case she loses balance.

9. Help the person to put her shoes or slippers on and help her to get into a robe. Apply a transfer belt.

10. Help the person to stand.

   a. Stand facing the person.

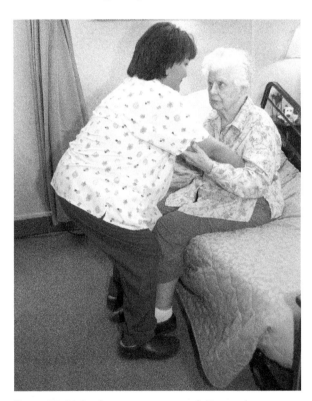

Step 10 Help the person to stand. Brace the person's knees with your knees, and the person's feet with your feet.

   b. Have the person put her hands on the edge of the bed, alongside each thigh.

   c. Make sure the person's feet are flat on the floor.

   d. Have the person lean forward.

   e. Grasp the transfer belt at each side, using an underhand grasp. (If you are not using a transfer belt, pass your arms under the

person's arms and rest your hands on her upper back.)

   f. Position your feet alongside the person's feet, flexing your knees. Place your shins against the person's shins to block the person's feet and keep her knees from buckling as she stands up.

   g. Have the person push down on the bed with her hands and stand on the count of "three." Assist the person into a standing position by pulling on the transfer belt as you straighten your knees. (If you are not using a transfer belt, assist the person into a standing position by gently pulling her up and forward as you straighten your knees.) Remember to keep your back straight.

11. Support the person in the standing position by holding the transfer belt or by keeping your hands on her upper back. Continue to block the person's feet and knees with your feet and knees.

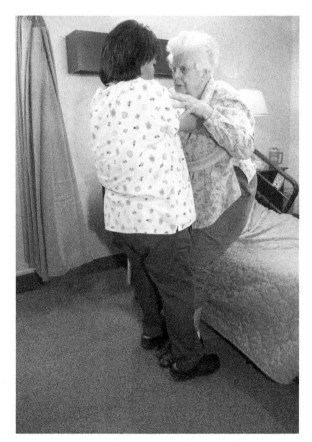

Step 11 Support the person in the standing position.

12. Help the person to turn by pivoting on the stronger leg toward the chair. This will allow the person to grasp the far arm of the wheelchair.

(continued)

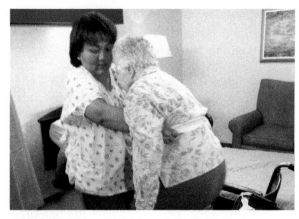

Step 12 Help the person to turn so that she can grasp the arms of the wheelchair and sit down.

13. Continue to assist the person with turning until she is able to grasp the other armrest. The backs of the person's legs should touch the edge of the chair.

14. Lower the person into the wheelchair by bending your hips and knees.

15. Make sure the person's buttocks are at the back of the chair. Make sure the person is comfortable and in good body alignment.

16. Remove the transfer belt.

17. Position the person's feet on the footrests of the wheelchair. Buckle the wheelchair safety belt (if ordered) and cover the person's lap and legs with a lap blanket, if desired. Make sure that the lap blanket does not drag on the floor.

Finishing Up CLSOWR

18. Position the wheelchair according to the person's preference.

19. Complete the "Finishing Up" steps.

PROCEDURE 11-10

Transferring a Person From a Bed to a Wheelchair (Two Workers)

WHY YOU DO IT   Wheelchairs are used to transport people who have trouble walking. Using proper technique helps to keep both you and the person safe during the transfer from bed to wheelchair.

Getting Ready WCKIEPS

1. Complete the "Getting Ready" steps.

Supplies

- wheelchair
- lap blanket (optional)
- person's robe
- person's slippers or shoes

Procedure

2. Place the wheelchair alongside the bed, facing the foot of the bed.

3. Lock the wheelchair wheels and either remove the footrests or swing them to the side.

4. Fanfold the top linens to the foot of the bed.

5. Make sure that the bed is positioned at a comfortable working height (to promote good body mechanics) and that the wheels are locked. Raise the head of the bed as tolerated.

6. Help the person to move toward the side of the bed where the wheelchair is located.

7. Help the person to put his shoes or slippers on, and help him get into a robe.

8. Stand by the side of the bed, behind the wheelchair. Standing behind the person, pass your arms under the person's arms and grasp his forearms. The other worker grasps the person's thighs and calves.

9. Working in unison with the other worker, lift the person from the bed and bring him toward the wheelchair on the count of "three." Lower the person into the wheelchair.

10. Make sure the person's buttocks are at the back of the chair. Make sure the person is comfortable and in good body alignment.

11. Position the person's feet on the footrests of the wheelchair. Buckle the wheelchair safety belt (if ordered) and cover the person's lap and legs with a lap blanket, if desired. Make sure that the lap blanket does not drag on the floor.

Finishing Up CLSOWR

12. Position the wheelchair according to the person's preference.

13. Complete the "Finishing Up" steps.

PROCEDURE 11-11

Transferring a Person From a Wheelchair to a Bed

WHY YOU DO IT   Wheelchairs are used to transport people who have trouble walking. Using proper technique helps to keep both you and the person safe during the transfer from wheelchair to bed.

Getting Ready WGKTEPS

1. Complete the "Getting Ready" steps.

Supplies

● transfer belt

Procedure

2. Make sure that the bed is lowered to its lowest position and that the wheels are locked. Raise the head of the bed, fanfold the top linens to the foot of the bed, and raise the opposite side rail.

3. Position the wheelchair close to the side of the bed so that the person's strong side is next to the bed. Lock the wheelchair wheels and either remove the footrests or swing them to the side.

4. Remove the person's lap blanket (if one was used) and release the wheelchair safety belt, if in use. Apply a transfer belt.

5. Stand facing the person with your feet spread about 30.5 cm apart and with your knees slightly bent to protect your back. With your back straight, slide the person to the front of the wheelchair seat.

6. Grasp the transfer belt (or pass your arms under the person's arms, placing your hands on her upper back). Position your feet alongside the person's feet, flexing your knees. Place your shins against the person's shins to block the person's feet and keep her knees from buckling as she stands up.

7. Have the person rest her hands on your arms and assist her to stand by pulling on the transfer belt as you straighten your knees. (If you are not using a transfer belt, assist the person into a standing position by gently pulling her up and forward as you straighten your knees.) Remember to keep your back straight. Alternatively, a person who requires less assistance can place her hands on the wheelchair arms for support and "push off" while you offer support.

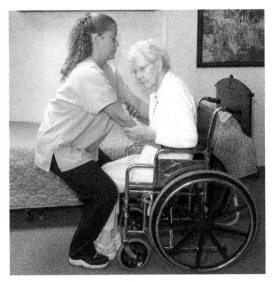

Step 7 Help the person to stand.

8. Slowly help the person to turn toward the bed by pivoting on her strong leg. Help the person to sit on the edge of the bed.

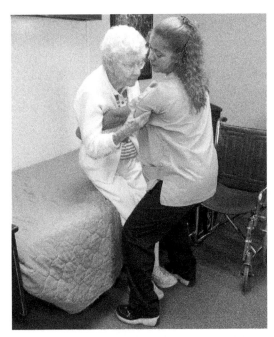

Step 8 Help the person to sit on the edge of the bed.

(continued)

9. Remove the person's robe and slippers, if appropriate.

10. Move the wheelchair out of the way.

11. Place one of your arms around the person's shoulders and one arm under her legs. Swing the person's legs onto the bed.

12. Help the person to move to the center of the bed and position her comfortably.

13. Straighten the bottom linens and make sure the person is comfortable and in good body alignment. Draw the top linens over the person.

14. If the side rails are in use, return them to the raised position.

Finishing Up   CLSOWR

15. Complete the "Finishing Up" steps.

PROCEDURE 11-12

Transferring a Person From a Bed to a Stretcher (Four Workers)

WHY YOU DO IT   Stretchers are used to transport people to other parts of the facility for surgery or diagnostic testing. Critically ill and comatose people are also transported on stretchers. Using proper technique helps to keep both you and the person safe during the transfer from bed to stretcher.

Getting Ready   WCKIEPS

1. Complete the "Getting Ready" steps.

Supplies

- stretcher
- lift sheet (if one is not already on the bed)
- blanket

Procedure

2. Raise the bed to its highest level. (The stretcher should be slightly lower than the bed.) Lower the head of the bed so that the bed is flat. Make sure that the bed wheels are locked. Lower the side rails. Fanfold the top linens to the side of the bed opposite the stretcher.

3. If the lift sheet is already on the bed, make sure that it is positioned so that it is under the person's shoulders and hips. (If a lift sheet is not already on the bed, position one under the person's shoulders and hips.)

4. Position the stretcher alongside the bed. Lock the stretcher wheels and move the stretcher safety belts out of the way.

5. Two workers stand at the side of the bed facing their co-workers, who are positioned along the outside edge of the stretcher.

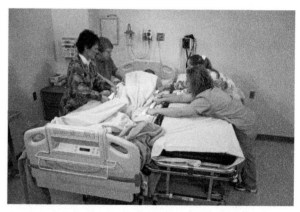

Step 5 Stand at the side of the bed facing your co-worker, who is positioned along the outside edge of the stretcher. Another pair of workers does the same.

6. Grasp the edge of the lift sheet and roll it over as close to the person's body as possible. This will provide for a better grip. (Your co-workers do the same.)

7. On the count of "three," all four workers slowly and carefully lift up on the lift sheet in unison and move the person to the side of the bed.

8. On the count of "three," all four workers slowly and carefully lift up on the transfer sheet in unison and move the person to the side of the stretcher.

9. Position the person on the stretcher and make sure he or she is in good body alignment. Reposition the pillow under the person's head and cover the person with a blanket for modesty and warmth. Buckle the stretcher safety belts across the person and raise the side rails on the stretcher. Raise the head of the stretcher as the person requests.

Finishing Up CLSOWR

10. Transport the person to the appropriate site. A person on a stretcher should always be transported "feet first." Remain with the person; never leave someone alone on a stretcher.

11. Complete the "Finishing Up" steps.

PROCEDURE 11-13

Transferring a Person From a Stretcher to a Bed (Four Workers)

WHY YOU DO IT   Stretchers are used to transport people to other parts of the facility for surgery or diagnostic testing. Critically ill and comatose people are also transported on stretchers. Using proper technique helps to keep both you and the person safe during the transfer from stretcher to bed.

Getting Ready WGKIEDS

1. Complete the "Getting Ready" steps.

Supplies

- lift sheet (if one is not already on the stretcher)

Procedure

2. Raise or lower the bed so that it is slightly lower than the stretcher. Lower the head of the bed so that the bed is flat. Make sure that the bed wheels are locked. Lower the side rails. Fanfold the top linens to the side of the bed opposite the stretcher.

3. If the lift sheet is already on the stretcher, make sure that it is positioned so that it is under the person's shoulders and hips. (If a lift sheet is not already on the stretcher, position one under the person's shoulders and hips.)

4. Unbuckle the stretcher safety belts and lower the side rails on the stretcher.

5. Position the stretcher against the bed and lock the stretcher wheels.

6. Two workers stand at the far side of the bed facing their co-workers, who are positioned along the outside edge of the stretcher. (Some facilities allow the workers on the far side of the bed to kneel on the bed to complete the transfer; follow your facility's policy.)

7. Grasp the edge of the lift sheet and roll it over as close to the person's body as possible. This will provide for a better grip. (Your co-workers do the same.)

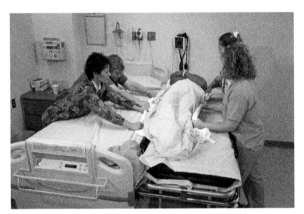

Step 6 Stand at the side of the bed facing your co-worker, who is positioned along the outside edge of the stretcher. Another pair of workers does the same.

8. On the count of "three," all four workers slowly and carefully lift up on the lift sheet in unison and move the person to the bed. Move the stretcher away from the bed.

9. Help the person to move to the center of the bed and, if desired, remove the lift sheet by turning the person first to one side, then the other. Position the person comfortably.

10. Straighten the bottom linens and make sure the person is comfortable and in good body alignment. Draw the top linens over the person.

11. Make sure the bed is lowered to its lowest position and that the wheels are locked. If the side rails are in use, return them to the raised position.

Finishing Up CLSOWR

12. Complete the "Finishing Up" steps.

PROCEDURE 11-14

Transferring a Person Using a Mechanical Lift (Two Workers)

WHY YOU DO IT   Using a mechanical lift to move a person who is helpless or very heavy is safer for both you and the person.

Getting Ready WCKIEPS

1. Complete the "Getting Ready" steps.

Supplies

- wheelchair
- mechanical lift
- sling in proper size
- lap blanket (optional)
- lap restraint (if ordered)

Procedure

2. Make sure that the bed is positioned at a comfortable working height (to promote good body mechanics) and that the wheels are locked.

3. If the side rails are in use, lower the side rails.

4. Fanfold the top linens to the foot of the bed.

5. Center the sling under the person. (To get the sling under the person, move the person as if you were making an occupied bed.) The lower edge of the sling should be positioned underneath the person's knees.

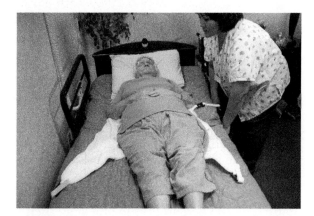

Step 5 Center the sling under the person.

6. Raise the head of the bed as tolerated.

7. Move the release valve on the lift to the closed position.

8. Raise the lift so that it can be positioned over the person.

9. Spread the legs of the lift to provide a solid base of support. The legs must be locked in this position, or the lift could tip over,

injuring you, the person you are trying to transfer, or both.

10. Move the lift into position over the person.

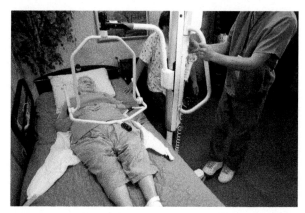

Step 10 Move the lift into position over the person.

11. Fasten the sling to the straps or chains of the lift. Make sure the hooks face away from the person.

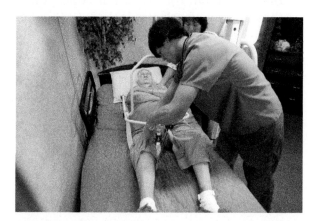

Step 11 Fasten the sling to the lift according to the manufacturer's instructions.

12. Attach the sling to the swivel bar with the short side attached to the top of the sling and the long side attached to the bottom of the sling.

13. Cross the person's arms across her chest. The person may hold onto the straps, but do not let her hold onto the swivel bar.

14. Raise the lift until the person and the sling are clear of the bed.

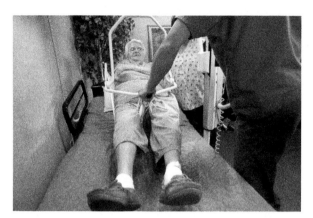

Step 14 Raise the lift until the person and the sling are clear of the bed.

15. Place the wheelchair alongside the bed, facing the foot of the bed. Lock the wheelchair wheels.

16. Have your co-worker support the person's legs as you move the lift into position over the wheelchair.

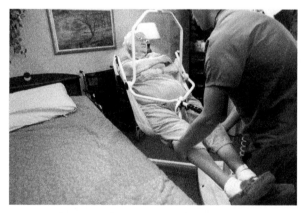

Step 16 A co-worker supports the person's legs as you move her into position over the wheelchair.

17. Turn the person so that she is facing the mast of the lift and is centered over the base. (The person's back should be facing the wheelchair.)

18. Move the lift so that the person is over the seat of the wheelchair.

19. Slowly open the release valve on the lift. Gently lower the person into the wheelchair. Make sure the person's buttocks are at the back of the chair.

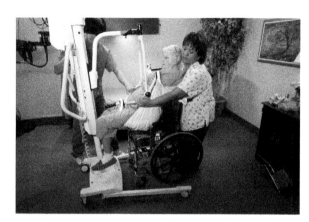

Step 19 Gently lower the person into the wheelchair.

20. Lower the swivel bar so that you can unhook the sling. Leave the sling under the person.

21. Make sure the person's buttocks are at the back of the chair. Make sure the person is comfortable and in good body alignment.

22. Position the person's feet on the footrests of the wheelchair. Buckle the wheelchair safety belt (or place a lap restraint, if ordered). Cover the person's lap and legs with a lap blanket, if desired. Make sure that the lap blanket does not drag on the floor.

Finishing Up   CLSOWR

23. Position the wheelchair according to the person's preference.

24. Follow the "Finishing Up" steps.

25. When the person is ready to return to bed, reverse the procedure.

PROCEDURE 11-15

Assisting a Person With Sitting on the Edge of the Bed ("Dangling")

WHY YOU DO IT   Allowing a person time to "dangle" before getting out of bed reduces the person's risk of falling due to dizziness or loss of consciousness.

Getting Ready   WORKERS

1. Complete the "Getting Ready" steps.

Procedure

2. Make sure that the bed is lowered to its lowest position and that the wheels are locked.

3. If the side rails are in use, lower the side rail on the working side of the bed. The side rail on the opposite side of the bed should remain up. Raise the head of the bed as tolerated. Fanfold the top linens to the foot of the bed.

4. **Method "A":**

   a. Stand at the side of the bed with your feet spread about 30 cm apart and with your knees slightly bent to protect your back.

   b. Have the person bend her knees and plant her feet on the bed.

   c. Gently slide one arm behind the person's upper back. Slide the other arm under her knees and rest your hand on the side of her thigh.

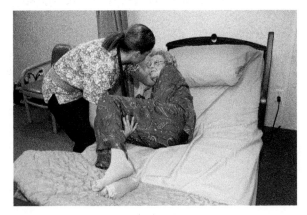

Step 4c Slide one arm behind the person's upper back. Slide the other arm under her knees.

d. With a single smooth movement, slide the person's legs over the side of the bed while moving her head and shoulders upward so that she is sitting on the edge of the bed.

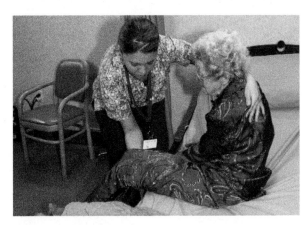

Step 4d Help the person to sit on the edge of the bed.

5. **Method "B":**

   a. Help the person to move toward the side of the bed.

   b. Have the person roll over onto her side, facing the side of the bed. Have the person flex her knees and bend the arm she is lying on in preparation for using it to prop her upper body up. Have the person bend her top arm so that her hand is in a position that will enable her to push off the bed.

   c. Instruct the person to rise to a sitting position by using the elbow of her bottom arm to raise her upper body while pushing against the mattress with her other hand. Advise the person to allow her legs to swing over the edge of the bed while you help to guide her into an upright position.

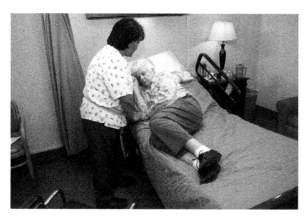

Step 5b Have the person roll onto her side, facing the side of the bed.

6. Have the person put her hands on the edge of the bed, alongside each thigh, for support. Watch for signs of dizziness or fainting. If the person feels faint, help her to lie down and call for the nurse.

7. Allow the person to "dangle" her legs over the side of the bed for the specified period of time, and then either take her vital signs (if indicated), help her to lie back down, or assist her to a standing position. Stay with her during the entire time.

Finishing Up CLSOWR

8. Complete the "Finishing Up" steps.

PROCEDURE 11-16

Assisting a Person With Walking (Ambulating)

WHY YOU DO IT   Assisting a person to ambulate regularly helps to meet the person's need for exercise and helps prevent complications of immobility. It also helps to keep a person as independent as possible for as long as possible.

Getting Ready WGKIEDS

1. Complete the "Getting Ready" steps.

Supplies

- transfer belt
- cane or walker (if indicated)
- person's robe
- person's slippers or shoes (nonskid soles)

Procedure

2. If the person is in bed, make sure that the bed is lowered to its lowest position and that the wheels are locked.

3. Assist the person to "dangle." Check the person's pulse; a weak pulse could lead to light-headedness. If the person's pulse is weak, stay with her and alert the nurse before attempting ambulation.

4. Help the person put her shoes or slippers on and help her into a robe. Apply a transfer belt.

5. Help the person to stand.

   a. Stand facing the person.

   b. Have the person put her hands on the edge of the bed, alongside each thigh.

   c. Make sure the person's feet are flat on the floor.

   d. Have the person lean forward.

   e. Grasp the transfer belt at each side, using an underhand grasp. (If you are not using a transfer belt, pass your arms under the person's arms and rest your hands on her upper back.)

   f. Position your feet alongside the person's feet, flexing your knees. Place your shins against the person's shins to block the person's feet and keep her knees from buckling as she stands up.

   g. Have the person push down on the bed with her hands and stand on the count of "three." Assist the person into a standing position by pulling on the transfer belt as you straighten your knees. (If you are not using a transfer belt, assist the person into a standing position by gently pulling her up and forward as you straighten your knees.) Remember to keep your back straight.

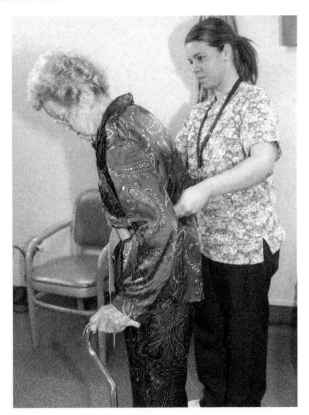

Step 7 Grasp the transfer belt with an underhand grip from the back.

6. Have the person grasp the cane or walker, if she is using one, in order to maintain balance. The person should hold the cane on her strong side.

7. Help the person to walk. Stand slightly behind the person on her weaker side. Grasp the transfer belt with an underhand grip from the back. If the person is using an ambulation device, make sure she is using it correctly.

8. After returning to the person's room, help her back into bed or a chair.

Finishing Up CLSOWR

9. Complete the "Finishing Up" steps.

WHAT DID YOU LEARN?

Multiple Choice

Select the single best answer for each of the following questions.

1. Which of the following describes good standing posture when helping to reposition or transfer a person?
   a. Feet 12 inches apart
   b. Abdominal muscles relaxed
   c. Arms out straight
   d. Feet close together

2. When assisting a person to move to the head of the bed, you should:
   a. Face the head of the bed
   b. Unlock the bed wheels
   c. Place a pillow under the person's head
   d. Place the foot that is farthest away from the bed edge behind the other foot

3. Which person is likely to need help moving and turning in bed?
   a. A person who is ambulatory
   b. A person who has Alzheimer's disease
   c. A sleeping person
   d. An unconscious person

4. To transfer a person correctly from a bed to a stretcher, you must:
   a. Use a mechanical lift
   b. Get help from at least five co-workers
   c. Use good body mechanics
   d. Raise the far side rail of the stretcher first

5. When moving and positioning people, you should:
   a. Avoid friction and shearing
   b. Use good body mechanics
   c. Use pillows and rolled towels to maintain the position
   d. All of the above

6. Sitting a person on the side of the bed is called:
   a. Semi-sitting
   b. Proning
   c. Supining
   d. Dangling

7. When transferring a person from one place to another, you should:
   a. Use a transfer belt (unless the person has a condition that prevents the use of a transfer belt)
   b. Adjust the bed to the lowest possible height
   c. Lock the brakes of the bed, wheelchair, or stretcher
   d. All of the above

8. A person in the prone position is lying on his:
   a. Right side
   b. Left side
   c. Abdomen
   d. Back

9. When moving a person by yourself and the person is wearing a transfer belt:
   a. Lift from the side
   b. Use an underhand grasp
   c. Use an overhand grasp
   d. Stand behind the person

10. A nurse asks you to place a patient in the semi-Fowler's position while his tube feeding is running. You know the head of the bed should be elevated:
    a. 90 degrees
    b. 60 degrees
    c. 30 degrees
    d. 15 degrees

11. A mechanical lift can be used to:
    a. Move a patient or resident who is very heavy
    b. Move a patient or resident who is very weak
    c. Help a personal support worker carry out her duties without injuring herself
    d. All of the above

12. When transferring a person from a bed to a stretcher, you should position the bed:
    a. At its lowest level
    b. At its highest level
    c. In the high Fowler's position
    d. In the supine position

13. A person who cannot reposition himself independently is at risk for developing:
    a. Pressure ulcers
    b. Blood clots
    c. Pneumonia
    d. All of the above

14. What is it called when a joint is held in one position for too long, and the tendons shorten?
    a. A pressure ulcer
    b. A bed sore
    c. A contracture
    d. A shearing injury

15. Why is it important to ensure that your patients or residents are in good body alignment every time you reposition them?
    a. Good body alignment is most comfortable for the patient or resident
    b. Good body alignment helps prevent complications, such as pressure ulcers and contractures
    c. Good body alignment helps the person to breathe easier and improves blood flow to tissues
    d. All of the above

16. What technique would you use to move Rosemary, a 15-year-old patient who has just had spinal surgery?
    a. Logrolling
    b. A mechanical lift
    c. Dangling
    d. Turning

STOP and Think!

Cynthia, a new personal support worker, has been assigned to take care of Mrs. Adkins. Mrs. Adkins weighs more than 250 pounds and has had a stroke, so she is paralyzed completely on her left side. Cynthia has to transfer Mrs. Adkins from her bed to a wheelchair so she can go to the shower room. What steps should Cynthia take to help ensure a safe transfer for Mrs. Adkins?

You have been assigned to the north hall and have five residents you must assist to the dining room for breakfast. Mr. Clark is recovering nicely from a fractured hip and is eager to walk to the dining room with the aid of his new walker. What words of advice can you give Mr. Clark to help him use his walker more efficiently?

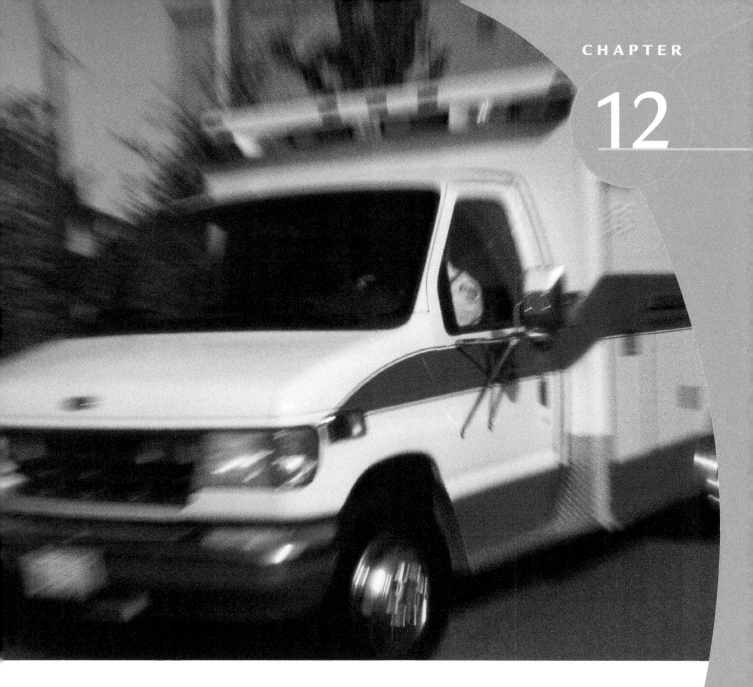

Basic First Aid and Emergency Care

WHAT WILL YOU LEARN?

Any condition that requires immediate medical attention to prevent a person from dying or having a permanent disability is an **emergency.** An emergency can occur as a result of an accident (such as a fall) or as a result of a medical condition (such as a heart attack or stroke). Emergency situations can occur anywhere, even in a health care setting.

Photo: An ambulance speeds through the streets to aid a person in need.

As a personal support worker, you must be prepared to provide safe, compassionate care for a person in an emergency situation. When you are finished with this chapter, you will be able to:

1. Discuss your role in an emergency situation.
2. Define terms used to describe a person's condition in an emergency situation.
3. List and discuss the ABCs of emergency care.
4. List some of the organizations that offer approved training in first aid and basic life support (BLS) measures.
5. List the signs and symptoms of a "heart attack" and describe the actions that a personal support worker would take to assist a person with these signs and symptoms.
6. List the signs and symptoms of a stroke.
7. Describe how you would assist a person who complains of feeling faint, or who has fainted.
8. Describe how you would assist a person who is having a seizure.
9. Describe how you would assist a person who is bleeding uncontrollably (hemorrhaging).
10. Describe some of the types and causes of shock, and describe how you would assist a person who is in shock.
11. Demonstrate how to clear the airway of a choking adult or child older than 1 year by using the Heimlich manoeuvre.
12. Demonstrate the method used to clear the airway of a choking infant.
13. Describe the steps of the chain of survival.

Vocabulary

Emergency	Respiratory arrest	Syncope	Hemorrhagic shock
Oriented to person, place, and time	Cardiac arrest	Grand mal seizure	Septic shock
	Clinical death	Petit mal (absence) seizure	Anaphylactic shock
Disoriented	Biological death		Aspiration
Unresponsive	Basic life support (BLS)	Hemorrhage	Heimlich manoeuvre
Emergency medical services (EMS) system	Rescue breathing	Pulse points	Chain of survival
	Cardiopulmonary resuscitation (CPR)	Shock	
First aid		Cardiogenic shock	

RESPONDING TO AN EMERGENCY

As you learned in Chapter 5, the nature of your daily duties will bring you in close and frequent contact with your patients or residents. This unique relationship gives you insight that others might not have. Through your interactions with your patients or residents, you become aware of their individual qualities, personalities, and habits. For example, you know that Mrs. Smith typically has an above-average blood pressure reading, even though she is taking medication. You know that Mr. Martin complains about his arthritis, especially in the morning. You know that Mr. Allen always says that he is starving after eating a full meal. You know which of your patients or residents are "morning people," and which are grumpy and slow until after they have had their first cup of coffee. Your familiarity with your patients or residents makes you more likely to notice when something is not quite right.

For example, the first sign of a stroke is often just a slight slurring of speech or a small change in a person's personality. Heart attacks may be signaled by complaints of fatigue or indigestion. Other emergency situations are recognized by changes in vital signs (such as respiratory rate, heart rate, and blood pressure) or behaviour. The people you care for will have varying levels of ability and awareness, and you will come to learn what is normal for each person. A change in a person's usual abilities or level of awareness

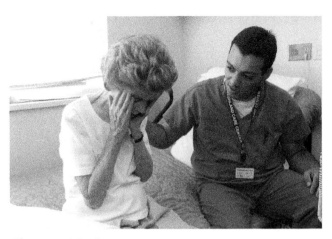

Figure 12-1
Being able to recognize an impending emergency is a life-saving skill.

can be a sign that something is wrong. A person who is usually alert and **oriented to person** (able to tell you who he is and who you are), **place** (able to tell you where he is), and **time** (able to tell you the year, the day of the week, and the time of day) can suddenly become **disoriented,** or unable to answer those basic questions. A person is said to be **unresponsive** if she is unconscious and cannot be aroused, or conscious but not responsive when spoken to or touched. Either of these conditions should be reported to the nurse immediately. By conscientiously reporting to the nurse any signs or symptoms that seem unusual or give you cause for alarm, you may prevent an emergency situation from worsening (Fig. 12-1).

In an emergency situation, your responsibilities as a personal support worker are clear. You should:

1. **Recognize that an emergency exists.** Use your observation skills and familiarity with the patient or resident to detect changes in behaviour or physical condition.
2. **Decide to act.** Stay calm and organize your thoughts. Check the scene to make sure that you are not entering a situation that is potentially dangerous for you, or for other members of the health care team. For example, a person who has been electrocuted may still be tangled in live electrical wires, which could shock you. Or, you could be entering an area that is contaminated with hazardous materials or gases. Acting hastily can make the problem worse in some situations. For example, someone who has fallen from a ladder may have injuries to the spinal column

that would be made worse if the person were moved.
3. **Check for consciousness.** If it is safe to do so, gently shake the person and call to him. The person may have just fainted ("passed out"), in which case you will need to call the nurse for help. Keep the person lying down, and stay with the person until the nurse arrives. The nurse will make sure that no other injuries are present and work to find out why the person fainted. If the person does not respond when you gently shake his arm and call to him, then you will need to . . .
4. **Activate the emergency medical services (EMS) system.** An **EMS system** is a network of resources (including people, equipment, and facilities) that is organized to respond to an emergency. Hospitals typically have a code or procedure for calling EMS assistance from within the facility. Home health care agencies, assisted-living facilities, and long-term care facilities may require you to dial "911" or some other emergency telephone number. Know your facility's or agency's policy so that you can get help quickly. Early activation of the EMS system allows a person in an emergency situation to get advanced medical care as soon as possible. This greatly increases the person's chances of survival. When you call, be prepared to give accurate information about your location and the condition of your patient or resident. If you work in a long-term care facility, an assisted-living facility, or for a home health care agency, the people who respond to your call may be emergency medical technicians (EMTs) or paramedics. In an acute-care facility, such as a hospital, the people who respond will be a specially trained group of nurses, doctors, and other health care workers.
5. **Provide appropriate care until the EMS personnel arrive.** Provide **first aid** (the care given to an injured or sick person while waiting for more advanced help to arrive) according to the situation and your level of training. (As in any situation, you should perform only those procedures that you have been trained to do and that are within your scope of practice.) Speak gently and calmly to the person, and reassure him that more help is on the way.
6. **Record the care you provided.** As always when you provide care, you must accurately record your observations and the care that you provided.

Helping Hands and a Caring Heart

FOCUS ON HUMANISTIC HEALTH CARE

An emergency can be very frightening for the person experiencing it. Although you will be focused on the person's physical needs, try not to forget about the other needs that the person and his or her family members have. Remain calm. Reassure the person and family members that more help is on the way. While the situation may be too serious to say something like, "Everything will be OK," you can certainly tell the person that you will "do everything you can to help."

BASIC LIFE SUPPORT MEASURES

Emergency situations often result when something occurs that affects breathing or circulation. The body's cells need oxygen to live. When we inhale, we take air, which contains oxygen, into our lungs. Once in the lungs, the oxygen in the air passes from the tiny air sacs of the lungs (called the *alveoli*) into the blood in the blood vessels that surround the alveoli. Each time the heart beats, the oxygen-containing blood is sent to all of the cells in the body.

Any process that affects our ability to take air into our lungs or to send oxygen-containing blood to the cells of the body is an emergency. Without oxygen, the cells of the body begin to die. Humans can live for days without food and water but only for a few minutes without oxygen.

Respiratory arrest means that breathing has stopped (*arrest* means "stop"). When breathing stops, the oxygen content of the blood decreases, and there is not enough oxygen for the cells of the body to function properly. Soon, key organs such as the brain and the heart stop functioning. A person who is in respiratory arrest may have a heartbeat initially, but if breathing is not started again soon, his heart will stop beating. The condition is called **cardiac arrest.** A person who has no pulse or is not breathing is said to be *clinically dead.* **Clinical death** can sometimes be reversed with prompt emergency treatment that restarts the heart and breathing. However, if clinical death is not promptly reversed, allowing oxygen-containing blood to reach the brain and the heart, **biological death** soon follows. Biological death is not reversible.

Basic life support (BLS) measures are taken to prevent respiratory arrest, cardiac arrest, or both. BLS techniques include **rescue breathing** and **cardiopulmonary resuscitation (CPR).** If the person is already in respiratory or cardiac arrest, BLS is used to keep the person alive until advanced medical assistance arrives. The ABCs of emergency care (Box 12-1) are used to determine whether a person needs BLS measures.

Your facility may require first aid and BLS training as a requirement for employment. In some states, first aid and BLS training are provided as part of personal support worker training. However, because improvements are periodically made in the way some of these techniques, such as CPR, are taught, we have not provided specific instructions for all first aid and BLS techniques in this book. If training in first aid and BLS is not included as part of your personal support worker training course, you can learn these techniques in courses offered by organizations such as the Canadian Red Cross (CRC) the Heart and Stroke Foundation, and St. John Ambulance. The programs offered by these organizations are taught by certified instructors, using approved teaching methods (Fig. 12-2). This additional training will allow you to be better prepared for emergency situations that may arise in your workplace, home, or community.

If you are trained in BLS measures and you find one of your patients or residents in a state of respiratory or cardiac arrest, be sure you know

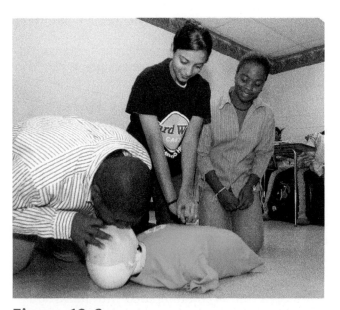

Figure 12-2
Students practice rescue breathing and cardiopulmonary resuscitation (CPR) on a mannequin during a basic life support (BLS) training course. (*AP Photo/The Commercial Dispatch, Kelly Tippett.*)

The ABCs of Emergency Care

"A" is for "airway." Open the person's airway by tilting her head back and lifting her chin. This prevents the person's tongue from falling backward against the back of the throat, blocking the flow of air to the lungs.

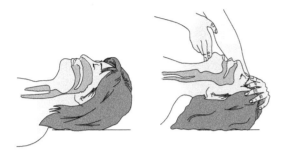

"B" is for "breathing." Check to see if the person is breathing by leaning close and placing your ear over her mouth and nose. Listen for the sounds of breathing, feel the person's breath moving against your cheek, and look for the rise and fall of the person's chest. The person is not breathing unless there is air movement as well as chest movement!

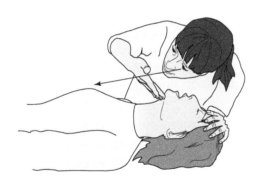

- If the person is breathing, keep her airway open or position her on her side. Continue to monitor the person's condition closely while waiting for assistance.
- If the person is not breathing, start rescue breathing according to your training. Remember that if an airway is not established and oxygen is not sent to the person's lungs, the person will not survive the incident, no matter what additional measures are taken.

"C" is for "circulation." Check the person's pulse. You can feel an adult's or child's pulse by placing your fingers on either side of the Adam's apple, over the carotid artery in the neck. An infant's pulse is felt over the brachial artery, in the upper arm. A person in an emergency situation may have a rapid, weak, erratic (irregular), or very slow pulse. A person with no pulse is in cardiac arrest and needs immediate CPR.

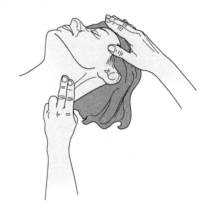

the person's wishes for resuscitation before beginning BLS. For example, a person who is terminally ill may not want to be resuscitated if she goes into respiratory or cardiac arrest. In this case, the person's chart would carry a no-code or do not resuscitate (DNR) order. (See Chapter 21, where the subject of advance directives is covered more fully.) If a person is on DNR status, follow your facility's or agency's policy accordingly.

EMERGENCY SITUATIONS

Many different emergency situations can occur, both in the home and community and in the health care setting. In this section, we will review some of the most common emergency situations, as well as what you should do to help a person in one of these situations.

"HEART ATTACKS" AND STROKES

Both heart attacks and strokes can occur suddenly. These are life-threatening situations that require emergency care. Perhaps the classic emergency situation is that of a "heart attack," or myocardial infarction (MI). The myocardium is the muscular wall of the heart. An infarction occurs when blood flow to a part of the body is blocked, depriving the cells of oxygen and causing them to die. So when a person has an MI, blood flow to the muscular wall of the heart is blocked, and part of the heart muscle dies. As a result, the heart is unable to pump blood effectively throughout the body, creating an emergency situation. If the damaged area of the heart is large enough, cardiac arrest can occur.

The signs and symptoms of a heart attack can vary greatly from one person to the next. Signs and symptoms of a heart attack may include:

- Pain or tightness in the chest, which may extend to the neck, back, or arm
- Pale or greyish skin
- Excessive sweating
- Trouble breathing
- Nausea or heartburn-like pain

If you observe that a person is having signs or symptoms of a heart attack, have the person lie down. Raise the person's head to help make breathing easier, and call the nurse or activate the EMS system immediately. Prompt medical intervention can help to minimize damage to the heart muscle. If the person goes into respiratory or cardiac arrest, you will need to begin BLS.

Strokes, also known as "brain attacks" or cerebrovascular accidents (CVAs), are also caused by blocked blood flow to a body part. In the case of a stroke, the affected body part is the brain, rather than the heart. Like a heart attack, a stroke can cause different signs and symptoms in different people. For example, a stroke might cause only mild physical changes in some people. In others, it might cause loss of consciousness or a coma. Signs and symptoms of a stroke could include any of the following:

- A change in a person's level of orientation or consciousness
- Slurred speech
- Muscle weakness or paralysis
- Drooping of the eyelid or a corner of the mouth
- Severe headache

If you think that a person is having or has had a stroke, report your observations to the nurse and activate the EMS system. Keep the person lying down and watch for signs of respiratory arrest until advanced care arrives. New advances in the treatment of stroke have resulted in improved outcomes for some patients, when treatment is started early.

FAINTING (SYNCOPE)

Fainting (also called **syncope**) occurs when the blood supply to the brain suddenly decreases, resulting in a loss of consciousness. Although fainting may be an early sign of a serious medical condition, such as a heart problem, it can also be the result of hunger ("low blood sugar"), pain, extreme emotion, fatigue, medication side effects, a "stuffy" room (poor ventilation), excessive heat, or standing for a long time. Fainting is not life-threatening in and of itself, but because a person who faints is at risk for injury from falling, it is important to act quickly if you believe a person is about to faint. A person who is about to faint may complain of dizziness or a temporary loss of vision. His skin may be pale and clammy and he may sweat excessively. He may breathe shallowly, and his pulse may be weak.

If you think that a person is about to faint, have the person lie down in the supine position and elevate his legs, or ask him to sit down and bend forward, placing his head between his knees (Fig. 12-3). These actions will increase blood flow to the brain, which may prevent the person from losing consciousness. Loosen any restraints or tight clothing (such as a belt or necktie), and have the person remain in the supine or sitting position (with his head between his knees) for at least 5 minutes. Do not leave the person unattended during this time. If necessary, use the call light control to call the nurse.

If a person you are assisting does faint, lower him to the floor or other flat surface, remembering to use good body mechanics (see Chapter 9,

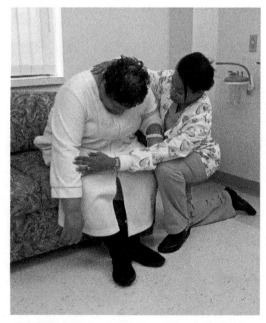

Figure 12-3
Having a person sit with her head between her knees increases blood flow to the brain and may prevent a fainting episode.

Box 9-1). Position the person on his back with his head turned to the side, in case he vomits. If you are sure that the person does not have any injuries to the head, neck, or spinal cord, raise his legs, and loosen any tight clothing or restraints. Make sure the person is breathing, and call for help. Then check the person's vital signs. Even if the person recovers from the episode quickly, have him continue to lie down until the nurse arrives.

> ## TELL THE NURSE ❗
>
> *Because fainting may be a sign of a serious medical condition, it is important to report and record the following for the nurse:*
>
> - What time the person fainted
> - Whether there was a change in the person's level of consciousness, and if so, how long this change lasted
> - Whether the person vomited
> - The person's appearance at the time of the incident (for example: overheated, pale, sweaty)
> - Whether the person complained of anything before the incident (for example, loss of vision, dizziness, nausea)
> - The actions you took to assist the person

SEIZURES

Seizures, also known as *convulsions*, occur when brain activity is interrupted. Seizures can result from head injuries (either recent or past), strokes, infections, high fevers, low blood sugar, poisonings, brain tumors, and epilepsy.

The severity of a seizure can vary. **Grand mal seizures** are characterized by violent jerking of the muscles all over the body. A person who is having a **petit mal (absence) seizure,** however, may simply stop speaking in mid-sentence and stare into space.

Although petit mal seizures are not an emergency situation, grand mal seizures usually are. Grand mal seizures cause a loss of consciousness and, because of the violent jerking of the muscles, place the person who is having the seizure at risk for injuring herself. If a person is standing or sitting when a seizure begins, she could be injured when she falls as the result of losing consciousness. A person who is having a

seizure is also at risk for injuring herself by striking nearby objects or by severely biting her own tongue and lips. A grand mal seizure may last for just a few seconds, or it may go on for as long as 5 to 10 minutes.

First aid for a person having a grand mal seizure involves protecting the person until the seizure is over, and keeping the airway open during the period of unconsciousness afterward. If a person is standing or sitting when a seizure begins, gently help the person to the floor and move furniture or other objects that might cause injury out of the way. Protect the person's head by placing a pillow or folded towel underneath it and call for help while allowing the seizure to run its course. Although in the past, it was common practice to insert a tongue blade into the person's mouth to prevent the person from biting her own tongue, you should not do this. Never attempt to place anything in the person's mouth or between the teeth. You may hurt the person or get bitten. It is common for a person who is having a grand mal seizure to lose control of her bladder or bowels. Because the gag reflex may also be temporarily lost, saliva may pool in the mouth. After the seizure is over, turn the person to her side (place her in the recovery position) and allow any secretions to drain from her mouth to prevent choking. Provide warmth and a quiet environment (Fig. 12-4). A person who has just had a seizure may be very disoriented, tired, or both, and she may have no memory of the episode at all.

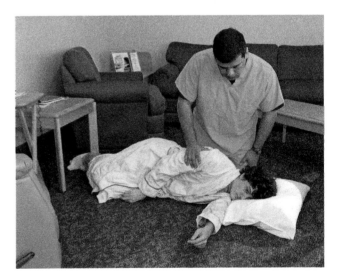

Figure 12-4
After the seizure has passed, place the person in the recovery position and allow secretions to drain from the mouth.

HEMORRHAGE

Hemorrhage (severe, uncontrolled bleeding) can be caused by trauma to a blood vessel or by certain illnesses, such as gastric ulcers. Ordinarily, when a blood vessel wall is injured, a blood clot forms to prevent the loss of blood. However, if the trauma to the blood vessel wall is major, or if the person lacks the clotting factors needed to form blood clots, the bleeding will not stop. It should be noted that people who are taking medications to prevent blood clotting are at high risk for hemorrhage as well, because the medication decreases the body's normal clotting response.

Hemorrhage can be either external (plainly visible) or internal (occurring within the body). Internal hemorrhage may be hidden unless the person vomits blood or passes blood through the rectum. Hemorrhage can be either venous or arterial, depending on the type of blood vessel that is injured. Venous hemorrhage flows steadily. Arterial hemorrhage spurts or pulses with the heartbeat. If hemorrhage is not controlled quickly, death will result.

If a person is hemorrhaging, call for help and make sure the person is lying down. Take standard precautions to protect yourself from exposure to bloodborne pathogens. Apply firm, steady pressure directly to the wound using a sterile dressing, a clean towel, or whatever else is clean and available for use as a compress. Continue to apply pressure to the wound until more advanced medical help comes. If the direct pressure does not stop or slow the flow of blood, raise the affected body part (if it is an arm or leg) and apply pressure to a pulse point above the wound. **Pulse points** are the points where large arteries run close enough to the surface of the skin to be felt as a pulse (see Chapter 16, Fig. 16-8). At these points, the artery can be compressed against a bone by applying direct pressure, helping to slow blood loss from a wound. A tourniquet is a device that is placed tightly around an arm or leg to cut off nearly all blood supply. A tourniquet is only used as a last resort to control bleeding, and should always be applied by a specially trained emergency responder.

SHOCK

Shock results when the organs and tissues of the body do not receive enough oxygen-containing blood. There are many different causes and types of shock. For example:

- **Cardiogenic shock** can occur when the heart is unable to pump enough blood throughout the body to meet the tissues' need for oxygen.
- **Hemorrhagic shock** results from massive blood loss, which means that there is not enough blood in the vessels to supply the tissues of the body.
- **Septic shock** is caused by severe bacterial infections that involve the entire body. The toxins produced by the bacteria cause the blood vessels to dilate (widen), leading to pooling of blood away from the heart and poor circulation.
- **Anaphylactic shock** is caused by a severe allergic reaction (for example, to medications, bee stings, or certain foods, such as nuts). As in septic shock, widening of the blood vessels occurs, causing the blood to pool away from the heart. In addition, the tiniest tubes in the lungs (called bronchioles) close off, preventing the oxygen in the air from passing into the lungs and reaching the blood.

To treat shock, the underlying cause of the shock must be addressed. For example, if a person is in shock because of hemorrhage, the bleeding must be stopped and the fluid replaced intravenously to prevent death. If the pumping action of the heart is too weak or erratic to circulate blood to the organs and tissues, the heart's ability to pump must be restored through medications or other measures, such as the implantation of a pacemaker.

A person entering a state of shock will have low blood pressure that continues to decrease. His pulse will be rapid and weak. His skin will be cool, clammy, and pale. He will be confused or disoriented. He will breathe rapidly, and if he is conscious, he may complain of thirst. Make sure that advanced emergency medical care has been called and keep the person warm and calm. The treatment for anaphylactic shock is the immediate administration of a medication called epinephrine (adrenaline). People who know that they are allergic to something that could cause them to go into anaphylactic shock (for example, bee stings) often carry this medication with them (Fig. 12-5). If a person who is in anaphylactic shock is unable to give himself this medication, someone else will need to do this for him.

AIRWAY OBSTRUCTIONS ("CHOKING")

Foreign material, such as food or vomitus, can become lodged in the airway ("windpipe"), blocking the flow of air to the lungs. The accidental

Figure 12-5
The EpiPen Auto-Injector, a self-injectable cartridge of epinephrine, is used to treat anaphylactic shock. The yellow EpiPen is for adults. The green one is for children. (*Photo courtesy of Dey, L.P.*)

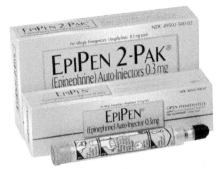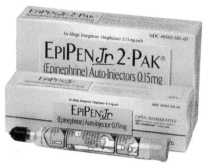

inhalation of foreign material into the airway is called **aspiration.** Aspiration is very common during meal times. People with poorly fitting dentures or who are missing teeth cannot chew their food properly, which puts them at risk for aspiration. In addition, talking or laughing with food in the mouth can lead to aspiration.

Children are at high risk for aspiration. Children often do not chew their food well, and they can choke on very small pieces of food. Foods that do not usually cause problems for adults, such as hard candies, hot dogs, popcorn, apples, grapes, carrots, and nuts, can be choking hazards for children. Children may put small toys or other objects in their mouths. They often try to eat while running, playing, laughing, or crying. All of these actions increase the risk for aspiration.

People who are not conscious or who have weak coughing or swallowing reflexes as a result of paralysis or the effects of a medication (for example, some pain medications) are also at an increased risk for aspiration. Most people who are vomiting can keep their airway clear and will choke and gag easily, but people with an impaired gag reflex may aspirate vomitus. This is why, when you are assisting a person who is vomiting or at risk for vomiting, you turn the person's head to the side to help keep the airway clear.

An airway obstruction can be either partial or complete. In a partial airway obstruction, the object is not totally blocking the airway and some air can pass through. A person who is coughing strongly and has good skin color most likely has a partial airway obstruction with good air exchange (that is, an adequate ability to breathe). Stay with the person and allow him to continue to cough. If the person is not already sitting up, help him to sit up to make breathing easier. If the person does not quickly cough up the object, call for help because advanced emergency medical assistance may be necessary to remove the item. Also, there is the risk that the item will move and totally obstruct the airway, in which case the person will need immediate assistance. A partial airway obstruction

with poor air exchange (that is, an inadequate ability to breathe) is demonstrated by a weak, ineffective coughing effort; high-pitched, "crowing" sounds as the person tries to breathe; and a bluish skin color (cyanosis). A person with this type of airway obstruction needs immediate help.

A complete airway obstruction is one that totally blocks all airflow to the lungs. The person cannot cough, speak, or breathe and will lose consciousness quickly if the object that is blocking airflow is not removed. The person will be frightened, and may run to the bathroom if the obstruction occurs in a public place, such as in a restaurant or dining room. (If you suspect that someone who has left the table is choking, please follow him.) The person may grab his throat in what is considered the universal choking sign (Fig. 12-6).

Clearing the Airway in Adults and Children Older Than 1 Year

Abdominal thrusts, commonly called the **Heimlich manoeuvre,** are used to clear an obstructed airway in an adult or a child older than 1 year who is choking. The thoracic (chest) cavity, which contains the heart and lungs, is separated from the abdominal cavity, which contains the stomach and other organs, by the diaphragm, a flat muscle. During the Heimlich manoeuvre, the area beneath the diaphragm (the abdominal cavity) is compressed, forcing the air out of the lungs. This dislodges the object that is blocking the airway (Fig. 12-7). The procedure for performing the Heimlich manoeuvre on a person who is conscious is given in Procedure 12-1. In 2005, the Canadian Heart and Stroke Association made revisions on how to relieve foreign-body airway obstructions in an unconscious person. The changes have been included in Procedure 12-2.

The Heimlich manoeuvre is done the same way in children older than 1 year and in adults, except that in children, less force is applied to the

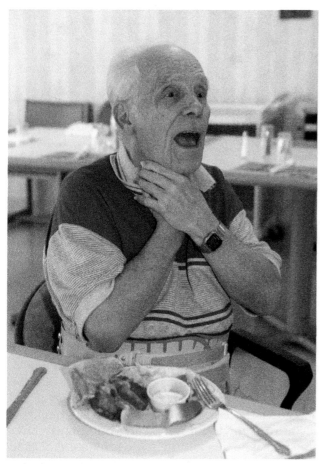

Figure 12-6
Grasping the throat is the universal sign for "I'm choking!"

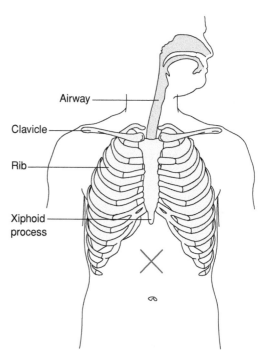

Figure 12-7
Applying pressure to the abdominal cavity (*red X*) forces the air out of the lungs, which in turn forces the object out of the person's airway.

abdomen. This is to avoid injuring the child's ribs, sternum (breastbone), and internal organs. In very heavy people or pregnant women, the Heimlich manoeuvre is modified so that chest thrusts, rather than abdominal thrusts, are used. This is because in these situations, giving abdominal thrusts would be either impossible or dangerous. In the case of a very heavy person, it is too hard to get your arms around the person. In the case of a pregnant woman, applying pressure to the abdomen could harm the baby. Procedure 12-3 explains how to give chest thrusts to both conscious and unconscious people.

When a person is choking, the EMS system should be activated as soon as possible. While you wait for help, perform the Heimlich manoeuvre repeatedly, until the airway is open again and the person starts breathing on his own. If the person does not start breathing on his own, perform rescue breathing after the airway is cleared. You may need to start CPR if the person goes into cardiac arrest. However, you must understand that until the obstruction has been removed and air is sent to the lungs, CPR will not be effective.

Clearing the Airway in Infants

In children younger than 1 year, the Heimlich manoeuvre is not used because of the risk for damaging the baby's internal organs. Instead, a combination of back blows and chest thrusts is used. Clearing the airway in a conscious infant is described in Procedure 12-4. Clearing the airway in an unconscious infant is described in Procedure 12-5. You can give back blows and chest thrusts while standing or sitting. If the infant is large or your hands are small, you may prefer to sit.

THE CHAIN OF SURVIVAL

A person's ability to survive an emergency, and to survive it without any permanent damage, relies on a series of events called the **chain of survival:**

1. Someone must recognize that an emergency situation exists, and activate the EMS system.
2. First responder care (basic first aid, including BLS if applicable) must be given by able people at the scene of the emergency.

3. Medical intervention, such as that provided by an EMT, a paramedic, a nurse, or a doctor, must be provided as soon as possible.
4. After the immediate crisis passes, hospital care may be needed to help the person survive. As the person's condition improves, she may be transferred to a subacute care unit or return to a long-term care facility or private home for further recovery.
5. Rehabilitation, the final step in the chain of survival, focuses on improving the general health status of the person. One goal of rehabilitation may be to help the person to recover abilities that may have been lost as a

result of the emergency. For example, a person who has suffered a stroke may need to relearn skills such as walking or speaking. Another goal of rehabilitation may be to help the person learn how to prevent further progression of a disease. For example, a person who has had a heart attack may be taught new diet management skills, and started on an exercise program.

As a personal support worker, you can play a vital role in helping to see a person through the immediate crisis (steps 1 and 2). You may also care for someone who is in the recovery phase (steps 4 and 5).

SUMMARY

- Any situation in which a person needs immediate medical attention to prevent death or permanent disability is considered an emergency. Emergencies can result from medical conditions (such as a heart attack or stroke) or from an accident (such as a fall).
  - Your knowledge of your patient's or resident's usual condition may allow you to recognize a potential emergency situation. By communicating what you have observed to the nurse, you may be able to prevent the emergency from getting worse.
  - In an emergency situation, you will be responsible for (1) recognizing that an emergency exists (2) deciding to act, (3) checking for consciousness, (4) activating the facility's emergency response system, (5) providing appropriate care per your training and scope of practice until the emergency personnel arrive, and (6) recording your observations and the care you provided.
- The ABCs of emergency care involve maintaining the person's airway, making sure that the person is breathing, and checking the person's pulse to make sure that the heart is beating and blood is circulating throughout the body.
  - Basic life support (BLS) measures support the ABCs: **a**irway, **b**reathing, and **c**irculation. BLS measures include rescue breathing and cardiopulmonary resuscitation (CPR).
  - Training in first aid and BLS measures, whether required by your employer or not,

will prepare you for emergency situations that may arise in your workplace, home, or community.
- Common emergency situations include fainting, seizures, hemorrhage, shock, and choking.
  - Although fainting is not life-threatening, it could put the person at risk for injury from falling. If a person complains of feeling faint, have her lie down or place her head between her knees to increase blood flow to the brain.
  - First aid for a person who is having a seizure involves protecting the person from injury during the seizure and keeping the airway open after the seizure.
  - Hemorrhage is controlled by applying direct pressure to the wound or to a pulse point above the wound.
  - Shock results when the organs and tissues of the body do not receive enough oxygen-rich blood. Keep a person who is in shock warm and calm until emergency personnel arrive.
  - Airway obstructions block the flow of oxygen into the lungs and can quickly result in death if the obstruction is not cleared.
- Receiving skilled first aid, along with early medical intervention, increases a person's chance of surviving an emergency and minimizes the person's chances of having permanent disabilities as a result of the incident.

PROCEDURE 12-1

Performing Abdominal Thrusts in Conscious Adults and Children Older Than 1 Year

WHY YOU DO IT   If the object is not removed from the airway, allowing air to get to the lungs, the person will die.

1. Check the person's ability to breathe and speak by tapping him or her on the shoulder and saying, "Are you okay? Can you talk? I can help you." A person who cannot breathe or speak needs immediate help.

2. If the person starts to cough, wait and see whether the coughing will dislodge the object. If the person's cough is weak and ineffective, or if the person is in obvious distress, continue with step 3.

3. Stay with the person and call for help. Have the person who is helping you activate the facility's emergency response system.

4. Stand behind the person with the obstructed airway and wrap your arms around his or her waist.

5. Make a fist with one hand and place the thumb of the fist against the person's abdomen, just above the navel and below the sternum (breastbone). Grasp your fist with the other hand. (Do not tuck your thumb inside your fist.)

6. Being careful not to put pressure on the person's ribs or sternum with your forearms, press your fist inward and pull upward, using quick thrusting motions, until the object is expelled, the person begins to cough forcefully, or the person loses consciousness.

   a. If the object is expelled, stay with the person, and follow the nurse's directions.

   b. If the person begins to cough, wait and see whether the coughing results in expulsion of the object. If it does not, continue giving abdominal thrusts.

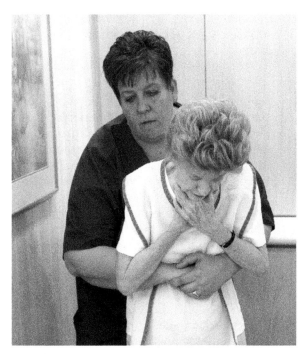

Step 5 Place your fist just above the person's navel and below the sternum.

   c. If the person loses consciousness, lower the person to the floor and begin Procedure 12-2, beginning with step 3.

7. The person should be evaluated by a doctor following the choking incident.

8. Record your observations and actions according to your facility's policy.

PROCEDURE 12-2

Relieving a Foreign-body Airway Obstruction in Unconscious Adults and Children Older Than 1 Year

WHY YOU DO IT   If the object is not removed from the airway, allowing air to get to the lungs, the person will die.

1. Check the person's state of consciousness by gently shaking or tapping him or her. An unresponsive person needs immediate help.

2. Stay with the person and call for help. Have the person who is helping you activate the facility's emergency response system.

3. **Head tilt/chin lift maneuver.** Position the person on his or her back on a hard, flat surface. Open the person's airway by tilting the head back and lifting the chin. Look, feel, and listen for signs of breathing.

4. **Rescue breathing.** If the person is not breathing, keep his or her head tilted back and the chin lifted. Blow two breaths into the person's mouth through a ventilation barrier device, removing your mouth from the device and inhaling between each breath. If the air does not go in, repeat the head tilt/chin lift maneuver and attempt rescue breathing once again.

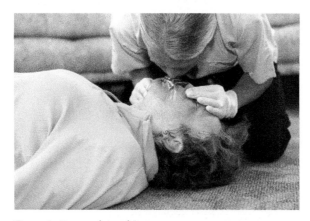

Step 4 Rescue breathing.

5. **Object check.** If no air enters the person's lungs after the second attempt, perform an object check. Kneel beside the person's head and open the airway using the head tilt/chin lift maneuver. Look for the object. If you see the object, remove it. If you cannot see the object, continue to step 6.

6. Repeat the head tilt/chin lift maneuver. Blow two breaths into the person's mouth through a ventilation barrier device, removing your mouth from the device and inhaling between each breath. If the air does not go in, repeat the head tilt/chin lift maneuver and attempt rescue breathing once again.

7. **Chest compressions.** If no air enters the person's lungs after the second attempt, begin chest compressions. To give chest compressions to an unconscious person:

   a. Kneel beside the person.

   b. Place the heel of your hand closest to the person's head on his sternum (breastbone) and place your other hand on top and interlock your fingers.

   c. Position your body forward so that your shoulders are over the center of the person's chest and your arms are straight. You will want to compress straight down and up. Do not rock back and forth.

   d. Compress the chest 3 to 5 cm on an adult (2.5 to 4 cm on a child) quickly at a rate of 100 compressions per minute for 30 compressions.

8. Perform an object check.

9. Repeat the head tilt/chin lift maneuver. Blow two breaths into the person's mouth through a ventilation barrier device, removing your mouth from the device and inhaling between each breath. If the air does not go in, repeat the head tilt/chin lift maneuver and attempt rescue breathing once again.

10. Repeat the chest compression–object check–rescue breathing sequence until the object is expelled, rescue breathing is successful, or other trained personnel arrive and take over.

11. The person should be evaluated by a doctor following the choking incident.

12. Record your observations and actions according to facility policy.

PROCEDURE 12-3

Performing Chest Thrusts in Conscious Adults and Children Older Than 1 Year

WHY YOU DO IT   If the object is not removed from the airway, allowing air to get to the lungs, the person will die.

If the Person Is Conscious

1. Stand behind the person and place your arms under the person's armpits and around his or her chest.
2. Make a fist with one hand and place the thumb of the fist against the center of the person's sternum. Be sure that your thumb is centered on the sternum, not on the lower tip of the sternum (the xiphoid process) and not on the ribs.

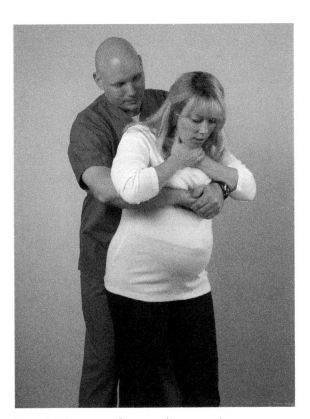

Step 2 Place your fist over the person's sternum.

3. Give up to five quick chest thrusts by grasping your fist with your other hand and pressing inward five times. Each thrust should compress the chest 3 to 5 cm.
4. Continue to give chest thrusts until the object is expelled, the person begins to cough forcefully, or the person loses consciousness.
   a. If the object is expelled, stay with the person, and follow the nurse's directions.
   b. If the person begins to cough, wait and see whether the coughing results in expulsion of the object. If it does not, continue giving chest thrusts in groups of five.
   c. If the person loses consciousness, lower the person to the floor and initiate the procedure below.
5. The person should be evaluated by a doctor following the choking incident.
6. Record your observations and actions according to facility policy.

If the person becomes unconscious, follow the steps in Procedure 12-2.

PROCEDURE / 12-4

Clearing the Airway in a Conscious Infant

WHY YOU DO IT   If the object is not removed from the airway, allowing air to get to the lungs, the infant will die.

1. Check the infant's ability to breathe and cry. An infant who cannot breathe or cry needs immediate help.
2. Stay with the infant. Call for help and have the person who is helping you activate the emergency medical services (EMS) system.
3. Position the infant on his or her back on your forearm. Place your other arm on top of the infant, using your thumb and forefinger to hold the infant's jaw while sandwiching the infant between your forearms.

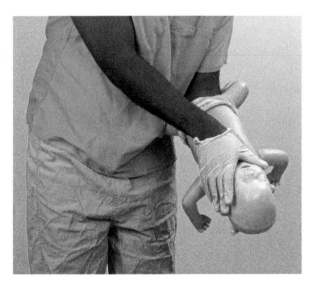

Step 3 Hold the infant on his back between your forearms.

4. Rotate your arms, so that the infant is facing downward, still sandwiched between your forearms. Lower your arm onto your thigh so that the infant's head is lower than his or her chest.
5. Give five firm blows to the back (between the infant's shoulder blades), using the heel of your hand. Be sure that you continue to support the infant's head and neck by firmly holding the baby's jaw between your thumb and forefinger.

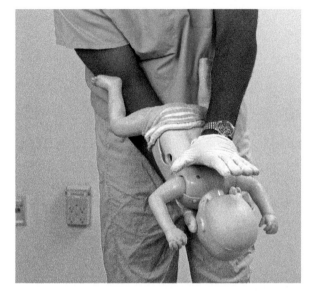

Step 5 Use the heel of your hand to deliver back blows while supporting the infant's head and neck.

6. If the back blows do not dislodge the foreign body, you must turn the infant over in preparation for administering chest thrusts. Turn the infant over by placing your free hand and forearm along the infant's head and back so that the infant is sandwiched between your hands and forearms. Continue to support the infant's head between your thumb and forefinger from the front, while you cradle the back of the head with your other hand. Turn the infant onto his or her back. Lower your arm onto your thigh so that the infant's head is lower than his or her chest.
7. To locate the correct place to give chest thrusts, imagine a line running across the infant's chest between the nipples. Place the pads of your first three fingers on the infant's sternum (breastbone), even with this imaginary line. If you feel the notch at the end of the infant's sternum, move your fingers toward the infant's head so that your fingers are over the center of the sternum.

(continued)

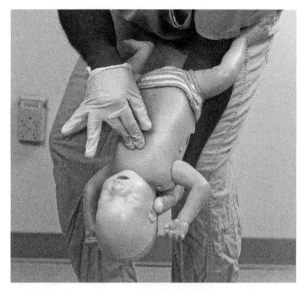

Step 7 Place the pads of your first three fingers on the infant's sternum to give chest thrusts.

8. Lift your ring finger off the chest, and using the pads of the two remaining fingers, com-

press the sternum 1.3 to 2.54 cm, and then let the sternum return to its normal position. Give five chest thrusts.

9. Repeat the back blow–chest thrust sequence until the foreign body is expelled, the infant begins to cough forcefully, or the infant loses consciousness.

   a. If the foreign body is expelled, stay with the infant, and follow the nurse's directions.

   b. If the infant begins to cough, wait and see if the coughing results in expulsion of the object. If it does not, continue giving five back blows followed by five chest thrusts.

   c. If the infant loses consciousness, initiate the procedure described in Procedure 12-5, beginning with step 4.

10. The infant should be evaluated by a doctor following the choking incident.

11. Record your observations and actions according to facility policy.

PROCEDURE 12-5

Clearing the Airway in an Unconscious Infant

WHY YOU DO IT   If the object is not removed from the airway, allowing air to get to the lungs, the infant will die.

---

1. Check the infant's responsiveness by gently shaking the infant and speaking to him. An unresponsive infant needs immediate help.

2. Stay with the infant and call for help. Have the person who is helping you activate the emergency medical services (EMS) system.

3. **Head tilt/chin lift maneuver.** Position the infant on his or her back on a hard, flat surface. Open the infant's airway by tilting the head back slightly and lifting the chin until the infant's nose points toward the ceiling. Look, feel, and listen for signs of breathing.

4. **Rescue breathing.** If the infant is not breathing, keep his or her head tilted back and the chin lifted. Cover the infant's nose and mouth with your mouth or an airway device and blow two slow breaths into the infant's mouth, removing your mouth from

the infant's nose and mouth and inhaling between each breath. If the air does not go in, repeat the head tilt/chin lift maneuver and attempt rescue breathing once again.

5. If no air enters the infant's lungs after the second attempt, assume that the infant's airway is blocked.

6. **Chest compressions**

   a. Place the infant on a flat surface.

   b. Open his airway and look for a foreign object in his throat. If an object is visible, remove it using a "pincer"-type motion with your fingers.

   c. Begin quick downward chest compressions by placing two fingers in the center of the infant's chest, just below the nipple line. Compress 1.3 cm deep with each compressions at a rate of 100 per minute for 30 compressions.

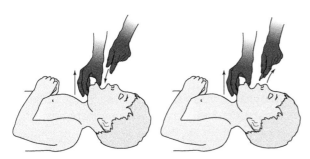

Step 6 If you see a foreign body in the infant's mouth, try to remove it using a "pincer"-type motion.

7. **Foreign body check**

   a. After completing a cycle of 30 chest compressions, open the infant's airway and look for a foreign object.

   b. If you see an object, remove it.

8. Blow two slow breaths into the infant's nose and mouth, removing your nose and mouth from the infant's mouth and inhaling between each breath. If the air does not go in, repeat the head tilt/chin lift maneuver and attempt rescue breathing once again.

9. Repeat steps 6 through 8 until the foreign body is expelled, rescue breathing is successful, or other trained personnel arrive and take over.

10. The infant should be evaluated by a doctor following the choking incident.

11. Record your observations and actions according to facility policy.

WHAT DID YOU LEARN?

Multiple Choice

Select the single best answer for each of the following questions.

1. A person with an airway obstruction will usually:
   a. Have a seizure
   b. Vomit
   c. Be able to speak and breathe normally
   d. Clutch at his or her throat

2. The first step in the chain of survival is:
   a. Rehabilitation
   b. Recognizing that an emergency exists and calling for help
   c. Giving first aid
   d. Initiating basic life support (BLS) measures

3. In the ABCs of emergency care, the "C" stands for:
   a. Cardiac
   b. Consciousness
   c. Circulation
   d. Check for bleeding

4. You are helping to prepare a holiday dinner at your mother's house, when suddenly your sister misses the vegetable she is trying to slice and cuts deeply into her finger instead. Blood is spurting from the cut, which indicates to you that your sister:
   a. Is hemorrhaging internally
   b. Has cut a vein
   c. Has cut an artery
   d. Requires the application of a tourniquet

5. Where do you place your fist while clearing an obstructed airway in a conscious adult?
   a. On the person's back
   b. Above the person's navel
   c. On the person's chest
   d. Below the person's navel

6. If a person is coughing but able to breathe, you should:
   a. Administer oxygen
   b. Use a finger sweep to remove the object that is obstructing the person's airway
   c. Perform the Heimlich manoeuvre
   d. Stay with the person and allow him or her to continue coughing

7. Which is a sign or symptom of shock?
   a. Low blood pressure
   b. A weak, rapid pulse
   c. Cool, clammy, pale skin
   d. All of the above

8. Which of the following actions should you take to assist a person who is having a grand mal seizure?
   a. Protect the person's head by placing a pillow underneath it
   b. Clear the area by moving furniture out of the way
   c. Avoid placing anything in the person's mouth
   d. All of the above

Matching

Match each numbered item with its appropriate lettered description.

_____ 1. Emergency medical services (EMS) system

_____ 2. First aid

_____ 3. Basic life support (BLS)

_____ 4. Clinically dead

_____ 5. Respiratory arrest

_____ 6. Cardiac arrest

_____ 7. Grand mal seizure

_____ 8. Petit mal (absence) seizure

_____ 9. Anaphylactic shock

_____ 10. Fainting (syncope)

a. Occurs when the blood supply to the brain suddenly decreases, resulting in a loss of consciousness

b. Condition of a person who has no pulse or is not breathing

c. Breathing has stopped

d. A potentially deadly allergic reaction (for example, to a bee sting or certain foods, such as nuts)

e. Heart has stopped

f. Care given to an injured person before more advanced medical assistance arrives

g. A network of resources, including people, equipment, and facilities, that is organized to respond to an emergency

h. The person stares off into space or stops speaking for a moment

i. Measures taken to prevent respiratory arrest, cardiac arrest, or both

j. Generalized and violent contraction and relaxation of the body's muscles

STOP and Think!

You work as a personal support worker in a nursing home. One of your responsibilities is to check on the residents while the nurses are attending the change-of-shift report. You enter Mrs. Oblonsky's room and find her on the floor. She has no roommate, so no one witnessed what happened. It does not appear that Mrs. Oblonsky fell out of bed. Her color is pale, and her lips are turning blue. What should you do first?

One of your responsibilities is to oversee the residents of the long-term care facility where you work while they are in the recreation room. Today, the residents are gathered and getting ready for an activity. Everyone is busy talking, selecting teams, and generally having fun. Everyone, that is, except for Mr. Grant. Normally outgoing and friendly, today Mr. Grant is just sitting in his wheelchair, staring into space without moving. You speak to Mr. Grant and notice that he seems confused and is having difficulty forming his words. The left side of his mouth looks droopy and he's drooling a bit. These observations may be signs of what emergency situation? What should you do?

Personal Support Workers Make a Difference!

"My name is Henrietta, and I have been a resident of the Sunnydale Nursing Facility for the past 6 years. I came to live here after a stroke partially paralyzed my left side and left me unable to walk. I am well cared for, and have grown to care for most of the people who work here like my own family. I've also made many new friends. It's funny—since coming to live here, I actually get to see more people and do more things than when I lived at home, alone. There are always planned activities—such as bingo games, poetry readings, jigsaw puzzle get-togethers, and card games—that allow us residents to get together and socialize. Perhaps my favorite social activity of all is dinner in the large dining room. The dining room has large bay windows and French doors that look westward out over the mountains, giving us "front row seats" for the sunset. There is also a piano, and on most nights, Mitch, a volunteer from the community, comes and plays wonderful music on the piano as we eat.

One night not too long ago, however, I had a horrible scare in the dining room. I was chewing a piece of chicken when I laughed at a joke one of my friends told. The chicken slid down my throat the wrong way, and got stuck in my windpipe. I couldn't breathe or speak. . . . I was so frightened! I was convinced that after working so hard to survive my stroke, I would die from choking on a stupid piece of chicken! Fortunately for me, one of the personal support workers, Paula, saw my terrified expression from across the room and rushed to my aid. She asked if I was choking and told me that she could help. As she positioned herself behind me, she called to another personal support worker that I was choking, and asked him to call the nurse. In the meantime, Paula performed that manoeuvre—the Heimlich, I think they call it—and the piece of chicken flew right out of my mouth!

After the excitement had died down, Paula stayed with me for a while just to make sure I was okay. I didn't want to admit how scared I was, but secretly, I was really glad to have her company. I actually slept well that night, knowing that angels disguised as personal support workers like Paula were watching over me. Although I still love having dinner in the dining room with my friends, I now try to pay a little bit more attention to my food. I never want to experience the feeling of choking again!"

You can listen to more stories about how personal support workers make a difference on the CD in the front of your book.

3

BASIC PATIENT AND RESIDENT CARE

13 The Patient or Resident Environment
14 Admissions, Transfers, and Discharges
15 Bedmaking
16 Vital Signs, Height, and Weight
17 Cleanliness and Hygiene
18 Grooming
19 Basic Nutrition
20 Assisting With Urinary and Bowel Elimination

You may have chosen to pursue a career as a personal support worker for many reasons, but chances are good that at least one of those reasons had to do with a desire to help and care for others. As a personal support worker, you will have the chance to fulfill this desire many times over! In Unit 3, we will explore the skills and responsibilities that form the basis for the daily care you will provide for your patients and residents.

Photo: Taking blood pressures is a skill you will use every day.

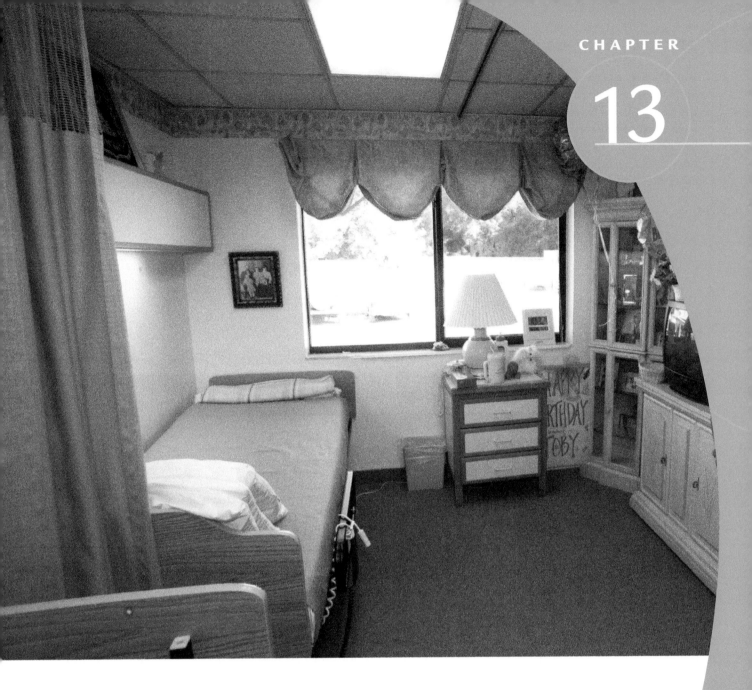

The Patient or Resident Environment

WHAT WILL YOU LEARN?

Have you ever moved into a new house or apartment? If so, you probably remember how strange the place felt, until you managed to get some boxes unpacked and make it your own. After you had added your own personal touch, even if it was just to hang a picture, then the place probably felt more like "home." For a person who is entering a health

Photo: Residents of long-term care facilities are encouraged to make their rooms as "home-like" as possible.

235

care facility, whether just for a few nights' stay or for the rest of his or her life, the idea of "home" takes on a whole new meaning. Suddenly, "home" may only be one room, or even half of one room, and everything that the person has always associated with "home" is gone, except for perhaps a few select items. Items that were never part of the person's home environment before, such as special beds and medical equipment, may now be present. In this chapter, we will take a closer look at the physical environment in a health care facility, and how that environment can affect a person's well-being. We will also provide an overview of the standard equipment and furniture that is typically found in a patient's or resident's room. When you are finished with this chapter, you will be able to:

1. Describe the types of rooms that are commonly found in different health care settings.
2. List the provincial/territorial regulations relating to the physical environment in long-term care facilities.
3. Explain your role in helping to keep the patient's or resident's environment clean and comfortable.
4. Describe the standard equipment and furniture found in a person's room in a health care facility.
5. Discuss the importance of allowing a person to have and display personal items.

Vocabulary

Unit	Task lighting	Reverse Trendelenburg's	Over-bed table
Ventilation system	Gatches	position	Call light system
General lighting	Trendelenburg's position		

THE PATIENT OR RESIDENT UNIT

In Chapter 1, you learned about the many different types of health care facilities, such as hospitals, long-term care facilities, and assisted-living facilities. You also learned that some people receive health care in their homes, from home health care agencies or hospice organizations. A patient's or resident's room, also referred to as a patient's or resident's **unit,** will vary in the way it is set up according to the type of facility and the needs of the person. However, no matter what form the person's room takes—whether it is a single room, a room shared with a roommate, or an apartment-like suite of rooms—the room is considered the person's home.

HOSPITALS

Several different types of rooms are usually found within a hospital (Fig. 13-1). Patients who are recovering from an illness or surgery may stay in double-occupancy rooms (rooms that can accommodate two people). Patients who are very ill may have private rooms in the intensive care unit (ICU) or critical care unit (CCU). These rooms contain special equipment that helps the health care team monitor and care for very ill patients. On the maternity ward, new mothers and babies may receive care before, during, and after the birthing process in a room called a birthing suite. A birthing suite is typically very home-like, with curtains, attractive furniture, and attractive cabinets that contain monitoring equipment and an entertainment center. Other special accommodations include an attached room for waiting family members, a special bed designed to make the process of labor and delivery easier, and possibly even a whirlpool bath! Some hospitals have sub-acute care (skilled nursing) units for patients who are not quite well enough to go home, but not quite sick enough to be in a typical hospital room. The sub-acute care unit is usually designed to be more home-like, and may include a common (communal) dining room and activity rooms for the patients.

All patient rooms have some form of bathroom. However, the setup varies according to the type of room. Usually, the bathroom is attached to the patient's room and will include a shower or bathtub, a toilet, and a sink. Some attached bathrooms may contain only a sink and a toilet, with communal bathing facilities located down the hall. The bathrooms in health care facilities usually have special features, such as handrails and a toilet that is higher than a regular toilet, to help people who may be unsteady or have limited mobility. There may also be more "open space," to accommodate a wheelchair. Finally, there will be a call light or an intercom system to ensure that a person can obtain help if necessary (Fig. 13-2).

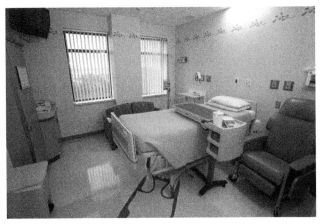

A. Typical hospital room

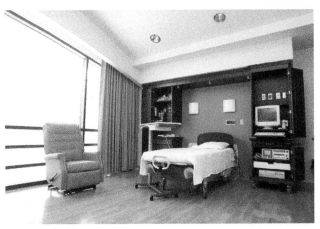

C. Birthing suite

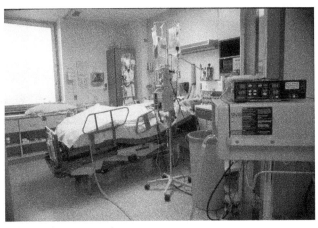

B. Intensive care unit

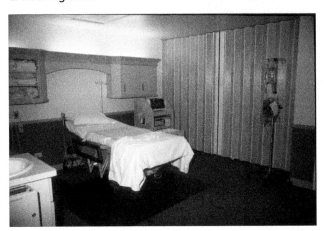

D. Sub-acute care unit

Figure 13-1
Patient rooms in the hospital vary, depending on the needs of the patient. (**A**) A typical hospital room. (**B**) A room in the intensive care unit (ICU). (**C**) A birthing suite in the maternity ward. (**D**) A room in the sub-acute care unit. (**B**, *Custom Medical Stock Photo*; **D**, *Ron Gould/Custom Medical Stock Photo.*)

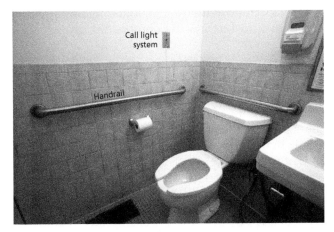

Figure 13-2
Most bathrooms in health care facilities have modifications for people who have trouble with mobility. For example, the bathroom usually has handrails, an elevated toilet, or both to make it easier for a person to get up and sit down. The bathroom also has a call light or intercom system, so that a person can call for help if necessary.

LONG-TERM CARE FACILITIES

As you will recall, long-term care facilities provide care for people who are not able to care for themselves independently. In most cases, a person moving into a long-term care facility is making a permanent move into what is truly a new home. For most people, moving into a long-term care facility represents a major change. For example, a person who once enjoyed an apartment or home with several rooms would now have to adjust to living in a single room, possibly with a roommate. To help ease the transition, people who are moving into a long-term care facility are usually allowed to furnish their rooms with one or two favourite pieces of furniture and various personal items (Fig. 13-3).

Each room in a long-term care facility may have a full private bath, consisting of a shower or tub, a toilet, and a sink. Or it may have a partial bath, consisting of a toilet and a sink, that is

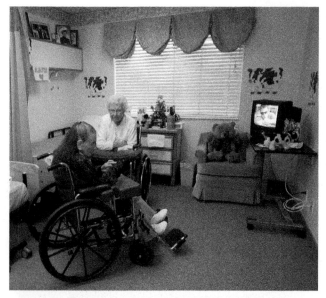

Figure 13-3
People moving into a long-term care facility are often encouraged to bring one or two favourite pieces of furniture, as well as small decorative items, to furnish their new home.

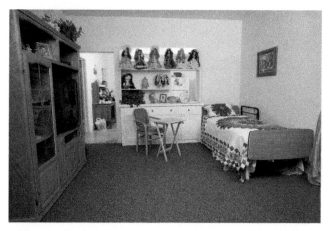

Figure 13-5
When a person is receiving health care at home from a home health care agency, the bedroom, living room, or dining room becomes the person's "unit."

shared between two rooms. In this case, a communal bath area, designed to accommodate the bathing of several residents at the same time, is located down the hall. Like a bathroom in a patient room, a bathroom in a resident room will have special modifications, such as handrails and a means of calling for help.

In addition to resident rooms, long-term care facilities usually have common rooms where residents gather to socialize, such as the dining room, day (or activity) rooms, and a small chapel

where religious services are held. Long-term care facilities may also be designed with patios and gardens to allow the residents access to outdoor activities.

ASSISTED-LIVING FACILITIES

Assisted-living facilities are a type of long-term care facility. However, the residents of assisted-living facilities are usually still somewhat independent. In some assisted-living facilities, residents live in private apartments consisting of a common area, one (or maybe even two) bedrooms, a bathroom, and possibly even a small kitchen (Fig. 13-4). In other assisted-living facilities, residents live in suites consisting of a private bedroom and bath, with communal dining and activity rooms.

HOME HEALTH CARE

Some people receive health care services in their homes. Usually in this situation, the person's bedroom, living room, or dining room becomes the patient care unit (Fig. 13-5). The home health care setting is discussed in more detail in Unit 8.

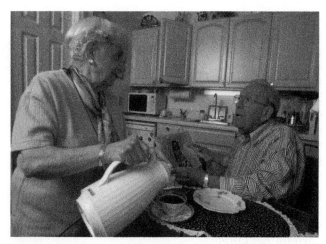

Figure 13-4
Residents of assisted-living facilities may have an apartment with a kitchen. (*Catrina Genovese/Index Stock Imagery, Inc.*)

ENSURING COMFORT

Environmental conditions, such as a room's cleanliness, temperature, noise level, and quality of light, affect how we feel. Imagine what it would be like if you were confined to bed in a dirty room, or one that smelled bad or was too hot or too noisy or too dark. To enhance the comfort and well-being of patients and residents, hospitals and long-term care facilities have policies designed to regulate the environment within the health care facility. In long-term care facilities, these policies are set by the province or territory. Facilities that receive federal funding from Medicare must follow these regulations. Aspects of the resident's environment that are regulated include:

- The size of the room
- The lighting that must be available
- The temperature at which the facility must be maintained
- The measures that must be taken to maintain air quality
- The measures that must be taken to control noise
- The types of furnishings and equipment that must be present
- The types of modifications to the room that must be present to ensure safety (such as handrails and a call light or intercom system in the bathroom)
- The minimal amount of personal space for storage of belongings that each resident is allowed to have
- The ability to provide privacy for each resident

CLEANLINESS

Cleanliness is essential for controlling the spread of infection and odours. In addition, a facility's cleanliness and overall appearance is something that people who are receiving health care at the facility, as well as their family members and other visitors, notice. The appearance of the facility is a reflection on the quality of service provided. To make a good impression, a facility does not need to be new or filled with state-of-the-art equipment—but it does need to be kept clean and neat.

Each member of the health care team is responsible for keeping the facility clean (Fig. 13-6). The housekeeping or custodial staff does major, routine cleaning of the facility (such as mopping floors, emptying waste containers, and cleaning bathrooms). However, each member of the health care team also has specific duties related to maintaining cleanliness. For example, personal support workers are responsible for changing the bed linens according to facility policy and for helping patients and residents to keep their personal belongings neat and clean. In addition, if you notice something out of place, then it is your

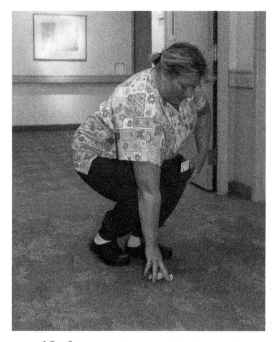

Figure 13-6
Keeping the facility neat and clean is the responsibility of each member of the health care team.

responsibility to correct the problem. For example, if you notice something spilled on the floor or a countertop, you should wipe it up. If you see a piece of garbage on the floor, you should pick it up and dispose of it properly. If you notice that there is an ongoing problem, such as wastebaskets not being emptied or bathrooms not being cleaned properly, you should report this observation to the nurse, so that she can follow up with the appropriate people.

ODOUR CONTROL

There are many potential sources of bad odours in a health care setting. The smell of vomit (emesis), wound drainage, urine, or feces can make any environment unpleasant! However, there are things you can do to help minimize odours and maintain a pleasant environment:

- Follow your facility's policy regarding the handling of waste and soiled linens.
- Keep the lids on laundry and waste receptacles closed.
- Empty and clean emesis basins, urinals, bedside commodes, and bedpans promptly.
- Use a facility-approved air freshener when appropriate.
- Assist your patients and residents with routine personal care. Clean skin and good oral hygiene are essential for controlling odours.

- Pay attention to your personal hygiene (see Chapter 3). Scented products, such as cologne, aftershave, or perfume, can be nice, but they must be used sparingly. If you apply too much, the scent may be overpowering, and many people are sensitive to strong scents. If you are a smoker, be aware that the odours from smoking can cling to your clothes and hair and are considered unpleasant by many people. Make sure you wash your hands after smoking and use a mint or breath freshener before continuing your patient or resident care duties.

VENTILATION

A **ventilation system** provides fresh air and keeps air circulating. A well-functioning ventilation system is essential for carrying away unpleasant odours, for keeping the air from seeming stale, and for preventing rooms from feeling stuffy. However, good ventilation systems can also create drafts (chilly currents of air), especially near the circulation vents. Infants, elderly people, and people who are ill may become easily chilled and may require an extra blanket, a sweater, or a lap robe to stay warm (Fig. 13-7).

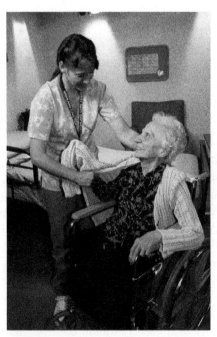

Figure 13-7
Although good ventilation is essential for health and comfort, elderly people, infants, and people who are ill often "catch a chill." Provide additional layers as needed, and be sure to position people away from drafts created by the ventilation system.

Also, be sure to position chairs and beds so that your patient or resident is not in a drafty area. For example, avoid placing furniture and wheelchairs right underneath a circulation vent.

ROOM TEMPERATURE

Most people prefer a room temperature that is somewhere between 20°C (68°F) and 22°C (74°F). However, people who are ill, elderly, or relatively inactive may prefer a warmer room temperature. Be sure to follow your facility's policy with regard to room temperature. Remember that the temperature regulations are intended to ensure the comfort of the people you care for.

LIGHTING

There are two major types of lighting used in the health care setting: general lighting and task lighting. Usually, both lighting types are used in a single room. **General lighting** provides overall illumination (light), allowing a person to see and move about safely. Sunlight is one common source of general lighting. Usually the general light provided by an uncovered window is supplemented by light from a ceiling fixture. Many people prefer to have the drapes or blinds covering the windows in a room opened during the day, to allow natural light in. Others may prefer a darkened room, or to illuminate the room with light from a ceiling fixture instead of sunlight. You should ask each of your patients or residents what he or she prefers, and act accordingly (Fig. 13-8).

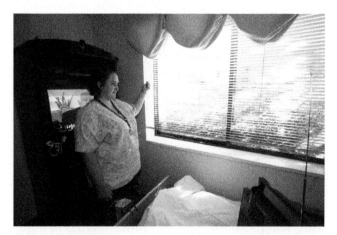

Figure 13-8
Some people prefer to have the blinds or drapes opened during the day to let in the sunlight. Others prefer a darkened room and will want to have the blinds or drapes drawn. Always ask the patient or resident about his or her preference.

Task lighting directs bright light toward a specific area. In a patient or resident room, task lighting is usually provided by a fixture mounted over the head of the bed. Some of these fixtures provide both general and task lighting with dual switches. The patient or resident may use task lighting for activities that require good light to prevent eyestrain, such as reading, needlework, or doing a crossword puzzle. You would use task lighting when providing patient or resident care, so that you could see clearly while carrying out the procedure. The focused illumination provided by task lighting also helps you to notice changes that should be reported to the nurse. For example, you may notice a change in a person's skin tone or a strange new rash that might otherwise go unnoticed.

NOISE CONTROL

Health care facilities can be such busy, noisy places! Imagine that you are a patient on a typical floor in a hospital. It is about 11:30 in the morning, and there is a lot of activity. The telephone is ringing at the nurse's station. Here comes the man with the cart carrying the food trays up from the kitchen. You know he is coming because his cart has a squeaky wheel. A nurse and a personal support worker are having a conversation in the hallway about what needs to be done that afternoon. A patient down the hall, who is a little bit hard of hearing, has the volume turned all the way up on his television set. He is watching a talk show, and every once in a while, you can hear the audience clapping. Several visitors are going down the hallway to visit a friend who is recovering from surgery, and they are laughing and talking as they go. A radio is playing somewhere. You are not feeling very well, and you wonder if things will ever quiet down enough for you to get some rest!

Although a certain level of noise in a busy place is to be expected, too much noise can affect the comfort of patients and residents. Because a quiet environment is known to promote rest and sleep and aid healing, many health care facilities have programs designed to remind people of the importance of keeping noise levels down inside the facility (Fig. 13-9). As a personal support worker, there are many things you can do to help minimize noise and maintain a pleasant environment:

- Encourage patients or residents to use headsets or earphones when watching television or listening to the radio

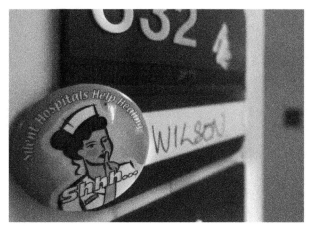

Figure 13-9
A quiet environment is so important for the well-being of patients or residents that some health care facilities post signs designed to remind staff and visitors to keep quiet. "Shhh" is an acronym for Silent Hospitals Help Healing. (*Frank Franklin II/AP.*)

- Answer telephones promptly
- Report noisy equipment that needs to be adjusted or oiled
- Be aware of the volume of your voice

FURNITURE AND EQUIPMENT

The furniture and equipment that is considered "standard" for a patient's or resident's room will differ according to the facility and to the specific needs of the patient or resident. To ensure your own safety, as well as that of your patients or residents, you must make sure that you know how to operate and adjust any furniture and equipment that is considered standard in the facility where you work. The furniture and equipment described in this section would be considered standard for a typical room in a hospital or a long-term care facility. In a facility that offers specialized care (for example, a burn unit or rehabilitation center), items considered standard might vary from this list.

BEDS

An adjustable bed, commonly referred to as a *hospital bed*, is used in most health care settings (Fig. 13-10). The frame of an adjustable bed can be raised or lowered, moving the entire bed either farther away from, or closer to, the floor. This

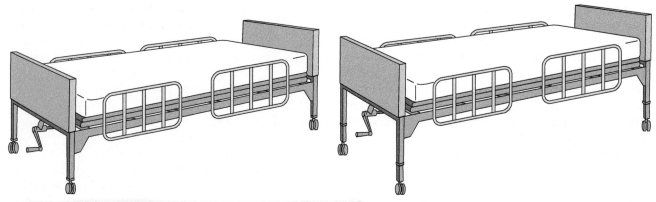

A. The bed can be moved up or down in terms of distance from the floor.

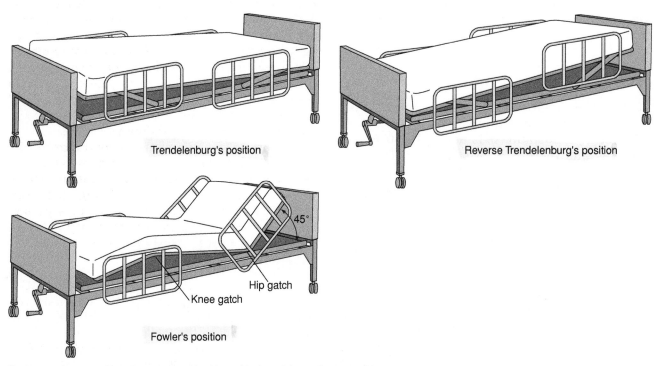

Trendelenburg's position

Reverse Trendelenburg's position

45°

Hip gatch

Knee gatch

Fowler's position

B. The mattress can be adjusted to assist with positioning of the patient or resident.

Figure 13-10
Most beds used in health care settings are adjustable, both in terms of **(A)** their height from the floor and **(B)** the position of the mattress.

helps health care workers maintain good body mechanics when performing care procedures. It also helps the patient or resident to get into or out of the bed. The mattress platform on an adjustable bed can also be positioned in a variety of ways to keep the patient or resident comfortable. Sometimes, the doctor will order a specific mattress position for a patient or resident.

The mattress platforms of most adjustable beds have joints at the hips and knees, which allow the mattress to "break." These joints are called **gatches,** named after Willis Gatch, the surgeon who developed the first bed that was adjustable at the hips and knees. The hip gatch raises the person's upper body to a semi-sitting position (Fowler's position; see also Chapter 11). The knee gatch raises the person's knees to help prevent the person from sliding toward the end of the bed while in the Fowler's position. In addition to having hip and knee gatches, most adjustable beds permit the mattress to be "tilted" without bending the person at the waist. In **Trendelenburg's position,** the foot of the mattress is raised so that the person's head is lower than her feet.

Trendelenburg's position is sometimes used for a person who has gone into shock and has a very low blood pressure, to encourage blood flow to the heart. In the **reverse Trendelenburg's position,** the head of the mattress is raised so the person's head is higher than her feet. The reverse Trendelenburg's position is useful for people who are recovering from spinal cord injury or back surgery, or who are in traction.

Adjustable beds are adjusted either electrically, using control buttons located on or near the side rails, or manually, using a system of cranks located at the foot of the bed (Fig. 13-11). One advantage of electrically operated beds is that the control buttons are located in a place that is accessible to the patient or resident, as well as to members of the health care team. When using an electrically operated bed, remember that it is a piece of electrical equipment. Appropriate safety precautions should be taken when operating it to avoid electrical shock (see Chapter 9). When using a manually operated bed, remember to fold the cranks down and away under the bed after you are finished using them, so that people who are walking near the foot of the bed do not bump into them.

In addition to being adjustable, adjustable beds usually have two other features that regular beds do not—side rails and wheels (casters). The side rails on a bed are raised to help prevent a person from falling out of the bed. Always remember, however, that side rails can be considered a form of restraint, and should only be used according to your facility's policies and the care plan. Some of your patients or residents may want to have one of the side rails raised, so that they can use it as an assistive device for repositioning. The patient or resident can grab the side rail and use it to reposition himself in bed or to get up.

Wheels make the bed easier to move from place to place, which is sometimes necessary when a person needs to be moved from one part of the facility to another without leaving his or her bed. Wheels are also useful when it is necessary to move the bed to clean underneath it. The wheels have locking devices that are used to keep the bed steady and prevent it from rolling. Always make sure the bed's wheels are locked, unless you are moving it (Fig. 13-12)! A person could be injured while getting into or out of the bed if the bed shifts out from underneath him. Additionally, you may be injured if the bed suddenly shifts away from you while you are providing care to a patient or resident.

In some cases, you may care for a person who is in a regular bed, instead of an adjustable bed. For example, some assisted-living and long-term care facilities allow people to bring their own beds from home, if they prefer. Also, a person who is being cared for in her home may not have an adjustable bed. When you are caring for a

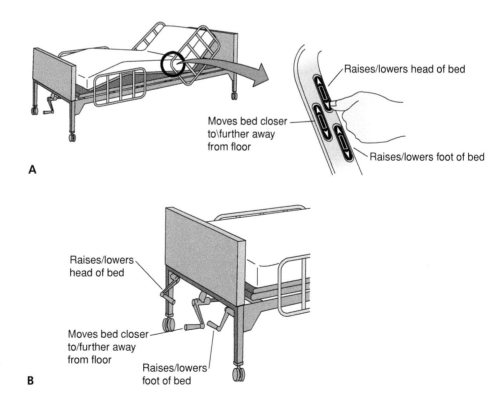

Figure 13-11
Adjustable beds may be adjusted electrically **(A)** or by hand **(B)**.

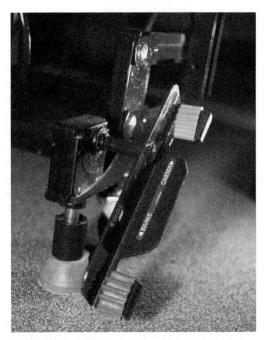

Figure 13-12
Wheel locks help to prevent unintentional movement of the bed. There are different types of wheel locks. In the type shown here, the red pedal locks the wheel, and the green pedal unlocks it.

person in a regular bed, you can use blocks to elevate the head of the bed. Positioning devices, such as pillows shaped to support a person in a sitting position, are available to help achieve the other positions.

CHAIRS

A person's room should be furnished with one or two chairs that are comfortable for the person and will accommodate any visitors. Some people with disabilities require special chairs, such as geri-chairs (a cushioned chair with a high back and foot rest), wheelchairs, or chairs with special lifting devices that help the person to get in and out of the chair easily. A person who is recovering from hip or spinal surgery may need a chair that has firm upholstery, a straight back, and no armrests. Many residents of long-term care facilities will bring a favourite chair or two from home. These chairs may recline or have a rocking action that the person finds very comfortable.

OVER-BED TABLES

Most health care facilities furnish patient and resident rooms with **over-bed tables,** which fit over the bed or a chair and can be raised or lowered as

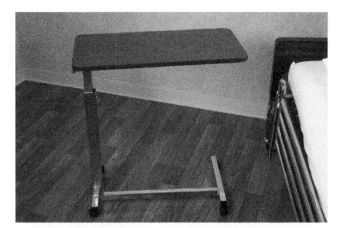

Figure 13-13
The over-bed table fits over the bed or a chair.

needed (Fig. 13-13). You will use the over-bed table to hold basins and other articles when carrying out personal care for a patient or resident. The patient or resident may use the over-bed table as a surface for writing a letter, or for eating a meal or snack. When kept in easy reach of the person, the over-bed table is an excellent place to keep a water pitcher or any other items the person may want close by. Because the over-bed table is considered a "clean" area, items placed there should be either sterile or clean. One way to help remember this is to consider the over-bed table the person's dining room table—you would never place dirty items, such as bedpans or soiled linens, there.

STORAGE UNITS

Various types of storage units are used to house a patient's or resident's belongings. A bedside table is often placed next to the bed and used to store personal care items. Most bedside tables have drawers or a combination of drawers and closed shelves. The person's toothpaste and toothbrush, lotion, soap, deodorant, and other personal hygiene items are usually stored in the top drawer, while basins, bedpans, and other care equipment are stored neatly underneath in the lower drawers or shelves. The telephone, a flower arrangement, and other personal items may be placed on top of the bedside table (Fig. 13-14).

Additional storage for a person's personal items may be provided in the form of a closet, a wardrobe, or a chest of drawers. Provincial/territorial regulations require long-term care facilities to provide each resident with enough storage space for his or her clothing and other personal

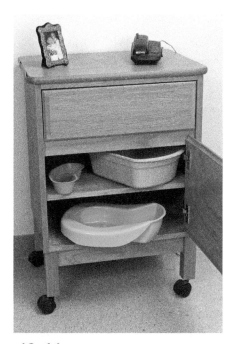

Figure 13-14
Personal care items are usually stored in the bedside table.

items. The resident must have free access to this storage space and the items it contains. Because the resident's closet, wardrobe, or chest of drawers is considered private, personal property, you must have the person's permission to remove items from it (Fig. 13-15).

Occasionally, you will need to inspect a resident's personal storage area. For example, you

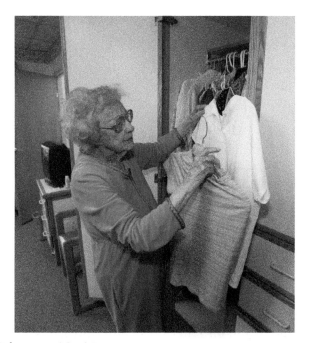

Figure 13-15
The resident's closet is considered private, personal property.

may suspect that a resident is keeping something in the storage area that is not permitted, such as food. Food can spoil and may attract insects and rodents. In this situation, you would be permitted to inspect the personal storage space, but first you must inform the resident of your intent to do so, and the search must be conducted in the resident's presence. If you must carry out an inspection of a resident's personal storage space, it may be a good idea to have another staff member present during the inspection to verify that you acted appropriately and within the regulations.

CALL LIGHT AND INTERCOM SYSTEMS

Patients and residents must have a way of communicating with the health care staff at all times. Most health care facilities have a **call light system,** which patients or residents can use to alert a staff member that they need help. Many also have an intercom system, which allows staff members to speak to a patient or resident in his room from the nurses' station.

A call light system consists of a call light control (usually either a cord that is pulled or a hand-held button device), a light in the hall (over the doorway of the patient's or resident's room), and a panel of lights at the nurses' station or some other central location. When the person pulls the cord or pushes the button on the call light control, the light over the doorway blinks and the light on the panel at the nurses' station lights, alerting the staff that the person needs help. A staff member who is at the nurses' station could then use the intercom system to communicate with the patient or resident before going to the person's room (Fig. 13-16).

The call light control must always be within a person's reach, whether the person is in the bed or in a chair. An unconscious or comatose person will be unable to call for help and should be checked on very frequently. It is also important to note that a person who is hearing impaired will have difficulty communicating with an intercom system. The person will not be able to understand what you are saying, so remember to respond in person to a hearing-impaired person's calls. Answer all requests for assistance promptly, even though it can be frustrating to respond to numerous, seemingly silly requests from any particular person, especially when you are very busy. Sometimes people who use the call light system excessively are feeling scared and lonely. What they

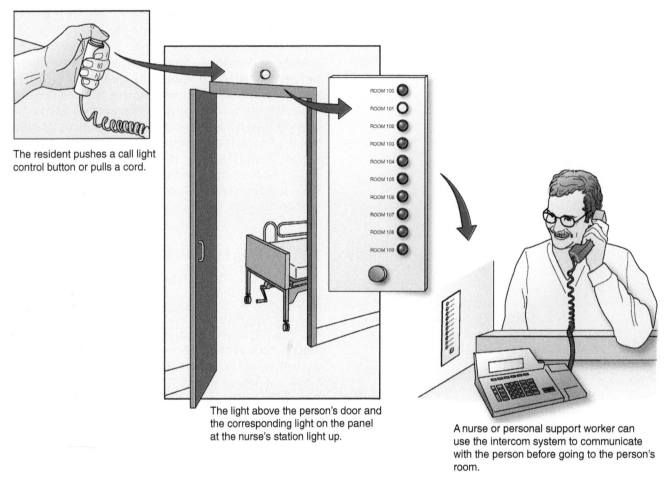

The resident pushes a call light control button or pulls a cord.

The light above the person's door and the corresponding light on the panel at the nurse's station light up.

A nurse or personal support worker can use the intercom system to communicate with the person before going to the person's room.

ROOM 100
ROOM 101
ROOM 102
ROOM 103
ROOM 104
ROOM 105
ROOM 106
ROOM 107
ROOM 108
ROOM 109

Figure 13-16
Call light and intercom systems allow patients and residents to communicate with members of the health care team.

are really seeking is reassurance that if a problem actually does occur, someone will come quickly to their aid. Part of helping to meet a person's safety and security needs is your quick response to a request for help.

PRIVACY CURTAINS AND ROOM DIVIDERS

Each patient or resident unit will have privacy curtains (which are usually hung from the ceiling) or room dividers. The privacy curtain should be closed, or a room divider used, when you are providing care for your patients or residents. The door to the room should also be closed, as the privacy curtains do little to keep voices and other sounds private. Provincial/territorial regulations require long-term care facilities to use privacy curtains or room dividers to protect the privacy of each resident.

OTHER EQUIPMENT

Depending on the type of facility and the purpose of the room, other equipment may be present. For example, many rooms have hanging intravenous (IV) poles and outlets for oxygen and suction devices. The Canadian Centre for Occupational Health and Safety (CCOHS) requires personal protective equipment (PPE), such as gloves, and disposal equipment, such as sharps containers, to be kept in every patient or resident care area for your use. Therefore, the room may be equipped with a wall-mounted sharps disposal box and a wall-mounted box of disposable gloves.

PERSONAL ITEMS

When a person enters a health care facility, he may bring personal items along to add a "touch of home." Usually the number and type of personal items depends on whether the stay at the health care facility is temporary or permanent. For example, a person entering the hospital for a brief stay may just bring along a favourite photograph or a religious item. A person who is moving into a long-term care facility may bring along furniture and larger decorative items.

Many residents in long-term care facilities bring their own bedspreads or comforters to make up the standard facility bed. They may have their own clothing, jewelry, books, and favourite wall hangings. Some residents bring a television, a stereo, or even a personal computer to their new home, and many have a private telephone line installed in their rooms so that they can keep in touch with loved ones and friends. You may see plants, drawings from grandchildren, and maybe even a small pet, such as a bird or a fish, in your residents' rooms!

The CCOHS regulations state that a resident's unit must be safe, clean, orderly, and free from obstacles where people must walk. You should help your residents to decorate their rooms according to their own individual taste and preference, while making sure that they stay within the safety standards established by CCOHS regulations and your facility.

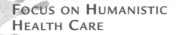

Helping Hands and a Caring Heart

Focus on Humanistic Health Care

Our homes are decorated with things that have special meaning to us. In the same way, many of the items a patient or resident chooses to bring to a long-term care facility will hold special meaning. You may notice items in a person's room that represent the person's cultural background, spiritual beliefs, or mementos from a career or a hobby. Take an interest in these things. Ask the resident to tell you about them. This lets the resident know that you care about him as an individual.

Always respect a person's personal items as if they belonged to you. Remember that even a small scrap of paper can be very precious to a resident, especially if it is a note from someone the person loves. While you may consider a resident's personal things quite a bit of clutter, especially if you have to help keep these things neat, remember that each one of those items represents a piece of that person's life. When you show respect for, and take an interest in, a patient's or resident's personal belongings, you are letting the person know that you truly care for him.

TELL THE NURSE

You are responsible for making sure that the patient's or resident's room is home-like, clean, and safe. Report the following situations to a nurse immediately:

- You notice that a piece of equipment or furniture in the room is not working properly

- A patient or resident has been injured by a piece of equipment or furniture in the room

- You have been injured by a piece of equipment or furniture in the room

- You suspect that a patient or resident is storing unwrapped food in a drawer or closet area

- A patient or resident, or one of his family members, complains that personal items are missing from the room

- You accidentally break a personal item belonging to a patient or resident

- Bathroom fixtures and floors do not appear to be properly cleaned or wastebaskets are not emptied

- There is an odour in the room that cannot be eliminated

SUMMARY

- Patient or resident rooms in a health care facility will vary according to the purpose of the facility and the needs of the person being cared for in the room.
  - A patient room in a hospital is a person's temporary home.

- A resident room in a long-term care or assisted-living facility usually becomes a person's permanent home.
- The physical environment of a health care facility contributes to a person's overall comfort, health, and well-being. Long-term care

facilities that receive federal funding must follow provincial/territorial regulations concerning the physical environment of the resident's room.

- A clean environment is essential for odour and infection control. In addition, many people judge a facility according to its level of cleanliness.
  - All members of the health care team are responsible for providing a clean and comfortable environment for patients and residents.
  - Personal support workers are responsible for helping patients and residents keep their rooms neat and clean.
- Odour control is achieved by promptly removing and cleaning dirty emesis basins, urinals, bedpans, and linens. Assisting patients and residents with bathing and brushing their teeth also helps to prevent odours.
- Good ventilation helps carry away unpleasant odours and prevents stale air. However, it is important to protect your patients and residents from becoming chilled as a result of the drafts created by the ventilation system.
- The temperature of a patient's or resident's room should be maintained between 20°C (68°F) and 22°C (74°F), according to your facility's policy.
- Adequate light must be provided for all activities that take place in a person's room.
  - General lighting, such as that provided by sunlight or an overhead ceiling fixture, provides overall illumination.
  - Task lighting focuses bright light on one particular area.

- Too much noise interferes with a person's ability to rest.
- Most patient and resident rooms contain the same basic furniture and equipment.
  - All patient or resident rooms contain a bed. In most cases, the bed will be an electrically or manually operated adjustable bed.
  - All patient or resident rooms contain at least one chair, to accommodate a visitor and to provide a "change of scenery" for the patient or resident. Many residents in long-term care facilities bring a favourite chair from home to furnish their rooms.
  - Over-bed tables fit over a person's bed to provide a work surface for both the patient or resident and the health care worker. The over-bed table is considered a "clean" area.
  - Personal care items, such as toiletries, are usually stored in the bedside table.
  - In long-term care facilities, a closet, wardrobe, or chest of drawers is used to provide private storage space for the resident's personal belongings.
  - Call light and intercom systems are used for communication.
    - The call light system allows patients or residents to signal that they need help.
    - The intercom system allows members of the health care team to communicate with patients or residents without leaving the nurses' station.
  - Privacy curtains or room dividers are used to help maintain a resident's or patient's privacy when care is being given.
- People entering a health care facility may want to bring personal items to add a "touch of home." Always show as much care for a person's personal items as you would for your own most treasured belongings.

WHAT DID YOU LEARN?

Multiple Choice

Select the single best answer for each of the following questions.

1. How should a resident's room look?
   a. Functional and sparsely decorated
   b. Like a hospital room
   c. As home-like as possible
   d. Like a hotel room
2. You show respect to a patient or resident when you:

   a. Knock before entering his or her room
   b. Close the door and pull the privacy curtain when you are providing care
   c. Handle the person's personal belongings with care
   d. All of the above

3. The nurse tells you that Mr. Haskill's bed-side table is looking a little bit disorderly, and asks you to clean it up a bit. You should:
   a. Search the shelves for hidden food and throw anything that you find away
   b. Remove the bedpan and washbasin, because these items do not belong there
   c. Straighten the items on the top of the table and on the shelves, removing any dirty items so that they can be cleaned and returned
   d. All of the above

4. Which regulations state that a resident's unit must be clean, safe, orderly, and free of obstacles in the pathway?
   a. Canadian Centre for Occupational Health and Safety (CCOHS) regulations
   b. Provincial long-term care legislation
   c. Medicare regulations
   d. Medicaid regulations

5. One of your patients has had back surgery, and the nurse asks you to position his bed so that the head of the bed is elevated. The patient's body needs to remain flat against the mattress. What position would the nurse tell you to put the patient in?
   a. Reverse Trendelenburg's position
   b. Fowler's position
   c. Prone position
   d. Trendelenburg's position✗

6. Each member of the health care team has specific duties related to maintaining a clean patient or resident environment. You have noticed that your residents' bathrooms have been less well kept than usual lately. The sinks are not being cleaned thoroughly, and sometimes the wastebaskets are not emptied. Who has fallen down on the job?
   a. The residents—routine upkeep of the bathroom is their responsibility
   b. You—routine upkeep of the bathroom is your responsibility
   c. The housekeeping staff—routine upkeep of the bathroom is their responsibility
   d. The nurse—routine upkeep of the bathroom is her responsibility

7. How can you help to control unpleasant odours in the workplace?
   a. Empty emesis basins promptly
   b. Assist your patients or residents with skin care and oral hygiene
   c. Use facility-approved air fresheners as necessary
   d. All of the above

Matching

Match each numbered item with its appropriate lettered description.

_____ 1. Side rails

_____ 2. Patient or resident unit

_____ 3. Over-bed table

a. The patient's or resident's pitcher and meal trays may be placed here
b. The space where a patient or resident lives in a health care facility
c. Used to prevent a person from falling out of bed, and as an assistive device; may also be considered a form of restraint

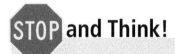

STOP and Think!

One of your residents, Mrs. Grant, is complaining that she is cold even though you are feeling a bit too warm. What are some measures that you can take to help make Mrs. Grant more comfortable?

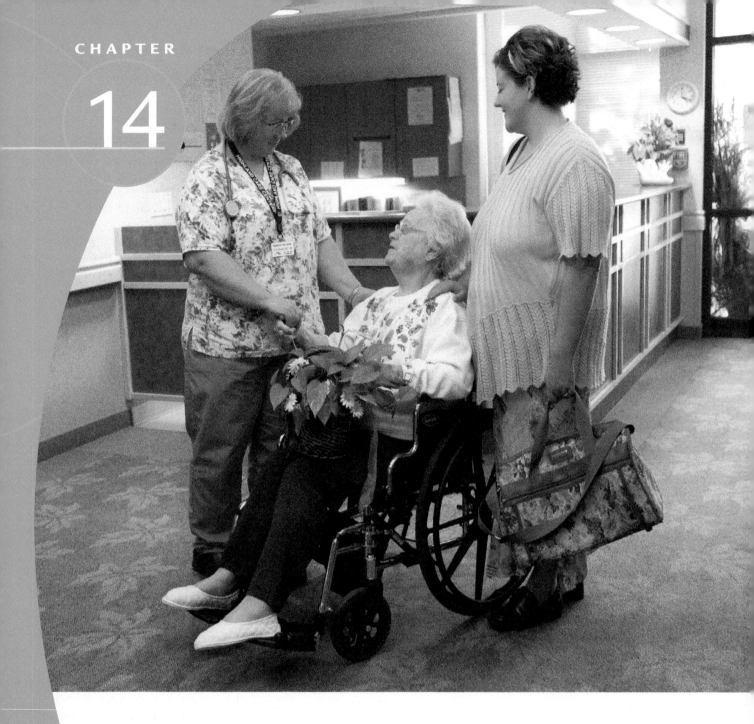

Admissions, Transfers, and Discharges

WHAT WILL YOU LEARN?

Checking people into and out of a health care facility is a routine event in many health care settings. Routine, that is, unless you are the person being admitted ("checked in"), discharged ("checked out"), or transferred (moved from one room in the facility to

Photo: A new resident arrives at a long-term care facility.

another, or moved to another facility altogether). All of these events cause a major change to the patient's or resident's daily routine and normal lifestyle. For many people, this is very upsetting. In this chapter, you will learn how admissions, transfers, and discharges are carried out. You will also learn about things you can do to help make these times of change easier for your patients or residents. When you are finished with this chapter, you will be able to:

1. Explain why admission to a health care facility may be emotionally difficult for a person and his or her family members.
2. Discuss how the personal support worker can help to make a person's admission into a health care facility a more pleasant experience.
3. List the personal support worker's responsibilities during the admission process.
4. Describe some of the reasons a person in a health care facility might need to be moved to another room, or to another facility.
5. List the personal support worker's responsibilities when assisting with the transfer of a patient or resident.
6. Discuss the purpose of discharge planning.
7. List the personal support worker's responsibilities during the discharge process.

Vocabulary

Admission	Resident inventory	Discharge	Discharge planning
Admission sheet	sheet	Against medical advice	
Nursing history	Transfer	(AMA)	

ADMISSIONS

An **admission** is the official entry of a person into a health care setting. A person who needs health care must be formally admitted by his or her attending physician to the health care facility that will be providing the care, whether the length of the stay is:

- A few hours (for example, a person entering an outpatient surgical unit for same-day surgery)
- A few days or weeks (for example, a person entering a hospital to receive treatment for a complication of diabetes)
- A few months
- The rest of the person's life (for example, a person entering a long-term care facility because of advanced Alzheimer's disease)

In the case of a home health care agency, the health care setting is the client's home, but there may still be an admissions process. This is because admission is a time of orientation, for both the new patient, resident, or client and the health care team. During the admissions process, the patient, resident, or client is informed of her

rights and the policies of the facility or agency, and introduced to the people who will be caring for her. At the same time, the members of the health care team are introduced to the person and her family, and the process of gathering the information that the health care team needs to care for the person properly begins.

The members of the health care team may regard the process of admitting a person to the facility as routine. To the person being admitted, however, this "routine" event can be very stressful. A person being admitted for health care services must take on a new role—that of a patient, resident, or client. Taking on this new role can be stressful because most people are used to thinking of themselves as independent, unique individuals, not as dependent people in need of the services of the health care industry. The person may feel a loss of identity, as the illness or condition takes "center stage," with all of the other qualities that make the person unique to fading into the background. This is why the members of the health care team must always make an effort to treat each new patient or resident as if he is a guest in the facility. Make the person feel welcome, not like he is just another body to wash. Ask the person how he prefers to be addressed.

This helps maintain the person's sense of identity and individuality. Never refer to a patient or resident as "the gallbladder in room 212." If you cannot remember the person's name, at least say "the person in room 212 who has gallbladder problems."

In addition to feeling stressed by the need to adjust to a new role, a person who is being admitted to a health care facility may also be feeling fear and anxiety about the future. For example, a person who is entering a long-term care facility may worry that she will not like her new home, and she may be sad about giving up her old one. A person who is being admitted to the hospital may worry that diagnostic tests will reveal bad news, or that a surgery will not be successful. Even if the reason for the admission to a health care facility is joyous (for example, to deliver a baby), there may still be some lingering fear and anxiety (for example, about what labor and delivery will actually be like, or whether the baby will be healthy). The health care setting itself may be frightening. Imagine how you would feel if you were entering an environment filled with strangers asking personal questions about your life and poking and prodding your body with strange equipments! One way to help ease the fear and anxiety felt by patients or residents is to include their family members in the admissions process. Make sure that family members know that they are welcome, and that their support of the patient or resident is beneficial (Fig. 14-1).

Admitting a loved one to a health care facility is stressful for family members, too. Family members will have many of the same fears and worries about the future as the person being admitted. They may feel helpless. If the person is being admitted to a health care facility because family members are no longer able to provide the proper care at home, the family members may feel guilty. Stress can make people behave differently from how they would under normal circumstances. Some family members may become demanding, bossy, or critical when they are under stress. Understanding the feelings that might cause a person to act this way can help you make allowances for the person's behavior. Showing empathy and kindness and involving family members in the admissions process can help family members feel better about the situation.

THE ADMISSIONS PROCESS

Because the admissions process is an emotional time for the patient or resident and his family members, you must focus on the person and his needs, as well as on the process and the paperwork. Most admissions follow a process established by the health care facility:

1. The admissions process usually begins in a doctor's office, unless the admission is caused by an emergency. In the case of an emergency, the person may arrive at the health care facility without seeing his doctor first. Normally, however, the admissions process begins when a doctor writes orders regarding the specific needs of the person. These orders usually include the doctor's diagnosis of the person's condition, and specify dietary orders, activity status, medications, diagnostic tests, and the type of room required by the person.

2. On arrival at the health care facility, the person first goes to the admissions office, where he meets with an admissions clerk or a nurse who is responsible for admissions. The health care team member who is handling the admission will help the person to complete an **admission sheet,** which gathers standard information about the person, such as his name, address, date of birth and age, Social Insurance number, gender, insurance and employment information, emergency notification information, and advance directive information (Fig. 14-2). The admissions clerk or nurse will also have the person sign a consent form giving the facility permission to treat the person's medical condition. When the admissions paperwork is completed, the admissions clerk or nurse will provide the

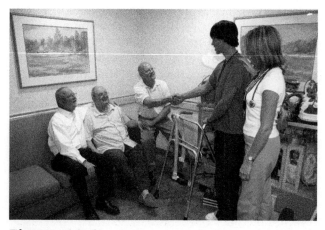

Figure 14-1

Being admitted to a health care facility is often stressful for the patient or resident, as well as his or her family members. Involving family members in the admissions process can help to put everyone at ease.

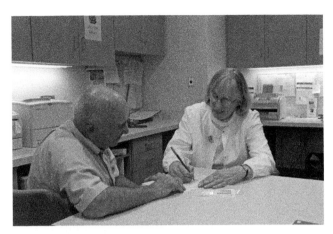

Figure 14-2
The admissions clerk or nurse helps the patient or resident to fill out the admission sheet.

patient or resident with a way of being identified. In a hospital, an identification bracelet will be issued (Fig. 14-3). In a long-term care facility, a photograph of the person will be taken for identification purposes.

3. After completing the admissions paperwork, the person will be escorted to his room by the admissions clerk or nurse, a volunteer, or a personal support worker. Depending on the situation, the person may be able to walk to his room, or he may be taken there in a wheelchair or on a stretcher.

4. A personal support worker is usually responsible for helping the person to unpack and for taking and recording the person's vital signs, height, and weight. If you work in a hospital, you may need to help the person change into a hospital gown or pajamas.

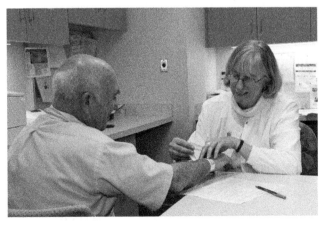

Figure 14-3
Each patient receives an identification bracelet in the admissions office.

Make sure that the person is comfortable by helping him into bed or a chair. Next, a nurse will come to the patient's or resident's room to complete the **nursing history.** As you will remember from Chapter 5, the nursing history is used to gather information about the person's preferences, abilities, disabilities, and habits (Fig. 14-4). The nurse completes this document by interviewing the patient or resident (or, in some cases, a family member of the patient or resident).

TACTICS FOR MAKING A NEW PATIENT OR RESIDENT FEEL WELCOME

When a new patient is being admitted to a hospital, the admissions staff will usually notify the nursing staff as soon as the person arrives in the admissions office. This gives the nursing team time to prepare for the person's arrival. When a person is being admitted to a long-term care facility, the nursing staff typically has a few days' advance notice of the new arrival. As a member of the nursing team, you will play a very important role in making sure that the person feels expected and welcomed when he arrives at the health care facility. A good first impression can go a long way toward easing a person's anxiety, especially if one of the things the person is anxious about is the quality of care that he will be receiving while staying at your facility. As a personal support worker, you will use the following tactics to make sure that the admission goes as smoothly as possible.

Prepare the Person's Room in Advance of His or Her Arrival

Ask the nurse about any special requirements that your new patient or resident may have. Does the person use a walker or some other ambulation device, or will he be arriving in a wheelchair or on a stretcher? If so, you will want to check the placement of the furniture in the room and move it as necessary to ensure easy entry into the room. If necessary, adjust the lighting and temperature of the room. Open the blinds or drapes and prepare the bed by turning the sheets back, lowering the bed to the lowest position, and making sure the wheels are locked (see Chapter 15). If the person is arriving by stretcher, you would prepare the bed in a slightly different manner (also described in Chapter 15).

(Text continued on page 256)

Admission Database

NURSING ADMISSION DATA

CURRENT MEDICATIONS, SUPPLEMENTS, NON-PRESCRIPTION DRUGS:

NAME	DOSE/FREQUENCY	LAST DOSE
Aspirin	2 prn	1 month
Maalox	prn	this Am

☐ MEDICATION TO PHARMACY ☐ MEDICATION SENT HOME

ALLERGEN: (DRUGS, FOOD, TAPES, DYES, OTHERS)

ALLERGEN	SYMPTOMS
Penicillin	rash

DATE __1-16-07__ TIME __0900__

ADMISSION   ☐ OBSERVATION

☒ AMBULATORY ☐ WHEELCHAIR ☐ STRETCHER
☐ CORRECT IDENTIFICATION BAND
ADMITTED FROM: ☒ HOME ☐ NURSING FACILITY
          ☐ EMERGENCY ROOM ☐ OTHER_____
INFORMATION GIVEN BY: ☐ FAMILY MEMBER ☐ FRIEND ☒ PATIENT
     ☐ UNABLE TO TAKE HISTORY - PATIENT UNRESPONSIVE/CONFUSED
       NOT ACCOMPANIED BY FAMILY OR FRIEND
     ☐ PREVIOUS MEDICAL RECORD

ORIENTATION TO ROOM
☒ VISITING HOURS ☒ CALL LIGHT IN REACH: ☒ EXPLAINED
☒ OPERATION OF BED AND SIDE RAILS ☒ USE OF PHONE
☒ VALUABLES SENT HOME ☐ IN SAFE ☐ IN POSSESSION
     SPECIFY _____
☒ PATIENT HANDBOOK   ☒ INTRODUCED TO ROOMMATE

MEDICAL HISTORY
ADMITTED MEDICAL DIAGNOSIS __Peptic Ulcer__

PAST HOSPITALIZATIONS AND/OR ILLNESS: (MEDICAL, SURGICAL, EMOTIONAL PROBLEMS) __1986 - Appendectomy__

WHAT IS REASON FOR ADMISSION? (PATIENT'S OWN WORDS) __"My doctor says I have An ulcer"__

LEGAL GUARDIAN (NAME/PHONE) _____
CONTACT PERSON (NAME/PHONE) __Mrs. Jolle, 335-4001__
PHYSICIAN NOTIFIED __✓__ TIME __0830__
PRIMARY CARE PHYSICIAN __Dr. Wills__

*OBJECTIVE DATA:
1. **CLINICAL DATA**
AGE __36__ HEIGHT __5'6"__
WEIGHT __122__ ☒ BEDSCALE ☐ STANDING APPROXIMATE ____
TEMP: __98.4__ PULSE: __118__ RESPIRATIONS __16__
BLOOD PRESSURE (RIGHT ARM) __120/68__ (LEFT ARM) __122/70__
          ☒ SITTING ☐ LYING
N.T./N.A. INITIALS __O.B.__

2. **NUTRITIONAL/METABOLIC PATTERN**
ORAL MUCOSA: ☒ HEALTHY COLOR ____
     ☐ MOIST ☐ DRY ☐ LESIONS____
TEETH: ☒ NO PROBLEM CONDITION:____
     ☐ DENTURES ☐ UPPER ☐ LOWER ☐ PARTIAL
     ☐ MISSING TEETH ☐ CAPS/CROWNS
☒ WELL NOURISHED ☐ OBESE ☐ EMACIATED
SKIN: ☒ TURGOR NORMAL ☐ OTHER____
     ☒ INTACT ☐ OTHER ____
     TEMP __Warm__ COLOR __brown__ ☐ DIAPHORESIS
☐ TUBES

3. **RESPIRATION/CIRCULATION PATTERN**
BREATH SOUNDS __Clear__
LIP COLOR __pink__ ☐ USE OF ACCESSORY MUSCLES
COUGH: ☐ NON-PRODUCTIVE ☐ PRODUCTIVE SPUTUM COLOR____
APICAL RATE __120__ RHYTHM: ☒ REGULAR ☐ IRREGULAR
ABNORMAL HEART SOUNDS NOTED __No__
NECK VEIN DISTENTION AT 45 DEGREES: ☐ PRESENT ☒ ABSENT
☐ EDEMA: LOCATION____
RIGHT DORSALIS PEDAL PULSE: ☒ STRONG ☐ WEAK ☐ ABSENT
LEFT DORSALIS PEDAL PULSE: ☒ STRONG ☐ WEAK ☐ ABSENT
CALF TENDERNESS ☒ NO ☐ YES ☐ N/A
EXTREMITIES COLOR __brown__
          TEMP __Warm__

4. **ELIMINATION PATTERN**
ABDOMEN: ☒ SOFT   ☐ FIRM
          ☐ NON-TENDER   ☐ TENDER
          ☐ NON-DISTENDED ☐ DISTENDED ____Girth
☐ OSTOMIES/TUBES: TYPE____
☐ NORMAL BOWEL SOUNDS ☐ HYPOACTIVE ☒ HYPERACTIVE ☐ ABSENT

*SUBJECTIVE DATA:
1. **HEALTH PERCEPTIONS/HEALTH MANAGEMENT PATTERN**
GENERAL HEALTH __Excellent__
USE OF: ☐ TOBACCO: HOW MUCH/HOW LONG? __No__
     ☐ ALCOHOL: HOW MUCH/HOW LONG? __No__
     ☐ OTHER DRUGS TYPE(s) __None__
2. **NUTRITIONAL/METABOLIC PATTERN**
DIET/RESTRICTIONS/SUPPLEMENTS: __Regular diet__

☐ INSTRUCTED IN DIET PREVIOUSLY BY:____
TIME OF LAST P.O. INTAKE: __0700__
FLUID INTAKE (AMOUNT/DAY) __5-6 glasses__
WEIGHT: ☐ NO PROBLEMS____
☐ GAIN ☒ LOSS/HOW MUCH/HOW LONG __10 lbs / 1 month__
☒ SKIN NORMAL ☐ HEALING PROBLEMS
     ☐ COLOR CHANGE OF SKIN
     ☐ SKIN LESIONS/RASH____
3. **RESPIRATION/CIRCULATION PATTERN**
HISTORY OF: ☐ COUGH ☐ SPUTUM ____
☐ SHORTNESS OF BREATH ☐ WITHOUT EXERCISE ☐ WITH EXERCISE

HISTORY OF: ☐ PACEMAKER ☐ RATE____
          ☐ BLOOD CLOTS ☐ CHEST PAIN ☐ PEDAL EDEMA

☒ CHECK BOX IF DATA IS PERTINENT
*SEE NURSES NOTES FOR FURTHER NOTATIONS OR ANY CHANGES.

(continued)

Figure 14-4

The nursing history is used to gather information about the person's preferences, abilities, disabilities, and habits. The nurse completes the nursing history. (*Courtesy of Southeast Missouri Hospital, Cape Girardeau, MO.*)

Admission Database (continued)

*SUBJECTIVE DATA (Cont'd) LBM_____

4. ELIMINATION PATTERN
BOWEL HABITS: STOOLS/DAY _2_ COLOR _dk. brown_ ☒ SOFT/FORMED
⬜ CONSTIPATION: ⬜ LAXATIVE ⬜ ENEMA
⬜ DIARRHEA ⬜ INCONTINENCE
BLADDER HABITS: URINATES/DAY _5-6_ ☒ NO PROBLEM ⬜ SELF-CATH
⬜ URGENCY ⬜ FREQUENCY ⬜ NOCTURIA
⬜ DYSURIA ⬜ HEMATURIA ⬜ INCONTINENCE

5. SEXUALITY/REPRODUCTIVE PATTERN (IF APPROPRIATE)
LAST MENSTRUAL PERIOD _1-10-00_ MENSTRUAL PROBLEMS ⬜ YES ☒ NO
BIRTH CONTROL MEASURES _None_ # PREGNANCIES _2_
COMPLICATIONS OF PREGNANCIES _None_
HX VENEREAL DISEASE _No_
SEXUAL CONCERNS: _None_

6. ACTIVITY/EXERCISE PATTERN
ENERGY LEVEL: ⬜ TIRES EASILY ⬜ AVERAGE ☒ HIGH/ENERGY
ABLE TO: ☒ FEED SELF ☒ BATHE SELF
⬜ BATHE/FEED SELF WITH ASSISTANCE
☒ AMBULATE ☒ CLIMB STAIRS !
☒ CAN DO HOUSEHOLD CHORES
AIDS: ⬜ CANE ⬜ WALKER ⬜ WHEELCHAIR ⬜ OTHER _____
GAIT: ⬜ STEADY ⬜ UNSTEADY ⬜ LIMP ⬜ UNABLE TO WALK
PROTHESIS_____

7. SLEEP/REST PATTERN
DO YOU FEEL RESTED AFTER SLEEP? ☒ YES ⬜ NO ⬜ NO PROBLEM
SLEEP PROBLEMS: ⬜ TROUBLE FALLING ASLEEP ⬜ EARLY AM WAKING
⬜ OTHER_____

8. COGNITIVE/PERCEPTUAL PATTERN
HEARING: ☒ NORMAL ⬜ IMPAIRED: ⬜ LEFT EAR ⬜ RIGHT EAR ⬜ AID
VISION: ⬜ NORMAL ⬜ IMPAIRED ☒ GLASSES ⬜ PROTHESIS
⬜ FARSIGHTED ⬜ NEARSIGHTED
OTHER PROBLEMS_____
COMMUNICATION: LANGUAGE SPOKEN _English_
UNDERSTANDS_____ UNABLE TO: ⬜ READ ⬜ WRITE
ABLE TO: ☒ READ ☒ WRITE ⬜ LIP READ
COGNITION: ☒ NO PROBLEMS ⬜ RECENT MEMORY CHANGE
⬜ DIFFICULTY LEARNING
DISCOMFORT/PAIN: ⬜ NO ☒ YES DESCRIBE _Epigastric_
HOW DO YOU MANAGE YOUR PAIN? _Bland food, Maalox_

9. COPING/STRESS TOLERANCE PATTERN
SPECIAL CONCERNS REGARDING HOSPITALIZATION? ⬜ NO ☒ YES
Care of Children

10. SELF-PERCEPTION/SELF-CONCEPT PATTERN
CONCERNS ABOUT HOW YOUR ILLNESS AFFECTS YOU? ⬜ NO ☒ YES
Concerned about health

11. ROLE/RELATIONSHIP PATTERN
MARITAL STATUS: ⬜ MARRIED ⬜ SINGLE ⬜ WIDOWED ☒ DIVORCED
CHILDREN (#) _2_ OTHER DEPENDENT(S) _0_
OCCUPATION _Secretary_
RESIDENCY (TYPE) _apartment_
WHO LIVES AT HOME WITH YOU? _Children_
SUPPORT SYSTEM (CLOSE FRIEND/FAMILY MEMBER) _yes_
FAMILY CONCERNS ABOUT HOSPITALIZATION? _yes_

12. VALUE/BELIEF PATTERN
RELIGIOUS AFFILIATION _Baptist_
RELIGIOUS RESTRICTIONS _0_
⬜ WOULD LIKE CHAPLAIN TO VISIT (IF YES, NOTIFY CHAPLAIN)

☒ WOULD LIKE FAMILY MINISTER TO VISIT
NAME _Mr. Ame_ PHONE _314-6000_
RELIGIOUS ACTIVITIES IMPORTANT TO YOU _Bible_
SUBJECTIVE DATA SIGNATURE _P. LeMone RN_ _____ (Nurse)

6. ACTIVITY/EXERCISE PATTERN
ROM: ☒ FULL ⬜ OTHER_____
BALANCE AND GAIT: ☒ STEADY ⬜ UNSTEADY ⬜ LIMP_____
HAND GRASPS: ☒ EQUAL ☒ STRONG
⬜ WEAKNESS/PARALYSIS ⬜ RIGHT ⬜ LEFT
LEG MUSCLES: ☒ EQUAL ☒ STRONG
WEAKNESS/PARALYSIS ⬜ RIGHT ⬜ LEFT

8. COGNITIVE/PERCEPTUAL PATTERN
LEVEL OF CONSCIOUSNESS: ☒ ALERT ☒ RESPONDS TO PAIN
ORIENTED TO: ☒ TIME ☒ PLACE ☒ PERSON
MOOD: ☒ CALM ⬜ SAD ⬜ ANGRY
⬜ WITHDRAWN ⬜ OTHER_____
PUPILS: ☒ EQUAL ☒ REACTIVE ⬜ OTHER_____
COGNITION: ☒ ABLE TO FOLLOW SIMPLE COMMANDS
☒ RESPONDS APPROPRIATELY TO QUESTIONS
⬜ UNABLE TO FOLLOW COMMANDS
⬜ OTHER_____
HEARING: ☒ NORMAL ⬜ OTHER_____
VISION: ☒ NORMAL ⬜ OTHER_____
MANIFESTATIONS OF PAIN_____

10. SELF-PERCEPTION/SELF-CONCEPT PATTERN
EYE CONTACT: ☒ APPROPRIATE ⬜ DOWNCAST ⬜ STARING
BODY POSTURE: ☒ RELAXED ⬜ STOOPED ⬜ RIGID
BEHAVIOR: 1 ② 3 4 5 (CIRCLE)
RELAXED NERVOUS
OTHER_____

11. ROLE/RELATIONSHIP PATTERN
BEHAVIOR: ① 2 3 4 5 (CIRCLE)
PASSIVE ASSERTIVE AGGRESSIVE
INTERACTION WITH FAMILY/SIGNIFICANT OTHER: ⬜ N/A
☒ RELAXED ⬜ TENSE ⬜ ANGRY ⬜ WITHDRAWN ⬜ OTHER_____

COMMENTS:_____

Worried about effect of illness and possible surgery on care of Children, job, and income. Has strong support of family.

SIGNATURE _P. LeMone, RN_ _____ (Nurse)

Figure 14-4 (*Continued*)

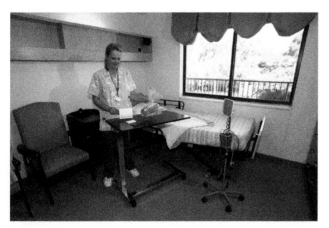

Figure 14-5
Turning the bed sheets down and opening the blinds or drapes to let the sunshine in says to a new patient or resident, "Welcome! We were expecting you!" Making sure the room is stocked with the necessary equipment and supplies, including personal toiletry items, also indicates to the new patient or resident that his or her arrival was planned for and expected.

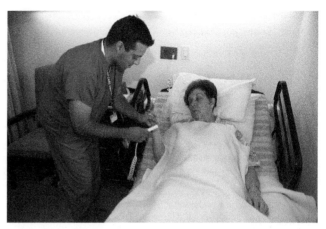

Figure 14-6
A new patient or resident must be taught how to operate the equipment in the room. Here, a personal support worker shows a new resident how to use the call light control.

Gather the equipment you will need for taking and recording the person's vital signs (see Chapter 16). Make sure any other equipment needed by the incoming patient or resident, such as oxygen tubing, a suctioning device, or an intravenous (IV) pole, is in the room before the person arrives. If your facility provides them, obtain an admissions pack for the person. A typical admissions pack would contain a basin, a water pitcher, a drinking cup, a package of tissues, and assorted personal care items (such as toothpaste, soap, and shampoo). Preparing the room in a thoughtful manner indicates to the new patient or resident that his arrival was anticipated and planned for (Fig. 14-5).

Greet the Person Warmly and Introduce Yourself

When you meet the person and his family members for the first time, be sure to introduce yourself. Give your title and explain how you will be involved in the care of the person. A warm, courteous, professional greeting helps to put people at ease and gives them confidence that they will be well taken care of by the health care team.

Help the Person Settle Into His or Her New Home

Always take the time to give a new patient or resident a "tour" of the room (Fig. 14-6). Point out the location of the bathroom. Show the person

how to use the call light control, how to adjust the bed, how to adjust the lights, and how to operate any other appliances or pieces of equipment in the room. For example, in a hospital setting, you may need to show the person how to get an outside line on the telephone, or how to turn the television on and off and adjust the volume.

You should also help the person unpack and find appropriate places for her personal belongings (Fig. 14-7). If you work in a long-term care facility, you will need to complete a resident inventory sheet as part of the unpacking process. The **resident inventory sheet** is a document that lists and briefly describes all of the resident's personal belongings. When completing the

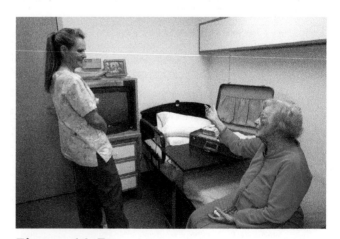

Figure 14-7
Helping the person to unpack and find suitable spots for personal items can make a new environment feel more "home-like" instantly.

resident inventory sheet, make sure that you describe each item objectively. For example, when describing a resident's ring, you would write, "yellow metal ring with two blue stones" instead of "gold ring with two sapphires" because you do not know for sure that the ring is gold or the stones are sapphires. The resident inventory sheet is used to help make sure that a resident leaves the facility with all of her belongings, in the event of a transfer or discharge (Fig. 14-8). It is also used to assist with tracking if belongings are misplaced or borrowed. Some long-term care facilities require each resident to write her name inside each article of clothing to help with laundry sorting. You may need to help the resident do this if it has not been done already.

If the person has brought personal items to decorate with, let the person know that you will be willing to assist in any way you can. For example, a resident of a long-term care facility may need your help with hanging a favorite picture on the wall, or obtaining a bulletin board to display treasured cards and pieces of art.

Practice Good Communication Skills

While you are helping the person to get settled, talk to him! Involving the person in conversation will indicate to the person that you are interested in him, personally, and it will let you get to know the person a little bit better. You know your own duties better than anyone else, and questions that you ask the patient or resident will help you to plan each person's care. For example, you might ask the person when he likes to bathe, whether he likes to take a nap between lunch and dinner, or whether he would prefer to take meals in the dining room or in his room. Be sure to listen to what the person is saying to you, both on his own and in response to your questions. Is the person asking questions or expressing feelings that suggest that he is scared, worried, or upset? Answer questions about your specific responsibilities to the best of your ability. Questions the patient or resident may have about his medical care should be directed to the nurse. Report to the nurse any concerns you may have about the person's ability to adjust to the new environment.

Inventory of Personal Effects

Resident _____ Room No. _____

Description :	
Bathrobe	Cane
Bed Jackets	Comb Brush
Belts	Crutches
Blouses	Dentures-Full Upper ( ) Lower ( )
Bras	Partial Upper ( ) Lower ( )
Coat	Furniture
Dresses	Glasses-Rimmed ( ) Rimless ( )
Girdles	Luggage
Hat	Other
Hose	Prosthesis
Nightgowns	Purse
Pajamas	Radio
Panties	Razors - Electric ( ) Safety ( )
Shirts	Rings
Shoes	Toothbrush
Skirts	Walker
Slips	Watch
Slippers	Wheelchair
Sweaters	
Ties	
Trousers	
Undershirts	
Undershorts	
Wallet	

I certify that the above is a correct list of my personal belongings. I take full responsibility for retaining in my possession the articles listed above and any others brought to me while a resident in this facility.

ALL ITEMS BROUGHT FOR THE PERSONAL USE OF THE RESIDENT MUST BE PROPERLY MARKED AND LISTED AS ARE THE ABOVE. Please bring additional items to the Nurses' Station for proper handling.

Resident's washable clothing to be: _____ taken home for laundering _____ laundered here at the center.

I understand the Management will not be responsible for any valuables, money, or clothing left in the possession of the resident._____ Date_____

Signature of Resident (or Relative) _____ Date _____
Signature of Nurse _____ Date _____

Disposition on Discharge   *Upon Discharge, all personal items are sent with resident or picked up by responsible party. Upon transfer, all personal items are to be boxed and placed in designated storage area for safekeeping.

Signature of Nurse _____   Signature of Resident/Relative _____
Date _____   Date _____

Figure 14-8

A resident inventory sheet is completed when a person is admitted to a long-term care facility. This document is used to keep track of each person's belongings.

TRANSFERS

A **transfer** occurs whenever a patient or resident is moved within or between health care settings. A transfer can be:

- From one room to another (for example, from a semi-private to a private room)
- From one unit to another (for example, from the intensive care unit [ICU] to a standard care floor)
- From one health care facility to another (for example, from a long-term care facility to a hospital for the treatment of an acute illness)

Transfers can occur when a person's medical condition improves, or when it worsens. Transfers can also occur when a preferred room becomes available for a person on a waiting list, or when it is necessary to move people to resolve conflicts between roommates.

As is the case with admissions, transfers can be stressful for the patient or resident, as well as her family members. The reason for the transfer may cause anxiety, especially if the person's condition has worsened or if the person is being transferred from a hospital to a long-term care facility. These transfers may not be expected or desired by either the person or the person's family members. They are usually the result of necessity. Even if the transfer is expected and desirable (for example, a resident in a long-term care facility is moving from one room to another because the view is better), the person being transferred may still experience some stress as a result of the change.

The physical transfer can be carried out in a number of ways. The patient or resident may simply walk, or she may be transported in a wheelchair or on a stretcher. Sometimes, the person does not even need to get out of bed. The bed (with the person in it) is simply moved to another room or unit. An ambulance may be used when a person is being moved from one health care facility to another. However, many people are transferred from one facility to another by their regular means of transportation, such as a car or taxi.

Your duties related to assisting with transfers will vary according to the type of facility where you work. In a hospital or acute care setting, you will be responsible for gathering and packing the person's belongings. It is very important that you help to make sure that all of the person's belongings are packed and sent along with her, so that nothing gets lost. You may also need to assist the nurse in transporting the person to the new room or unit, or to the waiting ambulance, car, or taxi. The nurse is usually responsible for reporting information about the person's medical condition and medications or other treatments to the receiving nurse. If the transfer is taking place within the hospital, you may be asked to report information about the person's preferences and habits to the receiving personal support worker.

In a long-term care facility, the assistance you provide will be more personal. Although the nurse will report medical information about the resident to the receiving nurse, you will be responsible for

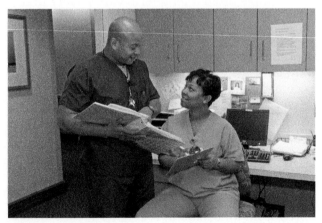

Figure 14-9
Two personal support workers meet to discuss the personal care needs of a resident who is being transferred from one part of the facility to another.

reporting personal care information about the resident to the receiving personal support worker (Fig. 14-9). This is appropriate because you are the caregiver who is most likely to know the most about your resident's personal preferences. For example, you would know that Mr. Vasquez does not like overcooked vegetables, that he requires minimal assistance in the bathroom, and that he likes to read the paper after breakfast. By providing the new personal support worker with this information, you are helping to ensure that the transition from one caregiver to another is as seamless as possible for your resident.

DISCHARGES

A **discharge** is the official release of a patient or a resident from a health care facility to her home. A patient's or resident's discharge is ordered by the doctor. Occasionally, a person will insist on leaving a health care setting without a doctor's order, or **against medical advice (AMA).** A person who is mentally competent may choose to leave a facility if she wants to. However, that person must sign certain documents first. By signing these documents, the person states that she understands that leaving the facility without a doctor's order releases the doctor and the health care facility from any legal responsibility regarding her health status because she has refused to follow the recommendations for her care. If a person tells you that she is leaving the facility, you must report this to the nurse immediately. The nurse will follow the facility's policy for ensuring that a person who is leaving AMA is aware of the consequences of her actions.

Although some people initiate their own departure from a health care facility, most people wait to be officially discharged. Many times, the official discharge is a happy event, but sometimes, people have mixed emotions about leaving. As you will recall from Chapter 1, the ever-increasing costs of health care have created a situation where patients are being discharged from hospitals before they are fully recovered. Many patients are still acutely ill or need complicated treatment and care at the time of their discharge from the hospital. For these people and their family members, leaving behind the safe, professional care provided by the hospital staff can be a frightening experience.

To help ease the transition from a health care facility to home for patients and residents, preparations for discharge begin as soon as a person is admitted to the health care facility. **Discharge planning** is the process used by the members of the health care team to help prepare a patient or resident to leave the facility. Discharge planning helps to ensure that the person continues to receive quality care, either from a home health care agency or from family members, after the discharge. The purpose of discharge planning is to identify the needs that a person will have after his discharge and to make arrangements for meeting these needs after the person goes home. For example, as a result of discharge planning:

- A patient's family members may be taught how to change a wound dressing before the patient is sent home
- A resident and his family may receive help in planning a special diet before the resident is sent home
- Arrangements may be made to transfer a patient from the hospital to a long-term care facility for a short recovery period
- The services of a home health care agency may be obtained

The ultimate goal of discharge planning is to help the patient or resident achieve the best health status possible after he leaves the health care facility (Fig. 14-10).

When a patient or resident is discharged from a health care facility, the nurse is responsible for making sure that the person and his family members have been taught what they need to know about the person's condition and how to monitor or care for it. Your responsibilities when a person is discharged are related more to helping the person to gather and pack his belongings and say good-bye to friends and caregivers. Ask the nurse or the person about the estimated time of discharge so that you can have the person ready to leave on time, taking into account the time the person needs to pack and say his good-byes. You may need to assist the person out of the facility or help to carry his belongings.

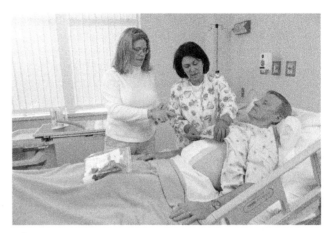

Figure 14-10

Nurses are responsible for discharge planning, a process that helps to ensure a continuation of care for people after they leave a health care facility. Here, a nurse is showing a patient's family member how to change a wound dressing.

TELL THE NURSE

The changes that accompany discharges, transfers, and admissions to health care facilities can be very stressful for a person and for his family members. Often, a lot of information is communicated in a very short period of time, and the patient or resident (as well as his family members) may have trouble absorbing and understanding everything. Make sure you observe and listen carefully to your patient or resident and to his family members during these transitions. Report any of the following to the nurse immediately:

- Any questions that have to do with a person's medical condition or transfer
- Any comments that would indicate that the person or a family member does not fully understand what she has been told by a doctor or nurse
- Any signs of anxiety, such as crying, confusion, agitation, or other unexplained behavior
- Any changes in the person's vital signs or mental status
- Any mention of leaving the facility against medical advice (AMA)

SUMMARY

- Admission to a health care facility is a time of orientation. The patient or resident must learn to accept his new environment and his new status as a "patient" or "resident," and

the members of the health care team must learn about their new patient or resident.

- Assuming the role of a patient or resident can be stressful for a person. Therefore, the person's physical and emotional needs must always remain the focus of the admissions process.

- Newly admitted patients or residents should be welcomed as if they are guests in your facility.
- A smooth admissions process helps to reduce a person's anxiety about entering the health care facility. Many of the personal support worker's duties revolve around making the admissions process easier for the patient or resident and his family members.
  - Personal support workers are responsible for preparing the person's room, taking the person's vital signs and measuring his height and weight, helping the person to unpack, and teaching the person how to use the equipment in the room.
  - By actively listening to the comments made by the person and his family members during the admissions process, the personal support worker can notify the nurse of any specific concerns that may need to be addressed.

- Transfers occur when a patient or resident is moved, either within a health care setting or between health care settings.
  - Transfers can occur when a person's medical condition improves, or when it worsens.
  - When a person is transferred within a hospital or long-term care facility, the personal support worker is responsible for passing vital information about the resident's care to the receiving personal support worker.
- Although many people look forward to going home after being discharged from a health care facility, some might wonder whether they will be able to manage on their own, or with only the help of family members.
  - Discharge planning helps to ensure that a patient or resident continues to receive quality health care, even after being released from a health care facility. Discharge planning begins at the time of admission and is the responsibility of the nurse.
  - The personal support worker is responsible for helping a person prepare for discharge by gathering and packing all of a person's personal items.

WHAT DID YOU LEARN?

Multiple Choice

Select the single best answer for each of the following questions.

1. One of your patients is being transferred to another unit in the hospital. What would you pack for him to take along?
   a. His bed linens
   b. His medical record
   c. His personal belongings
   d. All of the above
2. One of your patients, Mrs. Sarandis, mentions to you that she is leaving the hospital, and her son is coming to pick her up. Before Mrs. Sarandis can be permitted to leave the premises, she must have:
   a. A nurse's order for discharge
   b. A doctor's order for discharge
   c. An admissions sheet on record
   d. A completed resident inventory sheet
3. As a personal support worker, one of your tasks during the admission process will be to:

   a. Take and record the new patient's or resident's vital signs
   b. Assess the new patient's or resident's medical condition
   c. Hurry the new patient or resident through the admissions process to keep things running smoothly
   d. Reassure the new patient or resident by telling him or her that everything will be fine
4. Who writes the orders on admission for a person's diet, medications, level of activity, and type of room?
   a. The admissions clerk
   b. The patient or resident, or one of his or her family members
   c. The director of nursing
   d. The person's doctor

5. Discharge planning begins:
   a. A couple of days before the patient or resident is scheduled to be discharged
   b. When the patient or resident is admitted to the health care facility
   c. The day the patient or resident is scheduled to be discharged
   d. Before the patient or resident is admitted to the health care facility
6. The ultimate goal of discharge planning is to:
   a. Make sure that the room is clean and ready for the next patient or resident
   b. Close out the care plan
   c. Help the person who is being discharged achieve his or her best level of health
   d. Make sure that all of the patient's or resident's belongings are accounted for
7. Who is responsible for carrying out the actions prescribed by the discharge plan (for example, teaching a patient's family member how to change a dressing)?
   a. The doctor
   b. The hospital social worker
   c. The nurse
   d. The personal support worker
8. Mr. Singer, one of your patients, tells you that he hates the food at the hospital and feels that being hospitalized is actually doing him more harm than good. He says that he has called his wife, and she is coming that afternoon to take him home. As far as you know, Mr. Singer's discharge has not been ordered. What should you do?
   a. Apply a restraint
   b. Help Mr. Singer pack; it is his right to leave if he wants to
   c. Tell the nurse immediately
   d. Remind Mr. Singer's roommate that the door to the room must be kept shut and locked at all times
9. Why should a newly admitted patient or resident be given a warm welcome?
   a. Because he represents more revenue for the facility
   b. Because he will be a good roommate for another lonely patient or resident
   c. Because he may be feeling scared and uncomfortable about entering a health care facility
   d. He should not be given a warm welcome; after all, admissions happen every day and a "business as usual" attitude is best to avoid upsetting the other patients or residents

STOP and Think!

Mr. Gardner has lived in his own home for the last 50 years. He now requires some assistance with his meal preparation, dressing, and reminders to take his oral medication. Mr. Gardner's son is transferring him to an assisted-living facility for supervision reasons. Mr. Gardner tells you that he is uncomfortable and scared about the new facility, since he does not know anyone there. How can you help Mr. Gardner?

Mrs. Becker is being admitted as a new resident to the long-term care facility where you work.

Mrs. Becker's daughter, Rhonda, has accompanied her mother to her room. Rhonda mentions to you that she is feeling "like a bad daughter" because she is unable to care for her mother in her own home. She goes on to explain that both she and her husband travel extensively for work, and there would be periods when no one would be around to help care for Mom. Describe some things you could do to help both Mrs. Becker and Rhonda feel more comfortable about Mrs. Becker coming to live at the long-term care facility.

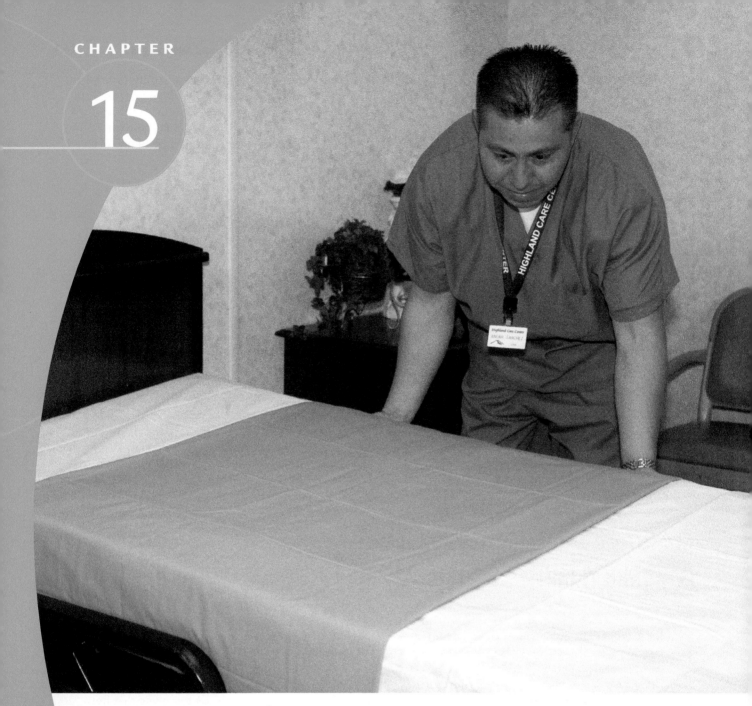

Bedmaking

WHAT WILL YOU LEARN?

For someone who is tired or ill, nothing is quite as comforting as clean, crisp linens on the bed. Clean linens are essential not only for your patient's or resident's comfort, but also for infection control and the prevention of skin breakdown and pressure ulcers. A neat,

Photo: A well-made bed is essential to a person's mental and physical well-being. Here, a personal support worker tucks in a draw sheet.

well-made bed is a sign that the facility provides capable, competent care to its patients or residents. When you are finished with this chapter, you will be able to:

1. Describe ways that a properly made bed can increase a person's comfort and well-being.
2. List the different types of linens and their uses.
3. Demonstrate the proper way to handle and care for linens.
4. Explain the infection control measures that are used during bedmaking.
5. Demonstrate techniques of proper bedmaking, including making a closed bed, opening a bed, preparing a surgical bed, and making an occupied bed.

Vocabulary

Draw sheet	Pressure-relieving	Footboard	Open bed
Lift sheet	mattress	Mitered corner	Surgical bed
Bed protector	Bed board	Closed bed	Occupied bed
Bath blanket	Bed cradle	Fanfolded	Toe pleat

LINENS AND OTHER SUPPLIES FOR BEDMAKING

LINENS

Many types of linens are used to make a bed. On your bed at home, you probably have a mattress pad, a bottom (or fitted) sheet, a top (or flat) sheet, a pillow covered in a pillowcase, and a bedspread or comforter. If you live in a cold climate, you may add a blanket to your bed during the winter months to provide extra warmth. In a health care facility, all of these basic linens are used, and some special ones may be added, depending on the needs of the patient or resident. Linens that you may see in use in a health care facility include the following.

Mattress Pads

A mattress pad is a thick layer of padding that is placed on the mattress to help make the bed more comfortable for the patient or resident, and to protect the mattress from moisture and soiling. The mattress pad may be "fitted." In this case, it will have elasticized sides that wrap around and underneath the mattress, holding the pad securely to the mattress. Or, the mattress pad may be "flat" (non-fitted).

Often, in health care facilities, the mattress has a rubber coating that helps to keep the mattress dry. When no mattress pad is used, and a bottom sheet is placed directly on the rubberized mattress, the person may become very warm and start to sweat because the rubber retains the person's body heat. The bottom sheet becomes damp and stays damp, because the rubberized mattress does not absorb the extra moisture. Lying on a damp sheet is uncomfortable for the patient or resident. In addition, lying on a damp sheet can cause the skin to become reddened and irritated, which can lead to skin breakdown and pressure ulcers. Therefore, when a rubberized mattress is in use, a mattress pad may be used to help pull moisture away from the person's skin.

In a home environment or a long-term care facility, the person may use a standard mattress on his own bed. In this situation, a waterproof mattress pad can be used to help protect the mattress, especially if the person is incontinent (unable to control his bladder or bowels).

Bottom and Top Sheets

The sheets used to make a bed may be white or colored, plain or print. Regardless of their other characteristics, however, sheets need to be clean and wrinkle-free. A bed is made with two sheets, a bottom sheet and a top sheet. Some facilities use flat, or non-fitted, sheets as bottom sheets, or the bottom sheet may be fitted. When you are using a flat sheet as the bottom sheet, it is important to tuck the sheet tightly so that movement does not cause the sheet to loosen and wrinkle underneath the person. Wrinkled sheets are uncomfortable and can create areas of pressure on a person's skin, which can lead to skin breakdown. The top sheet is a flat sheet.

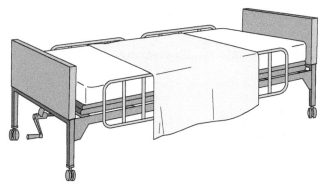

Figure 15-1

A draw sheet is a small sheet that is placed over the middle of the bottom sheet to absorb extra moisture when a mattress pad is not used. Sometimes, draw sheets are used to assist with turning or lifting a person. When a draw sheet is used for this purpose, it is called a "lift sheet."

Draw Sheets

A **draw sheet** is a small, flat sheet that is placed over the middle of the bottom sheet, covering the area of the bed from above the person's shoulders to below his or her buttocks (Fig. 15-1). When a rubberized mattress is in use, a draw sheet may be used instead of a mattress pad to form a protective, moisture-absorbing barrier between the person's body and the rubberized mattress. Some facilities use rubberized or plastic draw sheets to protect the mattress from soiling. If a rubberized draw sheet is used, it is always covered with a cotton draw sheet to protect the person's skin from contact with the rubber. The sides of the draw sheet are tucked tightly under the mattress to prevent wrinkling.

A **lift sheet** is simply a draw sheet that is used to help lift or reposition a person who needs assistance with moving in bed (see Chapter 11). A draw sheet or a lift sheet can be made easily by folding a flat sheet in half. Make sure that the seams are folded toward the inside so that they do not rub against the person's skin. If a folded flat sheet is being used as a lift sheet, the folded edge of the sheet is positioned above the person's shoulders and the loose ends are positioned below the buttocks. When a draw sheet is to be used as a lift sheet, the sides are usually allowed to hang free, although some facilities may require you to tuck the sides of the lift sheet under the mattress after lifting or repositioning the person, to reduce wrinkling.

Bed Protectors

A **bed protector** is a square of quilted absorbent fabric backed with waterproof material. The bed protector measures approximately 91 cm by 91 cm. Bed protectors may be disposable, or they may be laundered and reused.

Some facilities may call bed protectors "incontinence pads" or "soaker pads." In addition to being used for people who are incontinent, bed protectors are often used for people with draining wounds. The urine, feces, or wound drainage is pulled away from the person's body by the absorbent layers of the bed protector, and the waterproof layer keeps the liquid from soiling the rest of the linens on the bed. Sometimes, only the bed protector needs to be changed, resulting in more efficient and economical care.

Blankets

Blankets provided by a facility are usually woven cotton and should be available as requested by a person for his or her comfort. Residents of long-term care facilities or home health care clients may use their own blankets, which may be wool, cotton, or synthetic, depending on the person's preference and the climate. Because wool blankets can create static and sparks, they should be used with caution if the patient or resident is receiving supplemental oxygen. Electric blankets should be checked for faulty wiring or plugs and may not be safe to use if the person is incontinent or unable to adjust the controls independently (for example, if the person is very old or very young). Electric blankets should only be used according to facility policy.

Bedspreads

A bedspread adds the finishing touch to a well-made bed and can add a decorative touch to a person's room. Hospitals and sub-acute care facilities may supply bedspreads for their patients to use. Other types of health care facilities may encourage their residents to use their own bed coverings. Allowing a person to use her bedspread from home is one way that long-term care facilities help to foster a sense of independence and individuality in residents.

Pillows and Pillowcases

Pillows are used for comfort and to aid in positioning. They may be available in many sizes and are made from a variety of materials. Some pillows are covered with waterproof material or treated with a waterproofing substance to protect them from moisture and to aid with cleaning. Pillows are always covered with clean pillowcases. Care for pillows that become wet or soiled will vary according to facility.

Bath Blankets

A **bath blanket** is a lightweight cotton blanket or flannel sheet that is used to provide modesty and warmth during a bed bath or a linen change. A flat sheet may also be used for this purpose if the facility does not provide a special bath blanket. The bath blanket is not made into the bed, but because it is used during bed baths and linen changes, it is gathered along with the other linens.

OTHER BEDMAKING SUPPLIES

Occasionally, other equipment or supplies are used on a person's bed, depending on the specific needs of the patient or resident. Some of the items used include the following:

- A **pressure-relieving mattress** may be placed on top of the regular mattress to help prevent skin breakdown in patients and residents who must stay in bed for long periods of time. Thin foam pads that resemble the inside of an egg carton, called "egg crate mattresses," were used in the past to help relieve pressure, but now are used only for comfort. Use of foam pads is decreasing because the foam is difficult to keep clean and dry, especially if the person is incontinent. Newer versions of pressure-relieving mattresses may be filled with air or water, and are made out of a material that is easily cleaned. Special beds used to prevent skin breakdown are described in Chapter 24.
- A **bed board** is a piece of wood (usually plywood) that is placed under the mattress to

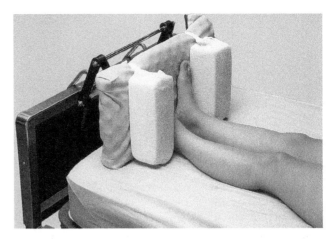

Figure 15-3
A footboard is placed against the end of the bed to keep the person's feet in proper alignment. (*Courtesy of the Posey Company.*)

provide extra support. The bed board keeps the mattress from sagging, helping to keep the person's body properly aligned. Bed boards are most commonly used in the home health care and long-term care settings.

- A **bed cradle** is a metal frame that is placed between the bottom and top sheets to keep the top sheet, the blanket, and the bedspread away from the person's feet (Fig. 15-2). Bed cradles are often used for people who are recovering from burns to prevent the top sheet from touching the burned skin, which would be very painful. They are also often used for people who are at risk for developing pressure ulcers on their feet.
- A **footboard** is a padded board that is placed upright at the foot of the bed (Fig. 15-3). The person's feet rest flat against the footboard, helping to keep the feet in proper alignment.

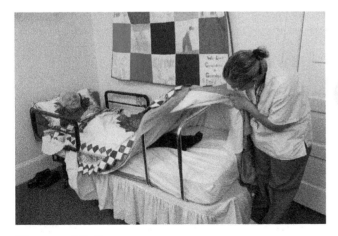

Figure 15-2
A bed cradle is used to keep the top sheet, the blanket, and the bedspread off the patient's or resident's feet. The linens are tucked in at the end of the bed and along the sides to keep the person from getting cold.

HANDLING OF LINENS

The types of linens used for bedmaking will vary, depending on the facility and the needs of the patient or resident. During your employee orientation, you will learn which linens to use to make the beds. Additional information specific to each patient or resident will be provided on the care plan.

No matter which linens are used in your facility, you should always collect the linens in the order that they will be used—mattress pad, bottom sheet, draw sheet, top sheet, blanket, bedspread, pillowcases. Once you have collected your

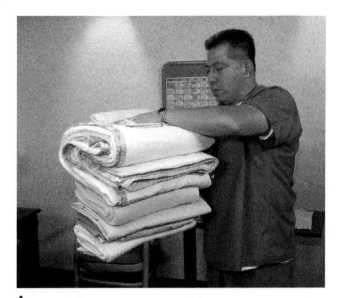
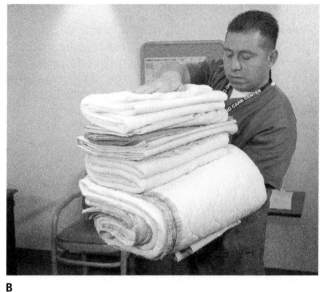

A   **B**

Figure 15-4
Handling linens. **(A)** First, collect the linens in the order that they will be used. Here, the personal support worker has gathered a mattress pad, a bottom sheet, a draw sheet, a top sheet, a blanket, a bedspread, and two pillowcases. The mattress pad is on the bottom of the stack and the pillowcases are on the top. Note that the personal support worker is holding the linens away from his body.
(B) Next, flip the stack of linens over so that the item you will need first is on top. Now the pillowcases are on the bottom of the stack and the mattress pad is on top, ready to be put on the bed.

stack of linens, flip the stack over so that the item you will need first is on the top of the stack (Fig. 15-4). Collecting linens in the order that they will be put on the bed helps you to remember which linens you need to collect. In addition, because the linens will be arranged in order of use, you will be able to make the bed more efficiently, without searching through the stack for the proper item.

Always remember that linens can act as fomites, or objects capable of spreading infection. For this reason, you should always use infection control practices when handling linens. Always wash your hands before collecting clean linens, and avoid letting clean linens come in contact with dirty surfaces, such as your uniform or the floor. When removing used linens from the bed, wear gloves, and roll the linens toward the center of the bed (down from the top and up from the bottom) to confine any soiled areas on the inside (Fig. 15-5). You may be required to place the used linen in a plastic bag as it is removed from the bed to help prevent the spread of pathogens. The linen bag is then removed from the room and taken to a designated area. If a linen bag is not used, then the used linens are placed in the linen hamper

immediately, as per your facility's policy. Do not place dirty linens on the floor, or hold them against your uniform.

Guidelines Box 15-1 summarizes some general guidelines for the handling of linens. These guidelines apply no matter where you work.

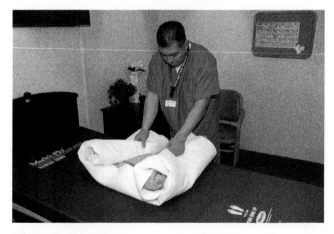

Figure 15-5
Gloves are worn to remove linens from the bed, because the linens may be soiled with body fluids. The soiled area is rolled toward the center of the bed.

Guidelines Box 15-1 Guidelines for Handling Linens

WHAT YOU DO	WHY YOU DO IT
Always wash your hands before collecting clean linens.	Washing your hands prevents microbes on your hands from being transferred to the clean linens.
Do not hold linens, clean or dirty, against your uniform.	If you hold clean linens against your uniform, microbes on your uniform could be transferred to the linens. If you hold dirty linens against your uniform, then microbes from the dirty linens could be transferred to your uniform.
When collecting linens, collect only those that you will need for that person's bed. For example, if a draw sheet is not needed, do not collect one.	Extra linens brought into a person's room are considered soiled, and therefore must not be returned to the clean linen cart or used for another person. These linens must now be laundered, which costs the facility extra money and manpower and creates additional wear on the linens, shortening their lifetime of use.
Collect linens in the order that they will be used. Once you have collected your stack of linens, flip the stack over so that the item you will need first is on the top of the stack.	Collecting linens in the order that they will be put on the bed helps you to remember which linens you need to collect. In addition, because the linens will be arranged in order of use, you will be able to make the bed more efficiently, without searching through the stack for the proper item.
Place clean linens on a clean surface in the room, such as the over-bed table or a chair. Do not place clean linens on the floor.	Clean linens can become contaminated with microbes if you place them on a "dirty" surface, such as the floor.
Wear gloves when removing used linens from a bed. Roll the linens toward the center of the bed to confine the soiled area inside.	Any item contaminated with blood or other body substances is a potential source of exposure to pathogens for the health care worker. Following the standard precautions and wearing proper personal protective equipment (PPE) will help to minimize your exposure. Confining the soiled area to the inside of the linens helps to ensure that other people, such as the people in the laundry, do not come in contact with the potentially infectious material.
If body fluids or substances leak through the linens to the mattress or bed frame, the mattress or bed frame should be wiped with an appropriate cleaning solution before placing clean linens on the bed. Remove your gloves and wash your hands before handling the clean linens.	These infection control methods help to prevent the clean sheets from becoming contaminated.

(continued)

Guidelines Box 15-1 Guidelines for Handling Linens (continued)	
WHAT YOU DO	*WHY YOU DO IT*
After removing the dirty linens from the bed, place them in the linen hamper immediately. Your facility may require you to place dirty linens in a plastic bag or pillowcase before placing them in the linen hamper. Do not place dirty linens on the floor or on any other surface.	Placing the dirty linens in the linen hamper immediately helps to control the spread of infection.

STANDARD BEDMAKING TECHNIQUES

Routine bedmaking is usually done in the morning, before visiting hours, while your patients or residents are bathing or dressing. How often the linens on a person's bed are changed will vary according to the type of health care facility and the person's needs. For example, in a hospital, the policy may be to change each person's linens completely on a daily basis. In a long-term care setting, the policy may call for less frequent linen changes. However,

a person's bed must be remade each time any of the linens become soiled or excessively wrinkled, regardless of the time of day. Soiling of the sheets can occur as a result of spilled food or drink or as a result of excessive sweating, vomit, urine, feces, wound drainage, or leakage from a feeding tube. In each of these instances, a linen change would be required. Change as many of the bed linens as necessary to ensure a clean, dry, wrinkle-free bed for your patient or resident. General guidelines for bedmaking are given in Guidelines Box 15-2.

To make a bed, you will need to know how to make a **mitered corner** (Fig. 15-6). Mitering

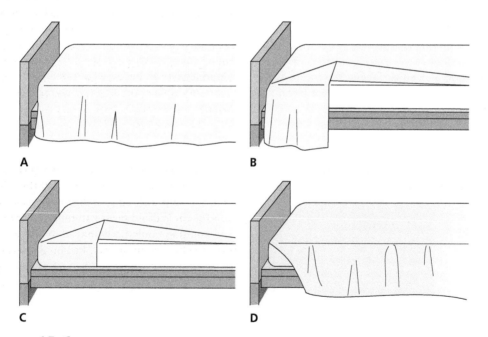

Figure 15-6

How to make a mitered corner. Here, a mitered corner is being made on a top sheet. **(A)** The bottom of the sheet has been tucked under the end of the mattress. The side of the sheet is hanging over the side of the bed. **(B)** Grasp the edge of the sheet about 30 centimetres from the foot of the bed and lift it up, forming a triangle. Lay the triangular fold on the top of the bed, and smooth the hanging portion of the sheet against the side of the mattress. **(C)** Tuck the hanging portion of the sheet underneath the mattress, while holding the triangular fold taut against the top of the bed. **(D)** Bring the triangular fold back down over the edge of the mattress, and leave the side hanging loose.

Guidelines Box 15-2 Guidelines for Bedmaking

WHAT YOU DO	WHY YOU DO IT
Always place linens on the bed so that the seams of the sheets face away from the person's skin.	The seams of the sheets can rub the person's skin, causing irritation and leading to skin breakdown.
Linens must be pulled tightly to avoid wrinkling. Layering should be kept to a minimum.	The wrinkles and extra layers of linens can cause skin breakdown and contribute to the formation of pressure ulcers.
Linens should be changed whenever they become soiled or wet, regardless of the time of day.	Besides causing discomfort, soiled or wet sheets can cause skin breakdown and contribute to the formation of pressure ulcers.
Do not shake linens when placing them on the bed.	Dust is a transport mechanism for microbes. Shaking linens stirs up dust from the floor. The dust then settles on surfaces in the room and can be easily transferred onto eating utensils or into a wound, causing an infection.
When you need to change the linens on a person's bed with the person still in the bed, always be sure to explain what you are doing throughout the procedure. Talk reassuringly to the person, even if the person is unconscious and you think that the person cannot hear you. Close the door, pull the privacy curtain, and keep the person covered at all times.	Having the bed linens changed while still in the bed can be a frightening experience for a bedridden person, particularly if the person is unconscious. Even if the person is conscious, movement may cause pain, and incontinence (the involuntary loss of urine or feces) can be embarrassing if it occurs. If the person is mentally impaired, he or she may become combative. Explaining what you are doing and taking care to preserve the person's modesty during the procedure will make the procedure more pleasant for the person.
Check the bed linens for personal items before removing the linens from the bed.	Personal items, such as dentures, eyeglasses, or jewelry, may become lost in the bed linens. If these linens are removed from the bed, bundled up, and sent to the laundry, the mislaid personal items may not be discovered and they could be damaged in the wash cycle, or they may be lost altogether. Personal items may be expensive and inconvenient to replace. If they hold sentimental value, they may be irreplaceable.

is a way of folding and tucking the sheet so that it lies flat and neat against the mattress. When a flat sheet is used as the bottom sheet, the mitered corners are made at the top of the bed to help secure the sheet to the mattress. Mitered corners are made at the foot of the bed to hold the top sheet, blanket, and bedspread in place.

CLOSED (UNOCCUPIED) BEDS

A **closed bed** is an empty bed (Fig. 15-7A). A bed that is unoccupied because the previous patient or resident has been discharged from the facility and a new patient or resident has yet to arrive is considered a closed bed. Similarly, a bed that is unoccupied because the patient or resident is

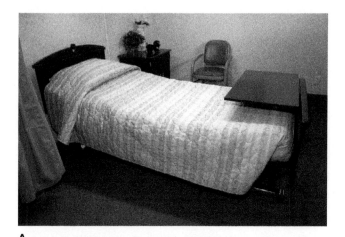

A

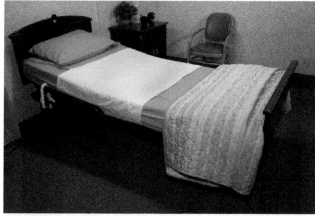

B

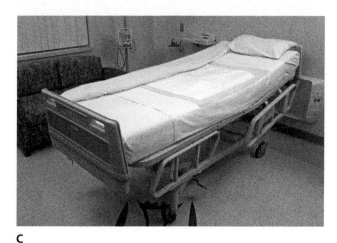

C

Figure 15-7
Types of beds. **(A)** A closed bed is an unoccupied bed.
(B) When a closed bed is "opened," the top sheet, blanket, and bedspread are "fanfolded" to the foot of the bed.
(C) A surgical bed is a closed bed that has been "opened" to receive a person on a stretcher. The top linens are fanfolded to the side of the bed.

simply not in it at the moment (and is not expected back any time soon) is also considered a closed bed. For example, many long-term care facilities make closed beds each day for residents who are not bedridden. Procedure 15-1 explains how to make a closed bed.

When the top sheet, blanket, and bedspread of a closed bed are turned back, or **fanfolded,** the closed bed becomes an **open bed,** or a bed ready to receive a patient or resident. For example, you would open a bed in preparation for a new admission, or after you have changed the linens while a patient or resident is bathing or out of the room for a diagnostic test. Because the patient or resident would be expected to return to the bed shortly, you would fanfold the linens back in anticipation of his return. Similarly, in some long-term care facilities, the linens on the beds of residents who are not bedridden are folded back in the evening, before the residents return to their rooms. To open a closed bed, you first grasp the bedspread, blanket, and top sheet and fold them back to the foot of the bed, creat-

ing a fanfold (Fig. 15-7B). Finish by making sure that the bed is in the lowest position and the bed wheels are locked. Place the call light control near the head of the bed, clipping it to the bottom sheet.

A **surgical bed** is a closed bed that has been opened to receive a patient or resident who will be arriving by stretcher. A surgical bed may be prepared for a patient who is returning to the room following surgery or a diagnostic procedure, or for one who is being transferred from another unit (such as the emergency room). When preparing a surgical bed, instead of folding the top sheet, blanket, and bedspread to the foot of the bed, you loosen these linens from the foot of the bed and fold them toward the side of the bed, leaving one side open and ready to receive the person (Fig. 15-7C). After folding the linens to the side, raise the bed so that the stretcher will be slightly higher than the bed. Make sure that the bed wheels are locked, and ensure a clear path by moving any furniture away from the bed.

OCCUPIED BEDS

"She went out of the room and came back with the old nurse of the early morning. Together they made the bed with me in it. That was new to me and an admirable proceeding."

—*A Farewell to Arms*, Ernest Hemingway

Some conditions make it difficult or impossible for a person to get out of bed for a linen change. When this is the case, it is necessary to change the linens while the person is still in the bed. This is called making an **occupied bed** (Procedure 15-2). In most facilities, this procedure is carried out on a routine basis after the person has been bathed. However, as always, if the linens become wet or soiled in between scheduled linen changes, then they must be changed. Because it can be frightening for a bedridden person to have the linens changed while he or she is still in the bed, remember to explain to the person what you are doing throughout this procedure. Keep the privacy curtain and the door closed during the procedure, to help maintain the person's modesty. If the linens you are removing from the bed are soiled with blood or other body substances, you must wear gloves. Remember to remove the soiled gloves and put on clean ones before handling the clean linens.

Helping Hands and a Caring Heart

FOCUS ON HUMANISTIC HEALTH CARE

All of us can probably remember a time when we were really sick and someone came and freshened us up and changed our sheets. Think about how loved and well cared-for you felt! That is how your patients or residents will feel when you replace their hot, wrinkled, soiled linens with cool, ironed, clean ones. When a complete linen change is not necessary, the simple act of pulling the wrinkles out of the linens and plumping up the pillow can be very comforting to a patient or resident.

SUMMARY

- A well-made bed is essential to a person's mental and physical well-being.
  - Clean, dry, wrinkle-free linens help make a person who is ill feel cared for and more comfortable.
  - Clean, dry, wrinkle-free linens help to prevent complications, such as pressure ulcers. Dampness contributes to skin breakdown and wrinkled sheets can cause friction, both of which are factors in the development of pressure ulcers.
  - Clean, dry linens are important for odour and infection control.
- A variety of linens are used to make a bed. Facility policy and the patient's or resident's particular needs dictate which linens are used to make the bed.
- Special devices, such as pressure-relieving mattresses and bed cradles, are used to improve the patient's or resident's comfort and to prevent the development of complications related to spending long periods of time in bed, such as pressure ulcers.

- Because linens soiled with body fluids and substances can act as fomites, it is important to use good infection control practices when handling soiled linens.
  - Never hold dirty linens against your uniform, or place them on the floor or other surface in the room. Dirty linens must be placed in the linen hamper or linen bag immediately.
  - Always wash your hands before handling clean linens. Never hold clean linens against your uniform, or place them on the floor. Clean linens may be placed on a clean surface in the room, such as the over-bed table.
  - Always wear gloves when it is possible you will be handling linens soiled with body fluids or other substances.
- A bed is either unoccupied ("closed") or occupied. A closed bed may be "opened" in anticipation of receiving a patient or resident by fanfolding the sheets to allow easier access.

Making an Unoccupied (Closed) Bed

WHY YOU DO IT Clean, dry, wrinkle-free linens promote comfort, help to prevent complications (such as pressure ulcers), and are important for odour and infection control.

Getting Ready WORKIEPS

1. Complete the "Getting Ready" steps.*

Supplies

- mattress pad
- bottom sheet
- lift (draw) sheet (if necessary)
- bed protector (if necessary)
- top sheet
- blanket
- bedspread
- pillowcase

Procedure

2. Place the linens on a clean surface close to the bed (for example, the over-bed table).

3. Make sure that the bed is positioned at a comfortable working height (to promote good body mechanics) and that the wheels are locked.

4. Lower the side rails and move the mattress to the head of the bed (it may have shifted toward the foot of the bed if the occupant of the bed had the head of the bed elevated).

   Note: The mattress pad, bottom sheet, and draw sheet are positioned and tucked in on one side of the bed before moving to the other side to complete these actions. This is most efficient in terms of energy and time.

5. Place the mattress pad on the bed and unfold it so that only one vertical crease remains. Make sure that this crease is centered on the mattress. If the mattress pad is fitted, carefully pull the corners of the near side over the corners of the mattress and smooth down the sides. If the mattress pad is flat, make sure the top of the pad is even with the head of the mattress. Open the mattress pad across the bed, taking care to keep it centered.

6. Place the bottom sheet on the bed. If the bottom sheet is fitted, carefully pull the corners of the near side over the corners of the mattress and smooth down the sides. If the bottom sheet is flat:

   a. Place the sheet so that when you unfold it, the wide hem will be at the head of the bed and the hem stitching will be against the mattress, away from the person who will be occupying the bed.

   b. Unfold the sheet so that only one vertical crease remains. Make sure that this crease is vertically centered on the mattress.

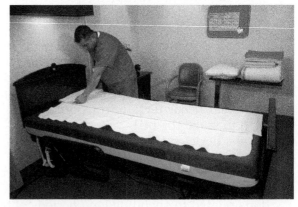

Step 6b Unfold the sheet so that only one vertical crease remains.

---

*It is assumed that the dirty linens have been removed from the bed, and the bed frame has been cleaned, as per facility policy, prior to beginning this procedure.

c. Open the sheet across the bed, taking care to keep it centered. The same length of sheet (approximately 30 to 46 centimetres) should hang over each side of the bed. Make sure that the lower edge of the sheet is even with the foot of the mattress.

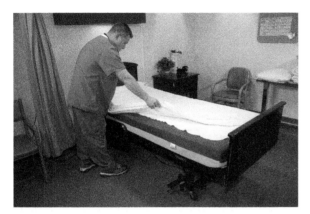

Step 6c Open the sheet across the bed, taking care to keep it centered.

d. Tuck the sheet under the mattress at the head of the bed and miter the corner.

e. Tuck the near side of the sheet underneath the mattress, working from the head of the bed toward the foot. As you tuck, make sure there are no wrinkles in the sheet and that the mattress pad remains smooth and in place.

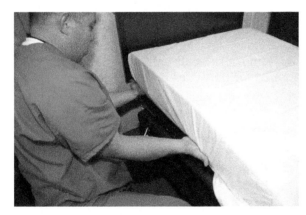

Step 6e After mitering the corner at the head of the bed, tuck the side of the sheet underneath the mattress.

7. Place the lift sheet on the bed so that the top of the sheet is approximately 30 centimetres from the head of the mattress. If you are using a plastic or rubberized lift sheet, place a cotton lift sheet on top of it. Smooth the lift sheet across the bed and tuck the near side under the mattress.

8. Now, move to the other side of the bed and repeat the process of aligning the mattress pad, mitering the corner, and tucking in the bottom sheet and lift sheet.

9. Place the top sheet on the bed so that when you unfold it, the wide hem will be at the head of the bed and the hem stitching will be facing upward, away from the person who will be occupying the bed.

   a. Unfold the sheet so that only one vertical crease remains. Make sure that this crease is centered vertically on the mattress.

   b. Open the sheet across the bed, taking care to keep it centered. The same length of sheet (approximately 30 to 46 centimetres) should hang over each side of the bed. Make sure that the top edge of the sheet is even with the head of the mattress. Pull the bottom of the sheet over the foot of the bed, but do not tuck it in yet (it will be tucked in with the blanket and bedspread).

10. Place the blanket on the bed and unfold it in the same manner as the sheet, keeping the center crease in the center of the bed. The same length of blanket (approximately 30 to 46 centimetres) should hang over each side of the bed. Make sure that the top edge of the blanket is approximately 15 to 20 centimetres from the head of the mattress. Fold the top edge of the sheet back over the top edge of the blanket, creating a cuff. Pull the bottom edge of the blanket over the sheet at the foot of the bed, but do not tuck anything in yet.

11. Place the bedspread on the bed and unfold it in the same manner as the sheet, keeping the center crease in the center of the bed. The sides of the bedspread should be even and cover all of the other bed linens. Make sure that the top of the bedspread is even with the head of the mattress, unless the pillow is to be tucked under the bedspread (in which case you will need to allow more length at the top). Pull the bottom of the bedspread over the blanket and sheet at the foot of the bed.

12. Together, tuck the bedspread, the blanket, and the top sheet under the foot of the mattress. Make a mitered corner at the foot of the bed on both sides.

13. Fold the top of the bedspread back over the blanket to make a cuff.

(continued)

14. Rest the pillow on the bed. Grasping the closed end of the pillowcase, turn the pillowcase inside out over your hand and arm. Grasp the pillow through the pillowcase and pull the pillowcase down over the pillow. Make sure any tags or zippers are on the inside of the pillowcase.

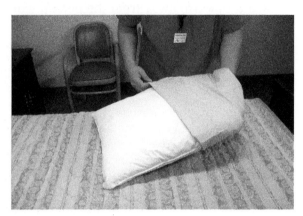

Step 14 Grasp the pillow through the pillowcase and pull the pillowcase down over the pillow.

15. Place the pillow on the bed with the open end of the pillowcase facing away from the door.

Finishing Up CLSOWR

16. Complete the "Finishing Up" steps.

PROCEDURE 15-2

Making an Occupied Bed

WHY YOU DO IT   Clean, dry, wrinkle-free linens promote comfort, help to prevent complications (such as pressure ulcers), and are important for odour and infection control.

Getting Ready WGKIEpS

1. Complete the "Getting Ready" steps.

Supplies

- gloves
- bath blanket
- mattress pad
- bottom sheet
- lift (draw) sheet
- bed protector (if necessary)
- top sheet
- blanket
- bedspread
- pillowcase

Procedure

2. Place the linens on a clean surface close to the bed (for example, the over-bed table).

3. Make sure that the bed is positioned at a comfortable working height (to promote good body mechanics) and that the wheels are locked.

4. Remove the call-light control and check the bed for dentures or any other personal items.

5. Lower the head of the bed so that the bed is flat (as tolerated).

6. Put on the gloves (the linens may be wet or soiled).

7. Remove the bedspread and blanket from the bed. If they are to be reused, fold them and place them on a clean surface, such as a chair.

8. Loosen the top sheet at the foot of the bed and spread a bath blanket over the top sheet (and the person).

9. If the person is able, have her hold the bath blanket. If not, tuck the corners under the person's shoulders. Remove the top sheet by pulling it out from underneath the bath

blanket, being careful not to expose the person.

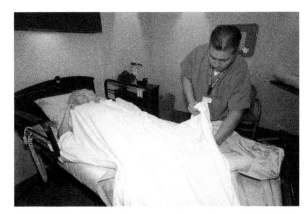

Step 9 Remove the top sheet by pulling it out from underneath the bath blanket.

10. Place the top sheet in the linen hamper or linen bag.

11. If the side rails are in use, lower the side rail on the working side of the bed. The side rail on the opposite side of the bed should remain up. Turn the person onto her side so that she is facing away from you. Reposition the pillow under the person's head, and adjust the bath blanket to keep the person covered.

12. Loosen the lift sheet, bottom sheet, and (if necessary) the mattress pad.

13. Fanfold the bottom linens toward the person's back, tucking them slightly underneath her.

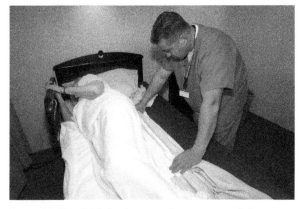

Step 13 Fanfold the bottom linens toward the person's back.

14. Straighten the mattress pad (if it is not being changed). If the mattress pad is being changed, place the clean mattress pad on the bed and unfold it so that only one

vertical crease remains. Make sure that this crease is centered vertically on the mattress. If the mattress pad is fitted, carefully pull the corners of the near side over the corners of the mattress and smooth down the sides. If the mattress pad is flat, make sure the top of the pad is even with the head of the mattress. Fanfold the opposite side of the mattress pad close to the patient or resident.

15. Place the clean bottom sheet on the bed. If the bottom sheet is fitted, carefully pull the corners over the corners of the mattress and smooth down the sides. If the bottom sheet is flat:

a. Place the sheet so that when you unfold it, the wide hem will be at the head of the bed and the hem stitching will be against the mattress, away from the person who will be occupying the bed.

b. Unfold the sheet so that only one vertical crease remains. Make sure that this crease is centered vertically on the mattress.

c. Open the sheet across the bed, taking care to keep it centered. The same length of sheet (approximately 30 to 46 centimetres) should hang over each side of the bed. Make sure that the lower edge of the sheet is even with the foot of the mattress. Fanfold the opposite side of the sheet close to the patient or resident.

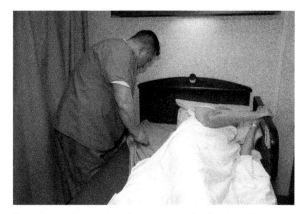

Step 15c Open the sheet across the bed, taking care to keep it centered.

d. Tuck the sheet under the mattress at the head of the bed and miter the corner.

e. Tuck the near side of the sheet underneath the mattress, working from the head of the bed toward the foot. As you tuck, make sure there are no wrinkles in

(continued)

the sheet and that the mattress pad remains smooth and in place.

16. Place the lift sheet on the bed so that the top of the sheet is approximately 30 centimetres from the head of the mattress. If you are using a plastic or rubberized lift sheet, place a cotton lift sheet on top of it. Fanfold the opposite side of the lift sheet close to the patient or resident. Smooth the lift sheet across the bed and tuck the near side under the mattress.

17. Raise the side rail on the working side of the bed. Help the person to roll toward you, over the folded linens. Reposition the pillow under the person's head and adjust the bath blanket to keep the person covered.

18. Move to the other side of the bed and lower the side rail.

19. Loosen and remove the soiled bottom linens and place them in the linen hamper or linen bag. Change your gloves if they become soiled.

20. Now, repeat the process of aligning the mattress pad, mitering the corner, and tucking in the bottom sheet and lift sheet.

21. Help the person to move to the center of the bed and position her comfortably. Raise the side rail on the working side of the bed.

22. Change the pillowcase and place the pillow under the person's head.

23. Place the clean top sheet over the person (who is still covered with the bath blanket), being careful not to cover her face. The sheet should be placed so that when you unfold it, the wide hem will be at the head of the bed and the hem stitching will be facing upward, away from the person who will be occupying the bed.

    a. Unfold the sheet so that only one vertical crease remains. Make sure that this crease is centered vertically on the mattress.

    b. Open the sheet across the bed, taking care to keep it centered. The same length of sheet (approximately 30 to 46 centimetres) should hang over each side of the bed.

    c. If the person is able, have her hold the top sheet. If not, tuck the corners under her shoulders. Remove the bath blanket by pulling it out from underneath the top sheet, being careful not to expose the person. Place the bath blanket in the linen hamper or linen bag.

24. Place the blanket and then the bedspread over the top sheet. Together, tuck the bedspread, the blanket, and the top sheet under the foot of the mattress. Make a mitered corner at the foot of the bed on both sides.

25. Make a toe pleat by grasping the top sheet, the blanket, and the bedspread over the person's feet and pulling the linens straight up. The toe pleat allows the person to move her feet and helps to relieve pressure on the feet from tightly tucked linens.

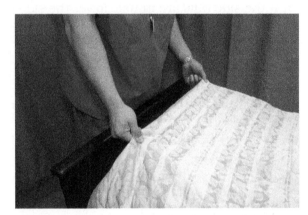

Step 25 Make a toe pleat by pulling straight up on the top linens.

26. Lower the bed to its lowest position and make sure that the wheels are locked. Raise the head of the bed as the person requests.

27. Remove your gloves and dispose of them in a facility-approved waste container.

Finishing Up

28. Complete the "Finishing Up" steps.

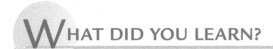

WHAT DID YOU LEARN?

Multiple Choice

Select the single best answer for each of the following questions.

1. What is a draw sheet?
   a. A fitted bottom sheet
   b. A half-sized sheet that is placed over the middle of the bottom sheet and has varied uses, including protecting the mattress from soiling
   c. A half-sized sheet that is placed over the middle of the top sheet and used to make toe pleats
   d. A sheet used to add a decorative touch to the person's room

2. What is a bed that has a person in it called?
   a. An open bed
   b. A closed bed
   c. A surgical bed
   d. An occupied bed

3. A bed that has the top linens fanfolded to the side has been prepared for what type of patient?
   a. A patient who is paraplegic
   b. A patient who is incontinent
   c. A patient who will be arriving on a stretcher
   d. A patient who will be returning to bed in the evening

4. A sheet of wood that is placed under the mattress for extra support is called:
   a. A bed cradle
   b. A bed board

   c. A stretcher
   d. An egg crate mattress

5. When you are handling linens, always remember to:
   a. Shake the bedspread to remove dust
   b. Place the dirty linens on the floor, to get them out of your way
   c. Hold the linens away from your body
   d. All of the above

6. What do you call a metal frame that is placed between the bottom and top sheets to keep the bed linens from resting on the person's feet?
   a. A bed board
   b. A pressure-relieving mattress
   c. A bed cradle
   d. A footboard

7. What personal protective equipment (PPE) should be worn when removing used bed linens?
   a. Gloves
   b. A gown
   c. Eye goggles
   d. No PPE is necessary

8. When are bed linens changed?
   a. When they become wet or soiled
   b. According to facility policy
   c. When they become excessively wrinkled
   d. All of the above

STOP and Think!

You are making an occupied bed. There is no linen hamper in the room and you have already removed the soiled linens from the bed. What should you do with the soiled linens until you can take them to the linen room or hallway hamper? Mrs. O'Shea, the resident, is lying on her side in the bed, covered with a bath blanket.

Barbara is a personal support worker on 3 West. She has already changed the bed linens twice dur-

ing her shift for one of her patients, Mrs. Bridges. Mrs. Bridges is receiving chemotherapy for cancer, and one of the side effects of the medication is uncontrollable diarrhea. Now Mrs. Bridges' call light is on again. When Barbara goes to check on her, she discovers that Mrs. Bridges has soiled the bed again. Barbara tells Mrs. Bridges she'll be right back, and leaves to go get supplies from the linen closet. What are some items Barbara should collect, along with clean sheets?

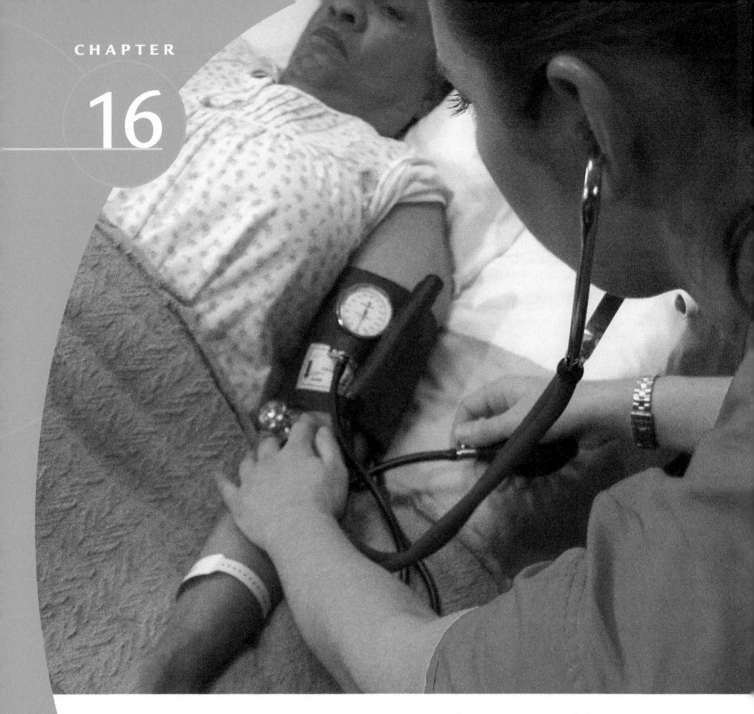

Vital Signs, Height, and Weight

WHAT WILL YOU LEARN?

The word "vital" means "necessary to life." This is why those in the health care field refer to certain key measurements that provide essential information about a person's health as **vital signs.** When we evaluate a person's vital signs, we look at the person's body temperature, heartbeat (pulse), breathing (respirations), and blood pressure. One of the many important duties you will perform as a personal support worker will be to routinely

Photo: A personal support worker takes a resident's blood pressure.

measure and record your patients' or residents' vital signs. A person's height and weight, although not technically vital signs, also provide insight into a person's overall health status. Therefore, you will also be responsible for obtaining and recording these measurements (although not as frequently as the vital sign measurements). Because a change in a person's normal vital sign measurements can be a sign of illness, your ability to detect a change and report this to the nurse promptly is essential to the well-being of your patients or residents. When you are finished with this chapter, you will be able to:

1. Define the term *vital signs* and discuss how the vital signs reflect changes in a person's medical condition.
2. Understand the importance of accurately measuring and recording vital signs, and of reporting any changes to the nurse.
3. Describe the factors affecting a person's body temperature.
4. Discuss various terms used to describe an abnormal body temperature.
5. List common sites used for measuring a person's body temperature, and the advantages and disadvantages associated with each site.
6. Demonstrate the proper use of a glass thermometer, an electronic or digital thermometer, and a tympanic thermometer.
7. Define the term *pulse* and describe factors that may affect a person's pulse.
8. Describe the different qualities of the pulse that a personal support worker should be aware of when taking a person's pulse.
9. List common sites used for taking a person's pulse.
10. Diagram the parts of the stethoscope and explain how this tool is used.
11. Demonstrate the proper way to measure and record a radial pulse and an apical pulse.
12. Describe the factors that may affect a person's respirations.
13. Explain the terms used to describe a person's respirations.
14. Demonstrate the proper way to measure and record a person's respirations.
15. Define the term *blood pressure* and describe factors that may affect a person's blood pressure.
16. Discuss various terms used to describe an abnormal blood pressure.
17. Discuss the various methods used to measure a person's blood pressure.
18. Explain how a sphygmomanometer works, and demonstrate how to use this tool to measure a person's blood pressure.
19. List and describe the Korotkoff sounds, which are heard while taking a person's blood pressure.
20. Discuss factors that can lead to a change in a person's weight.
21. Demonstrate the proper way to measure a person's height and weight using an upright scale.
22. Demonstrate the proper way to measure a person's weight using a chair scale.
23. Demonstrate the proper way to measure a person's height when the person is in bed.

Vocabulary

Vital signs	Stethoscope	Respiratory rhythm	Systolic pressure
Body temperature	Diaphragm	Depth of respiration	Diastolic pressure
Metabolism	Bell	Eupnea	Pulse pressure
Febrile	Pulse deficit	Tachypnea	Sphygmomanometer
Pulse	Tachycardia	Bradypnea	Korotkoff sounds
Pulse rate	Bradycardia	Dyspnea	Hypertension
Pulse rhythm	Inhalation (inspiration)	Hyperventilation	Hypotension
Dysrhythmia	Exhalation (expiration)	Hypoventilation	Orthostatic
Pulse amplitude	Respiratory rate	Blood pressure	hypotension

WHAT DO VITAL SIGNS TELL US?

Vital signs reflect functions that are regulated automatically by the body, such as:

- How fast the heart beats
- The internal temperature of the body
- The rate at which a person breathes

Because the body is always trying to maintain a state of balance, "control centres" (located mostly in the brain) regulate what is going on inside the body and make adjustments as necessary to keep things within the range of normal. Therefore, a change in a vital sign may indicate that something has put the body out of balance, and the body is trying to get that balance back.

There are many factors that can cause changes in a person's vital sign measurements. A person's vital sign measurements may vary over the course of a day (for example, in response to emotional or physical stress or a change in position), while still staying within the range of "normal." However, a major or a long-lasting change in one or more of a person's vital sign measurements may be a response to illness or injury. As you read this chapter, pay attention to the ranges that are considered "normal" for each vital sign. Knowing these ranges will allow you to quickly recognize measurements that are not within the range of normal. Also remember that your definition of "normal" will vary according to the person. For example, you may come to know that Ms. Goldblum's blood pressure tends to be at the low end of the normal range, while Mr. Hanson's tends to be a little bit higher than average. Your knowledge of your patient or resident will allow you to know whether the vital sign measurements you have obtained are normal readings for that person.

MEASURING AND RECORDING VITAL SIGNS

Vital signs are measured and compared with normal values (as well as the values that are considered normal for the individual) under many different circumstances. For example, it is routine for vital signs to be taken each time a person visits the doctor, and when a person is admitted to a hospital or long-term care facility. It may also be necessary to check a person's vital signs:

- Before and after certain medications are given

- Before, during, and after a surgical or diagnostic procedure
- In an emergency situation

Patients in a hospital may have their vital signs taken every shift or every few hours, while residents of a long-term care facility may have their vital signs taken only once daily or even weekly. A patient who is critically ill may be attached to machines that measure his vital signs continuously and display the results on a monitor. The care plan, the doctor's order sheet, or both will specify how often each of your patient's or resident's vital signs are to be measured and recorded. However, it is also within your scope of practice to take a person's vital signs if the person complains of dizziness, nausea, or pain, or if you notice that the person just is not looking or acting like he or she normally does. If a person has been participating in an activity that may affect her vital signs (for example, walking, drinking, eating) you should give the person a few minutes to sit and relax before taking her vital signs.

Facilities will have different policies regarding how vital signs are recorded. Some facilities will record vital sign measurements on one flow sheet for the unit, which lists the names of all of the patients or residents on a particular unit. Other facilities will use one flow sheet per patient or resident. This flow sheet may be kept in the person's medical record, or at the person's bedside. If you take a person's vital signs and get a measurement that is abnormal (either higher or lower than normal for that particular person), you should take the measurement again for the sake of accuracy and then report your findings to the nurse immediately.

The skills you will use to measure a person's vital signs may seem difficult when you are first learning them, but practice will make you more comfortable with taking vital sign measurements. Measuring and recording vital sign measurements accurately is critical because many people rely on this information to make important decisions about the patient's or resident's care. In addition, a problem may go unnoticed if a vital sign measurement is measured or recorded inaccurately. Always ask for assistance, either from another personal support worker or a nurse, if you are having difficulty when checking a person's vital signs. Asking for help when you need it is not a sign of failure or an inability to do your job—rather, it demonstrates that you are responsible and interested in seeing that your patient or resident receives the best possible care. Let's take a look now at the individual vital signs, starting with body temperature.

BODY TEMPERATURE

The **body temperature** is simply how hot the body is. When we measure someone's body temperature, what we are measuring is the difference between the heat produced by the person's body and the heat lost by the person's body. The human body produces heat as a normal process of metabolism. **Metabolism** is the word used to describe the physical and chemical changes that occur when the cells of the body change the food that we eat into energy. Muscle movement also produces heat. This is why we become hotter when we exercise, and why we shiver when we are cold (shivering moves the muscles, producing heat). Heat loss occurs normally through the skin, through the passing of urine and feces, and through the process of breathing, and is increased by bodily responses such as sweating. The body temperature is regulated by a "control centre" that is located in the brain.

FACTORS AFFECTING THE BODY TEMPERATURE

Although a healthy person's body temperature is usually fairly constant, small changes may occur as a result of physical or emotional stress, the environmental temperature, or even the time of day. For example, it is typical for a person's body temperature to be lower in the morning and increase slightly throughout the day, probably from an increase in activity levels. Stress causes the release of hormones that increase metabolism and the heart rate, readying the body to respond to the source of the stress. This response, called the "fight or flight" response, is discussed in detail in Chapter 30. The increase in metabolism and heart rate can lead to an increase in body temperature as well. Finally, exposure to either very hot or very cold environmental temperatures can cause changes in a person's body temperature.

A person's age and gender also play a role in determining body temperature. Very young people and very old people tend to be more sensitive to environmental temperature changes. Infants often have immature control centres, which means that their bodies are slower to adjust to changes in temperature. In addition, infants usually lose body heat through their skin more easily. An elderly person's body may not produce as

much heat as it did in younger years, due to muscle loss as a result of normal aging. Finally, a woman's body temperature tends to change more frequently than a man's, because of the hormonal changes that occur with the menstrual cycle and during pregnancy and menopause.

MEASURING THE BODY TEMPERATURE

The body temperature can be measured from several different areas of the body:

- The mouth (an *oral temperature*)
- The rectum (a *rectal temperature*)
- The armpit (an *axillary temperature*)
- The ear (a *tympanic temperature*)
- The forehead (a *temporal temperature*)

Where the body temperature is measured depends on facility policy and the needs of the patient or resident. Because the method used to measure the temperature affects the accuracy of the measurement, you should note which method was used when you record the temperature, as per your facility's policy. For example, many facilities use "O" for oral, "R" for rectal, "T" for tympanic, and "A" for axillary. The body temperature is measured in either degrees Celsius (°C) or degrees Fahrenheit (°F) using a clinical thermometer.

Types of Thermometers

There are many different types of thermometers in use.

Glass thermometers

When most of us think of a thermometer, we think of a glass thermometer (Fig. 16-1). Glass

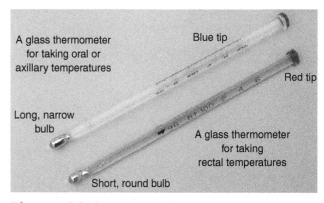

Figure 16-1

Glass thermometers may vary slightly in appearance depending on their intended use.

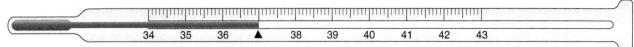

A **Celsius (C°) thermometer** is scaled from 34°C to 43°C. Each long line indicates 1 degree and each short line indicates $1/10$ (0.1) of a degree. This thermometer is reading 37°C.

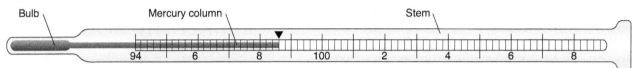

A **Fahrenheit (F°) thermometer** is scaled from 94°F to 108°F. Each long line indicates 1 degree and each short line indicates $2/10$ (0.2) of a degree. This thermometer is reading 98.6°F.

Figure 16-2
Temperature scales on glass thermometers.

thermometers consist of a glass bulb attached to a thin glass tube that is marked with a temperature scale and filled with mercury (a metallic substance). The mercury inside the thermometer expands with heat and moves up the glass tube, showing the temperature on the scale. The Celsius thermometer is scaled from 34°C to 43°C, while the Fahrenheit thermometer is scaled from 94°F to 108°F (Fig. 16-2). Before you use a glass thermometer, the mercury must be "shaken down" to below the 34° mark on a Celsius thermometer or the 94° mark on a Fahrenheit thermometer (Fig. 16-3). To read a glass thermometer, hold it horizontally by the stem at eye level and rotate it until the line of mercury becomes visible (Fig. 16-4).

In most facilities that use glass thermometers, each patient or resident has her own thermometer, which is kept in a case at the person's bedside. Because glass thermometers are not disposable, they must be cleaned properly after each use, according to facility policy. Sometimes, a clear plastic cover called a *sheath* is used to cover the thermometer, and then the sheath is discarded. The thermometer is washed with warm water and soap (never hot water, which can cause the thermometer to shatter), rinsed with cool water, and placed in a disinfectant solution. The amount of time that the thermometer must soak in the disinfectant will vary, depending on the type of disinfectant solution used. If a glass thermometer breaks while you are cleaning it (or at any other time), avoid touching the mercury and the broken glass, and prevent others from doing so as well. Call the nurse immediately. Mercury is toxic and must be cleaned up according to facility policy.

Because of the dangers associated with breakage and spilled mercury, many facilities have stopped using glass thermometers. Some facilities still use glass thermometers, but have switched to using newer models, which contain a

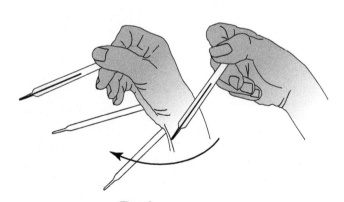

Figure 16-3
A glass thermometer is "shaken down" before use by holding the thermometer firmly by the stem and snapping your wrist downward.

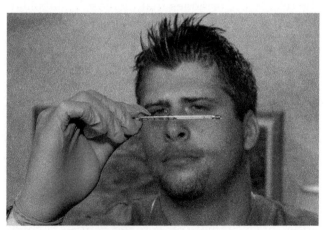

Figure 16-4
To read a glass thermometer, hold it horizontally by the stem at eye level.

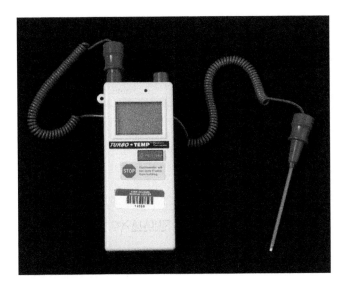

Figure 16-5
Battery-operated electronic thermometers display the person's temperature on a screen. (*Courtesy of Medline Industries, Inc.*)

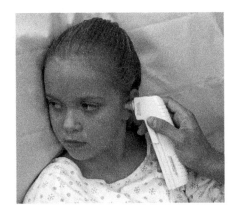

Figure 16-6
A tympanic thermometer is inserted into the ear canal.

substance that behaves the same way as mercury but is less toxic.

Electronic thermometers

Because glass thermometers can break, posing a danger to both the patient or resident and the health care worker, more and more facilities are using electronic thermometers instead (Fig. 16-5). Electronic thermometers are powered by batteries, and the temperature is displayed on a screen on the front of the instrument. A probe, covered with a disposable sheath, is placed in the patient's or resident's mouth, rectum, or armpit to measure the temperature. A blue probe is used for taking oral or axillary temperatures. A red probe is used for taking rectal temperatures. After the probe is used, the disposable sheath is discarded.

Tympanic thermometers

A tympanic thermometer (Fig. 16-6) is used to measure the body temperature in the ear. The probe of this battery-operated instrument is inserted into the ear canal, where it rests near the eardrum (tympanic membrane). The person's temperature is displayed on a screen after a few seconds. Tympanic thermometers are often used for children because they allow a temperature to be measured in a safe, quick, and relatively painless manner.

Temporal artery thermometers

The temporal artery thermometer represents the latest development in thermometer technology

(Fig. 16-7). Remember how your mother used to place her cool hand on your hot forehead to check for a fever? The temporal artery thermometer is simply a "high-tech" version of Mom's gesture. As the device is passed over a person's forehead, it detects the body temperature at numerous points. It then performs a series of calculations on the readings to arrive at the person's peak body temperature. The temporal artery thermometer is even more accurate than a tympanic thermometer, and it is considered the least invasive of all of the thermometers available (because it does not have to be inserted into any body opening).

Sites for Measuring Body Temperature
Mouth (oral temperature)

Measuring a person's body temperature by placing the thermometer in his or her mouth is simple and causes the person minimal discomfort. Because the thermometer is being placed in the

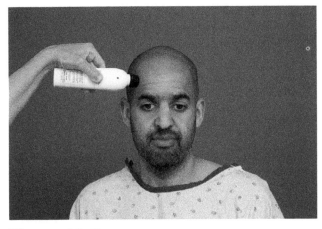

Figure 16-7
A temporal artery thermometer is placed in the middle of the person's forehead and swept toward the ear, stopping in front of the ear.

mouth, which is not an entirely enclosed space, the temperature reading may not be as accurate as with some of the other methods. For example, measuring the temperature in the rectum or ear gives a more accurate reading, because the thermometer is placed into a tightly closed space. However, many times, the reading provided by placing the thermometer in the mouth is accurate enough. An oral temperature may be measured using a glass thermometer or an electronic thermometer (Procedure 16-1).

If a person eats, drinks, smokes, or chews gum within 15 minutes of having an oral temperature taken, the measurement may not be accurate. If one of your patients or residents has done any of these things shortly before you intend to take his temperature orally, then you must either use a different method or wait for a period of time as specified by your facility's policy (usually 15 to 30 minutes). In certain situations, an oral temperature should not be taken. For example, an oral temperature should not be taken if the patient or resident:

- Is unconscious
- Is unable to keep his mouth closed (necessary in order to keep the thermometer in place)
- Is unable to breathe through his nose
- Is likely to bite the oral thermometer (for example, a child younger than 5 years, a disoriented person, or a person with a history of seizures)
- Is coughing or sneezing
- Has recently had mouth surgery or an injury to the mouth
- Is receiving oxygen by a face mask (because the oxygen may cause the temperature measurement to be inaccurate)

Rectum (rectal temperature)

Measuring a person's body temperature by placing the thermometer in the rectum provides a more accurate measurement of the person's body temperature because the thermometer is placed in an enclosed space. However, placing the thermometer rectally is also the most risky method of taking a temperature, and it can be uncomfortable and embarrassing for the patient or resident.

A rectal temperature may be obtained using a glass thermometer or an electronic thermometer (Procedure 16-2). The thermometer must be lubricated and inserted carefully into the rectum, not more than 2.5 centimetres in a child or 3 to 4 centimetres in an adult.

When you are taking a temperature rectally, it is important that you stay with the patient or resident during the entire procedure, both to hold the thermometer in place and to make sure that the person is all right. The thermometer could stimulate the vagus nerve, an important nerve that begins in the brain and sends branches to the heart, lungs, stomach, and rectum. Stimulation of the vagus nerve may temporarily decrease the person's heart rate and blood pressure, which can be dangerous. A different method of measuring the temperature should be used if the person:

- Has hemorrhoids, rectal bleeding, or a disease involving the rectum
- Has diarrhea
- Has had rectal surgery
- Has certain heart conditions

Armpit (axillary temperature)

An axillary temperature is measured by placing the thermometer under the person's arm and then having the person hold his arm close to his body. The axillary method provides the least reliable measurement of body temperature, but if the oral and rectal methods are not safe, and a tympanic or temporal thermometer is not available, then the axillary method can be used. The axillary temperature may be taken using a glass thermometer or an electronic thermometer (Procedure 16-3). If the person has just washed under her arms, or applied deodorant or antiperspirant, then you must wait for at least 15 minutes before taking the axillary temperature. Also, if the person has recently had chest or breast surgery, and it is necessary to take the person's temperature using the axillary method, then the thermometer should be placed on the unaffected side of the body.

Ear (tympanic temperature)

Because a tympanic thermometer measures the temperature of the blood in the small vessels in the eardrum, the temperature it gives is very accurate. Procedure 16-4 describes how to take a tympanic temperature.

Forehead (temporal temperature)

A temporal artery thermometer is swept across a person's forehead to obtain a body temperature measurement.

NORMAL AND ABNORMAL FINDINGS

The normal body temperature varies slightly from person to person. In fact, a person's normal body temperature may be anywhere from

Table 16-1	Normal Adult Temperature Ranges	
METHOD USED TO OBTAIN TEMPERATURE	CELSIUS (°C)	FAHRENHEIT (°F)
Oral	36.5 to 37.5	97.6 to 99.6
Rectal	37 to 38.1	98.6 to 100.6
Axillary	36 to 37	96.6 to 98.6
Tympanic	37	98.6
Temporal	37	98.6

0.1 degree Celsius to 1 degree Celsius higher or lower than the range generally considered normal. The normal range also varies according to which method is used to measure the body temperature (Table 16-1).

A person who has an increased body temperature is said to have a fever, or be **febrile.** Fever is a common finding with illness and is the body's normal response to infection. However, an elderly person's temperature may actually decrease, or only slightly increase, in response to illness or infection. For this reason, even a very slight change in an older person's temperature should be reported to the nurse.

TELL THE NURSE

Changes in a person's temperature can be a sign that something is wrong. Be sure to report the following observations to the nurse immediately:

● The person's temperature is higher than normal

● The person's temperature is lower than normal

Figure 16-8
The pulse points are places where the arteries run close to the surface of the skin, allowing the pulse to be felt. When taking a person's pulse, it is common to place your fingers on the radial artery (in the wrist). An apical pulse can be taken by placing a stethoscope on the person's chest, over the apex of the heart.

PULSE

Each time the heart beats, it sends a wave, or **pulse,** of blood through the arteries. The arteries are the blood vessels that carry oxygen-containing blood away from the heart to all of the tissues of the body. The pulse, a throbbing sensation just underneath the skin, can be felt (palpated) by placing your fingers gently over an artery that runs close to the surface of the skin, such as the carotid artery in the neck or the radial artery in the wrist (Fig. 16-8). Although we can only feel the pulse in a few of the body's arteries (those

that run closest to the surface of the skin), all of the arteries in the body have a pulse. The pulse tells us many things:

• By feeling for and counting the pulse, we are able to measure the **pulse rate,** or the number of pulsations that can be felt in 1 minute. The pulse rate tells us the heart rate, or how fast the heart is beating.

• In addition to measuring the pulse rate, we can detect the **pulse rhythm,** or the pattern of the pulsations and the pauses between them. Normally, the pulse rhythm is smooth and regular, with the same amount of time in between each pulsation. An irregular pulse rhythm is called a **dysrhythmia** (*dys*- means "bad" or "difficult").

- Finally, we can evaluate the force or quality of the pulse, known as the **pulse amplitude** or the pulse character. Each pulsation should be strong, and easy to feel. Pulses that are difficult to feel may be described as "weak" or "thready." A weak or thready pulse usually means that the heart is having trouble circulating blood throughout the body.

FACTORS AFFECTING THE PULSE

The rate at which the heart beats is controlled automatically by the body's central nervous system. When the nervous system senses that the tissues need more oxygen and nutrients (for example, when a person is exercising), it increases the heart rate so that blood reaches the tissues faster. A person's heart rate will also increase during times of anger and anxiety, illness, pain, fever, and excitement, and when taking certain medications.

MEASURING THE PULSE

Radial Pulse

One common way of measuring the pulse rate is by placing the middle two or three fingers over the radial artery, which is located on the inside of the wrist (see Fig. 16-8), and counting the number of pulses that occur in either 30 seconds or 1 minute. The thumb is not used to palpate the artery because the thumb has its own pulse. Although the pulse may be taken at other pulse points, taking the pulse at the radial artery is easiest for the patient or resident. The carotid or femoral arteries may be used to assess the pulse during an emergency situation when cardiopulmonary resuscitation (CPR) is being administered. Procedure 16-5 describes how to take a radial pulse.

Apical Pulse

The apical pulse is measured by listening (auscultating) over the apex of the heart with a stethoscope. The apex of the heart (that is, the lower tip of the heart) is located approximately 5 centimetres below the level of the left nipple (see Fig. 16-8). An apical pulse is taken when a person has a weak or irregular pulse that may be difficult to feel in the radial artery. An apical pulse

may also be used to measure heart rate in infants and in people with known heart disease.

A **stethoscope,** a device that makes sound louder and transfers it to the listener's ears, is used to take an apical pulse. The stethoscope allows you to hear, rather than feel, each beat of the person's heart. The stethoscope has the following parts (Fig. 16-9):

- Earpieces, which are placed in your ears
- A brace and binaurals, which connect the earpieces to the rubber or plastic tubing that conducts the sound
- An amplifying device, which makes the sound louder

The amplifying device, which is the part of the stethoscope that is placed against the person's skin, is usually two-sided. One side, called the **diaphragm,** is a large flat surface that is used to

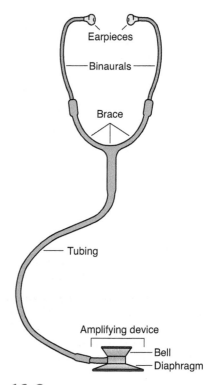

Figure 16-9

A stethoscope is used to listen to the heartbeat (when taking an apical pulse) or blood moving through the arteries (when taking a blood pressure). The sound is made louder by the amplifying device and transmitted by the rubber tubing to the earpieces, which fit snugly in the user's ear canals. The brace and binaurals, which are usually made of metal, connect the rubber or plastic tubing to the earpieces and prevent it from twisting or kinking, which could distort the sound. The rubber or plastic tubing may be single (as shown) or double.

hear loud, harsh sounds like an apical pulse, blood rushing through the arteries, or respiratory sounds. The other side, called the **bell,** is a small rounded surface that is designed to pick up faint sounds like heart murmurs or difficult-to-hear blood pressures. The bell side is also commonly used to listen to apical pulses in infants and small children. The amplifying device rotates so that the sound comes from either the diaphragm or the bell, but not both at the same time.

Before using a stethoscope, clean both the earpieces and the diaphragm or bell by wiping them with alcohol wipes. Place the earpieces in each ear canal. You will know that the earpieces are placed correctly when they fit snugly, yet comfortably, and block out any outside sound. Next, tap lightly on the diaphragm. You should be able to hear the tapping. If you cannot hear the tapping, rotate the amplifying device and tap again. When you can hear the tapping, you are ready to go! Procedure 16-6 describes how to take an apical pulse using a stethoscope.

The apical pulse rate and the radial pulse rate should be the same in any single person. Occasionally, however, the heart does not pump strongly enough to send enough blood through the arteries with each beat. This means that while each beat of the heart may be heard over the apex of the heart using a stethoscope, it may not be felt in the wrist. This difference between the apical pulse rate and the radial pulse rate is known as the **pulse deficit.** The pulse deficit is measured by having one member of the nursing team take the person's apical pulse while another team member takes the person's radial pulse. The two counts are then compared to determine the pulse deficit. For example, if the apical pulse is 84 beats/min and the radial pulse is 80 beats/min, the difference between the apical pulse and the radial pulse (that is, the pulse deficit) is 4 beats/min (84 − 80 = 4). The apical pulse rate will always be higher than the radial pulse rate, because it is easier to hear a heartbeat at the source than it is to feel it.

NORMAL AND ABNORMAL FINDINGS

As with temperature, there is an accepted normal pulse rate. The pulse rate is faster in infants and small children and gradually slows as a person reaches adulthood. **Tachycardia** is a rapid heart rate, or a pulse rate of more than 100 beats/min for an adult (*tachy-* means "fast" and *cardia*

means "heart"). A heart rate that is slower than normal (that is, a pulse rate of less than 60 beats/min) is called **bradycardia** (*brady-* means "slow"). Certain illnesses or conditions can cause bradycardia. Bradycardia may also be a normal finding in a young, athletic person who is very physically fit, because the person's physical conditioning allows the heart to pump stronger and more effectively, which slows the heart rate.

TELL THE NURSE

Changes in a person's pulse rate, rhythm, or amplitude can be a sign that something is wrong. Be sure to report the following observations to the nurse immediately:

- The person's pulse rate is higher than normal
- The person's pulse rate is lower than normal
- The person's pulse rhythm is irregular
- The person's pulse is weak or "thready"

RESPIRATION

Respiration is the process of breathing. To live, we must have oxygen. We must also get rid of waste products that are created as a result of normal cellular function (metabolism). One of these waste products is carbon dioxide.

When we inhale, we take oxygen-containing air into the body. Once in the lungs, the oxygen in the air passes across a thin membrane into the bloodstream, where it is carried by the red blood cells to all of the cells in the body by the action of the heart, which pumps the oxygen-rich blood throughout the body. As the body's cells use the oxygen and nutrients delivered to them by the blood, they give off carbon dioxide, which the blood takes back to the lungs. There, the carbon dioxide crosses the same thin membrane, moving from the blood into the air still remaining in the lungs. When we exhale, we breathe out the carbon dioxide in the lungs. So, the process of breathing performs two vital functions—it brings oxygen, a substance necessary for life, into the body, and it removes carbon dioxide, a waste product that is not necessary for life, from the body.

During the **inhalation (inspiration)** phase of respiration, the chest expands (rises) as air is brought into the lungs. During the **exhalation (expiration)** phase of respiration, the chest deflates (falls) as air moves out of the lungs. When we measure a person's respirations, we look at the person's:

- **Respiratory rate,** or the number of times the person breathes in 1 minute (one breath is both an inhalation and an exhalation)
- **Respiratory rhythm,** or the regularity with which the person breathes
- **Depth of respiration,** or the quality of each breath (for example, is it deep or shallow?)

FACTORS AFFECTING RESPIRATION

As with other vital functions, the process of breathing is controlled mainly by the central nervous system, in a part of the brain called the medulla. Control centres, called chemoreceptors, are located in the medulla and in some of the major arteries. These control centres monitor the carbon dioxide and oxygen content of the blood and adjust the rate and depth of breathing accordingly. For example, exercise increases the body's use of oxygen as well as its production of carbon dioxide and will increase both the rate and depth of a person's respirations. Other factors that may affect respiration rate, depth, and regularity include anxiety, pain, fear, fever, infections and diseases of the heart and lungs, stroke or head injury, and certain medications.

In addition to being controlled automatically by the nervous system, breathing can also be controlled to a certain extent by the individual (for example, when we "hold our breath" while swimming). In this respect, breathing is different from the other vital signs.

MEASURING RESPIRATION

Many tests are available to evaluate a person's respiratory function. The simplest approach involves no equipment, other than a watch. The respiratory rate is easily determined by watching the rise and fall of a person's chest and counting the number of breaths that occur in either 30 seconds or 1 minute. (Remember that one breath consists of both an inhalation and an exhalation.) Usually, the rise and fall of the chest can be easily observed by standing beside the person, or by watching her back. In some situations, you may need to stand slightly behind the person while she is seated and look down at the chest to detect the movement. Or, you can actually place your hand either near the collarbone or

on the person's side to feel her breathing if it is not easily seen. Most small children and some older adults use their abdominal muscles to assist with breathing. In these people, breathing can be easily seen by watching the abdomen move instead of the chest.

Because a person can consciously control her respirations if she is aware that she is being observed, a more accurate measurement may be obtained if you measure the respiratory rate right after you take the person's pulse, with your fingers still on the person's wrist as if you were still counting the pulse. It is also easy to count a person's respirations while she sleeps, before you have awakened her to measure other vital signs. This is the one instance where it is acceptable to carry out a task without telling the patient or resident exactly what you are doing! Procedure 16-7 describes how to measure a person's respiratory rate.

NORMAL AND ABNORMAL FINDINGS

Under normal conditions, a healthy, resting adult will breathe about 16 to 20 times a minute, while infants and children may have a significantly higher respiratory rate. A normal respiratory rate is called **eupnea.** (The prefix *eu-* means "good" and the suffix *-pnea* means "breathing.") A respiratory rate that is higher than normal (greater than 24 breaths/min in an adult) is called **tachypnea,** while a respiratory rate that is lower than normal (less than 10 breaths/min) is called **bradypnea.** (Recall that *tachy-* means "fast," and *brady-* means "slow.")

Normally, the chest should rise and fall evenly, in a regular rhythm. Breathing should be quiet and easy. Laboured or difficult respirations are termed **dyspnea** (recall that *dys-* means "bad" or "difficult"). Other notable respiratory patterns are **hyperventilation** (increased rate and depth of breathing) and **hypoventilation** (decreased rate and depth of breathing).

TELL THE NURSE

Changes in a person's respiratory rate, respiratory rhythm, or depth of respirations can be a sign that something is wrong. Be sure to report the following observations to the nurse immediately:

- The person's respiratory rate is greater than 24 breaths/min

- The person's respiratory rate is less than 10 breaths/min
- The person's respiratory rhythm is irregular
- The person's breaths are either very deep or very shallow
- The person's breathing is difficult or painful
- The person's chest does not rise equally on both sides

BLOOD PRESSURE

The force of the blood pushing against the arterial walls is known as the **blood pressure.** There are two pressure levels that are measured when taking a person's blood pressure measurement. The first, known as the **systolic pressure,** is the pressure that is caused by the blood when the heart muscle contracts, sending a wave of blood through the artery. The second, known as the **diastolic pressure,** occurs when the heart muscle relaxes. Although the heart is relaxed, there is still pressure as the blood flows through the arteries.

Blood pressure is measured in millimetres of mercury (mm Hg) and is recorded as a fraction. The systolic pressure, which is higher, is recorded first, followed by the diastolic pressure, which is lower. For instance, if a person's systolic measurement is 110 mm Hg and his diastolic measurement is 72 mm Hg, then the blood pressure would be recorded as 110/72 mm Hg. The difference between the systolic and diastolic pressures is known as the **pulse pressure,** which in this case would be 38 mm Hg (110 − 72 = 38).

Blood pressure is considered a vital sign because it gives us important information about a person's health and risk for disease. Adequate blood pressure is necessary to keep blood flow constant to all of the tissues of the body. A blood pressure that is too low is a bad sign because it means the tissues of the body are not receiving enough oxygen and nutrients. On the other hand, a blood pressure that is too high forces the heart to do extra work, which, over time, damages the heart. High blood pressure also places stress on the kidneys, which can lead to kidney failure, and on the blood vessels, which can lead to stroke. Blood pressure measurements allow health care workers to monitor existing problems and possibly prevent future ones.

FACTORS AFFECTING BLOOD PRESSURE

The pressure that the blood puts on the arterial walls is controlled by three factors:

- **Cardiac output.** The cardiac output is the amount of blood that the heart is able to pump with each beat. If the heart is able to pump more blood into the vessel with each beat, then blood flow increases, leading to an increase in blood pressure. On the other hand, if the cardiac output is weak, then blood flow decreases, leading to a decrease in blood pressure.
- **Blood volume.** The amount of blood in the vessels at any given time influences the blood pressure. If the blood volume is low, for example, as a result of hemorrhage (see Chapter 12), then the blood pressure will decrease. Similarly, an increase in blood volume leads to an increase in blood pressure. In some people, a salty meal is enough to increase blood pressure, because the salt causes the body to store water, which increases the blood volume.
- **Resistance to blood flow.** Resistance is how hard it is for the blood to flow through the vessels. If the vessels are narrowed (for example, as a result of arteriosclerosis, or "hardening of the arteries"), then the resistance will be high and so will the blood pressure. Resistance is also increased when the blood is thick.

Blood pressure is also influenced by certain factors that we cannot do anything about, such as age, gender, and race:

- **Age.** Young people tend to have lower blood pressures than older people. Aging causes a decrease in the elasticity of the blood vessels (that is, the blood vessels' ability to stretch and bounce back as the blood pulses through). Decreased elasticity results in increased resistance and a higher blood pressure.
- **Gender.** Women tend to have lower blood pressures than men. However, women who take oral contraceptives ("birth control pills") may have a slightly increased blood pressure.
- **Race.** People of certain races (for example, African Americans) tend to have higher blood pressures than people of other races.

MEASURING BLOOD PRESSURE

Manually Operated Sphygmomanometers

Measuring and recording a person's blood pressure is a routine task for personal support workers. There are many ways to measure a person's blood pressure. The most common method is by using a manually operated **sphygmomanometer** and a stethoscope. *Sphygmo-* is from the Greek word for "pulse," and *-manometer* means "a flat instrument used to measure pressure." A manual sphygmomanometer consists of:

- A cuff (a flat, cloth-covered inflatable pouch)
- A bulb, which is squeezed or pumped to fill the cuff with air
- A manometer (the device that measures the air pressure in the inflatable pouch)

Cuffs come in various sizes. The cuff must fit the person properly, or the blood pressure measurement will not be accurate. To find out what size cuff to use, measure around the person's upper arm, halfway between his elbow and shoulder. Cuff sizes are given in Table 16-2.

Two tubes are attached to the pouch within the cuff—one is attached to the bulb used to inflate the pouch, and the other is attached to the manometer. The manometer may be either aneroid or mercury (Fig. 16-10). An aneroid manometer is a small, round dial with a needle

Table 16-2 Blood Pressure Cuff Sizes

ARM MEASUREMENT (cm)	NAME OF CUFF TO USE
13 to 20	Child
24 to 32	Adult
32 to 42	Large Adult
42 to 50	Thigh

that indicates the pressure. A mercury manometer is a column of mercury that may be mounted on a wall or placed on a table. The manometer measures the pressure of the air in the cuff in millimetres of mercury (mm Hg). Long dashes mark increments of 10 mm Hg and the short dashes in between mark increments of 2 mm Hg.

The most common place to measure a person's blood pressure is in the brachial artery of the upper arm. However, the popliteal artery (which can be felt at the back of the person's knee) can be used as well. Measuring a blood pressure is quite simple, once you have had some practice. The cuff is wrapped around the person's upper arm where the brachial artery is located. You can feel the brachial artery pulse in the antecubital space (the inner bend of the elbow) by straightening the person's arm and placing your fingers across the inside of the joint. After positioning the cuff, place the diaphragm of your stethoscope directly over where you felt the brachial

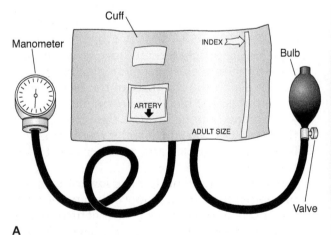
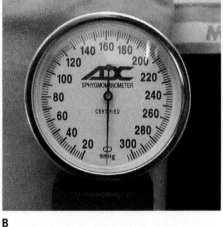
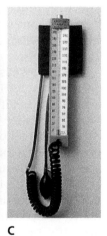

A   B   C

Figure 16-10
(A) A manual sphygmomanometer consists of a cuff, a bulb, and a manometer. The manometer may be either aneroid or mercury. Do you know which type of manometer is shown here? The tubes attach the inflatable pouch inside the cuff to the bulb and to the manometer.
(B) An aneroid manometer. **(C)** A mercury manometer.

artery in the antecubital space, and close the valve on the pumping bulb by turning it clockwise. Do not close the valve too tightly, or it will be difficult to release the air when you are ready. As you pump the bulb, air will enter the pouch in the cuff and you will see the needle (on an aneroid manometer) or the column of mercury (on a mercury manometer) move, indicating that the pressure of the air in the cuff is increasing.

Remember that you have two pressures that are measured within an artery, the systolic pressure (when the heart pumps) and the diastolic pressure (when the heart relaxes). When the pressure within the cuff becomes higher than the systolic pressure in the artery, it will essentially cut off the circulation and not allow any blood to flow through the brachial artery past the cuff. Continue pumping the bulb until the pressure in the cuff is 30 mm Hg higher than the systolic pressure. There are two ways to do this:

- Place the stethoscope over the brachial artery, and inflate the cuff slowly. After you have inflated the cuff a bit, you will start to hear the pulse through your stethoscope. Continue inflating the cuff until you hear the pulse stop (this is the person's systolic pressure) and continue inflating the cuff 30 mm Hg more.
- Or, with your fingers on the person's radial pulse, you can inflate the cuff until you no longer can feel the pulse. The reading on the manometer will indicate the person's systolic pressure. Continue inflating the cuff 30 mm Hg more.

When the pressure in the cuff is 30 mm Hg higher than the systolic pressure, open the valve slightly (by turning it counter clockwise). Opening the valve slightly allows the slow release of air from the cuff, which lowers the pressure in the cuff. Under normal conditions, you may not be able to hear the brachial pulse, but under pressure, you will be able to hear the pulse through the stethoscope. As the pressure in the cuff falls (as indicated by the needle on the aneroid dial or the column of mercury) you listen for sounds, called **Korotkoff sounds** (Box 16-1), through the stethoscope. When the pressure in the cuff is equal to or slightly lower than the systolic pressure in the artery, blood will suddenly begin to flow through the brachial artery and you will start hearing the pulse. When you hear the first sound of the pulse, note the reading on the manometer. This is your systolic pressure. Now continue to listen to the pulse. When the pressure inside the cuff is less than the lowest arterial pressure, or diastolic pressure, the sound of the pulse will stop, because the

---

BOX 16-1 **Korotkoff Sounds**

In some people, you will only be able to hear the beginning and ending sounds while auscultating the blood pressure, but in others, all of these sounds will be distinct.

Phase I: Faint but clear tapping sounds that gradually become louder. The first tapping sound is the systolic pressure.

Phase II: Muffled or swishing sounds that may actually disappear if a person has significant hypertension.

Phase III: Distinct, loud tapping sounds as the blood begins to flow more freely through the artery.

Phase IV: The sound may abruptly become muffled and soft. Keep listening.*

Phase V: The last sound heard before a period of continuous silence. This is the diastolic pressure.

---

*Occasionally, the tapping sounds of the pulse will be heard all the way down to zero. In this case, listening for the abrupt softening of phase IV will give you an approximate diastolic reading.

---

artery is no longer under pressure. The last sound that you hear is the diastolic pressure, and it is shown by the reading on the manometer.

Procedure 16-8 summarizes how to take a blood pressure. Guidelines for taking a blood pressure are given in Guidelines Box 16-1. Learning to take blood pressures takes time and practice. At first, you will need to concentrate on how to operate the equipment and control the rate at which the air leaves the cuff. Next, you will need to become familiar with the sounds that you will hear as the cuff deflates, and learn to recognize the beginning and ending sounds. Each person's blood pressure will sound slightly different. In some people, the blood pressure is easy to measure. In others, measuring the blood pressure will challenge even the most experienced personal support worker. A good rule of thumb is if a person's brachial or radial pulse feels stronger in one arm over the other, you will have an easier time taking the blood pressure in the arm with the stronger pulse. Do not get discouraged if taking blood pressures is difficult at first. The more you practice, the more competent and confident you will become. As with any skill you will learn, if you have difficulty taking a person's blood pressure or if you are unsure of a reading you get, always ask for a second opinion or help from another personal support worker or a nurse. Your responsibility to the people you care for takes priority over your pride.

Guidelines Box 16-1   Guidelines for Taking a Person's Blood Pressure

WHAT YOU DO	WHY YOU DO IT
Allow the person time to relax prior to taking the blood pressure.	Recent exercise and emotions (such as fear) can cause a blood pressure reading to be falsely elevated.
Make sure the manometer is properly calibrated (that is, it reads "0" when there is no air in the cuff).	A manometer that is not properly calibrated will not give an accurate pressure reading.
Use a cuff that is properly sized for the patient or resident.	A cuff that does not fit will not allow you to accurately measure the person's blood pressure. A cuff that is too small will result in a high reading, while a cuff that is too large will result in a low reading.
Make sure the cuff fits snugly around the person's arm before inflating it.	A cuff that is too loose can cause the skin to "pinch" under the cuff when the cuff is inflated, damaging the skin.
Do not place the cuff over a person's clothing.	Clothing will distort the Korotkoff sounds.
Do not take a blood pressure on an arm where an intravenous (IV) line is placed, or on an arm that is injured or in a cast.	Inflating the cuff can cause pain and swelling, and it may dislodge an IV line if one is present.
In a person who has had a mastectomy, do not take a blood pressure on the arm that is on the same side of the body as the breast that was removed.	Some people who have mastectomies also have the lymph nodes in the armpit removed, which disrupts fluid flow from the tissues in the hand and lower arm. This can lead to an inaccurate blood pressure reading.
Do not partially deflate the cuff and then reinflate it while taking a blood pressure measurement. If you make a mistake, release all of the air from the cuff and wait at least 30 seconds before trying again.	Partially deflating and then reinflating the cuff is uncomfortable for the patient or resident, and it will result in an inaccurate reading.
If you are unable to hear the Korotkoff sounds, make sure the room is quiet and check your equipment: ● Make sure the diaphragm of the stethoscope is active by gently tapping on it. ● Make sure the diaphragm of the stethoscope is placed directly over the brachial pulse. ● Make sure the earpieces of the stethoscope are seated properly in your ears.	Most difficulties with measuring blood pressure result from operator error. However, if you have checked your equipment and you still cannot hear the Korotkoff sounds, notify the nurse immediately. The person may have severe hypotension.

Automated Sphygmomanometers and Other Means of Measuring Blood Pressure

Your facility may use automated (electronic) sphygmomanometers instead of manual ones. Some automated models feature automatic inflation and deflation of the cuff, while others require the cuff to be manually inflated but will deflate it automatically. The blood pressure is displayed digitally.

A person's blood pressure can also be measured directly, by inserting a catheter into an artery, or possibly even the heart. Because this procedure is invasive (that is, something is inserted into a normally enclosed part of the person's body), it carries some risk for the person. This method of assessing blood pressure might be used when continuous blood pressure monitoring is required, such as during a surgical procedure or when a patient is critically ill.

NORMAL AND ABNORMAL FINDINGS

Normally, a person's blood pressure moves up and down within the range of normal during the course of a day. For example:

- Blood pressure readings are usually lowest in the morning, and can increase by as much as 10 mm Hg later in the day.
- Blood pressure is generally lower when a person is lying down, as compared to when he is sitting or standing.
- Blood pressure readings are usually slightly higher after a meal, especially a meal with a high salt content.
- Exercise will temporarily increase the systolic blood pressure.
- Stress, anxiety, fear, and pain will also temporarily raise a person's blood pressure.

Much medical research has been done related to blood pressure and its effects on health. Studies have shown that for any individual, there is a wide range of blood pressure readings that can be considered "normal." When you are taking a person's blood pressure, it is important to allow that person time to relax or rest for a bit so that the blood pressure reading reflects the person's normal pressure, and not the changes that can occur from exertion or being emotionally upset. Also, as a personal support worker, you must learn to recognize the range of blood pressure measurements that can be considered "normal" for each of your patients or residents, so that you will be able to recognize any changes. A person's blood pressure

could rise or fall 20 to 30 mm Hg and still be within the range of what is considered normal for that person. However, a change in a person's blood pressure that is that large should be recognized and reported immediately to the nurse.

TELL THE NURSE

Changes in a person's blood pressure can be a sign that something is wrong. Be sure to report the following observations to the nurse immediately:

- The person's blood pressure is higher than normal
- The person's blood pressure is lower than normal

Accepted normal ranges for the systolic pressure are between 100 and 140 mm Hg, and for the diastolic pressure, between 60 and 90 mm Hg. If a person has a blood pressure that is consistently higher than 140 mm Hg (systolic) and/or 90 mm Hg (diastolic), then that person is said to have **hypertension** (high blood pressure). To diagnose a person with hypertension and start treatment for this condition, the person's blood pressure measurements must be taken and recorded over a period of time to show a pattern of constant elevation. Medications for hypertension should be taken as ordered. If the person stops taking the medication or does not take it according to the prescribed schedule, the person's hypertension will usually return. Too often, a patient or resident will tell you that "I used to take medicine for my blood pressure, but the medicine brought my pressure back to normal, so I don't need to take it anymore." Measuring that person's blood pressure will usually tell a completely different story! Hypertension is often called the "silent killer" because a person with this condition does not feel ill, yet is at great risk for complications (and possibly even death) as a result of it.

A person who has a blood pressure that is consistently lower than 90 mm Hg (systolic) and/or 60 mm Hg (diastolic) is said to have **hypotension** (low blood pressure). Some people may have **orthostatic hypotension,** which is a sudden decrease in blood pressure that occurs when a person stands up from a sitting or lying position. When a person is sitting or lying down, the heart does not need to work as hard to pump blood throughout the body and the blood vessels are relaxed, so resistance is low. However, when the person stands up, the body needs to make up for the change in position. The heart pumps harder and the vessels constrict to bring the blood pressure back up to a normal level.

Until the body manages to make up for the sudden change in position, the person may feel lightheaded and faint. Some medications and aging can increase the time the body needs to adjust. The lack of blood flow to the brain can cause the person to feel dizzy. This is why, when you are assisting a person to "dangle" (see Chapter 11), you must give the person a minute to adjust before proceeding. Always remind your patients or residents to first sit for a moment before standing up, to allow time for the body to adjust. Helping a person who experiences orthostatic hypotension to remember to take those extra few moments for the body to adjust can help prevent a fall.

For some patients or residents, you may be asked to take a sequence of blood pressures—usually first with the person lying down, then sitting, then standing. This is done to evaluate how well the person's body adapts to changes in position. Facility policy will state the order of the blood pressure measurements when a sequence of measurements is needed.

HEIGHT AND WEIGHT

Although height and weight are not technically vital signs, these measurements are taken periodically while a person is receiving care. The relationship of a person's weight to his height can provide insight into the person's overall health and nutritional status. In addition, a person's weight is often used to calculate medication dosages. In some cases, a change in a person's weight might indicate that the person's condition is getting worse, or that it is getting better. For all of these reasons, it is useful to obtain a "baseline" height and weight for each patient or resident, and to measure the person's weight periodically thereafter.

A person's height is measured only on admission. A person's weight is measured on admission, and on transfer or discharge. It may also be necessary to measure a person's weight at regular intervals throughout the person's stay. A person's weight is rechecked periodically for various reasons:

- Weight is an indicator of nutritional status.
- Weight is an indicator of heart and kidney function. If the heart or kidneys are not functioning well, the person will retain fluid, which will cause an increase in weight.
- Changes in weight can be a sign of disease. For example, one of the signs of some types of cancer is major, unexplained weight loss.
- Many medications are prescribed according to body weight. If a person gains or loses a

great deal of weight, it may be necessary to adjust the person's medication dosages.

MEASURING HEIGHT AND WEIGHT

Height is measured in centimetres (cm) or in feet (') and inches ("). Weight is measured in kilograms (kg) or pounds (lb). You may need to convert your patient's or resident's height and weight into measurements the person will understand:

- 1 inch = 2.54 cm
- 2.2 lb = 1 kg

The type of scale you will use to measure a person's weight will depend on the person's ability to get out of bed and stand. Common types of scales include upright scales, chair scales, and sling scales.

Scales may be mechanical or digital. If you are using a mechanical scale to measure a person's weight, you must slide weights along a bar by hand until the bar is balanced (Fig. 16-11). If you are using a digital scale, you simply turn the scale on. The digital scale measures the person's weight automatically and displays it on a screen.

Measuring Height and Weight Using an Upright Scale

An upright scale is used to obtain height and weight measurements for a person who is able to stand on her own. Procedure 16-9 describes how to use an upright scale to measure a person's height and weight.

Measuring Weight Using a Chair Scale

A chair scale (Fig. 16-12) is used to obtain a weight measurement for a person who cannot stand independently, but is able to get out of bed. One type of chair scale is for use with a wheelchair. The wheelchair is first weighed without the person in it to determine its weight. Next, the wheelchair, with the person in it, is rolled onto the scale. The weight of the empty wheelchair is subtracted from the weight of the wheelchair with the person in it to determine the person's weight. The other type of chair scale is simply a chair-like device that allows the person to sit while having his weight measured. Procedure 16-10 describes how to use a chair scale.

Measuring Height and Weight Using a Tape Measure and a Sling Scale

If a person is unable to get out of bed at all, the person will have to be weighed in bed. Some

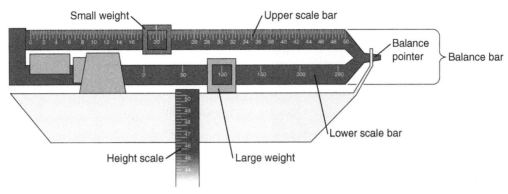

Figure 16-11

A mechanical scale. Most scales have a rotating *balance bar* that measures in both kilograms and pounds. The *large weight* slides along the *lower scale bar*. The *small weight* slides along the *upper scale bar*. The *balance pointer* is centered between the two scale bars when the weight on the scale bars equals the person's weight.

acute care facilities have beds with built-in scales. If this type of bed is not available where you work, then you will have to weigh the person using a sling scale (Fig. 16-13). The person's height is measured using a tape measure.

Procedure 16-11 describes how to obtain height and weight measurements using a tape measure and a sling scale. Because sling scales from different manufacturers may vary greatly in their procedures for use, do not attempt to use

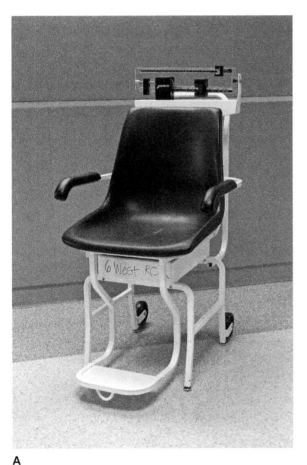

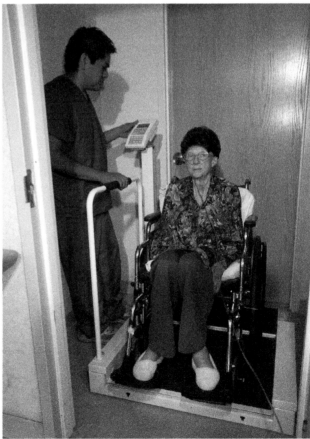

A   **B**

Figure 16-12

A chair scale is used to obtain weight measurements for a person who cannot stand up independently but is able to get out of bed. **(A)** A chair scale. **(B)** A chair scale for use with a wheelchair.

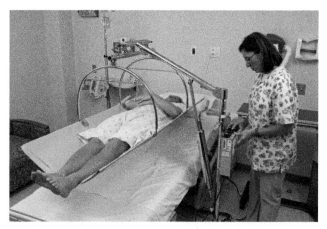

Figure 16-13
A sling scale is used to obtain weight measurements for a person who cannot get out of bed.

Table 16-3 Normal Pediatric Temperature Ranges

METHOD USED TO OBTAIN TEMPERATURE	CELSIUS (°C)	FAHRENHEIT (°F)
Oral	36–37	97–99
Rectal	37–38	98–100
Axillary	35–36	96–98
Tympanic	37–38	98–100

a sling scale unless you have been trained in its use.

MEASURING VITAL SIGNS IN CHILDREN

The procedures for measuring vital signs are the same whether you are caring for children or adults. However, when you are measuring vital signs in a child, you will need to adjust your approach somewhat. Children can present their own challenges, depending on their age and ability to cooperate. For example, a toddler will prefer to remain seated in his parent's lap while you are measuring his vital signs. He will be fascinated by your equipment and reach out to touch parts of it, such as the shiny stethoscope bell. Older children will expect a simple explanation of what you are going to do and how the procedure will feel. An adolescent will be very impressed that you are treating her as an adult if you tell her what the readings are as you take the vital signs.

Children who are younger than 5 years of age may not be able to cooperate fully for the measurement of an oral temperature, so a tympanic or axillary measurement will work best. Measure the child's pulse and respirations first, while the child is still cooperative, calm, and not suspicious of what you are doing. Make sure that you measure the pulse rate and respiratory rate for a full minute on children younger than 12 years. Blood pressure may be measured manually or with an electronic blood pressure device. The weight and age of the child determine cuff size. A cuff that is not the appropriate size will affect the accuracy of the reading.

The normal ranges for vital signs in children are given in Tables 16-3 and 16-4.

Table 16-4 Normal Pediatric Pulse, Respiration, and Blood Pressure Ranges

AGE OF CHILD	PULSE RATE (beats/min)*	RESPIRATION RATE (breaths/min)*	BLOOD PRESSURE (mm Hg)
Infant (0–1 year)	120–160	30–60	73/55
Toddler (1–3 years)	80–130	24–40	90/55
Preschooler (3–5 years)	80–120	22–34	94/60
School-aged child (5–12 years)	75–110	15–25	100/75
Adolescent (12–20 years)	60–100	15–20	102/80

*The pulse and respiration rates are always measured for a full minute in children younger than 12 years.

SUMMARY

- Vital signs provide essential information about a person's health.
  - The vital signs are body temperature, pulse, respirations, and blood pressure. A person's height and weight, although not technically vital signs, also provide insight into a person's overall health.
  - Measuring and recording vital signs is a routine part of a personal support worker's daily duties.
    - Vital signs must be measured and recorded accurately because many people rely on this information to make decisions about the person's care. In addition, a change in vital signs can be an important early sign that something is wrong.
    - Personal support workers must be familiar with accepted normal ranges for all of the vital signs. In addition, personal support workers must come to recognize what is "normal" for each of the patients or residents in their care.
    - Learning the skills associated with taking vital signs takes practice. With practice, comes confidence.
- Body temperature is a measure of how hot the body is.
  - The body temperature can be measured using a number of devices in a number of places.
    - Types of thermometers include glass (mercury) thermometers, electronic thermometers, tympanic thermometers, and temporal artery thermometers.
    - A person's temperature may be measured in the mouth, rectum, ear, armpit, or forehead.
  - An elevated temperature may be a sign of infection. Extreme changes in the environmental temperature can also affect a person's body temperature.
- The pulse reflects the rate, rhythm, and strength of the heartbeat, and therefore is a vital sign.
  - The pulse can be measured by feeling the radial artery (in the wrist) or by listening to the apical pulse (in the chest) with a stethoscope.
  - Tachycardia is an excessively rapid heartbeat. Bradycardia is an excessively slow heartbeat.

- The respiratory rate, rhythm, and depth are a reflection of how well the person is breathing.
  - The respiratory rate is measured by counting the number of times the person inhales and exhales in 30 seconds (or 1 minute, if the respirations are irregular).
    - The chest rises with each inhalation and falls with each exhalation.
    - One respiration = one inhalation + one exhalation.
  - Dyspnea is laboured breathing. Tachypnea is a respiratory rate that is too fast, and bradypnea is a respiratory rate that is too slow.
- The blood pressure reflects the force the blood exerts against the arterial walls. Cardiac output, blood volume, and resistance affect the blood pressure.
  - Blood pressure is most often measured in the brachial artery using a sphygmomanometer and a stethoscope.
  - Korotkoff sounds are the sounds the blood makes as it rushes through the artery.
    - Phase I Korotkoff sounds signal the systolic pressure, or the pressure when the heart beats.
    - Phase V Korotkoff sounds signal the diastolic pressure, or the pressure when the heart relaxes.
    - Listening for and interpreting the Korotkoff sounds take practice.
  - Hypertension, or a consistently high blood pressure, can have serious long-term consequences if not treated.
  - Orthostatic hypotension, or low blood pressure on changing positions, affects many people and is the reason people are encouraged to sit for a minute before standing up from a lying position.
- Height and weight are measured when a person enters a health care facility.
  - Weight is measured periodically. Major weight loss or gain can be an early sign of disease. In addition, many medication dosages are calculated according to a person's body weight.
  - A variety of devices, including upright scales, chair scales, and sling scales, can be used to measure a person's weight, depending on the person's situation.

PROCEDURE 16-1

Measuring an Oral Temperature (Glass or Electronic Thermometer)

WHY YOU DO IT   A change in a person's normal temperature may be a sign of illness. Taking an oral temperature is fast and causes the patient or resident minimal discomfort.

Getting Ready WGKIEPS

1. Complete the "Getting Ready" steps.

Supplies

If using a glass thermometer:

- paper towels
- tissues
- thermometer sheath
- oral glass thermometer

If using an electronic thermometer:

- probe sheath
- electronic thermometer with oral (blue) probe

Procedure

2. Ask the person if he or she has eaten, consumed a beverage, chewed gum, or smoked within the last 15 minutes. If so, wait 15 to 30 minutes before proceeding (or follow facility policy).

3. Prepare the thermometer.

   a. **Glass thermometer:** Run cool water over the thermometer to rinse away the disinfectant. Dry the thermometer with a paper towel and inspect it for cracks or chips. Carefully shake down the glass thermometer so that the indicator material is below the 34° mark (if using a Celsius thermometer) or the 94° mark (if using a Fahrenheit thermometer). Cover the end of the glass thermometer with the thermometer sheath.

   b. **Electronic thermometer:** Cover the electronic probe with the probe sheath. Turn the thermometer on and wait until the "ready" sign appears on the display screen.

4. Ask the person to open his or her mouth. Slowly and carefully insert the thermometer, placing the tip under the person's tongue and to one side.

5. Ask the person to gently close his or her mouth around the thermometer without biting down. If necessary, hold the thermometer in place. Ask the person to breathe through his or her nose.

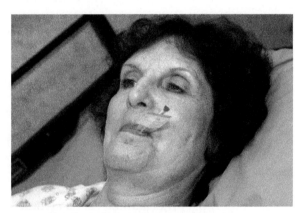

Step 5 The person breathes through her nose while holding the thermometer in her mouth.

6. Leave the thermometer in place for the specified amount of time:

   a. **Glass thermometer:** 3 to 5 minutes (or follow facility policy)

   b. **Electronic thermometer:** until the instrument blinks or beeps (usually just a few seconds)

7. Ask the person to open his or her mouth. Remove the thermometer from the person's mouth.

8. Read the temperature measurement.

   a. **Glass thermometer:** Using a tissue, remove the thermometer sheath from the glass thermometer, being careful not to touch the bulb end of the thermometer. Dispose of the tissue and the thermometer sheath in a facility-approved waste container. Hold the thermometer horizontally by the stem at eye level while facing a light source. Rotate the thermometer until you can see the level of the indicator material. Read the temperature.

b. Electronic thermometer: Read the temperature on the electronic thermometer's display screen. Remove the probe sheath from the probe by pushing the button on the top of the probe. Direct the probe sheath into a facility-approved waste container.

9. Prepare the thermometer for its next use.

a. Glass thermometer: Shake down the glass thermometer, clean it according to facility policy, and return it to its disinfectant-filled case.

b. Electronic thermometer: Replace the probe into the electronic thermometer. (Always read the temperature before placing the probe in the instrument because this action clears the display screen.) Turn the instrument off if it does not automatically turn itself off. Place the thermometer in its charger.

10. Note the person's name, the time, the temperature, and the method on your notepad (or record the temperature and the method on the person's medical record if it is kept at the bedside). Place an "O" (or the notation designated by your facility) next to the measurement to indicate that the measurement was taken orally. Report an abnormal temperature to the nurse immediately.

Finishing Up CLSOWR

11. Complete the "Finishing Up" steps.

PROCEDURE 16-2

Measuring a Rectal Temperature (Glass or Electronic Thermometer)

WHY YOU DO IT   A change in a person's normal temperature may be a sign of illness. The rectal temperature measurement is a very accurate measurement of the body's temperature.

Getting Ready WCKIEPS

1. Complete the "Getting Ready" steps.

Supplies
- gloves
- paper towels
- tissues
- lubricant jelly

If using a glass thermometer:
- thermometer sheath
- rectal glass thermometer

If using an electronic thermometer:
- probe sheath
- electronic thermometer with rectal (red) probe

Procedure

2. Make sure that the bed is positioned at a comfortable working height (to promote good body mechanics) and that the wheels are locked.

3. Prepare the thermometer.

a. Glass thermometer: Run cool water over the thermometer to rinse away the disinfectant. Dry the thermometer with a paper towel and inspect it for cracks or chips. Carefully shake down the glass thermometer so that the indicator material is below the 34° mark (if using a Celsius thermometer) or the 94° mark (if using a Fahrenheit thermometer). Cover the end of the glass thermometer with the thermometer sheath.

b. Electronic thermometer: Cover the electronic probe with the probe sheath. Turn the thermometer on and wait until the "ready" sign appears on the display screen.

4. Place the thermometer on a clean paper towel on the over-bed table. Open the lubricant package and squeeze a small amount of

(continued)

lubricant onto the paper towel. Lubricate the tip of the thermometer to ease insertion.

5. If the side rails are in use, lower the side rail on the working side of the bed. The side rail on the opposite side of the bed should remain up. Lower the head of the bed so that the bed is flat (as tolerated).

6. Ask the person to lie on his or her side, facing away from you, in Sims' position. Help the person into this position, if necessary.

7. Fanfold the top linens to below the person's buttocks. Adjust the person's hospital gown or pajama bottoms as necessary to expose the person's buttocks.

8. Put on the gloves.

9. With one hand, raise the person's upper buttock to expose the anus. Suggest that the person take a deep breath and slowly exhale as the thermometer is inserted. Using your other hand, gently and carefully insert the lubricated end of the thermometer into the person's rectum (not more than 3 to 4 centimetres for adults, or 2.5 centimetres for children). Never force the thermometer into the rectum. If you are unable to insert the thermometer, stop and call the nurse.

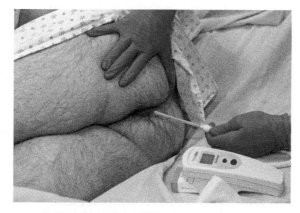

Step 9 Gently and carefully insert the lubricated end of the thermometer into the person's rectum.

10. Hold the thermometer in place for the specified amount of time:

    a. **Glass thermometer:** 3 to 5 minutes (or follow facility policy)

    b. **Electronic thermometer:** until the instrument blinks or beeps (usually just a few seconds)

11. Remove the thermometer from the person's rectum. Wipe the person's anal area with a tissue to remove the lubricant, and adjust the person's hospital gown or pajama bottoms as necessary to cover the buttocks.

12. Read the temperature measurement.

    a. **Glass thermometer:** Using a tissue, remove the thermometer sheath from the glass thermometer, being careful not to touch the bulb end of the thermometer. Dispose of the tissue and the thermometer sheath in a facility-approved waste container. Hold the thermometer horizontally by the stem at eye level while facing a light source. Rotate the thermometer until you can see the level of the indicator material. Read the temperature.

    b. **Electronic thermometer:** Read the temperature on the electronic thermometer's display screen. Remove the probe sheath from the probe by pushing the button on the top of the probe. Direct the probe sheath into a facility-approved waste container.

13. Remove your gloves and dispose of them according to facility policy. Wash your hands.

14. Note the person's name, the time, the temperature, and the method on your notepad (or record the temperature and the method on the person's medical record if it is kept at the bedside). Place an "R" (or the notation designated by your facility) next to the measurement to indicate that the measurement was taken rectally. Report an abnormal temperature to the nurse immediately.

15. Help the person back into a comfortable position, straighten the bottom linens, and draw the top linens over the person. Raise the head of the bed, as the person requests.

16. Make sure that the bed is lowered to its lowest position and that the wheels are locked. If the side rails are in use, return the side rails to the raised position.

17. Prepare the thermometer for its next use.

    a. **Glass thermometer:** Shake down the glass thermometer, clean it according to facility policy, and return it to its disinfectant-filled case.

    b. **Electronic thermometer:** Replace the probe into the electronic thermometer. (Always read the temperature before placing the probe in the instrument because this action clears the display screen.) Turn the instrument off if it does not automatically turn itself off. Place the thermometer in its charger.

Finishing Up   CLSOWR

18. Complete the "Finishing Up" steps.

PROCEDURE 16-3

Measuring an Axillary Temperature (Glass or Electronic Thermometer)

WHY YOU DO IT A change in a person's normal temperature may be a sign of illness. The axillary method is used when other methods cannot be used.

Getting Ready WORKTEPS

1. Complete the "Getting Ready" steps.

Supplies

- paper towels
- tissues

If using a glass thermometer:

- thermometer sheath
- oral glass thermometer

If using an electronic thermometer:

- probe sheath
- electronic thermometer with oral (blue) probe

Procedure

2. Ask the person if he or she has bathed or applied deodorant or antiperspirant within the last 15 minutes. If so, wait 15 to 30 minutes before proceeding (or follow facility policy).

3. Prepare the thermometer.

   a. **Glass thermometer:** Run cool water over the thermometer to rinse away the disinfectant. Dry the thermometer with a paper towel and inspect it for cracks or chips. Carefully shake down the glass thermometer so that the indicator material is below the 34° mark (if using a Celsius thermometer) or the 94° mark (if using a Fahrenheit thermometer). Cover the end of the glass thermometer with the thermometer sheath.

   b. **Electronic thermometer:** Cover the electronic probe with the probe sheath. Turn the thermometer on and wait until the "ready" sign appears on the display screen.

4. Assist the person with removing his or her arm from the sleeve of his or her hospital gown or pajama top.

5. Pat the axilla (underarm area) gently with a paper towel.

6. Ask the person to lift his or her arm slightly. Position the tip of the thermometer in the center of the axilla and ask the person to hold the thermometer in place by holding his or her arm close to the body (or by grasping the arm with the opposite hand).

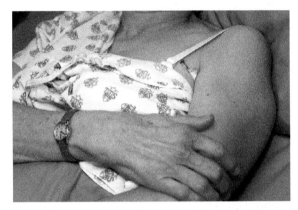

Step 6 The person holds the thermometer in place by grasping her arm with the opposite hand.

7. Leave the thermometer in place for the specified amount of time:

   a. **Glass thermometer:** 10 minutes (or follow facility policy)

   b. **Electronic thermometer:** until the instrument blinks or beeps (usually just a few seconds)

8. Ask the person to lift his or her arm slightly. Remove the thermometer.

9. Read the temperature measurement.

   a. **Glass thermometer:** Using a tissue, remove the thermometer sheath from the glass thermometer, being careful not to touch the bulb end of the thermometer. Dispose of the tissue and the thermometer sheath in a facility-approved waste container. Hold the thermometer horizontally by the stem at eye level while facing a light source. Rotate the thermometer until you can see the level of the indicator material. Read the temperature.

   b. **Electronic thermometer:** Read the temperature on the electronic thermometer's

(continued)

display screen. Remove the probe sheath from the probe by pushing the button on the top of the probe. Direct the probe sheath into a facility-approved waste container.

10. Note the person's name, the time, the temperature, and the method on your notepad (or record the temperature and the method on the person's medical record, if it is kept at the bedside). Place an "A" (or the notation designated by your facility) next to the measurement to indicate that the measurement was taken in the axilla. Report an abnormal temperature to the nurse immediately.

11. Help the person back into his or her hospital gown or pajama top.

12. Prepare the thermometer for its next use:
    a. **Glass thermometer:** Shake down the glass thermometer, clean it according to facility policy, and return it to its disinfectant-filled case.
    b. **Electronic thermometer:** Replace the probe into the electronic thermometer. (Always read the temperature before placing the probe in the instrument because this action clears the display screen.) Turn the instrument off, if it does not automatically turn itself off. Place the thermometer in its charger.

Finishing Up CLSOWR

13. Complete the "Finishing Up" steps.

PROCEDURE 16-4

Measuring a Tympanic Temperature (Tympanic Thermometer)

WHY YOU DO IT   A change in a person's normal temperature may be a sign of illness. Taking a tympanic temperature is fast and causes the patient or resident minimal discomfort.

Getting Ready WCKIEpS

1. Complete the "Getting Ready" steps.

Supplies
- tympanic probe sheath (cover)
- tympanic thermometer

Procedure

2. If the person wears a hearing aid, remove it carefully and wait 2 minutes before taking the person's temperature.

3. Inspect the ear canal for excessive cerumen (ear wax). If you see excessive wax build-up in the ear canal, gently wipe the ear canal with a warm, moist washcloth.

4. Cover the cone-shaped end of the thermometer with the probe sheath. Turn the thermometer on and wait until the "ready" sign appears on the display screen.

5. Stand slightly to the front of, and facing, the person. To straighten the ear canal (which will ease insertion of the thermometer), grasp the top portion of the person's ear and gently pull:

a. Up and back (in an adult)
b. Straight back (in a child)

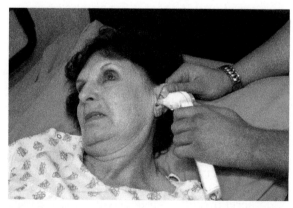

Step 5a In an adult, grasp the top portion of the person's ear and gently pull up and back to insert the thermometer.

6. Insert the covered probe into the person's ear canal, pointing the probe down and toward the front of the ear canal (pretend that you are aiming for the person's nose). This will seal off the ear canal by seating the probe

properly, leading to a more accurate temperature reading.

7. To take the temperature, press the button on the instrument. Keep the button depressed and the probe in place until the instrument blinks or beeps (usually 1 second).

8. Remove the probe and read the temperature on the display screen.

9. Remove the probe sheath from the probe by pushing the button on the side of the instrument. Direct the probe sheath into a facility-approved waste container.

10. Note the person's name, the time, the temperature, and the method on your notepad (or record the temperature and method on the person's medical record if it is kept at the bedside). Place a "T" (or the notation designated by your facility) next to the measurement to indicate that the measurement was taken in the ear (i.e., using a tympanic thermometer). Report an abnormal temperature to the nurse immediately.

11. If your facility requires a tympanic temperature to be taken in both ears, repeat the procedure, using a clean probe cover for the other ear.

12. Turn the instrument off if it does not automatically turn itself off. Place the thermometer in its charger.

Finishing Up CLSOWR

13. Complete the "Finishing Up" steps.

PROCEDURE 16-5

Taking a Radial Pulse

WHY YOU DO IT   A change in a person's normal pulse rate, rhythm, or amplitude may be a sign of illness. Taking the pulse at the radial artery is easiest for the patient or resident.

Getting Ready WGKIEPS

1. Complete the "Getting Ready" steps.

Supplies

● watch with second hand

Procedure

2. Rest the person's arm on the over-bed table or on the bed. Locate the radial pulse in the person's wrist using your middle two or three fingers. (TIP: The radial pulse will be on the person's "thumb" side.)

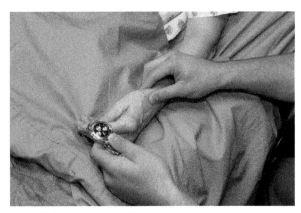

Step 2 Locate the radial pulse in the person's wrist using your middle two or three fingers.

3. Note the strength and regularity of the pulse. Look at your watch and wait until the second hand gets to the "12" or "6." When the second hand reaches the "12" or the "6," begin counting the pulse.

   a. If the pulse rhythm is regular, count the number of pulses that occur in 30 seconds and multiply the result by 2 to arrive at the pulse rate.

   b. If the pulse rhythm is irregular, count the number of pulses that occur in 60 seconds. Counting each pulse that occurs over the course of 1 full minute is the only way to obtain a truly accurate pulse rate when the pulse is irregular.

4. Note the person's name; the time; and the pulse rate, rhythm, and amplitude on your notepad (or record the pulse rate, rhythm, and amplitude on the person's medical record if it is kept at the bedside). Report an abnormal pulse rate, rhythm, or amplitude to the nurse immediately.

Finishing Up CLSOWR

5. Complete the "Finishing Up" steps.

PROCEDURE 16-6

Taking an Apical Pulse

WHY YOU DO IT An apical pulse is taken when a person has a weak or irregular pulse that may be difficult to feel in the redial artery. An apical pulse may also be used to measure heart rate in infants and in people with known heart disease.

Getting Ready WGKIEPS

1. Complete the "Getting Ready" steps.

Supplies

- alcohol wipes
- dual-sided stethoscope
- watch with second hand

Procedure

2. Help the person to a sitting position by raising the head of the bed.

3. Using alcohol wipes, clean the earpieces, the diaphragm, and the bell of the stethoscope. Place the earpieces in your ears.

4. Place the diaphragm (or the bell, if the person is a child or infant) of the stethoscope under the person's clothing, on the apical pulse site (located approximately 5 centimetres below the person's left nipple). The diaphragm or bell must be placed directly on the person's skin because clothing will distort the sound.

5. Using two fingers, hold the diaphragm or bell firmly against the person's chest. Look at your watch and wait until the second hand gets to the "12" or "6." When the second hand reaches the "12" or the "6," begin counting the heartbeat.

6. Count the number of heartbeats that occur in 60 seconds. Each time the heart beats, you will hear two sounds, best described as a "lubb" and a "dupp." Both sounds make up one beat of the heart and should be counted as such.

7. After 60 seconds, remove the diaphragm of the stethoscope from the person's chest. Adjust the person's clothing as necessary and help the person back into a comfortable position. Lower the head of the bed, as the person requests.

8. Note the person's name; the time; the pulse rate, rhythm, and amplitude; and the method on your notepad (or record the pulse rate, rhythm, and amplitude and the method on the person's medical record if it is kept at the bedside). Place an "a" (or the notation designated by your facility) next to the measurement to indicate that the measurement was taken apically. Report an abnormal pulse to the nurse immediately.

9. Using alcohol wipes, clean the earpieces, the diaphragm, and the bell of the stethoscope.

Finishing Up CLSOWR

10. Complete the "Finishing Up" steps.

Step 5 Hold the diaphragm or bell firmly against the person's chest.

PROCEDURE 16-7

Counting Respirations

WHY YOU DO IT   A change in a person's normal respiratory rate, rhythm, or depth of breathing may be a sign of illness.

Getting Ready   WCKIEPS
1. Complete the "Getting Ready" steps.

Supplies
- watch with second hand

Procedure
2. Look at your watch and wait until the second hand gets to the "12" or "6." When the second hand reaches the "12" or the "6," look at the person's chest (or place your hand near the person's collarbone or on his or her side) and begin counting each rise and fall of the chest as one breath.

   a. If the respiratory rhythm is regular, count the number of breaths that occur in 30 seconds and multiply the result by 2 to arrive at the respiratory rate.

   b. If the respiratory rhythm is irregular, count the number of breaths that occur in 60 seconds. Counting each respiration that occurs over the course of 1 full minute is the only way to obtain a truly accurate respiratory rate when the person's breathing is irregular.

3. Note the person's name, the time, and the respiratory rate on your notepad (or record the respiratory rate on the person's medical record if it is kept at the bedside). Report abnormal respirations to the nurse immediately.

Finishing Up   CLSOWR
4. Complete the "Finishing Up" steps.

PROCEDURE 16-8

Measuring Blood Pressure

WHY YOU DO IT   Blood pressure measurements allow health care workers to monitor existing problems and possibly even prevent future ones.

Getting Ready   WCKIEPS
1. Complete the "Getting Ready" steps.

Supplies
- alcohol wipes
- stethoscope
- sphygmomanometer

Procedure
2. Assist the person into a sitting or lying position. Position the person's arm so that the forearm is level with the heart and the palm of the hand is facing upward. Assist the person with rolling up his or her sleeve so that the upper arm is exposed.

3. Using alcohol wipes, clean the earpieces, the diaphragm, and the bell of the stethoscope.

4. Stand no more than 1 metre away from the manometer. If it is not mounted on the wall, stand a mercury manometer upright on a flat surface, at eye level. Lay an aneroid manometer on a flat surface directly in front of you or leave it attached to the blood pressure cuff.

5. Squeeze the cuff to empty it of any remaining air. Turn the valve on the bulb clockwise to close it; this will cause the cuff to inflate when you pump the bulb.

6. Locate the person's brachial artery in the antecubital space by placing your fingers at the inner aspect of the elbow.

(continued)

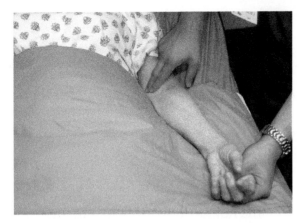

Step 6 Locate the person's brachial artery in the antecubital space (inner aspect of the elbow).

7. Place the arrow mark on the cuff over the brachial artery. Wrap the cuff around the person's upper arm so that the bottom of the cuff is at least 2.54 cm above the person's elbow. The cuff must be even and snug.

8. Place the stethoscope earpieces in your ears.

9. Pump the bulb until the pressure in the cuff is 30 mm Hg higher than the systolic pressure. There are two ways to do this:

   Method "A." Hold the bulb in one hand and position the diaphragm of the stethoscope over the brachial artery with the other hand. Inflate the cuff until you hear the pulse stop and then inflate the cuff 30 mm Hg more.

   Method "B." Hold the bulb in one hand and feel for the person's radial pulse (in his or her wrist) with the other hand. Inflate the cuff until you are no longer able to feel the radial pulse and then inflate the cuff 30 mm Hg more.

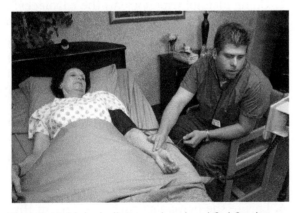

Step 9 Hold the bulb in one hand and feel for the person's radial pulse (in the wrist) with the other hand.

10. Position the diaphragm of the stethoscope over the brachial artery (or continue to hold it there if you used method "A" to inflate the cuff).

11. Turn the valve on the bulb slightly counterclockwise to allow air to escape from the cuff slowly.

12. Note the reading on the manometer where the first Korotkoff sound is heard. This is the systolic reading.

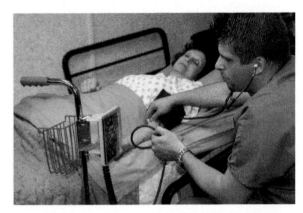

Step 12 With the diaphragm of the stethoscope over the person's brachial artery, allow the air to leave the cuff slowly while listening for the beginning and ending sounds of the brachial pulse and watching the manometer.

13. Continue to deflate the cuff. Note the reading on the manometer where the last Korotkoff sound is heard. This is the diastolic reading.

14. Deflate the cuff completely and remove it from the person's arm. Remove the stethoscope from your ears.

15. Note the person's name, the time, and the blood pressure on your notepad (or record the blood pressure on the person's medical record if it is kept at the bedside). Report an abnormal blood pressure to the nurse immediately.

16. Return the sphygmomanometer to its case or wall holder.

17. Using alcohol wipes, clean the earpieces, the diaphragm, and the bell of the stethoscope.

Finishing Up

18. Complete the "Finishing Up" steps.

PROCEDURE 16-9

Measuring Height and Weight Using an Upright Scale

WHY YOU DO IT   An upright scale is used to measure the height and weight of a person who can stand independently. A person's weight is often used to calculate medication doses. In some cases, a change in a person's weight might indicate that the person's condition is getting worse or that it is getting better.

Getting Ready   WORKBOOK

1. Complete the "Getting Ready" steps.

Supplies

- upright scale

Procedure

2. Ask the person to urinate. If necessary, assist the person to the bathroom or offer the bedpan or urinal.

3. Move the weights all the way to the left of the balance bar.

4. Help the person onto the scale platform so that she is facing the balance bar. Once the person is on the scale platform, do not allow her to hold on to you or to the scale.

5. Move the large weight on the lower scale bar to the right to the weight closest to the person's prior weight. For example, if the person weighed 70 kilograms the last time you weighed her, you would move the large weight to the "70" mark.

6. Move the small weight on the upper scale bar to the right until the balance pointer is centered between the two scale bars.

7. Read the numbers on the upper and the lower scale bars where each weight has settled and add these two numbers together. This is the person's weight.

8. Have the person carefully turn around to face away from the scale bar. Slide the height scale up so that you can pull out the height rod, which extends from the top of the height scale. Be careful not to hit the person in the head with the height rod.

9. Slide the height rod down so that it lightly touches the top of the person's head. Read the number at the point where the height rod meets the height scale. This is the person's height.

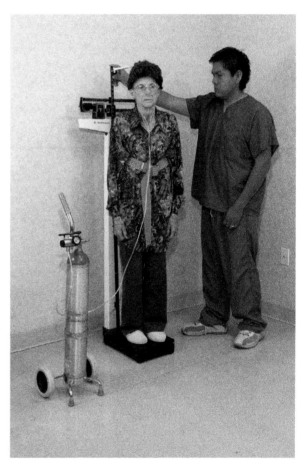

Step 9 Slide the height rod down so that it lightly touches the top of the person's head.

(continued)

10. Hold the height rod in your hand, and help the person step down from the scale.

11. Assist the person back to her room.

12. Note the person's name, the time, and the weight and height on your notepad (or record the weight and height on the person's med-

ical record if it is kept at the bedside). Report a change in the person's weight to the nurse.

Finishing Up CLSOWR

13. Complete the "Finishing Up" steps.

PROCEDURE 16-10

Measuring Weight Using a Chair Scale

WHY YOU DO IT A chair scale is used to measure the weight of a person who cannot stand independently but is able to get out of bed. A person's weight is often used to calculate medication doses. In some cases, a change in a person's weight might indicate that the person's condition is getting worse or that it is getting better.

Getting Ready WCKIEpS

1. Complete the "Getting Ready" steps.

Supplies

- transfer belt
- wheelchair*

Procedure

2. Ask the person to urinate. If necessary, assist the person to the bathroom or offer the bedpan or urinal.

3. Assist or wheel the person to the scale, using a transfer belt, a wheelchair, or both.

4. Reset the scale to "0" by turning it on.

5. Help the person onto the scale.

   a. If a regular chair scale is being used, help the person to sit in the chair on the scale. Make sure the person is seated properly, with his or her buttocks against the back of the chair and feet on the footrests.

   b. If a wheelchair scale is being used, roll the occupied wheelchair onto the platform and lock the wheels.

6. Read the weight on the display screen. If a wheelchair scale is being used, you must subtract the weight of the unoccupied wheel-

chair from this figure to determine the person's weight.

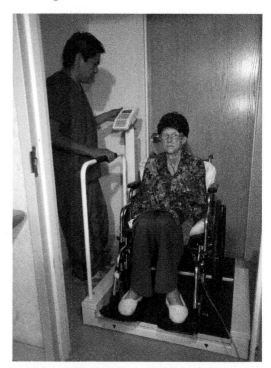

Step 6 Read the weight on the display screen.

7. Help the person off of the scale.

   a. If a regular chair scale is being used, assist the person out of the chair and back into a wheelchair if one was used for the transfer.

   b. If a wheelchair scale is being used, unlock the wheels and roll the wheelchair off the platform.

---

*If you will be using a wheelchair scale to weigh the person, take the empty wheelchair to the wheelchair scale and weigh it before taking it to the person's room. Be sure to write down the weight of the empty wheelchair.

8. Assist the person back to his or her room.

9. Note the person's name, the time, and the weight on your notepad (or record the weight on the person's medical record if it is kept at the bedside). Report a change in the person's weight to the nurse.

Finishing Up   CLSOWR

10. Complete the "Finishing Up" steps.

PROCEDURE 16-11

Measuring Height and Weight Using a Tape Measure and a Sling Scale

WHY YOU DO IT   A tape measure and a sling scale are used to obtain a person's height and weight when the person cannot get out of bed at all. A person's weight is often used to calculate medication doses. In some cases, change in a person's weight might indicate that the person's condition is getting worse or that it is getting better.

Getting Ready   WCKIEPS

1. Complete the "Getting Ready" steps.

Supplies

- sling scale
- tape measure

Procedure

2. Ask the person to urinate. If necessary, assist the person to the bathroom or offer the bedpan or urinal.

3. Position the sling scale next to the bed. Make sure that the bed is positioned at a comfortable working height (to promote good body mechanics) and that the wheels are locked. If the side rails are in use, lower the side rail on the working side of the bed. The side rail on the opposite side of the bed should remain up.

4. Fanfold the top linens to the foot of the bed.

5. Centre the sling under the person. (To get the sling under the person, move the person as if you were making an occupied bed.)

6. Position the person in the supine position, or according to the manufacturer's instructions.

7. Move the release valve on the sling scale to the closed position.

8. Raise the sling scale so that it can be positioned over the person.

9. Spread the legs of the sling scale to provide a solid base of support. The legs must be locked in this position, or the scale could tip over, injuring you, the person you are trying to weigh, or both.

10. Move the scale into position over the person.

11. Fasten the sling to the straps or chains of the scale. Make sure the hooks face away from the person.

12. Cross the person's arms over her chest.

13. Slowly raise the sling until the person is clear of the bed.

14. Read the weight on the display screen. Note the person's name, the time, and the weight on your notepad (or record the weight on the person's medical record, if it is kept at the bedside). Report a change in the person's weight to the nurse.

15. Gently lower the person to the bed and remove the sling by gently rolling the person first to one side, then the other.

16. Position the person in the supine position, with her arms by her sides and her legs straight.

(continued)

17. Using a pencil, make a small mark on the bottom sheet at the top of the person's head. Make another small mark at her heels.

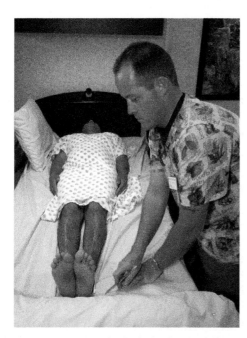

Step 17 Using a pencil, mark the bottom sheet at the top of the person's head and at his heels.

18. Using the tape measure, measure the distance between the pencil marks. This is the person's height.

19. Note the person's name, the time, and the height on your notepad (or record the height on the person's medical record, if it is kept at the bedside).

20. Make sure that the bed is lowered to its lowest position and that the wheels are locked. If the side rails are in use, return the side rails to the raised position.

Finishing Up CLSOWR

21. Complete the "Finishing Up" steps.

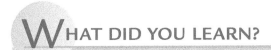

WHAT DID YOU LEARN?

Multiple Choice

Select the single best answer for each of the following questions.

1. A stethoscope is used to determine the:
   a. Brachial pulse rate
   b. Carotid pulse rate
   c. Apical pulse rate
   d. Popliteal pulse rate

2. Which one of the following is the pressure exerted by the blood flowing through the arteries when the heart muscle relaxes?
   a. Diastolic pressure
   b. Pulse pressure
   c. Pulse deficit
   d. Systolic pressure

3. The most common site for counting the pulse is the:
   a. Brachial artery
   b. Radial artery
   c. Carotid artery
   d. Apex of the heart

4. When counting respirations, you should:
   a. Have the person exercise first to get a true reading
   b. Count five respirations and then check your watch
   c. Avoid telling the person what you are going to do
   d. Have the person count respirations while you take her pulse

5. You are using a glass Celsius thermometer. When you shake it down, the mercury should be below the:
   a. 37.5 mark
   b. Arrow
   c. 100°F mark
   d. 34°C mark

6. Which of the following can cause an inaccurate oral temperature reading?
   a. The person exercised vigorously 15 minutes prior to having his temperature taken
   b. The personal support worker failed to shake down the mercury thermometer
   c. The person drank a cup of hot coffee 15 minutes prior to having his temperature taken
   d. All of the above

7. One of your patients, Ms. Jones, has a temperature of 45°C, a pulse rate of 80 beats/min, and a respiratory rate of 30 breaths/min. Which finding should be reported to the nurse immediately?
   a. Ms. Jones' respiratory rate
   b. Ms. Jones' pulse rate
   c. Ms. Jones' temperature
   d. None of these findings needs to be reported to the nurse

8. Which one of the following could cause a decreased pulse rate?
   a. Pain
   b. Anger
   c. Certain medications
   d. Fever

9. What should you observe when taking a person's pulse?
   a. The rhythm and regularity of the pulse
   b. The number of beats per minute
   c. The strength of the pulse
   d. All of the above

10. If you notice a significant change in a person's vital signs, what should you do?
    a. Record the change with a special notation to indicate that the reading was different
    b. Mention the change to the nurse at the end of your shift
    c. Tell the patient or resident about the change
    d. Report the change to a nurse immediately

11. Which instrument is used to measure blood pressure?
    a. A temporal artery thermometer
    b. A sphygmomanometer
    c. An upright scale
    d. A watch with a second hand

12. Which one of the following conditions would prevent you from taking an oral temperature?
    a. The person has diarrhea
    b. The person has just had a mastectomy
    c. The person is unconscious
    d. The person is a 10-year-old child

STOP and Think!

You are assigned to take vital signs on all the residents in the north hall of your facility. Mrs. Tito, in room 102, has a cast on her left arm and an intravenous (IV) line in her right arm. How are you going to take Mrs. Tito's blood pressure?

Vital sign measurements are routinely taken once daily at the long-term care facility where you work. Today, as you take Mr. Hayes' pulse, you notice that it does not feel as strong as usual, and although his rate is about what it always is, the rhythm is irregular. What should you do?

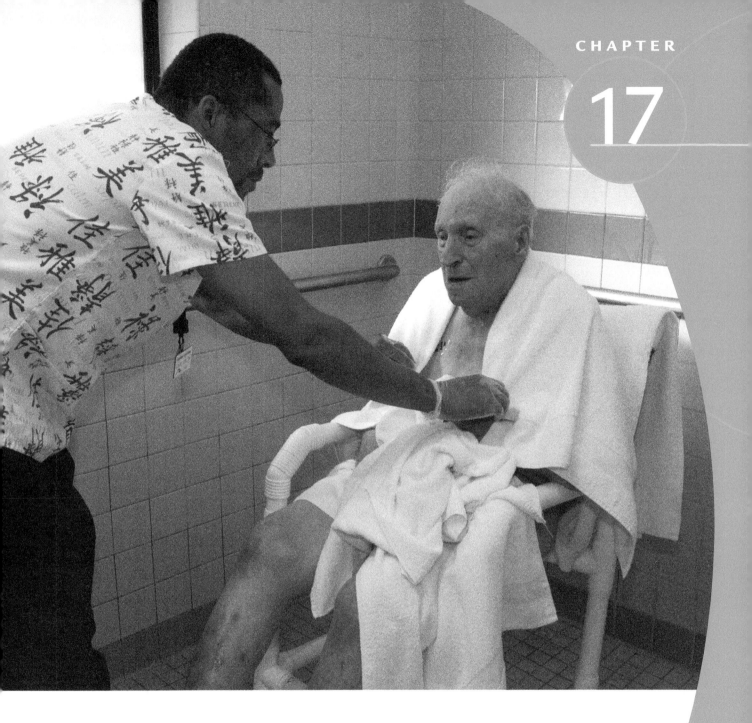

Cleanliness and Hygiene

WHAT WILL YOU LEARN?

In this chapter, we will begin to explore the personal support worker's role in helping people with **activities of daily living (ADLs),** or the routine tasks of daily life (such as bathing, eating, and grooming). Most people handle these tasks easily on their own, but people who are sick, injured, or otherwise disabled often need help with these basic activities. You will recall the discussion in Chapter 3 about how important good personal hygiene

Photo: A personal support worker assists a resident in the tub room, following a shower.

313

(cleanliness) is for both physical and emotional health. In this chapter, you will learn how to assist your patients or residents with keeping their skin and mouths clean, two activities that are key to maintaining personal hygiene. When you are finished with this chapter, you will be able to:

1. Describe the practices that make up personal hygiene.
2. Understand the importance of good hygiene in relation to a person's physical and emotional well-being.
3. Discuss how personal and cultural preferences influence a person's hygiene practices.
4. Describe practices that are considered to be a part of oral care.
5. Explain situations that may require a person to need more frequent oral care.
6. Discuss actions that promote the safe handling of a person's dentures.
7. Demonstrate proper technique for providing oral care for a person with natural teeth, for a person with dentures, and for an unconscious person.
8. Explain why perineal care is an essential aspect of daily hygiene.
9. Discuss sensitivity issues that a personal support worker should be aware of when assisting with perineal care.
10. Demonstrate proper technique for providing perineal care for males and for females.
11. Explain how bathing and skin care benefit a person's health.
12. List the methods of bathing a personal support worker may be asked to assist with.
13. Describe observations that a personal support worker should make while assisting a person with bathing and skin care.
14. Explain the benefits of massage.
15. Demonstrate proper technique for bathing a person (in bed or in a shower or bathtub), and giving a back massage.

Vocabulary

Activities of daily living (ADLs)	Evening (hour of sleep, hs) care	Halitosis	Perineum
Early morning care	PRN (as-needed) care	Gingivitis	Circumcision
Morning (A.M.) care	Diaphoretic	Periodontitis	Foreskin
Afternoon care	Dental caries	Edentulous	Deodorant
		Perineal care (peri-care)	Antiperspirant

THE BENEFITS OF PERSONAL HYGIENE

Personal hygiene (cleanliness) helps to promote both physical and emotional health. The practices associated with personal hygiene—skin care (including bathing and moisturizing) and oral care (including brushing the teeth and flossing)—keep the skin and the mucous membranes of the mouth healthy. As you will remember from Chapter 7, the skin and mucous membranes of the body act as the first line of defense against infection. Caring for the skin and the mouth helps to prevent conditions such as rashes, dry skin, and cracked lips, which interrupt the body's first line of defense by creating a portal of entry for microbes. In addition, keeping the skin and mouth clean helps to reduce the number of microbes on these surfaces, which also helps to minimize the risk of infection.

In addition to promoting physical health, good personal hygiene promotes emotional health by helping a person to feel relaxed and well cared for. A person who feels relaxed and comfortable is able to rest better. Being clean and refreshed also helps a person meet his or her need for self-esteem (see Chapter 6) by preventing body and breath odours and making the person feel attractive to others.

SCHEDULING OF ROUTINE CARE

In many health care facilities, routine activities associated with personal hygiene are carried out at specific times throughout the day:

- **Early morning care** is provided after a person wakes up to prepare him or her for breakfast or early diagnostic testing or treatment. The person is assisted with using the toilet, washing the face and hands, and mouth care. Dentures may need to be inserted prior to eating. Many people will want to have their hair brushed or combed. Residents of long-term care facilities may need help with dressing, in preparation for breakfast in the dining room.
- **Morning (A.M.)** care is when the morning personal hygiene routine is completed, to prepare the person for the day. During morning care, patients and residents are assisted with using the toilet, bathing, oral care, shaving, hair care, dressing, and putting on makeup. The amount of assistance each patient or resident will need in carrying out these activities will vary. In some facilities, the morning bath is followed by a back massage. General housekeeping duties, such as tidying the person's room and changing the bed linens, are also performed during morning care. Facility policies differ regarding the frequency of bathing and linen changes.
- **Afternoon care** is care that is provided before and after lunch and dinner. Many people rest or receive visitors in the early afternoon. A general "freshening up" involves assistance with using the toilet, washing of the hands and face, and oral care.
- **Evening (hour of sleep, hs) care** is provided in preparation for sleep. During evening care, patients or residents are assisted with washing their hands and face, brushing their teeth, changing into pajamas, and using the toilet. Other bedtime preparations include straightening the bed linens and fluffing the pillows. Many residents in long-term care facilities may prefer to bathe in the evening instead of in the morning. "Extras," such as a bath, soft music, and a back massage, or reading in bed for a while before turning out the light can help a

person fall into a restful sleep. Allowing for these "extras" when providing evening care to your patients or residents shows a caring and compassionate attitude, because you are considering the person's preferences and honoring these wishes whenever possible.

The scheduling of routine personal care promotes efficiency and allows the nursing staff to plan these activities around other scheduled activities, such as meals, treatments, visiting hours, and social events. Sometimes, however, it is necessary to break from the schedule in order to accommodate a person's needs. **PRN (as-needed) care** is personal hygiene care that is provided whenever a patient or resident needs it, throughout the day or night. For example, a person in a coma needs frequent mouth care because he tends to breathe through his mouth and he cannot take food or liquids orally, situations that put him at risk for a dry mouth. An incontinent person requires perineal care (peri-care), or cleansing of the genital and anal region, each time she loses control of her bowel or bladder. If her clothing or bedding is wet or soiled, these items will need to be changed as well. A person who is **diaphoretic** (that is, a person who has a medical condition that causes him to sweat a great deal) may need partial sponge baths, fresh linens, and a change of clothes frequently throughout the day. Any situation or condition that causes wetness or soiling of the skin, clothing, or bedding needs immediate attention.

Helping Hands and a Caring Heart

FOCUS ON HUMANISTIC HEALTH CARE

Care is provided according to the facility's or agency's schedule, but adjustments can be made to take into account the patient's or resident's personal preferences. For example, many long-term care facilities schedule baths as a routine part of the morning care, but some residents may prefer a bath later in the day or in the evening. Whenever possible, the resident's request should be granted. If you had always bathed in the evening, before bed, and then after entering a nursing home were told you had to bathe in the morning, how would you feel? Patients and residents may be required to change their normal routines to a certain extent to conform to the policies of the hospital or long-term care facility, but you can look for ways to accommodate each of your patient's or resident's personal preferences, while still following the rules of the facility. For example, asking a person whether he prefers to bathe in the morning or in the evening, allowing him to choose either bar soap or liquid soap, and permitting him to use the type of deodorant he prefers will show that you care about the person as an individual. These actions will also help the person to maintain a sense of familiarity in an otherwise changed life. Certain cultural and religious beliefs may discourage bathing during certain times or may promote ritualistic bathing as part of a ceremony or spiritual service. Whenever possible, you should make an effort to accommodate these preferences as well.

ASSISTING WITH ORAL CARE

Keeping the mouth and teeth clean and healthy is an important part of personal hygiene. A clean, healthy mouth feels good and makes food taste better, and contributes to overall health. **Dental caries** (cavities) and **halitosis** (bad breath that does not go away) are caused by poor oral hygiene. Poor oral hygiene can also cause **gingivitis** (inflammation of the gums), which can lead to **periodontitis** (infection and inflammation of the soft tissue and bones that support the teeth). Periodontitis is the main cause of tooth loss in people older than 35 years, and it may be associated with other serious health problems as well, such as atherosclerosis ("hardening of the arteries"). Assisting your patients or residents with regular oral care is an important responsibility because healthy teeth and gums are important for a person's overall health and well-being.

A person who has lost one or more natural teeth may have dental implants (prosthetic teeth that are surgically placed in the jaw bone), dentures (prosthetic teeth that can be taken in and out), or a combination of these. A person may have a partial denture or a full denture. Partial dentures are used when only some teeth are missing. Full dentures are used when a person is missing all of his top teeth or all of his bottom teeth. A person who has no teeth at all is said to be **edentulous** (without teeth).

Oral care is usually provided on awakening, after meals, and before bed. People who are unable or not allowed to take food or fluids by mouth will need oral care as often as every 1 or 2 hours to keep their mouths fresh and moist. Most people can manage their own oral care, with assistance as needed. A person who is not allowed out of bed may still be able to brush and floss her own teeth, if you provide the necessary supplies. Occasionally a person will be too ill or weak to provide oral care for himself, and you will need to provide this care for him. Because the gums sometimes bleed as a result of routine oral

care, it is important to practice standard precautions when assisting with brushing and flossing the teeth or cleaning dentures.

Helping your patients or residents with oral care presents many opportunities for observation.

TELL THE NURSE

While assisting a person with oral care, pay attention to the following:

- Dry, red, cracked, or bleeding lips, gums, or mucous membranes
- Cold sores on the lips or mucous membranes
- Red, irritated, swollen, or bleeding gums
- Cracked, chipped, or broken teeth; loose teeth; blackened teeth
- Chipped, cracked, or poorly fitting full or partial dentures
- Red sores or canker sores inside the mouth; white spots inside the mouth; any areas of pus or infection
- Bad breath that does not improve after oral care
- Fruity-smelling breath (possibly a sign of diabetes mellitus)
- A red or swollen tongue or a white coating on the tongue

PROVIDING ORAL CARE FOR A PERSON WITH NATURAL TEETH

Natural teeth are best cleaned with a toothbrush and toothpaste, followed by flossing. Because bacteria in the mouth do the most damage to the teeth and gums after eating, the best time to brush is after meals. Brushing alone is not enough to remove food that lodges between the teeth, so flossing once a day is recommended as part of good oral hygiene. Many people like to use a mouthwash after brushing to complete their oral care routine. The use of mouthwash can further reduce harmful bacteria in the mouth.

Toothbrushes should have soft bristles and be small enough to reach all of the teeth. Electric toothbrushes are simple to use and effective, especially for people who have limited strength or use of their hands.

Procedure 17-1 describes how to assist a person with brushing and flossing the teeth.

PROVIDING ORAL CARE FOR A PERSON WITH DENTURES

Dentures take the place of a person's natural teeth, allowing the person to chew his or her food properly. Dentures that do not fit properly or that hurt the mouth when worn are not very useful for chewing. Proper care of the gums and dentures helps to keep the dentures fitting properly and comfortably.

Some people wear their dentures all of the time. Others may leave their dentures out at night or only wear them for meals. Personal preference for wearing dentures is to be respected.

Remember that people are more likely to wear their dentures if they are kept clean.

A denture brush (or a toothbrush) and denture cleaner (or toothpaste) are used to clean all surfaces of the denture. Some people use a denture adhesive to help keep the denture in place better. Be sure to remove all of the adhesive material when cleaning the denture. Rinse the denture with lukewarm water. Hot water should not be used because it can damage the dentures.

General guidelines for providing oral care for a person with dentures are given in Guidelines Box 17-1. Procedure 17-2 describes how to provide oral care for a person who wears dentures.

Guidelines Box 17-1 Guidelines for Providing Oral Care for a Person With Dentures

WHAT YOU DO	WHY YOU DO IT
Handle a person's dentures with care.	Dentures are expensive and difficult to replace.
When a person is not wearing his or her dentures, store them in a denture cup filled with lukewarm water or a denture solution.	The water or solution prevents the dentures from drying out and warping. If the dentures warp, they will not fit properly.
When cleaning dentures, use lukewarm (not hot) water.	Hot water can damage the dentures.
When cleaning dentures, line the sink with a washcloth or paper towels.	The washcloth or towels help to prevent breaking or chipping of the denture if you accidentally drop it into the sink.
Have the person rinse his or her dentures after eating.	Rinsing the dentures after eating removes food trapped between the gums and dentures. Trapped food can cause discomfort and promotes the growth of bacteria.
Before placing the dentures in the person's mouth, allow the person to rinse with water or mouthwash or use a moist, foam-tipped applicator to clean the surfaces inside the person's mouth. Wet the dentures before placing them in the person's mouth.	Placing dentures inside the mouth is more difficult when the mouth and dentures are dry. In addition, the moisture helps to create the suction that is needed to hold the dentures in place.
Label the person's denture cup with the person's name and room number.	Putting the person's name and room number on the denture cup helps prevent the dentures from being misplaced.

PROVIDING ORAL CARE FOR AN UNCONSCIOUS PERSON

A person who is unconscious needs frequent mouth care to keep the mucous membranes of the mouth moist and healthy. An unconscious person breathes with her mouth open, which causes secretions to thicken and dry on the lips and in the mouth. These dried secretions, along with the intake of air through the mouth, can lead to cracking of the lips and tongue. Cracked, dry lips are very uncomfortable and they create a portal of entry for microbes.

Natural teeth are gently brushed with either a small amount of toothpaste or saline (salt water). If the person is edentulous, the gums, tongue, and inside of the cheeks are cleaned using a sponge-tipped swab moistened with saline or mouthwash. The mouth can be rinsed with a small amount of saline or water to clean out dried secretions. You may need to place a padded tongue blade between the upper and lower back teeth to keep the mouth open during oral care (Fig. 17-1). General guidelines for providing oral care for a person who is unconscious are given in Guidelines Box 17-2. Procedure 17-3 describes how to provide oral care for a person who is unconscious.

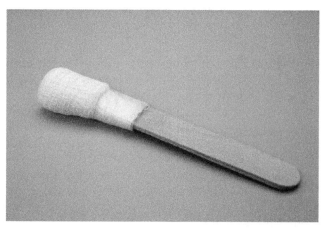

Figure 17-1
It may be necessary to use a padded tongue blade to keep an unconscious person's mouth open while providing oral care. A padded tongue blade is made by folding a gauze square around two wooden tongue blades and taping the gauze in place.

ASSISTING WITH PERINEAL CARE

Perineal care (peri-care) is the cleaning of the **perineum** and associated structures (Fig. 17-2). In women, the perineum extends from the bottom

Guidelines Box 17-2	Guidelines for Providing Oral Care for a Person Who Is Unconscious
WHAT YOU DO	*WHY YOU DO IT*
Turn the person on his or her side (or turn the person's head to the side) so that fluids run out of the mouth, not back toward the throat.	Turning the person onto his or her side (or turning the head to the side) helps to prevent aspiration (the accidental inhalation of foreign material into the airway). Aspiration can lead to complications such as choking or pneumonia.
Never place your fingers in the person's mouth.	An unconscious person may bite down involuntarily and without warning.
Explain what you are doing throughout the procedure, even though the person may not seem to be able to hear you or respond to you.	The person may be aware on some level that someone is doing something to him or her. Telling the person what you are doing reassures the person and helps the person to feel safe.
Apply lip lubricant to the person's lips as needed.	This helps to prevent drying and cracking of the lips, which is uncomfortable for the person and can lead to infection.

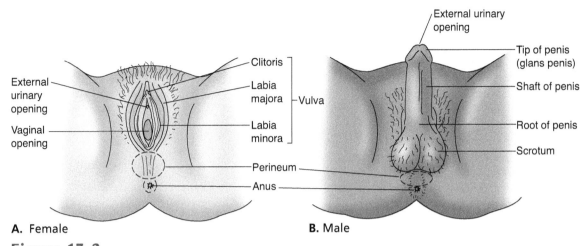

A. Female   **B.** Male

Figure 17-2
Perineal care refers to care of the perineum and associated structures. **(A)** The female perineum and associated structures. **(B)** The male perineum and associated structures.

of the vagina to the anus. In men, the perineum extends from the root of the penis to the anus. When nurses talk about "providing perineal care," they mean cleaning the perineum and anus, as well as the vulva (in women) and the penis (in men).

Making sure that the perineum, the vulva (in women), and the penis (in men) are clean is important for two main reasons:

- **Prevention of infection.** Because many microbes live in our digestive tracts and are passed from the body in the feces, there are always large numbers of microbes in and around the anus. The perineal area provides the perfect environment to support the growth of these microbes, because it is warm, dark, and moist. Because the perineum is close to the vulva (in women) and the penis (in men), these microbes can easily enter the vagina or urethra, causing infection. Therefore, inadequate hygiene in the perineal area puts the person at risk for infection.
- **Prevention of skin breakdown and odour.** The perineum, vulva, and penis are delicate, with many folds of skin. Feces, urine, and other body fluids, such as menstrual blood, can become trapped in these folds, leading to skin irritation and odour if they are not properly removed.

Perineal care is routinely performed at least once daily, as part of the bath. People with diarrhea or who are incontinent of urine or feces will need perineal care performed more frequently. Women with vaginal bleeding (from surgery,

childbirth, or menses) or vaginal discharge will also need more frequent perineal care. Any person who can manage her own perineal care should be encouraged to do so to the best of her ability. A person who is unable to provide for her own self-care will need your help. When helping your patients and residents with perineal care, be aware of signs and symptoms that could indicate a health problem.

TELL THE NURSE

Tell the nurse immediately if you observe any of the following signs when providing perineal care for one of your patients or residents:

- Any unusual redness, inflammation, or skin rashes in the perineal area
- Any unusual discharge from the vagina or penis
- Any bleeding from the vagina (especially in a postmenopausal woman) or the anus
- Any abnormal odour

When you are providing perineal care for a person, you must have the person's consent for the procedure before beginning. For example, while helping a person with a bath, you may explain what you are about to do and ask the person's permission to go further. Make sure to explain the procedure completely, using professional yet understandable words (such as "crotch," "privates," "bottom," or "the area between your legs"). When there is a language barrier, stop and think. You may need an interpreter.

For many reasons (such as cultural or religious beliefs, or a history of physical abuse), some people may object strongly to being touched by a member of the opposite sex, or even by a member of the same sex. Please respect your patient's or resident's wishes and work to find a suitable compromise, if at all possible. Perineal care can be embarrassing, both for the person receiving it and for the person providing it. Very few people are comfortable exposing their most private body parts to strangers, or seeing the private body parts of strangers. Draping the person's body with a bath blanket so that only the area to be cleaned is exposed helps to preserve the person's sense of modesty (Fig. 17-3). Another potential source of embarrassment for both the patient or resident and the personal support worker is the fact that male patients or residents may become aroused during perineal care, simply from stimulation of the penis during washing. Acting in a professional, competent manner and

using a gentle touch will help to ease embarrassment on the part of the patient or resident. Guidelines for providing perineal care are given in Guidelines Box 17-3.

Helping Hands and a Caring Heart

FOCUS ON HUMANISTIC HEALTH CARE

Having to help another person with perineal care may seem very unpleasant or embarrassing to you. But think of it this way—what if you were sick or injured to the point that you had wet yourself or had a bowel movement in the bed? Think of how wonderful it would feel to have someone clean you up, help you change your clothes, and give you fresh bed linens. You would feel clean and cared for.

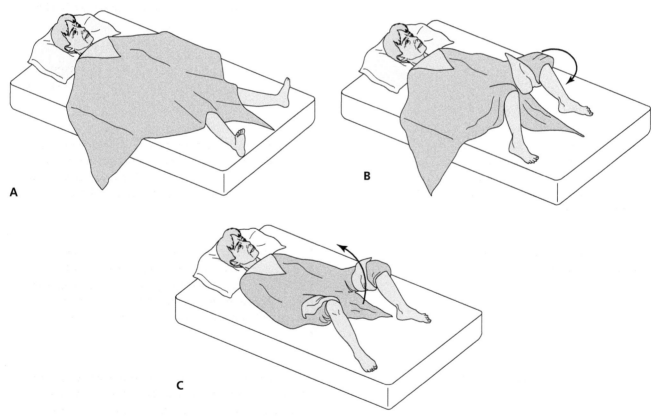

Figure 17-3
A bath blanket is used to preserve the person's modesty during perineal care. **(A)** The bath blanket is placed over the person's body so that one corner is pointing toward the person's head and the other is between the person's legs, covering the perineum. The other two corners are to the right and to the left, respectively. **(B)** The right corner is brought under and around the person's right leg, and then the same is done on the left. **(C)** The top corner is lifted up to expose only the perineal area.

Guidelines Box 17-3 Guidelines for Providing Perineal Care

WHAT YOU DO	WHY YOU DO IT
Explain the procedure to the person, even if he or she is unconscious.	Many people find being touched in an intimate area by a stranger embarrassing, frightening, or even offensive. Explaining the procedure in a professional way helps to put the person at ease and reassures the person that he or she will be treated with respect.
Take care to protect the person's modesty.	Receiving perineal care can be very embarrassing. Properly draping the person may help to relieve some of the person's discomfort and feeling of being "exposed."
Always check the temperature of the water using a bath thermometer. The water temperature should be between 43.3°C (110°F) and 46.1°C (115°F).*	Water that is too cold is uncomfortable, and water that is too hot could scald the person. A bath thermometer provides *objective* information. Testing the water with your hand provides *subjective* information. (In other words, water that "feels all right" to your touch may, in reality, be much too hot or too cold. The only way to know that the water temperature is within the safe range is to measure it.)
Follow standard precautions when providing perineal care.	Providing perineal care places you at risk for exposure to urine, feces, and other body substances (for example, blood, vaginal secretions, semen).
Perineal care is the last part of a person's bathing routine. Washcloths, towels, and the water in the wash basin (if a bed bath is being given) are discarded and not used on any other body parts after the perineal care is completed.	The anus is a source of microbes and the perineum provides an environment that supports their growth. To prevent spread of these microbes to other parts of the body, where they may gain access and cause infection, the perineal area is washed last.
The vulva (in women) or the penis (in men) is cleaned before the perineum.	Because the anus opens onto the perineum, the perineum is often contaminated with microbes from the digestive tract. Therefore, this area is washed last to prevent microbes from the digestive tract from being introduced into the vagina or urethra, where they can cause infection.
Rinse the skin thoroughly to remove all soap.	The skin of the perineum and surrounding structures is delicate. Soap is drying and can irritate the skin if not rinsed away. Squeezing clean, warm water from a washcloth held over the perineal area is an effective method of rinsing when giving a bed bath.

(continued)

Guidelines Box 17-3 Guidelines for Providing Perineal Care (continued)

WHAT YOU DO	WHY YOU DO IT
Gently pat the skin dry. Do not rub vigorously. Dry the skin thoroughly.	The skin of the perineum and surrounding structures is delicate. Vigorously rubbing the skin with a towel is uncomfortable for the person and can create friction, which in turn can cause skin breakdown. Moisture in areas where skin comes in contact with skin can also lead to skin breakdown.
Remove your gloves and wash your hands before touching clean clothing or linens.	Gloves worn while providing perineal care are considered contaminated.

*The water in the basin can be slightly hotter [43.3°C (110°F)] than the water in a tub or shower [40.5°C (105°F)] because it cools off quickly and the person will not be immersed in it.

PROVIDING PERINEAL CARE FOR FEMALE PATIENTS AND RESIDENTS

Procedure 17-4 describes how to assist a female patient or resident with perineal care.

PROVIDING PERINEAL CARE FOR MALE PATIENTS AND RESIDENTS

Male patients or residents may be circumcised or uncircumcised (Fig. 17-4). **Circumcision** is a procedure involving the removal of the **foreskin,** the fold of loose skin that covers the head of the penis. Male infants are often circumcised for religious or cultural reasons. When you are assisting an uncircumcised man with perineal care, it is important to pull the foreskin back so that the head of the penis can be cleaned thoroughly. After cleaning and rinsing the penis, always remember to pull the foreskin back up over the head of the penis. If the foreskin is not pulled back into place, it can create a band around the penis, causing pain and swelling. Procedure 17-5 describes how to assist a male patient or resident with perineal care.

ASSISTING WITH SKIN CARE

BATHING

Bathing serves many purposes. The act of bathing:

- Helps a person feel relaxed and refreshed
- Cleans the skin and eliminates body odours
- Exercises muscles that might otherwise not be used
- Stimulates blood flow to the skin (through touching and massaging of the skin), which helps to prevent skin breakdown
- Helps the patient or resident meet the needs of love and belonging and self-esteem
- Gives the personal support worker an opportunity to observe for skin problems and to communicate and bond with the patient or resident

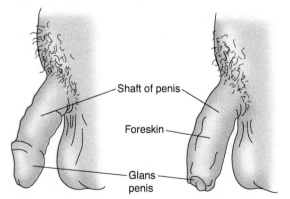

A. Circumcised   **B.** Uncircumcised

Figure 17-4
Male patients or residents may have a circumcised or uncircumcised penis. **(A)** A circumcised penis. **(B)** An uncircumcised penis.

The frequency and method of bathing are determined by many factors, including:
- Personal choice
- The person's state of health
- The weather
- The person's level of activity
- The person's ability to care for himself
- The policies and procedures of the facility

For example, people may bathe more often during the warmer months or when they are most active, and less often during the winter months or periods of physical inactivity. Hospital policy may state that patients receive daily baths, while the policy of a long-term care facility may call for residents to receive complete baths or showers two or three times weekly with partial baths on days in between.

Some patients or residents may refuse a bath, and they do have the right to refuse. For example, a resident may ask to skip his or her bath for many reasons: "I'm tired and I want to sleep." "I feel a cold coming on," "I don't feel up to it today." You could insist that the person bathe, creating tension and causing the person to feel unappreciated and disrespected. Or, you could offer to help the person "just freshen up a bit instead" and actually achieve the goal of bathing in a different manner. For example, you could assist the person with a partial bath at the sink instead of a complete bath in a tub or shower. With this approach, the person is clean but was allowed to refuse his or her bath (so to speak), and you have fulfilled your responsibility while also respecting the person's wishes.

For some patients and residents, such as those who have dementia or are confused, bath time can be very frightening. People who are confused or demented simply do not understand what you intend to do to them and they cannot remember what bathing is all about. Extra help from your co-workers and a calm, efficient attitude will help. Sometimes, singing to a confused person or playing soothing music will help to calm the person a bit. If a person refuses personal hygienic care consistently, report this to the nurse. If a person is unable to understand the consequences that can result from a lack of bathing or skin care, the decision may be made to bathe the person against his or her wishes out of respect for the person's health.

Supplies for Bathing

Various supplies are used for bathing and skin care, many of which you are already familiar with:

- **Soap,** available in liquid or cake form, is used to clean the skin. The lather lifts away dirt,

oil, microbes, and sweat. Because soap is drying to the skin, it is important to rinse it away completely. For people with dry, fragile skin (such as elderly people), it may be better to use a soapless cleanser or just plain water.
- **Soapless cleansers.** Often, these products are supplied on premoistened disposable cloths. Many soapless cleansers do not need to be rinsed away. These products clean, moisturize, and protect the skin. Some of these products are for use specifically in the perineal area.
- **Bath oils** are added to the bath water to scent and moisten the skin. Because bath oils make the surface of the bathtub slippery, these products should be used with caution.
- **Lotions** and **creams,** which may be perfumed or unscented, are applied to skin that is still slightly damp to create a moisture barrier that helps to prevent drying and chapping. Lotions and creams are an especially important part of skin care for elderly people, because with aging, the skin secretes a reduced amount of natural oil, resulting in dryness and a loss of elasticity.
- **Body powder** can help absorb moisture and sweat and reduces friction between skin surfaces that touch. Powder should only be applied to skin that has been dried thoroughly. When using powder, sprinkle a small amount into the palm of your hand, and then gently pat it on to the person's skin. Avoid big clouds of powder—too much powder can irritate the skin, and if the person inhales it, then it can irritate the airways too. In addition, powder spilled on the floor can be very slippery.
- **Deodorants** and **antiperspirants** are often applied after bathing to help prevent body odour. **Deodorants** are products that cover or mask odour. **Antiperspirants** contain ingredients that stop or slow sweating. Most antiperspirant products also contain a deodorant. Application of an antiperspirant or deodorant should be included as part of a person's hygiene routine if the person requests it.

Most people are particular about the skin care products they use. Some people are sensitive or allergic to ingredients commonly used in skin care products. If you notice that one of your patients or residents develops itching, redness, or a rash after using a skin care product, please report this observation to the nurse and stop use of that particular product until the source of the

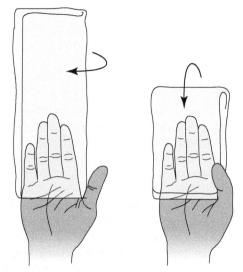

Figure 17-5
Making a bath mitt from a washcloth.

skin irritation has been determined. Always ask new patients or residents if they have particular preferences in skin care products, or if there are any products that cause problems for them.

In addition to skin care products, a variety of linens are used for bathing. Bath blankets are used to preserve a person's modesty during a bed bath or when providing perineal care. A washcloth is wrapped around the hand to form a "mitt" for cleansing the body (Fig. 17-5). A towel is used to dry the body, and can also be used to help preserve the person's modesty. A clean gown, pajamas, or change of clothes should be available for the patient or resident to put on after the bath.

Standard Bathing Techniques

A complete bath, or one that involves the entire body, is not always necessary. In some cases, a complete bath may not be allowed for medical reasons. For example, a person who has just had surgery may not be able to take a complete bath until her incision has healed. When a complete bath is not possible, a partial bath will provide many of the same health benefits and achieve the same goals of odour and infection control. During a partial bath, only the face, hands, axillae (armpits), back, buttocks, and perineal area are washed. A partial bath can be done at the sink or, if the person cannot get out of bed, at the bedside. In long-term care facilities, a partial bath is often part of the morning care on days that the resident is not scheduled to have a complete bath. A partial bath can also be provided anytime a person needs to "freshen up."

The amount of assistance each resident or patient will need to bathe will vary according to the person's degree of disability. For people who can bathe themselves, you will only need to see that they have bathing supplies and clean clothes. Some people will only need your help to clean hard-to-reach areas, such as the back or feet. Others will need your help throughout the bath. You should encourage your patients or residents to do as much for themselves as possible during bathing and other personal care routines. Allowing a person to perform as much of her personal hygiene routine as possible on her own encourages feelings of independence and self-worth. It also provides a form of exercise, increasing the person's muscle tone, mobility, and circulation. General guidelines for assisting patients and residents with bathing are given in Guidelines Box 17-4.

Assisting your patients or residents with bathing provides an excellent opportunity for you to observe the patient's or resident's skin and body for any changes in condition that should be reported to the nurse. Because you will be caring for the person regularly, you will be more likely to notice changes that might go unnoticed by others.

TELL THE NURSE

Tell the nurse immediately if you observe any of the following signs or symptoms while assisting a person with his or her bath:

- New rashes, bruises, broken skin, bleeding, or unusual odours
- Areas that are red, pale, or have a bluish cast (cyanosis)
- Areas that are swollen or tender
- Any complaints of burning or itching
- New hair loss (anywhere on the body, not just on the head)
- A flaking, itchy, or sore scalp or the presence of nits (head lice)
- Redness or yellow discolouration of the sclera (that is, the whites of the eyes)
- Yellowing or thickening of the fingernails or toenails
- Changes in mental status and alertness (for example, disorientation, confusion)

Guidelines Box 17-4 Guidelines for Bathing

WHAT YOU DO	WHY YOU DO IT
Follow the doctor's orders or the care plan when determining what type of bath the person is to receive.	A person's medical condition may dictate the type of bath he or she can have. For example, a person with a spinal injury may not be permitted to have a whirlpool bath, while for a person with poor skin circulation, a whirlpool bath may be considered a type of therapy.
Before beginning the bath, explain to the person how the bathing procedure will be carried out (and how the person can assist in the process). In addition, explain the benefits of bathing (such as comfort, healthy skin).	Explaining the details of the bathing process may help to relieve the person's fears (for example, about potential exposure), and will help the person to see how he or she can participate in the process. Explaining the procedure is particularly important for people with memory problems, who may find the bathing experience frightening because they cannot remember what bathing is or why it is important.
Collect all necessary equipment, linens, bath products, and clothing before beginning the bath. If the person will be taking a tub bath, check the tub room for cleanliness and prepare the tub before bringing the person into the room.	Being prepared and having all necessary supplies and equipment at hand will allow the bath to proceed efficiently. Efficiency is necessary to protect the person's modesty and to prevent chills.
Close all doors and windows in the room, and make sure the blinds are down or the curtains are drawn.	Closing doors and windows eliminates drafts in the room, which could cause the person to become chilled. In addition, closing doors and covering the windows protect the person's modesty and privacy.
Place a nonskid mat in the bathtub or on the shower floor. Encourage the person to use handrails. Provide a shower chair for people who are weak or unsteady.	These measures help to protect the person from falling.
Never lock the bathroom door.	Because you should never leave a person alone in the bathtub or shower, if you need help for any reason, you will have to call for someone to come to you. This person will need to be able to access the bathroom without your help.
Always check the temperature of the water using a bath thermometer. The water temperature should be between 40.5°C (105°F) and 46.1°C (115°F).	Water that is too cold is uncomfortable, and water that is too hot could scald the person. A bath thermometer provides *objective* information. Testing the water with your hand provides *subjective* information. (In other words, water that "feels all right" to your touch may, in reality, be much too hot or too cold. The only way to know that the water temperature is within the safe range is to measure it.)

(continued)

Guidelines Box 17-4   Guidelines for Bathing (continued)

WHAT YOU DO	WHY YOU DO IT
When assisting a person to and from the tub room, always make sure that he or she is adequately covered.	The person's privacy and modesty must be protected at all times.
Always help the person into and out of the bathtub or shower.	A wet bathroom floor can be slippery, and can place the person at risk for falling.
Follow standard precautions when bathing a person.	Bathing a person places you at risk for coming into contact with non-intact skin or body fluids.
Wash from the cleanest to the dirtiest areas.	This approach prevents contamination of clean areas.
Touch the person's body gently yet deliberately, using long, firm strokes.	A gentle yet firm touch conveys to the person that this is a routine procedure being carried out by a professional, ensures that the skin is properly cleaned, and stimulates skin circulation.
Rinse the skin thoroughly to remove all soap.	Soap is drying and can irritate the skin if not rinsed away.
Gently pat the skin dry. Do not rub vigorously. Dry the skin thoroughly, especially in areas where skin touches skin (for example, underneath the breasts, between the legs).	The skin, especially that of elderly people, is fragile. Vigorously rubbing the skin with a towel is uncomfortable for the person and can create friction, which in turn can cause skin breakdown. Moisture in areas where skin comes in contact with skin can also lead to skin breakdown.

Shower or tub baths

A shower or tub bath is the preferred method of bathing, because it allows for thorough cleaning and rinsing of the skin. Showers in many facilities have stalls that are large enough for a shower chair to fit inside, allowing a weak or unsteady person to sit down while taking a shower (Fig. 17-6). Some long-term facilities have whirlpool tubs that stimulate blood flow and relax muscles by the action of the water (Fig. 17-7). These tubs usually have chair-lift devices to allow for easy and safe transfer of residents into and out of the tub. The lift devices also allow people who are in a coma or who are severely physically disabled to receive the comfort and benefit of a whirlpool bath. Most tubs have a shower attachment so that hair can be washed during the bath. Many modern tub and shower units also have controls that pre-set the water temperature, ensuring that it is not too hot or too cold.

Procedure 17-6 describes how to assist with a tub bath or shower. After each use, the tub or shower stall (and the shower chair, if one was used) is disinfected. This is important to prevent the spread of infection. Facility policy will state who is responsible for cleaning and disinfecting the bathing equipment.

Bed baths

Some patients and residents are simply too weak or ill to take a shower or tub bath. In this situation, bath supplies and a basin of warm water are

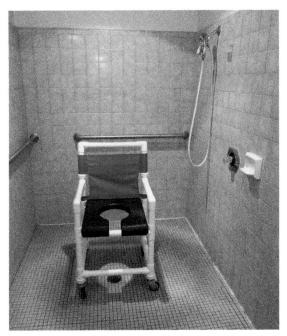

Figure 17-6
Shower stalls in health care facilities are usually wide enough to accommodate a shower chair. Use of a shower chair helps to reduce the risk of falling.

brought to the bedside, and the person is assisted with bathing in bed (Fig. 17-8). A complete or partial bed bath is given, depending on the needs of the patient or resident (Procedures 17-7 and 17-8, respectively).

An alternative to the traditional bed bath is the use of a "bag bath." With this method, a plastic bag containing 8 to 10 washcloths soaked in a soapless cleanser is warmed in the microwave, and a different cloth is used to clean each main body part. "Bag baths" are very comfortable and refreshing for the patient or resident, and they are efficient and effective for the nursing staff (Fig. 17-9).

Helping Hands and a Caring Heart

FOCUS ON HUMANISTIC HEALTH CARE

When assisting a patient or resident with bathing, think about how you would feel if you were in that person's situation. You might feel embarrassed because you have

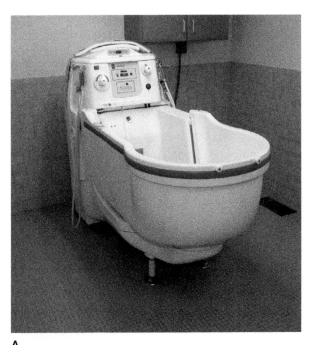

A   B

Figure 17-7
(A) Many long-term care facilities have whirlpool tubs, which help to stimulate circulation and massage the skin. **(B)** On this model, the front of the tub swings open to make it easier for the patient or resident to get into and out of the tub.

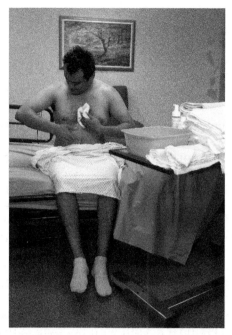

Figure 17-8
When a shower or tub bath is not possible, a bed bath can be given. Some patients or residents, like the man shown here, will be able to bathe themselves with minimal assistance, while others will require a great deal of assistance.

to rely on someone else to help you with one of life's most basic tasks. You might also feel exposed because another person (possibly of the opposite sex) is seeing and touching your body. Acknowledge your patient's or resident's feelings by providing as much privacy as possible during the procedure and by maintaining a professional attitude at all times.

MASSAGE

Illness, disability that results in loss of mobility, and aging all contribute to a loss of blood flow (circulation) to the skin. A person who sits in a chair or wheelchair for long periods of time or who must remain in bed is at an increased risk for developing pressure ulcers (see Chapter 24) as a result of that lack of blood flow. Massaging the skin regularly helps to stimulate the circulation. It is also very relaxing for the patient or resident. A back massage is usually performed after a person's bath while rubbing lotion or cream into the skin, when repositioning a helpless person, or as a part of evening care to promote relaxation and sleep. Some studies have shown that slow, gentle massage can calm sick babies and confused or demented elderly people who become agitated easily.

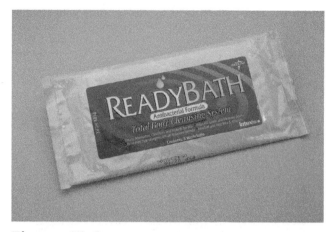

Figure 17-9
Many facilities use "bag baths" as a quick and efficient alternative to a traditional bed bath.

An effective back massage takes approximately 4 to 6 minutes to complete and can be performed with the person in either the prone or the lateral position. The extra minutes spent massaging a patient's or resident's back are well worth the effort and are beneficial for both physical and emotional health. While performing a back massage, you have an excellent opportunity to observe the person's skin for potential problems.

TELL THE NURSE

Skin breakdown can lead to pressure ulcers. Tell the nurse immediately if you observe any of the following early signs of skin breakdown:

- Reddened skin, especially over a bony area, that does not return to its normal colour after a gentle massage

- Pale, white, or shiny skin over a bony area

- Areas of skin that are hot to the touch

- Areas of skin that are painful or tender

As with any personal care procedure, always check with a nurse or read the person's care plan before beginning—a back massage should not be performed on a person with fractured ribs or a back injury, nor should it be performed on a person who has recently had back surgery. Procedure 17-9 describes how to give a back massage.

SUMMARY

- Cleanliness of the body is essential for a person's physical and emotional well-being.
  - Healthy skin and mucous membranes help protect the body from being invaded by infection-causing microbes.
  - Feeling clean also improves a person's self-esteem and increases comfort.
- Allowing people to participate in their own self-care helps to maintain independence, but assisting as necessary helps to ensure that hygiene is performed thoroughly. Assisting a person with personal hygiene activities provides many opportunities for observation.
- Activities associated with personal hygiene are usually carried out at scheduled times throughout the day.
  - When possible, adjustments are made to the schedule to accommodate personal preferences (for example, bathing in the evening versus the morning).
  - Assistance with personal hygiene is provided any time that a patient's or resident's condition warrants it. Wet or soiled skin, clothing, or bedding requires immediate attention.
- Oral care involves caring for the teeth, gums, lips, and mucous membranes of the mouth. A clean, healthy mouth makes food taste better, provides a line of defense against infection, and allows a person to chew his or her food properly.
  - Natural teeth should be brushed and flossed daily.
  - Dentures must be handled with care because they are expensive.
  - Standard precautions should be taken when providing oral care because contact

with body fluids is possible. Droplet precautions should be taken if the patient or resident is known to have an infection caused by exposure to droplets released from the mouth or nose.
- Perineal care involves cleansing of the perineum, the anus, the vulva (in women), and the penis (in men).
  - Inadequate hygiene in the perineal area places a person at risk for infection and skin breakdown, and can lead to unpleasant odours.
  - Because receiving assistance with perineal care is embarrassing for most people, take extra care to preserve the person's modesty. Having a professional attitude when assisting a person with perineal care also demonstrates competence and helps to ease embarrassment on the part of the patient or resident.
  - Standard precautions should be taken when providing perineal care because contact with body fluids is likely.
  - Always wash toward the anus, away from the urethra. This helps to prevent the spread of microbes from the anus and perineum into the urethra or vagina, where they could cause infection.
- Skin care involves keeping the skin clean and moisturized. Skin care may also involve massage to enhance blood flow to the skin.
  - Bathing may be accomplished in a bathtub or shower, at the sink, or in bed.
  - During a partial bath, only the face, hands, axillae, back, buttocks, and perineum are washed.
  - A back massage is relaxing for the patient or resident and helps to prevent the development of pressure ulcers.

Brushing and Flossing the Teeth

WHY YOU DO IT Brushing and flossing the teeth helps to keep the teeth and gums healthy, makes the mouth feel better and food taste better, and prevents bad breath.

Getting Ready WCKIEps

1. Complete the "Getting Ready" steps.

Supplies

- gloves
- paper towels
- straw (optional)
- paper cups
- emesis basin
- toothbrush
- toothpaste
- dental floss
- lip lubricant (optional)
- mouthwash (optional)
- towel

Procedure

2. Cover the over-bed table with paper towels. Place the oral care supplies on the over-bed table. Fill a paper cup with water.

3. Make sure that the bed is positioned at a comfortable working height (to promote good body mechanics) and that the wheels are locked.

4. If the side rails are in use, lower the side rail on the working side of the bed. The side rail on the opposite side of the bed should remain up.

5. Raise the head of the bed as tolerated. Place a towel under the person's chin.

6. Put on the gloves.

7. Wet the toothbrush. Put a small amount of toothpaste on the toothbrush.

8. Brush the person's teeth as follows:

   a. Position the toothbrush at a 45-degree angle to the gums, against the outer surface of the top teeth. Starting at the back of the mouth, brush the outer surface of each tooth using a gentle circular motion. Repeat for the lower teeth. Allow the person to spit toothpaste into the emesis basin as necessary.

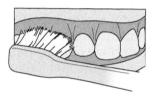

Step 8a Clean the outer surfaces of the teeth.

   b. Position the toothbrush at a 45-degree angle to the gums, against the inner surface of the top teeth. Starting at the back of the mouth, brush the inner surface of each tooth using a gentle circular motion. Repeat for the lower teeth.

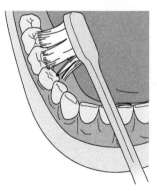

Step 8b Clean the inner surfaces of the teeth.

   c. Brush the chewing surfaces of the upper and lower teeth using a gentle circular motion.

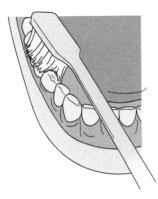

Step 8c Clean the chewing surfaces of the teeth.

   d. Brush the tongue.

9. Offer the person the cup of water (and a straw, if desired) and ask her to rinse her mouth completely. Hold the emesis basin underneath the person's chin so that she can spit the water into the basin.

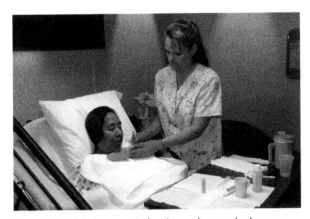

Step 9 Hold the emesis basin underneath the person's chin so that she can spit.

10. Place the emesis basin on the over-bed table and dry the person's mouth and chin thoroughly using a towel.

11. Cut a piece of dental floss measuring about 45 centimetres. Wrap the dental floss around the middle finger of each hand. Hold the dental floss between your thumb and index finger on each hand and stretch it tight.

12. Insert a segment of dental floss between two teeth, starting with the back upper teeth. Move the floss up and down gently, and then remove the dental floss from the person's mouth. Advance the floss a bit by releasing it from one middle finger and wrapping it

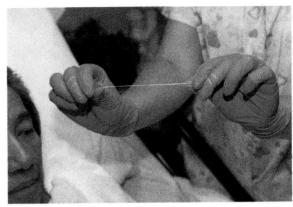

Step 11 Hold the dental floss between your thumb and index finger on each hand and stretch it tight.

around the other, and move on to the next two teeth. Use a new strand of dental floss as necessary. Offer the person the glass of water (and the straw, if desired) to rinse as necessary. Floss all of the person's teeth.

13. Offer the person the cup of water (and the straw, if desired) and ask her to rinse her mouth completely. Hold the emesis basin underneath the person's chin so that she can spit the water into the basin.

14. Place the emesis basin on the over-bed table and dry the person's mouth and chin thoroughly using a towel.

15. Pour a small amount of mouthwash (approximately ¼ cup) into another paper cup and help the person to rinse, as the person requests.

16. Apply lip lubricant to the lips, as the person requests.

17. If the side rails are in use, return the side rails to the raised position. Lower the head of the bed as the person requests. Make sure that the bed is lowered to its lowest position and that the wheels are locked.

18. Gather the soiled linens and place them in the linen hamper or linen bag. Dispose of disposable items in a facility-approved waste container. Clean equipment and return it to the storage area.

19. Remove your gloves and dispose of them in a facility-approved waste container.

Finishing Up CLSOWR

20. Complete the "Finishing Up" steps.

PROCEDURE 17-2

Providing Oral Care for a Person With Dentures

WHY YOU DO IT   Proper care of the gums and dentures helps to keep the mouth healthy and the dentures fitting properly and comfortably. It also makes the mouth feel better and food taste better and prevents bad breath.

Getting Ready WORKSTEPS

1. Complete the "Getting Ready" steps.

Supplies

- gloves
- paper towels
- gauze squares (4" × 4")
- straw (optional)
- foam-tipped applicators (optional)
- emesis basin
- paper cups
- denture cup
- denture brush or toothbrush
- denture cleaner or toothpaste
- denture solution (optional)
- mouthwash (optional)
- lip lubricant (optional)
- towel
- washcloth

Procedure

2. Cover the over-bed table with paper towels. Place the oral care supplies on the over-bed table. Fill a paper cup with water.

3. Make sure that the bed is positioned at a comfortable working height (to promote good body mechanics) and that the wheels are locked. Raise the head of the bed as tolerated. Place a towel under the person's chin.

4. Put on the gloves.

5. Ask the person to remove his dentures and place them in the emesis basin. If the person needs assistance with removing his dentures:

   a. Ask the person to open his mouth.

   b. Holding a gauze square between your thumb and index finger, grasp the upper denture, moving it up and down slightly to break the seal. Ease the denture down, forward, and out of the mouth. Place the denture in the emesis basin.

   c. Holding a gauze square between your thumb and index finger, grasp the lower denture. Turn the denture slightly, lifting it out of the mouth. Place the denture in the emesis basin.

6. Take the emesis basin, the washcloth, the denture cup, the denture brush or toothbrush, and the denture cleaner or toothpaste to the sink. Line the sink with the washcloth to provide extra cushioning. Fill the sink partially with lukewarm water. Do not place the dentures in the sink.

7. Wet the denture brush or the toothbrush. Put a small amount of toothpaste or denture cleaner on the denture brush or toothbrush. Working with one denture at a time, hold the denture in the palm of your hand and brush it on all surfaces until it is clean. Rinse the denture thoroughly under lukewarm running water and place it in the denture cup. Repeat with the other denture.

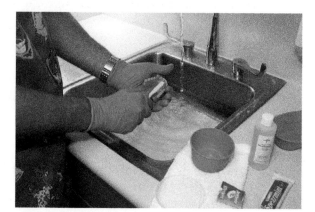

Step 7 Hold the denture in the palm of your hand, and brush it on all surfaces until it is clean.

8. If the dentures are to be stored, fill the denture cup with lukewarm water, a mixture of one part mouthwash to one part lukewarm water, or a denture solution so that the dentures are covered. Put the lid on the denture cup. Return the denture cup to the person's bedside table, making sure that it is within easy reach.

9. If the dentures are to be reinserted in the person's mouth, take the emesis basin, the denture cup, and the toothbrush to the over-bed table. If the side rails are in use,

lower the side rail on the working side of the bed. The side rail on the opposite side of the bed should remain up.

   a. Offer the person the cup of water (and a straw, if desired) and ask him to rinse his mouth completely. Some people may wish to use mouthwash instead of water. Hold the emesis basin underneath the person's chin so that he can spit the water or mouthwash into the basin.

   b. Place the emesis basin on the over-bed table and dry the person's mouth and chin thoroughly using a face towel.

   c. Gently clean the person's gums and tongue and the insides of the cheeks with the toothbrush or a foam-tipped applicator moistened with water or mouthwash. Use fresh applicators as needed.

   d. Ask the person to insert his dentures. If the person needs assistance with inserting his dentures:

      ● Ask the person to open his mouth.

      ● Gently lift the person's upper lip up. Grasp the upper denture between your thumb and index finger and insert it in the person's mouth. Press gently on

the denture to be sure that it is seated properly.

      ● Gently pull the person's lower lip down. Grasp the lower denture between your thumb and index finger and insert it in the person's mouth.

   e. Return the denture cup to the person's bedside table, making sure that it is within easy reach.

10. Dry the person's mouth and chin thoroughly using a towel. Apply lip lubricant to the lips, as the person requests.

11. Reposition the person comfortably and lower the head of the bed if necessary. If the side rails are in use, return the side rails to the raised position. Make sure that the bed is lowered to its lowest position and that the wheels are locked.

12. Gather the soiled linens and place them in the linen hamper or linen bag. Dispose of disposable items in a facility-approved waste container. Clean equipment and return it to the storage area.

13. Remove your gloves and dispose of them in a facility-approved waste container.

Finishing Up

14. Complete the "Finishing Up" steps.

PROCEDURE 17-3

Providing Oral Care for an Unconscious Person

WHY YOU DO IT   An unconscious person breathes through the mouth, causing the lips and mucous membranes to dry out. Frequent mouth care keeps the mucous membranes of the mouth moist and healthy and promotes comfort.

Getting Ready

1. Complete the "Getting Ready" steps.

Supplies

- gloves
- paper towels
- sponge-tipped applicators
- padded tongue blade
- paper cups
- emesis basin
- toothbrush and toothpaste (if the person has natural teeth)
- lip lubricant
- saline (optional)
- mouthwash (optional)
- towels

Procedure

2. Cover the over-bed table with paper towels. Place the oral care supplies on the over-bed table. Fill the paper cup with water.

(continued)

3. Make sure that the bed is positioned at a comfortable working height (to promote good body mechanics) and that the wheels are locked. If the side rails are in use, lower the side rail on the working side of the bed. The side rail on the opposite side of the bed should remain up.

4. Raise the head of the bed as tolerated. Turn the person's head to the side facing you. If it is difficult to keep the person's head turned to the side, roll the person onto his or her side.

5. If the person's condition permits, gently lift the person's head and place a towel on the pillow. Place the emesis basin on the towel, level with the person's chin.

6. Put on the gloves.

7. Open the person's mouth using the padded tongue blade. Be gentle; do not force the mouth open. Insert the tongue blade between the upper and lower teeth at the back of the mouth to hold the person's mouth open.

8. Clean the inside of the mouth:

   a. If the person has natural teeth, they should be gently brushed as described in Procedure 18-1.

   b. If the person is edentulous, gently clean the person's gums and tongue and the insides of the cheeks with the toothbrush or a foam-tipped applicator moistened with water, saline, or mouthwash. Use fresh applicators as needed.

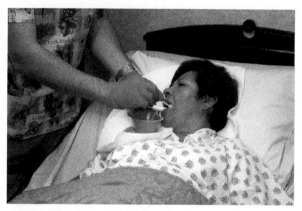

Step 8 Clean the inside of the person's mouth, using a padded tongue blade to keep the mouth open.

9. Dry the person's mouth and chin thoroughly using a towel. Apply lip lubricant to the lips. Reposition the person comfortably.

10. If the side rails are in use, return the side rails to the raised position. Lower the head of the bed. Make sure that the bed is lowered to its lowest position and that the wheels are locked.

11. Gather the soiled linens and place them in the linen hamper or linen bag. Dispose of disposable items in a facility-approved waste container. Clean equipment and return it to the storage area.

12. Remove your gloves and dispose of them in a facility-approved waste container.

Finishing Up CLSOWR

13. Complete the "Finishing Up" steps.

PROCEDURE 17-4

Providing Female Perineal Care

WHY YOU DO IT   Proper perineal care helps to prevent skin breakdown (which can lead to pressure ulcers), infection, and odour.

Getting Ready WGKIEpS

1. Complete the "Getting Ready" steps.

Supplies

- gloves
- paper towels
- bed protector
- bath thermometer
- wash basin
- bedpan
- soap
- bath blanket
- washcloths
- towel
- clean clothing
- clean linens (if necessary)

Procedure

2. Cover the over-bed table with paper towels. Place the wash basin, toiletries, clean clothing, and clean linens on the over-bed table.

3. Make sure that the bed is positioned at a comfortable working height (to promote good body mechanics) and that the wheels are locked.

4. Put on the gloves.

5. Because bathing often stimulates the urge to urinate, offer the bedpan. If the person uses the bedpan, empty and clean it before proceeding with the perineal care. Remove your gloves and dispose of them in a facility-approved waste container. Wash your hands and put on a clean pair of gloves.

6. Lower the head of the bed to a flat position (as tolerated).

7. Fill the wash basin with warm water [43.3°C (110°F) to 46.1°C (115°F) on the bath thermometer]. Place the basin on the over-bed table.

8. If the side rails are in use, lower the side rail on the working side. The side rail on the opposite side of the bed should remain up.

9. Spread the bath blanket over the top linens (and the person). If the person is able, have her hold the bath blanket. If not, tuck the corners under the person's shoulders. Fanfold the top linens to the foot of the bed.

10. Assist the person with undressing.

11. Ask the person to open her legs and bend her knees, if possible. If she is not able to bend her knees, help her spread her legs as much as possible.

12. Position the bath blanket over the person so that one corner can be wrapped under and around each leg.

13. Position the bed protector under the person's buttocks to keep the bed linens dry.

14. Lift the corner of the bath blanket that is between the person's legs upward, exposing only the perineal area.

15. Form a mitt around your hand with one of the washcloths. Wet the mitt with warm, clean water and apply soap.

16. Using the other hand, separate the labia. Clean the vulva by placing your washcloth-covered hand at the top of the vulva and stroking downward to the anus. Use a different part of the washcloth for each stroke. Repeat until the area is clean.

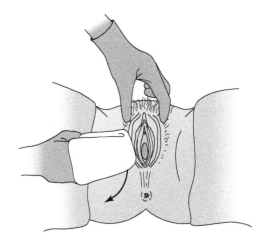

Step 16 Clean the vulva by placing your washcloth-covered hand at the top of the vulva and stroking downward to the anus.

17. Rinse the vulva and perineum thoroughly:

    Method "A": Form a mitt around your hand with a clean, wet washcloth. Using the other hand, separate the labia. Rinse the vulva by placing your washcloth-covered hand at the top of the vulva and stroking downward to the anus. Use a different part of the washcloth for each stroke. Repeat until the area is free of soap.

    Method "B": Hold a clean washcloth saturated with clean, warm water over the vulva. Squeeze the water from the washcloth onto the vulva and allow it to run over the vulva and perineum. Repeat until the area is free of soap.

18. Dry the perineal area thoroughly using a towel.

19. Turn the person onto her side so that she is facing away from you. Help the person toward the working side of the bed so that her buttocks are within easy reach. Adjust the bath blanket to keep the person covered.

20. Form a mitt around your hand with one of the washcloths. Wet the mitt with warm, clean water and apply soap.

21. Using the other hand, separate the buttocks. Place your washcloth-covered hand at the front of the body and stroke toward the back. First clean one side, then the other side, and finally the middle, using a different part of the washcloth each time, until the anal area is clean.

(continued)

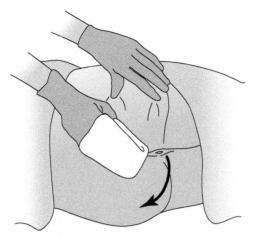

Step 21 Clean the anal area by placing your wash-cloth-covered hand at the front of the body and stroking toward the back.

22. Rinse and dry the anal area thoroughly. Remove the bed protector from underneath the person.

23. Remove your gloves and dispose of them in a facility-approved waste container. Put on a clean pair of gloves.

24. Assist the person into the supine position. Reposition the pillow under her head. Remove the bath blanket and help the person into the clean clothing.

25. If the bedding is wet or soiled, change the bed linens.

26. If the side rails are in use, return the side rail to the raised position. Raise the head of the bed as the person requests. Make sure that the bed is lowered to its lowest position and that the wheels are locked.

27. Gather the soiled linens and place them in the linen hamper or linen bag. Dispose of disposable items in a facility-approved waste container. Clean equipment and return it to the storage area.

28. Remove your gloves and dispose of them in a facility-approved waste container.

Finishing Up CLSOWR

29. Complete the "Finishing Up" steps.

PROCEDURE 17-5

Providing Male Perineal Care

WHY YOU DO IT Proper perineal care helps to prevent skin breakdown (which can lead to pressure ulcers), infection, and odour.

Getting Ready WCKIEPS

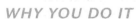

1. Complete the "Getting Ready" steps.

Supplies

- gloves
- paper towels
- bed protector
- bath thermometer
- wash basin
- bedpan or urinal
- soap
- bath blanket
- washcloths
- towel
- clean clothing
- clean linens (if necessary)

Procedure

2. Cover the over-bed table with paper towels. Place the wash basin, toiletries, clean clothing, and clean linens on the over-bed table.

3. Make sure that the bed is positioned at a comfortable working height (to promote good body mechanics) and that the wheels are locked.

4. Put on the gloves.

5. Because bathing often stimulates the urge to urinate, offer the bedpan or urinal. If the person uses the bedpan or urinal, empty and clean it before proceeding with the perineal care. Remove your gloves and dispose of them in a facility-approved waste container. Wash your hands and put on a clean pair of gloves.

6. Lower the head of the bed to a flat position (as tolerated).

7. Fill the wash basin with warm water [43.3°C (110°F) to 46.1°C (115°F) on the bath thermometer]. Place the basin on the over-bed table.

8. If the side rails are in use, lower the side rail on the working side. The side rail

on the opposite side of the bed should remain up.

9. Spread the bath blanket over the top linens (and the person). If the person is able, have him hold the bath blanket. If not, tuck the corners under the person's shoulders. Fanfold the top linens to the foot of the bed.

10. Assist the person with undressing.

11. Ask the person to open his legs and bend his knees, if possible. If he is not able to bend his knees, help him spread his legs as much as possible.

12. Position the bath blanket over the person so that one corner can be wrapped under and around each leg.

13. Position the bed protector under the person's buttocks to keep the bed linens dry.

14. Lift the corner of the bath blanket that is between the person's legs upward, exposing only the perineal area.

15. Form a mitt around your hand with one of the washcloths. Wet the mitt with warm, clean water and apply soap.

16. Using the other hand, hold the penis slightly away from the body.

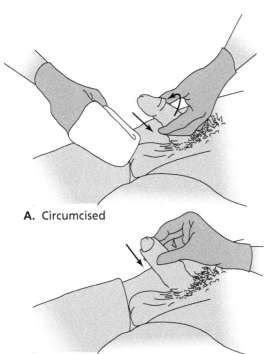

A. Circumcised

B. Uncircumcised

Step 16 To wash the penis, pass the washcloth in a circular motion, moving from the tip of the penis to the base. **(A)** circumcised penis; **(B)** uncircumcised penis.

a. If the person is circumcised: Place your washcloth-covered hand at the tip of the penis and wash in a circular motion, downward to the base of the penis. Repeat, using a different part of the washcloth each time, until the area is clean. Rinse and dry the tip and the shaft of the penis thoroughly:

   Method "A": Form a mitt around your hand with a clean, wet washcloth. Using the other hand, hold the penis slightly away from the body. Place your washcloth-covered hand at the tip of the penis and wipe in a circular motion, downward to the base of the penis. Repeat, using a different part of the washcloth each time, until the area is rinsed. Dry the penis thoroughly.

   Method "B": Hold a clean washcloth saturated with clean, warm water over the area. Squeeze the water from the washcloth onto the area. Dry the penis thoroughly.

b. If the person is uncircumcised: Retract the foreskin by gently pushing the skin toward the base of the penis. Place your washcloth-covered hand at the tip of the penis and wash in a circular motion, downward to the base of the penis. Repeat using a different part of the washcloth each time until the area is clean. Rinse and dry the tip and shaft of the penis thoroughly before gently pulling the foreskin back into its normal position.

17. Form a mitt around your hand with one of the washcloths. Wet the mitt with warm, clean water and apply soap. Wash the scrotum and perineum. Rinse and dry the scrotum and perineum thoroughly.

18. Turn the person onto his side so that he is facing away from you. Help the person toward the working side of the bed so that his buttocks are within easy reach. Adjust the bath blanket to keep the person covered.

19. Form a mitt around your hand with one of the washcloths. Wet the mitt with warm, clean water and apply soap.

20. Using the other hand, separate the buttocks. Place your washcloth-covered hand at the front of the body and stroke toward the back. First clean one side, then the other side, and finally the middle, using a different part of

(continued)

the washcloth each time, until the anal area is clean.

21. Rinse and dry the anal area thoroughly. Remove the bed protector from underneath the person.

22. Remove your gloves and dispose of them in a facility-approved waste container. Put on a clean pair of gloves.

23. Assist the person into the supine position. Reposition the pillow under the person's head. Remove the bath blanket and help the person into the clean clothing.

24. If the bedding is wet or soiled, change the bed linens.

25. If the side rails are in use, return the side rail to the raised position. Make sure that the bed is lowered to its lowest position and that the wheels are locked.

26. Gather the soiled linens and place them in the linen hamper or linen bag. Dispose of disposable items in a facility-approved waste container. Clean equipment and return it to the storage area.

27. Remove your gloves and dispose of them in a facility-approved waste container.

Finishing Up   CLSOWR
28. Complete the "Finishing Up" steps.

PROCEDURE 17-6

Assisting With a Tub Bath or Shower

WHY YOU DO IT   Cleansing of the skin helps to prevent skin breakdown (which can lead to pressure ulcers), infection, and odor. A shower or tub bath allows for thorough cleaning and rinsing of the skin.

Getting Ready   WCKIEPS

1. Prepare the tub room. Place a nonskid mat on the floor of the tub or shower. If the person will be taking a tub bath, fill the tub halfway with warm water (43.3°C [105°F] to 46.1°C [115°F] on the bath thermometer). Obtain a shower chair if necessary and place it in the shower. Place a towel on the chair in the tub room where the person will sit while drying off.

2. Complete the "Getting Ready" steps.

Supplies

- gloves
- bath thermometer
- soap
- washcloths
- towels
- lotion (optional)
- powder (optional)
- deodorant or antiperspirant (optional)
- clean clothing

Procedure

3. Ask the person if she needs to use the bathroom before bathing.

4. Assist the person to the tub room.

5. If the person will be taking a tub bath, check the temperature of the water and make sure

the nonskid mat is secure. If the person will be taking a shower, turn on the water and adjust the temperature until the water is comfortable.

6. Assist the person with undressing. Assist the person into the bathtub or shower.

7. If the person is able to bathe herself, either partially or completely:

    a. Place bathing supplies within easy reach.

    b. Many facilities require you to remain in the room while the person bathes or showers. If facility policy permits you to leave the room, explain how to use the call-light control and ask the person to signal when bathing is complete or when she has done as much as she can on her own and needs help completing the bath. Stay nearby and check on the person every 5 minutes. The person should not remain in the bathtub or shower for longer than 20 minutes. Return when the person signals. Remember to knock before entering.

8. If the person is unable to bathe herself or requires assistance:

    a. Put on the gloves and form a mitt around your hand with one of the washcloths.

b. If necessary, ask the person what parts of the body were not washed. Assist the person as needed with completing the bath. Wash the cleanest areas first and the dirtiest areas last:

- **Eyes.** Wet the mitt with warm, clean water. Ask the person to close her eyes. Place your washcloth-covered hand at the inner corner of the eye and stroke gently outward, toward the outer corner. Use a different part of the washcloth for each eye.
- **Face, neck, and ears.** Ask the person if you should use soap on the face. Rinse the washcloth and apply soap, if requested. Wash the face, neck, and ears, moving from the top of the head to the bottom (so that the nose and mouth are washed last). Rinse thoroughly.
- **Arms and axillae (armpits).** Rinse the washcloth and apply soap. Place your washcloth-covered hand at the shoulder and stroke downward, toward the hand, using long, firm strokes. Wash the hand. If necessary, assist the person with raising her arm so that you can wash the axilla. Repeat for the other arm and axilla.
- **Chest and abdomen.** Using long, firm strokes, wash the person's chest and abdomen.
- **Legs and feet.** Place your washcloth-covered hand at the top of the thigh and stroke downward, toward the foot, using long, firm strokes. Wash the foot. Repeat for the other leg.
- **Back and buttocks:** Wash the person's back and buttocks, moving from top to bottom and using long, firm strokes.
- **Perineal area:** Complete perineal care.

9. Make sure that soap is thoroughly rinsed from all parts of the body.

10. Remove your gloves and dispose of them in a facility-approved waste container. Put on a clean pair of gloves.

11. If the person is taking a tub bath, drain the water and carefully assist the person out of the tub and into the towel-covered chair. If the person is taking a shower, turn the water off and assist the person into the towel-covered chair.

12. Wrap a towel around the person. Using another bath towel, help the person to dry off, patting the skin dry. Take care to ensure that areas where "skin meets skin" are dried thoroughly (for example, in between the toes and underneath the breasts).

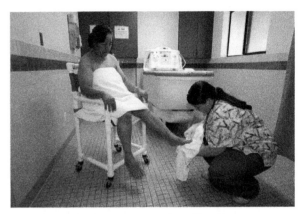

Step 12 Help the person to dry off, taking extra care to dry areas where "skin meets skin."

13. Help the person to apply lotion, powder, deodorant, antiperspirant, or other personal care products as the person requests.

14. Help the person into the clean clothing. If the person is wearing nightwear, help her into a robe. Help the person into her slippers.

15. Remove your gloves and dispose of them in a facility-approved waste container.

16. Assist the person back to her room.

Finishing Up CLSOWR

17. Complete the "Finishing Up" steps.

18. Gather the soiled linens and place them in the linen hamper or linen bag. Dispose of disposable items in a facility-approved waste container. Clean equipment and return it to the storage area.

19. Clean the tub room and shower chair (if used), if housekeeping is not responsible for this task at your facility.

PROCEDURE 17-7

Giving a Complete Bed Bath

WHY YOU DO IT   Cleansing of the skin helps to prevent skin breakdown (which can lead to pressure ulcers), infection, and odour. A bed bath is given when a person is too weak or ill to take a shower or tub bath.

Getting Ready WORKERS

1. Complete the "Getting Ready" steps.

Supplies

- gloves
- paper towels
- bed protectors
- oral hygiene supplies (see Procedures 18-1 through 18-3)
- bath thermometer
- wash basin
- bedpan or urinal
- soap
- lotion (optional)
- powder (optional)
- deodorant or antiperspirant (optional)
- washcloths
- towels
- bath blanket
- clean clothing
- clean linens (if necessary)

Procedure

2. Cover the over-bed table with paper towels. Place the wash basin, toiletries, clean clothing, and clean linens on the over-bed table.

3. Make sure that the bed is positioned at a comfortable working height (to promote good body mechanics) and that the wheels are locked.

4. Put on the gloves.

5. Because bathing often stimulates the urge to urinate, offer the bedpan or urinal. If the person uses the bedpan or urinal, empty and clean it before proceeding with the bath. Remove your gloves and dispose of them in a facility-approved waste container. Wash your hands and put on a clean pair of gloves.

6. Assist the person with oral care.

7. Remove the bedspread and blanket from the bed. If they are to be reused, fold them and place them on a clean surface, such as the chair.

8. Spread the bath blanket over the top linens (and the person). If the person is able, have him hold the bath blanket. If not, tuck the corners under the person's shoulders. Fanfold the top linens to the foot of the bed.

9. Assist the person with undressing.

10. Lower the head of the bed so that the bed is flat (as tolerated). Position the pillow under the person's head.

11. Fill the wash basin with warm water (43.3°C [110°F] to 46.1°C [115°F] on the bath thermometer). Place the basin on the over-bed table.

12. If the side rails are in use, lower the side rail on the working side of the bed. The side rail on the opposite side of the bed should remain up.

13. Place a towel over the person's chest to keep the bath blanket dry.

14. To keep the bath water from becoming soapy too quickly, you can use two washcloths—one with soap, for washing; and one without soap, for rinsing. Form a mitt around your hand with one of the washcloths. Wet the mitt with warm, clean water. Ask the person to close his eyes. Place your washcloth-covered hand at the inner corner of the eye and stroke gently outward, toward the outer corner. Use a different part of the washcloth for each eye. Using a towel, dry the person's eyes.

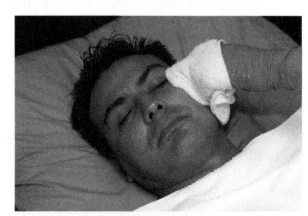

Step 14 Wash the person's eyes, moving from the inside corner toward the outer corner.

15. Ask the person if you should use soap on the face. Rinse the washcloth and apply soap, if requested. Wash the face, neck, and ears, moving from the top of the head to the bottom (so that the nose and mouth are washed last). Using the clean washcloth,

rinse thoroughly, and pat the person's face, neck, and ears dry with a towel.

16. Place a bed protector under the person's far arm, to keep the linens dry. Form a mitt around your hand with the washcloth. Wet the mitt and apply soap. Place your wash-cloth-covered hand at the shoulder and stroke downward, toward the hand, using long, firm strokes. Wash the hand. If necessary, assist the person with raising his arm so that you can wash the axilla. Rinse thoroughly, and pat the person's arm, hand, and axilla dry with a towel. Remove the bed protector from underneath the person's arm.

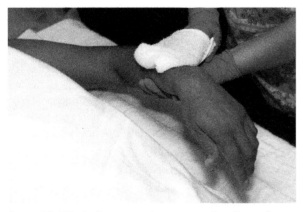

Step 16 Wash the person's arm, moving from the shoulder to the wrist.

17. Repeat for the other arm.

18. Place a towel horizontally across the person's chest. (The person is now covered with both a bath blanket and a towel.) With the towel in place, fold the bath blanket down to the person's waist. Wet the mitt and apply soap. Reach under the towel and wash the person's chest, using long, firm strokes. Using the clean washcloth, rinse thoroughly, and pat the person's chest dry with a towel.

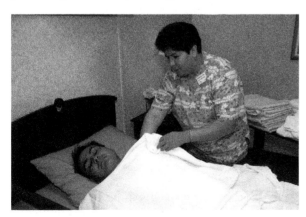

Step 18 Reach under the towel and wash the person's chest.

19. With the towel still in place, fold the bath blanket down to the pubic area. Form a mitt around your hand with the washcloth. Wet the mitt and apply soap. Reach under the towel and wash the person's abdomen, using long, firm strokes. Rinse thoroughly and pat the person's abdomen dry with a towel.

20. Replace the bath blanket by unfolding it back over the towel and the person's body. Slide the towel out from underneath the bath blanket.

21. Change the water in the wash basin if it is cool or soapy. (If the side rails are in use, raise the side rails before leaving the bedside.)

22. Fold the bath blanket so that the far leg is completely exposed. Place a bed protector under the person's far leg to keep the linens dry. Wet the mitt and apply soap. Place your washcloth-covered hand at the top of the thigh and stroke downward, toward the foot, using long, firm strokes. Rinse thoroughly and pat the person's leg dry with a bath towel.

23. Put the wash basin on the bed protector and place the person's foot in the basin. Wash the entire foot, including between the toes, with the soapy washcloth. Rinse thoroughly and pat the person's foot dry with a towel. Be sure to dry between the toes. Remove the wash basin. Remove the bed protector from underneath the person's leg.

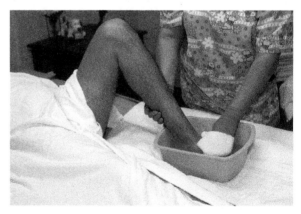

Step 23 Put the wash basin on the bed protector and place the person's foot in the basin.

24. Repeat for the other leg and foot.

25. Change the water in the wash basin. (If the side rails are in use, raise the side rails before leaving the bedside.)

(continued)

26. Turn the person onto his or her side so that he or she is facing away from you. Help the person toward the working side of the bed so that his back is within easy reach. Adjust the bath blanket to keep the front of the person covered (exposing only the back and buttocks). Place a bed protector on the bed alongside the person's back to keep the linens dry.

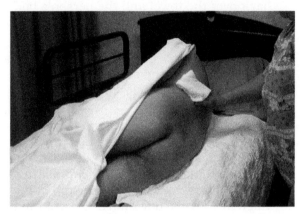

Step 26 Wash the person's back and buttocks using long, firm strokes.

27. Form a mitt around your hand with the washcloth. Wet the mitt and apply soap. Wash the person's back and buttocks, moving from top to bottom and using long, firm strokes. Rinse thoroughly and pat the person's back and buttocks dry using a bath towel. At this point, a back massage may be given.

28. If the person is able to perform perineal care, assist the person into Fowler's position and adjust the over-bed table so that the bathing supplies are within easy reach. Place the call-light control within easy reach and ask the person to signal when perineal care is complete. If the person is unable to perform perineal care, assist the person onto his back and complete perineal care.

29. Remove your gloves and dispose of them in a facility-approved waste container. Put on a clean pair of gloves.

30. Help the person to apply lotion, powder, deodorant, antiperspirant, or other personal care products as the person requests.

31. Help the person into the clean clothing.

32. If the bedding is wet or soiled, change the bed linens.

33. Carry out range-of-motion exercises as ordered.

34. If the side rails are in use, return the side rails to the raised position. Raise or lower the head of the bed as the person requests. Make sure that the bed is lowered to its lowest position and that the wheels are locked.

35. Gather the soiled linens and place them in the linen hamper or linen bag. Dispose of disposable items in a facility-approved waste container. Clean equipment and return it to the storage area.

36. Remove your gloves and dispose of them in a facility-approved waste container.

Finishing Up CLSOWR

37. Complete the "Finishing Up" steps.

PROCEDURE 17-8

Giving a Partial Bed Bath

WHY YOU DO IT Cleansing of the skin helps to prevent skin breakdown (which can lead to pressure ulcers), infection, and odour. A partial bed bath is given when a complete bath or shower is not allowed for medical reasons, or when a patient or resident does not feel up to a complete bath or shower.

Getting Ready WCKIEPS

1. Complete the "Getting Ready" steps.

Supplies

- gloves
- paper towels
- bed protectors
- oral hygiene supplies (see Procedures 17-1 through 17-3)
- bath thermometer
- wash basin
- bedpan or urinal
- soap
- lotion (optional)
- powder (optional)
- washcloths
- towels
- bath blanket
- clean clothing
- clean linens (if necessary)

Procedure

2. Cover the over-bed table with paper towels. Place the wash basin, toiletries, clean clothing, and clean linens on the over-bed table. Put on the gloves.

3. Because bathing often stimulates the urge to urinate, offer the bedpan or urinal. If the person uses the bedpan or urinal, empty and clean it before proceeding with the bath. Remove your gloves and dispose of them in a facility-approved waste container. Wash your hands and put on a clean pair of gloves.

4. Assist the person with oral hygiene. Remove your gloves and dispose of them in a facility-approved waste container. Wash your hands.

5. Fill the wash basin with warm water (43.3°C [110°F] to 46.1°C [115°F] on the bath thermometer). Place the basin on the over-bed table.

6. If the person will be bathing independently, make sure that the bed is lowered to its lowest position and that the wheels are locked. If you will be assisting the person with bathing, make sure that the bed is positioned at a comfortable working height (to promote good body mechanics) and that the wheels are locked. If the side rails are in use, lower the side rail on the working side. The side rails on the opposite side of the bed should remain up.

7. The bath may either be carried out with the person in Fowler's position, or the person can be assisted to sit on the edge of the bed. Help the person to undress as necessary.

8. If the person is able to bathe herself, either partially or completely:

   a. Place bathing supplies within easy reach.

   b. Many facilities require you to remain in the room while the person bathes. If facility policy permits you to leave the room, explain how to use the call light control and ask the person to signal when bathing is complete or when she has done as much as she can on her own and needs help completing the bath. Stay nearby and check on the person every 5 minutes. Return when the person signals. Remember to knock before entering.

9. If the person is unable to bathe herself, or requires assistance:

   a. Put on the gloves and form a mitt around your hand with one of the washcloths.

   b. If necessary, ask the person what parts of the body were not washed. Assist the person as needed with completing the bath.

Wash the cleanest areas first and the dirtiest areas last:
- **Face, neck, and ears.** Ask the person if you should use soap on the face. Rinse the washcloth and apply soap, if requested. Wash the face, neck, and ears, moving from the top of the head to the bottom (so that the nose and mouth are washed last). Rinse thoroughly, and pat the person's face, neck, and ears dry with a towel.
- **Hands.** Wash the hand. Rinse thoroughly, and pat the hand dry with a towel. Repeat for the other hand.
- **Axillae (armpits).** If necessary, assist the person with raising her arm so that you can wash the axilla. Rinse thoroughly, and pat the axilla dry with a towel. Repeat for the other axilla.
- **Back and buttocks.** Rinse the washcloth and apply soap. Wash the person's back and buttocks, moving from top to bottom and using long, firm strokes. Rinse thoroughly, and pat the back and buttocks dry with a towel.
- **Perineal area.** Complete male or female perineal care.

10. Remove your gloves and dispose of them in a facility-approved waste container. Put on a clean pair of gloves.

11. Help the person to apply lotion, powder, deodorant, antiperspirant, or other personal care products as the person requests.

12. Help the person into the clean clothing.

13. If the bedding is wet or soiled, change the bed linens.

14. Carry out range-of-motion exercises as ordered.

15. If the side rails are in use, return the side rails to the raised position. Raise or lower the head of the bed as the person requests. Make sure that the bed is lowered to its lowest position and that the wheels are locked.

16. Gather the soiled linens and place them in the linen hamper or linen bag. Dispose of disposable items in a facility-approved waste container. Clean equipment and return it to the storage area.

17. Remove your gloves and dispose of them in a facility-approved waste container.

Finishing Up CLSOWR

18. Complete the "Finishing Up" steps.

PROCEDURE 17-9

Giving a Back Massage

WHY YOU DO IT   A back message promotes comfort and relaxation. Massage also stimulates blood flow to the skin, which helps to prevent pressure ulcers.

Getting Ready WORKBOOK

1. Complete the "Getting Ready" steps.

Supplies

- gloves (if contact with broken skin is likely)
- wash basin
- lotion
- bath blanket
- towel

Procedure

2. Fill the wash basin with warm water. Place the bottle of lotion in the basin of warm water to warm it.

3. Make sure that the bed is positioned at a comfortable working height (to promote good body mechanics) and that the wheels are locked.

4. Lower the head of the bed so that the bed is flat (as tolerated). If the side rails are in use, lower the side rail on the working side of the bed. The side rail on the opposite side of the bed should remain up.

5. Help the person into the prone position, or turn the person onto his or her side so that he or she is facing away from you.

6. Reposition the pillow under the person's head and adjust the bath blanket to keep the person covered, exposing only the back and buttocks.

7. Put on the gloves if contact with broken skin is likely.

8. Pour some lotion into your cupped palm and rub your hands together to distribute the lotion onto both palms.

9. Apply the lotion to the person's back with the palms of your hands. Massage the lotion into the person's skin, using long, gliding strokes (*effleurage*), moving up the center of the back from the buttocks to the shoulders, and then back down along the outside of the back. Do not directly rub any reddened areas. Repeat four times.

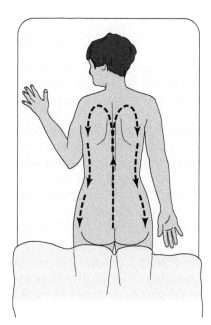

Step 9 Move up the center of the back from the buttocks to the shoulders, and then back down along the outside of the back.

10. For the next set of strokes, move up the center of the back from the buttocks to the shoulders and then back down along the outside of the back. On the downstroke, massage the person's shoulders and back using a small circular motion. Repeat four times.

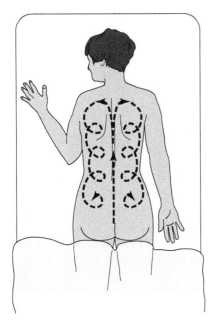

Step 10 For the next set of strokes, massage the person's shoulders and back using a small circular motion on the downstroke.

11. For the next set of strokes, move up the center of the back from the buttocks to the shoulders, and then back down along the outside of the back. On the downstroke, massage the person's shoulders, back, and buttocks using a small circular motion, paying special attention to the area at the base of the spine. Repeat four times.

12. Finish with long, gliding strokes (*effleurage*), moving up the center of the back from the buttocks to the shoulders and then back down along the outside of the back. Repeat four times.

13. Remove your gloves and dispose of them in a facility-approved waste container.

14. If the back massage is being given as part of a bath, assist the person onto his or her

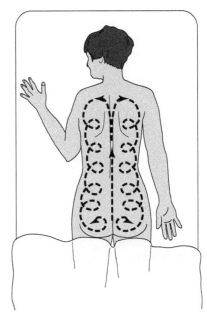

Step 11 For the final set of strokes, massage the person's shoulders, back, and buttocks using a small circular motion on the downstroke.

back and continue with the bath. If the back massage is being given before bed or at any other time, help the person back into his or her pajamas, nightgown, or hospital gown.

15. If the side rails are in use, return the side rails to the raised position. Make sure that the bed is lowered to its lowest position and that the wheels are locked.

16. Gather the soiled linens and place them in the linen hamper or linen bag. Dispose of disposable items in a facility-approved waste container. Clean equipment and return it to the storage area.

Finishing Up CLSOWR

17. Complete the "Finishing Up" steps.

WHAT DID YOU LEARN?

Multiple Choice

Select the single best answer for each of the following questions.

1. As a safety measure, when you give mouth care to an unconscious person, you should position the person in which position?
   a. Semi-Fowler's position with head turned to side
   b. Supine position
   c. Fowler's position
   d. Prone position

2. Why do you line the sink with a washcloth when cleaning a person's dentures?
   a. To ensure that you always have a wet washcloth handy when you need one
   b. To protect the sink from scratches
   c. To guard against breaking the dentures
   d. To prevent contamination of the dentures

3. Which one of the following is within the range of appropriate temperatures for bath water?
   a. 36.6°C (98°F)
   b. 100°C (212°F)
   c. 48.9°C (120°F)
   d. 40.5°C (105°F)

4. When giving a complete bed bath, you should:
   a. Position yourself on one side of the bed and stay there
   b. Use the same water throughout the bath to minimize trips to the sink
   c. Avoid washing the person's perineal area because the person may be embarrassed
   d. Keep the person covered as much as possible

5. When assisting a man with perineal care, you should always:
   a. Hold the penis at a 90 degree angle to the body
   b. Wash from the base of the penis toward the tip
   c. Retract the foreskin if the man is uncircumcised
   d. Clean the scrotum first

6. When assisting a person with a shower, you should:
   a. Use a bath blanket to prevent falls
   b. Run the water until the temperature reaches 51.6°C (125°F)
   c. Wear waterproof personal protective equipment (PPE) to protect yourself from getting wet

   d. Use a shower chair if the person is weak or unsteady

7. Which one of the following actions must be taken to keep the skin healthy?
   a. Apply generous amounts of lotion after the bath
   b. Rinse the skin well and dry it thoroughly, especially in areas where "skin meets skin"
   c. Apply generous amounts of powder after the bath
   d. Rub the skin vigorously with the washcloth

8. How are natural teeth brushed?
   a. Using a circular motion
   b. For at least 10 minutes on each side
   c. Using an "up and down" motion
   d. All of the above

9. When assisting a woman with perineal care, you should always:
   a. Gently yet thoroughly dry the perineal area and vulva
   b. Clean the rectal area last
   c. Move the washcloth in a downward direction, from the urethra to the anus
   d. All of the above

10. What is the first thing you should do before assisting a person with a tub bath?
    a. Gather the necessary supplies
    b. Make sure the tub is clean
    c. Check the temperature of the water
    d. Check the care plan to make sure the person is allowed to have a tub bath

11. Which of the following observations made while assisting with mouth care would you report to the nurse?
    a. Lips that are dry, cracked, swollen, or blistered
    b. Irritations, sores, or white patches in the mouth or on the tongue
    c. Bleeding, swelling, or redness of the gums
    d. All of the above

12. How long should a back massage last?
    a. 2 minutes
    b. 1 minute
    c. 4 to 6 minutes
    d. 15 minutes

Matching

Match each numbered item with its appropriate lettered description.

_____ **1.** Perineal care (peri-care)

_____ **2.** Activities of daily living (ADLs)

_____ **3.** Evening (hour of sleep, hs) care

_____ **4.** Gingivitis

_____ **5.** PRN (as-needed) care

_____ **6.** Antiperspirant

_____ **7.** Edentulous

a. Without teeth

b. Routine tasks of daily life, such as bathing, eating, and grooming

c. Care that is provided at any time of the day or night, when the person's condition warrants it

d. Inflammation of the gums, caused by poor oral hygiene

e. Stops or slows secretion of sweat

f. Care that is routinely provided at bedtime

g. Cleaning of the perineum, the anus, and the vulva or penis

STOP and Think!

Mrs. Davis is a resident at your facility, which specializes in caring for people with Alzheimer's disease. As Mrs. Davis' disease has progressed, she has become progressively more lax about matters related to personal hygiene. She dislikes bathing, and if you do not remove her soiled clothes from her room she will continue to wear them every day. Today Mrs. Davis is scheduled to have a shower, and as you might have predicted, she tells you that she "will not take a shower today." What should you do?

Jaxon is a 15-year-old who was recently admitted to your rehabilitation unit following an accident. The doctor ordered complete bed rest for Jaxon until his condition stabilizes. You need to give Jaxon a bed bath, and you can tell that he is very embarrassed at the prospect. What can you do to make the situation more comfortable for Jaxon?

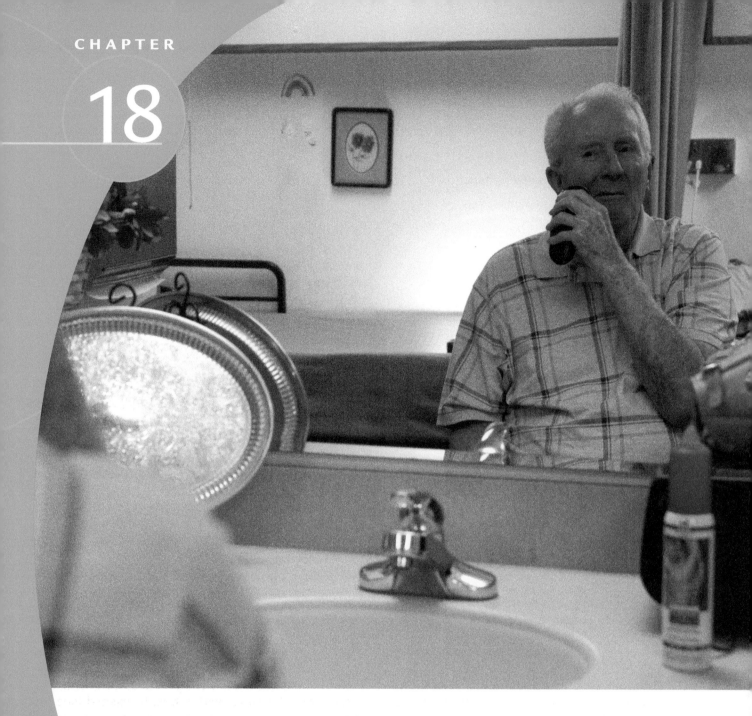

Grooming

WHAT WILL YOU LEARN?

In the previous chapter, you learned how to help people with their most basic aspects of personal care, those activities related to keeping the body clean and healthy. **Grooming,** or activities related to maintaining a neat and attractive appearance, goes beyond basic personal hygiene. The routine care of the hands and feet (including the nails), shampooing and styling of the hair, the application of makeup, and shaving are all

Photo: Grooming practices help people to feel more attractive and confident.

grooming practices that play a role in maintaining both physical and emotional health. Imagine that you are a patient or a resident, and you are unable to complete your regular grooming activities. Your hair is uncombed, you have not applied makeup (if you are a woman) or shaved (if you are a man), and you are not dressed for visitors, yet company arrives anyway. How would you feel? Would you be able to fully enjoy your guests, or would you be worried about your appearance? Helping your patients and residents with "putting their best face forward," the subject of this chapter, is part of providing holistic care. When you are finished with this chapter, you will be able to:

1. Describe factors that influence a person's grooming habits.
2. Explain the effect that illness or disability may have on a person's grooming habits.
3. Understand the importance of proper hand and foot care.
4. List changes that occur in a person's feet as a result of aging or illness.
5. Demonstrate proper technique for assisting with hand and foot care.
6. Discuss the various dressing needs that a patient or resident may have.
7. Demonstrate proper technique for helping a person to dress and undress.
8. Discuss disorders a personal support worker may observe when assisting with hair care.
9. Describe the different methods used to assist a person with shampooing his or her hair.
10. Describe methods used to style a person's hair.
11. Demonstrate proper technique for shampooing a bedridden person's hair and combing a person's hair.
12. Describe the tools and supplies used for shaving.
13. Demonstrate how to safely shave a man's face.
14. Explain how the use of makeup can affect a person's sense of well-being.

Vocabulary

Grooming	Tinea pedis	Tinea capitis	Alopecia
Cuticle	Podiatrist	Seborrheic dermatitis	Pediculosis capitis
Hangnails	Dandruff	(cradle cap)	Nits

A person's grooming practices may be very simple (for example, washing and combing the hair and applying a bit of moisturizing lotion to the skin). Or they may be very complex (for example, styling the hair with a blow dryer and curlers, applying makeup, applying perfume or cologne, and polishing the nails). Think for a moment about the routine grooming practices that you perform each day before you leave home to face the world. Have you ever overslept and had to go to school or work without your routine grooming accomplished? How did you feel? Did it affect your self-esteem?

Patients and residents have personal grooming routines, just as you do. Like yours, their personal grooming practices are influenced by cultural and religious beliefs, upbringing, current fashion, and their feelings about their own sexuality. Many women feel more feminine if they are wearing lipstick and have polished nails, while others are quite happy with a freshly washed face and a ponytail. Men also have grooming routines that make them feel attractive and self-confident, such as shaving and applying cologne or aftershave, or caring for a beard or moustache. Illness or disability can affect a person's ability to complete his or her grooming practices, causing the person to feel unattractive and "not quite himself."

Many patients or residents can use assistive devices to complete grooming tasks independently. However, some patients or residents will need your help to complete their grooming routine. As with any aspect of care, check with the nurse or check the person's care plan to find out about any limitations or specifics related to grooming.

Helping Hands and a Caring Heart

FOCUS ON HUMANISTIC HEALTH CARE

As a personal support worker, you must provide humanistic, holistic care for your patients and residents. This means looking after their physical needs, as well as their emotional needs. Helping a person to complete his or her routine grooming practices meets many of the person's emotional needs, as well as some physical ones. When you take the time and make the effort to style a person's hair attractively, polish her nails, or help apply makeup as part of morning care, you make that person feel extra special. Your actions help the person to meet the needs of love and belonging, because she feels cared for as the unique individual that she is. You also help the person to meet her need for self-esteem. Not only is she clean and comfortable, but she feels attractive too.

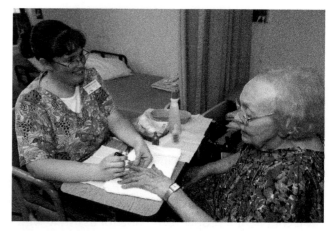

Figure 18-1
Giving a person a manicure gives you the opportunity to spend "quality time" with a patient or resident.

ASSISTING WITH HAND AND FOOT CARE

CARE OF THE HANDS

Soft, smooth skin and trimmed, filed fingernails feel wonderful and are important for overall health and comfort. Dryness and chapping of the skin on the hands is uncomfortable and creates a portal of entry for microbes. Poorly cared for fingernails can become long and rough, placing the person at risk for accidentally scratching himself. For example, a person who is disoriented can hurt himself if his fingernails are not kept short and smooth. For people who are alert and oriented, fingernail length is a personal choice, but the edges should be kept smooth.

A simple care routine is used to keep the skin of the hands healthy and the fingernails neat (Procedure 18-1). Even if the person can care for her own hands and fingernails, getting a manicure from someone else can really lift the person's spirits, especially if the person is not feeling her best (Fig. 18-1). In addition to making the person feel cared for, helping a patient or resident with hand and nail care gives you the chance to observe for signs of health. In a healthy person, the nailbed is pink. There is no gap between the nail and the nailbed. When viewed

from the side, the nail is convex (it curves slightly). The **cuticle** (the skin along the edges of the nail) is smooth and unbroken.

Nail care is usually easiest to perform on nails that have been soaked for a short time in warm water. During or immediately following a bath is an ideal time to perform nail care, because the water makes the nails soft and flexible. When nail care is provided at a time other than bath time, the nails can be softened by soaking the ends of the fingers for a short time in a small basin of warm water.

Fingernails are trimmed with clippers, not scissors, to a length no shorter than even with the ends of the fingers (Fig. 18-2). In some states and facilities, trimming a patient's or resident's fingernails is outside of the scope of practice for personal support workers, so be sure to follow the policy at the facility where you work. After

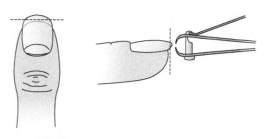

Figure 18-2
Nails are cut using nail clippers. Cut the nails straight across, being careful not to cut too close to the skin. Always make sure that it is within your scope of practice to trim a patient's or resident's fingernails or toenails. In many facilities, this task must be performed by a nurse.

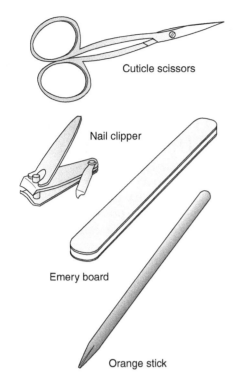

Figure 18-3
Tools used during hand and foot care.

Cuticle scissors

Nail clipper

Emery board

Orange stick

trimming, the nails are filed into an oval shape using an emery board. Pain or tenderness can result from **hangnails** (broken pieces of cuticle). Hangnails may need to be trimmed using cuticle scissors so that they do not rub or snag on clothing or linens. Torn hangnails can cause bleeding and inflammation of the cuticle.

The blunt end of an orange stick (Fig. 18-3) or the edge of a washcloth is used to gently push the cuticles back, and then the orange stick is used to clean underneath the tips of the nails.

Some people like to use nail polish. If nail polish is not used, then the surfaces of the nails can be lightly buffed to give them shine. Applying hand cream helps to seal in moisture and prevent dryness of the skin and cuticles.

CARE OF THE FEET

Care of the feet is essential for good grooming as well as for good health. The feet tend to sweat, especially when slippers or shoes and socks are worn, leading to odours and a warm, moist environment that encourages the growth of microbes. For example, the disorder commonly known as "athlete's foot" **(tinea pedis)** is a fungal infection of the skin and nails. ("Pedis" comes from the Latin word for foot, *pedalis*.) Toenails that are allowed to grow too long can make wearing footwear uncomfortable, and the nails may become ingrown (a condition where the nail curves down and back into the skin, causing injury and pain). Finally, the feet are at risk for injury—how many times have you had your foot stepped on, stubbed your toes against a piece of furniture, or developed a blister as a result of shoes that did not fit properly?

Injuries such as cuts and blisters are painful for a person with normal blood flow to the feet and toes. For a person with poor blood flow (for example, as a result of the normal aging process, a heart problem, or diabetes mellitus), a cut or a blister might develop into a life-threatening condition. Because the wounded area is not receiving the normal amount of blood, the area receives less oxygen and nutrients and fewer infection-fighting white blood cells. Healing is delayed, and the risk of infection is increased. In addition, people with poor blood flow often have reduced sensation as well. While you would certainly notice if a new pair of shoes made a blister on your heel, a person with reduced blood flow and sensation might not be aware of the blister, and a small blister could quickly become a dangerous infection. Helping a person with foot care allows you to observe the person's feet for small blisters, cracks in the skin, peeling of the skin between the toes or on the soles of the feet, ingrown toenails, and other problems. Red or tender areas should also be reported to the nurse immediately.

Like hand care, foot care is a grooming task that is easily added to the bathing routine. If foot care is done at a time other than bath time, the feet should first be bathed, rinsed, and dried thoroughly (especially between the toes). Prolonged soaking is not recommended. In most facilities, personal support workers are not allowed to trim the toenails of patients or residents, because a small injury could cause a life-threatening infection. This task is usually performed by a nurse or a **podiatrist,** a doctor who specializes in the care of the feet. The attention of a podiatrist is especially necessary when the toenails are thick and difficult to trim (as a result of aging or poor blood flow; Fig. 18-4). If you are allowed to trim your patients' or residents' toenails, use clippers and cut the toenails straight across. Never try to trim or file corns or calluses.

After the toenails are trimmed, they are filed to remove rough edges. Applying foot powder or

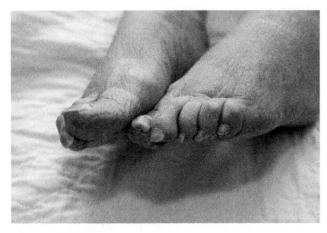

Figure 18-4
Many elderly people have thick, yellowed toenails as a result of age or poor circulation. Because thickened toenails may be difficult to trim and an accidental injury can have serious consequences, many health care facilities require that a nurse or a podiatrist trim patients' or residents' toenails.

lotion to dry feet is refreshing and comforting. Cotton socks help to keep the feet warm and will absorb sweat. (Be careful when helping an elderly person to put on socks—roll the cuff of the sock down before putting it on the person's foot and take care not to accidentally scratch the person with your fingernails or jewelry when pulling the sock up over the heel.) Encourage your patients or residents to wear appropriate footwear. Well-fitting, supportive shoes with nonskid soles help to protect the feet and make walking safer by helping to prevent falls and slipping. Procedure 18-2 describes how to assist a patient or resident with foot care.

TELL THE NURSE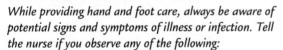

While providing hand and foot care, always be aware of potential signs and symptoms of illness or infection. Tell the nurse if you observe any of the following:

- Nailbeds that are either very pale or blue, or bruised
- Nails that are unusually yellow or white
- Nails that are unusually thick
- Nails that are broken or have been cut too short (especially if there is also bleeding or tenderness)
- Nails that are ingrown
- Cuticles that are torn, red, or swollen

- Skin that is blistered, red, or tender (especially on the feet)
- Any unusual rashes or odours

ASSISTING WITH DRESSING AND UNDRESSING

As a personal support worker, you will be responsible for helping your patients or residents to change their clothes, possibly several times a day. Dressing is usually a routine part of morning and evening care. However, clothing should be changed any time that it becomes wet or soiled. The type of clothing worn by people receiving health care services differs according to the type of facility and the abilities of the person. If a resident of a long-term care facility is able to be out of bed during the day, he or she may wear street clothes during the day and a hospital gown, a nightgown, or pajamas at night. Procedure 18-3 describes how to assist a person with dressing in street clothes and nightwear. A patient in a hospital or acute care setting or a resident who has a specific physical disability or medical condition may wear a hospital gown or nightwear day and night. Procedure 18-4 describes how to change a hospital gown.

As with other personal care routines, the amount of help that each person needs for dressing will vary. Some people will need no assistance, except perhaps for some help tying their shoes or zipping a back zipper. Others may need a lot of assistance with every part of the process, from selecting clothes to putting them on. Allowing a person to choose the clothing he or she wishes to wear is a top priority when assisting with dressing (Fig. 18-5). When a person is unable to choose his or her own clothes, use good taste and common sense when choosing items for the person to wear. Dressing appropriately for the day's activities and with consideration for the season and environment will help residents and patients stay comfortable. If a person chooses an item of clothing that is not appropriate for the weather or the day's planned activities, gently suggest a more appropriate choice. Remember that some elderly or ill people may chill more easily than others and may need a sweater or jacket to remain warm, especially if there is air conditioning.

Comfort and ease of dressing help determine many wardrobe choices for the residents of long-term care facilities. Many residents are undergoing

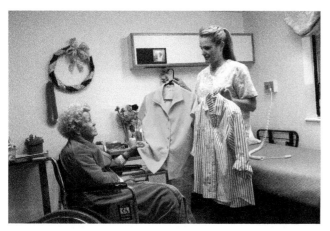

Figure 18-5
Whenever possible, a person should be permitted to choose which articles of clothing he or she will wear.

rehabilitation following an accident or a disabling illness, such as a stroke. The goal of rehabilitation is to return the person to the highest level of independent functioning as possible. In addition to selecting clothes that are easy to take on and off, a weak or disabled person may use one or more of the many assistive devices that are available to make dressing easier. For example, clothing that closes with a Velcro™ fastener instead of zippers or buttons allows a person with limited use of his or her fingers to manage dressing and toileting with little or no assistance (Fig. 18-6A). Long-handled shoehorns and graspers allow a person to put on his or her own socks and shoes (Fig. 18-6B). The use of these assistive devices

can allow a person to maintain a large amount of personal independence in spite of disabilities.

Some patients or residents will, however, need your help with dressing and undressing. For example, consider the following situations:

- A person has an extremity (an arm or a leg) that is weak, paralyzed, in a cast, or splinted.
- A person has recently had surgery on an arm or a leg.
- A person has an intravenous (IV) line (Fig. 18-7).

These conditions may make helping the person to dress or undress a bit more challenging, but good planning on your part can simplify the situation. For example, if you place the garment's sleeve or leg onto the affected extremity first, dressing becomes much easier for both you and the person being dressed. (When it comes time to remove the garment, reverse the procedure—work with the strong arm or leg first and undress the affected extremity last.) If the person has an IV line, bring the IV bag and tubing through the sleeve first and then follow with the arm (see Fig. 18-7). Some hospitals and acute care units may have special hospital gowns with openings in the shoulder that make dressing and undressing with IV lines in place easier. You should not remove an IV line from an infusion pump or disconnect IV tubing when assisting a person to dress or undress. If you are unsure about how to manage an IV line or a bandage while helping a person to dress or undress, ask a nurse for assistance.

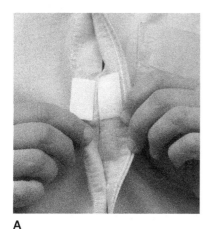

A

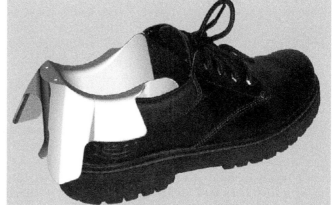

B

Figure 18-6
Assistive devices are available to help people with disabilities dress themselves independently.
(A) Velcro™ fasteners on this shirt replace buttons or a zipper, which require more use of the fingers to manage. **(B)** A shoehorn makes it easier to put on shoes. (*Photos courtesy of Sammons Preston Rolyan, Bolingbrook, IL.*)

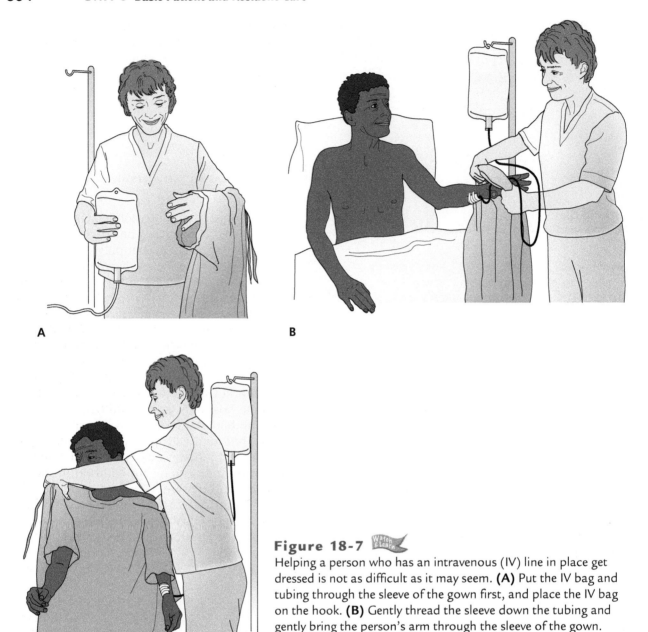

A

B

C

Figure 18-7 Watch & Learn

Helping a person who has an intravenous (IV) line in place get dressed is not as difficult as it may seem. **(A)** Put the IV bag and tubing through the sleeve of the gown first, and place the IV bag on the hook. **(B)** Gently thread the sleeve down the tubing and gently bring the person's arm through the sleeve of the gown. **(C)** Bring the gown across the person's chest and guide the other arm through the other sleeve.

ASSISTING WITH HAIR CARE

Routine care is necessary to keep the hair clean and neat. For many people, the appearance of their hair affects how they feel about themselves. Have you ever had a "bad hair day"? Did you feel like you would rather walk around with a paper bag on your head than have other people see your hair dirty or poorly styled? Helping with hair care is an essential part of providing care for those who need you. Routine grooming of the hair involves daily brushing, combing, and styling and is usually accomplished as part of early morning care, when a person arises. Additional grooming may be necessary throughout the day, for example, after napping or before visiting times. Some health care facilities have on-site salons and barbershops where patients and residents can have their hair cut, washed, and professionally styled (Fig. 18-8).

The texture and length of the hair affect how a person cares for it. Hair that is straight and fine can be as hard to manage as hair that is curly and coarse. The hair of elderly people tends to be

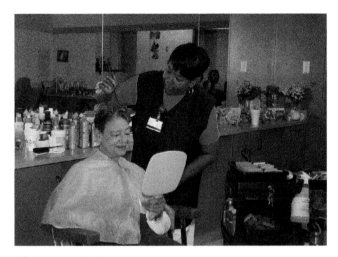

Figure 18-8
Some facilities have on-site salons and barbershops for the convenience of residents.

fragile. Personal preferences regarding hairstyle and the products used when grooming the hair vary and should be respected whenever possible. Asking a person about his or her usual hair care routine and preferred products will provide you with much useful information. Patients and residents should be encouraged to participate in caring for their own hair to their fullest ability. For example, a person with a paralyzed or injured arm can be encouraged to brush her hair on her "strong" side, and then you can complete the job on the other side (Fig. 18-9).

When assisting with grooming of the hair, it is important to observe the hair and scalp for any abnormalities. Common conditions of the hair and scalp that you may see in your patients or residents include the following:

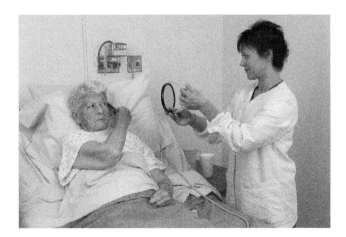

Figure 18-9
To foster independence and self-esteem, encourage your patients or residents to do as much as possible for themselves, while you stand by ready to offer assistance as needed.

- **Dandruff** is itching and flaking of the scalp. Daily brushing and using a medicated shampoo may be all that is needed to control dandruff.
- **Tinea capitis,** a fungal infection of the scalp, may also cause itching and flaking of the scalp. ("Capitis" comes from the Latin word for head, *caput.*)
- **Seborrheic dermatitis** (commonly referred to as **"cradle cap"** when it occurs in infants) causes severe scaling of the scalp. Thick, yellow, crusty patches are seen. The nurse may ask you to help shampoo the person daily with a medicated shampoo until the scaling is cleared up.
- **Alopecia,** or baldness, can be caused by many conditions. Alopecia is most commonly the result of an inherited trait in men and is rarely seen in women, although women may experience thinning of the hair with aging. Medications used to treat cancer (chemotherapy) and certain forms of radiation treatment can cause total baldness in both men and women. Stress, illness, and poor nutrition can also cause the hair to thin.
- **Pediculosis capitis,** or head lice, is particularly common in children. Lice, as you will recall from Chapter 7, are very small parasitic insects that feed on the blood of the host, or the person who is infected. The insects lay their eggs (called **nits**) on the hair shaft, near the root. The nits look like dandruff flakes or small pieces of lint, but cannot be brushed or shaken off the hair. Head lice are transmitted from person to person by direct contact with an infected person's hair. They may also be transmitted indirectly, through contact with clothing, bed linens, brushes and combs, and cloth-covered furniture (for example, the back of a sofa or chair where an infected person has rested his or her head). Pediculosis is treated with medicated creams and shampoos. The person's clothing and bed linens must be washed in very hot water to prevent reinfection.

TELL THE NURSE

When providing hair care, it is important to observe the condition of the person's hair and scalp. Make sure to report any of the following findings to the nurse immediately:

- Flaking, crusting, or scaling of the scalp
- Redness, itching, or tenderness of the scalp

- Unusual hair loss, especially if it is occurring in patches
- A foul smell
- Severely matted or tangled hair
- Nits ("flakes" that cannot be brushed or shaken off the hair)

SHAMPOOING THE HAIR

Hair should be washed as often as is necessary to keep it clean. The frequency of shampooing will vary according to personal preference and health status. People who are feverish or who have been sweating due to illness or from physical activity may welcome a non-scheduled shampoo to help them feel fresh and clean. Other people may only need their hair washed once or twice a week.

Many people in health care facilities can shampoo their own hair when they bathe. Others will need help. There are several ways to help a person shampoo his or her hair. Many bathtubs and showers have hand-held showerheads that make it easy to shampoo the hair during a person's bath. The hair can also be shampooed in a sink, either by having the person sit with his back to the sink and tilt his head backward, or by having the person face the sink and bend his head forward (Fig. 18-10). However, remember that for many elderly people, shampooing at the sink is either uncomfortable or impossible because it is more difficult for an older person to bend his or her neck to the degree required. When a person cannot get out of bed, a shampoo trough is used to wash the hair (Procedure 18-5).

As any trip down a drugstore or grocery store aisle will reveal, there are many different types of shampoos and conditioners to choose from. (Conditioners are used by many people to improve the hair's texture and reduce tangles.) Respecting personal preference in products is important. When a person is too ill to have regular shampoos, a "dry shampoo" product may be used instead. Before shampooing a patient's or resident's hair, always check with the nurse or the care plan to find out necessary details, such as the frequency of shampoos, the method used, and the products preferred.

STYLING THE HAIR

After the hair has been washed and towel-dried, the hair is dried and styled according to the person's wishes (Fig. 18-11). Most men and some women with shorter hair may prefer to allow their hair to air dry. Others may want to have their hair styled and dried with a blow dryer, or they may want their hair rolled on curlers and dried under a salon-style dryer. If you are using electric appliances to dry and style a person's hair, be sure to follow the safety precautions related to the use of electrical items as described in Chapter 9—for example, check for frayed cords and never use an electrical appliance near water. Be very careful not to burn the person's scalp with the dryer or curling iron. It is best to use a low heat setting.

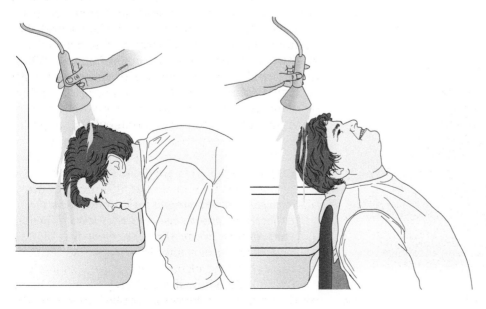

Figure 18-10
A person's hair can be shampooed at the sink, provided the person does not have neck or back problems.

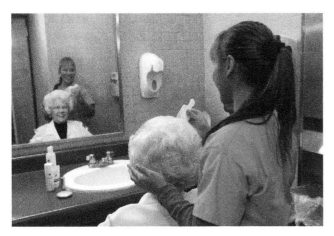

Figure 18-11
After shampooing, some people may like to have their hair dried and styled.

The time and attention you spend helping your patients or residents style their hair will help to make those in your care feel and look attractive, which will certainly have a positive effect on their well-being. Stop and think for a moment how you felt the last time you had your hair professionally done, or a friend offered to wash and style your hair. That is how well-cared for and pampered your patients or residents will feel when you provide these services for them!

PREVENTING TANGLES

Regular brushing and combing of the hair helps to keep hair soft and tangle-free. The scalp produces oil that keeps the hair shiny and soft. Brushing distributes this oil throughout the hair. Hair that is long or curly may need to be braided after it is brushed to help prevent tangling (Fig. 18-12).

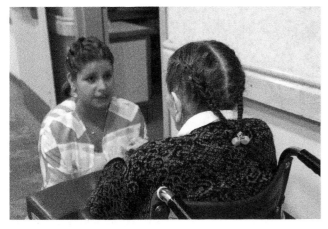

Figure 18-12
Braiding helps to prevent tangles in hair that is long or curly.

Many African Caribbean people have curly hair and a very dry scalp. African Caribbean hair may require braiding and the application of a moisturizing product to keep the hair soft and pliable. The use of barrettes, headbands, and clips can be both functional (by keeping hair out of the face) and decorative.

Sometimes the hair becomes tangled, especially if the person has been restricted to bed for a period of time. To remove tangles from the hair, use a wide-tooth comb and start at the ends of the hair, one section at a time, gently working up toward the scalp (Procedure 18-6). Hair that is very tangled or matted may need to be cut, but the nurse must first obtain permission from the person or his or her legal guardian to cut the hair.

ASSISTING WITH SHAVING

ASSISTING MEN

Shaving is a routine grooming practice among most men. Shaving a man's face should be a part of either morning or evening care, depending on the person's preference (some men prefer to shave before going to bed). Prior to shaving, the face should be cleaned and the beard softened, making bath time an ideal time to complete the shave. The frequency of shaving depends on how fast the beard grows and personal preference.

The type of shaving tool used also varies (Fig. 18-13). Many men prefer to use a safety razor, which may be disposable or have a changeable blade unit. Blades that are dull pull at the beard and do not cut the hair smoothly and should be changed. Disposable razors are used once and then discarded. Used blades and disposable razors should always be disposed of in a sharps container, not in a wastebasket. When using a safety razor, the beard is softened with warm water and a shaving cream or gel is applied to retain the moisture and reduce the friction of the blade against the skin. Some men may prefer to use shaving soap instead of a shaving cream or gel. In this case, a shaving brush is used to lather the soap and apply it to the beard. Procedure 18-7 describes how to shave a man's face using a blade razor and shaving cream, gel, or soap.

Other men like to use electric razors. People who are taking drugs that decrease the blood's ability to form a clot should always use an electric razor, because electric razors are less likely to cut or nick the skin. If an electric razor is being used, a pre-shave lotion is applied to soften the

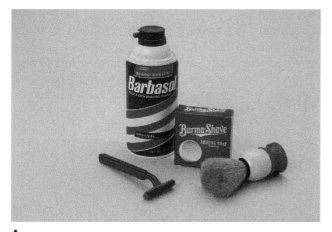

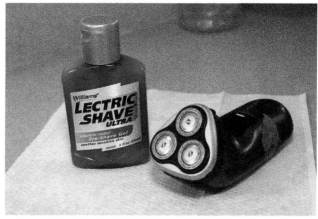

A

B

Figure 18-13
Shaving supplies. **(A)** A safety razor is used with shaving cream or gel or shaving soap. **(B)** An electric razor is used with a pre-shave lotion. An electric razor carries less risk of cuts or nicks, and therefore is preferred for a person who is taking medications that affect the blood's ability to clot.

beard and allow the razor to glide smoothly across the face. The usual safety precautions that are taken with all electrical appliances should be taken when using an electric razor. The electric razor is cleaned after each use.

If a person is able, he should be encouraged to do his own shaving. You should provide whatever assistance is necessary, which may range from placing a chair and a mirror near the sink or bringing supplies and water to the bedside, to completing the shave in full. When shaving a person, always remember to wear gloves because a cut or a nick will put you at risk for exposure to bloodborne pathogens. Always ask the nurse or check the care plan to determine if there are any limitations or special instructions for a person's shave.

A man may prefer to have a beard or mustache instead of being clean-shaven. Beards and mustaches need routine grooming care also. They must be kept clean and free of food and drink and will need to be combed or brushed and trimmed regularly. Never shave off a person's beard or mustache unless the person requests that you do so. Be careful when shaving near the mustache or beard to avoid accidentally shaving part of the facial hair off.

ASSISTING WOMEN

Shaving the legs, underarms, or both makes many women feel feminine and attractive. In addition, some women experience the growth of coarse facial hair as they age and may request your help with removing this unwanted hair. If a woman is unable to shave her legs, armpits, or

face and wants to do so, you should help her as necessary.

Many of the same principles used when assisting men to shave apply to women as well. The hair should be softened with warm water first, making bath time the ideal time to shave. A safety razor or an electric razor may be used. If a safety razor is used, shaving cream or gel should be applied first. Like men, many women will have clear preferences regarding the type of razor and shaving products that are used, and respecting the person's preferences is important. A woman's face is shaved in the same manner as a man's. When shaving the armpits, it is best to move in the direction of hair growth. When shaving the legs, start at the ankle and move upward, against the direction of hair growth. Many women shave their legs only below the knee, while others may shave the thigh as well.

ASSISTING WITH THE APPLICATION OF MAKE-UP

Many women, and some men, wear makeup because it helps them to feel more confident and attractive. A person's culture, religion, age, and feelings about his or her own sexuality all contribute to that person's feelings about, and use of, makeup. Many times, the types of makeup a person likes and the way she applies them are influenced by the time in that person's life when she felt most attractive. For example, many of your elderly ladies will insist on wearing dark lipstick and heavy face powder because that was the style that was popular during their younger years. Other women may insist that a certain type of mascara or a certain shade of eye shadow is an essential grooming item.

Helping a person to continue with her normal personal grooming routine has an enormous impact on the person's continued well-being. For some people, wearing makeup increases their self-esteem and feelings of self-worth. When you help a person who likes to wear makeup to complete this part of her grooming routine, the person will feel that you take special care of her and that you value her as the unique human being that she is. This idea is at the heart of humanistic care.

Summary

- Caring for the hands and feet (especially the fingernails and toenails), selecting an outfit to wear, shampooing and styling the hair, shaving, and applying makeup are grooming practices that people may engage in to make themselves feel more attractive and confident.
  - Grooming practices differ from hygiene practices in that grooming practices are performed mainly for the sake of appearance. Therefore, good grooming is more essential for emotional health than for physical health. However, grooming practices do benefit physical health as well.
  - Personal grooming practices are highly variable and are influenced by many factors, including culture, religion, upbringing, current fashion, and a person's feelings about his or her own sexuality. Respecting your patient's or resident's personal preferences is an important part of providing holistic care. Remembering this is very important when assisting with grooming.
- Care of the hands and feet focuses on keeping the skin and nails clean and healthy.
  - Assisting with hand and foot care gives the personal support worker the chance to observe for potential health problems, including poor blood flow and fungal infections.
  - Poor blood flow to the feet is associated with many health problems, including decreased sensation and an increased risk for a life-threatening infection. Poor blood flow may be caused by heart disease, diabetes mellitus, or the normal aging process.
  - Trimming a person's toenails is usually beyond the personal support worker's scope of practice. Instead, this task is performed by a nurse or a podiatrist.
- Dressing daily is necessary for warmth and modesty, and it gives people a sense of purpose.
- For many people, dressing is a way of expressing themselves. Therefore, a person's preferences regarding outfit selection should be followed whenever possible. Sometimes, due to disability or illness, a person will be required to wear a hospital gown or nightwear during the day.
  - Wet or soiled garments must be exchanged for dry, clean ones as often as necessary.
  - Assistive devices, such as Velcro™ fasteners, shoehorns, and graspers, increase a disabled person's independence. With increased independence comes increased self-esteem.
  - Certain conditions (for example, a weak, paralyzed, or injured arm or leg or an IV line) can make dressing more challenging but by no means impossible.
- Most people feel best when their hair is clean, free of tangles, and styled in a familiar style.
  - Assisting with hair care gives the personal support worker a chance to observe for conditions of the scalp and hair, including dandruff, tinea capitis, seborrheic dermatitis (cradle cap), alopecia, and pediculosis capitis (head lice).
  - Hair may be shampooed as part of a tub or shower bath, at the sink, or in bed, using a shampoo trough.
  - Styling tools include blow dryers, curling irons, hot curlers, and salon-style hairdryers. Caution must be used when operating these electrical appliances.
  - Regular brushing and combing keeps the hair shiny and tangle-free.
- Most men shave their faces daily, either completely or partially. Many women shave their legs, their underarms, or both.
- Many women, and some men, consider the application of makeup to be an essential grooming activity.

PROCEDURE 18-1

Assisting With Hand Care

WHY YOU DO IT   Soft, smooth skin and trimmed, filed fingernails are important for overall health and comfort.

Getting Ready WORKSTEPS

1. Complete the "Getting Ready" steps.

Supplies

- gloves (if contact with broken skin is likely)
- paper towels
- orange stick
- nail clippers
- emery board (nail file)
- bath thermometer
- emesis basin
- soap
- lotion
- nail polish remover (optional)
- nail polish (optional)
- cotton balls (optional)
- washcloth
- towel

Procedure

2. Make sure that the bed is lowered to its lowest position and that the wheels are locked.

3. Cover the over-bed table with paper towels. Pour some liquid soap into the emesis basin and fill the basin with warm water (37.7°C [100°F] to 46.1°C [115°F] on the bath thermometer). Place the emesis basin on the over-bed table, along with the nail care supplies and clean linens.

4. If the side rails are in use, lower the side rail on the working side of the bed. The side rail on the opposite side of the bed should remain up.

5. Help the person to transfer from the bed to a bedside chair, assist the person to sit on the edge of the bed, or raise the head of the bed as tolerated.

6. Put on the gloves if contact with broken skin is likely.

7. If the person is wearing nail polish and wants it removed, remove the nail polish by putting a small amount of nail polish remover on a cotton ball and gently rubbing each nail.

8. Help the person to position the tips of his or her fingers in the basin to soak. Let the person soak his or her fingers for about 5 minutes.

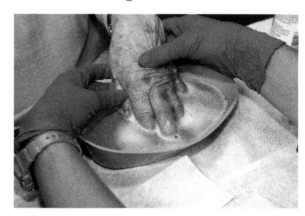

Step 8 Soak the nails to soften them.

9. Working with one hand at a time, lift the person's hand out of the basin and wash the entire hand, including between the fingers, with the soapy washcloth. Use the orange stick to gently clean underneath the person's fingernails. Rinse thoroughly and pat the person's hand dry with a towel. Be sure to dry between the fingers. Repeat with the other hand.

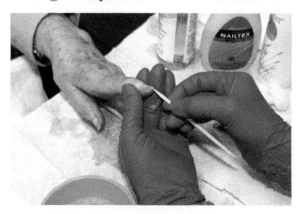

Step 9 Clean under the person's nails using the orange stick.

10. Remove the emesis basin and dry the person's hands thoroughly. If facility policy allows it, gently push the cuticles back with the orange stick.

11. If facility policy allows it, use the nail clippers to cut the person's fingernails. If the person's nails need to be trimmed but this task is outside of your scope of practice, report this need to the nurse.

12. Use the emery board to file the fingernails into an oval shape and smooth the rough edges.

13. Apply lotion to the person's hands and gently massage it into the skin.

14. Apply nail polish as the person requests.

15. If necessary, help the person return to bed. If the side rails are in use, return the side rails to the raised position. Lower the head of the bed as the person requests.

16. Gather the soiled linens and place them in the linen hamper or linen bag. Dispose of disposable items in a facility-approved waste container. Clean equipment and return it to the storage area.

17. Remove your gloves and dispose of them in a facility-approved waste container.

Finishing Up CLSOWR

18. Complete the "Finishing Up" steps.

PROCEDURE 18-2

Assisting With Foot Care

WHY YOU DO IT   Soft, smooth skin and trimmed, filed toenails are important for overall health and comfort.

Getting Ready WGKIEPS

1. Complete the "Getting Ready" steps.

Supplies

- gloves (if contact with broken skin is likely)
- paper towels
- bed protector
- orange stick
- nailbrush
- nail clippers
- emery board (nail file)
- wash basin
- bath thermometer
- soap
- lotion
- nail polish remover (optional)
- nail polish (optional)
- cotton balls (optional)
- washcloth
- towels

Procedure

2. Make sure that the bed is lowered to its lowest position and that the wheels are locked.

3. Cover the over-bed table with paper towels. Pour some liquid soap into the wash basin and fill the basin with warm water (37.7°C [100°F] to 46.1°C [115°F] on the bath thermometer). Place the wash basin on the over-bed table, along with the nail care supplies and clean linens.

4. If the side rails are in use, lower the side rail on the working side of the bed. The side rail on the opposite side of the bed should remain up.

5. If the person is able to get out of bed, help the person to transfer from the bed to a bedside chair. If the person is not able to get out of bed, raise the head of the bed as tolerated. Fanfold the top linens to the foot of the bed.

6. Put on the gloves if contact with broken skin is likely.

7. If the person is wearing nail polish and wants it removed, remove the nail polish by putting a small amount of nail polish remover on a cotton ball and gently rubbing each nail.

8. Place a bed protector on the floor in front of the chair (if the person is out of bed) or on the bottom sheet (if the person is in bed). Place the wash basin on the bed protector.

9. Help the person to position his or her feet in the basin to soak. Let the person soak his or her feet for about 5 minutes.

10. Remove the emesis basin and dry the person's hands thoroughly. If facility policy allows it, gently push the cuticles back with the orange stick.

11. If facility policy allows it, use the nail clippers to cut the person's toenails. If the

(continued)

11. person's nails need to be trimmed but this task is outside of your scope of practice, report this need to the nurse.

12. Use the emery board to smooth the rough edges of the toenails.

13. Apply lotion to the person's feet and gently massage it into the skin.

14. Apply nail polish as the person requests.

15. If necessary, help the person return to bed. If the side rails are in use, return the side rails to the raised position. Lower the head of the bed as the person requests.

16. Gather the soiled linens and place them in the linen hamper or linen bag. Dispose of disposable items in a facility-approved waste container. Clean equipment and return it to the storage area.

17. Remove your gloves and dispose of them in a facility-approved waste container.

Finishing Up CL30WR

18. Complete the "Finishing Up" steps.

PROCEDURE 18-3

Assisting a Person With Dressing

WHY YOU DO IT People who are able to be out of bed during the day usually wear regular clothing during the day and pajamas or nightgowns at night. Getting dressed in the morning helps people to feel better about themselves. Clothing must be changed every time it becomes wet or soiled.

Getting Ready WCKIEPS

1. Complete the "Getting Ready" steps.

Supplies

- gloves (if contact with broken skin is likely)
- bath blanket
- clean clothing

Procedure

2. Make sure that the bed is positioned at a comfortable working height (to promote good body mechanics) and that the wheels are locked.

3. Lower the head of the bed so that the bed is flat (as tolerated). If the side rails are in use, lower the side rail on the working side of the bed. The side rail on the opposite side of the bed should remain up.

4. Put on the gloves if contact with broken skin is likely.

5. Spread the bath blanket over the top linens (and the person). If the person is able, have him or her hold the bath blanket. If not, tuck the corners under the person's shoulders. Fanfold the top linens to the foot of the bed.

6. Assist the person with undressing:

   a. **Garments that fasten in the back.** Undo any fasteners, such as buttons, zippers, snaps, or ties. Gently lift the person's head and shoulders and gather the garment around the person's neck. Working with the person's strongest side first, gently remove the arm from the garment by sliding the garment down the arm. Repeat with the other arm. (If it is not possible to lift the person's head and shoulders, roll the person onto his or her side facing away from you. Working with the person's strongest side first, gently remove the arm from the garment. Roll the person onto his or her other side, facing you and remove the other arm from the garment.) Remove the garment completely by lifting it over the person's head.

   b. **Garments that fasten in the front.** Undo any fasteners, such as buttons, zippers, snaps, or ties. To remove the top, gently lift the person's head and shoulders. Working with the person's strongest side first, gently remove the arm from the garment by sliding the garment over the shoulder and down the arm. Gather the garment behind the person and remove the garment completely by sliding the other sleeve over the weak shoulder and arm. To remove the bottoms, undo any fasteners, such as buttons, zippers, or snaps. Ask the person to lift his or her buttocks off the bed and gently slide the pants down to the ankles and over the feet. (If the person cannot raise his or her buttocks off the bed, help the person to roll first to his or her strong side, allowing you to pull the bottoms down on the weak side. Then roll the person to his or her weak side and finish pulling the bottoms down.)

7. Assist the person with putting on his or her undergarments:

   a. **Underpants.** Facing the foot of the bed, gather the underpants together at the leg opening and at the waistband. Working with one foot at a time, slip first one foot and then the other through the waistband and into the leg openings. Slide the underpants up the person's legs as far as they will go, and then ask the person to lift his or her buttocks off the bed. Gently slide the underpants up over the buttocks. (If the person cannot raise his or her buttocks off the bed, help the person to roll first to his or her strong side, allowing you to pull the underpants up on the weak side. Then roll the person to his or her weak side and finish pulling the underpants up.) Adjust the underpants so that they fit comfortably.

   b. **Bra.** Working with the person's weak side first, slip the arms through the straps and position the straps on the shoulders so that the front of the bra is covering the person's chest. Adjust the cups of the bra over the person's breasts. Raise the person's head and shoulders and help the person to lean forward so that you can fasten the bra in the back.

   c. **Undershirt.** Facing the head of the bed, gather the top and the bottom of the undershirt together at the neck opening. Place the undershirt over the person's head. Working with the person's weak side first, slip the arms through the arm openings. Raise the person's head and shoulders and help the person to lean forward so that you can pull the undershirt down, smoothing out any wrinkles.

8. Assist the person with putting on his or her outerwear:

   a. **Pants.** Assist the person with putting on his or her pants by following the same procedure as that used for putting on underpants (see step 7a). Fasten any buttons, zippers, snaps, or ties.

   b. **Shirts and sweaters that fasten in the front.** Facing the head of the bed, place your hand and arm through the wristband of the garment. Working with the person's weak side first, grasp the person's hand and slip the garment off of your hand and arm, gently guiding the person's arm into the sleeve. Pull the sleeve up, adjusting it at the shoulder. Raise the person's head and shoulders and help the person to lean forward so that you can bring the other side of the garment around the back of the person's body. Guide the person's strong arm into the sleeve of the garment. Fasten any buttons, zippers, snaps, or ties.

   c. **Sweatshirts and pullover sweaters.** Assist the person with putting on a sweatshirt or pullover sweater by following the same procedure as that used for putting on an undershirt (see step 7c). Fasten any buttons, zippers, snaps, or ties.

   d. **Blouses that fasten in the back.** Facing the head of the bed, place your hand and arm through the wristband of the garment. Working with the person's weak side first, grasp the person's hand and slip the garment off of your hand and arm, gently guiding the person's arm into the sleeve. Pull the sleeve up, adjusting it at the shoulder. Repeat for the other side. Raise the person's head and shoulders and help the person to lean forward so that you can bring the sides of the garment around to the back. Fasten any buttons, zippers, snaps, or ties.

9. Assist the person with putting on footwear:

   a. **Socks or knee-high stockings.** Gather the sock or stocking, bringing the toe area and the opening together. With the toe area facing up, slip the sock or stocking over the person's foot. Smooth the heel of the sock or stocking over the person's heel, and pull the sock or stocking up into position. Adjust the sock or stocking so that it fits comfortably. Repeat for the other foot.

   b. **Shoes or slippers.** If the shoe has laces, loosen them completely to make it easier to slip the shoe onto the foot. Guide the person's foot into the shoe or slipper. A shoehorn may be used to help ease the person's heel into the shoe. Make sure that the foot

(continued)

is seated properly in the shoe. Socks or stockings should not be bunched at the toe. If necessary, tie the shoe or fasten the Velcro™ fasteners securely.

10. If the person will be remaining in bed and the side rails are in use, return the side rails to the raised position. Raise the head of the bed as the person requests.

11. Gather the soiled garments and place them in the linen hamper or linen bag.

12. Remove your gloves and dispose of them in a facility-approved waste container.

Finishing Up CLSOWR

13. Complete the "Finishing Up" steps.

PROCEDURE 18-4

Changing a Hospital Gown

WHY YOU DO IT   People who are too ill to get out of bed may wear a hospital gown. The gown must be changed every time it becomes wet or soiled.

Getting Ready WGKIEPS

1. Complete the "Getting Ready" steps.

Supplies

- gloves (if contact with broken skin is likely)
- clean hospital gown

Procedure

2. Make sure that the bed is positioned at a comfortable working height (to promote good body mechanics) and that the wheels are locked.

3. Lower the head of the bed so that the bed is flat (as tolerated). If the side rails are in use, lower them on the working side of the bed. The side rails on the opposite side of the bed should remain up.

4. Put on the gloves if contact with broken skin is likely.

5. Have the person turn onto his or her side facing away from you so that you can untie the gown at the neck and waist. Assist the person back into the supine position. If the person cannot turn onto his or her side, reach under the person and untie the gown.

6. Loosen the gown from around the person's body.

7. Unfold the clean gown and lay it over the person's chest.

8. Working with the person's strongest side first, remove one sleeve at a time, leaving the old gown draped over the person's body.

9. Working with the person's weakest side first, slide the arm through the sleeve of the clean gown. Repeat for the other arm.

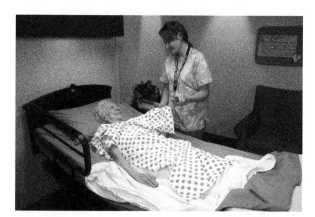

Step 9 Slide the person's arm through the sleeve of the clean gown.

10. Remove the soiled gown from underneath the clean gown and place it in the linen hamper or linen bag.

11. Have the person turn onto his or her side, facing away from you, so that you can tie the gown at the neck and waist (or reach under the person and tie the gown). Adjust the gown so that it fits comfortably.

12. If the side rails are in use, return the side rails to the raised position. Raise the head of the bed as the person requests.

13. Remove your gloves and dispose of them in a facility-approved waste container.

Finishing Up CLSOWR

14. Complete the "Finishing Up" steps.

PROCEDURE 18-5

Shampooing a Person's Hair in Bed

WHY YOU DO IT   Clean hair helps a person to look and feel attractive and is important for a person's self-esteem.

Getting Ready WGKIEᴅS

1. Complete the "Getting Ready" steps.

Supplies

- gloves (if contact with broken skin is likely)
- paper towels
- bed protector
- wash basin
- water pitcher
- bath thermometer
- shampoo trough
- comb
- brush
- blow dryer (optional)
- shampoo
- conditioner (optional)
- washcloth
- towels

Procedure

2. Make sure that the bed is positioned at a comfortable working height (to promote good body mechanics) and that the wheels are locked.

3. Fill the water pitcher with warm water (37.7°C [100°F] to 46.1°C [115°F] on the bath thermometer).

4. Cover the over-bed table with paper towels. Place the hair care supplies and clean linens on the over-bed table.

5. Raise the head of the bed as tolerated. Comb the person's hair to remove snarls and tangles.

6. Lower the head of the bed so that the bed is flat (as tolerated). If the side rails are in use, lower the side rail on the working side of the bed. The side rail on the opposite side of the bed should remain up.

7. Put on the gloves if contact with broken skin is likely.

8. Gently lift the person's head and shoulders and reposition the pillow under the person's shoulders. Cover the head of the bed and the pillow with the bed protector and place the shampoo trough on the bed protector. Help the person to rest his or her head on the shampoo trough. Place a towel across the person's shoulders and chest.

9. Place the wash basin on the floor beside the bed to catch the water as it drains from the shampoo trough.

10. Ask the person to hold the washcloth over his or her eyes.

11. Holding the water pitcher in one hand, slowly pour water over the person's hair until the hair is completely wet. Use your other hand to help direct the flow of water away from the person's eyes and ears.

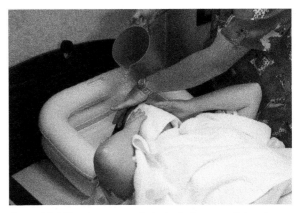

Step 11 Wet the person's hair, being careful to keep the water out of her eyes.

12. Apply a small amount of shampoo to the wet hair. Lather the hair and massage the scalp to help stimulate the circulation.

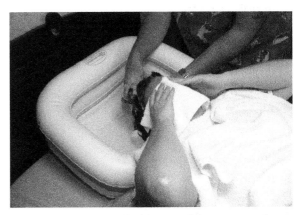

Step 12 Apply a small amount of shampoo and work it into a lather.

13. Using the water pitcher, rinse the hair thoroughly.

(continued)

14. Apply conditioner, as the person requests. Rinse the hair thoroughly.

15. Gently lift the person's head and shoulders and remove the shampoo trough and bed protector. Wrap the person's hair in a towel.

16. Raise the head of the bed as tolerated. Gently pat the person's face, neck, and ears dry and finish towel drying the hair.

17. Replace any wet or soiled linens. (If the side rails are in use, raise the side rails before leaving the bedside to get the necessary replacement linens.)

18. Comb the person's hair to remove snarls and tangles.

19. Dry and style the hair with the brush and blow dryer, as the person requests. Use the cool setting and take care not to burn the person's scalp or face.

20. Reposition the pillow under the person's head and straighten the bed linens. If the side rails are in use, return the side rails to the raised position. Lower the head of the bed as the person requests.

21. Gather the soiled linens and place them in the linen hamper or linen bag. Dispose of disposable items in a facility-approved waste container. Clean equipment and return it to the storage area.

22. Remove your gloves and dispose of them in a facility-approved waste container.

Finishing Up CLSOWR

23. Complete the "Finishing Up" steps.

PROCEDURE 18-6

Combing a Person's Hair

WHY YOU DO IT   Combing the hair helps to prevent tangles and gives the hair a neat appearance.

Getting Ready WGKJEPS

1. Complete the "Getting Ready" steps.

Supplies

- paper towels
- wide-toothed comb or pick
- brush
- mirror
- hair accessories (optional)
- detangler or leave-in conditioner (optional)
- towels

Procedure

2. Make sure that the bed is positioned at a comfortable working height (to promote good body mechanics) and that the wheels are locked.

3. Cover the over-bed table with paper towels. Place the hair care supplies and clean linens on the over-bed table.

4. Raise the head of the bed as tolerated. Gently lift the person's head and shoulders and cover the pillow with a towel. Drape another towel across the person's back and shoulders.

5. If the side rails are in use, lower the side rail on the working side of the bed. The side rail on the opposite side of the bed should remain up.

6. If the hair is tangled, work on the tangles first. Put a small amount of detangler or leave-in conditioner on the tangled hair. Begin at the ends of the hair and work toward the scalp. Hold the lock of hair just above the tangle (closest to the scalp) and use the wide-tooth comb to gently work through the tangle.

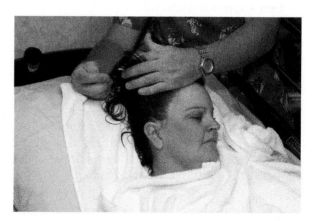

Step 6 Hold the lock of hair just above the tangle.

7. Using the brush and working with one 5 centimetres section at a time, gently brush the hair, moving from the roots of the hair toward the ends.

8. Secure the hair using barrettes, clips, or pins or braid the hair, as the person requests. Offer the person the mirror to check his or her appearance when you are finished.

9. Reposition the pillow under the person's head and straighten the bed linens. If the side rails are in use, return the side rails to the raised position. Lower the head of the bed as the person requests.

10. Gather the soiled linens and place them in the linen hamper or linen bag. Dispose of disposable items in a facility-approved waste container. Clean equipment and return it to the storage area.

Finishing Up CLSOWR

11. Complete the "Finishing Up" steps.

PROCEDURE 18-7

Shaving a Person's Face

WHY YOU DO IT   Shaving removes unwanted hair and is a routine grooming practice for many patients and residents.

Getting Ready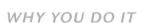

1. Complete the "Getting Ready" steps.

Supplies

- gloves
- paper towels
- safety razor
- shaving cream/gel/ soap
- shaving brush (if using shaving soap)
- aftershave lotion (optional)
- wash basin
- bath thermometer
- mirror
- washcloth
- towels

Procedure

2. Make sure that the bed is lowered to its lowest position and that the wheels are locked.

3. Fill the wash basin with warm water (37.7°C [100°F] to 46.1°C [115°F] on the bath thermometer).

4. Cover the over-bed table with paper towels. Place the wash basin, shaving supplies, and clean linens on the over-bed table.

5. If the side rails are in use, lower the side rail on the working side of the bed. The side rail on the opposite side of the bed should remain up.

6. Help the person to transfer from the bed to a bedside chair, assist the person to sit on the edge of the bed, or raise the head of the bed as tolerated.

7. Place a towel across the person's shoulders and chest.

8. Put on the gloves.

9. Wet the washcloth with warm, clean water. Soften the beard by holding the washcloth against the person's face for 2 to 3 minutes.

10. Apply shaving cream, gel, or soap to the beard.

11. Shave the person's cheeks:

    a. Stand facing the person.

    b. Gently pull the skin tight and shave downward, in the direction of hair growth (that is, toward the chin). Use short, even strokes, rinsing the razor frequently in the wash basin. Repeat until all of the lather on the cheek has been removed.

    c. Repeat for the other cheek.

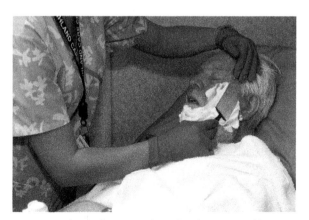

Step 11 Shave downward, in the direction of hair growth.

(continued)

12. Shave the person's chin:

   a. Ask the person to "tighten the chin" by drawing the lower lip over the teeth.

   b. Shave the chin using short, even, downward strokes. Repeat until all of the lather on the chin has been removed, rinsing the razor frequently in the wash basin.

13. Shave the person's neck:

   a. Ask the person to tip his head back.

   b. Gently pull the skin tight and shave upward, in the direction of hair growth (that is, toward the chin). Use short, even strokes, rinsing the razor frequently in the wash basin. Repeat until all of the lather on the neck has been removed.

14. Shave the area between the person's nose and upper lip:

   a. Ask the person to "tighten his upper lip" by drawing the upper lip over the teeth.

   b. Shave the area between the nose and the upper lip using short, even downward strokes. Repeat until all of the lather has been removed, rinsing the razor frequently in the wash basin.

15. Change the water in the wash basin. (If the side rails are in use, raise the side rails

before leaving the bedside.) Form a mitt around your hand with the washcloth and wet the mitt with warm, clean water. Wash the person's face and neck. Rinse thoroughly and pat the person's face, neck, and ears dry with the face towel.

16. Apply aftershave lotion, as the person requests.

17. If you have accidentally nicked the skin and the person is bleeding, apply direct pressure with a tissue until the bleeding stops. Report the incident to the nurse.

18. If necessary, help the person return to bed. If the side rails are in use, return the side rails to the raised position.

19. Gather the soiled linens and place them in the linen hamper or linen bag. Dispose of disposable items in a facility-approved waste container. Clean equipment and return it to the storage area.

20. Remove your gloves and dispose of them in a facility-approved waste container.

Finishing Up CLSOWR

21. Complete the "Finishing Up" steps.

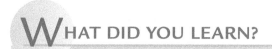

WHAT DID YOU LEARN?

Multiple Choice

Select the single best answer for each of the following questions.

1. You are a personal support worker in a long-term care facility. Which one of the following procedures may be beyond your scope of practice?
   a. Assisting a resident with bathing
   b. Polishing a female resident's fingernails
   c. Trimming the toenails of a resident with diabetes
   d. Assisting a resident with oral hygiene

2. When helping a person to dress, which item of clothing would you put on first?
   a. Underpants
   b. Socks
   c. Slacks
   d. Sweater

3. Mrs. Dinksley, one of your residents, had a stroke that caused her left side to become weak. You are helping Mrs. Dinksley put on a cardigan sweater. Which arm should you put in the sleeve first?
   a. The left arm
   b. The right arm
   c. Either arm; it makes no difference
   d. Neither arm; Mrs. Dinksley should wear a hospital gown

4. Mr. Bush has just been admitted to the long-term care facility where you work. You are telling him about the facility's policies. One of these policies is that residents are bathed on Monday, Wednesday, and Friday mornings. Mr. Bush looks worried, and says that he always bathes and shaves before he goes to bed, and he likes to do this every night. How do you react to this?
   a. You tell Mr. Bush that you're sorry, but he has to follow facility policy.
   b. You tell Mr. Bush "OK" but then schedule him for a bath every Monday, Wednesday, and Friday morning, just like everyone else.
   c. You respect Mr. Bush's choice and ask the nurse if you can schedule him for a bath and a shave as part of evening care, every evening.
   d. You report Mr. Bush to the nurse because he is being difficult.

5. Brushing the hair is important to:
   a. Make it grow faster
   b. Make it soft and shiny and prevent tangles
   c. Keep it clean
   d. Keep it free from lice

6. When shaving a man's face with a safety razor and shaving cream, you should:
   a. Soften the beard with warm water before applying the shaving cream
   b. Apply aftershave lotion after the shave is complete, if the man requests it
   c. Give the man a mirror so that he can check his appearance when you are finished
   d. All of the above

7. When shaving a man's face, you should:
   a. Apply shaving cream sparingly
   b. Use upward strokes when shaving the cheeks
   c. Apply an antiseptic to any cuts or nicks
   d. Use downward strokes to shave the chin

8. Which one of the following statements about nail care is true?
   a. Scissors are used to trim the nails.
   b. Elderly people do not need nail care because their nails do not grow as fast.
   c. Providing nail care allows you to examine the hands and feet for signs of health and disease.
   d. Nail care is an activity that can be skipped if there is not enough time.

9. Which one of the following benefits does a patient or resident enjoy when you shampoo his or her hair?
   a. Improved circulation (blood flow) to the scalp
   b. A clean, neat appearance
   c. Increased feelings of well-being
   d. All of the above

10. Which one of the following statements about helping a resident to dress is true?
    a. Residents like staff members to decide what they are going to wear.
    b. Residents are used to being dressed in front of others.

c. Residents care about how they look.

d. Residents who are disabled do not need to dress in street clothes.

11. One of your residents, Mrs. Ament, has diabetes. Why is providing foot care an important part of caring for Mrs. Ament?

a. The circulation to her feet is likely to be poor, which puts her at risk for infection and other complications.

b. Diabetes makes the toenails grow faster.

c. People with diabetes usually do not take good care of their feet.

d. All of the above.

12. You must remove a soiled gown from a patient who has an intravenous (IV) line. What is the best way to do this?

a. Remove the gown from the arm with the IV first.

b. Ask the nurse to disconnect the bag and tubing before beginning.

c. Disconnect the bag and tubing before beginning.

d. Remove the opposite arm from the gown first.

Matching

Match each numbered item with its appropriate lettered description.

_____ 1. Pediculosis capitis

_____ 2. Alopecia

_____ 3. Podiatrist

_____ 4. Tinea pedis

_____ 5. Tinea capitis

a. A fungal infection of the scalp

b. Loss of hair

c. A fungal infection of the feet

d. Head lice

e. A doctor who specializes in care of the feet

STOP and Think!

Today you are helping Mrs. Wiseman get dressed. She is especially excited this morning because it is Saturday and her son is coming to visit. Since her son's favourite color is blue, Mrs. Wiseman has picked out a lightweight blue blouse to wear. You know that Mrs. Wisemen tends to chill easily, and you don't think she is going to be comfortable wearing the blouse that she has picked out. You suggest a different blouse, but Mrs. Wiseman tells you that she would rather wear the blouse that she picked out originally. How can you provide Mrs. Wiseman with her choice of clothing and still make sure that she is warm enough? What other grooming tasks can you help Mrs. Wiseman with so that she feels presentable for her son's visit?

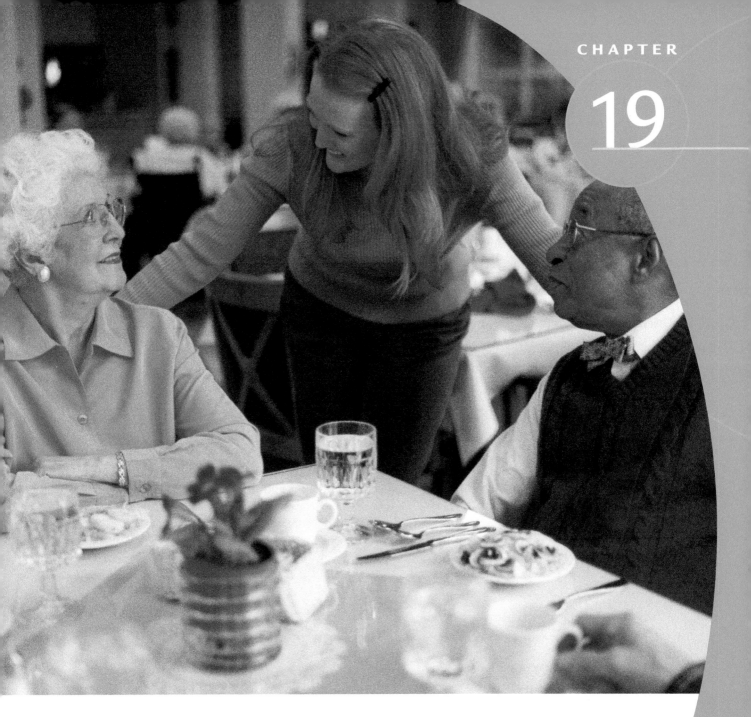

Basic Nutrition

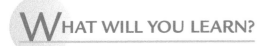
WHAT WILL YOU LEARN?

Few things are more satisfying than a good meal—you know, one that is made up of your favourite foods, all cooked to perfection, just like Mom's home cooking. Eating meets many needs for people, both emotionally and physically. In this chapter, you will learn about what we need to eat to keep our bodies healthy. You will also learn how to help your

Photo: Meal time is as much about socializing as it is about eating. (Punchstock)

371

patients and residents to meet their own nutritional needs. When you are finished with this chapter, you will be able to:

1. Define the term *nutrition* and explain why our bodies need adequate nutrition.
2. List the general types of nutrients and describe how the body uses them.
3. Discuss how Canada's Food Guide can be used to help plan and provide better nutrition for a person.
4. Explain factors that influence a person's food preferences.
5. List and describe common special diets.
6. Discuss the importance of making meals attractive and the dining experience pleasant.
7. Explain the steps that are taken to help prepare a person for meal time.
8. Describe ways that a personal support worker may need to help a person during meal time.
9. Demonstrate proper technique for feeding a person who cannot feed herself.
10. Describe how the amount of solid food eaten is recorded.
11. Discuss other ways of providing nutrition for people who are unable to take food by mouth.
12. Explain the fluid needs of the body and factors that affect the body's fluid balance.
13. Demonstrate methods used to measure and record fluid intake and output.

Vocabulary

Nutrients	Fat-soluble	Nasogastric tube	Fluid balance
Nutrition	Water-soluble	Nasointestinal tube	Dehydration
Ingestion	Obese	Gastrostomy tube	Edema
Digestion	Appetite	Jejunostomy tube	NPO status
Absorption	Anorexia	Percutaneous endoscopic	Intake and output (I&O)
Metabolism	Dietitian	gastrostomy (PEG) tube	flow sheet
Calories	Nutritional supplement	Total parenteral	Graduate
Glucose	Intravenous (IV) therapy	nutrition (TPN,	
Amino acids	Enteral nutrition	hyperalimentation)	

FOOD AND HOW OUR BODIES USE IT

All living things eat. The food that we take into our bodies is broken down into essential elements, called **nutrients.** The body uses these nutrients to grow, to repair itself, and to carry out processes essential for living. **Nutrition,** or the process of taking in and using food, involves the following steps:

- **Ingestion,** the intake of food
- **Digestion,** the breaking down of food into simple elements (nutrients)
- **Absorption,** the transfer of these nutrients from the digestive tract into the bloodstream
- **Metabolism,** the process that occurs in cells to convert the nutrients into energy

To function, the body needs a continuous supply of energy, which it gets from the metabolism of food. You know that your body uses energy when you run to catch a bus, reposition a patient or resident, or climb a flight of stairs. But did you also know that your body uses energy even when you are sitting perfectly still? Every time you blink, or your heart beats, or your lungs expand to take in air, you are using energy. The energy to power our bodies comes from food, especially food that is high in carbohydrates, protein, or fat. Energy is measured in units called kilocalories, more commonly known as **calories.**

In addition to providing us with energy, food provides us with other substances our bodies need to function properly. Other substances found in food that benefit us include vitamins and minerals, fibre, and water:

- **Vitamins** and **minerals** are small molecules that help to regulate body processes and form structures within the body. For example, vitamin K helps the blood to clot, and calcium, a mineral, helps to build strong bones. Table 19-1 lists some of the common vitamins and minerals and describes how they benefit the body.

- **Fibre** is found in fruits, vegetables, and whole grain cereals and breads. Fibre may be soluble, which means that it can be broken down (digested). Or it may be insoluble, which means that it cannot be digested. Insoluble fibre helps to prevent problems with bowel movements by adding bulk to the feces.

Table 19-1 Vitamins and Minerals

NUTRIENT	SOURCES	FUNCTION
VITAMINS		
Vitamin A	Liver, carrots, egg yolks, fortified milk	Helps us to see in dim light Keeps skin and mucous membranes healthy
Vitamin B_1 (thiamin)	Pork, liver, whole and enriched grains, legumes	Helps produce energy from glucose Assists with nerve function
Vitamin B_2 (riboflavin)	Milk, organ meats (for example, brain, kidneys, liver), enriched grains, green vegetables	Assists with the metabolism of carbohydrates, protein, and fat
Vitamin B_3 (niacin)	Kidneys, grains, lean meats, nuts	Assists with the metabolism of carbohydrates, protein, and fat
Vitamin B_{12}	Meat (including organ meats), eggs, milk, cheese	Assists with the formation of hemoglobin (the molecule that carries oxygen throughout the body) and red blood cells
Folic acid	Green leafy vegetables, meats, and whole grains	Assists with protein metabolism and the formation of red blood cells
Vitamin C (ascorbic acid)	Citrus fruits, broccoli, green peppers, strawberries, green leafy vegetables	Assists with tissue healing, building red blood cells, and iron absorption
Vitamin D	Sunlight, fortified milk, fish liver oils	Assists with the absorption of calcium and phosphorus to strengthen bones
Vitamin E	Vegetable oils, wheat germ, whole grains	Assists with the formation of red blood cells Assists with the reproductive system
Vitamin K	Vegetable oils, wheat germ, whole grains, liver, green leafy vegetables, eggs	Assists with metabolism of the proteins necessary for normal blood clotting
MINERALS		
Calcium	Milk, cheese, canned fish with bones, green leafy vegetables	Keeps the teeth and bones strong Assists with blood clotting Assists with nerve function and contraction of the heart and skeletal muscles
Phosphorus	Milk, soft drinks, meat, nuts, peas, beans	Keeps the teeth and bones strong Assists with the metabolism of carbohydrates, protein, and fat
Iron	Liver, lean meats, enriched and whole grain breads, cheese, green leafy vegetables	Used to produce hemoglobin (the molecule that carries oxygen throughout the body)
Iodine	Table salt and seafood	Used by the thyroid gland to produce hormones for cell metabolism
Sodium	Table salt	Assists with fluid balance, nerve function, and contraction of the heart and skeletal muscles
Potassium	Whole grains, fruits, green leafy vegetables	Assists with fluid balance, nerve function, and contraction of the heart and skeletal muscles

- **Water,** which will be discussed in more detail later in this chapter, plays many important roles in helping the body to function well.

TYPES OF NUTRIENTS

There are six general types of nutrients. Three of these nutrient types (carbohydrates, proteins, and fat) supply energy. The remaining three (minerals, vitamins, and water) regulate body processes.

Carbohydrates

Foods containing carbohydrates form the basis of many diets throughout the world because these foods tend to be plentiful and inexpensive. Carbohydrates are found in bread, cereal, fruit, vegetables, and table sugar. Carbohydrates are the source of the body's most basic type of fuel, **glucose.** Glucose, sometimes called "blood sugar," is carried in the blood and rapidly absorbed by every cell in the body. The cells use the glucose to "run," much like your car uses gas. Glucose is a simple carbohydrate, or sugar, which means that it passes quickly from the digestive tract into the bloodstream. Other carbohydrates, known as complex carbohydrates, or starches, must be broken down into simple sugars before the body can use them. Extra carbohydrates that are not used immediately as fuel are either stored in the liver or converted to fat and stored elsewhere in the body. Each gram of carbohydrate provides the body with 4 calories, or energy units.

Protein

Protein is found in foods such as milk and cheese, meat, poultry, fish, eggs, nuts, and dried peas and beans. Proteins contain **amino acids,** small molecules that are the "building blocks" of all of the body's cells. Therefore, foods containing protein help the body to rebuild tissue that breaks down from normal use and to grow new tissue after illness or injury. In addition to providing amino acids, protein is a source of fuel. Like carbohydrates, protein provides the body with 4 calories per gram.

Fats (Lipids)

Fats are found in butter, cooking oils, whole milk, cheese, meat, egg yolks, nuts, shortening, and lard. Fats make food taste better and satisfy the appetite longer because they take longer to digest than most other food sources. Although a "low-fat" diet is recommended for most people to maintain health, not all fats are bad. In fact, the body requires a certain amount of dietary fat to function properly. For example, some vitamins will dissolve only in fat, not water (that is, they are **fat-soluble**). This means that fat must be present in order for the body to use the vitamins. Fat also protects our organs and helps us to stay warm. Finally, fats are the most concentrated source of energy, providing 9 calories per gram.

Vitamins

Vitamins, as described earlier and in Table 19-1, play a key role in many body processes. Vitamins are classified as water-soluble or fat-soluble. **Water-soluble** vitamins dissolve in water. Water-soluble vitamins (vitamin C and the B-complex vitamins) are absorbed directly from the digestive tract into the bloodstream. The body cannot store water-soluble vitamins. Instead, any extra amounts of these vitamins are passed from the body in the urine. This means that water-soluble vitamins must be replenished daily for use by the body.

Fat-soluble vitamins (vitamins A, D, E, and K) are absorbed and stored in the body's fat, where they can be used as needed. Unlike water-soluble vitamins, fat-soluble vitamins are not easily passed from the body. For this reason, consuming too much of a fat-soluble vitamin can be as harmful as not consuming enough, because the vitamin builds up in the body. In some cases, this build-up may actually be harmful.

Minerals

Minerals help provide structure within the body. For example, fluoride strengthens the teeth and calcium strengthens the bones. Minerals also regulate body processes. For example, red blood cells need iron to do their job of carrying oxygen to all of the cells in the body. Key minerals that the body needs to function properly are summarized in Table 19-1.

Water

Water is provided in the diet in the form of beverages, such as juice, soda, milk, coffee, tea, and, of course, water! Water is also found in many foods, such as fruits and vegetables. Water provides no calories or nutrition, but may be more essential to life than food. You can live for quite a long time without food, but only for 3 to 7 days without water. Every cell in your body contains water, which is why water accounts for approximately 50% to 60% of your body weight! Water does the following things for our bodies:

- The nutrients found in food must be dissolved in fluid and circulated throughout the body. Water forms the basis for this fluid.
- Water transports waste products out of the body, by way of the urine and feces.
- Water keeps us cool when it evaporates from our skin in the form of sweat.
- Water keeps the mucous membranes moist.
- Water forms the basis of the fluid that helps our joints to move smoothly.

A BALANCED DIET

For the best health, you must follow a diet that provides your body with a balanced amount of the essential nutrients. Two tools are available to help you achieve this goal—Canada's Food Guide and the nutrition labels on food.

Canada's Food Guide

In Canada, the number of children and adults who are overweight or **obese** (extremely overweight) is increasing every year. Unhealthy eating habits, combined with a lack of physical activity, are the primary reasons we are seeing an increase in obesity. As a result, we are also seeing a significant increase in health problems related to being overweight or obese, such as cardiovascular disease and diabetes.

To help Canadians plan a healthy diet, the Canadian government developed Canada's Food Guide (Fig. 19-1). Because many different cultural groups are represented in Canada, Canada's Food Guide includes food choices that are representative of different cultures. Canada's Food Guide emphasizes the importance of getting enough physical activity and eating a healthy, balanced diet. Some foods contain many nutrients that our bodies need to remain healthy, but other foods have little or no nutritional value. The best way to get the nutrients you need is to eat a variety of healthy food every day. Canada's Food Guide describes a healthy diet as one that:

- Emphasizes fruits, vegetables, whole grains, and fat-free or low-fat milk products
- Includes lean meats, poultry, fish, beans, eggs, and nuts
- Is low in saturated fats, *trans* fats, cholesterol, salt (sodium), and added sugars

In general, the recommendations in Canada's Food Guide apply for all healthy people older than 2 years. However, nutritional requirements vary at different times throughout a person's life. For example:

- Infants and young children have an increased need for calories and iron because they are growing rapidly.
- Teenagers experiencing "growth spurts" have increased caloric and nutritional needs.
- Pregnant and breast-feeding women need more protein and calcium.
- People who are recovering from physical trauma, such as that caused by burns or surgery, have different nutritional requirements than healthy people. Similarly, some illnesses change the nutritional requirements of the body, including chronic conditions such as diabetes, kidney disease, or alcoholism.
- Older people have different nutritional requirements, because of the physical changes that occur with normal aging. Older people do not need as many calories as younger people because they are usually less active. They also may not feel thirsty as often, although the need for water and other fluids increases with age.

Food Labels

There is a second tool available to help you plan a balanced diet—the nutrition labels that appear on most foods offered for sale at the grocery store. Education about proper nutrition and diet planning is one of the most effective ways of promoting health and helping to prevent some illnesses. The labels of all packaged foods include information about the food's nutritional value, approximate serving size, and any related health claims (Fig. 19-2). By reading the nutrition label, you can see how the food can help you to achieve your nutrition goals for the day.

FACTORS THAT AFFECT FOOD CHOICES AND EATING HABITS

Canada's Food Guide and food labels help us to make wise food choices. However, factors other than the nutritional content of a food often affect the choices we make about what we eat and when we eat it. Some people prefer a hot, hearty breakfast to start the day, while others may want only a bowl of cereal or coffee and toast. Some

(Text continued on page 378)

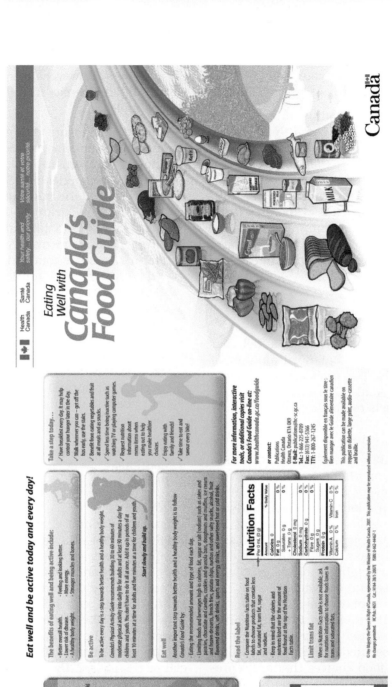

Health Canada / Santé Canada

Your health and safety... our priority. / Votre santé et votre sécurité... notre priorité.

Eating Well with Canada's Food Guide

Canada

Advice for different ages and stages...

Children
Following Canada's Food Guide helps children grow and thrive.

Young children have small appetites and need calories for growth and development.

- Serve small nutritious meals and snacks each day.
- Do not restrict nutritious foods because of their fat content. Offer a variety of foods from the four food groups.
- Most of all... be a good role model.

Women of childbearing age
All women who could become pregnant and those who are pregnant or breastfeeding need a multivitamin containing folic acid every day.

Pregnant women need to ensure that their multivitamin also contains iron. A health care professional can help you find the multivitamin that's right for you.

Pregnant and breastfeeding women need more calories. Include an extra 2 to 3 Food Guide Servings each day.

Here are two examples:
- Have fruit and yogurt for a snack, or
- Have an extra slice of toast at breakfast and an extra glass of milk at supper.

Men and women over 50
The need for vitamin D increases after the age of 50.

In addition to following Canada's Food Guide, everyone over the age of 50 should take a daily vitamin D supplement of 10 µg (400 IU).

How do I count Food Guide Servings in a meal?

Here is an example:

Vegetable and beef stir-fry with rice, a glass of milk and an apple for dessert

250 mL (1 cup) mixed broccoli, carrot and sweet red pepper	=	2 Vegetables and Fruit Food Guide Servings
75 g (2½ oz.) lean beef	=	1 Meat and Alternatives Food Guide Serving
250 mL (1 cup) brown rice	=	2 Grain Products Food Guide Servings
5 mL (1 tsp) canola oil	=	part of your Oils and Fats intake for the day
250 mL (1 cup) 1% milk	=	1 Milk and Alternatives Food Guide Serving
1 apple	=	1 Vegetables and Fruit Food Guide Serving

Eat well and be active today and every day!

The benefits of eating well and being active include:
- Better overall health.
- Lower risk of disease.
- A healthy body weight.
- Feeling and looking better.
- More energy.
- Stronger muscles and bones.

Be active
To be active every day is a step towards better health and a healthy body weight.

Canada's Physical Activity Guide recommends building 30 to 60 minutes of moderate physical activity into daily life for adults and at least 90 minutes a day for children and youth. You don't have to do it all at once. Add it up in periods of at least 10 minutes at a time for adults and five minutes at a time for children and youth.

Start slowly and build up.

Eat well
Another important step towards better health and a healthy body weight is to follow Canada's Food Guide by:

- Eating the recommended amount and type of food each day.
- Limiting foods and beverages high in calories, fat, sugar or salt (sodium) such as cakes and pastries, chocolate and candies, cookies and granola bars, doughnuts and muffins, ice cream and frozen desserts, french fries, potato chips, nachos and other salty snacks, alcohol, fruit flavoured drinks, soft drinks, sports and energy drinks, and sweetened hot or cold drinks.

Read the label
- Compare the Nutrition Facts table on food labels to choose products that contain less fat, saturated fat, trans fat, sugar and sodium.
- Keep in mind that the calories and nutrients listed are for the amount of food found at the top of the Nutrition Facts table.

Nutrition Facts
Per 0 mL (0 g)

Amount	% Daily Value
Calories 0	
Fat 0 g	0 %
Saturated 0 g	0 %
+ Trans 0 g	
Cholesterol 0 mg	
Sodium 0 mg	0 %
Carbohydrate 0 g	0 %
Fibre 0 g	0 %
Sugars 0 g	
Protein 0 g	
Vitamin A 0 %	Vitamin C 0 %
Calcium 0 %	Iron 0 %

Limit trans fat
When a Nutrition Facts table is not available, ask for nutrition information to choose foods lower in trans and saturated fats.

Take a step today...
- Have breakfast every day. It may help control your hunger later in the day.
- Walk wherever you can — get off the bus early, use the stairs.
- Benefit from eating vegetables and fruit at all meals and as snacks.
- Spend less time being inactive such as watching TV or playing computer games.
- Request nutrition information about menu items when eating out to help you make healthier choices.
- Enjoy eating with family and friends!
- Take time to eat and savour every bite!

For more information, interactive tools, or additional copies visit Canada's Food Guide on-line at:
www.healthcanada.gc.ca/foodguide

or contact:
Publications
Health Canada
Ottawa, Ontario K1A 0K9
E-mail: publications@hc-sc.gc.ca
Tel.: 1-866-225-0709
Fax: (613) 941-5366
TTY: 1-800-267-1245

Également disponible en français sous le titre :
Bien manger avec le Guide alimentaire canadien

This publication can be made available on request on diskette, large print, audio-cassette and braille.

376

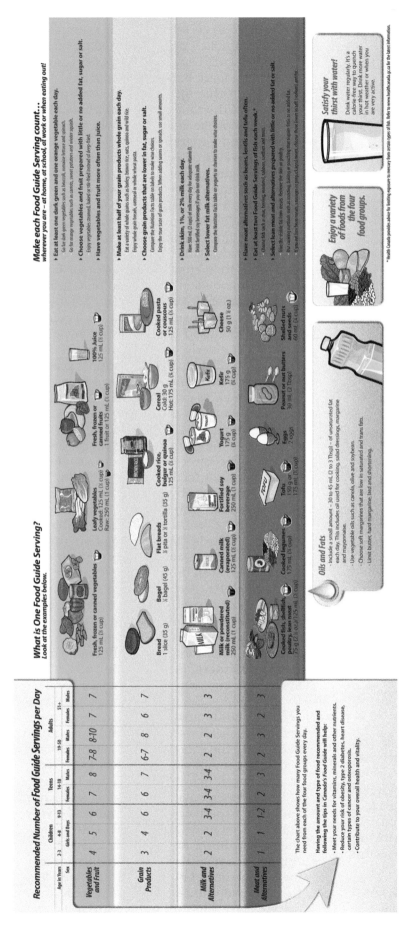

Figure 19-1

Canada's Food Guide was developed by the Canadian government to help Canadians plan a healthy diet. Canada Food Guide recommends balancing food intake and physical activity, and choosing foods that have high nutritional value.

Nutrition Facts
Serving Size 1 1/2 oz (40 g/about 5 dried plums)
Servings Per Container About 9

Amount Per Serving

Calories 100   Calories from Fat 0

	% Daily Value*
Total Fat 0 g	**0%**
Saturated Fat 0 g	**0%**
Cholesterol 0 mg	**0%**
Sodium 5 mg	**0%**
Potassium 290 mg	**8%**
Total Carbohydrate 24 g	**8%**
Dietary Fiber 3 g	**11%**
Soluble Fiber 1 g	
Insoluble Fiber 1 g	
Sugars 12 g	
Protein 1 g	

Vitamin A 10% (100% as beta carotene)

Vitamin C 0%   •   Iron 2%

Calcium 2%

*Percent Daily Values are based on a 2,000 calorie diet. Your daily values may be higher or lower depending on your calorie needs:

		Calories:	2,000	2,500
Total Fat	Less than		65 g	80 g
Sat Fat	Less than		20 g	25 g
Cholesterol	Less than		300 mg	300 mg
Sodium	Less than		2,400 mg	2,400 mg
Potassium			3,500 mg	3,500 mg
Total Carbohydrate			300 g	375 g
Dietary Fiber			25 g	30 g

INGREDIENTS: PITTED CALIFORNIA DRIED PLUMS (PRUNES), NATURAL AND ARTIFICIAL FLAVOR, POTASSIUM SORBATE AS A PRESERVATIVE.
PACKED BY: SUNSWEET GROWERS INC. YUBA CITY, CA 95993-9370 U.S.A.
® SUNSWEET and THE SMART SNACK are Registered Trademarks of Sunsweet Growers Inc. in the U.S. and Other Countries
© SUNSWEET GROWERS INC.
FOR QUESTIONS OR COMMENTS CALL:
1-800-417-2253, 9 A.M.-6 P.M. (E.T.), MON.-FRI.
OR VISIT OUR WEB SITE: WWW.SUNSWEET.COM

☀ *Look for the Sun to See*
Sunsweet Dried Plums Healthy Facts

Exchange: 1 1/2 fruit. Exchange calculations based on the Exchange Lists for Meal Planning. © 1995 The American Dietetic Association, the American Diabetes Association.

Figure 19-2
The law requires all packaged foods to have a nutrition label like this one. (*Courtesy of Sunsweet Growers, Inc.*)

people like a light meal at lunch time, while others eat their main meal at mid-day. Dinner may consist of a light snack for some while others routinely have a seven-course meal. Listed below are some of the factors that affect a person's food choices and eating habits. Think about your own eating habits and food likes and dislikes. Are any of your personal preferences related to the factors listed here?

- **Religion.** Dietary restrictions are a part of many religions. Some of these restrictions are specific to certain days (for example, the Roman Catholic custom of avoiding meat on Fridays during Lent, or the Jewish tradition of avoiding flour-based foods during Passover). Other dietary restrictions are in effect all of the time (for example, some Jewish people keep a kosher kitchen).

- **Culture and geography.** People often like certain foods because they are associated with their culture, or the area where they grew up. Cultural preferences are a combination of heritage, religion, geography, and all of the characteristics that make a person unique. Some people are willing to try new foods, while others prefer to stay with what they know. This desire for familiar foods is one reason why chain restaurants are so popular in Canada.

- **Finances.** Food can be expensive. People who are on a fixed income, especially disabled or elderly people, may find it difficult to afford foods that supply good nutrition. Often, fresh fruits and vegetables and lean cuts of meat are among the most expensive items in the grocery cart. Milk and cheese, which are also nutritious, may also be out of many people's price range. Instead, people in the lower economic levels often rely on cheaper foods that are high in calories and carbohydrates, but low in many nutrients. Fortunately, a small food budget does not necessarily make it impossible to eat healthy foods. With information and planning, it is possible to afford nutritionally sound food, even on a fixed income.

- **Kitchen skills.** People who do not know how to cook, do not like to cook, or do not have time to cook may choose to eat in restaurants more often. They may also rely on convenience foods and packaged foods.

- **Individual taste.** Some people find certain foods delicious, while others could barely swallow a bite. Some people may not like a certain food because of its texture, or the degree of spiciness. Others will avoid a food because of the way it looks or smells. Many people are unable to eat certain foods, no matter how much they love them, because of food allergies. As you certainly know from your own experience, individual tastes vary greatly, even among people who belong to the same culture (or the same family)!

- **Appetite.** Appetite is simply the desire for food. Appetite is both physically driven (by the feeling of hunger) and emotionally driven. Have you ever had your television show interrupted by a commercial for some type of food, where the food looked so good you actually started to feel hungry? You may not have actually been physically hungry, but the sight of the food and the thought of how it would taste stimulated your appetite. The opposite can be true as well. For example, a person who is ill or under emotional stress may be physically hungry, but have no appetite for any food. This loss of appetite is called **anorexia.**

Helping Hands and a Caring Heart

FOCUS ON HUMANISTIC HEALTH CARE

Meal times can be difficult for people who are receiving health care. The person may miss his or her family members. Foods that the person used to love may no longer be on the person's diet. Pain, anxiety, illness, and medication side effects can cause the person to have little or no appetite. Part of providing humanistic care is encouraging your patients to eat adequate amounts of food, even when they have no appetite. Actions such as making sure the food is served at the appropriate temperature, providing pleasant conversation, and assisting the person to be physically comfortable help the person to relax and enjoy the meal.

SPECIAL DIETS

Meals prepared for people in health care facilities are specific to each person's individual needs. Personal preferences are taken into account when planning meals. To find out as much as possible about the patient's or resident's eating habits and food likes and dislikes, a nurse completes a dietary assessment as part of the admissions process. During the assessment, the nurse asks the person (or his family members, if the person cannot answer for himself) about eating habits, favourite foods, and foods that should be avoided. This information is shared with the **dietitian,** a person who has a degree in nutrition. The dietitian uses the information from the dietary assessment, as well as her knowledge of nutrition, to plan a diet for the person that he will enjoy eating and that will keep him healthy.

The type of diet that is ordered for a person in a health care setting is determined by many factors. People with illnesses such as diabetes, heart disease, or kidney disease require special diets.

People who are recovering from surgery or trauma may require liquid or high-calorie diets for a period of time. Just the normal changes in the digestive system that accompany aging may require foods that are easier to chew, easier to digest, and have added fibre to help prevent constipation. Specific diets are ordered by a doctor and prepared by a dietitian.

Brief descriptions of some of the special diets that you may see ordered in a health care facility are provided here. It is important for you to familiarize yourself with your facility's specific diets and the foods that they include. That way, if a mistake is made in the kitchen and the wrong meal is delivered for one of your patients or residents, you will be able to recognize that an error has been made. Diets that are commonly seen in health care facilities include the following:

- **Regular ("house") diet.** This is simply a well-balanced diet. There are no restrictions on specific foods or condiments (for example, salt, pepper, ketchup, salad dressing). A person on a regular diet is usually allowed to eat foods prepared and brought by friends and family members. There are many variations to the regular diet. For example, a high-calorie or low-calorie version may be ordered to promote weight gain or weight loss. A low-residue or high-fibre version may be ordered to either decrease or increase dietary fibre for people with certain digestive problems. A bland diet contains foods that are easy to digest and will not irritate the digestive tract.
- **Clear liquid diet.** Clear liquids are substances that can be poured at room or body temperature and that you can see through. Foods that are considered clear liquids include water, gelatin, fat-free broth or bouillon, popsicles, clear juices (for example, apple, cranberry, grape), clear carbonated sodas, and coffee and tea (without cream). A person who is nauseous or vomiting, or who has just had surgery or is recovering from an acute illness or trauma, may be given a clear liquid diet initially. Clear liquids do not contain enough nutrients to maintain health for very long, so a person is usually progressed into a more nutritious diet as soon as the body can tolerate it.
- **Full liquid diet.** A full liquid diet is the clear liquid diet, plus any food that can be poured at room or body temperature. For example, milk, plain frozen desserts (such as popsicles, ice cream, or frozen yogurt),

pasteurized eggs (egg custard or eggnog), cereal gruels, and strained soups and juices are all considered full liquids. Full liquids contain more nutrition than clear liquids, but a high-calorie, high-protein liquid dietary supplement may be added if the person must be on a full-liquid diet for more than 3 days.

- **Soft diet.** Soft diets are usually regular diets that have been changed slightly to remove foods that are hard to chew or digest. The soft diet is used for people who have difficulty chewing or swallowing their food. The soft diet is not highly seasoned and does not contain foods that are fried or high in fibre. Soft diets contain adequate nutrition. Therefore, a person can remain on a soft diet for as long as is necessary.

- **Diabetic diet (consistent-carbohydrate diabetes meal plan).** This diet regulates the amount of fat, carbohydrates, and protein that a person with diabetes mellitus consumes. The person's specific energy and nutritional requirements determine the amounts of fat, carbohydrates, and protein that are permitted. The diet is different for each person. A person with diabetes who is receiving insulin injections must eat enough to prevent her blood sugar levels from dropping. When caring for patients or residents who have diabetes, you must make special note of the amount of food the person eats at each meal.

- **Sodium-restricted diet.** Sodium restriction is helpful for the treatment of certain types of heart disease, hypertension (high blood pressure), and kidney disease. A person on a sodium-restricted diet may be allowed to have a small amount of salt, or none at all. For example, some people may be able to eat foods that have some salt in them, but they will not be allowed to add extra salt at the table or eat very salty foods, such as pickles. Other people may have severe restrictions placed on their salt intake. For these people, food will be prepared without any salt at all, and of course, the person will not be able to add salt to the food at the table. Some people on sodium-restricted diets may use salt substitutes. If you have a patient or resident who has been placed on a sodium-restricted diet, make sure you know whether he is allowed to use a little bit of salt or a salt substitute, or none at all.

- **Low-cholesterol diet.** Following a diet that is low in saturated fats and cholesterol is

good advice for everybody, but it is especially good advice for a person with heart disease. Foods are chosen that are lower in animal fat and prepared in ways that do not add additional fats. The addition of butter, shortening, and margarine to foods is avoided, and foods such as fruits and vegetables, whole grains, and skim milk are encouraged.

Some of your patients or residents will have **nutritional supplements** that are either offered with the meal or as an in-between meal snack. These nutritional supplements, which can be used to supply extra calories or protein, often take the form of a flavored shake or drink. These drinks are convenient and easy to serve. People with diabetes mellitus may require snacks in between meals to keep their blood sugar levels stable. The dietitian will plan for the nutritional supplements. It is usually the personal support worker's responsibility to serve these nutritional supplements at specific times throughout the day and record that the supplements have been consumed. If your patient or resident refuses to eat an ordered supplement, report this to a nurse.

As you can see, the people you are caring for could be placed on any number of special diets for a variety of reasons. Take the time to learn about a person's medical condition, and the reason a particular diet was ordered for that person. For example, you could ask the nurse if she knows of any articles you could read about the person's condition. This additional information will give you the insight you need to make good observations about a person's dietary habits. Your patients or residents will benefit, and so will you, because you will become a more effective member of the health care team.

MEAL TIME

A tasty meal, good company, and a relaxed dining atmosphere satisfy physical needs (hunger) as well as emotional ones (the need for love and belonging). In most cultures, eating is a social event. We eat at parties and celebrations, we eat on dates, we eat certain foods on certain holidays, and we look forward to catching up with family members and friends over the dinner table (Fig. 19-3). Now imagine that you have just moved into a long-term care facility or been admitted to the hospital. Who will you share your meals with? Would you miss one special dish that your family always has for Sunday dinner?

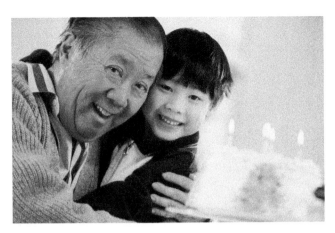

Figure 19-3
In most cultures, food plays a central role at social events.

You might find yourself feeling a little lonely and homesick.

Meal time for people in a health care setting can be difficult for many reasons:

- The person may miss family members or familiar foods.
- Food choices may be limited or the food may not be prepared the way the person likes it.
- Meals are usually served at specific times, not just when the person feels like eating.
- Meal time can be lonely, especially if the person must stay in his or her room to eat.
- Physical problems (such as pain or nausea) and emotional problems (such as anxiety) can affect a person's appetite.
- The person may be embarrassed if he or she needs help to eat.

Long-term care facilities have policies that relate to the resident's dining experience (Box 19-1). These regulations ensure that each resident's

---

BOX 19-1 **Standards Relating to the Resident's Dining Experience**

- Meals must meet the individual nutritional needs of each resident.
- Food must be served at the proper temperature.
- Food must be appealing to look at and seasoned to the individual resident's preference.
- Special diets, such as those followed for religious reasons, must be provided.
- Dining in the company of other residents is recommended.
- Residents in rehabilitation who are learning how to eat independently again must have a private area in which to eat.

---

rights are respected. They help to ensure that meal time is as enjoyable as possible for the resident. By providing companionship and assistance as needed, you can help to make sure that meal time remains a pleasant part of your patient's or resident's daily routine. Food should be presented in a way that will stimulate the appetite. Offering small portions of favourite foods frequently throughout the day can help increase a person's desire to eat. A clean, fresh mouth makes food taste better. A comfortable position, whether the person is using an over-bed table in bed or is seated at a regular table in the dining room, keeps the person focused on the food. If the person uses glasses or a hearing aid, make sure that these aids are in place. Provide pleasant conversation. All of these measures help to set a relaxed overall atmosphere and stimulate the appetite.

PREPARING FOR MEAL TIME

You will need to help your patients and residents get ready for each meal. Be sure to give your patients or residents enough time to prepare for meals. Allowing time to prepare is especially important before breakfast, because early morning care must be completed before the meal. In a long-term care facility, the residents are assisted to the dining room to eat. In a hospital, the patients usually take their meals in their rooms. The assistance you provide will vary, depending on the person you are helping. Some people only need to be reminded that it is "almost time for lunch" and they will prepare themselves to eat. Others will need your help to get ready for the meal. The following actions are taken to help prepare a person for meal time:

- Assist the person with toileting. Help him to the bathroom, or offer the bedpan or urinal.
- Assist the person with basic hygiene. Help him to wash his hands and face, and brush his teeth. If the person wears dentures, glasses, or a hearing aid, make sure these items are clean and in place.
- Position the person for eating. Residents in long-term care facilities are walked to the dining room, or taken in a wheelchair. In many facilities, the resident is helped from the wheelchair into a standard dining chair for the meal. If the person will be eating his meal in bed, smooth the bed linens and position the bed in a high Fowler's position if permitted. Clear the over-bed table of clutter and wipe down the surface if necessary.

- Provide a pleasant environment. Remove any offensive or odourous items, such as bedpans or emesis basins, from the room. Adjust the lighting for comfort and turn on the radio or television if the person asks you to. Many people like to listen to music or watch a favourite program while they eat.

ASSISTING THE PERSON TO EAT

Once these preparations are completed, it is time to eat! Meals should be served as soon as they are delivered from the kitchen. This helps to ensure that hot foods are hot and cold foods are cold. Check that the name on the meal tray matches the name of the resident or patient who will be receiving it (Fig. 19-4). Also make sure that the diet noted on the tray matches the diet noted on the person's medical chart or care plan. If the meal is not as ordered, ask a nurse to confirm that a mistake has been made, and then return the meal to the kitchen. The kitchen will replace the meal with the correct one.

In many facilities, especially long-term care facilities, a cloth or paper clothing protector is used. This protector is placed over the person's chest to prevent the clothing from being soiled with food during the meal. Wearing a clothing protector is a matter of personal choice, so always ask the resident if it is all right for you to put the clothing protector on her before the meal. Please do not refer to the clothing protector as a "bib." An adult, especially one who is already feeling self-conscious because she needs help eating, will not appreciate being likened to a helpless baby!

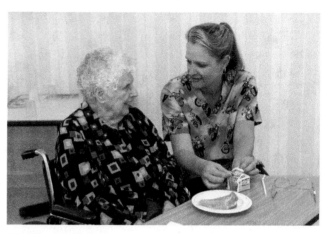

Figure 19-5
Some people will be able to eat on their own if you give them a little bit of assistance.

Help the person to eat as necessary. Encourage your patients or residents to do as much for themselves as possible to help promote their independence. The care plan will have basic information about the type of assistance the person needs, or you can ask the nurse. First, remove the cover from the tray and tell the person what foods are on the tray. No one likes "mystery meat" for dinner! Depending on the situation, you may also need to help the person with opening milk cartons or removing silverware from its wrapper, buttering bread, or cutting up meat (Fig. 19-5). If the person needs help seasoning the food, make sure that you add salt, pepper, and condiments according to the patient's or resident's tastes, not your own. If the person has poor eyesight, you will need to tell her where items are on the tray. Describe the food and help the person to find it on the plate by referencing a clock face (Fig. 19-6). For example,

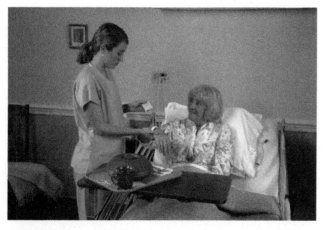

Figure 19-4
Always make sure that the right meal tray is being delivered to the right person.

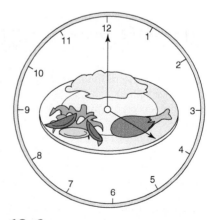

Figure 19-6
You can help a person with poor eyesight locate food on the plate by describing its location in terms of a clock face.

you might say, "Okay, Mr. Diaz—your pork chop is at 12 o'clock. The potatoes are at 3 o'clock, the green beans are at 6 o'clock, and the corn is at 9 o'clock. Your milk is on the upper right corner of the tray and your roll is on a bread plate to the left of your dinner plate."

Many of the people in your care will have some sort of physical disability that affects their ability to feed themselves. Special forks, knives, spoons, plates, and cups can help people with physical disabilities regain their independence. For example, many people who have had a stroke may have limited use of their hands and arms. They may be able to make big, sweeping movements, but small, delicate movements, such as those needed to hold and use regular silverware, are difficult. Specially made eating utensils, like those shown in Figure 19-7, allow the person to overcome these difficulties and feed himself. A person who has lost the use of one hand will have

to learn to eat using only the other hand. In this situation, a plate with a raised rim is very helpful. The rim is used to help guide food, much as you would use a knife to guide peas onto your fork. Special holders that fit around drinking glasses make it easier to hold the glass. All of these assistive devices help a disabled person regain independence, which is important for self-esteem.

FEEDING DEPENDENT PATIENTS AND RESIDENTS

Some people may not be able to feed themselves at all (Fig. 19-8). Even though these patients and residents will depend on you to do most of the work, it is very important that you involve them as much as possible in the process of eating. For example, you might ask the patient or resident to

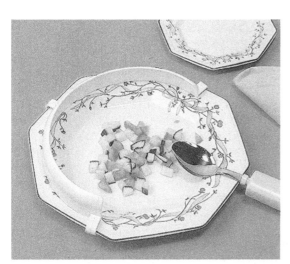

A. Plate guard

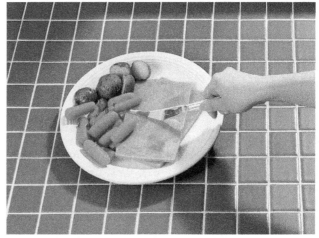

B. Knife with a rounded blade

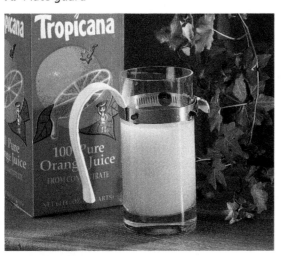

C. Cup holder

Figure 19-7
Assistive eating utensils help people with physical disabilities feed themselves. **(A)** Plate guards help to keep food on the plate and provide an "extra hand" for pushing food onto the fork. **(B)** A knife with a rounded blade can be rocked back and forth to cut food. This knife prevents the food from sliding on the plate. **(C)** A cup holder fits around a drinking glass, giving the person a firmer grip. (*Photos courtesy of Sammons Preston Rolyan, Bolingbrook, IL.*)

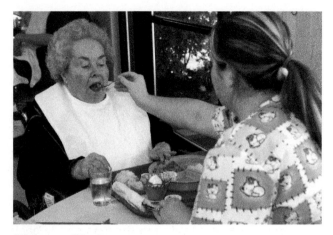

Figure 19-8
Some people may not be able to feed themselves.

help you by holding her own napkin. Remember that meal time is a very social time in a person's day. It is important to talk to the person you are feeding, even if the person does not answer you. Hearing your voice and knowing that you care about him or her will increase the person's appetite and aid digestion.

The types of food served will differ according to the person's chewing and swallowing abilities. Some people may be able to eat solid food, while others will require semi-solid or liquid food. When feeding another person, always use a spoon, not a fork, because the blunt edge of the spoon is safer than the sharp tines of the fork. Fill the spoon only about one-third full for each bite, and offer the bites slowly to prevent choking. Never rush the person through eating. Be sure to tell the person what foods you are offering her. If the person is alert and able to respond, ask her in what order she would like to try the food on the plate. Make sure you have seasoned the food according to the person's preference. If she is unable to tell you her preference, season the food mildly. Give the person enough time to chew and swallow each bite. You may need to gently remind the person to chew and swallow, especially if the person has dementia.

Offer liquids frequently, between bites. Some people find drinking through a straw to be easiest. Some people may have difficulty swallowing as the result of a stroke, injury, or dementia. These people can choke easily on liquids, so always offer liquids slowly. Sometimes the doctor orders the use of an additive that thickens the liquid, making it easier to swallow. The nurse or therapist will show you how to use these additives to thicken liquids if this is necessary for one of your patients or residents.

Procedure 19-1 gives the steps for feeding a patient or resident who needs complete assistance with eating.

Helping Hands and a Caring Heart

FOCUS ON HUMANISTIC HEALTH CARE

Think for a moment—when you are hungry, you sit down and eat. You cut your juicy steak, butter your hot rolls, and never give the act of eating a second thought. How would it feel to have to rely on another person to feed you, or cut up your food? Would you feel like a small child again, or a burden, or just useless? Be sensitive to your patients' or residents' feelings as you assist them with meals. Realize how very much they would like to be able to perform routine activities like eating without a second thought, just like you do.

MEASURING AND RECORDING FOOD INTAKE

Most long-term care facilities and some hospitals will require you to record the amount of food that the person eats. In some facilities, you will just have to note the portion of the total meal that was consumed (for example, Mrs. Wells ate 60% of her breakfast, 80% of her lunch, and 30% of her dinner). Many facilities will want you to tell the nurse if one of your patients or residents eats less than 70% of his or her meal.

In other facilities, you will have to note what percentage of *each* food was eaten (for example, At dinner, Mr. Sommers ate 100% of his mashed potatoes, 50% of his salad, and 75% of his chicken breast). The nurse or dietitian will then convert the percentages that you provide into "total calories consumed," and this number is recorded on the person's chart.

As a personal support worker, you will play a key role in the ongoing evaluation of your patients' or residents' dietary status. Of all the nursing team members, you will have the most contact with your patients or residents during meal times. You will see which foods are eaten readily and which are left on the tray. When you notice that a food has not been eaten, you might talk to the person about it. For example:

Personal support worker: Hi, Mr. Wheeling! How was your lunch? (*Noticing that the dessert has not been eaten*) Oh! I see you

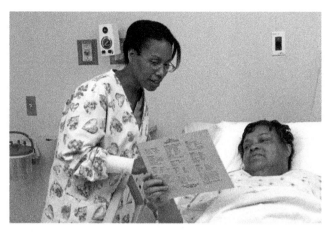

Figure 19-9
Respecting a person's preferences when it comes to food lets the person know that you care about him or her as an individual.

didn't eat your dessert. Are you full, or do you just not like vanilla tapioca?
Mr. Wheeling: Well, actually, I am pretty full, so I decided to skip the tapioca today. It's not my favourite anyway. (*Wrinkling nose*) I don't like the lumps.
Personal support worker: Well, I'm glad you told me! We ought to be able to avoid "lumpy" desserts in the future . . . maybe vanilla pudding or ice cream would be better instead?
Mr. Wheeling (*smiling*): Thanks, Nancy. That would be great. I do look forward to dessert!

Talking with the person about why a food was not eaten serves two purposes. First, it allows you to give the nurse information that she and the dietitian can use to plan future meals for the person. Second, when you notice that a food has gone untouched and take the time to ask the person about it, you let the person know that you care about him as an individual (Fig. 19-9).

OTHER WAYS OF PROVIDING FLUIDS AND NUTRITION

Drinking water and chewing, swallowing, and digesting food are the best ways to obtain fluids and nutrients. However, sometimes drinking and eating "the regular way" are simply not possible. For people who have problems chewing, swallowing, or digesting their food, fluids and nutrients must be provided another way. Three alternate

methods of providing fluids and nutrition include intravenous (IV) therapy, enteral nutrition, and total parenteral nutrition (TPN, hyperalimentation).

INTRAVENOUS (IV) THERAPY

In **intravenous (IV) therapy,** fluids are given through a small catheter (tube) that is inserted into a vein (*intra* = in; *venous* = vein). The IV tubing (sometimes called an "IV line") is connected to a bag that contains the IV fluid (Fig. 19-10). The fluid slowly drips through the tubing and into the vein. Usually the IV line, which is thin, is inserted into one of the small veins in the arm or the back of the hand.

IV therapy is not a source of complete nutrition, but it is useful when a person needs fluids. In addition to water, the IV fluid usually contains glucose, vitamins, and minerals. Drugs, such as pain medications or antibiotics, may also be added to the IV fluid. Sometimes, blood is given through an IV line.

You will not be responsible for managing IV therapy, but you may care for many people who have an IV line in place.

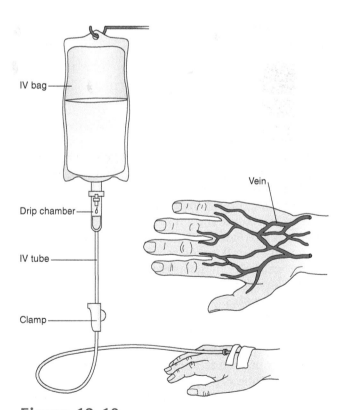

Figure 19-10
Intravenous (IV) therapy is used to give fluids. The IV fluid drips from the bag, into the tubing, and into the person's vein. The nurse uses the clamp to control the rate of flow.

TELL THE NURSE ❗

When caring for a person with an IV line, report any of the following observations to the nurse immediately:

● The tubing has become disconnected

● The fluid bag is empty

● The IV fluid is not dripping into the drip chamber

● Blood has backed up into the IV tubing

● The person complains of pain at the IV site

● There is swelling or redness at the IV site

ENTERAL NUTRITION

The word "enteral" comes from the Greek word for "intestines," *enteron*. **Enteral nutrition** involves placing food directly into the stomach or intestines, which eliminates the need for the person to chew or swallow. For example, a person who is in a coma is not able to chew and swallow. Certain injuries to the head and neck may prevent a person from chewing and swallowing, as might certain cancers. Sometimes people in the advanced stages of dementia "forget" how to swallow. All of these people may require enteral nutrition.

Enteral nutrition is sometimes called "tube feeding" because food, in the form of a formula-like fluid, is delivered through a tube that has been passed into the digestive tract. There are many ways to access the digestive tract with the feeding tube (Fig. 19-11):

- A **nasogastric tube** is inserted through the nose (*naso-*), down the throat, and into the stomach (*gastric*).
- A **nasointestinal** tube is inserted through the nose (*naso-*), down the throat, and into the small intestine (*intestinal*).
- A **gastrostomy tube** is inserted into the stomach (*gastro-*) through a surgical incision (*stoma*). The incision is made in the abdomen.
- A **jejunostomy tube** is inserted into the jejunum (part of the small intestine) through a surgical incision (*stoma*). The incision is made in the abdomen.
- A **percutaneous endoscopic gastrostomy (PEG) tube** is a special type of gastrostomy tube that is inserted into the stomach with the aid of an *endoscope*, a lighted, flexible tool that allows the doctor to see inside the body. The endoscope is passed through the mouth, down the throat, and into the stomach to help

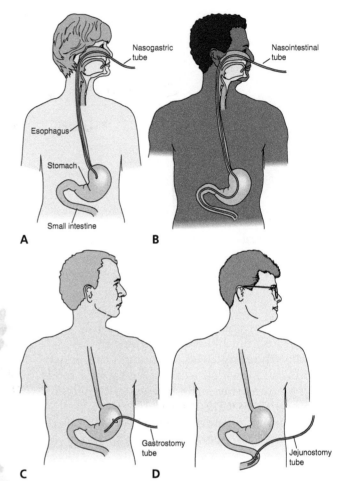

Figure 19-11
Enteral feeding tubes are inserted directly into the stomach or intestines. **(A)** A nasogastric tube is passed through the nose, down the throat, and into the stomach. **(B)** A nasointestinal tube is passed through the nose, down the throat, and into the small intestine. **(C)** A gastrostomy tube is inserted into the stomach through a surgical incision. **(D)** A jejunostomy tube is inserted into the small intestine through a surgical incision.

the doctor determine where to make the incision for the PEG tube (Fig. 19-12). Placement of a PEG tube is faster, cheaper, and less risky for the patient than placement of a regular gastrostomy tube because open abdominal surgery is not needed.

When a person needs enteral nutrition for only a short time, a nasogastric or nasointestinal tube is usually used. These tubes do not require a surgical incision for placement. However, they can cause irritation of the nose and the back of the throat and may be difficult for the person to tolerate. The tube can be easily displaced, especially if the person vomits, coughs, or pulls on the tube. Because it is possible for the tube to

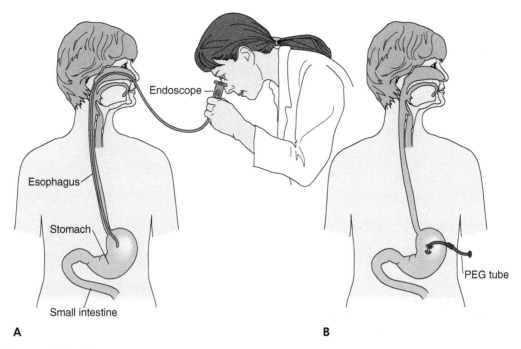

Esophagus

Stomach

Endoscope

Small intestine

PEG tube

A **B**

Figure 19-12
A percutaneous endoscopic gastrostomy (PEG) tube is a type of gastrostomy tube that is placed using an endoscope. **(A)** The endoscope is passed through the nose, down the throat, and into the stomach. A small incision is made for inserting the PEG tube, and then the endoscope is withdrawn. **(B)** The PEG tube in place.

become displaced during feeding, nurses are responsible for feeding people with nasogastric or nasointestinal tubes.

When a person needs enteral nutrition for more than a few days, a gastrostomy, jejunostomy, or PEG tube is used. These tubes are inserted through an incision in the abdomen, so irritation of the nose and throat is not a problem. Gastrostomy, jejunostomy, and PEG tubes are not as easily dislodged from their position as nasogastric or nasointestinal tubes are. However, they can come loose when a person moves, or during repositioning. People who are disoriented or confused may also pull them out by accident.

Enteral feedings may be given at scheduled times, or continuously by an infusion pump (Fig. 19-13). A person who is receiving nourishment through an enteral tube is at high risk for aspiration (inhalation of foreign material into the lungs). Aspiration can occur if the person regurgitates (vomits) the feeding formula and it goes down the windpipe and into the lungs. To help avoid regurgitation and aspiration, the head of the bed is raised during the feeding and for a period of time afterward.

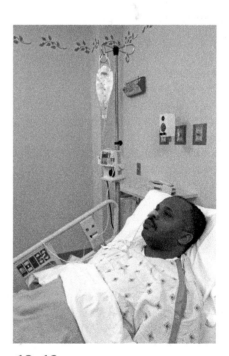

Figure 19-13
This patient is receiving enteral nutrition through a continuous infusion pump.

TELL THE NURSE ❗

Notify the nurse if you suspect that a person who is receiving enteral nutrition has regurgitated or aspirated the feeding or if you think that the feeding tube has become displaced. (Remember that only nurses can reconnect tubing that has been displaced.) Signs and symptoms of problems with enteral feeding devices include:

● Nausea, bloating, or pain during the feeding

● Coughing, gagging, or vomiting during the feeding

● Abdominal distention (a swollen abdomen)

● Diarrhea

● Drainage from around the tube insertion site

● Disconnected tubing

TOTAL PARENTERAL NUTRITION (HYPERALIMENTATION)

People who are very ill, injured, or recovering from surgery, especially gastrointestinal surgery, may not be able to tolerate food in the digestive tract. For these people, nourishment is delivered directly into the bloodstream through a large catheter (tube) inserted into a large vein near the heart (Fig. 19-14). This method of nutrient delivery is called **total parenteral nutrition (TPN)** or **hyperalimentation.** *Parenteral* means "by some way other than through the digestive tract." And *hyperalimentation* means "above (*hyper*) the alimentary (or digestive) tract." So you can see that both terms refer to a method of feeding that does not involve the digestive tract.

As you will recall from the beginning of the chapter, the digestive tract breaks food down into nutrients, and then these nutrients are absorbed into the bloodstream. If a person is receiving TPN, then the nutrients must be delivered to the bloodstream in their smallest form, because digestion does not occur. Water, glucose, vitamins, and minerals are small molecules. But proteins and fats are bigger. This is why a large catheter is used for TPN, instead of an IV line. The large catheter used for TPN is wider and allows the bigger fat and protein molecules to pass through. An IV line is smaller and only allows smaller molecules, such as water, glucose, vitamins, minerals, and medications to pass. The ability to administer fats and proteins, as well as the other four classes of nutrients, is where the "total" comes from in the term *total parenteral nutrition.*

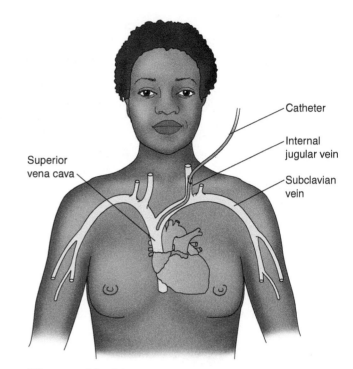

Figure 19-14
Total parenteral nutrition (TPN) delivers nutrients directly to the bloodstream. A large catheter (or "central line") is inserted into a large vein near the heart.

As a personal support worker, you will not be responsible for giving TPN feedings, but you may care for people receiving them.

FLUIDS AND HYDRATION

FLUID BALANCE

As you learned earlier, water is just as necessary to life as food, if not more so. A healthy adult needs to drink between 6 to 8 glasses (1500 to 2000 mL) of fluid each day just to keep up with the fluid that normally leaves the body in urine, feces, sweat, and the air we exhale. Most of these fluid needs are met by drinking water, juice, milk, and other beverages. However, certain foods, such as cucumbers, watermelon, grapes, and soup, have high water contents as well and provide some of the fluid needed by the body.

When the amount of fluid taken into the body equals the amount of fluid that leaves the body, a state of **fluid balance** occurs. Fluid balance is important for health. **Dehydration** occurs when there is too little fluid in the tissues of the body. Causes of dehydration include diarrhea, vomiting, hemorrhage, severe burns, diaphoresis (excessive sweating), and simply not drinking enough fluids. In all of these situations, the amount of fluid that leaves the body is greater than the amount of fluid taken in. Older people are often at risk for dehydration because they do not feel thirsty as often as younger people do. People in comas and people with dementia are also at risk for dehydration because they may not be able to ask for a drink.

The opposite of dehydration, **edema,** occurs when there is too much fluid in the tissues of the body. Kidney disease and certain types of heart disease can make it hard for the body to get rid of extra water, resulting in edema. In these situations, the amount of fluid that leaves the body is less than the amount of fluid taken in. For a person with edema, the doctor may restrict the person's fluid intake or order certain medications to help the body rid itself of the excess fluid.

OFFERING FLUIDS

Personal support workers are responsible for providing fresh drinking water and other fluids to patients and residents. Many of your patients or residents will be allowed to have as much water as they like, and should be encouraged to drink (Fig. 19-15). If a person is allowed to have ice water, make sure that the water pitcher is filled with fresh, cold water. Replace the water when the ice melts or when the pitcher is almost empty. People are more likely to drink fluids that taste good and are served at the appropriate temperature. Remember to also offer a drink regularly to people who are elderly, bed-bound, confused, or taking pain medications. These people might not remember to drink fluids often enough, or they may feel that they are being a burden to you by asking for a drink.

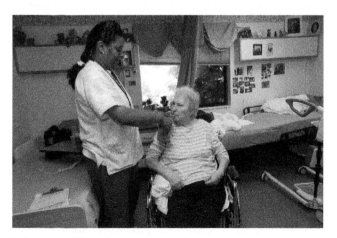

Figure 19-15
Water is essential to life.

Sometimes, the doctor may either increase or restrict a person's fluid intake. An order to encourage fluids (sometimes called "force fluids") means that the person should increase his or her fluid intake. The nurse will give you information about the amount and type of fluids that should be offered. Most people do not like having to drink a large amount of liquid all at once. Offering small amounts of a drink that the person likes frequently throughout the day is a better approach. Make sure that the fluids you offer are cold or hot, and fresh. Not many people like room-temperature water, flat soda, or lukewarm tea.

Offering small amounts of fluids at regular times throughout the day is also a good approach when the doctor has restricted a person's fluid intake. This approach helps to make sure that the person is never too thirsty, by spreading out his or her fluid intake over the course of the day. Frequent oral hygiene also helps to keep the person comfortable and prevent "dry mouth." Recording the amount of fluid taken in is an important part of your duties when you are either encouraging or restricting fluids for a person.

Some patients or residents will not be allowed to have any fluids at all in preparation for surgery or a diagnostic procedure. A person who is not allowed to have any fluids at all is said to be on **"NPO status."** *NPO* stands for *nils per os,* or "nothing by mouth" in Latin. NPO means exactly what it stands for—no fluids (not even water or ice chips), no food, no hard candy, no gum. If one of your patients or residents has been placed on NPO status, empty his water pitcher and store it out of sight. You might also want to gently remind visitors that the person is not allowed to have anything to eat or drink, and suggest that they enjoy their own snacks and beverages in another room. Being on NPO status can be extremely uncomfortable. Think of all of those cartoons where a man lost in a hot desert keeps imagining that he sees a big frosty glass of water "just ahead." Being thirsty and not being able to drink is difficult. Frequent oral care helps to relieve some of the discomfort until the person is allowed to have fluids again.

MEASURING AND RECORDING INTAKE AND OUTPUT

Certain medical conditions can make monitoring a person's fluid balance very important. For those people, an order to "maintain intake and output measurements" will be followed. All of the fluids that enter and leave the body are measured and recorded on an **intake and output**

(I&O) flow sheet. In health care facilities, fluids are measured and recorded in millilitres (mL) or cubic centimetres (cc): 1 mL is the same as 1 cc. One fluid ounce is equal to 30 mL or 30 cc.

Each time the person takes in fluids, or fluids leave the body, the amount is recorded. The amounts are totalled at the end of the shift and again at the end of the 24-hour reporting period. The amount of intake can then be compared with the amount of output to monitor the person's fluid balance.

Measuring Fluid Intake

Fluid intake includes all of the fluids that a person drinks, including those foods that are liquid at room or body temperature (such as gelatin, ice cream, pudding, and popsicles). Other fluids that are considered as part of a person's total intake include enteral or TPN feedings and IV fluids, but the nurse will be responsible for recording these amounts. The health care facility where you work will have a listing of the amount of fluid in common servings, and you will need to become familiar with the amount of fluid contained by the cups, glasses, and bowls used in your facility. Remember that 30 mL (30 cc) is equal to 1 fluid ounce, so an 8-ounce carton of milk would equal 240 mL (8 × 30 = 240). But what if the person did not drink the entire carton of milk? In this case, you can estimate how much fluid was taken in. For example, if the person drank half of the carton of milk, then half of 8 ounces is 4, so 4 × 30 would be 120 mL. (Another way to arrive at this figure is to calculate what the total carton is worth in millilitres, and then divide by the amount consumed: 240/2 = 120 mL.)

Sometimes it is necessary to calculate intake exactly. In this situation, you would calculate how many fluids were offered to the person before he or she started to eat. For example, let's say a person's meal tray contained 150 mL of orange juice, 240 mL of milk, and 90 mL of water at the beginning of the meal. This would mean that 480 mL of fluid were offered (150 + 240 + 90 = 480). After the person has finished with the meal, you would take all of the fluids left in the glasses and pour them into a **graduate** (a measuring device) to measure the amount left (Fig. 19-16). Let's say that 40 mL of fluid are left. You would subtract the amount left (40 mL) from the total amount offered (480 mL) and record the total consumed as 440 mL.

Measuring Fluid Output

Fluids that are considered output are urine, vomit, blood, wound drainage, and diarrhea. Output is

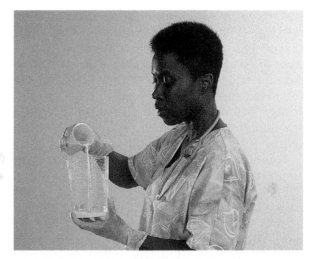

Figure 19-16
A graduate is a measuring device that is used to measure fluids. The graduate is marked with lines that indicate millilitres (mL) on the left and ounces (oz) on the right. (*Copyright B. Proud.*)

measured and recorded the same way that intake is. A person who is on I&O status will need to be reminded to urinate into a measuring device. The urine cannot be discarded until you have measured and recorded the amount. Urine collection devices are available that can be used on a regular toilet, or with a bedside commode (Fig. 19-17). Urinals have measurements marked on the side so that you can easily see the amount that they contain. Urine from a bedpan or a urinary catheter drainage bag is poured into a graduate for measurement. (Urinary catheters are discussed in detail in Chapter 20.)

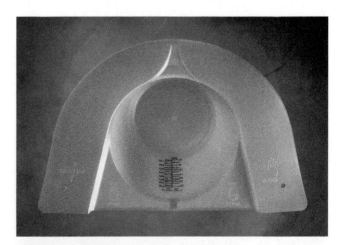

Figure 19-17
A collection device (sometimes called a "commode hat") is placed over the toilet seat before the person urinates, to contain and measure the amount of urine. (*Photograph courtesy of Medline Industries, Inc.*)

If a person vomits, the amount can be measured using the markings on the emesis basin. If the person vomited somewhere other than in the emesis basin (for example, on the floor or bed linens), then the nurse will estimate the amount of vomit. Blood and wound drainage is either estimated by the nurse or measured in a graduate if it is collected into a drainage device. Diarrhea is estimated for amount also.

Always remember to wear gloves when measuring output.

Summary

- Food and fluids are necessary for life.
  - Food provides us with energy and nutrients that our bodies need to work properly.
  - The six types of nutrients are carbohydrates, proteins, fats, vitamins, minerals, and water.
    - Carbohydrates, proteins, and fat provide energy.
    - Vitamins, minerals, and water regulate body processes.
- To be healthy, we need to eat a variety of nutritious foods every day.
  - Not all foods are equally nutritious.
  - Nutrients work best in combination with other nutrients.
  - Canada's Food Guide and nutrition labels on packaged foods can be used to plan a healthy diet.
  - People in health care settings often have special needs as far as nutrition is concerned.
- Factors that influence a person's eating habits include religion, culture, geography, finances, kitchen skills, food likes and dislikes, and appetite.
- Eating helps us to meet both physical and emotional needs.
  - Helping a person to prepare for meal time and serving meals promptly contributes to comfort and a relaxed atmosphere.
  - Respecting the individual's preferences is important when it comes to food.
  - Talking with the person as you assist with the meal is important, even if the person cannot answer you.
  - When our emotional needs are met, it is easier for us to meet our physical needs. Ensuring that meal time is pleasant can help improve a person's appetite.
- Personal support workers assist people with meals as necessary.
  - Patients and residents are encouraged to do as much as they can for themselves.

- Assistive devices are available to help people with physical impairments to eat on their own.
  - Some people will need to be fed.
- When a person cannot take food or fluids by mouth, nutrition and fluids are provided in other ways.
  - Intravenous (IV) therapy provides fluids, glucose, vitamins, and minerals through a small catheter inserted into one of the small veins of the arm or hand. IV therapy does not provide complete nutrition.
  - Enteral nutrition is provided by a tube that is placed directly into the stomach or intestines.
    - Nasogastric tubes, nasointestinal tubes, gastrostomy tubes, jejunostomy tubes, and percutaneous endoscopic gastrostomy (PEG) tubes are used for enteral feeding.
    - Formula-like food is usually delivered through an infusion device, either continuously or at specified times.
  - Total parenteral nutrition (TPN, hyperalimentation) involves the delivery of all six classes of nutrients through a catheter inserted into a large vein near the heart.
- Maintaining proper fluid balance is important for health.
  - The amount of fluids taken into the body should equal the amount of fluids that leave the body.
    - If the amount of fluid leaving the body is greater than the amount taken in, dehydration can occur.
    - If the amount of fluid leaving the body is less than the amount taken in, edema can occur.
  - A doctor may order a person's fluid intake to be increased or restricted. People who have no fluid restrictions should be encouraged to drink frequently.
  - A person's fluid balance is monitored by measuring and recording fluid intake and output. One fluid ounce = 30 millilitres (mL) = 30 cubic centimetres (cc).

PROCEDURE   **19-1**

Feeding a Dependent Person

WHY YOU DO IT   A person who cannot feed himself or herself will need to be fed to ensure that he or she receives proper nutrition. Providing companionship during the meal is just as important as providing assistance with the actual task of eating.

Getting Ready

1. Complete the "Getting Ready" steps.

Supplies

- gloves
- paper towels
- clothing protector
- oral hygiene supplies
- wash basin
- bedpan or urinal
- towel
- washcloth

Procedure

2. Cover the over-bed table with paper towels. Place the oral hygiene supplies on the over-bed table. Fill the wash basin with warm water (37.7°C [110°F] to 46.1°C [115°F] on the bath thermometer). Place the basin on the over-bed table.

3. If the side rails are in use, lower the side rail on the working side of the bed. The side rail on the opposite side of the bed should remain up. Raise the head of the bed. Make sure that the bed is positioned at a comfortable working height (to promote good body mechanics) and that the wheels are locked.

4. Put on the gloves.

5. Assist the person with oral hygiene.

6. Offer the bedpan or urinal. If the person uses the bedpan or urinal, empty and clean it before proceeding with the meal. Remove your gloves and dispose of them in a facility-approved waste container. Wash your hands.

7. Wash the person's hands and face.

8. Clear the over-bed table and position it over the bed at the proper height for the person.

9. Get the meal tray from the dietary cart. (If the side rails are in use, raise the side rails before leaving the bedside.) Check the meal tray to make sure that it has the person's name on it and that it contains the correct diet for the person. Place the meal tray on the over-bed table.

10. Ask the person if he or she would like to use a clothing protector. Put the clothing protector on the person, if desired.

11. Uncover the meal tray, and prepare the food for eating (for example, cut the meat, butter the bread, open any containers). Tell the person what is on the tray.

12. Take a seat.

13. Allow the person to choose what he or she would like to taste first. Using a spoon, offer a small bite to the person (fill the spoon no more than one-third full). Allow the person enough time to swallow the food.

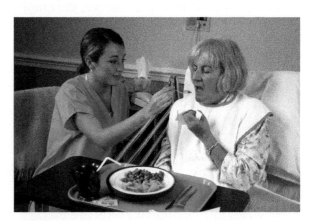

Step 13 Using a spoon, offer a small bite to the person.

14. Offer the person something to drink every few bites. Use the napkin to wipe the person's mouth and chin as often as necessary. Allow the person to assist with the eating process to the best of his or her ability.

15. Continue in this manner until the person is finished. Encourage the person to finish the food on the tray, but do not force the person to eat.

16. Remove the tray and the clothing protector when the person has finished eating.

17. Put on a clean pair of gloves. Assist the person with oral hygiene.

18. If the side rails are in use, return the side rails to the raised position. Lower the head of the bed as the person requests. Make sure that the bed is lowered to its lowest position and that the wheels are locked.

19. Gather the soiled linens and place them in the linen hamper or linen bag. Dispose of disposable items in a facility-approved waste container. Clean equipment and return it to the storage area.

20. Remove your gloves and dispose of them in a facility-approved waste container.

21. Record the percentage of food eaten and the amount of fluid intake in the person's medical record, per your facility's policy. Report an abnormal appetite to the nurse (for example, less than 70% of the total meal consumed).

Finishing Up CLSOWR

22. Complete the "Finishing Up" steps.

WHAT DID YOU LEARN?

Multiple Choice

Select the single best answer for each of the following questions.

1. When assisting a person with eating, one of the first things you should do is:
   a. Provide the person with privacy
   b. Butter the person's bread
   c. Wash your hands and the person's hands
   d. Cut the food into large pieces

2. Mrs. Wellington is blind. Which one of the following should she have during meal time?
   a. A soft diet
   b. Help identifying the location of the food on the plate
   c. A large spoon
   d. A cup holder

3. Mr. Jones is 98 years old and has no food restrictions on his diet. However, he is missing several teeth. Which one of the following menus would be the best choice for Mr. Jones?
   a. Spare ribs, macaroni and cheese, coleslaw, and fruit cocktail
   b. Hamburger, french fries, corn on the cob, and ice cream
   c. Baked fish, mashed potatoes, spinach soufflé, and tapioca
   d. Fried chicken, baked potato, green beans, and chocolate chip cookies

4. Which one of the following lists only items that would be included in fluid intake?
   a. Orange juice, soft boiled egg, toast
   b. Milk, soup, gelatin
   c. Water, mashed potatoes, egg custard
   d. Milk, ham sandwich, ice cream bar

5. Miss Lee drank one-third of an 8-ounce glass of iced tea. How many millilitres of fluid did Miss Lee drink?
   a. 60 mL
   b. 80 mL
   c. 100 mL
   d. 240 mL

6. Which one of the following lists foods that are good sources of protein?
   a. Steak, chicken, fish
   b. Spinach, carrots, beets
   c. Bread, cereal, rice
   d. Apples, oranges, bananas

7. Which one of the following nutrients accounts for 50% to 60% of our total body weight?
   a. Vitamin A
   b. Glucose
   c. Water
   d. Calcium

8. At the beginning of your shift, you give Mr. Gibson a water pitcher containing 270 mL of water. At the end of your shift, you note that 35 mL of water are left in the pitcher. How much water did Mr. Gibson drink?
   a. 35 mL
   b. 175 mL
   c. 235 mL
   d. 140 mL

9. Which of the following lists foods that are good sources of carbohydrates?
   a. Liver, fish, chicken
   b. Cereal, fruit, bread
   c. Milk, beans, cheese
   d. Water, soda, butter

10. Which one of the following can be harmful if too much is consumed?
    a. Folic acid
    b. Water-soluble vitamins (for example, vitamins C and B_{12})
    c. Fat-soluble vitamins (for example, vitamins A, D, E, and K)
    d. None of the above

11. Which health care professional is specially trained to plan for the patient's or resident's nutritional needs and teach about good nutrition?
    a. The nurse
    b. The dietitian
    c. The personal support worker
    d. The doctor

12. Which one of the following can affect a person's food likes and dislikes?
    a. The person's religious beliefs
    b. The person's culture
    c. Where the person lives
    d. All of the above

Matching

Match the amount of fluid in millilitres (mL) with the same amount in ounces (oz).

_____ **1.** 240 mL

_____ **2.** 180 mL

_____ **3.** 300 mL

_____ **4.** 30 mL

_____ **5.** 120 mL

_____ **6.** 150 mL

a. 10 oz

b. 5 oz

c. 8 oz

d. 4 oz

e. 1 oz

f. 6 oz

STOP and Think!

Mrs. Giovanni was recently admitted to your long-term care facility. She is a bit underweight and her doctor wants her to consume more calories each day. The problem is Mrs. Giovanni will only eat about half of her meal at meal time. She says, "I just get full quickly." What are some ways you may be able to help Mrs. Giovanni improve her nutritional intake?

You work in an assisted-living facility, and one of your residents, Mr. Wayne, has severe arthritis in his hands. The arthritis makes it hard for Mr. Wayne to use his silverware, but he refuses to let you help him eat. He says that he'll let you feed him "if and when they cut off both of my hands!" Lately, the arthritis has gotten much worse and Mr. Wayne is having more and more difficulty eating. Most of the food winds up beside the plate, instead of in his mouth, and what little food makes it to his mouth is cold by the time it gets there. You know that Mr. Wayne has to eat to maintain his health. What can you do to assist Mr. Wayne in feeding himself? What member of the staff could you ask to assist you?

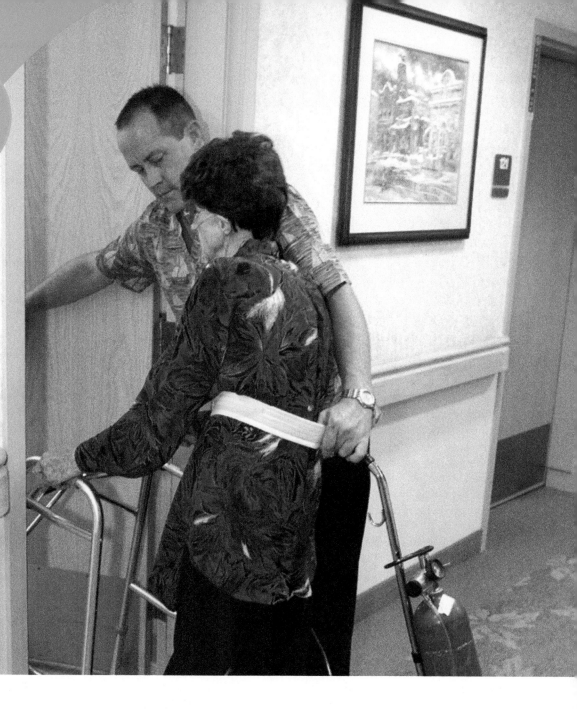

Assisting With Urinary and Bowel Elimination

WHAT WILL YOU LEARN?

In Chapter 19, you learned about how we take in food and convert it to energy in a process called *metabolism*. During this conversion process, waste materials (or by-products) are created. These waste products must be removed from our bodies,

Photo: Personal support workers help their patients or residents to meet their elimination needs by providing assistance as necessary.

or we will become sick. Wastes are eliminated from the body in various forms. The urinary system rids the body of waste products that have been filtered from the bloodstream, along with excess fluid, in the form of urine. The digestive system rids the body of the solid waste that is left over from the foods that we eat, in the form of feces, or bowel movements. Although there are other ways the body rids itself of waste, urinary and bowel elimination is the subject of this chapter.

Your patients or residents may have physical or mental difficulties that affect their ability to manage urinary or bowel elimination, or both. As a personal support worker, you will need to assist your patients or residents with elimination as necessary. When you are finished with this chapter, you will be able to:

1. Describe two methods the body uses to eliminate waste products.
2. Discuss attitudes that people may have regarding the processes of urinary or bowel elimination.
3. Discuss actions the personal support worker can take to promote normal urinary and bowel elimination, and explain why normal urinary and bowel elimination is essential to health.
4. List normal characteristics of urine and describe observations that a personal support worker may make when assisting a person with urinary elimination that should be reported to the nurse.
5. Demonstrate methods used to measure and record urinary output.
6. Describe the use of urinary catheters and demonstrate how to provide routine catheter care.
7. Describe five types of urinary incontinence and methods the personal support worker uses to assist people who are incontinent of urine.
8. Understand the underlying principles of bladder training.
9. Discuss the process of bowel elimination and characteristics of normal stool.
10. Define problems with bowel elimination that are often seen in the health care setting.
11. List the types of enemas and discuss reasons why a person may require an enema.
12. Demonstrate proper technique for assisting with urinary and bowel elimination, obtaining urine and stool samples, providing catheter care, and administering enemas.

Vocabulary

Bedside commode	Occult	Suprapubic catheter	Constipation
Bedpan	Frequency	Catheter care	Laxative
Fracture pan	Urgency	Urinary incontinence	Stool softener
Urinal	Nocturia	Urinary retention	Fibre supplement
Urinalysis	Dysuria	Condom catheter	Fecal impaction
Midstream ("clean catch") urine specimen	Oliguria	Chyme	Digital examination
	Polyuria	Peristalsis	Flatulence
	Diuresis	Feces	Fecal (bowel) incontinence
Urination	Anuria	Defecate	
Voiding	Catheter	Stool	Enema
Micturition	Straight catheter	Flatus	Rectal suppository
Hematuria	Indwelling catheter	Diarrhea	

ASSISTING WITH ELIMINATION

ELIMINATION EQUIPMENT

Many of your patients or residents will need no more assistance with elimination than a steady arm to lean on during the trip to the bathroom.

The bathrooms in many health care facilities have special features that make them easier for people with physical disabilities to use (Fig. 20-1A). For example, hand rails attached to the walls alongside the toilet or onto the toilet itself make it easier for the person to sit down and get back up. Some toilets have higher seats, so the person does not have to bend her knees as much to sit

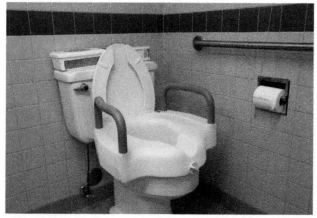

A

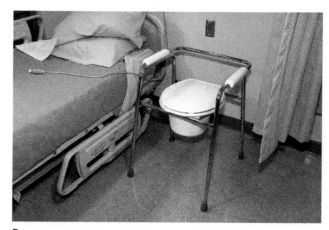

B

Figure 20-1
(A) Many toilets in health care facilities have special modifications that make them easier to use.
(B) A bedside commode can be used if a person can get out of bed but is not capable of walking the distance to the bathroom.

down and get back up. Modifications like these allow many patients or residents to use the toilet in the bathroom with very little assistance from you. However, some of your patients or residents may not be able to get out of bed at all, or they may be too weak or ill to walk to the bathroom. These people will need more help with elimination, and special equipment.

Bedside Commodes

For a person who is able to get out of bed, but who is not able to walk to the bathroom, a bedside commode can make toileting easier (see Fig. 20-1B). The **bedside commode** is a chair frame with a toilet seat and a removable collection bucket. If the person is weak or unsteady, you will need to help her get out of bed and over to the bedside commode.

Bedpans

A **bedpan** is used for elimination when a person is unable to get out of bed at all (Fig. 20-2A). A woman who cannot get out of bed uses a bedpan to urinate, and for bowel movements. A man who cannot get out of bed uses a bedpan for bowel movements, and a urinal to urinate (see next section).

Bedpans, while sometimes necessary, must be used with extreme care. It is very easy to bruise or tear the fragile skin of an elderly or disabled person. In addition to causing immediate pain to the person, an injury like this can also lead to the formation of a pressure ulcer later on. Arthritis can make using a bedpan very painful, as can fractures of the back or legs. If a

person has an injury or disability that makes it too uncomfortable or dangerous to use a regular bedpan, a special bedpan called a fracture pan is used. The **fracture pan,** which is wedge-shaped, is placed underneath the person's buttocks with the thin edge toward the person's back (Fig. 20-2B).

Using a bedpan is uncomfortable, and the discomfort alone can cause the person to have difficulty using it. Many facilities use disposable bedpans that are made from molded plastic. However, some facilities still use bedpans made from stainless steel. If the facility where you work uses metal bedpans, be sure to warm the bedpan before offering it to the patient or resident. You can do this by wrapping the bedpan in a warm towel, or running warm water over the seat area and then drying it before use. Rubbing a small amount of powder on the rim of the bedpan can make it easier to slide under the person. If the person's condition allows, raise the head of the bed to promote a more natural elimination position. Provide as much privacy as safely possible. Procedure 20-1 describes how to help a person to use a bedpan.

Urinals

A man uses a **urinal** to urinate when he cannot get out of bed (Fig. 20-3). The urinal is designed to fit between the man's legs. To urinate, the man puts his penis in the opening of the urinal. If the man is very weak or disabled, you may need to place his penis inside the opening of the urinal for him. Procedure 20-2 describes how to help a man use a urinal.

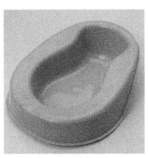

A. Regular bedpan

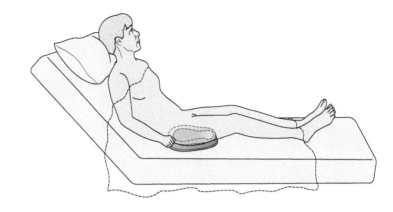

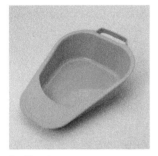

B. Fracture pan

Figure 20-2

Bedpans are used for women who cannot get out of bed to urinate. A bedridden man also uses a bedpan for bowel movements. **(A)** A standard bedpan. Position a standard bedpan like a regular toilet seat—the buttocks are placed on the wide, rounded shelf, with the open end pointed toward the foot of the bed. **(B)** A fracture pan. Position a fracture pan with the thin edge toward the head of the bed.

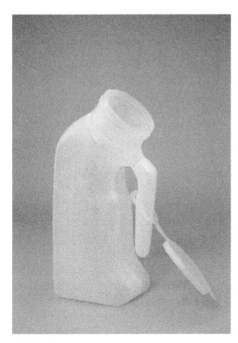

Figure 20-3

Men who cannot get out of bed to urinate can use a urinal.

PROMOTING NORMAL ELIMINATION

Being in a health care facility can change a person's normal elimination patterns, which can cause health problems. The most effective method of treating urinary and bowel problems is to prevent them from happening in the first place. As a personal support worker, you can help promote normal urinary and bowel function for your patients or residents. The following tips are simple, but effective:

- Encourage plenty of fluids, unless a person has a medical condition that requires fluid restriction. Drinking plenty of fluids helps the kidneys to work properly, and regular urination flushes harmful bacteria from the bladder, helping to prevent urinary tract infections. In addition, drinking enough fluids helps to keep the feces soft, making bowel movements easier.

- Answer call lights promptly and take people to the bathroom or provide them with a bedpan or urinal as soon as they ask you to. Many residents and patients do not want to "bother" the nursing staff and will wait until the last minute to call for assistance with the bedpan or for help getting to the bathroom. If the person must wait too long for help to arrive, he or she may have an accident.

- Encourage your patients or residents to call when they first feel the urge to void. This can help to prevent accidents. In addition, "holding" urine or feces is not only uncomfortable, it can lead to problems such as constipation.
- Offer patients or residents the chance to eliminate frequently, especially if they are bed-bound or require assistance. Some people may find it easier to accept an offer of assistance than to ask for help.
- Provide for privacy and comfort. A person is able to urinate or have a bowel movement much more easily if she is warm enough, in a comfortable position, and ensured of as much privacy as possible. Most women urinate and have bowel movements in a sitting or squatting position. Help a woman to sit upright by elevating the head of the bed (if she is using a bedpan), or have her lean forward a bit while seated on the toilet or bedside commode. Most men stand up to urinate and sit down to have a bowel movement. Some men have no difficulty using a urinal while lying down, but others will need to sit up or even to stand. In this case, you may need to help the man to sit or stand up.

Helping Hands and a Caring Heart

FOCUS ON HUMANISTIC HEALTH CARE

Everyone urinates and has bowel movements. However, most people consider elimination a private activity and would prefer not to discuss it with others. In a health care facility, people may be forced to think about and discuss elimination much more than they would normally care to! Think about how it would affect you to be a patient or a resident in a health care facility. Nurses and personal support workers ask you about your bathroom patterns. They want to know if you have had a bowel movement today, how big it was, and what it looked like. They want you to urinate into a cup and then carry the sample to the nurses' station in full view of everyone. You may have to share a bathroom, or worse yet, use a bedpan while being separated from other people in the room by only a

curtain! Elimination, especially when it must take place in a fairly public way, is very embarrassing for many people.

A person who is a patient or a resident in a health care facility may have difficulty with elimination, especially if elimination must occur under conditions that are not as private as the person would like. Regardless of the amount of assistance that your patients or residents need, privacy and consideration for individual preferences are essential. Provide privacy to the extent possible with regard to the safety of the person. Close the bathroom door, or close the privacy curtains and the door to the room, if the person cannot use the regular toilet. Always make sure the call light is in reach so that the person can call you when he is ready for assistance. Some people are too weak or unsteady to be left alone while they urinate or have a bowel movement. In fact, some people will actually need for you to help hold them in the correct position during elimination. Being professional, kind, and straightforward about the "business at hand" will help to ease your patient's or resident's embarrassment.

Similarly, it is important to help your residents or patients keep their sense of dignity. For many people, needing assistance with this most private of bodily functions is humiliating. Feelings of embarrassment and shame are made worse when patients or residents accidentally soil themselves, their bed linens, or their clothing with urine or feces. This is a fairly common occurrence in health care facilities. The effects of medications, being in a strange place, reluctance to ask for help, and physical or mental disabilities can all lead to accidents. Again, kindness, empathy, and a professional attitude can go a long way toward easing the patient's or resident's embarrassment.

If a person is having difficulty urinating, there are some things you can do to help. For example, try turning on the faucet and allowing water to run into the sink. The sound of running water, which accompanied many of our early toilet training lessons, can help a person relax enough to start the urine stream. The sound of the running water also helps to cover up the sounds of urination, which may put some people more at ease. Putting the person's fingers in a basin of warm water can also help stimulate urination.

If a person is having difficulty moving his bowels, make sure that the person does not feel rushed. Many people like to read while having a bowel movement. Some people find that drinking warm fluids (such as coffee, tea, or warm water with lemon) helps stimulate the bowels to empty. Finally, regular exercise and foods that contain insoluble fibre help to promote regular bowel movements.

General guidelines for assisting a person with elimination are given in Guidelines Box 20-1.

Guidelines Box 20-1 Guidelines for Assisting With Elimination

WHAT YOU DO	WHY YOU DO IT
Always honour a person's request for assistance with elimination as quickly as possible.	Answering call lights quickly builds trust and prevents accidents. If a person who is bed-bound must wait too long for assistance, he could have an accident in the bed. A weak or unsteady person may try to walk to the bathroom on her own, rather than waiting for help to arrive. This puts the person at risk for a fall. Finally, it is very uncomfortable to "hold" urine or feces for a long time, and doing so can change the normal elimination patterns, causing health problems.
Always provide the person with as much privacy as safety considerations will allow.	Regular elimination is essential to health, so it is important to make this process as normal as possible for your patients or residents. Many people have difficulty urinating or having a bowel movement if they think that someone else can hear them, or if someone else is in the bathroom with them.
If you leave the person alone, always make sure that the call light control is within easy reach of the person.	The person will need the call light control to let you know when she is finished, or if she needs help.
Make sure the toilet paper is within easy reach of the person. If the person is unable to wipe himself, assist with this task.	Wiping promotes comfort and helps to prevent irritation, odours, and infection.
Be sure to provide good perineal care as necessary, especially after bowel movements (see Chapter 17).	Good perineal care promotes comfort and helps to prevent irritation, odours, and infection.
Provide the person with the chance to wash his hands after elimination. This can be accomplished by stopping by the sink if the person is in the bathroom, or by providing a warm, wet washcloth after assisting the person from the bedside commode or removing the bedpan or urinal.	Most people prefer to wash their hands after using the toilet. Allowing people to follow their normal routines whenever possible is important, especially when other aspects of the routine need to be altered. In addition, handwashing is important for hygiene.
Always wear gloves when assisting a person with elimination, or when handling a bedpan, bedside commode bucket, or urinal that contains waste.	Urine and feces are considered body fluids and may contain pathogens.
Before disposing of waste, observe the feces or urine for amount and any unusual characteristics. Report and record your observations.	Abnormalities in the urine or feces could indicate a health problem.

(continued)

Guidelines Box 20-1	Guidelines for Assisting With Elimination (continued)
WHAT YOU DO	**WHY YOU DO IT**
Never place a bedpan or urinal on an over-bed table or bedside table, even if the bedpan or urinal is clean. Dirty bedpans and urinals are taken to the bathroom immediately after use and cleaned and disinfected according to facility policy. Clean bedpans are either stored in a cabinet underneath the bedside table or returned to the equipment room. Clean urinals may be hung over the side rail, stored in a cabinet, or returned to the equipment room.	The over-bed table and bedside table are considered "clean" areas. Even if the bedpan or urinal is clean, most people do not want items associated with elimination placed on surfaces where they eat or have personal items displayed.
If there are odours in the room as a result of elimination, use an air freshener.	Most people will appreciate the use of an air freshener to make the air in the room smell fresher. Just be professional in any remarks you may make about the odour.
Disinfect equipment used for elimination carefully, according to facility policy.	Bedpans, urinals, and bedside commode buckets can act as fomites (that is, non-living objects that can transmit pathogens and cause infection) if they are not properly disinfected.

OBTAINING URINE AND STOOL SPECIMENS

Because the contents of a person's urine or feces can provide a doctor with clues about the person's overall health status, you may be asked to obtain a urine or stool specimen (sample) for laboratory study. When assisting with specimen collection, it is very important to make sure that the specimen container is properly labeled with the person's name and room number. Otherwise, a person may be diagnosed with, and receive treatment for, a condition he or she does not have! It is also important to make sure that the specimen is handled correctly after you obtain it. For example, in certain situations, the specimen may need to be delivered to the laboratory while it is still warm, or placed in a special plastic transport bag. If a specimen is not being delivered to the laboratory right away, then it needs to be stored properly until the scheduled pick-up time. Before collecting *any* specimen—of urine, feces, or any other body fluid—always ask yourself the following questions:

- Do I have the right person?
- Do I have the right laboratory requisition slip? (The laboratory requisition slip states the person's name, the date, and the type of test to be done. It is filled out by the nurse and sent with the specimen to the laboratory.)
- What method is to be used to collect the specimen?
- Do I have the right type of specimen container?
- Is the specimen container properly labeled?
- What is the correct date and time?
- What storage and delivery method must I use?

Finally, always remember to wear gloves when assisting with specimen collection and when handling the specimen containers.

Obtaining a Urine Specimen

Urinalysis, or examination of the urine under a microscope and by chemical means, is a commonly used diagnostic tool in the health care setting. Substances found in urine during urinalysis can help doctors diagnose kidney disease, certain metabolic diseases, and infections. The collection and analysis of urine over the course of 24 hours allows for evaluation of kidney function. To perform urinalysis, a urine specimen must be obtained.

Depending on the situation, the method of collecting a urine specimen may vary. For routine urinalysis, no special collection procedures are necessary. The person is asked to urinate directly into the specimen cup, if possible. If this is difficult for the person, he or she can urinate into a specimen collection device ("commode hat"; see Chapter 19, Fig. 19-17), or into a bedpan or urinal. The person must not have a bowel movement at the same time the urine is being collected, or place toilet paper in the collection device, because these actions will change the urinalysis results. The urine is then poured from the collection device, bedpan, or urinal into the specimen cup. The procedure for obtaining a routine urine sample is described in Procedure 20-3.

In some situations, it may be necessary to obtain a **midstream ("clean catch") urine specimen** using a sterile specimen container. This method of collecting urine prevents contamination of the urine by the bacteria that normally live in and around the urethra. A midstream ("clean catch") urine specimen is usually ordered when the doctor suspects a urinary tract infection. This way, if any bacteria are found in the urine sample, the doctor knows that they are the ones most likely responsible for the infection. When a midstream ("clean catch") urine specimen is requested, the person is asked to clean the area around the urethral opening with a special cleansing wipe. The urine flow is started, then stopped, then started again. The urine sample is collected from the restarted flow. Procedure 20-4 describes how to assist a person with obtaining a midstream ("clean catch") urine specimen.

Your facility or agency may train you to do a type of routine urine testing that involves dipping chemically treated paper strips into a urine sample. Chemicals on the paper react with certain substances that may be found in the urine, causing the chemical blocks on the paper to change colour if these substances are present in the urine. The paper is then compared with a colour chart that comes with the strips (Fig. 20-4), and the results are recorded in the person's chart and reported to the nurse.

Obtaining a Stool Sample

Stool can be analyzed for the presence of blood, pathogens (such as parasites or bacteria), fat, and other things that are not normally found in feces. Because people do not have bowel movements as often as they urinate, if a stool sample is needed, the person should be notified well in advance so that the specimen can be collected when it becomes available. Ask the nurse if there are any particular collection methods that should be used. Stool can be collected in a bedpan, bedside commode, or in a collection device placed

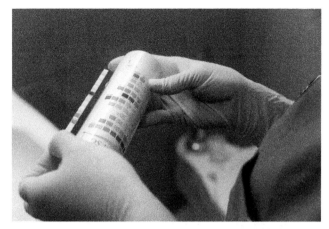

Figure 20-4
Chemically treated reagent strips are used to test urine for some substances. Your facility may train you to do this type of urinalysis.

onto a regular toilet. The person must not urinate at the same time the stool sample is being collected, or place toilet paper in the collection device, because these actions will change the test results. The procedure for collecting a stool sample is given in Procedure 20-5.

URINARY ELIMINATION

The urinary system, which is discussed in more detail in Chapter 32, is made up of the kidneys, ureters, urinary bladder, and urethra (Fig. 20-5). Blood passes through the kidneys, which remove waste products and excess fluid, forming urine. It takes the kidneys approximately one half hour to process the body's total blood volume. As it forms, the urine flows from the kidneys through the ureters and is stored in the urinary bladder. As the bladder fills, we begin to feel the urge to urinate. Urine leaves the body through the urethra.

The process of passing urine from the body is known by several terms, including **urination, voiding,** and **micturition.** Many of your patients or residents will have their own terms for urinating, such as "peeing" or "passing water." When talking about urination with a patient or resident, you should use words that the person is familiar with. This is especially important when talking with children.

In healthy people, urine is clear, without cloudiness or particles. Sometimes urine that has been in a container for a while will become cloudy as it cools. Healthy urine is pale yellow, straw-coloured, or dark gold (amber) in colour, with a slight odour. A slight red tinge to the urine may

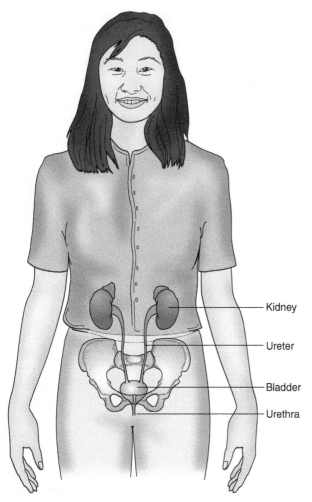

Figure 20-5
The urinary system.

occur. For example, **frequency** is the term used to describe voiding that occurs more often than usual. Frequency is often accompanied by a feeling of **urgency,** or the need to urinate immediately. A person with a urinary tract infection may experience frequency and urgency. **Nocturia** is the need to get up more than once or twice during the night to urinate, to the point where sleep is disrupted. Nocturia can be a sign of pain or depression, a prostate or bladder disorder, or heart failure.

Urination should not cause discomfort. **Dysuria** is difficulty voiding that may or may not be associated with pain. Some people describe the discomfort they feel during urination as a "burning" or "cramping" sensation. Dysuria is often associated with bladder infections, prostate problems, and some sexually transmitted infections (STIs).

TELL THE NURSE

Changes in the quality of a person's urine or urination habits can be a sign that something is wrong. Be sure to report the following observations to the nurse immediately:

- The urine is cloudy or contains particles, is an abnormal colour, or has an abnormal odour

- The person complains that the urine is difficult or painful to pass (that is, the person has dysuria)

- The person is experiencing frequency, urgency, or both

- The person needs to get up more frequently than usual to use the bathroom during the night

indicate **hematuria,** or the presence of blood in the urine. This is an abnormal finding. Sometimes hematuria is **occult** (that is, hidden) and must be detected using urinalysis. Some foods and drugs can also affect the colour and odour of urine. When you are helping a patient or resident with urination, observe the urine and report any abnormalities to the nurse. Urine with an unusual odour or appearance could be a sign of illness or infection.

The frequency of voiding, and the amount of urine voided each time, will differ from person to person. Many factors influence a person's urination habits, including the amount of fluids the person drinks, the types of medications the person takes, the person's age, and the person's lifelong tendencies. For example, some people void quite frequently, at the first urge, while others may hold their urine for as long as possible, even if a bathroom is readily available. You will soon become aware of the urination habits that are normal for each person in your care. This knowledge will allow you to recognize any changes that may

MEASURING URINE OUTPUT

As you learned in Chapter 19, urine output is a key indicator of fluid balance. In a person who is maintaining a good fluid balance, urine output is neither too high nor too low.

- **Oliguria** is the state of voiding a very small amount of urine over a given period of time (for example, voiding only 100 to 400 mL of urine over 24 hours). *Olig-* means "few" and *-uria* means "urine." A person who is dehydrated might become oliguric (that is, have a urine output that is well below normal).

- **Polyuria** (*poly-* means "many") is excessive urine output. Polyuria, also known as **diuresis,** can be a sign of a health problem. For example, polyuria can be a symptom of poorly controlled diabetes. Or, polyuria may be the desired effect of a medication. For example, a person who is retaining excessive amounts of fluid (for example, as the result of a heart disorder) may be put on a medication called a diuretic to help rid the body of the extra fluid. The polyuria that results is a sign that the medication is having the desired effect.

Evaluating a person's urine output is also a good way to determine how well a person's kidneys are working. **Anuria** (*an-* means "none") is defined as the state of voiding less than 100 mL of urine over the course of 24 hours. Anuria usually indicates that a person is in kidney failure.

Not all of the people you care for will need to have their urine output measured and recorded, but people who have illnesses or take medications that may alter their body's ability to maintain a healthy fluid balance will need to have their urine output measured regularly. Some people who are critically ill will have their urine output measured and recorded every hour, but most people in the health care setting have routine orders for their urine output to be measured and recorded each shift.

If a person uses a regular toilet, you will need to remind the person to void into a specimen collection device ("commode hat") and to call you after he or she has finished voiding so that you can measure and record the amount of urine. Specimen collection devices, urinals, and the drainage bags used with urinary catheters often have markings that make measuring urine output easy. If they do not, then the urine output can be measured by pouring it into a graduate (Fig. 20-6). A graduate is also used to measure urine output if a person voids into a bedpan or bedside commode bucket.

If the urine output of one of your residents or patients is being monitored, you will need to keep a record of the amount of urine passed at each voiding. Some intake and output (I&O) flow sheets will have spaces to record the amount of each individual voiding, while others may only have a space to record the end-of-shift amount. To obtain the end-of-shift amount, simply add the individual amounts together and record the total in the appropriate space.

URINARY CATHETERIZATION

Sometimes a person is unable to urinate using a toilet, bedpan, urinal, or bedside commode, due to disability or illness. In these situations, a

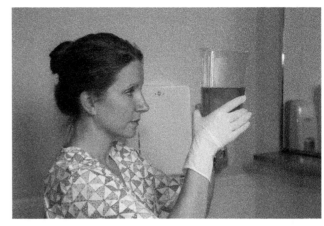

Figure 20-6
To measure urine output, the urine is poured into a measuring device called a graduate. The graduate is held at eye level to properly determine the amount of fluid it contains.

urinary catheter is used. A **catheter** is a tube that is inserted into the body for the purpose of administering or removing fluids. A urinary catheter is inserted into the bladder through the urethra (or through an incision made in the abdominal wall) to allow the urine in the bladder to drain out. A urinary catheter is used in many different situations:

- A urinary catheter may be inserted to drain the bladder before or during a surgical procedure, during recovery from a serious illness or injury, or to collect urine for testing.
- A urinary catheter may be used for a person who is incontinent of urine, if the person has wounds or pressure ulcers that would be made worse by contact with urine.
- A urinary catheter is necessary when a person is unable to urinate because of an obstruction in the urethra.

Usually, inserting a urinary catheter is beyond the scope of practice for a personal support worker, although in some facilities, personal support workers are provided with additional training that allows them to catheterize residents or patients. Inserting a catheter is a procedure that requires sterile technique because it involves putting a foreign object (that is, the catheter) into a person's body. If sterile technique is not used, the catheter can introduce infection-causing bacteria into the bladder. Regardless of whether or not you are trained to actually insert urinary catheters, caring for people who have urinary catheters in place will almost certainly be a part of your daily duties.

Types of Urinary Catheters

You will see many different types of urinary catheters in use.

Straight catheters

A **straight catheter,** also known as a Robinson, Rob-Nel, or Red Rubber catheter, is used when the catheter is to be inserted and removed immediately. The catheter is introduced into the bladder, the urine is allowed to drain out, and the catheter is removed (Fig. 20-7A). This type of catheterization is commonly used to obtain a sterile urine specimen from a woman, before or after surgery, after a vaginal delivery, or when a person needs to empty his bladder

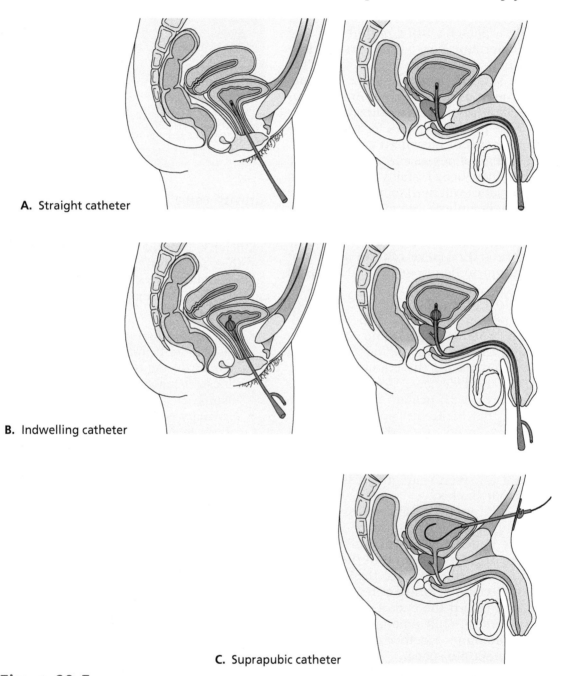

A. Straight catheter

B. Indwelling catheter

C. Suprapubic catheter

Figure 20-7
Types of catheters. **(A)** A straight catheter is inserted into the bladder, the urine is drained, and then the catheter is removed. **(B)** An indwelling catheter, also known as a Foley catheter or a retention catheter, remains in the body and urine drains continuously into a drainage bag. **(C)** A suprapubic catheter is inserted into the bladder through a surgical incision made above the pubic bone (*supra-* means "above"). A suprapubic catheter is a bit less likely to promote urinary infections because its location keeps the opening away from the contaminated perineal area.

but cannot as a result of pain or swelling that is temporary.

Indwelling catheters

An **indwelling catheter,** also known as a retention or Foley catheter, is left inside the bladder to provide continuous urine drainage. An indwelling catheter has a soft balloon that is inflated inside the bladder to keep the catheter from sliding out of the urethra (see Fig. 20-7B). Urine collects in a drainage bag, which is attached to the indwelling catheter by a length of tubing.

An indwelling catheter may have two lumens or three lumens (Fig. 20-8). A double-lumen indwelling catheter has two lumens. One lumen, which connects to the catheter tubing, is for urine drainage. The other is used to inflate the balloon that holds the catheter in place. A triple-lumen indwelling catheter has three lumens. The extra lumen is used to flush the bladder with irrigation fluid. Regular flushing of the bladder with irrigation fluid helps to keep blood clots from forming inside the bladder. This is important in certain situations, such as when a man has just had prostate surgery.

Suprapubic catheters

A **suprapubic catheter** is a type of indwelling catheter. The suprapubic catheter is inserted into the bladder through a surgical incision made in the abdominal wall, right above the pubic bone (see Fig. 20-7C). This type of catheter is most often used for people with blocked urethras, and for men. Men typically are not able to use an indwelling urinary catheter that is inserted through the urethra for long periods of time due to the anatomy of the male urethra. While a woman's urethra is straight and only about 5 cm long, a man's urethra is curved in an "S" shape and is about 15 cm long (see Fig. 20-7B). In men, the pressure of the indwelling catheter can cause erosion of the mucous membrane that lines the urethra in the curved areas.

Caring for a Person With an Indwelling Urinary Catheter

Indwelling urinary catheters are connected by a length of tubing to a urine drainage bag. Urine drains continuously from the bladder, through

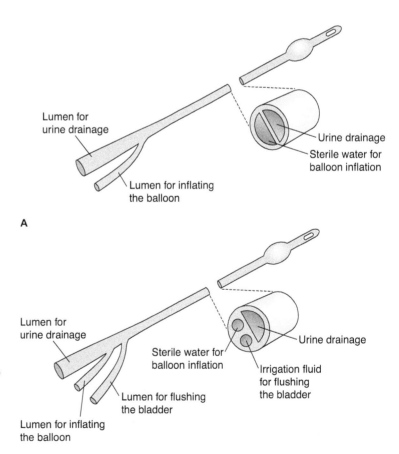

Figure 20-8

(A) A double-lumen indwelling catheter has two lumens. One lumen is for urine drainage. The other is used to inflate the balloon that holds the catheter in place. **(B)** A triple-lumen indwelling catheter has three lumens. The additional lumen is used to flush the bladder with irrigation fluid.

Lumen for urine drainage
Lumen for inflating the balloon
Urine drainage
Sterile water for balloon inflation

A

Lumen for urine drainage
Sterile water for balloon inflation
Urine drainage
Irrigation fluid for flushing the bladder
Lumen for flushing the bladder
Lumen for inflating the balloon

B

the catheter, down the tubing, and into the drainage bag (Fig. 20-9). There are several different types of urine drainage bags that you will see in the health care setting. Some urine drainage bags have a long length of tubing that allows them to be carried or secured to a bed frame or the back of a wheelchair. Other urine drainage bags, called "leg bags," are connected to the catheter by a short length of tubing and secured to the person's thigh with straps. Leg bags are useful because they can be concealed underneath a person's clothing and they allow the person to move around freely.

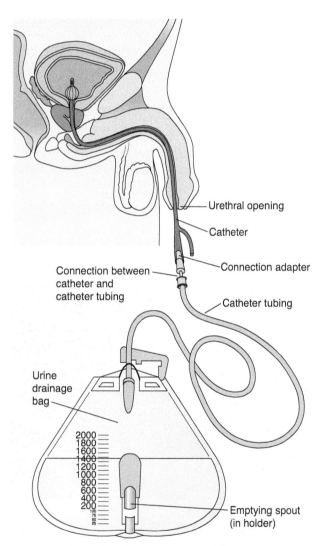

Figure 20-9
The indwelling urinary catheter drainage system consists of a catheter that is connected to a urine drainage bag by way of a length of tubing. The urine drainage bag has a connection adapter, where the tubing attaches, and an emptying spout, which is unclamped to allow the urine to drain from the bag. When not in use, the emptying spout is stored in a holder that is part of the bag.

When a regular urine drainage bag with a long length of tubing is being used, the tubing is secured loosely to the person's body near the insertion site using a catheter strap or adhesive tape. Securing the tubing to the person's body prevents the catheter from being accidentally pulled out during repositioning. In women, the tubing is attached to the thigh. In men, the tubing is attached to the thigh or lower abdomen (Fig. 20-10). A little bit of slack is left in the tubing to prevent the catheter from pulling against the bladder outlet and the urethral opening. The remaining length of tubing is then gently coiled and secured to the bed linens using a plastic clip (Fig. 20-11). Coiling the tubing prevents the tubing from becoming bent or kinked, which would stop the free flow of urine into the drainage bag. Coiling the tubing and securing it to the bed linens also keep the weight of the tubing from pulling against the person's body. The drainage bag is then secured to the bed frame or the back of the person's wheelchair, at a level lower than the person's bladder (Fig. 20-12). If the drainage bag and tubing are higher than the person's bladder, then gravity could cause old, contaminated urine to run back down the tubing and into the person's bladder, causing an infection.

All urine drainage bags have a connection adapter (where the catheter tubing attaches) and an emptying spout that is opened to allow urine to drain from the bag. Because the inside of the catheter and tubing are sterile, it is safer for the person if the bag is not disconnected from the tubing once the catheter is in place. Disconnecting the bag from the tubing can allow harmful bacteria to enter the catheter. Occasionally, the tubing has to be disconnected from the bag (for example, to change the bag if it is leaking, to replace a regular drainage bag with a leg bag, or to perform certain procedures). If you must disconnect the tubing from the bag, be sure to prevent the end of the tubing from touching anything, and wipe the exposed tubing with an antibacterial wipe before reconnecting the drainage bag. General guidelines for caring for a person with an indwelling catheter are given in Guidelines Box 20-2.

Providing catheter care

Although you may not be permitted to catheterize your patients or residents, you will most likely be responsible for providing catheter care. **Catheter care** involves thorough cleaning of the perineal area (especially around the urethra) and the catheter tubing that extends outside of the body, to prevent infection. Providing good catheter care

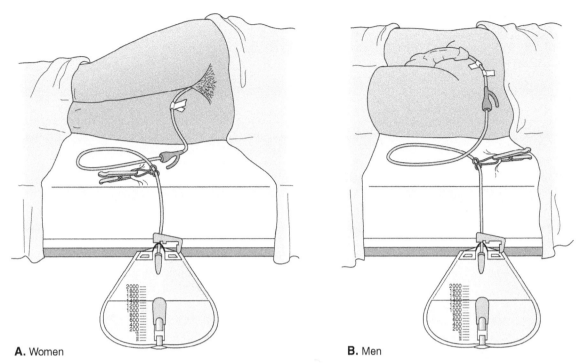

A. Women   **B.** Men

Figure 20-10
The catheter tubing is secured loosely to the person's body to prevent tension on the tubing and catheter, which could cause discomfort. Securing the tubing also prevents the catheter from accidentally being pulled out of the body during repositioning. **(A)** In women, the tubing is secured to the inner thigh. **(B)** In men, the tubing is connected either to the inner thigh or the lower abdomen.

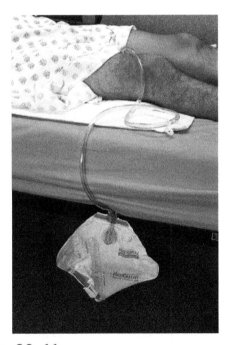

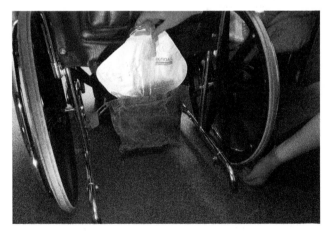

Figure 20-12
When a person with an indwelling urinary catheter is in a wheelchair, the urine drainage bag is attached to the back of the person's wheelchair, away from the wheels and at a level that is lower than the person's bladder. When the person is in bed, the urine drainage bag is attached to the bed frame (see Fig. 20-11).

Figure 20-11
The catheter tubing is gently coiled (to prevent it from kinking) and secured to the bed linens with a plastic clip.

Guidelines Box 20-2 — Guidelines for Caring for People With Indwelling Catheters

WHAT YOU DO	WHY YOU DO IT
Loosely secure the catheter tubing to the person near the insertion site, using a catheter strap or adhesive tape.	Securing the catheter tubing helps to prevent the catheter from being pulled out during repositioning. Allowing a little bit of slack helps to prevent the catheter from pulling against the bladder outlet and the urethral opening.
Gently coil the remaining length of tubing and secure it to the bed linens using a plastic clip.	Coiling the tubing helps to prevent kinking, which could stop the free flow of urine into the drainage bag. It also keeps the weight of the tubing from pulling against the area where the tubing is secured to the person's body.
When repositioning a person who has an indwelling catheter, always make sure to unclip the coiled tubing from the linens before beginning the procedure. When you are finished with the procedure, secure the coiled tubing to the linens again.	The person needs to be able to move freely during procedures such as repositioning. If you try to move a person in the direction opposite from the length of tubing, and the length of tubing is still attached to the bed linens, then the catheter could be pulled out of the person's body.
Make sure that the person is not lying on the coiled tubing.	This would be uncomfortable for the person. In addition, the weight of the person's body on the tubing could stop the free flow of urine into the drainage bag.
Always make sure the urine drainage bag is placed at a level lower than that of the person's bladder.	Raising the urine drainage bag up higher than the bladder can cause old, contaminated urine to run back into the bladder, which can lead to infection.
Never attach a urine drainage bag to a side rail. Instead, attach the drainage bag to the bed frame.	Raising the side rail would raise the drainage bag to a level that is higher than the person's bladder. The bed frame does not move; therefore, the level of the drainage bag cannot change.
Keep the drainage bag off the floor. When emptying the drainage bag, be sure that the open emptying spout does not touch anything.	Bacteria can enter the closed drainage system in this manner. The presence of bacteria in the system can lead to health care–associated urinary tract infections in people with indwelling catheters.
Always wear gloves when emptying the urine drainage bag.	Urine is a body fluid and may contain pathogens.

is important because the catheter provides a pathway for bacteria to travel up from the perineum into the bladder, where they can cause infection. In addition, having a catheter in place eliminates the "flushing" action of normal urination, which helps to remove bacteria from the urinary tract naturally. Because bacteria can be introduced into the body both when a urinary catheter is inserted and after it is in place, urinary tract infections in catheterized people are among the most common health care–associated infections (HAIs). (Remember that HAIs are acquired in the health care setting.)

In an effort to reduce the risk of HAIs in people who are catheterized, many facilities require catheter care to be provided routinely (for example, once or twice daily), and again whenever the perineal area becomes soiled (such as when a person is incontinent of feces). Soap and water or a special antibacterial solution may be used when providing catheter care. The procedure for providing catheter care is given in Procedure 20-6.

Emptying urine drainage bags

Urine drainage bags are routinely emptied and the urine measured at the end of each shift unless ordered otherwise. Urine drainage bags should also be emptied if they become too full. Leg bags need to be emptied frequently because they are smaller and hold less urine. The procedure for emptying a urine drainage bag is given in Procedure 20-7.

TELL THE NURSE

When caring for a catheterized person, make sure you report any of the following observations to the nurse immediately:

- Changes in the colour, clarity, or odour of the urine

- Failure of urine to flow freely through the tubing (make sure that the tubing is not kinked or bent)

- The person complains of pain or discomfort as a result of the catheter

- Redness, swelling, or discharge from the catheter insertion site

- Leaking of urine around the catheter insertion site

Preparing for removal of an indwelling catheter

Use of an indwelling catheter can lead to temporary urinary incontinence when the catheter is removed, because the catheter allows the bladder to become "lazy." While the catheter was in place, urine drained out of the body continuously. The bladder did not have to fill up and then empty itself. This lack of activity can decrease the muscle tone of the bladder, leading to incontinence. To prepare the bladder for removal of the catheter and prevent temporary incontinence from developing, it is common to clamp the tubing of the catheter for a period of time to allow the urine to fill the bladder. The tubing is then unclamped and the urine is allowed to drain from the bladder. This procedure is repeated over a period of time, with the time intervals between clamping and emptying becoming increasingly longer. Then the catheter is removed and the person is allowed to void normally. The nurse will let you know if you are to help prepare a person for removal of an indwelling catheter.

URINARY INCONTINENCE

Urinary incontinence is the inability to hold one's urine, or the involuntary loss of urine from the bladder. Urinary incontinence may be temporary or permanent. Temporary urinary incontinence can occur as a result of a bladder infection, or after an indwelling catheter that has been in place for a long time is removed. Permanent urinary incontinence can be caused by many things, including:

- Decreased muscle tone in the bladder or the muscles that support the bladder, such as occurs after childbirth or from obesity
- Injuries or illnesses that affect the spinal cord, the brain, or the nerves that control bladder function
- Dementia

Urinary incontinence can be emotionally devastating for both the incontinent person and the person's caregivers. For the person who is incontinent, having wet clothes or smelling like urine can be very embarrassing. In addition, being incontinent of urine places a person at risk for developing skin problems (such as rashes and pressure ulcers) and for falling (as the person rushes to the bathroom to avoid having an accident). For the caregiver, caring for a person who is incontinent of urine can be frustrating and emotionally draining. It is not uncommon to change a person's clothes or bedding, only to have the person wet herself all over again. Because caring for an incontinent person can be so emotionally trying and time-consuming, incontinence is the factor that most often leads family members to have a relative admitted to a long-term care facility.

Types of Urinary Incontinence

There are many types of urinary incontinence:

- *Stress incontinence* is probably the most common type of urinary incontinence. In stress incontinence, urine leaks from the bladder when the person coughs, sneezes, or exerts herself. Stress incontinence can also occur if a person delays voiding and the bladder becomes too full. Childbirth, obesity, and loss of muscle tone as a result of aging are all factors that can contribute to stress incontinence. Stress incontinence can also occur in men after prostate surgery. Stress incontinence can often be corrected with exercises or surgery.
- *Urge incontinence* is the involuntary release of urine right after feeling a strong urge to void. This type of incontinence is common in people with urinary tract infections because irritation of the bladder causes the bladder muscle to spasm, expelling the contents of the bladder with little warning. Other conditions that decrease the ability of the bladder to hold urine, such as an enlarged prostate gland or increased intake of caffeinated beverages or alcohol, can also cause urge incontinence.
- *Functional incontinence* occurs in the absence of physical or nervous system problems affecting the urinary tract. The person just cannot make it to the bathroom in enough time, or wait until a bedpan or urinal is provided. It is thought that being in a strange environment (as a hospital or long-term care facility would be to someone who has just been admitted) contributes to functional incontinence. Confusion, disorientation, and loss of mobility are also contributing factors.
- *Overflow incontinence* occurs when the bladder is too full of urine. Overflow incontinence is associated with **urinary retention,** which is the inability of the bladder to empty either completely during urination, or at all. Urinary retention can result from blockage of the bladder outlet (such as occurs with an enlarged prostate gland or from swelling of the urethra during labour or childbirth), or from pain following a surgical procedure. Some injuries that involve the spinal cord can also keep the bladder from emptying

fully, leading to urinary retention. Because the bladder does not empty completely when the person voids, it refills with urine quickly, and the urine simply overflows. A person with overflow incontinence may "dribble" urine in between visits to the bathroom. If a person cannot empty his bladder completely, it may be necessary to insert a catheter (either temporarily or permanently) to allow urine to drain from the bladder and prevent urinary retention and overflow incontinence from occurring.

- *Reflex incontinence* occurs when there is damage to the nerves that enable the person to control urination. The bladder fills, but the person does not feel the urge to urinate. When the bladder is completely full, it empties reflexively (that is, automatically). Some people with certain disorders of the nervous system, such as paralysis from a spinal cord injury, will catheterize themselves with a straight catheter on a regular basis to prevent reflex urinary incontinence.

Managing Urinary Incontinence

Many products are available to help manage urinary incontinence, including incontinence pads, incontinence briefs, and condom catheters. In addition, techniques such as bladder training may be used to help a person overcome certain types of incontinence. For some people, temporary or permanent catheterization may be necessary to manage the incontinence.

Incontinence pads and briefs

Products made for urinary incontinence are available to help prevent soiling of clothes and furniture (Fig. 20-13). Incontinence pads and briefs are specially made to absorb urine and hold it away from the person's skin. Keeping the skin dry helps to reduce the skin problems that can occur from prolonged contact with urine. Incontinence pads are placed inside the person's underpants to prevent wetting of the clothes and to draw the moisture away from the person's body. Incontinence briefs are worn instead of underpants. Incontinence pads and briefs are very useful for active people.

For a person who is confined to bed, special bed protectors are used to help to keep the bed linens and mattress dry and to wick urine away from the person's skin. Many facilities have policies that specify that incontinence briefs are to be

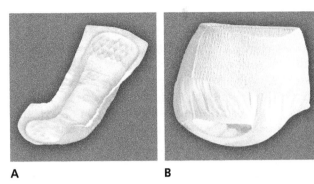

A   **B**

Figure 20-13
Incontinence pads and briefs are worn under clothing to absorb moisture and keep it away from the body. **(A)** DEPEND Guards for men. **(B)** DEPEND Extra Absorbency Underwear. (*Photographs courtesy of Kimberly-Clark Worldwide, Inc., Neenah, WI.*)

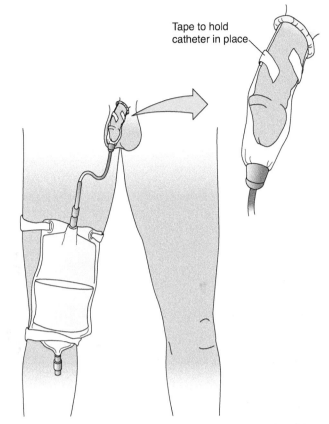

Tape to hold catheter in place

Figure 20-14
A condom catheter can be used to manage urinary incontinence in men. If tape is used to secure the condom catheter to the penis, it should be applied in a spiral fashion, not a circular fashion.

used only when the person is out of bed, and that bed protectors are to be used when the person is sleeping. Incontinence briefs tend to fit closely, which makes it difficult for air to reach the skin. Switching between briefs and bed protectors helps to prevent skin breakdown by allowing the skin to be exposed to the air at night. As a personal support worker, you must make sure that these incontinence products are changed frequently and that urine is cleaned from the skin whenever the change occurs. (See Chapter 17 for a discussion of providing perineal care, which is especially important in people who are incontinent of urine, feces, or both.)

Condom catheters

A **condom catheter** can be used to manage incontinence in men. A condom catheter is not a true catheter because it is not placed inside the body. It consists of a soft plastic or rubber sheath, tubing, and a collection bag for the urine (Fig. 20-14). The sheath is placed over the penis and the collection bag is attached to the leg. The urine flows through the tubing into the collection bag, allowing the man to urinate at will.

The condom must fit the penis. It should be fastened securely enough to prevent leaking, but not so snugly that it restricts circulation. Many condom catheters have adhesive material on the inside of the condom that allows for a good seal. Others must be secured with elastic tape. The tape strip is applied in a spiral fashion to allow for changes in the size of the penis (see Fig. 20-14). Applying the tape in an overlapping, circular fashion would compromise blood flow if

the man had an erection, possibly causing permanent damage to the penis.

Use of a condom catheter requires good skin care. The penis must be cleaned, and the condom apparatus changed, daily.

Bladder training

Bladder training is commonly used to help people relearn how to control their urinary elimination. For example, a person may be encouraged to use the bedpan, urinal, or commode at scheduled times. Scheduling helps promote regular emptying of the bladder. The primary goal is for the person to be able to control involuntary urination. If this is not possible, then the person may still at least be able to get to the bathroom in time to avoid accidents, because she will know when voiding is due to occur. The person's care plan will note any special bladder training techniques that are being used and the nurse will instruct you on any specific duties you will be assigned as part of that training.

BOWEL ELIMINATION

The digestive tract, which is discussed in more detail in Chapter 31, consists of the mouth, esophagus, stomach, small intestine, large intestine, rectum, and anus (Fig. 20-15). The rectum is actually part of the large intestine, and together, the large and small intestines are sometimes referred to as "bowels." Essentially, the digestive tract is a long, hollow tube. The food and fluids that we take in are broken down into smaller pieces and mixed together in the stomach, forming a partially digested food and fluid mixture known as **chyme.** From the stomach, the chyme passes slowly into the small intestine, where more digestion occurs and nutrients and fluid are absorbed, and then into the large intestine. Wave-like muscular movements, called **peristalsis,** move the chyme

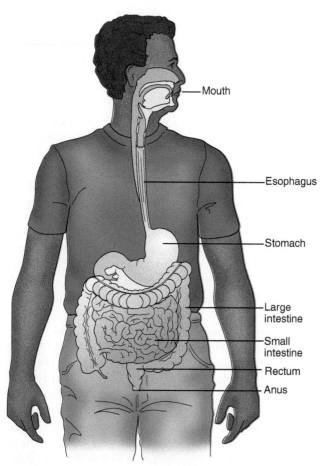

Figure 20-15
The digestive tract consists of the mouth, esophagus, stomach, small intestine, large intestine, rectum, and anus.

through the intestines. Finally, the chyme reaches the last part of the large intestine, called the rectum. At this point, all of the nutrients have been removed, and what remains is a semi-solid waste material, called **feces.** The presence of feces in the rectum stimulates the urge to **defecate** (that is, have a bowel movement), and the feces leave the body through the anus, the very end of the digestive tract. Sometimes fecal material is referred to as "**stool**" after it leaves the body.

Flatus (or gas) is a natural by-product of digestion, just as feces are. Eating certain foods, such as beans, broccoli, cabbage, cauliflower, and onions, can lead to the formation of flatus. The passing of flatus may be quite noisy and depending on what was eaten, the flatus may have a foul odour. For some people, passing flatus is very embarrassing.

In healthy people, feces are soft, brown, moist, and formed, with a distinct odour. Certain foods and medications can affect the colour and odour of feces. When you are helping a patient or resident with defecation, observe the feces and report any abnormalities to the nurse. Feces with an unusual odour or appearance could be a sign of illness or infection.

The frequency of a person's bowel movements, and the amount of feces passed each time, will differ from person to person. Many factors influence a person's bowel elimination pattern, including the amount of fluid the person drinks and the type of food he or she eats, the types of drugs the person takes, the person's age, the person's level of activity, and the person's lifelong elimination habits. For example, some people have a bowel movement every morning. Other people are not so predictable. For some people, one or two bowel movements a day is normal. For others, one bowel movement every 2 or 3 days is normal. You will soon become aware of the bowel elimination pattern that is normal for each person in your care. This knowledge will allow you to recognize any changes that may occur.

PROBLEMS WITH BOWEL ELIMINATION

Problems with bowel elimination that are often seen in the health care setting include diarrhea, constipation, fecal impaction, flatulence, and fecal incontinence.

Diarrhea

Diarrhea is the passage of liquid, unformed stool. Diarrhea may occur frequently and can be accompanied by abdominal cramping. If diarrhea is frequent or excessive, the loss of fluid from the body can quickly cause dehydration, especially in young or elderly people. When caring for a person with diarrhea:

- Practice good infection control techniques. A common cause of diarrhea is a bacterial or viral infection. Because the pathogen that caused the diarrhea will be present in the feces, it is important to use good infection control techniques when caring for a person with diarrhea.
- Answer the call light quickly to provide access to the toilet, commode, or bedpan. A normally continent person can have temporary fecal incontinence from diarrhea, which can be very humiliating. Being quick to respond, compassionate, and supportive can help the person to feel better.
- Provide gentle, thorough skin care after each bowel movement to prevent skin breakdown.
- Make sure to record and report the frequency and amount of each incident of diarrhea.

Constipation

The opposite of diarrhea is constipation. **Constipation** occurs when the feces remain in the intestines for too long. The delay allows too much fluid to be reabsorbed by the intestines, resulting in hard, dry feces that are difficult to pass. Constipation is fairly common among patients and residents. Risk factors for developing constipation include:

- Taking medications that slow peristalsis (for example, pain medications)
- Not taking in enough dietary fibre or fluids
- Not getting enough exercise
- Delaying having a bowel movement after the urge occurs
- Lack of privacy

As you learned earlier in this chapter, there are many things a personal support worker can do to help a patient or resident maintain normal bowel function and prevent constipation. For example, encouraging patients or residents to eat fibre-rich foods, drink plenty of fluids, and exercise regularly can help to keep bowel function regular. However, if a person is constipated and all other methods of promoting normal bowel function have failed, the doctor may order a laxative, stool softener, or fibre supplement.

- A **laxative** is a medication that chemically stimulates peristalsis so that material inside the intestines moves through at a faster pace. The resulting bowel movement is soft (or pos-

sibly liquid) and occurs within a few hours of taking the laxative, or overnight. Laxatives are acceptable for occasional use, but should not be used regularly. The problem with regular laxative use is that laxatives cause the chyme to pass through the intestines too quickly for nutrients and fluids to be absorbed. This can result in poor nutrition and dehydration. The intestines also become used to being chemically stimulated to move and can become dependent on the laxative.

- **Stool softeners** help to keep fluid in the feces and are used to help prevent constipation for some people. Unlike laxatives, stool softeners do not chemically stimulate the intestines to cause a bowel movement.
- **Fibre supplements,** in the form of tablets or drink additives, can add bulk to the feces, causing it to hold fluid and preventing constipation.

Fecal Impaction

A **fecal impaction** occurs when constipation is not relieved. The feces build up in the rectum and become harder and harder as more and more fluid is absorbed. Eventually, it becomes almost impossible to pass the feces normally. The impaction blocks the passage of normal stool, but liquid stool may go around the impacted mass. A person with an impaction is usually very uncomfortable, and may complain of abdominal or rectal pain or of liquid feces "seeping" out of the anus. The person's abdomen may be swollen.

If a person is thought to have a fecal impaction, a **digital examination** is done (Fig. 20-16). During the digital examination, a finger is inserted into the person's rectum to feel for the impacted mass (*digital* means "finger"). The impaction is then removed by using the finger to break the impacted feces apart and scoop it out of the rectum piece by piece. The doctor may also order the use of an oil retention enema or medication to help remove the impaction. Digital removal of a fecal impaction is very uncomfortable and embarrassing for most patients and residents. Many facilities require that a nurse remove an impaction, but your assistance will be necessary. If you are allowed to remove an impaction, make sure you have been adequately trained for the procedure and that it is part of your job description.

Flatulence

Flatulence is the presence of excessive amounts of flatus (gas) in the intestines, causing abdominal distension (swelling) and discomfort. Sometimes

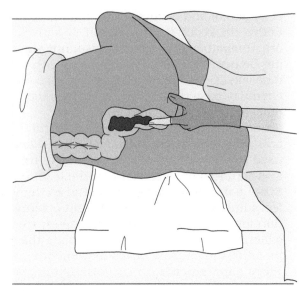

Figure 20-16
Digital examination. A finger is inserted into the person's rectum to check for a fecal impaction.

people have difficulty passing flatus because of a lack of activity or a recent surgical procedure. Getting out of bed and walking might be all that is needed to help the person to expel the gas. If walking is not allowed, positioning the person on her left side may help. If the flatulence cannot be relieved with these methods, a nurse may insert a rectal tube to help the gas escape (Fig. 20-17).

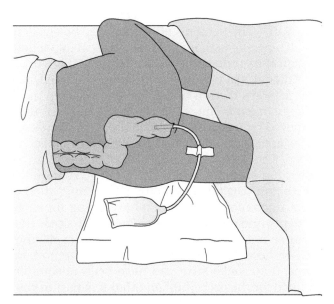

Figure 20-17
A rectal tube may be placed to relieve flatulence (excess gas in the intestines) if the gas cannot be passed naturally. The small bag connected to the end of the rectal tube is used to collect any liquid stool that may escape with the flatus.

Fecal Incontinence

Fecal (bowel) incontinence is the inability to hold one's feces, or the involuntary loss of feces from the bowel. Like urinary incontinence, fecal incontinence can be temporary or permanent. Temporary fecal incontinence can occur with a severe case of diarrhea, simply because the person might not be able to get to the bathroom quickly enough. Some people experience temporary fecal incontinence if the call light is not answered soon enough. Diseases or injuries that affect the nervous system can also result in temporary or permanent fecal incontinence. A person who is unconscious will be incontinent of feces. A person who has dementia will develop fecal incontinence as the disease progresses.

Bowel training is very similar to bladder training and works to promote regular, controlled bowel movements. Offering the commode or bedpan at regular scheduled intervals is a common method of bowel training. Bowel training is often started by keeping track of when an incontinent person usually has a bowel movement, then making sure to provide the appropriate toilet facilities during that time period.

TELL THE NURSE

Changes in the quality of a person's feces or pattern of defecation can be a sign that something is wrong. Be sure to report the following observations to the nurse immediately:

- The person has diarrhea or is constipated
- There is blood or mucus in the stool
- The stool is black or dark green
- The stool is foul-smelling
- The person complains that the feces are painful or difficult to pass
- There is bleeding from the anus during or after a bowel movement
- The person has a swollen abdomen or complains of abdominal pain
- The person complains of liquid feces "seeping" from the anus
- The person has excessive flatus (gas)

ENEMAS

An **enema** is the introduction of fluid into the large intestine by way of the anus for the purpose of removing stool from the rectum. There are several reasons a person would be given an enema. Enemas are used to relieve constipation and fecal impactions and to empty the intestine of fecal material before surgery or certain diagnostic tests. Sometimes enemas are used as part of a bowel training program.

Types of Enemas

Several types of enemas are used in the health care setting (Fig. 20-18). Some are prepared by the nurse or personal support worker, and others come prepackaged. The solution that is placed into the rectum varies according to the reason the enema was ordered.

- *Cleansing enemas* are primarily used to remove feces from the lower large intestine. *Tap water enemas* and *saline (salt water) enemas* help soften the stool and stimulate peristalsis. Enemas containing these solutions should not be given repeatedly because the intestine can absorb the solution, causing a fluid imbalance in the body. *Soapsuds enemas* consist of water and a small amount of a very gentle soap called *castile soap*. The soap solution irritates the lining of the bowel, stimulating peristalsis. These, too, must be used with caution

because too much soap can cause damage to the lining of the intestines.
- An *oil retention enema* contains mineral, olive, or cottonseed oil. The oil lubricates the inside of the intestine and any stool that is present, making the stool easier to pass or remove. Oil retention enemas are useful for helping to remove fecal impactions.
- *Commercially prepared and packaged enemas* usually contain 120 mL of a solution that irritates the intestinal mucosa to promote peristalsis. Some commercial enemas contain a solution that is absorbed into the stool to make it softer and easier to pass.

Administering Enemas

Enemas are ordered by a doctor and usually given by a nurse. Some facilities allow personal support workers to administer enemas after adequate training. Make sure you are familiar with your facility's policies on the administration of enemas. If you are permitted to give enemas, be sure to follow proper procedures and the doctor's orders closely. Make sure the solution is correct for the person, that you have the correct amount of solution, and that the solution is at the proper

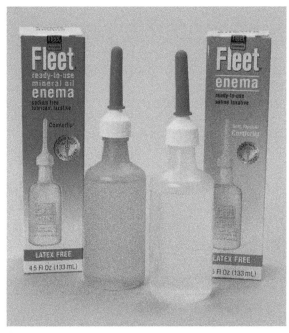

A

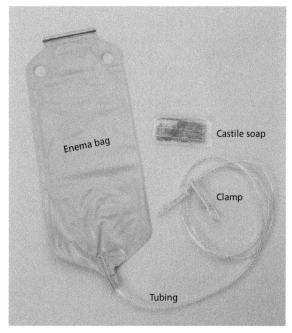

B

Figure 20-18
There are many different types of enema solutions. **(A)** Commercially prepared enema solutions. **(B)** A soapsuds enema is prepared using castile soap and water (not shown) and administered using an enema bag.

temperature. Enema solutions that are too cool can cause abdominal cramping and pain, while solutions that are too hot can cause serious injury and possibly even death. When you are assisting with the administration of an enema, make sure that a bed protector and bedpan are in place, or that the path to the bathroom is clear. When it comes time for the person to expel the enema, she will need immediate access to toilet facilities.

An enema is given with the person on her left side in Sims' position. When a person is lying on her left side in Sims' position, the intestine is positioned to take the best advantage of gravity. The solution will flow downward to clean a longer segment of bowel (Fig. 20-19). Having the person lie on her right side in Sims' position is not as effective because the enema solution flows only as far as the rectum and does not clean as much of the bowel. After the enema has been administered, the person is asked to hold the solution in the bowel for the specified amount of time, and then to expel the solution. The doctor may order a cleansing enema to be administered "until clear," which means that enemas are to be given until the enema return from the person does not contain any fecal material. If you are responsible for giving a cleansing enema, make sure to ask the nurse how many enemas are allowed to be given during a particular session.

Receiving an enema can be uncomfortable and embarrassing. To make the procedure easier for the person, keep the person covered as much as possible and ensure that she has as much privacy as possible. Having the person take a few slow, deep breaths as the enema tubing is inserted into the rectum may help to relax the person and make insertion easier. The procedure for administering an enema is given in Procedure 20-8.

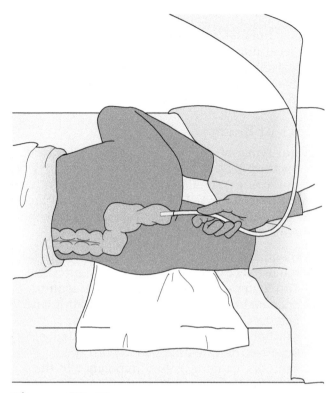

Figure 20-19
The left Sims' position is used when a person is to receive an enema. This position exposes the greatest amount of the bowel to the enema solution.

RECTAL SUPPOSITORIES

A **rectal suppository** is a small, wax-like cone or oval that is inserted into the anus. The wax-like substance dissolves at body temperature, stimulating peristalsis or lubricating and softening the stool. Glycerin rectal suppositories are often used to help with bowel elimination before resorting to an enema. Some rectal suppositories also contain medication. These should only be inserted by a nurse.

SUMMARY

- The elimination of waste products from the body is one of the most basic physical needs.
  - Although elimination is a natural function, many people are not comfortable discussing it or doing it in front of others. A person's culture and upbringing influence how comfortable he is with the body processes involved in elimination.
  - Normal urinary and bowel elimination can be promoted by encouraging fluids, answering the call light promptly, and

  providing for the person's privacy and comfort.
- Incontinence is the inability to hold one's urine, feces, or both until a suitable receptacle (for example, a toilet, bedside commode, or bedpan) is made available. Incontinence has many causes and may be temporary or permanent.
  - Incontinence is difficult emotionally for both the person who is incontinent and that person's caregiver.

- Being incontinent of urine or feces places a person at risk for skin breakdown. Providing good perineal care is essential when caring for a person who is incontinent of urine, feces, or both.
- The urinary system rids the body of waste products that have been filtered from the bloodstream.
  - Normal urine is clear, pale yellow to dark gold in colour, with a characteristic odour. Urinary patterns vary among individuals. Any abnormal observations should be reported to the nurse.
  - A person who is having trouble urinating for physical or emotional reasons may need to have a urinary catheter placed to remove the urine from the bladder.
    - Urinary catheters may be left in place for an extended period of time, or inserted and then removed as soon as the bladder has been drained.
    - Providing good catheter care is essential to prevent health care–associated infections (HAIs). The use of urinary catheters is the leading cause of HAIs.
- The digestive system rids the body of waste products that are left over from digestion.

- Normal stool is soft, brown, moist, formed, and has a distinct odour. Bowel elimination patterns vary among individuals. Any abnormal observations should be reported to the nurse.
  - Constipation occurs when feces remain in the intestine too long and excess fluid is absorbed, leaving the stool hard and difficult to pass. Fecal impaction can result if constipation is not relieved.
  - Diarrhea is the passage of liquid, unformed stool. Diarrhea can lead to dehydration.
- An enema is the introduction of solution into the large intestine. An enema is sometimes ordered by a doctor to treat or prevent bowel elimination problems.
  - The type of enema solution used is determined by the reason the enema has been ordered.
  - Enemas are usually given by a nurse. However, in some facilities, enema administration is within the scope of practice of the personal support worker. Enemas must be administered correctly, with special attention paid to the position of the person.

Assisting a Person With Using a Bedpan

WHY YOU DO IT   Bedpans are used for women who cannot get out of bed to urinate or have a bowel movement and for men who cannot get out of bed to have a bowel movement.

Getting Ready   WGKIEps

1. Complete the "Getting Ready" steps.

Supplies

- gloves
- bed protector
- toilet paper
- bedpan
- bedpan cover (or paper towels)
- perineal care supplies
- washcloth
- towel

Procedure

2. Make sure that the bed is positioned at a comfortable working height (to promote good body mechanics) and that the wheels are locked. If the side rails are in use, lower the side rail on the working side of the bed. The side rail on the opposite side of the bed should remain up. If necessary, lower the head of the bed so that the bed is flat (as tolerated).

3. Put on the gloves.

4. Fanfold the top linens to the foot of the bed. Place the bed protector on the bed. Adjust the person's hospital gown or pajama bottoms as necessary to expose the person's buttocks.

5. Place the bedpan underneath the person's buttocks. This can be accomplished by either helping the person to lie on her side, facing away from you, or by asking the person to bend her knees, press her heels into the mattress, and lift her buttocks. Slide the bedpan underneath the person (if the person is holding her buttocks away from the bed by bending her knees) or place the bedpan against her buttocks and help her to roll back onto it.

a. A standard bedpan is positioned like a regular toilet seat.

b. A fracture pan is positioned with the narrow end pointed toward the head of the bed.

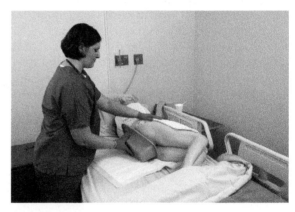

Step 5 Place the bedpan against the person's buttocks and help the person to roll back onto it.

6. Raise the head of the bed as tolerated. Draw the top linens over the person for modesty and warmth.

7. Make sure that the toilet paper and the call-light control are within reach. If the side rails are in use, return the side rails to the raised position.

8. Remove your gloves and wash your hands.

9. If safety permits, leave the room and ask the person to call you when she is finished. Remember to close the door on your way out.

10. Return when the person signals. Remember to knock before entering.

11. If the side rails are in use, lower the side rail on the working side of the bed. Lower the head of the bed so that the bed is flat (as tolerated).

12. Put on a clean pair of gloves.

13. Fanfold the top linens to the foot of the bed.

14. Ask the person to bend her knees, press her heels into the mattress, and lift her buttocks so that you can remove the bedpan and bed protector. (Or help the person to roll onto her side, facing away from you, while you hold the bedpan securely in place against the mattress to prevent the contents from spilling. Remove the bedpan and bed protector and then help the person to roll back.) If necessary, help the person to use the toilet paper.

15. Cover the bedpan with the bedpan cover or paper towels. Take the bedpan to the bathroom. (If the side rails are in use, raise them before leaving the bedside.)

16. Remove your gloves and dispose of them in a facility-approved waste container. Wash your hands.

17. Return to the bedside. Give the person a wet washcloth and help the person to wash her hands. Make sure the person's perineum is clean and dry. If necessary, provide perineal care.

18. Adjust the person's hospital gown or pajama bottoms as necessary to cover the buttocks.

Help the person back into a comfortable position, straighten the bottom linens, and draw the top linens over the person. Raise the head of the bed, as the person requests. Make sure that the bed is lowered to its lowest position and that the wheels are locked.

19. Return to the bathroom. Put on a clean pair of gloves. If the person is on intake and output (I&O) status, measure the urine. Note the colour, amount, and quality of the urine or feces before emptying the contents of the bedpan into the toilet. (If anything unusual is observed, do not empty the bedpan until a nurse has had a chance to look at its contents.)

20. Gather the soiled linens and place them in the linen hamper or linen bag. Dispose of disposable items in a facility-approved waste container. Clean equipment and return it to the storage area.

21. Remove your gloves and dispose of them in a facility-approved waste container.

Finishing Up CLSOWR

22. Complete the "Finishing Up" steps.

PROCEDURE 20-2

Assisting a Man With Using a Urinal

WHY YOU DO IT   Urinals are used for men who cannot get out of bed to urinate.

Getting Ready WCKIEDS

1. Complete the "Getting Ready" steps.

Supplies

- gloves
- toilet paper
- urinal
- washcloth
- towel

Procedure

2. Ask the man what position he prefers—lying, sitting, or standing. If necessary, raise the head of the bed as tolerated. If the man would prefer to stand, help him to sit on the edge of the bed and then to stand up.

3. Put on the gloves.

4. Hand the man the urinal. If necessary, assist him in positioning it correctly.

5. Make sure that the toilet paper and the call-light control are within reach.

6. Remove your gloves and wash your hands.

7. If safety permits, leave the room and ask the man to call you when he is finished. Remember to close the door on your way out.

8. Return when the man signals. Remember to knock before entering.

9. Put on a clean pair of gloves. Have the man hand you the urinal, or remove it if he is unable to hand it to you. Put the lid on the

(continued)

urinal and hang it on the side rail while you assist the man with handwashing and perineal care as needed. Lower the head of the bed as the man requests.

10. Take the urinal to the bathroom. If the man is on intake and output (I&O) status, measure the urine. Note the colour, amount, and quality of the urine before emptying the contents of the urinal into the toilet. (If anything unusual is observed, do not empty the urinal until a nurse has had a chance to look at its contents.)

11. Gather the soiled linens and place them in the linen hamper or linen bag. Dispose of disposable items in a facility-approved waste container. Clean equipment and return it to the storage area.

12. Remove your gloves and dispose of them in a facility-approved waste container.

Finishing Up CLSOWR

13. Complete the "Finishing Up" steps.

PROCEDURE 20-3

Collecting a Routine Urine Specimen

WHY YOU DO IT   A routine urine specimen is often requested for urinalysis. Proper collection and handling of the urine specimen helps to ensure that the urinalysis results are accurate.

Getting Ready WCKIEPS

1. Complete the "Getting Ready" steps.

Supplies
- gloves
- paper towel
- toilet paper
- specimen container and label
- plastic transport bag (if required at your facility)
- plastic bag or waste container
- specimen collection device ("commode hat"), bedpan, or urinal

Procedure

2. Complete the label with the person's name, room number, and other identifying information. Put the completed label on the specimen container. Take the specimen container to the bathroom. Place a paper towel on the counter. Open the specimen container and place the lid on the paper towel, with the inside of the lid facing up.

3. If the person will be using a regular toilet or bedside commode, fit the specimen collection device underneath the toilet or commode seat. Otherwise, provide the person with a bedpan or urinal, as applicable.

4. Assist the person with urination as necessary. Before leaving the room, remind the person not to have a bowel movement or place toilet paper into the specimen collection device, bedpan, or urinal. Provide a plastic bag or waste container for the used toilet paper.

5. Return when the person signals. Remember to knock before entering.

6. Put on the gloves.

7. If the person used a regular toilet or bedside commode, assist the person with handwashing and perineal care as necessary and then help the person to return to bed. If the person used a bedpan or urinal, cover and remove the bedpan or urinal and assist the person with handwashing and perineal care as necessary.

8. Take the covered bedpan, urinal, or specimen collection device (if the person used a bedside commode) to the bathroom. (If the side rails are in use, raise the side rails before leaving the bedside.)

9. If the person is on intake and output (I&O) status, measure the urine. Note the colour, amount, and quality of the urine.

10. Raise the toilet seat. While holding the specimen container over the toilet, carefully fill it about three-quarters full with urine from the

specimen collection device, bedpan, or urinal. Discard the rest of the urine into the toilet.

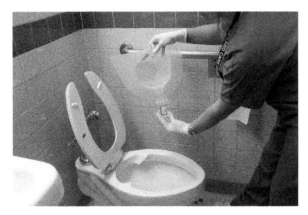

Step 10 Hold the specimen container over the toilet and fill it about three-quarters full with urine.

11. Put the lid on the specimen container. Make sure that the lid is tight. Put the specimen container on the paper towel on the counter.

12. Remove one glove and dispose of it in a facility-approved waste container. Holding the plastic transport bag in your ungloved hand, place the specimen container into the transport bag with your gloved hand. Avoid touching the outside of the transport bag with your glove.

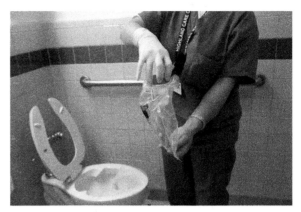

Step 12 Place the specimen container into the transport bag with your gloved hand.

13. Remove the other glove and dispose of it in a facility-approved waste container.

14. Gather the soiled linens and place them in the linen hamper or linen bag. Dispose of disposable items in a facility-approved waste container. Clean equipment and return it to the storage area.

15. Take the specimen container to the designated location.

Finishing Up CLSOWR

16. Complete the "Finishing Up" steps.

PROCEDURE 20-4

Collecting a Midstream ("Clean Catch") Urine Specimen

WHY YOU DO IT   A midstream ("clean catch") urine specimen is often requested for urinalysis when the doctor suspects a urinary tract infection. Proper collection and handling of the urine specimen helps to ensure that the urinalysis results are accurate.

Getting Ready WGKIEpS

1. Complete the "Getting Ready" steps.

Supplies

- gloves
- paper towel
- toilet paper
- specimen container and label
- "clean catch" kit
- plastic transport bag (if required at your facility)
- bedpan or urinal (if necessary)

Procedure

2. Complete the label with the person's name, room number, and other identifying information. Put the completed label on the specimen container.

3. If the person will be using a regular toilet or bedside commode, help the person to the bathroom or bedside commode. Otherwise, provide the person with a bedpan or urinal, as applicable.

(continued)

4. Put on the gloves.

5. Place a paper towel on the counter (if the person is in the bathroom) or on the over-bed table (if the person is using a bedside commode, bedpan, or urinal). Open the specimen container and place the lid on the paper towel, with the inside of the lid facing up.

6. Open the "clean catch" kit. Have the person clean his or her perineum using the wipes in the kit. Assist as necessary:

   a. **If the person is a woman:** Use one hand to separate the labia. Hold the wipe in the other hand. Place your wipe-covered hand at the top of the vulva and stroke downward to the anus.

   b. **If the person is a circumcised man:** Use one hand to hold the penis slightly away from the body. Hold the wipe in the other hand. Place your wipe-covered hand at the tip of the penis and wash in a circular motion, downward to the base of the penis.

   c. **If the person is an uncircumcised man:** Retract the foreskin by gently pushing the skin toward the base of the penis. Place your wipe-covered hand at the tip of the penis and wash in a circular motion, downward to the base of the penis.

7. Assist the person with urination as necessary. Before leaving the room:

   a. Make sure that the toilet paper, call-light control, and specimen container are within reach.

   b. Remind the person that he or she must start the stream of urine, then stop it, then restart it. The urine sample is to be collected from the restarted flow. If the person is a woman, she must hold the labia open until the specimen is collected. If the person is an uncircumcised man, he must keep the foreskin pulled back until the specimen is collected.

8. Remove your gloves and dispose of them in a facility-approved waste container.

9. Return when the person signals. Remember to knock before entering.

10. Put on a clean pair of gloves.

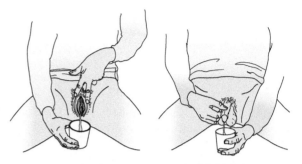

Steps 6a and 6c Women must hold the labia open while voiding to prevent contamination of the urine sample. Uncircumcised men must keep the foreskin pulled back.

11. If the person used a regular toilet or bedside commode, assist the person with handwashing and perineal care as necessary and then help the person to return to bed. If the person used a bedpan or urinal, remove the bedpan or urinal and assist the person with handwashing and perineal care as necessary.

12. Put the lid on the specimen container, being careful not to touch the inside of the lid or container. Make sure that the lid is tight. Put the specimen container on the paper towel on the counter or over-bed table.

13. Remove one glove and dispose of it in a facility-approved waste container. Holding the plastic transport bag in your ungloved hand, place the specimen container into the transport bag with your gloved hand. Avoid touching the outside of the transport bag with your glove.

14. Remove the other glove and dispose of it in a facility-approved waste container.

15. Gather the soiled linens and place them in the linen hamper or linen bag. Dispose of disposable items in a facility-approved waste container. Clean equipment and return it to the storage area.

16. Take the specimen container to the designated location.

Finishing Up CLSOWR

17. Complete the "Finishing Up" steps.

PROCEDURE 20-5

Collecting a Stool Specimen

WHY YOU DO IT A stool sample is often requested for analysis. Proper collection and handling of the stool sample helps to ensure that the test results are accurate.

Getting Ready WGKIEPS

1. Complete the "Getting Ready" steps.

Supplies

- gloves
- paper towel
- tongue depressor
- toilet paper
- specimen container and label
- plastic transport bag (if required at your facility)
- plastic bag or waste container
- specimen collection device ("commode hat") or bedpan

Procedure

2. Complete the label with the person's name, room number, and other identifying information. Put the completed label on the specimen container. Take the specimen container to the bathroom. Place a paper towel on the counter. Open the specimen container and place the lid on the paper towel with the inside of the lid facing up.

3. If the person will be using a regular toilet or bedside commode, fit the specimen collection device underneath the toilet or commode seat. Otherwise, provide the person with a bedpan.

4. Assist the person with defecation as necessary. Before leaving the room, remind the person not to urinate or place toilet paper into the specimen collection device or bedpan. Provide a plastic bag or waste container for the used toilet paper.

5. Return when the person signals. Remember to knock before entering.

6. Put on the gloves.

7. If the person used a regular toilet or bedside commode, assist the person with handwashing and then help the person to return to bed. Provide perineal care as necessary. If the person used a bedpan, cover and remove the bedpan and assist the person with handwashing and perineal care as necessary.

8. Take the covered bedpan or specimen collection device (if the person used a bedside commode) to the bathroom. (If the side rails are in use, raise the side rails before leaving the bedside.)

9. Note the colour, amount, and quality of the feces. Using the tongue depressor, take two tablespoons of feces from the bedpan or specimen collection device and put them into the specimen container. Dispose of the tongue depressor in a facility-approved waste container. Empty the remaining contents of the bedpan or specimen collection device into the toilet.

10. Put the lid on the specimen cup. Make sure that the lid is tight. Put the specimen container on the paper towel on the counter.

11. Remove one glove and dispose of it in a facility-approved waste container. Holding the plastic transport bag in your ungloved hand, place the specimen container into the transport bag with your gloved hand. Avoid touching the outside of the transport bag with your glove.

12. Remove the other glove and dispose of it in a facility-approved waste container.

13. Gather the soiled linens and place them in the linen hamper or linen bag. Dispose of disposable items in a facility-approved waste container. Clean equipment and return it to the storage area.

14. Take the specimen container to the designated location.

Finishing Up CLSOWR

15. Complete the "Finishing Up" steps.

PROCEDURE 20-6

Providing Catheter Care

WHY YOU DO IT Providing proper catheter care helps to prevent the person from getting a urinary tract infection.

Getting Ready WORKBOOK

1. Complete the "Getting Ready" steps.

Supplies

- gloves
- paper towels
- bed protector
- bath thermometer
- wash basin
- soap or antiseptic solution
- bath blanket
- washcloths
- towels
- clean clothing

Procedure

2. Cover the over-bed table with paper towels.

3. Lower the head of the bed so that the bed is flat (as tolerated). Make sure that the bed is positioned at a comfortable working height (to promote good body mechanics) and that the wheels are locked.

4. Fill the wash basin with warm water (43.3°C [110°F] to 46.1°C [115°F] on the bath thermometer). Place the wash basin, soap, towels, and washcloths on the over-bed table.

5. If the side rails are in use, lower the side rail on the working side of the bed. The side rail on the opposite side of the bed should remain up.

6. Put on the gloves.

7. Spread the bath blanket over the top linens (and the person). If the person is able, have him or her hold the bath blanket. If not, tuck the corners under the person's shoulders. Fanfold the top linens to the foot of the bed.

8. Adjust the person's hospital gown or pajama bottoms as necessary to expose the person's perineum.

9. Ask the person to open his legs and bend his knees, if possible. If the person is not able to bend his knees, help the person to spread his legs as much as possible.

10. Position the bath blanket over the person so that one corner can be wrapped under and around each leg.

11. Position a bed protector under the person's buttocks to keep the bed linens dry.

12. Lift the corner of the bath blanket that is between the person's legs upward, exposing only the perineal area.

13. Form a mitt around your hand with one of the washcloths. Wet the mitt with warm, clean water and apply soap or antiseptic solution.

    a. **If the person is a woman:** Using the other hand, separate the labia. Place your washcloth-covered hand at the top of the vulva and stroke downward to the anus. Repeat, using a different part of the washcloth each time, until the area is clean. Rinse and dry the vulva and perineum thoroughly.

    b. **If the person is a circumcised man:** Place your washcloth-covered hand at the tip of the penis and wash in a circular motion, downward to the base of the penis. Repeat, using a different part of the washcloth each time, until the area is clean. Rinse and dry the tip and the shaft of the penis thoroughly.

    c. **If the person is an uncircumcised man:** Retract the foreskin by gently pushing the skin toward the base of the penis. Place your washcloth-covered hand at the tip of the penis and wash in a circular motion, downward to the base of the penis. Repeat, using a different part of the washcloth each time, until the area is clean. Rinse and dry the tip and the shaft of the penis thoroughly before gently pulling the foreskin back into its normal position.

14. Using a clean part of the washcloth, clean the catheter tubing, starting at the body and moving outward from the body about four inches.* Hold the catheter near the opening

---

*In some facilities, disposable antiseptic wipes may be used instead of a washcloth to clean the catheter tubing.

of the urethra. This will help to prevent tugging on the catheter as you clean it.

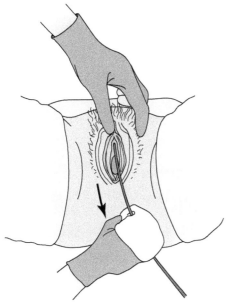

Step 14 Clean the catheter tubing, starting at the body and moving outward.

15. Dry the perineal area thoroughly using a towel.

16. Check that the catheter tubing is free from kinks. Make sure that it is securely taped to the person's leg.

17. Remove your gloves and dispose of them in a facility-approved waste container.

18. Assist the person into the supine position. Remove the bath blanket, and help the person into the clean clothing.

19. If the side rails are in use, return the side rails to the raised position. Raise the head of the bed as the person requests. Make sure that the bed is lowered to its lowest position and that the wheels are locked.

20. Gather the soiled linens and place them in the linen hamper or linen bag. Dispose of disposable items in a facility-approved waste container. Clean equipment and return it to the storage area.

Finishing Up CLSOWR

21. Complete the "Finishing Up" steps.

PROCEDURE 20-7

Emptying a Urine Drainage Bag

WHY YOU DO IT Urine drainage bags must be emptied whenever they are full and at the end of every shift (or as ordered).

Getting Ready WCKIEPS

1. Complete the "Getting Ready" steps.

Supplies
- gloves
- paper towels
- alcohol wipes (optional)
- graduate

Procedure

2. Put on the gloves.

3. Place a paper towel on the floor, underneath the urine drainage bag. Unhook the drainage bag emptying spout from its holder on the urine drainage bag. Position the graduate on the paper towel underneath the emptying spout.

4. Unclamp the emptying spout on the urine drainage bag and allow all of the urine to drain into the graduate. Avoid touching the

tip of the emptying spout with your hands or the side of the graduate.

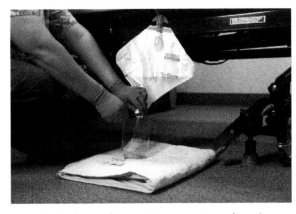

Step 4 Unclamp the emptying spout on the urine drainage bag and allow the urine to drain into the graduate.

(continued)

5. After the urine has drained into the graduate, wipe the emptying spout with an alcohol wipe (or follow facility policy). Reclamp the emptying spout and return it to its holder.

6. If the person is on intake and output (I&O) status, measure the urine. Note the colour, amount, and quality of the urine before emptying the contents of the graduate into the toilet. (If anything unusual is observed, do not empty the graduate until a nurse has had a chance to look at its contents.)

7. Dispose of disposable items in a facility-approved waste container. Clean equipment and return it to the storage area.

8. Remove your gloves and dispose of them in a facility-approved waste container.

Finishing Up CLSOWR

9. Complete the "Finishing Up" steps.

PROCEDURE 20-8

Administering a Soapsuds Enema

WHY YOU DO IT   A soapsuds enema may be ordered to remove feces from the large intestine prior to surgery or a diagnostic procedure. Proper administration of the enema is important to protect the person's safety and privacy during the procedure and to ensure that the enema is effective.

Getting Ready   WCKIEDS

1. Complete the "Getting Ready" steps.

Supplies

- gloves
- paper towel
- toilet paper
- bed protector
- lubricant jelly
- 5-mL packet of castile soap
- bedpan
- bedpan cover
- enema bag with tubing and clamp
- IV pole
- bath thermometer
- bath blanket
- perineal care supplies

Procedure

2. Make sure that the bed is positioned at a comfortable working height (to promote good body mechanics) and that the wheels are locked.

3. Prepare the enema solution in the bathroom or utility room. Clamp the tubing and then fill the enema bag with warm water (40.5°C [105°F] on the bath thermometer) in the specified amount (usually from 500 to 1500 mL). Add the castile soap packet and mix by gently rotating the enema bag. Do not shake the solution vigorously.

4. Release the clamp on the tubing and allow a little water to run through the tubing into the sink or bedpan. This will remove all of the air from the tubing. Reclamp the tubing.

5. Hang the enema bag on the IV pole and bring it to the person's bedside. Adjust the height of the IV pole so that the enema bag is hanging no more than 45 centimetres above the person's anus.

6. If the side rails are in use, lower the side rail on the working side of the bed. The side rail on the opposite side of the bed should remain up. Lower the head of the bed so that the bed is flat (as tolerated).

7. Spread the bath blanket over the top linens (and the person). If the person is able, have her hold the bath blanket. If not, tuck the corners under her shoulders. Fanfold the top linens to the foot of the bed.

8. Ask the person to lie on her left side, facing away from you, in Sims' position. Help her into this position, if necessary.

9. Put on the gloves.

10. Adjust the bath blanket and the person's hospital gown or pajama bottoms as necessary to expose the person's buttocks. Position the bed protector under the person's buttocks to keep the bed linens dry.

11. Open the lubricant package and squeeze a small amount of lubricant onto a paper

towel. Lubricate the tip of the enema tubing to ease insertion.

12. Suggest that the person take a deep breath and slowly exhale as the enema tubing is inserted. With one hand, raise the person's upper buttock to expose the anus. Using your other hand, gently and carefully insert the lubricated tip of the tubing into the person's rectum (not more than 8 to 10 centimetres for adults). Never force the tubing into the rectum. If you are unable to insert the tubing, stop and call the nurse.

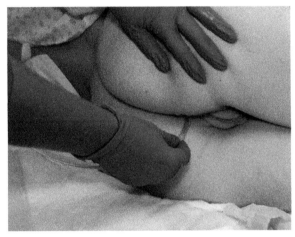

Step 12 Gently insert the top of the tubing into the person's rectum.

13. Unclamp the tubing and allow the solution to begin running. Hold the enema tubing firmly with one hand so that it does not slip out of the rectum. If the person complains of pain or cramping, slow down the rate of flow by tightening the clamp a bit. If the pain or cramping does not stop after slowing the rate of flow, stop the procedure and call the nurse.

14. When the fluid level reaches the bottom of the bag, clamp the tubing to avoid injecting air into the person's rectum.

15. Remove the tubing from the person's rectum and place it inside the enema bag. Gently place several thicknesses of toilet paper against the person's anus to absorb any fluid.

16. Ask the person to retain the enema solution for the specific amount of time.

17. Assist the person with expelling the enema as necessary, using the bedpan, bedside commode, or toilet. If the person is using a regular toilet, ask her not to flush the toilet after expelling the enema.

18. If the person used a regular toilet or bedside commode, assist her with handwashing and then help her to return to bed. Provide perineal care as necessary. If the person used a bedpan, cover and remove the bedpan and assist her with handwashing and perineal care as necessary.

19. Raise the head of the bed as the person requests. Make sure that the bed is lowered to its lowest position and that the wheels are locked. (If the side rails are in use, raise the side rails before leaving the bedside.)

20. Take the covered bedpan or commode bucket (if the person used a bedside commode) to the bathroom.

21. Note the colour, amount, and quality of feces before emptying the contents of the bedpan or commode bucket into the toilet. (If anything unusual is observed, do not empty the bedpan or commode bucket until a nurse has had a chance to look at its contents.)

22. Gather the soiled linens and place them in the linen hamper. Dispose of disposable items in a facility-approved waste container. Clean equipment and return it to the storage area.

23. Remove your gloves and dispose of them in a facility-approved waste container.

Finishing Up CLSOWR

24. Complete the "Finishing Up" steps.

WHAT DID YOU LEARN?

Multiple Choice

Select the single best answer for each of the following questions.

1. The perineum (perineal area) is cleaned before collecting a:
   a. 24-hour urine specimen
   b. Clean catch urine specimen
   c. Random urine specimen
   d. Stool specimen

2. The most comfortable position for using a bedpan is:
   a. Fowler's position
   b. Sims' position
   c. Prone position
   d. Supine position

3. How far is an enema tube inserted into the rectum in an adult?
   a. 8 to 10 centimetres
   b. 13 to 15 centimetres
   c. 18 to 20 centimetres
   d. 30 to 41 centimetres

4. One of your residents needs to have an enema administered. How should you position the resident in preparation for the enema?
   a. Left Sims' position
   b. Fowler's position
   c. Supine position
   d. Right Sims' position

5. In a person with an indwelling urinary catheter, why must the urine drainage bag be kept lower than the person's bladder?
   a. Keeping the drainage bag below bladder level will prevent a bedridden person from seeing the bag, which he or she might find embarrassing
   b. Keeping the drainage bag below bladder level will keep the person comfortable in bed
   c. Keeping the drainage bag below bladder level will prevent urine from returning to the bladder, where it could cause infection
   d. Keeping the drainage bag below bladder level will prevent the urine from leaking out

6. Which one of the following describes normal urine?
   a. Cloudy with a strong odour
   b. Well-formed
   c. Red-tinged
   d. Clear, light yellow, or golden with a slight odour

7. A healthy person's feces will be:
   a. Black and tarry
   b. Soft, brown, formed, and moist with a distinct odour
   c. Hard and pellet-like
   d. Long and stringy

8. To help your residents or patients to maintain healthy bowel function, it is important to:
   a. Answer call lights promptly
   b. Encourage them to eat a well-balanced diet and drink plenty of fluids
   c. Assist them with exercise
   d. All of the above

9. When caring for a person who is incontinent of urine or feces, it is important to:
   a. Provide good perineal care
   b. Let the person know that his or her behavior is inappropriate, so it will stop
   c. Take the person to the bathroom once daily
   d. Restrict fluids to reduce the chance of an accident

10. When caring for a person with an indwelling catheter, always remember to:
    a. Leave the drainage bag above the level of the bladder, while the person is in bed
    b. Tape any leaks at the connection site
    c. Wear gloves when providing daily catheter care
    d. Tape the drainage tube under the leg

Matching

Match each numbered item with its appropriate lettered description.

_____ 1. Hematuria

_____ 2. Peristalsis

_____ 3. Micturition

_____ 4. Defecation

_____ 5. Nocturia

_____ 6. Dysuria

_____ 7. Urinalysis

_____ 8. Anuria

_____ 9. Oliguria

_____ 10. Polyuria

a. Excessive urine production
b. Excessive urination at night
c. Difficulty urinating
d. No urine production
e. Urination
f. Passing of feces
g. Routine urine test
h. Inadequate urine production
i. Blood in the urine
j. Wave-like muscular movement of the intestines

STOP and Think!

You are a personal support worker in a hospital. One of your patients, Mrs. Walker, must use a bedpan because she is confined to bed, but she is having a hard time relaxing enough to urinate "in bed." What sorts of things could you do to help make using a bedpan easier for Mrs. Walker?

You are caring for Miss Smiley, who has an indwelling catheter. When you are making your end-of-shift rounds, you note that Miss Smiley's urinary drainage bag has very little urine in it. You know that the drainage bag was emptied right before you started your shift. That was almost 8 hours ago. What should you do?

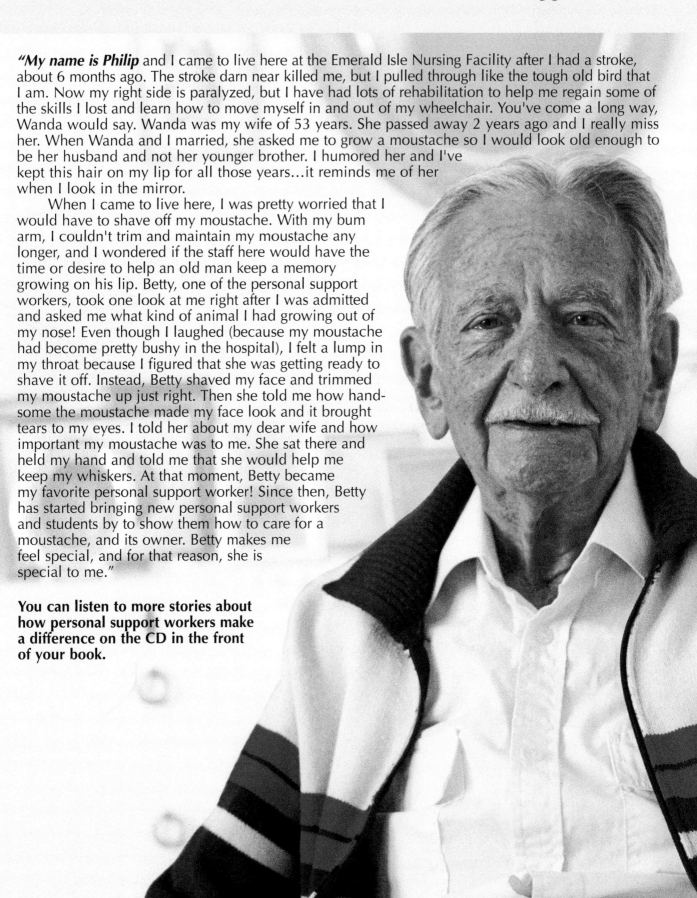

Personal Support Workers Make a Difference!

"My name is Philip and I came to live here at the Emerald Isle Nursing Facility after I had a stroke, about 6 months ago. The stroke darn near killed me, but I pulled through like the tough old bird that I am. Now my right side is paralyzed, but I have had lots of rehabilitation to help me regain some of the skills I lost and learn how to move myself in and out of my wheelchair. You've come a long way, Wanda would say. Wanda was my wife of 53 years. She passed away 2 years ago and I really miss her. When Wanda and I married, she asked me to grow a moustache so I would look old enough to be her husband and not her younger brother. I humored her and I've kept this hair on my lip for all those years...it reminds me of her when I look in the mirror.

When I came to live here, I was pretty worried that I would have to shave off my moustache. With my bum arm, I couldn't trim and maintain my moustache any longer, and I wondered if the staff here would have the time or desire to help an old man keep a memory growing on his lip. Betty, one of the personal support workers, took one look at me right after I was admitted and asked me what kind of animal I had growing out of my nose! Even though I laughed (because my moustache had become pretty bushy in the hospital), I felt a lump in my throat because I figured that she was getting ready to shave it off. Instead, Betty shaved my face and trimmed my moustache up just right. Then she told me how handsome the moustache made my face look and it brought tears to my eyes. I told her about my dear wife and how important my moustache was to me. She sat there and held my hand and told me that she would help me keep my whiskers. At that moment, Betty became my favorite personal support worker! Since then, Betty has started bringing new personal support workers and students by to show them how to care for a moustache, and its owner. Betty makes me feel special, and for that reason, she is special to me."

You can listen to more stories about how personal support workers make a difference on the CD in the front of your book.

4 DEATH AND DYING

21 Caring for People Who Are Terminally Ill
22 Caring for People Who Are Dying

Do not go gentle into that good night,
Old age should burn and rave at close of day
Rage, rage against the dying of the light.

—From *Do Not Go Gentle Into That Good Night*
by Dylan Thomas

In this poem by the Welsh poet Dylan Thomas (1914–1953), the speaker begs his father to fight, rather than accept, death. Although everyone who lives must die, accepting the certainty of our own death, or the death of someone we care about, is rarely easy. In Unit 4, we will look at the final stages of life and the role the personal support worker plays in providing compassionate care to those who are dying, and their families.

Photo: Sunset off the coast of Layang Layang Island, Malaysia. (Scubazoo/Photo Researchers, Inc.)

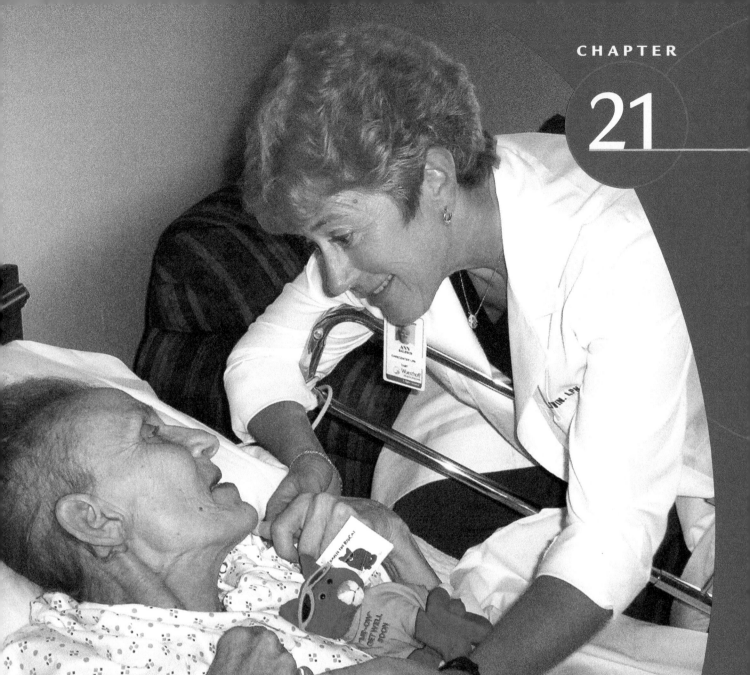

Caring for People Who Are Terminally Ill

WHAT WILL YOU LEARN?

This chapter focuses on caring for people with a terminal illness (an illness that will end in death). You will learn about the stages of grief a dying person experiences, and the role hospice workers play in caring for a dying person. You will also learn about care

Photo: A hospice nurse cares for one of her terminally ill patients. (Photograph courtesy of Wuesthoff Brevard Hospice & Palliative Care/Brenda Spakes.)

considerations for the terminally ill person's family, and the effects of caring for a terminally ill person on the caregiver. When you are finished with this chapter, you will be able to:

1. Define the term *terminal illness* and give examples of specific illnesses that are considered terminal.
2. List the stages of grief and discuss their effects on the terminally ill person.
3. Describe the effects of a terminal illness on the person's family.
4. Define the term *advance directives* and list examples of ways a terminally ill person specifies end-of-life care wishes.
5. Discuss the role of hospice in the care of the terminally ill person.
6. Describe care concerns when providing for the needs of the person with a terminal illness.
7. Explain how caring for terminally ill people can affect the personal support worker.

Vocabulary

Grief	Acceptance	Durable power of	No code or do not
Denial	Will	attorney for health care	resuscitate (DNR)
Anger	Advance	Supportive care	order
Bargaining	directive	Life-sustaining	Palliative care
Depression	Living will	treatment	

People die from many different causes and at many different ages. Some people die suddenly of accidents or acute illnesses; others die simply as a result of the natural aging process. Still others die from a terminal illness, an illness or condition for which there is no cure. There are many types of terminal illnesses. Acquired immunodeficiency syndrome (AIDS), as well as certain cancers, heart conditions, chronic respiratory disorders, kidney disorders, and liver disorders are all examples of conditions that can become terminal.

In years past, the person with a terminal illness was cared for in the home, surrounded by family and friends and treated by a family doctor or private-duty nurse (Fig. 21-1). Because modern technology and treatments did not exist, all caregivers could do was focus on making the person comfortable and filling his or her last days with love and compassion. Although the treatments that are available to us through modern medicine are certainly wonderful, we must be careful not to forget the "old-fashioned" aspect of caring for the terminally ill, which focused on allowing the person to live (and to die) with dignity. A primary focus of this book, and of the health care industry today, is holistic care—caring for the whole person by attending to the person's physical, as well as emotional and spiritual, needs. Applying the concept of holistic care

is very important when you are caring for people at the end of life's journey.

Some of you will have experienced life events, such as the death of someone close to you, that inspired you to enter the health care industry. However, many of you are entering the personal support worker profession with little or no exposure to death and the process of grieving. Caring for a terminally ill person can be very rewarding, but it can also be emotionally draining. To become emotionally secure enough to be supportive of a terminally ill person and her family members, you will need to explore your own feelings and emotions regarding death and dying. However, you must also remember that everyone has her own beliefs and ideas about death, and that these beliefs and ideas are just as important and meaningful to that person as yours are to you. (See Chapter 22 for a more detailed discussion of beliefs and practices related to death and dying across various religions and cultures.)

When you are caring for people who are dying, you should be aware of the power of listening and touch. In many cases, it is not necessary to say anything at all—your presence will be noticed and will be reassuring for the dying person. Listen to whatever the person needs to say, without imposing your own opinions or beliefs. Remember that this is your patient's or resident's

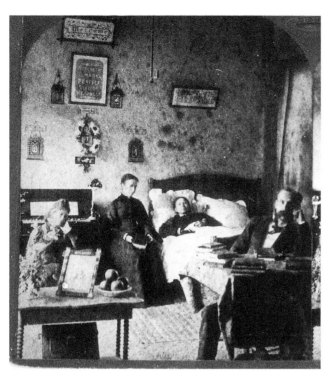

Figure 21-1
In the past, most people died at home, surrounded by family and friends. Today, we have many modern treatments available to us, but a humanistic, holistic approach to care is still necessary. (© *Stanley B. Burns, M.D./The Burns Archive.*)

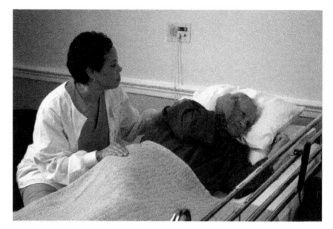

Figure 21-2
Denial helps to protect the person emotionally from overwhelming grief.

grief, and he or she must work through it on his or her own terms.

STAGES OF GRIEF

Anyone experiencing any type of loss, be it the loss of health, loss of a marriage, loss of a loved one, or the impending loss of his own life, will experience grief. **Grief** is defined as mental anguish, specifically associated with loss. Dr. Elisabeth Kübler-Ross (1926–2004), a Swiss-born doctor who came to the United States in the 1950s, is the author of a famous book called *On Death and Dying.* Dr. Kübler-Ross, a psychiatrist, chose to work with terminally ill people. During her conversations with her patients, they expressed to her their feelings about what they were going through. These conversations formed the basis for many of the ideas in *On Death and Dying.* One key idea Dr. Kübler-Ross outlined in *On Death and Dying* is the idea that dying people experience distinct stages of grief. These same stages are also seen to some degree in people who are diagnosed with chronic illnesses, especially

those illnesses that will greatly affect the person's way of living. For example, a person who has recently been told he has diabetes, heart disease, or hypertension may go through the same stages of grief that a person who has been told he is dying goes through. The stages of grief that Dr. Kübler-Ross identified are denial, anger, bargaining, depression, and acceptance.

Denial, the first stage of grief, occurs when a person is told that he has a terminal illness. The person refuses to accept the diagnosis or feels that a mistake has been made (Fig. 21-2). He may ask for a second opinion, or act as if nothing is wrong and avoid returning to the doctor for a period of time. Denial helps to protect a person emotionally from overwhelming grief. This stage of grief can last only a few minutes, or it may last until the person actually dies. As a personal support worker, it is not your place to convince the person that his illness exists, or to argue with the person about treatment or care issues. Instead, recognize that denial is a normal part of the grieving process, respond to the person in an honest yet neutral way, and communicate your observations to the nurse (Table 21-1). Be sure to tell the nurse if the person refuses medication or other medical treatment.

Anger occurs when the person realizes that he is actually going to die (Fig. 21-3). People may feel angry for different reasons, and each person handles anger differently. Some people may be angry with themselves for not seeking help sooner, or for making a lifestyle choice that contributed to the illness, such as smoking. People express anger differently. Some people become

Table 21-1   Stages of Grief

STAGE	SAMPLE DIALOGUE	APPROPRIATE RESPONSE FROM PERSONAL SUPPORT WORKER
Denial	**Patient:** "They don't know what they're talking about. I can't possibly have an incurable brain tumour." **Personal support worker:** "I'm sorry; it must have been very hard for you to learn the results of the MRI."	Acknowledges what the person is saying by responding in an honest, yet neutral way
Anger	**Patient:** "If you medical people weren't so incompetent, I wouldn't be so sick!" **Personal support worker:** "Mr. Smith, you seem so angry."	Acknowledges the person's anger and allows him to talk about it; by practicing empathy, avoids feeling defensive or taking the person's anger personally
Bargaining	**Patient:** "If I could just hang on until my sister arrives . . ." **Personal support worker:** "We'll do all we can to help you do that. But until then, I'll be with you."	Offers support that she can realistically provide, and reassures the person that he will be cared for
Depression	**Patient:** "I don't want to die. . . . I'm so sad." **Personal support worker** (sitting quietly and holding the patient's hand): "I'm here for you."	Offers comfort in the form of touch and silence; does not attempt to "cheer the person up"; if the person is refusing food or not sleeping, could offer to obtain whatever foods appeal to the person's appetite or to talk to the nurse about arranging for medication to aid sleep
Acceptance	**Patient:** "It won't be long until I'm going on to my reward." **Personal support worker:** "You're going on to your reward?"	Uses communication techniques that encourage the person to talk, such as rephrasing the person's statement as an open-ended question

moody and withdrawn, or uncooperative and hostile. Others may yell, or throw objects. If the person is religious, he may lose faith. Some people take their anger out on family members. Others may direct their anger toward health care professionals, feeling that the people they have placed so much trust in have somehow failed

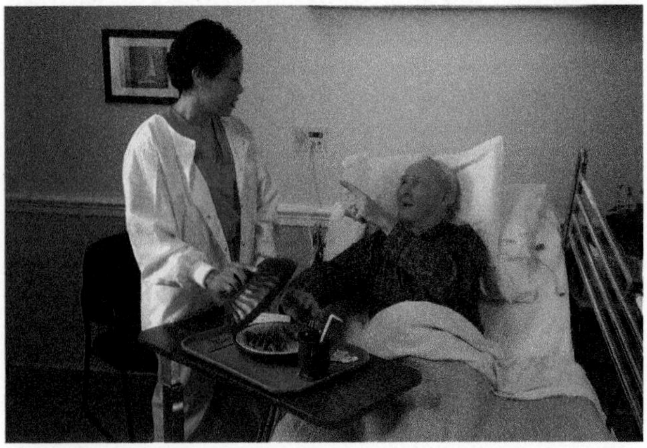

Figure 21-3
Many people who are grieving pass through a period of anger.

them. You must not take the anger personally—doing so can hurt your emotional well-being, as well as your ability to care for the person.

Bargaining is typically done on a very private basis by the terminally ill person. The person wants to "make a deal" with someone he feels has control over his fate, such as God or a health care provider (Fig. 21-4). The person may want to live long enough to accomplish a goal, or to witness a specific event, such as the birth of a child, a wedding, or an anniversary celebration. The will to live can be a very powerful force, and may, in fact, extend the person's life by a few months. As a personal support worker, it is important for you to allow the terminally ill person to experience the feeling of hope that accompanies this stage of grieving.

Depression is the stage in which the person fully realizes that death will be the end result of the illness (Fig. 21-5). The person will be sad and may have regrets about things he was not able to accomplish during his lifetime. Some people are quite withdrawn and may say little, while others may want to openly mourn for their loss. Recognize that depression is a normal part of the grieving process, and be supportive. Let the person

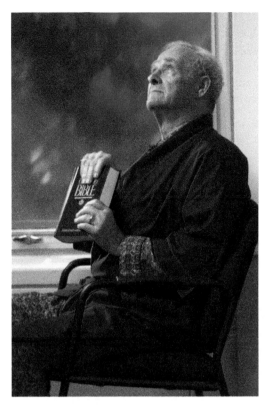

Figure 21-4
The bargaining stage is usually accompanied by a feeling of hope.

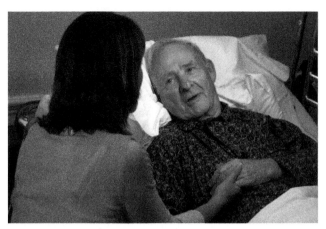

Figure 21-6
During the acceptance phase, the grieving person comes to terms with his death and begins to make plans for the future.

know that it is all right for him to be feeling the way he is feeling. Tell the nurse if a grieving person's depression causes the person to cry constantly, refuse food, or fail to sleep. Some people will require medical intervention to treat their depression.

Acceptance occurs when a terminally ill person comes to terms with the reality of his own

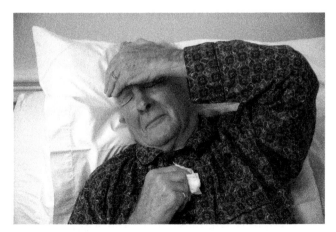

Figure 21-5
During the depression phase, the person realizes the full impact of his illness.

death, and is finally at peace with this knowledge (Fig. 21-6). Typically, people who have reached the acceptance stage will demonstrate their acceptance by completing unfinished business and saying their good-byes. Many will plan their funeral service or write a poem or letter to be read after they are gone. Often, they will want to talk about their death, in an effort to help family members accept it also. The acceptance stage does not necessarily occur when death is near; some people gain acceptance months or even years prior to their eventual death from the illness.

Terminally ill people may not pass through all the stages of grief, and they may not pass through them in order. Many people work through the first five stages of grief, only to "relapse" and experience some of the earlier stages again. Throughout the grieving process, the one thing that usually persists is hope. Even the most realistic and accepting patients hold on to the hope that a new drug will be developed, or that a new research project will yield a cure. Hope is what helps a terminally ill person face another day or another painful treatment. It is what drives the person to keep up with normal activities, such as eating and praying, when she might otherwise feel like giving up entirely. As a personal support worker, you must be responsive to, and nurture, a patient's hope, without being unrealistic.

One factor that influences how a person handles the grieving process is where the person is in his or her life in terms of responsibilities, commitments, accomplishments, hopes, and dreams. For example, a mother with young children will have different concerns than a mother whose children are grown and independent. A terminally ill person who is able to view her life with a feeling of satisfaction may act very differently from a person who has regrets about choices made, opportunities lost, or goals unmet. A child will handle a terminal illness very differently from an adult (often, children reach the acceptance stage faster than adults). It is important for you to recognize the stages of grief and understand that, although these stages have been identified, each person will experience them, and react to them, differently. Being able to recognize the stages of grief will enable you to provide better care to your patients or residents, because you will have a better understanding of what they are going through. This understanding will help you to be more effective in determining what your patients or residents need from you.

The family and loved ones of a terminally ill person will also go through the stages of grief as they prepare for their loss. Remembering this will help you to understand behavior that may not seem fair or appropriate. For example, a family member of a terminally ill person may direct her anger at you, but the family member is not necessarily angry with you—she is angry that she is losing someone she loves. Like the dying person, the family members will each pass through the stages of grief individually and at their own order and pace. Sometimes there is emotional upset within a family when the members of the family (including the person who is ill) are at different stages of the grieving process. Reporting your observations of this turmoil to the nurse will be helpful. Arranging for the assistance of clergy or other professionals experienced in grief counselling may be of great comfort to the person and the family (Fig. 21-7).

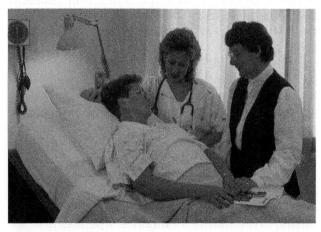

Figure 21-7
Grief counselling may be a comfort to the patient and the family. (*Mark Gibson.*)

TELL THE NURSE

When caring for a terminally ill person, pay attention to the person's emotional well-being, as well as his or her physical well-being. Report any of the following observations to the nurse immediately:

- The person refuses medications, or other medical treatment

- The person cries constantly, refuses food, or cannot sleep

- There is tension and disagreement within the family

- The person or a family member requests the assistance of clergy or a grief counsellor

- The person expresses interest in having a will made

WILLS

A **will** is a legal statement that expresses a person's wishes for the management of his or her affairs after death. For a will to be valid, the person must be deemed competent, or "of sound mind," at the time the will is made. If a patient or resident expresses a desire to make a will, you should relay this information to the nurse so that arrangements can be made for the person to talk with someone who is qualified to assist with preparing a will. Many health care facilities have people on site who are able to provide this kind of assistance. Or, the patient or resident may prefer to have the will prepared by his or her lawyer. As a personal support worker, you may be asked to sign a will as a witness. When you sign as a witness, your signature means that you saw the person sign the document and that, to the best of your knowledge, the document accurately expresses that person's wishes. You should never sign a will as a witness if you have been named as a benefactor of the will. A benefactor is a person who will receive money or other items belonging to the person who has died when the will is read.

DYING WITH DIGNITY
ADVANCE DIRECTIVES

All people have the right to die in a way that is as peaceful and dignified as possible. For many people, this means choosing to avoid "heroic measures" that will prolong life, if by taking these heroic measures, their quality of life will be compromised.

Many people make their wishes known through advance directives. An **advance directive** is a document that allows a person to make his wishes regarding health care known to family members and health care workers, in case the time comes when he is no longer able to make those wishes known himself. In Canada, there are different types of advance directives. Each province and territory uses different language and different laws for these documents. Examples of advance directives include living wills and durable powers of attorney for health care. A **living will** requests that death not be artificially postponed. A **durable power of attorney for health care** transfers the responsibility for handling a person's affairs and making medical decisions to a family member, friend, or other trusted individual, in the event that the person is no longer able to make these decisions on his or her own behalf. Many people, not just the terminally ill, arrange for living wills, durable powers of attorney, or both as a way of ensuring that their wishes regarding their own health care are known and honoured (Fig. 21-8).

Supportive care is offering treatments that will not prolong life, but will make a person more comfortable, such as oxygen therapy, nutritional supplementation, pain medication, range-of-motion exercises, grooming and hygiene, and positioning assistance. (Supportive care is discussed in detail in Chapter 22.) Examples of **life-sustaining treatments,** which tend to be more aggressive, include respiratory ventilation, cardiopulmonary resuscitation (CPR), and the placement of a feeding tube or intravenous (IV) line for the provision of nutrition. A terminally ill person who has made the decision to receive only supportive care at the end of her life will have a **no-code** or **do not resuscitate (DNR) order** written on her chart. This means that the usual efforts to save the person's life will not be made. The entire health care team should be aware of this order so that the person will be allowed to pass on with the compassion and dignity she has requested.

HOSPICE CARE

Hospice organizations have the mission of offering the terminally ill person the best quality of life possible, and ensuring his or her comfort and dignity as death approaches. Hospice care is provided by a multidisciplinary team (made up of nurses, personal support workers, clergy, social workers, doctors, mental health providers, and other professionals). The team seeks to meet the terminally ill person's, and his or her family members', physical, emotional, and spiritual needs. After the person's death, hospice provides grief counselling and other types of assistance for the family. Hospice care is available to patients and families 24 hours a day, 7 days a week, and can be provided to a terminally ill person in his or her home, a long-term care facility, or the hospital. In addition, some facilities specialize in providing hospice care. People become eligible for hospice care when their doctors tell them they have approximately 6 months left to live.

The first hospice program, St. Christopher's Hospice in London, was opened in 1974 to provide supportive care and palliative care to terminally ill people. **Palliative care** focuses on relieving uncomfortable symptoms, not on curing the problem that is causing the symptoms (Fig. 21-9). Examples of palliative treatments include the administration of medications to control pain, the use of chemotherapy or radiation to shrink a tumor (thereby making a person more comfortable), and the use of oxygen therapy to help keep a person with breathing problems comfortable. Surgical procedures can also be of a palliative nature. For example, surgery to remove a tumor that is blocking the intestines may be done primarily to increase the person's comfort, not to cure the cancer. Although hospice care focuses on pain and symptom control and not curative measures, it in no way asks that a terminally ill person give up hope for recovery or a cure from his or her illness.

In addition to providing palliative and supportive care, hospice organizations can assist

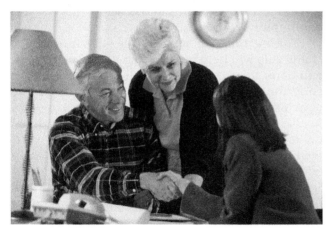

Figure 21-8

Having a living will, a durable power of attorney, or both helps to ensure that a person's wishes regarding his health care are known and honoured in case the person is not able to make these wishes known himself. Many people seek a lawyer's assistance in completing these documents, just so they have them in case they ever need them. Health care facilities also have staff members who are able to assist patients or residents with writing a living will or durable power of attorney. (© *Jupiter Images*)

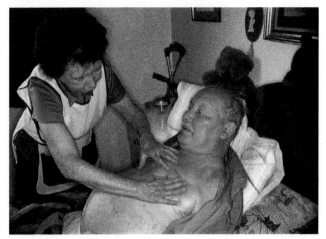

Figure 21-9
Hospice organizations can provide palliative care. Here, a nurse applies a skin patch used for pain control to the chest of a patient with cancer. (© *Samuel Ashfield/Photo Researchers, Inc.*)

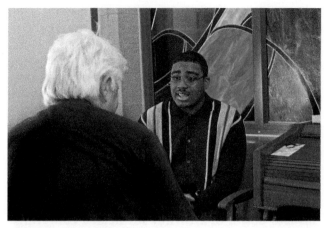

Figure 21-10
Clarifying your beliefs and confronting your fears about death and dying can help you to care for your patients and residents more effectively.

with having special equipment (such as a hospital bed or bedside commode) brought into a person's home. This special equipment often makes it easier for family members and other caregivers to meet the person's physical needs. The primary focus of the hospice team's efforts is to honour the wishes of the terminally ill person and the family. If a person wishes to die at home or at the hospital, the hospice organization will make every effort to honour these wishes. A terminally ill person can take much comfort in knowing that his or her wishes for a dignified and peaceful death will be honoured and that hospice is there to offer support and comfort to the family.

EFFECTS OF CARING FOR THE TERMINALLY ILL ON THE CAREGIVER

Caring for a terminally ill person will affect you. As we work with patients and residents, we become part of their lives and they become part of ours. When one of our patients or residents is diagnosed with a terminal illness, we go through a grief process very similar to that experienced by the person and the family. Additionally, because members of the health care profession feel a great need to be able to help others, we often feel inadequate when we must watch others suffer and grieve, and there is little we can do to relieve their pain. We may even question our professional calling. Regardless of how long you work in the medical profession, terminal illness and death will impact you emotionally.

Taking time for yourself is very important. Doing this will help you to keep your feelings and emotions in perspective and it will allow you to continue to give of yourself to others. Talking to your supervisor, a clergy member, or a mental health counsellor about questions and fears you have about death can help you to clarify your feelings about death and dying (Fig. 21-10). In addition, you might find seeking advice from an "expert" helpful when you are trying to work through feelings concerning a specific situation with a patient or resident.

SUMMARY

- As health care providers, we must strive to meet not only the physical needs, but also the spiritual and emotional needs, of the terminally ill people who trust us to care for them.
- Caring for people with a terminal illness requires an understanding of the ways in which people grieve.
  - Dr. Elisabeth Kübler-Ross, a noted authority on death and dying, identified five stages of grief that a person who is dying from a terminal illness experiences: denial, anger, bargaining, depression, and acceptance.
  - Having an understanding of these stages and what the person is feeling during each one enables us to be more compassionate and understanding toward both the person and the family.
- Advance directives and hospice care seek to preserve the terminally ill patient's right to die in as peaceful and dignified a manner as possible.
- Caring for a terminally ill person and his or her family members can be very rewarding. It can also be very difficult, emotionally.
  - Exploring your own feelings about death (with the help of a professional, if necessary) can help to prepare you for the loss of a patient or resident.
  - When caring for a terminally ill person, recognize that you will also go through the grieving process as part of caring for the person, and make allowance for this.

WHAT DID YOU LEARN?

Multiple Choice

Select the single best answer for each of the following questions.

1. Denial is:
   a. The stage of the grieving process in which the person becomes very depressed
   b. A form of bargaining with God for more time
   c. The final step of the grieving process
   d. The time during the grieving process when the person believes the diagnosis is incorrect

2. An organization that cares only for people who are dying is a:
   a. Skilled facility
   b. Sub-acute care unit
   c. Long-term care facility
   d. Hospice organization

3. The stage of grief when a person begins to say good-bye and make arrangements for his or her death is the:
   a. Bargaining stage
   b. Anger stage
   c. Denial stage
   d. Acceptance stage

4. Hospice care is designed to:
   a. Keep the person comfortable
   b. Prolong the person's life
   c. Treat the person aggressively
   d. All of the above

5. A patient with terminal cancer says he plans to live long enough to walk his daughter, who is getting married, down the aisle. This is an example of:
   a. Acceptance
   b. Depression
   c. Bargaining
   d. Denial

Matching

Match each numbered item with its appropriate lettered description.

__B__ 1. Durable power of attorney

__C__ 2. Living will

__A__ 3. Will

a. A legal document that expresses a person's wishes for the management of her affairs after her death

b. A legal document that transfers the responsibility for handling a person's affairs and making medical decisions to a family member, friend, or other trusted individual

c. A legal document that requests that death not be artificially postponed

STOP and Think!

Mrs. Brown, a resident in your long-term care facility, has a heart condition that is terminal. You have been caring for Mrs. Brown for a year or so now and have observed her working through the stages of grief as her condition has worsened. She seems to be in acceptance about her impending death and often talks about her funeral. The trouble is with Mrs. Brown's son. He used to visit quite often and was always friendly and courteous to the staff. Over the past few months, however, he has been visiting less often. When he has visited, he has been critical of you and the other caregivers, and once or twice he has even snapped at you. And just yesterday, you overheard him angrily telling his mother that he didn't want to hear anything else about a funeral! Why do you think Mrs. Brown's son is acting this way, and how can you help?

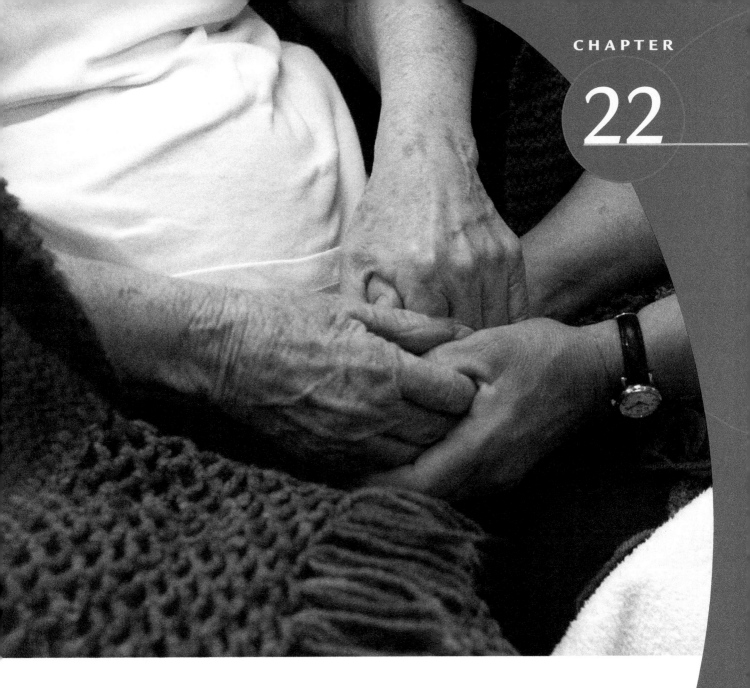

Caring for People Who Are Dying

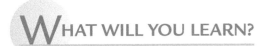HAT WILL YOU LEARN?

Each person is born to one possession which outvalues all his others—his last breath.

—Mark Twain

Most of us give little, if any, thought to what our "last breath" will be like. Sure, we read death notices in the newspaper and hear stories on the evening news about murders and fatal accidents, but do we ever really think about what the person who died

Photo: Sometimes, a simple gesture like holding someone's hand is the best thing you can do.

experienced during her last moments alive? Was the person in pain, was she lonely, did someone hold her hand, was someone there to hear the person's last words? In the quote above, the American writer Mark Twain (1835–1910) suggests that the very end of life is an important life experience, just like all of the experiences leading up to that moment. As a personal support worker, you will find yourself in the position of caring for a patient or resident who is dying. In this chapter, you will learn how you can help the dying person, and his or her family, in the time leading up to the person's "last breath," so that when the time comes, it is as peaceful as possible. You will also learn how to care for a person's body after death occurs. When you are finished with this chapter, you will be able to:

1. Describe the physical signs that frequently signal impending death.
2. Describe ways in which the personal support worker can provide comfort for the dying person.
3. Discuss how cultural and religious influences can affect how the dying person views death.
4. Describe the different ways in which family members may show grief.
5. Describe ways that a personal support worker can help the family of a dying person.
6. Discuss the various responsibilities that a personal support worker may have following the death of a patient or resident.

Vocabulary

Cyanotic	Afterlife	Postmortem care	Autopsy
Cheyne-Stokes respiration	Reincarnation	Rigor mortis	Shroud

Usually, we consider a person "dead" when the heart stops beating and cannot be started again. However, a doctor can also declare a person dead when there has been a permanent loss of brain function. To be declared "brain dead," a person must show no brain activity for a period of time specified by the law (usually 24 hours or more). Brain activity is monitored using sophisticated equipment, and several examinations are performed before the person is declared dead.

Many people die suddenly. However, often there is some warning of approaching death. As death draws near, a person may show certain characteristic physical signs, caused as the body begins to "shut down." These signs may appear over the course of a few hours or a few days, or within the space of a few minutes. Some people may not show these signs. However, recognizing these physical signs and understanding why they occur will help you to know what type of care to give the dying person. Family members may also notice these signs, and become concerned. In this case, you will need to reassure them that these signs are normal signs of dying. (Any specific questions regarding the person's condition should be directed to the nurse.) Physical signs of impending death include the following:

- As circulation fails, the blood pressure drops and the pulse becomes rapid and weak. The skin feels cool and clammy, even though the body temperature is rising. The person may perspire heavily and the skin may appear mottled (blotchy), very pale, **cyanotic** (blue-tinged), or greyish. Although you may be tempted to cover the person warmly, he or she will need only light bed coverings.
- The respiratory pattern changes. The person may take very irregular, shallow breaths, in an alternating fast–slow pattern. This pattern of breathing is called **Cheyne-Stokes respiration.** As the person weakens, fluid or mucus may collect in the air passages, causing the noisy, rattling breathing that is often known as the "death rattle."
- The digestive system slows down. The person may experience nausea, vomiting, abdominal swelling, fecal impaction, or bowel incontinence. The person may not want food or water. Offering ice chips and providing frequent oral care help to keep the mouth moist.
- Urine output decreases as the kidneys respond to the lack of blood flow. In addition, the person may become incontinent of urine.

- Nervous system changes result in decreased muscle tone and sensation. The muscles relax and the person may be too weak to reposition himself. Some people lose the ability to speak. The person may lose sensation in his arms or legs, and pain may decrease. Vision may become blurred. (You may notice that the person will turn toward a light in an effort to see better.) Hearing, however, usually remains normal until the moment of death.

- Consciousness may be altered. Some dying people lose consciousness and become comatose as death approaches. As consciousness decreases, pain usually does too. Some people remain conscious and oriented until the moment of death. It is common for a person who has drifted into and out of a semi-comatose state to become alert and oriented right before he or she dies.

When you are caring for a person who is dying, take note of any physical changes that you observe. Report these changes to the nurse and record them in the person's medical chart, per facility policy.

CARING FOR A DYING PERSON

A holistic approach to care is taken with a dying person, just as with any other person (Fig. 22-1) Dying people, like everyone else, have physical and emotional needs. These needs may change dramatically as the time of death approaches, and will vary greatly depending on the person. Every person has the right to die peacefully and with dignity (Box 22-1). As a personal support worker, it is your job to do everything you can to ensure that this right is honoured.

Many personal support workers (especially new personal support workers) compromise the

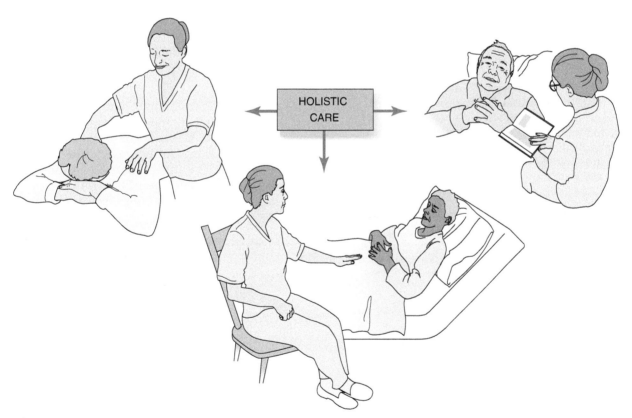

Figure 22-1
The personal support worker provides for the dying person's physical and emotional comfort. Examples of physical comfort measures include providing frequent oral care and back massages. Examples of emotional comfort measures include caring for the family, helping the person to meet spiritual needs (for example, by reading aloud from a book that has special meaning for the person), and simply spending quiet time with the person.

The Dying Person's Bill of Rights

I have the right to be treated as a living human being until I die.

I have the right to maintain a sense of hopefulness, however changing its focus may be.

I have the right to be cared for by those who can maintain a sense of hopefulness, however changing this might be.

I have the right to express my feelings and emotions about my approaching death in my own way.

I have the right to participate in decisions concerning my care.

I have the right to expect continuing medical and nursing attention even though "cure" goals must be changed to "comfort" goals.

I have the right not to die alone.

I have the right to be free from pain.

I have the right to have my questions answered honestly.

I have the right not to be deceived.

I have the right to have help from and for my family in accepting my death.

I have the right to die in peace and dignity.

I have a right to retain my individuality and not be judged for my decisions, which may be contrary to beliefs of others.

I have the right to discuss and enlarge my religious and/or spiritual experiences, whatever these may mean to others.

I have the right to expect that the sanctity of the human body will be respected after death.

I have the right to be cared for by caring, sensitive, knowledgeable people who will attempt to understand my needs and will be able to gain some satisfaction in helping me face my death.

(Created at the workshop *The Terminally Ill Patient and the Helping Person,* in Lansing, Michigan, sponsored by the Southwestern Michigan Inservice Education Council and conducted by Amelia J. Barbus, Associate Professor of Nursing, Wayne State University, Detroit.)

care they give to a dying patient or resident, without being fully aware that they are doing so. For example, a personal support worker might not check in on the dying person as often as he checks in on his other patients or residents. He might provide only the necessary care and then leave the person's room quickly, because he is afraid that if he stays, the person will want to talk about death. Or he may be overly cheerful around the person. These avoidance behaviours usually occur because the personal support worker has not yet explored his own feelings

about death. Many people who are new to the health care profession express concerns such as, "I'm afraid I'll cry if my resident dies," "I don't want to get too attached," or "I've never touched a dead person before and I'm scared." All of these are normal fears that new personal support workers have. As noted in Chapter 21, talking to your supervisor, a clergy member, or a mental health counsellor can help you to come to terms with your own feelings and beliefs about death. This knowledge of your own feelings will serve you well as you care for others who are dying.

Facing the death of a patient or resident never gets any easier. You will become very attached to your patients or residents. Although the relationship you have with your patient or resident can make providing end-of-life care very emotionally difficult for you, it is this relationship that will allow you to provide the holistic care that the dying person needs so much.

MEETING THE DYING PERSON'S PHYSICAL NEEDS

A dying person becomes more and more dependent on others for basic physical care as the time of death approaches. As the focus of care becomes comfort, the personal support worker has the opportunity to help the person feel that he is not alone in this last stage of life. Basic aspects of physical care for the dying person include the following:

- **Care of the skin.** More frequent skin care and linen changes are needed because of the urinary or bowel incontinence and the moist skin that often occur as the person nears death. The person will need to be checked regularly for incontinence of both urine and feces. His skin will need to be cleaned gently, and soiled clothing and linens must be changed. Bed protectors or indwelling urinary catheters may be needed to assist with incontinence problems.

- **Care of the mucous membranes.** Frequent oral care helps keep the mouth moist and more comfortable, especially if the person is comatose or not taking food or drink. Sometimes as death nears, the person does not blink as often, and a mucus crust may form around the eyelids. Gentle cleaning with a warm, wet washcloth helps to remove the dried mucus. The nurse may apply an ointment to keep the eyes moist. If the person is comatose, moist eye pads may be used for protection. Medical equipment, such as oxygen cannulas and nasogastric tubes, may cause irritation and crusting of mucus around the nostrils. Gently removing the mucus crust with a warm, wet washcloth and applying a lubricant can help to keep the person comfortable.

- **Positioning.** As the person's condition worsens, she may not be able to reposition herself without assistance. Frequent, regular position changes help to prevent pressure ulcers and promote comfort. The use of pillows or other positioning devices helps to maintain the body in proper alignment. If the person is in pain, you will need to be extra gentle and slow with position changes. Always tell the nurse if the person seems to be in pain so that necessary medications can be administered. A person who is having difficulty breathing will probably be more comfortable positioned with her head elevated.

- **Other comfort measures.** Receiving a back massage, listening to soft music, or being read to are all activities that can help a person to rest and feel better. Enemas may be necessary to assist with bowel elimination. Secretions may collect in the person's airways, making breathing difficult. If you notice that a person is having difficulty breathing, report this to the nurse. The nurse will provide suctioning and oxygen therapy, measures that can make breathing easier and more comfortable for the person. Keep the room well lit and ventilated. Remove soiled linens, bedpans, or emesis basins and use air freshener to help eliminate unpleasant odours.

As death nears, there may be changes in the dying person's ability to communicate with others. Therefore, when caring for a dying person, you must be very observant of the person's physical needs. As the person's ability to communicate pain, thirst, or other physical needs decreases, he will rely more and more on the care team to notice those needs and take care of them. In addition, you must take measures to make communication easier:

- Remember that as death approaches, the person's vision may become blurry. Keep the room well lit to help the person to see better. Also, make sure you introduce yourself when entering the room and encourage family members to do the same. Imagine how you would feel if you could no longer see well, and you could not tell who was entering and leaving your room!

- Speaking may become difficult for the person. In this case, asking simple "yes or no" questions will make communication more effective.

- Hearing usually remains quite sharp up until the time of death, even if the person is comatose. Always talk to the person as if he is able to hear you, even if he cannot respond. Explain procedures to the person and offer reassurance that you are there and will return soon when you must leave the room. Gently remind family members that the person may still be able to hear their conversations, and encourage them to talk to the person. Hearing the voices of family members can be comforting for the dying person. However, family members should be advised that potentially upsetting topics should be discussed elsewhere, out of earshot of the dying person.

A person's family members may wish to assist in providing physical care. If a family member says that she would like to be involved in caring for the dying person, encourage this by suggesting ways that the family member can help. For example, you might ask the family member if she would be willing to help you out by giving the person ice chips, and then show the family member how to do this (Fig. 22-2). Family members often

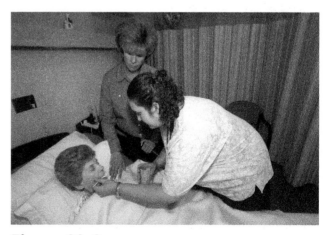

Figure 22-2
Sometimes, family members want to assist in meeting a dying person's physical needs. Here, a personal support worker is showing a family member how to ease the person's thirst by giving ice chips.

feel useless or helpless when it becomes clear that there is nothing left to do except wait for death to arrive. Participating in the care of a dying loved one can help a family member to feel better about the situation.

MEETING THE DYING PERSON'S EMOTIONAL NEEDS

Emotionally, people prepare for death very individually. People may have many fears regarding death, such as a fear of the unknown or a fear of losing dignity and self-control. Some may fear that death will be painful, or worry about the effects of their death on the people left behind. Some people have concerns about unfinished business. Another concern that many dying people have is a fear of facing death alone (Fig. 22-3). Some people are able to speak of their fears, while others remain silent, afraid to even speak of what frightens them the most.

Being a Good Listener

A personal support worker can help meet a dying person's emotional needs by being a good listener (Fig. 22-4). A dying person may want to talk about her fears related to dying, or what she expects the afterlife to be like. Or, the person might just want to remember significant events in her life, and share those memories with you now. If you sense that a person wants to talk, use the communication techniques you learned in Chapter 5 to encourage her and let her know that you are there to listen. Even though you may be uncomfortable

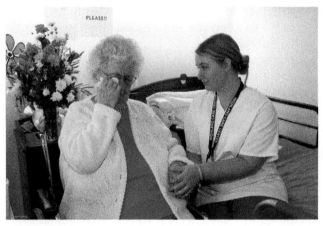

Figure 22-4
A personal support worker helps to meet a dying person's emotional needs by being a good listener. Although you may think that the dying person is the one who benefits the most from these times spent together, quite frequently you will find that you benefit too. These moments spent listening can help you to understand yourself better, as well as your patients or residents.

at first when a patient or resident brings up the subject of death, do not change the subject, make yourself "busy," or simply pat the person on the hand and say, "Oh, don't worry, honey; you've got lots of time left." Many dying people are very aware of their situation and they may tell you that their time here is very short. Do not avoid spending time with a dying person because you are afraid that the person will bring up a subject and you will not know what to say in response. You do not need to say anything—you just need to listen to what the person wants to tell you.

Other dying people do not want to talk and can become annoyed at your attempts to make small talk. Use your observation skills to note when a person would prefer not to talk. Although the person may not want to have a conversation, she will still want to know that you are nearby and watching out for her. Check on the person frequently and regularly and remind her that you are close by if she needs anything.

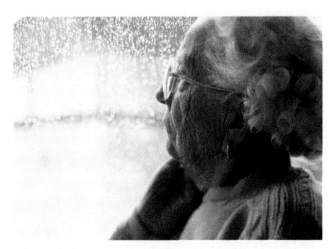

Figure 22-3
Many people have fears related to death, such as a fear of dying alone or of dying in pain. As a personal support worker, you can help to relieve some of these fears.

Helping Hands and a Caring Heart

FOCUS ON HUMANISTIC HEALTH CARE

Many dying people genuinely appreciate it when someone takes the time to sit near them quietly. Touch can convey so much more than words can in a situation like this.

Gently hold the person's hand or touch her shoulder when you are speaking to her. Gently smooth the person's hair after you have finished straightening the bed linens or repositioning the pillow, or comfort the person with a back massage. All of these actions let a person know that she is cared for and not alone.

Culture, Religion, and Spirituality

As you learned in Chapter 6, a person's culture and religion often influence how the person responds to illness and other life experiences, including death. Cultural and religious beliefs influence how a person feels about death and prepares for it. For example, some people may not feel comfortable talking about dying, because in their culture, death is considered a very private matter. On the other hand, some people may seem very accepting of death, because their culture or religion has taught them that death is not to be feared.

Many dying people find peace and comfort in their religious faith. They may wish to visit with clergy members, surround themselves with religious items, or spend time alone in prayer, meditation, and reading of religious texts. Some people may ask you to read to them. Although you may not share the person's religious beliefs, you should honour this request. For the dying person, hearing familiar words that reflect his or her deepest beliefs can bring great comfort. You must respect the beliefs of other people, even if you do not share these beliefs. Remember that your patient's or resident's faith is just as precious to her as yours is to you.

A dying person may request that you call a clergy member to administer religious blessings or "last rites." If such a request is made, report it immediately to the nurse so that the necessary arrangements can be made. When the clergy member arrives, make sure that there is a place for him or her to sit, and ensure privacy. As part of preparing for death, people often want to confess to a clergy member, and they will want privacy to do this.

Religion is but one aspect of spirituality and many people are very spiritual without belonging to any particular religious group. Most people who are "spiritual" believe that a higher being or spirit offers hope and peace, although this higher being may not necessarily be one that is recognized by the world's various religions. Spirituality gives a person inner strength to face life's challenges. It gives meaning to a person's life. Many people exhibit their inner spirituality by listening to music, reading poetry, or just watching a sunset.

When cultural and religious or spiritual beliefs provide an explanation for what happens to a person after death, they can be a source of comfort for the dying person (as well as for the person's family members). For example, many people believe in an **afterlife,** a state of being where the dead meet again with loved ones who have passed on before them. Other people believe in **reincarnation,** the idea that a person's spirit or soul will live again on Earth in the form of an animal or human being yet to be born.

Table 22-1 summarizes common religious practices related to death and dying. Remember that it is important to understand your patients or residents as individuals. While these general guidelines are good to know, they may not hold true for every patient or resident of a particular faith that you care for.

CARE OF THE FAMILY

Knowing that a loved one will die soon can be difficult for family members. Family members must cope with their own grief, and possibly that of other family members as well. Remember that the stress and grief experienced by family members can cause them to act in ways that may seem strange to you. For example, some people may treat you rudely, or snap at you in anger. Be polite and do not take offensive actions or words personally. Usually, these offensive behaviours are just a result of the person's grief. If a family member seems to be getting overly agitated or angry, or if arguing or aggression between family members occurs, notify the nurse immediately.

As a personal support worker, you may feel overwhelmed at the thought of caring for the family as well as for the patient or resident. However, there are many simple things you can do to comfort the family (Fig. 22-5).

- **Ensure good communication between the family members and the health care team.** Often, family members will have worries or fears related to the person's care or condition, and they may want to discuss these with you or another member of the health care team. If a family member asks you a question that you do not know the answer to or are not qualified to answer, make sure to relay this request for information to the nurse so that the family member's concerns can be addressed.

(Text continued on page 454)

Table 22-1 Religious Practices Related to Death and Dying*

	AS DEATH APPROACHES	WHEN DEATH IS IMMINENT	IMMEDIATELY AFTER DEATH	METHOD OF DISPOSAL	FUNERAL CUSTOMS	MOURNING PRACTICES
BUDDHISM	Dying person needs peace and quite to allow for meditation. A monk or religious teacher should be invited to talk to the dying person and chant passages of scripture.	The ideal is to die in a fully conscious and calm state of mind. If a monk is not available, a fellow Buddhist may chant to encourage a peaceful state of mind.	No special requirements relating to the care of the body. Buddhists from different countries will have their own traditions regarding care of the body. If a monk or religious teacher is not present, inform the monks of the appropriate school.	Buddhists bury or cremate according to local traditions.	Usually within 3 to 7 days a service may take place in the house prior to going to the cemetery or crematorium. Monks may be invited to remind the mourners of the impermanence of life.	There is great variation according to country of origin (for example, Sri Lankan Buddhist mourners may return to work in 3 or 4 days and place no religious restrictions on widows). Some Vietnamese have a series of rituals; mourning may last 100 days and mourning for a husband or father, 3 years.
CHRISTIANITY	Some Christians may wish for prayers and anointing with oil by a minister or priest.	Where appropriate, a priest or minister might be notified. Many Christians will wish to receive Communion (which will include some form of repentance and forgiveness). Prayers of commendation may also be said.	No special requirements.	Either burial or cremation. Increasingly only close family are present at the burial of the body or the ashes.	It is customary in some areas to hold a prayer service in the house of the dead person before the funeral. For Orthodox, Roman Catholics and some Anglicans the funeral involves a church service with a Mass or Communion. Sometimes the body is placed in the church the night before and in Orthodox funerals the casket remains open throughout the service. Protestant services are simpler and the body is usually not visible.	There is usually no official mourning period or mourning dress. There may be a service of memorial and thanksgiving some months after the funeral.
ISLAM	Other Muslims, usually family members, join the dying person in prayer and recite verses from the Quran. Dying person may wish to have face toward Mecca (south east).	The Declaration of Faith (Shahada) is said and, if possible, the dying person responds 'I bear witness that there is no God but God and Muhammad is His Messenger.'	Non-Muslim health workers should ask permission to touch the body, then use disposable gloves. The body must be kept covered. Soon after death, there is a ritual washing of the body by same-sex Muslims. Post-mortems are disliked.	Always burial.	Ideally burial is within 24 hours of death. Women are not included at the burial. Male family members carry the coffin either to the mosque or directly to the cemetery where the funeral prayer is said. The body is buried in a deep grave facing Mecca. In bigger cities there are special areas for Muslim burials and in some they are allowed to bury the shrouded body without a coffin. In some instances the body is embalmed and taken back to the country of origin for burial.	Islamic law requires friends and relatives to feed mourners for 3 days. After this the family should officially return to normal though unofficial mourning may continue until the 40th day. It is ended by Quranic readings and a meal.

JUDAISM	A rabbi may be called to join the dying Jew in prayer and facilitate the recitation of the Confession on a Death Bed.	The dying person should not be left alone. Jews present should recite psalms and when death occurs, the Declaration of Faith (Shema).	Health workers should handle the body as little as possible and cover with a white sheet. The Jewish Burial Society will collect the body and perform a ritual wash before burial. Post-mortems are disliked.	Burial as soon as possible in simple coffins. Some non-orthodox Jewish communities permit cremation. Funerals do not take place on the Sabbath or holy days.	The service takes place in designated Jewish burial grounds. Prayers are said in a chapel and at the graveside. Although women now attend funerals, the male mourners recite the prayers and place the coffin in the grave.
					After burial there are three periods of mourning throughout which designated mourners recite prayers thrice daily and refrain from certain activities. The first week (shiva) mourners remain at home; the 30 days following the burial (shloshim) concludes mourning for all but the children of the deceased who mourn for a year. When mourning is concluded the tombstone is consecrated with a ceremony at the cemetery.
HINDUISM	Hindus may receive comfort from hymns and readings from the Hindu holy books. Some may wish to lie on the floor. The family should be present.	The family may wish to call a Hindu priest to perform holy rites. A dying Hindu should be given Ganges water and the sacred Tulsi leaf in the mouth by the relatives. A person should die with the name of God being recited. Hindus often wish to die at home.	The family will usually want to wash the body themselves. If no family is available health workers should wear disposable gloves, close the eyes and straighten the limbs. Jewelry and religious objects should not be removed.	Cremation as soon as possible, with the exception of children younger than 3 years, who are buried.	Part of the service takes place at home. The pandit (priest) chants from scriptures and the chief mourner (usually the eldest son) performs the rituals. Mourners walk around the coffin which is then closed and taken to the crematorium for further prayers.
					Mourners and friends return to the deceased's house. In India the period of mourning and austerity (10 to 16 days) culminates in rituals enabling the dead person's soul to join the ancestors. In Britain these very important rituals occur soon after the funeral and involve gifts to priests or to charity. There may be further rituals at 1, 3, 6 and 12 months.
SIKHISM	A dying Sikh may receive comfort from reciting hymns from the Sikh holy book. A relative or any practicing Sikh may do so instead.	A Sikh person should die with the name of God, Waheguru (Wonderful Lord) being recited. Some Sikhs may want to have Amrit, holy water, in the mouth.	Health workers should not trim hair or beard. The body should be covered by plain white cloth. The 5Ks should remain on the body. Family members may wish to bathe the body themselves.	Cremation as soon as possible.	Similar to Hindus but dressing the person in the 5Ks. After a short ceremony in the home the body is taken to the gurdwara (temple) for a service and then to the crematorium for further prayer.
					Up to 10 days of readings from the scriptures attended by relatives and friends. At the conclusion the eldest son is given a turban as a sign that he is now head of the family.

*(Department of Health and Social Welfare, The Open University SUP 25176 8 Copyright © 1992 Reproduced for Carlisle & District PCT by Permission)
Produced by the North Cumbria Bereavement Forum

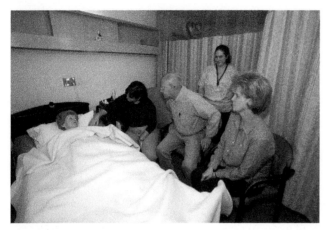

Figure 22-5
Family members will often seek reassurance and comfort from the nursing staff. As a personal support worker, there are many simple kindnesses you can extend to the family that will help make this ordeal easier for them. Here, a personal support worker has brought in an extra chair for a family member who has just arrived at the bedside.

- **Allow family members to stay with the dying person, and to participate in the person's care if they want to.** When a person is dying, many families wish to remain close by. Visiting hours are usually relaxed, allowing family members to stay with the dying person for as long as they like. Encourage family members to talk to the dying person and to help with the person's care. However, do not push family members to do this if they seem hesitant. Although you have responsibilities to the family, your first responsibility is to your patient or resident. When providing physical care to the dying person, please ask the family members to step outside for a moment (unless they have chosen to help you) and close the curtains to help maintain the person's dignity. Also, too many visitors for too long a period of time can be tiring for some patients or residents. If you suspect that the number of visitors or the length of time that they are staying is causing your patient or resident to become overly tired, please report your observations to the nurse.
- **Ensure that the family members' basic needs are met.** Make sure that there are enough chairs in the room, so that everyone can sit down. Encourage family members to rest and take meals as necessary. Show them how to find the restrooms, public telephones, vending machines, and cafeteria. If a family member is showing signs of weariness, offer to stay at the dying person's side while the

family member takes a short walk outside or down the hall to grab a cup of coffee.
- **Be readily available to provide needed care to the patient or resident without being intrusive of the family's privacy.** Often, the most comforting thing to family members is knowing that their loved one is receiving competent, compassionate care.

TELL THE NURSE

When you are caring for a person who is dying, be sure to report the following to the nurse immediately:

- The person seems to be in pain
- The person is having trouble breathing
- The person asks to see a clergy member
- The person seems overwhelmed by the number of visitors or the length of time that they are staying
- A family member has a question about the person's care or condition that you are not qualified to answer
- The person has died

POSTMORTEM CARE

If you are present when one of your patients or residents dies, you must notify the nurse that the person has died, and note the time. You may need to document the absence of vital signs. A doctor must be called to legally pronounce the person dead. The time of death is recorded on the person's death certificate. After the doctor has pronounced the person dead, you may be required to assist the nurse in giving postmortem care, depending on the policy at the facility or agency where you work.

Postmortem care is the care of a person's body after the person's death. Cultural and religious beliefs often dictate how the body is to be cared for after death (and by whom). In some cultures, family members help to clean and prepare the body for whatever lies ahead, in accordance with cultural and religious traditions.

Postmortem care is necessary to keep the body in proper alignment and to prevent skin damage and discoloration. The skin is cleaned of any mucus, urine, feces, or other fluids. Standard precautions are followed when performing postmortem care, because bodily fluids are still potentially infectious, even after death. The body is placed in proper alignment before rigor mortis occurs. **Rigor mortis** is the stiffening of the muscles that usually develops within 2 to 4 hours of death. Once rigor mortis occurs, it is difficult to reposition the body. It is not uncommon for air that has been trapped in the lungs or the digestive tract to be released from the body when the body is repositioned as part of postmortem care. It may sound like the person has sighed or moaned. This natural occurrence may frighten you, unless you are aware of its cause.

In some cases, an autopsy may be required to confirm or identify the cause of the person's death. An **autopsy** is an examination of the person's organs and tissues after the person has died. In most cases, the doctor is responsible for obtaining a family member's permission to perform an autopsy. If an autopsy is to be performed, medical devices such as tubes, drains, catheters, and intravenous (IV) lines are not removed as part of postmortem care. If an autopsy is not necessary, the nurse will usually remove these medical devices as part of the postmortem care procedure.

Many facilities only prepare the person's body for the family to view before sending it to the morgue or funeral home, where the funeral director completes the postmortem care procedure. In this case, the bed linens are straightened (or changed, if they are soiled). The body is cleaned, dressed in a clean gown or pajamas, and positioned in a natural position on the bed (Fig. 22-6). Draw the top sheet up to the person's shoulders and cuff it neatly. (Do not cover the person's face with the sheet. This can be very disturbing for family members.) Make sure that the room is neat, and adjust the lights so that they are not too bright. As always, provide for privacy. You will need to help collect the person's personal belongings to be sent with the family. Dentures are either placed in the person's mouth, or labelled and sent with the body to the funeral home.

After the family has viewed the body and left, the body may be wrapped in a **shroud** (a covering used to wrap the body of a person who has died) for transport to the morgue or funeral home. A shroud is contained in the preassembled postmortem kits used by many facilities (Fig. 22-7). The shroud may be a plastic sheet that is secured with pins, tapes, or ties (Fig. 22-8), or it may zip closed. The postmortem kit also usually contains safety pins or tape for securing the shroud, ties for holding the person's hands together, identification tags, a chin strap for securing the person's jaw, a plastic bag or envelope for the person's belongings, and 30 cm × 30 cm gauze pads to absorb drainage. It is important to know and follow your

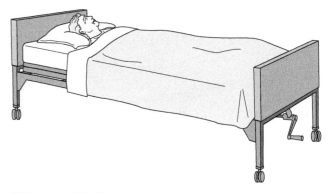

Figure 22-6
The body is placed in the supine position for viewing by the family. A pillow is placed under the person's head and shoulders.

facility's policies when providing postmortem care. An example of a standard procedure for providing postmortem care is given in Procedure 22-1. You show your respect for the person and the person's family by working quietly and preserving the person's privacy, even after death.

Providing postmortem care can be emotionally difficult. Health care workers often become very attached to their patients or residents and grieve when they die. It is not uncommon to feel frustrated at death when the focus of health care seems to be mostly on curing disease. It is perfectly

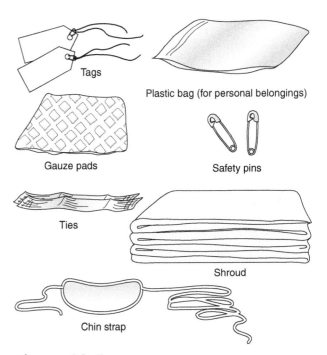

Figure 22-7
The contents of the postmortem kit vary, but most contain a shroud, something for securing the shroud, ties, gauze pads, a chin strap, identification tags, and a plastic bag or envelope for the person's belongings.

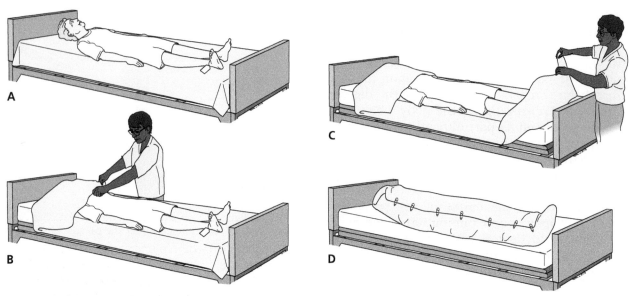

Figure 22-8
A shroud may be placed on the body after the family has left and before the body is taken to the morgue or funeral home. **(A)** The shroud is unfolded on the bed, and the body is placed on the shroud. **(B)** The top of the shroud is brought over the person's head. **(C)** The bottom of the shroud is brought over the person's feet. **(D)** The sides of the shroud are folded over the person's body and pinned, taped, or tied together. An identification tag is secured to the outside of the shroud.

acceptable to feel sad and cry at the passing of a patient or resident. You might be surprised to know that even the most experienced health care workers often seek a "shoulder to cry on." Talking about your feelings with a co-worker, supervisor, clergy member, or counsellor can help you work through your own grief. Allow yourself to be a human being and to feel emotions. It might also help to think of providing postmortem care as a way of paying your last respects to the dead person. In this way, the ritual of providing this care becomes a way of coping with your grief.

SUMMARY

- Providing holistic care is as important at the end of life as it is at any other time. Personal support workers must take steps to prevent their own discomfort with the subject of death from compromising their ability to care for dying people.
  - A dying person becomes very dependent on others for basic physical care. Recognizing the physical signs of impending death helps the personal support worker to provide the necessary care.
  - A dying person will need assistance to meet emotional and spiritual needs as well.
    - Emotionally, people prepare for death in their own individual ways. Cultural and religious beliefs and traditions greatly influence a person's response to illness and death.

  - Often, the best thing a personal support worker can do is listen if the person wants to talk, or spend quiet time with the person if he or she does not want to talk.
- Family members of a dying person require support as well.
  - Being respectful, thoughtful, and kind can do much to make family members feel better.
  - Some family members react poorly to grief and stress and may take out their frustrations on personal support workers or other members of the health care team.
- Postmortem care is done to prepare the body for the morgue or funeral home. In some facilities, the body is prepared for immediate viewing by the family, and then postmortem care is done at the morgue or funeral home.

PROCEDURE   22-1

Providing Postmortem Care

WHY YOU DO IT   Postmortem care keeps the body in proper alignment and prevents skin damage and discolouration.

Getting Ready   WCK IEPS

1. Complete the "Getting Ready" steps.

Supplies

- gloves
- paper towels
- cotton balls
- bed protector
- postmortem kit*
- wash basin
- soap
- comb
- bath blanket
- washcloth
- towel
- clean gown
- clean linens (if necessary)

Procedure

2. Cover the over-bed table with paper towels. Place your supplies on the over-bed table.

3. Make sure that the bed is positioned at a comfortable working height (to promote good body mechanics) and that the wheels are locked. Lower the head of the bed so that the bed is flat. Fanfold the top linens to the foot of the bed.

4. Put on the gloves.

5. If instructed to by the nurse, remove or turn off any medical equipment.

6. Place the body in the supine position. Position the pillow under the person's head and shoulders. Undress the body and cover it with the bath blanket.

7. Close the eyes. Put a moistened cotton ball on each eyelid if the eyes do not stay closed. If the person has an artificial eye, this should be in place, unless you are instructed otherwise.

8. Replace the person's dentures, unless you are instructed otherwise. Close the mouth and, if necessary, gently support the jaw with the chin strap, a light bandage, or a rolled hand towel.

9. Remove any jewelry and place it in a plastic bag or envelope for the family. List each piece of jewelry as you remove it. Do not remove engagement or wedding rings, unless it is your facility's policy to do so.

10. Fill the wash basin with warm water. Place the basin on the over-bed table. Wash the body and comb the hair.

11. If the family is to view the body, dress the body in a clean gown. If the bedding is wet or soiled, change the bed linens. Draw the top linens over the person, forming a cuff at the shoulders. (Do not cover the person's face.) Straighten the room, lower the lights, and provide for the family's privacy.

12. After the family leaves, collect all of the person's belongings, noting each item on your list.

13. Fill out three identification tags:

    a. Attach one to the right great toe or the right ankle.

    b. Attach one to the person's belongings.

    c. Save the last to be attached to the outside of the shroud (if used).

14. If a shroud is to be used, apply it now and attach the third identification tag to the outside of the shroud.

15. Gather the soiled linens and place them in the linen hamper. Dispose of disposable items in a facility-approved waste container. Clean equipment and return it to the storage area.

---

*The contents of the postmortem kit vary, but most contain a shroud, something for securing the shroud, ties, gauze pads, a chin strap, identification tags, and a plastic bag or envelope for the person's belongings.

(continued)

16. Remove your gloves and dispose of them in a facility-approved waste container.

17. Transfer the body from the bed to a stretcher for transport to the morgue, if appropriate. If the family has made funeral arrangements, leave the body in the room with the door or curtain closed.

18. Report the time the body was transported and the location of the person's belongings to the nurse.

Finishing Up CLSoWR

19. Complete the "Finishing Up" steps.

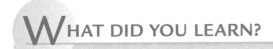

WHAT DID YOU LEARN?

Multiple Choice

Select the single best answer for each of the following questions.

1. When caring for a person who is dying, you should:
   a. Keep family members away from the dying person
   b. Keep the room dark
   c. Provide for the person's physical and emotional needs
   d. Change the subject if the person starts to talk about death or dying

2. A common sign of approaching death is:
   a. Severe pain that gets worse
   b. Normal or increased vital signs
   c. Cool, moist skin
   d. Increased appetite

3. Postmortem care is done:
   a. Right before the person dies
   b. After the doctor pronounces the person dead
   c. After rigor mortis sets in
   d. If there is time

4. As death approaches, the last sense to be lost is:
   a. Sight
   b. Hearing
   c. Smell
   d. Taste

5. Which one of the following is a true statement about providing postmortem care?
   a. Standard precautions are used because the body may be infectious
   b. Dentures are removed from the mouth and given to the family to take home
   c. There is no need for privacy because the person is dead
   d. All of the above

6. In caring for the dying person, the personal support worker also needs to care for the family. Which of the following can the personal support worker do to support the family?
   a. Allow family members to stay with the dying person
   b. Be respectful of the family
   c. Provide the family with privacy
   d. All of the above

7. You are helping to care for Mrs. Winger, who has a terminal illness. One day when you are in Mrs. Winger's room, she tells you that during difficult times she has always found comfort in reading poems by her favorite poets. What is this an example of?
   a. Culture
   b. Spirituality
   c. Religion
   d. Reincarnation

8. Which of the following meets a dying person's physical needs?
   a. Providing frequent skin care
   b. Listening if the person wants to talk
   c. Preventing rigor mortis
   d. All of the above

Matching

Match each numbered item with its appropriate lettered description.

D **1.** Reincarnation

E **2.** Cheyne-Stokes respiration

B **3.** Rigor mortis

C **4.** Postmortem care

A **5.** Autopsy

a. Examination of a person's tissues and organs after death

b. Stiffening of the muscles that occurs 2 to 4 hours after death

c. Care of a body after death

d. The belief that the soul of a dead person returns to Earth in the form of another human being or animal yet to be born

e. Pattern of rapid–slow respirations

STOP and Think!

You have been caring for Mr. Cole, who is dying. Now it appears that the time of death is rapidly approaching. Even though Mr. Cole is having trouble talking, he does manage to say to you, "I don't want to die alone." What can you do to help Mr. Cole?

Personal Support Workers Make a Difference!

"My mother recently passed away at Colchester County Nursing Home. Although Mom had been in poor health for some time, her death was hard on me. I must say, though, that the staff at Colchester County made this difficult time more bearable through their kindness and competence.

Last Monday, the phone rang and it was Elaine, one of the night nurses on duty. Elaine said that we needed to gather the family and come out, that Mom was dying. Soon, we had quite a crowd in Mom's room. I guess the staff was expecting us, because they had moved Mom's roommate to another room and brought in chairs so we would all have some place to sit. One of the personal support workers, Patty, was so great. She actually brought us a tray with a pot full of hot coffee, coffee cups, sugar, and creamer on it! We sat with Mom throughout the night and morning hours as she slowly weakened. Patty checked in with us often and would help turn Mom and change her when she soiled the bed. Sometimes she brought the nurse in to suction Mom when she started having trouble breathing. Although Mom could not talk to us, she regained consciousness about an hour before she died and looked us each in the eyes as we said our tearful good-byes.

When Mom took her last breath, we all knew what had happened. My sister went out into the hall to look for help. Luckily, Patty was nearby, and she quickly returned to the room to check Mom's vital signs. Then the doctor came in, and pronounced Mom dead. I asked Patty if I could help her wash Mom's body and get her into a clean gown, and Patty said that would be fine. Together, Patty and I prepared Mom for the funeral home. My family and I were allowed to stay in the room for a while after Mom died, just to reflect on things and finish making plans for the funeral.

Patty was really a godsend to me and my family during this difficult time. The excellent way Patty handled Mom's death spoke volumes about the care she gave to Mom while she was alive."

You can listen to more stories about how personal support workers make a difference on the CD in the front of your book.

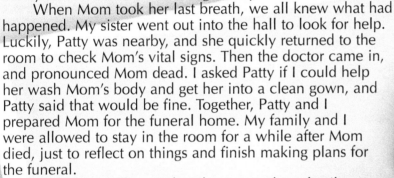
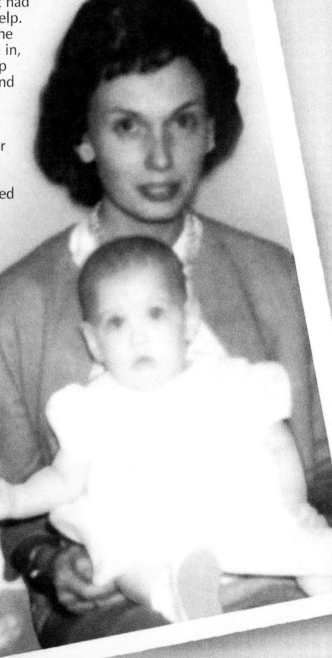

STRUCTURE AND FUNCTION OF THE HUMAN BODY

23 Basic Body Structure and Function
24 The Integumentary System
25 The Musculoskeletal System
26 The Respiratory System
27 The Cardiovascular System
28 The Nervous System
29 The Sensory System
30 The Endocrine System
31 The Digestive System
32 The Urinary System
33 The Reproductive System

The human body is truly remarkable in its ability to maintain health and to heal from disease. In this unit, we will explore how each organ system functions normally, as well as how disease or injury affects the function of the organ system. We will also explore the measures that are taken to help the body return to its best level of functioning after injury or illness. Knowing how the body works when it is healthy helps us to understand how to help the body heal and function more effectively during illness.

Photo: The human body has amazing capabilities. (AP Photo/The Canadian Press, Jonathan Hayward.)

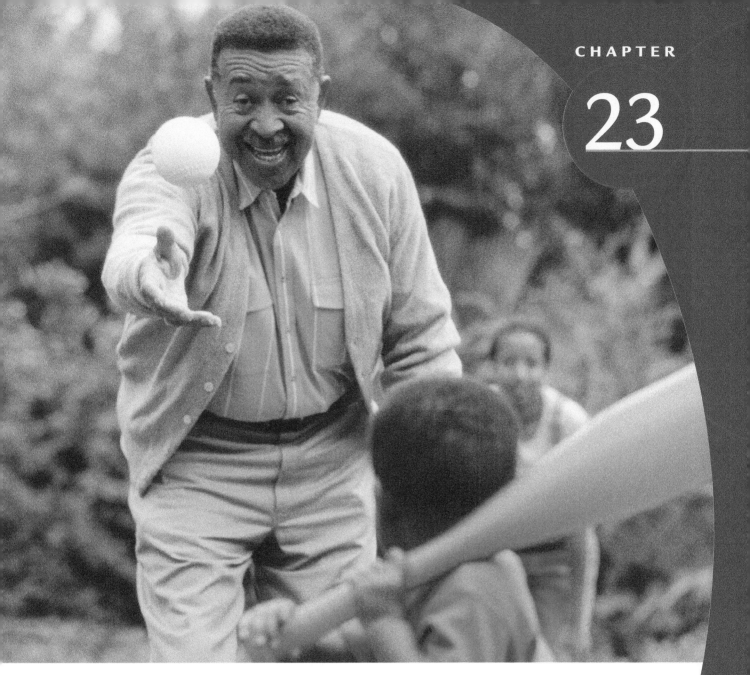

Basic Body Structure and Function

WHAT WILL YOU LEARN?

The human body is a wonder of design. In a healthy person, all of the body's parts work together effortlessly, like those of a highly efficient machine. To understand how a machine works, a mechanic studies the machine's parts and how they work together. The same is true of people who want to know how the human body works. **Anatomy** is the study of what body parts look like, where they are located, how big they are, and how they

Photo: When we are healthy, our bodies allow us to do the things we like to do.

465

connect to other body parts. **Physiology** is the study of how the body parts work. In this chapter, we will take a look at the body as a whole, functioning unit. You will learn about how changes in a person's normal anatomy or physiology can lead to disease or disabilities, and about the body's remarkable ability to correct small problems before they become large ones. In addition, you will learn about the important role the health care team plays in helping people to achieve their best possible level of functioning. When you are finished with this chapter, you will be able to:

1. Define the terms *anatomy* and *physiology.*
2. List and describe the basic levels of organization of the body.
3. Define the term *homeostasis* and give examples of how the body maintains the balance necessary for life.
4. Discuss how the body's inability to maintain homeostasis affects a person's health.
5. Describe the categories of disease and list some factors that may put a person at risk for developing a certain disease.
6. Explain the goal of rehabilitation.
7. Describe how the concept of humanistic care applies to rehabilitation.
8. Understand the personal support worker's responsibilities related to providing restorative care.

Vocabulary

Anatomy	Cytoplasm	Organ system	Restorative care
Physiology	Nucleus	Homeostasis	Supportive devices
Organism	Cell membrane	Disease	Assistive devices
Cell	Tissue	Disability	Prosthetic devices
Organelles	Organ	Rehabilitation	

HOW IS THE BODY ORGANIZED?

All living things, from a jellyfish that washes up on the beach to the largest elephant roaming the plains of Africa, share the same general organization. The basic unit of life is the cell. Cells group together to form tissues. Tissues group together to form organs, and organs group together to form organ systems. These levels of organization are shared by every living thing, or **organism,** whether it is an animal or a plant (Fig. 23-1). The reason not all living things look alike or function alike is because at each level, there are variations specific to the type of organism. Let's take a closer look now at the levels of organization that make up each organism—cells, tissues, organs, and organ systems.

CELLS

A **cell** is the basic unit of life. A cell is so small that it can only be seen with a microscope. A single cell, as small as it is, has all of the characteristics of life. It is capable of organization, which means

that it can join with other similar cells to perform a common function. It is capable of metabolism, which means that it takes in "raw materials" and converts them into the energy it needs to stay alive. It is capable of growth, which means that it changes in size over time. And finally, it is capable of reproduction, which means that it can make a copy of itself. Organization, metabolism, growth,

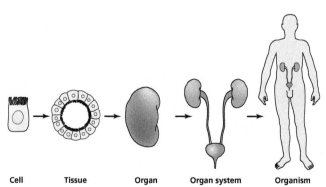

| Cell | Tissue | Organ | Organ system | Organism |

Figure 23-1

All living things (organisms) share the same basic levels of organization. Cells form tissues, tissues form organs, and organs form organ systems.

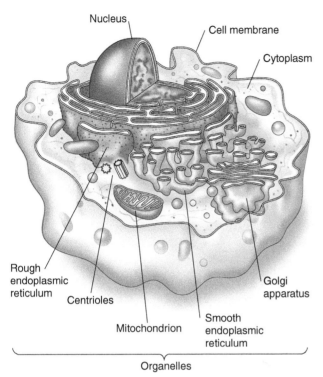

Figure 23-2
A cell contains organelles and a nucleus, which float in a jelly-like substance called cytoplasm. A cell membrane surrounds the cytoplasm and gives the cell its shape.

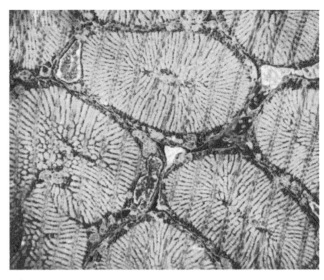

Figure 23-3
Cells join together to form tissues. (© *Scott Camazine/Photo Researchers, Inc.*)

and reproduction are basic qualities that make a living thing different from a non-living thing.

The human body is made up of millions of cells, of all different shapes, sizes, and functions. Each type of cell in the body has a specific duty. Our overall health depends on the ability of the cells of the body to do their jobs.

To function properly, cells require oxygen, water, nutrition, and the ability to eliminate waste products. Structures inside of the cell, called **organelles,** help the cell to make the energy it needs to stay alive and to rid itself of waste products (Fig. 23-2). The organelles float in a jelly-like substance called **cytoplasm.** In addition to organelles and cytoplasm, the cell contains a nucleus. The **nucleus** of the cell is like the cell's "brain." It contains all of the information the cell needs to do its job, grow, and reproduce. A **cell membrane** surrounds the cytoplasm and gives the cell its shape.

TISSUES

When cells that are similar in structure and specialized to perform a specific function join together, they form **tissue** (Fig. 23-3). There are four main types of tissue in the human body:

- **Epithelial tissue** covers the outside of the body, lines its internal structures, and forms glands. The purpose of epithelial tissue is protection. Epithelial tissue forms the outer part of the skin. It forms the mucous membranes that line our digestive, respiratory, urinary, and reproductive systems. It also covers organs such as the lungs and heart, and lines the inside of the blood vessels, abdominal cavity, and chest cavity.
- **Connective tissue** does what its name suggests—it connects other tissues together. Connective tissue supports and forms the framework for all of the parts of the body. Examples of connective tissue include bone, cartilage, ligaments, tendons, and fatty tissues. Blood is also considered a form of connective tissue.
- **Muscle tissue** produces movement. There are three types of muscle tissue found in the body (Table 23-1). Skeletal muscle allows you to move your arms, legs, and other parts of the body. Because you can decide when and how to move the parts of your body that contain skeletal muscle, skeletal muscle is said to be "voluntary," or under the control of the individual. The second type of muscle tissue, smooth muscle, lines the walls of organs such as the intestines, the stomach, and the blood vessels. The movement provided by smooth muscle is involuntary, or out of your control. For example, it is the smooth muscle in the walls of the intestines that produces peristalsis (the wave-like

Table 23-1 Types of Muscle Tissue

TYPE	FUNCTION	CONTROL
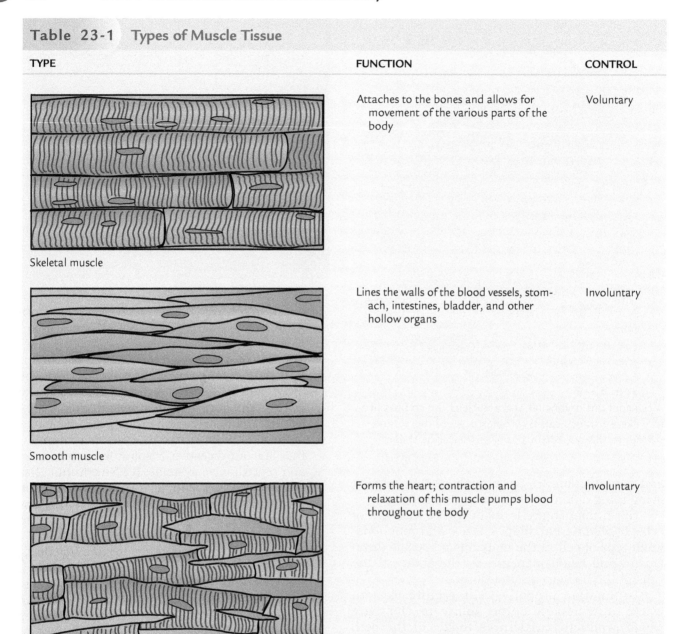Skeletal muscle	Attaches to the bones and allows for movement of the various parts of the body	Voluntary
Smooth muscle	Lines the walls of the blood vessels, stomach, intestines, bladder, and other hollow organs	Involuntary
Cardiac muscle	Forms the heart; contraction and relaxation of this muscle pumps blood throughout the body	Involuntary

movements that pass digested food through the intestines). You do not need to think about moving food through your intestines. Instead, this action occurs automatically. The third type of muscle tissue, cardiac muscle, forms the heart. Contraction and relaxation of the cardiac muscle pumps blood throughout the body. Like smooth muscle, cardiac muscle is involuntary.

- **Nervous tissue** conducts information. The brain, spinal cord, and nerves are made of nervous tissue. Nervous tissue allows one part of the body to "talk" to another part.

For example, nerves carry information to the brain to be processed and interpreted. In addition, the brain sends commands to other parts of the body through the nerves.

ORGANS

A group of tissues functioning together for a similar purpose form an **organ.** For example, the heart is made of all four tissue types, and its main function is to pump blood throughout the body. Other examples of organs include the stomach, liver, kidneys, and lungs. An organ may have one specific function, or it may have several.

ORGAN SYSTEMS

An **organ system** is a group of organs that work together to perform a specific function for the body. For the organ system to work properly, each organ within the system must function well. Human beings have 10 main organ systems (Fig. 23-4):

- The *integumentary system* includes the skin and its glands, the hair, and the nails. The function of the integumentary system is to protect the body.
- The *skeletal system* includes the bones. The function of the skeletal system is to provide a frame for the body and to give the body shape.
- The *muscular system* includes the muscles. The muscular system works along with the skeletal system to enable the body to move. Sometimes the muscular system and the skeletal system together are called the musculoskeletal system.
- The *respiratory system* includes the lungs and the airways. The respiratory system allows us to take in oxygen and get rid of carbon dioxide, a waste product of cellular metabolism.
- The *cardiovascular system* is made up of the blood, the heart, and the blood vessels. The cardiovascular system transports nutrients and oxygen to the cells of the body, and carries waste products away.
- The *nervous system* includes the brain, spinal cord, and nerves. The nervous system controls the functioning of the other organ systems. It also allows us to interact with our environment through the *special senses* (sight, hearing, smell, taste, and touch).
- The *endocrine system* is made up of glands found in specific locations throughout the body. These glands secrete chemical substances called *hormones*, which control the function of certain organs.
- The *digestive system* includes the teeth, salivary glands, tongue, esophagus, stomach, small intestine, large intestine, liver, pancreas, and gallbladder. The digestive system allows us to take in food and water, digest the food into nutrients, and absorb the nutrients into the bloodstream. The digestive system also removes solid waste from the body in the form of feces.
- The *urinary system* includes the kidneys, the bladder, the ureters, and the urethra. The urinary system removes liquid waste from the body in the form of urine.
- The *reproductive system* allows the human body to produce new life. Without a means of reproduction, human life would cease to exist.

As you can see, organ systems do not work alone. They work together to maintain the life of the organism.

HEALTH AND DISEASE

All of the organ systems work together to maintain **homeostasis,** or balance. Homeostasis is a basic concept in physiology. The word comes from the Greek words *homoios,* which means "same," and *stasis,* which means "standing." So homeostasis means "staying the same." For an organism to stay alive, certain conditions within the body must remain the same, within a range of normal limits. You were introduced to this idea in Chapter 16, when we discussed vital signs. For example, the body temperature must remain within a certain range. The blood pressure must remain within a certain range. The fluids that keep our cells moist and healthy must not be too acidic or too basic. Our blood must always contain the right amount of oxygen, nutrients, and other substances needed for metabolism.

All of the organ systems are constantly working together to maintain a state of balance. When the external or internal environment changes, the organ systems must make adjustments to compensate for the change. For example, imagine that you are playing basketball at the park with your friends on a very hot day. You begin to sweat. This is your body working to cool you down. As you continue to play and sweat, you begin to get thirsty. This is your body telling you that it needs more water. As you run back and forth on the court, you breathe harder and your heart rate increases, as your respiratory and circulatory systems work to send extra oxygen to your tissues. Your tissues need the extra oxygen because they use it to help produce the energy that allows you to keep playing.

Most of the time, you are not even aware of the adjustments your body is making to keep everything within the normal range. Even when you are sitting perfectly still, little adjustments are being made to keep the internal environment stable. Perhaps you are wondering how your

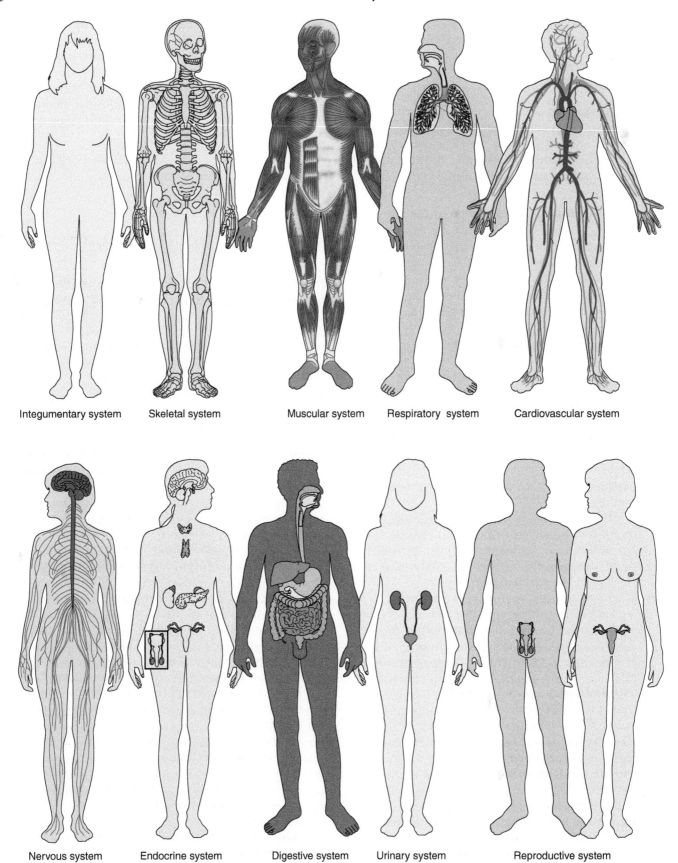

Integumentary system   Skeletal system   Muscular system   Respiratory system   Cardiovascular system

Nervous system   Endocrine system   Digestive system   Urinary system   Reproductive system

Figure 23-4

There are 10 organ systems in the human body.

body "knows" that an adjustment is needed. The answer is, through a feedback mechanism. Although all of the organ systems play a role in maintaining homeostasis, most of these feedback mechanisms are controlled by the nervous and endocrine systems.

The body's ability to maintain balance is an indicator of good health. There are times when the body's ability to maintain homeostasis is altered. This imbalance is usually the result of a disease. A **disease** (or a "disorder") occurs when the structure or function of an organ or an organ system is abnormal. Diseases can be acute (temporary) or chronic (long term). They can be mild or severe. Sometimes, the same disease may be severe in one person but mild in another.

CATEGORIES OF DISEASE

There are several common categories of disease. A disease may belong to more than one of these categories. Common categories of disease include:

- **Infectious.** Infections are believed to play a role in approximately half of all illnesses.
- **Degenerative.** To degenerate means to "break down." Degenerative diseases occur when the tissues of the body wear out or break down. Arthritis, muscular dystrophy, osteoporosis, and Alzheimer's disease are examples of degenerative diseases. These diseases can be inherited, or they can be caused by infection, injury, or aging. Sometimes there is no known cause.
- **Nutritional.** These disorders occur when a person's diet lacks certain nutrients. Consuming too much of any one nutrient (for example, vitamins) or too many calories can also cause nutritional disorders. For example, obesity is a nutritional disorder.
- **Metabolic (endocrine).** Metabolic disorders, such as diabetes, occur when the body is unable to metabolize or absorb certain nutrients. Metabolic disorders often occur when the body secretes either too much of one type of hormone, or not enough. Because the hormone is responsible for controlling the function of a particular organ, the organ does not function properly and an imbalance in homeostasis occurs.
- **Immune.** These disorders change the way the immune system behaves. Sometimes, as in acquired immunodeficiency syndrome (AIDS), the disease reduces the immune system's ability to fight off infection. Other times, the disease causes the immune

system to start attacking the body's own tissues.
- **Neoplastic.** The word *neoplasm* means "new growth." Many people use the word "cancer" or "tumor" when they are talking about neoplastic disease. Neoplasms cause problems by invading otherwise healthy tissues. The presence of the new growth prevents the tissues from functioning properly.
- **Psychiatric.** Mental disorders that affect a person's ability to function normally, such as depression, are also considered diseases.

RISK FACTORS FOR DISEASE

Why do some people get certain diseases and others do not? Why does a certain disease affect one person very mildly but totally destroy the health of another person? As a personal support worker, one of your many responsibilities will be to help improve or maintain the health of your patients or residents. To do that, you need to know about the factors that can put a person at risk for disease, or negatively affect his or her ability to recover from disease. Some of these factors include the following:

- **Age.** Some disorders are more likely to occur in certain age groups. For example, chickenpox, a viral infection, is more common in children. Age can also influence how a person reacts to disease. For example, when an adult gets the chickenpox, the infection is usually much more severe. In general, older people are more at risk for certain diseases because the process of aging causes a lot of wear and tear on the body's tissues and organs.
- **Gender.** A person's gender can put the person at risk for certain diseases. For instance, breast cancer is much more common in women than in men. Women are also more likely than men to develop diabetes. However, men are more likely to have heart disease.
- **Heredity.** The genes that we inherit from our parents may put us at risk for developing certain diseases. For example, scientists now know that some types of cancer, diabetes, and heart disease are inherited.
- **Lifestyle.** A person's living conditions and health habits play a major role in the person's overall health status. For example, a person who is homeless is more likely to get sick than a person who has shelter from

the weather. A person who gets too little rest and has poor nutritional habits is more likely to become ill than a person who gets enough sleep and eats well. A person who smokes is more likely to develop cancer, lung disease, or heart disease than a person who does not. A person who likes a deep, dark tan in the summer is more at risk for developing skin cancer than a person who uses sunscreen. These are just examples of the many ways in which lifestyle influences health.

- **Occupation.** Many jobs put a person at risk for certain diseases. For example, constant exposure to coal dust puts coal miners at risk for developing "black lung disease." Health care workers who do not take care to protect themselves are at risk for certain infections, such as human immunodeficiency virus (HIV) or hepatitis.

- **Chronic disease.** A person who has a chronic disease, such as diabetes or high blood pressure, is at increased risk for developing another disease. For example, a person who does not manage his diabetes well is likely to develop heart disease, blindness, or kidney failure. In addition, a person who has a chronic disease is often more likely to experience more severe problems from something that would not really affect a healthy person. For example, an ingrown toenail will cause discomfort and inconvenience in a healthy person. However, in a person with diabetes, the ingrown toenail could cause a severe infection, because diabetes changes the internal environment of the body, placing the person more at risk for infection.

- **Emotional health.** A person's emotional health can directly affect her physical health. Emotional stress can create physical problems such as headaches, digestive disorders, and muscle strain. In addition, stress makes the body more at risk for infection. If you remember from Chapter 14, just becoming a patient or resident of a health care facility can significantly increase a person's level of emotional stress and make coping with physical illness or disability more difficult.

Awareness of the factors that can put your patients or residents at risk for disease will help you to better meet their individual needs. When you meet your patient's or resident's specific needs, or observe and report signs that indicate that the person's body is struggling to return to a balanced state, you are making a very important contribution to the person's health.

REHABILITATION AND RESTORATIVE CARE

Many diseases and injuries leave the person with a **disability,** or impaired function. The disability can be physical, emotional, or both. Like diseases, some disabilities are acute while others are chronic. Some may be permanent (Fig. 23-5). A person with a disability may need minimal help with activities of daily living (ADLs) or total physical care, depending on how severe the disability is. One of the goals of the health care team is to help patients and residents learn to manage their disabilities and regain as much independence as possible.

Rehabilitation is the process of helping a person with a disability to return to his highest level of physical, emotional, or economic function. Rehabilitation is achieved through **restorative care,** or the measures that health care workers take to help a person regain health, strength, and function. Restorative care involves treatment, education, and the prevention of further disability. Like any other type of health care, restorative care is achieved through a team effort. Members of the team include the patient or resident and her family members, the nurse, the personal support worker, a doctor, and any number of other specialists, depending on the type of rehabilitation and the goals of the effort.

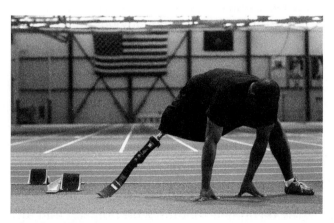

Figure 23-5

This young man has lost a leg, resulting in a permanent disability. However, he has adapted to the loss of the leg and is able to do everything that a person with two legs is able to do. Here, he is shown training to compete in the 100-meter dash at the U.S. Paralympics Track and Field National Championships. (*AP Photo/Carolyn Kaster.*)

The rehabilitative effort focuses on the individual needs and capabilities of the patient or resident. For example, following rehabilitation, some people will be able to leave the health care facility and live completely independently. Others will always be dependent to some degree on others for help with their ADLs, but following rehabilitation, they will be less dependent than they were before. Some people will require many months, or even years, of rehabilitation to return to their best level of functioning.

Rehabilitation services are offered by many types of facilities. Hospitals may offer a variety of rehabilitative services, from physical therapy to mental counselling. Some facilities provide only rehabilitative services for people with specific types of disabilities. For example, a facility may have the mission of helping people to cope with disabilities caused by head or spinal cord injuries, burns, or developmental disorders.

THE ROLE OF THE PERSONAL SUPPORT WORKER

The personal support worker plays a key role in the successful rehabilitation of a patient or resident. Although other health care professionals evaluate the person's rehabilitation needs and then plan the restorative care, the personal support worker plays a key role in helping to carry out the plan. Because of the unique relationship that develops between a personal support worker and the people he cares for, the personal support worker becomes the "eyes and ears" of the rehabilitation team.

You will be able to observe the patient or resident for any physical changes, positive or negative, that are related to the rehabilitation. You will be the one who notices that a new splint or supportive device has caused chafing or redness of the skin (Fig. 23-6). You will document the results of a bowel or bladder training plan, and it will be your responsibility to make sure that the person is taken to the bathroom on schedule. You will be the person responsible for adding the thickening powder to a person's liquids to help him swallow without choking. You will reassure, encourage, listen to, and praise the people you care for as they struggle with the challenges that rehabilitation brings.

Ask questions about new rehabilitation measures that have been planned for a resident or patient. Have the nurse or therapist explain how to use new equipment and show you how to help your patient or resident to use it (Fig. 23-7).

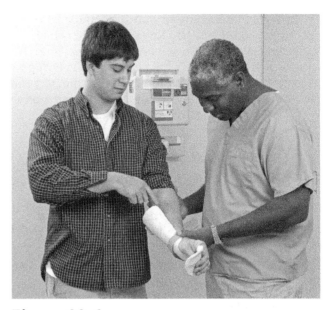

Figure 23-6
The personal support worker is the "eyes and ears" of the rehabilitation team.

Make sure you document and report your observations. If a new rehabilitation measure does not seem to be working for the person, perhaps a change is necessary. Your input can help initiate that change.

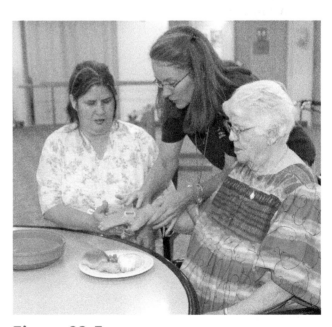

Figure 23-7
Ask the nurse or physical therapist to show you how to use assistive devices. This will allow you to help your patient or resident use the assistive device more effectively. Here, a physical therapist is showing a personal support worker how to assist a resident with using a wrist supporter with a spoon attached.

It is also important for you to monitor the person's emotional status. Rehabilitation, which in some cases can take a very long time, can be extremely frustrating for the person who is trying to overcome a disability. If you sense that one of your patients or residents is becoming depressed, angry, or frustrated, report this to the nurse. The nurse and the other members of the rehabilitation team will be able to help the person work through these feelings, so that he can again focus on recovery.

Guidelines for assisting with restorative care are given in Guidelines Box 23-1.

Guidelines Box 23-1	Assisting With Restorative Care
WHAT YOU DO	**WHY YOU DO IT**
Ask questions about new rehabilitation measures that have been planned for a resident or patient. Have the nurse or therapist explain to you how to use new equipment and show you how to help your patient or resident to use it.	Knowing about the special techniques that are being used with the person will allow you to help the person to practice these techniques. Knowing how to use any special equipment will allow you to help the person to use the equipment properly.
Monitor the person's emotional status.	Working to regain or maintain function, or learning to adjust to a loss of function, can be a long, difficult, and painful process. It is very easy for patients or residents to become frustrated and discouraged. Reporting your observations about the person's emotional status to the nurse will enable the rehabilitation team to help the person work through these feelings so that he or she can again focus on recovery.
Focus on the person's abilities, and celebrate all successes, no matter how small.	Achieving small goals gives the person an emotional boost and encourages him or her to keep working.
Encourage and reassure the person, but be realistic in your encouragement and be careful not to compare the person with someone else.	Each person will have individual responses to rehabilitation. Not all goals will be reached.
Give the person the time he or she needs to complete a task independently. Offer assistance only as needed and only if the person seems overly frustrated.	Although it may be faster or easier to just complete the task for the person, it is important for the person's self-esteem to let the person do as much for himself or herself as possible.
Be empathetic, but do not pity the person.	When you pity someone, it means that you recognize his or her loss. When you empathize with someone, it means that you can imagine how the person feels about the loss. Empathy will help you deal more effectively with the person's anger and frustration.
If you find yourself feeling frustrated with a patient or resident who is struggling with rehabilitation, talk to the nurse.	If you let the person's frustration and anger affect you, you may not be able to provide the person with the best care possible. You may need a break or a short reassignment from that person to continue to provide the best care possible.

TYPES OF REHABILITATION

There are many types of rehabilitation. The type of rehabilitation depends on the person's specific disability and the individual needs of that person. In many cases, a person may need a combination of different types of rehabilitation. For example, imagine a patient named Mr. Hayes. Mr. Hayes was involved in a car accident that killed his wife and resulted in the loss of his own leg. Mr. Hayes now needs to learn to walk with a prosthetic leg. He also needs to overcome the emotional crisis associated with the loss of his wife. Depending on what sort of job Mr. Hayes had before the accident, he may also need to learn new job skills so that he can work again. In this example, learning to walk with the prosthetic leg would be achieved through physical rehabilitation. Overcoming the grief and guilt caused by his wife's death would require emotional rehabilitation. Learning the skills needed to return to work would be achieved through vocational rehabilitation.

Physical Rehabilitation

Helping people to overcome physical disabilities is a common function of most health care facilities. Physical therapy helps to restore strength and function to limbs that have been affected by illness and injury. Exercise, combined with supportive

devices, assistive devices, prosthetic devices, or all three (Fig. 23-8), can help a person regain function.

- **Supportive devices,** such as splints and braces, help to stabilize a weak joint or limb.
- **Assistive devices** make certain tasks, such as transferring, walking, eating, or dressing, easier. You have already learned about many assistive devices in previous chapters.
- **Prosthetic devices** are artificial replacements for legs, feet, arms, or other body parts.

Although a person's disability may prevent him from ever doing some things again, there will be many things that he will be able to do independently following physical rehabilitation. The ability to function independently is very important for a person's self-esteem.

Another major focus of physical rehabilitation is to prevent complications that can result from the loss of function. When a person does not use a part of the body for a long time, he loses muscle mass in that part. As the muscle mass is lost, so too is the person's strength. For example, have you ever had a cast put on an arm or a leg for a long period of time? When the cast finally came off, your arm or leg probably looked skinny and felt weak. That was because during the time your arm or leg was in the cast, you were not able to move it, and your muscle mass decreased. When a person cannot use an arm or a leg, exercising the arm or leg helps to keep it working properly. Imagine that Mr. Gibbons has been in a coma for several months. Finally, after weeks of unconsciousness, Mr. Gibbons comes out of the coma. Fortunately, the people caring for Mr. Gibbons while he was in the coma took care to exercise his arms and legs for him. If they had not done this, complications associated with immobility, such as contractures and muscle atrophy, could have caused permanent disability. By preventing these complications from occurring, the health care team ensured that Mr. Gibbons would be able to be rehabilitated successfully.

Rehabilitative measures are also used to help people learn about and recover from chronic and acute illnesses. A person with diabetes will learn how to control her condition through a combination of exercise and diet. Cardiac rehabilitation involves the use of closely monitored exercise and dietary changes to help a person recover from a heart attack.

Emotional Rehabilitation

The stresses that accompany disability can interfere with a person's ability to cope emotionally.

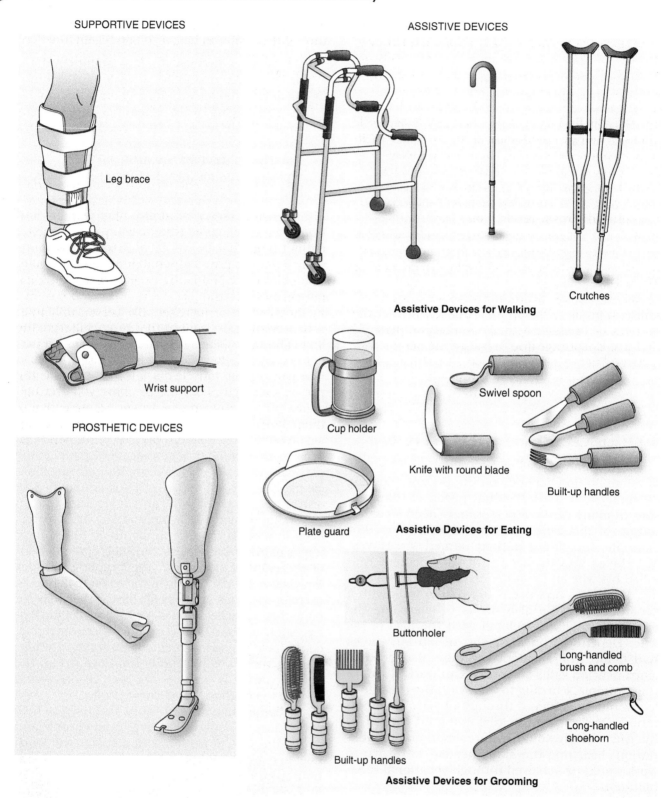

Figure 23-8
Supportive devices, assistive devices, prosthetic devices, or all three can help a person do certain tasks independently.

Feelings of despair and a loss of self-esteem often accompany conditions that cause a disability. The loss of ability, the loss of a "normal" appearance, the loss of income, and the loss of independence will affect each person differently. You will see some people rally in the face of disability and actually find a new focus for their lives, while others withdraw emotionally and use the disability as a reason not to try to improve. Some people who have experienced a devastating illness or injury may even talk of suicide. If you think that one of your patients or residents is experiencing emotional distress, report your concerns to the nurse. The nurse will arrange for emotional counselling to help the person overcome his grief and learn to accept and work with his disability (Fig. 23-9).

When you are caring for a person with a disability, there is a lot you can do to help meet the person's emotional needs. Focus on the person's abilities. Encourage and reassure the person, but be careful not to compare the person with someone else. For example, do not say, "Well, if Mr. Smith can learn to walk again, surely you can too!" Instead say, "Mr. Williams, I am so impressed by your progress! You've gone so much farther this week than you did last week!" Be realistic in your encouragement. Do not say things like, "Oh, keep on working and you'll be back to normal in no time" if it is unlikely that the person will ever be able to return to the level of function he had before the injury or illness. However, allow the person to hope for cures, new treatments, and advances in medical technology that can improve his quality of life.

Vocational Rehabilitation

A *vocation* is a job. The goal of vocational rehabilitation is to return a person to gainful employment. Gainful employment is a job or career that will provide enough income for the person to live, without being dependent on financial assistance to survive. Vocational rehabilitation is used when a person's disability causes her to lose the skills she needs to do the job she had prior to becoming disabled. In some cases, the person may just need vocational rehabilitation to relearn the skills she had before. In other cases, the person will need to learn a completely new set of skills that will enable her to get another type of job (Fig. 23-10). Assistance may also be available to help the person locate a new job, new living arrangements, or a new mode of transportation that will allow her to become independent again.

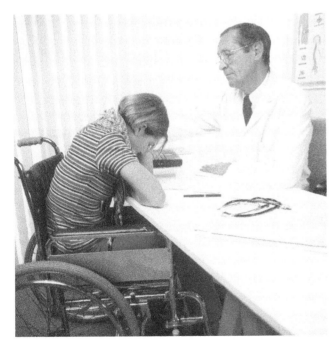

Figure 23-9
Emotional rehabilitation helps the person learn to cope with the losses caused by the disability. Many people with disabilities benefit from talking to a professional therapist or a clergy member. (© CC Studio/Photo Researchers, Inc.)

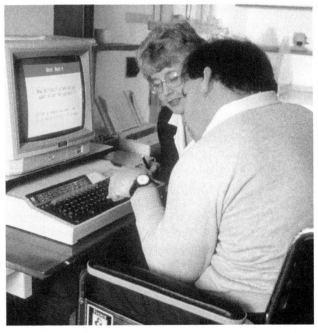

Figure 23-10
Vocational rehabilitation helps a person learn or re-learn the skills he will need to return to work. (© Simon Fraser/Disability Research, Hunters Moor Hospital/Photo Researchers, Inc.)

TELL THE NURSE

When you are caring for a person receiving rehabilitative therapy, you should report the following observations to the nurse immediately:

- A supportive device is broken or not working properly

- The person has a change in vital signs during or after the rehabilitation activity

- The person has pain, swelling, redness, or signs of inflammation around supportive devices or prosthetic devices

- The person is showing signs of depression or excessive frustration, such as crying, withdrawal, anger, or talk of suicide

- The person is having excessive difficulty with a new rehabilitation technique or treatment

SUMMARY

- Understanding how the healthy body works helps us to understand and treat disease.
- All living things share the same levels of organization.
  - A cell is the basic unit of life.
  - A group of cells that is similar in structure and specialized for a specific function forms tissue.
  - A group of tissues functioning together for a similar purpose forms an organ.
  - A group of organs that function together for the same general purpose forms an organ system.
  - A group of organ systems working together for the purpose of maintaining life forms an organism.
- All of the organ systems work together to maintain a state of homeostasis, or balance.
  - When the body's ability to maintain homeostasis is altered, disease or illness can result.
    - There are several common categories of disease. These categories often overlap.
    - Certain factors put some people more at risk for disease than others.
  - A personal support worker who is aware of the factors that put a person at risk for disease is able to provide better care for her patients or residents, because she has a better understanding of each individual's needs.

- A primary focus of the health care industry is to help a person recover from an illness or injury and regain independence. Rehabilitation is the process that helps a person with a disability return to the highest level of physical, emotional, and economic function possible.
  - Rehabilitation must focus on the whole person—his needs, well-being, and abilities—not just on the person's disabilities.
  - Rehabilitation involves a team of people working together to address the needs of the patient or resident. Because of the unique relationship that develops between a personal support worker and the people he cares for, the personal support worker becomes the "eyes and ears" of the rehabilitation team.
- Many types of rehabilitation are used to help a disabled person regain function.
  - Physical rehabilitation focuses on regaining physical function through the use of exercise, supportive devices, assistive devices, and prosthetic devices.
  - Emotional rehabilitation focuses on helping the person come to terms with the disability and cope with loss.
  - Vocational rehabilitation focuses on providing the person with the skills he or she needs in order to get a job and achieve financial independence.

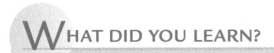

WHAT DID YOU LEARN?

Multiple Choice

Select the single best answer for each of the following questions.

1. The process that helps a person with a disability to return to her highest level of physical, emotional, or economic function is called:
   a. Homeostasis
   b. Metabolism
   c. Prosthetics
   d. Rehabilitation
2. Which of the following is a factor that might put a person at risk for disease?
   a. Age
   b. Heredity
   c. Gender
   d. All of the above
3. What is the purpose of epithelial tissue?
   a. To provide a frame for, and give shape to, the body

   b. To connect other types of tissue together
   c. To cover the body and line its cavities
   d. To conduct nerve impulses
4. Which one of the following would you be responsible for when providing a patient or resident with rehabilitative care?
   a. Adding a thickener to the person's drink to make the liquid easier to swallow
   b. Documenting the results of bladder training
   c. Observing the person for changes in ability, positive or negative
   d. All of the above

Matching

Match each numbered item with its appropriate lettered description.

__F__ 1. Anatomy

__J__ 2. Organ

__A__ 3. Vocational rehabilitation

__D__ 4. Cell

__E__ 5. Emotional rehabilitation

__C__ 6. Physical rehabilitation

__K__ 7. Tissue

__B__ 8. Physiology

__H__ 9. Homeostasis

__G__ 10. Organ system

__I__ 11. Organism

a. Used when a person's disability causes her to lose the skills she needs to do the job she had prior to becoming disabled
b. Study of how the body parts work
c. Used to restore strength and function to limbs that have been affected by illness and injury
d. Basic unit of life
e. Used to help a person manage the feelings caused by a disability
f. Study of what body parts look like, where they are located, how big they are, and how they connect to other body parts
g. A group of organs that work together to perform a specific function for the body
h. A state of balance
i. A living thing, formed by a group of organ systems working together for the purpose of maintaining life
j. A group of tissues functioning together for a similar purpose
k. Formed when cells that are similar in structure and specialized to perform a specific function join together

STOP and Think!

Jacob is working in the rehabilitation unit of his nursing facility. He has been assigned to care for Mr. Huff, who has recently had his right leg amputated (removed) above the knee. Jacob is to assist Mr. Huff in his transfers until he is able to do them himself. Mr. Huff is to do all of his own activities of daily living (ADLs), such as bathing, feeding, and dressing himself, with minimal help from Jacob. This morning when Jacob enters the room, he finds Mr. Huff on the floor between the bed and the wheelchair. Mr. Huff is struggling to climb into his wheelchair. When Jacob approaches him to help, Mr. Huff says angrily, "Leave me alone; I can do this. I'm OK, just leave me alone." What should Jacob do first? How might Jacob be able to help Mr. Huff maintain his independence and still be safe?

Amanda is assigned to care for Mrs. Webb, who recently had a stroke. When the stroke occurred, Mrs. Webb had been preparing dinner at the stove. As a result, when she fell, she also suffered severe burns on her arms. Now Mrs. Webb is receiving rehabilitation therapy for her left-sided weakness, in addition to recovering from the skin grafts used to treat the burns on her arms. Mrs. Webb is a widow and her children live out of state. She cries frequently because she says there is "no one to help her and she will probably end up staying in the nursing home for the rest of her life." Every time Amanda tries to get Mrs. Webb to participate in bathing and feeding herself, Mrs. Webb shakes her head and says she "just doesn't feel up to the effort today." Mrs. Webb's grafts are healing well and she is doing great in therapy. Is there anything Amanda can do to help Mrs. Webb not feel so helpless?

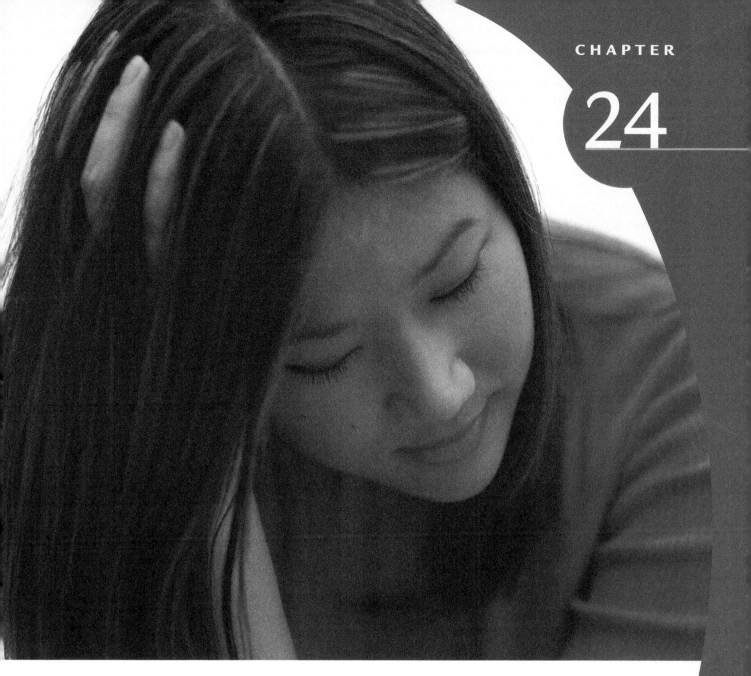

The Integumentary System

WHAT WILL YOU LEARN?

What is the largest organ in your body? Your skin! Just think—your body is covered in about 2 square metres of skin, and your skin alone weighs between 4 and 5 kilograms. You already know that a major function of this very large organ is to cover and protect your body. But did you also know that the skin gives us clues about what is going on inside a person's body? In this chapter, you will learn about the skin and the other organs that make up the integumentary system. You will learn about the importance of observing this organ system for changes

Photo: Your integumentary system includes your skin, hair, and nails.

that may indicate illness, and about actions you can take to help keep the skin (and its wearer!) healthy. When you are finished with this chapter, you will be able to:

1. List the layers of the skin.
2. Describe the accessory structures of the skin.
3. Discuss the major functions of the integumentary system.
4. Describe how normal aging processes affect the integumentary system.
5. Explain how pressure ulcers are formed and what conditions may increase a patient's or resident's risk of developing a pressure ulcer.
6. Describe how the personal support worker helps to prevent residents and patients from developing pressure ulcers.
7. Describe the different types of wounds that a patient or resident might have.
8. Discuss the personal support worker's duties regarding wound care.
9. Define terms used to describe skin lesions.

Vocabulary

Jaundice	Subcutaneous	Intentional wound	Macule
Pallor	tissue	Unintentional	Papule
Flushing	Sebum	wound	Vesicle
Cyanosis	Collagen	Lesion	Pustule
Epidermis	Bony prominences	Rash	Excoriation
Keratin	Necrosis	Dermatitis	Fissure
Melanin	Pressure points	Eczema	Ulcer
Dermis	Wound	Erythema	

The integumentary system gets its name from the Latin word *integumentum,* which means "a covering." The integumentary system is made up of the skin, which covers the body, and the structures that develop from it, called *accessory structures* or *appendages.* The accessory structures of the skin are the nails, the hair, the sebaceous glands (which secrete oils to keep the skin moist), and the sweat glands.

Of all the body's organ systems, the integumentary system is the most easily observed. Healthy skin is glowing and vibrant, and may range in colour from very light to very dark. A change in a person's normal skin colour can indicate a serious health problem and should be reported to the nurse immediately. For example:

- **Jaundice** is a yellow discolouration of the skin and the whites of the eyes. Jaundice is usually associated with liver disorders.
- **Pallor** is paleness, and **flushing** is redness. Some people appear pale or flushed most of the time. In these people, pallor or flushing would be considered "normal." However, if you notice pallor or flushing in a person who

is not normally pale or flushed, you should report this finding to the nurse.
- **Cyanosis** is a blue or grey discolouration of the skin, lips, and nail beds. Cyanosis develops when the skin does not receive enough oxygen. Cyanosis is a sign of a respiratory or circulatory disorder.

As you learned in Chapter 18, the condition of a person's hair and nails can also provide clues to the person's overall health. The hair should be shiny and soft, not brittle and dry, and the scalp should not be flaky or crusty. The nail beds of healthy nails are pink. The nails are flush with the nailbed and, when viewed from the side, the nails are slightly rounded.

TELL THE NURSE

The skin gives us many clues to a person's general health. Tell the nurse immediately if you observe any of the following:

- The person's skin looks abnormally pale or flushed, or has a bluish or yellowish hue

- The person has a new rash, or changes in an existing rash

- The person has a mole that has changed in appearance

STRUCTURE OF THE INTEGUMENTARY SYSTEM

SKIN

The skin is made up of two layers, the epidermis and the dermis (Fig. 24-1).

Epidermis

The **epidermis** is the outer layer of the skin. The epidermis is thickest on the soles of the feet and the palms of the hands, and very thin in areas such as the eyelids.

If you look at Figure 24-1, you will notice that the epidermis contains no blood vessels. You will also notice that it has two sublayers: a deep layer and a surface layer. New cells are produced in the deep layer of the epidermis. As the cells age, they work their way up, toward the surface of the body. As the maturing cells move toward the surface, they move farther away from the blood vessels, which are located in the dermis. This means that as the cells age, they move farther away from their supply of oxygen and nutrients. They also make **keratin,** a substance that causes them to thicken and become resistant to water. When the cells reach the surface of the body, they die and are shed. This process takes approximately 28 days—so, each month, you get a "new skin"!

In addition to continually producing new cells, the deep layer of the epidermis produces a substance called melanin. **Melanin,** from the Greek word *melas* ("black"), is a dark pigment that gives our skin, hair, and eyes colour. People with pale skin have less melanin than those with dark skin. Melanin helps to protect the skin from exposure to sunlight. In fact, continued exposure to sunlight causes the epidermis to produce more melanin, resulting in a tan. Sometimes melanin is deposited throughout the epidermis in an uneven pattern, resulting in freckles.

Dermis

The **dermis** is the deepest layer of the skin (see Fig. 24-1). The dermis consists of elastic connective tissue that allows it to stretch and move without damage. The dermis rests on a layer of fat called the **subcutaneous tissue.** Cutaneous is another word for "skin," and sub- means "below." Therefore, *subcutaneous* means "below the skin." The blood vessels and nerves that supply the skin start in the subcutaneous tissue and send branches into the dermis. Looking at Figure 24-1, you can see that the sensory receptors that allow us to feel pressure, pain, and temperature are located in the dermis. (The sense of touch will be discussed in more detail in Chapter 29.) The sebaceous glands, the sweat glands, and the hair follicles are also found in the dermis.

ACCESSORY STRUCTURES (APPENDAGES)

The skin's accessory structures include the sebaceous glands, the sweat glands, the hair, and the nails.

Sebaceous (Oil) Glands

The sebaceous glands secrete **sebum,** an oily substance that lubricates the skin and helps to prevent it from drying out. The sebum is also slightly acidic. This acidity helps to protect the skin from harmful bacteria that may be present on its surface. The sebaceous glands open into the hair follicles, and the sebum passes along the hair and onto the surface of the skin (see Fig. 24-1).

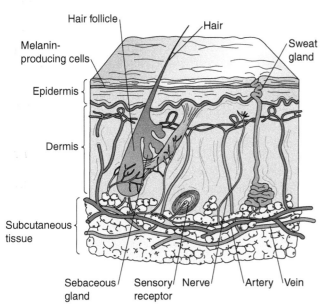

Figure 24-1
The skin has two layers, the dermis and epidermis. The skin rests on a layer of subcutaneous tissue.

Sweat Glands

There are two types of sweat glands: eccrine glands and apocrine glands. Eccrine glands are found in the skin that covers most parts of our bodies. Eccrine glands produce a thin, watery liquid that contains salt and small amounts of other bodily wastes. The purpose of the eccrine glands is to help cool the body through the process of evaporation. As the watery sweat leaves the surface of the skin, it takes heat with it, cooling the body down. Therefore, when you "work up a sweat," what you are experiencing is your eccrine glands at work! Another time you may have experienced your eccrine glands at work is when you have noticed your palms beginning to sweat as a result of being nervous. Many people sweat when they are nervous, and the palms of the hands contain a very large number of eccrine glands—hence, "sweaty palm syndrome."

The other type of sweat gland is the apocrine gland. Apocrine glands are found mostly in the skin of the armpits (axillae) and the perineum. The apocrine glands produce a thicker substance. When the bacteria that normally live on our skin mix with this substance, they produce what we know as "body odour." Apocrine glands become active when a person reaches puberty. As we age, the apocrine glands become less active.

Hair

Hair covers the entire body, except for the soles of the feet and the palms of the hands. Hair, especially that covering the scalp, helps to keep us warm. Most of the hair that covers the body is soft and fine, although in men, body hair tends to be thicker and more noticeable because of the action of certain hormones. In both men and women, the hair covering the scalp, armpits, and pubic area is thicker and coarser than the hair on the rest of the body.

Hair develops in the dermis of the skin from a sheath called a follicle (see Fig. 24-1). The part of the hair that we can see consists of dead cells that have been hardened by keratin. The living cells that produce new hair cells, causing the hair to grow, are found at the bottom of the follicle or hair root. Melanin gives the hair its colour. Blonde hair contains a small amount of melanin, while brunette hair contains much more.

Nails

Nails are made of special skin cells that have been hardened by the presence of keratin. Nail growth occurs from the nail root, the area where the nail emerges from the skin. Nails help to protect the ends of our fingers and toes.

FUNCTION OF THE INTEGUMENTARY SYSTEM

The integumentary system helps to maintain the body's homeostasis in three important ways. First, it offers a physical form of protection against microbes, chemicals, and other agents that could harm the body, if they gained access to the delicate organs inside. Second, the skin, which is water resistant, helps to maintain the body's fluid balance by preventing excessive loss or absorption of water. Finally, the integumentary system helps to regulate the temperature of the body, ensuring that the temperature stays within a tolerable range.

PROTECTION

As you learned in Chapter 7, the body's first line of defense against the invasion of harmful microbes is intact skin. The skin is a physical barrier that prevents microbes from entering the body. The skin also offers us some protection against harmful substances, such as chemicals, that may be encountered in the environment.

MAINTENANCE OF FLUID BALANCE

Imagine what would happen if your skin were not resistant to water! Every time it rained or you took a shower, you would soak up the water like a sponge. And every time you went out in the sun, you would run the risk of having all of your internal organs dry out. Needless to say, without your water-resistant skin, maintaining the proper fluid balance would be a constant struggle. Fortunately, the keratin-rich cells of the epidermis, combined with the oils secreted by the sebaceous glands, work very well to form a water-resistant protective barrier between your internal organs and the outside world.

REGULATION OF BODY TEMPERATURE

The skin plays an important role in regulating the body temperature. When a person gets warm—for example, after working outside in the sun—the blood vessels in the dermis of the skin dilate (widen), allowing more blood to flow close to the surface of the skin. As the blood passes just beneath the surface of the skin, the heat the blood contains radiates out from the body, lowering the temperature of the blood. The cooled blood then travels, carrying its coolness, back to the central areas of the body, thus lowering the body temperature. The production of sweat on the skin enhances this process by cooling the skin even more so that the blood cools more effectively. In essence, this process is the body's way of "opening the windows" to allow a cool breeze to circulate through the house (Fig. 24-2A).

The reverse is true when a person gets cold, for example, following exposure to cold air. The blood vessels in the skin constrict (become narrower), limiting the amount of blood that passes close to the surface of the skin. By keeping the blood in the warmer, central areas of the body, the amount of heat that is lost to the outside environment is kept to a minimum. You have seen how your skin becomes pale or bluish when you have been outside in the cold air. Your body is essentially "closing the windows" to stop the

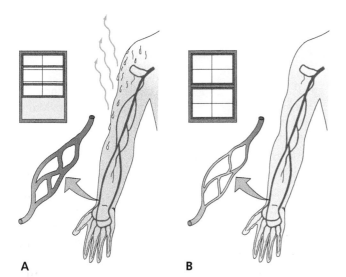

Figure 24-2
The skin plays an important role in maintaining the body's temperature within the proper range. **(A)** When the internal temperature is too high, the blood vessels in the skin dilate, causing more blood to pass near the surface of the skin and allowing heat to escape into the environment. Sweat evaporating from the surface of the skin also carries heat away from the body, contributing to the cooling process. **(B)** When the internal temperature is too low, the blood vessels in the skin constrict, causing less blood to pass near the surface of the skin and keeping the heat inside the body.

breeze from cooling the house too much (see Fig. 24-2B).

SENSATION

The skin contains millions of sensory receptors, special structures that allow us to detect pain, pressure, temperature, and touch. The sensory receptors and the role they play in sensation are discussed in detail in Chapter 29.

VITAMIN D PRODUCTION

As you remember from Chapter 19, vitamin D is a nutrient that helps our bodies absorb and use calcium, a mineral that keeps our bones healthy. The skin produces vitamin D when it is exposed to the sun. In fact, sun exposure is our main source of this important vitamin! Vitamin D is also obtained by eating foods such as milk and fish.

ELIMINATION AND ABSORPTION

The skin is an active organ that is capable of both removing substances from the body and taking substances into it. For example, sweat contains small amounts of waste materials, which leave the body when the sweat evaporates. The skin can also absorb some substances, such as chemicals. We use the ability of the skin to absorb chemicals when we give drugs using a "patch." An adhesive patch containing the drug is stuck to the skin, and the drug is slowly absorbed through the skin and into the blood vessels. You may be familiar with patches that prevent motion sickness, provide birth control, or help a person to stop smoking. In all of these cases, the medication on the patch is absorbed through the skin.

THE EFFECTS OF AGING ON THE INTEGUMENTARY SYSTEM

As we age, changes occur in all of our organ systems. These changes are not related to illness. Rather, they are normal changes that occur in everyone who reaches a certain age. These changes may just affect the person's appearance, or they may actually affect the way the person's body functions. Because there is a good chance that many of the people you will be caring for will be elderly, it is important for you to know about the changes that normally occur in each body system with aging. This knowledge will allow you to recognize age-related changes as normal. It will also allow you to provide better care for your elderly patients or residents, because you will be aware of their special needs.

CHANGES IN PHYSICAL APPEARANCE

Perhaps because the integumentary system is the most visible organ system, we have come to associate "getting old" with many of the physical changes that occur in the integumentary system as we age. Wrinkles, grey hair, and "age spots" are all very visible signs of aging (Fig. 24-3)! Wrinkles form due to the loss of **collagen,** a protein that supports connective tissue, such as that found in the dermis. In addition, the adipose (fatty) tissue in the subcutaneous layer that supports the dermis thins with age, making the subcutaneous layer less supportive of the dermis. As a result, the skin loses elasticity, leading to the formation of wrinkles. Melanin also is responsible for many of the changes typically associated with aging. Grey hair is caused by the loss of melanin from the hair. "Age spots" (sometimes called "liver spots") are caused by deposits of melanin in certain areas, such as the backs of the hands or the face. Whether or not a person's skin "shows his age" depends on many factors, such as heredity; the amount of time the person spends in the sun; the person's use of tobacco, drugs, or alcohol; and the person's overall state of health. Think about all of the people you know. Do any look much younger than their actual age, or much older? What factors do you think might be responsible for the person's remarkably youthful appearance, or unusually old appearance?

FRAGILE, DRY SKIN

There are many changes that occur to the integumentary system with aging that affect more than just our appearance. As collagen is lost from the dermis and the subcutaneous layer thins, the skin becomes thinner, more fragile, and more prone to injury (Fig. 24-4). Blood flow to the dermis decreases, and the cells of the epidermis do not replace themselves as rapidly. The decrease in blood flow to the skin means that when an

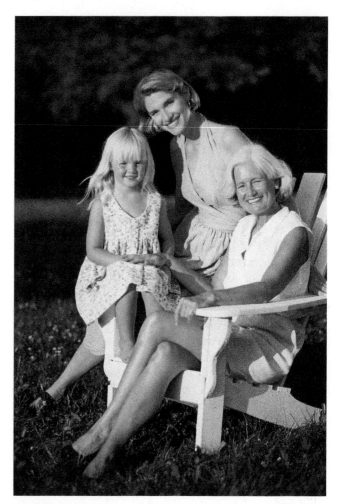

Figure 24-3
Wrinkles, grey hair, and "age spots" result from changes to the integumentary system that occur with aging. Many people view these normal signs of aging as signs of a life well lived! The woman on the right is pictured with her daughter (*middle*) and granddaughter (*left*). You can see how the skin changes in appearance over time.

injury occurs, the skin takes longer to heal itself, and the person is more at risk for developing an infection.

The number of sebaceous glands decreases, and as a result, so does the output of sebum. This leads to drying of the skin, which increases the risk for skin tears and injuries. In addition, with less sebum on the skin, the bacteria that normally live on the surface of our skin have more of a chance to cause trouble. (Recall that the acidity of sebum helps to keep these bacteria in check.)

When caring for an elderly person, keep the delicate nature of older skin in mind. Actions that would not cause harm in a younger person, such as gripping the person's arm to help her to

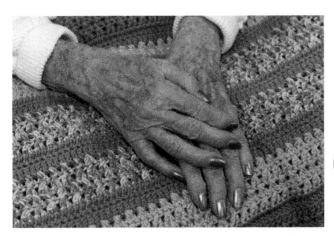

Figure 24-4
As skin ages, it becomes more delicate and prone
to injury.

stand or accidentally grazing her skin with your fingernails while helping her to put on her socks, can cause injury in an older person. It is very easy to tear an older person's skin, causing it to bleed. In addition, the skin of an older person is more sensitive to the drying effects of bathing than that of a younger person. In Chapter 17, you learned about some of the things that you can do to increase comfort and help to keep an older person's skin healthy, such as applying lotion after a bath to keep the skin soft and pliant.

THICKENING OF THE NAILS

As we age, our nails thicken and become yellow. This is especially true of the toenails. Because the nails are so tough, they are difficult to cut, and the person may be injured during the process. As you learned in Chapter 18, a nurse or a podiatrist is usually responsible for trimming an elderly person's toenails. The nurse or podiatrist may use a tool that looks like a sander to accomplish this task safely.

LESS EFFICIENT TEMPERATURE REGULATION

Changes to the integumentary system that occur with aging also affect the older person's ability to adjust to changes in the environmental temperature. The sweat glands decrease in number and the production of sweat decreases, making an older person more vulnerable to overheating. In addition, the decreased blood flow to the skin interferes with the skin's ability to participate

in temperature regulation. These changes must be considered when an older person is outside on a hot day, because they affect the ability of the body to cool itself and put the person at increased risk for heat-related problems, such as heat stroke.

DISORDERS OF THE INTEGUMENTARY SYSTEM

Many people in your care will have a disorder of the integumentary system. Sometimes, this disorder is the reason the person is in the health care facility. For example, this might be the case for a person who has suffered severe burns or trauma. Other times, the disorder develops after the person is already in the health care facility. For example, a person might develop a rash or a pressure ulcer, or have surgery that results in a surgical wound that must heal. As a personal support worker, you will play an important role in observing signs and symptoms of skin disorders, preventing the development of skin disorders, and helping people with skin disorders to heal.

PRESSURE ULCERS

Pressure ulcers, also known as *decubitus ulcers* or *bed sores,* form when a part of the body presses against a surface such as a mattress or chair for a long period of time. Lying on wrinkled bed linens or an object in the bed, sitting on a bedpan for a long period of time, or wearing a splint or brace that presses against the skin can also start the process of skin breakdown that leads to the formation of pressure ulcers.

Pressure ulcers are particularly likely to form over **bony prominences,** or parts of the body where there is very little fat between the bone and the skin. The weight of the person's body squeezes the soft tissue between the bony prominence and the surface the person is resting on, disrupting the flow of blood to the tissue. Lack of blood flow to the tissue deprives the tissue of oxygen and nutrients, causing it to die. Tissue death as a result of a lack of oxygen is called **necrosis.** The necrotic (dead) skin and underlying tissues peel off or break open, creating an open sore (Fig. 24-5). The sore is very painful and creates an opening for microbes to enter the body. Pressure ulcers may be very deep, extending all the way down to the bone. They are very difficult to heal once they have occurred.

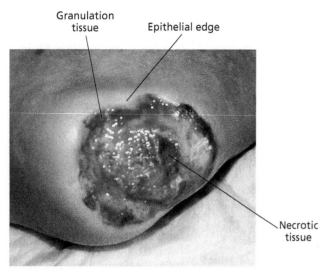

Granulation tissue   Epithelial edge

Necrotic tissue

Figure 24-5
Pressure ulcers are painful, difficult to treat, and potentially fatal. (Used with permission from Taylor, C., Lillis, C., LeMone, P., & Lynn, P. [2008]. *Fundamentals of nursing: The art and science of nursing care* [6th ed., p. 1023]. Philadelphia: Lippincott Williams & Wilkins.)

You will remember from Chapter 11 that many patients and residents are not able to change position easily, due to weakness, disability, or illness. This inability to change position without help places the person at high risk for developing a pressure ulcer. The most common sites for pressure ulcers to form are on the heels, ankles, knees, hips, toes, elbows, shoulder blades, ears, the back of the head, and along the spine (Fig. 24-6). These particular areas are referred to as **pressure points.**

The constant application of pressure on pressure points as a result of immobility is the basic cause of all pressure ulcers. Unfortunately, many people with limited mobility also have other risk factors for developing a pressure ulcer. The presence of any one of the following risk factors in a person with limited mobility makes it even more likely that the person will develop a pressure ulcer:

- **Advanced age.** As described earlier in this chapter, the normal aging process causes changes in a person's skin. The skin of an older person is fragile and thin, with less circulation. While a younger person may be able to tolerate staying in one position for 2 hours, an elderly person may need much more frequent position changes.
- **Poor nutrition and hydration.** For skin to remain healthy, good nutrition and proper hydration are essential. People who are not

receiving adequate nutrition or fluids because of illness, depression, or other conditions are more likely to develop pressure ulcers. Poor nutrition will also delay the healing of any pressure ulcers that have already formed.

- **Moisture.** Prolonged contact with water, urine, feces, or sweat causes the epidermis to soften and break down. Areas where skin touches skin (such as between the thighs, the folds of the abdomen, the armpits, and under the breasts) are places where sweat or bath water may become trapped on the skin, leading to skin breakdown. In addition to moisture, sweat, urine, and feces contain irritants such as salt, ammonia, and bacteria, which further contribute to the breakdown of the skin. Once skin breakdown begins, the door is wide open for a pressure ulcer to form.
- **Cardiovascular and respiratory problems.** A person with a heart or lung disorder often has problems getting adequate oxygen and nutrients to the tissues. In a person with a respiratory disorder, the blood that is delivered to the tissues may not contain enough oxygen. The heart of a person with a cardiovascular disorder may not be strong enough to deliver the blood to the tissues, even if it contains enough oxygen. Therefore, people with circulatory or respiratory problems are at even greater risk for developing pressure ulcers, because their tissues are already deprived of oxygen and nutrients.
- **Friction and shearing injuries.** In Chapter 11, you learned about how friction (rubbing) and shearing (pulling) forces can injure the skin and lead to skin breakdown. For example, shearing occurs when a person who is sitting up in bed slides down against the sheets. Shearing and friction injuries can also occur during repositioning.

Stages of Pressure Ulcers

Pressure ulcers develop in four stages (Fig. 24-7):

- **Stage 1.** Have you ever sat with your legs crossed for a long period of time? When you uncrossed your legs, the leg that had been on the bottom probably had a reddened area caused by the pressure of the leg that had been on top. There may even have been a slight "dent" in the skin. After a few minutes, the red area disappeared and the skin looked normal again. Every time you reposition a patient or resident, you should

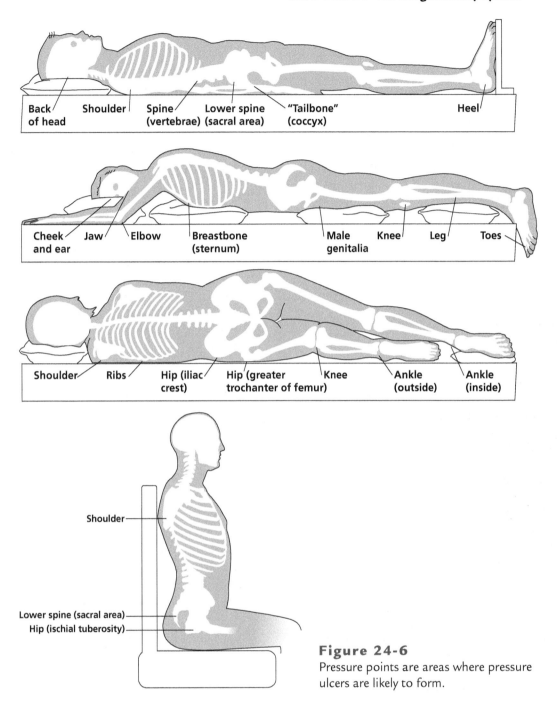

Figure 24-6
Pressure points are areas where pressure ulcers are likely to form.

look carefully for reddened areas. If the person's circulation is normal, the skin will return to its normal colour within a few minutes. If the skin stays red, feels hot to the touch, or is painful, you should report this finding to the nurse immediately. A reddened area that turns white means that blood flow has been compromised to the point that tissue damage has occurred. A stage 1 pressure ulcer is characterized by a

reddened area of skin that does not return to the normal colour after the pressure is removed. The reddened area may then become very pale or white and develop a shiny appearance.

- **Stage 2.** A stage 2 pressure ulcer looks like a blister, an abrasion, or a shallow crater. The epidermis peels away or cracks open, creating a portal of entry for microbes. The dermis may be partially worn away as well.

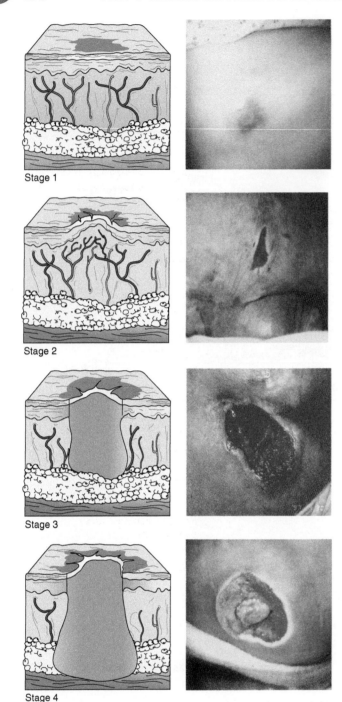

Stage 1

Stage 2

Stage 3

Stage 4

Figure 24-7
The four stages of pressure ulcer development.

- **Stage 3.** In a stage 3 pressure ulcer, the epidermis and dermis are gone, and the subcutaneous fat may be visible in the crater. There may be drainage from the wound.
- **Stage 4.** In a stage 4 pressure ulcer, the crater of damaged tissue extends all the way through the tissues to the muscle or bone.

The Personal Support Worker's Role in Preventing Pressure Ulcers

As you have already learned in previous chapters, the prevention of pressure ulcers is a major concern of the care team. Pressure ulcers are very painful and difficult to treat. Ultimately, they can cause a person to die. For these reasons, every effort must be made to prevent a pressure ulcer from forming in the first place. As a personal support worker, there are many things that you can do to help keep a person's skin healthy (Fig. 24-8).

- **Avoid allowing a person to remain in one position for a long period of time.** To prevent a pressure ulcer from forming, you must prevent any one part of a person's body from being under pressure for a long period of time. This means that you should not leave a person sitting on a bedpan for a long period of time, because the bedpan places a lot of pressure on the person's lower spine, one of the pressure points. It also means that a patient or resident who must stay in bed or in a wheelchair should be repositioned at least every 2 hours. A person who has additional risk factors for developing a pressure ulcer, as described earlier, may need to be repositioned even more often. The care plan will specify how often the person should be repositioned, and the sequence of positions.
- **Use your observation skills.** Look carefully at the skin of your patients or residents each and every time you provide care. After repositioning a person, move clothing and linens aside to check for reddened areas on the side of the body that had been bearing the person's weight. When assisting a person with bathing, changing wet or soiled linens, or giving a person a back massage, take that opportunity to look carefully at the person's skin.
- **Provide good skin care.** When assisting with a bath, clean skin gently and thoroughly and rinse off the soap well. Make sure the skin is dried well and use lotion to keep the skin's surface healthy and soft. Thoroughly clean and dry areas where skin touches skin, such as under the breasts or other skin folds, and apply a light dusting of a powder containing corn starch to help keep the skin dry. Provide frequent back massage to help stimulate circulation in the skin.

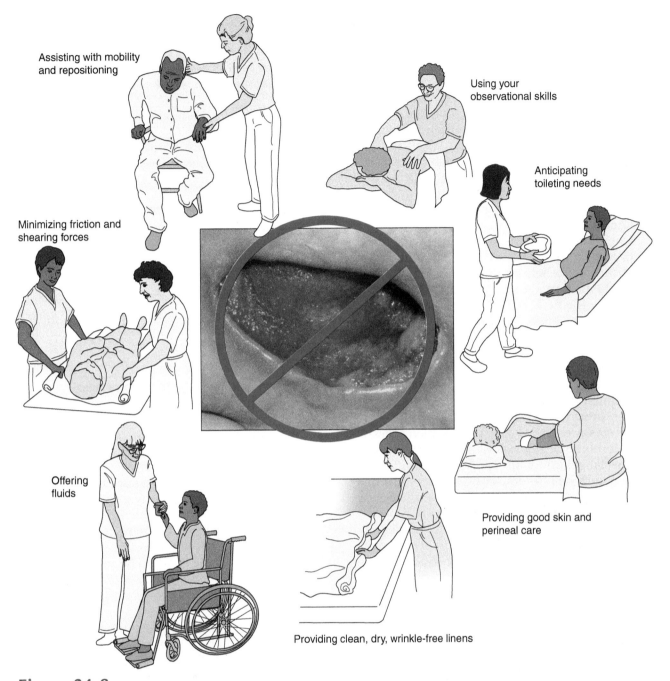

Assisting with mobility and repositioning

Using your observational skills

Anticipating toileting needs

Minimizing friction and shearing forces

Offering fluids

Providing clean, dry, wrinkle-free linens

Providing good skin and perineal care

Figure 24-8
There are many things you can do to help prevent a person from getting a pressure ulcer.
(*Photograph © Garry Watson/Photo Researchers, Inc.*)

- **Provide good perineal care.** Prompt removal of urine or feces from the skin is essential for the prevention of pressure ulcers. Good perineal care is especially important if a person is incontinent of urine or feces. Clean any urine or feces from the skin each time the person is incontinent. If the person is incontinent, the nurse may ask you to apply a product to the perineal area that helps to protect the skin from wet-

ness, such as Desitin ointment, after the perineal area has been cleaned and dried.
- **Anticipate toileting needs.** Assist your patients or residents to the bathroom (or provide a bedpan or urinal) frequently, to prevent soiling of the person's clothing or bed linens. If a person is incontinent, check on him or her every hour or so. This will allow you to detect and change wet, soiled linens promptly.

- **Encourage mobility.** Some patients or residents will sit in a chair or wheelchair all day long if you do not actively encourage them to get up and move around. Ask the patient or resident to take a walk with you every 2 hours, if she is able. The exercise helps to stimulate circulation and keeps the person from sitting in the same position for long periods of time. If a person is paralyzed, remind him to change positions in his chair or have him move between the chair and the bed to prevent skin breakdown.
- **Minimize skin injury caused by friction or shearing.** Use lift devices and lift sheets when moving and repositioning people to prevent injuries caused by friction and shearing. To help prevent shearing caused by the person sliding down in bed, do not elevate the head of the bed more than 30 degrees.
- **Encourage good nutrition and hydration.** Offer refreshing drinks frequently. Encourage your patients and residents to eat well. If a patient or resident is not eating, report this observation to the nurse.
- **Use pressure-reducing devices.** Many devices are available to help reduce pressure and minimize the risk of skin breakdown. Special gel and foam pads that fit on beds or in chairs help to distribute the person's body weight more evenly, preventing any one area from bearing most of the pressure. Elbow pads and booties may help prevent friction injuries caused by the skin rubbing against the sheets (Fig. 24-9).

TELL THE NURSE

When caring for a person who has a pressure ulcer or is at risk for developing a pressure ulcer, report the following observations immediately:

- The person has redness over a pressure point that does not go away within 5 minutes
- An area over a pressure point that was previously red has become pale, white, or shiny
- An area over a pressure point that was previously red is hot to the touch or painful
- A pressure ulcer has changed in size or depth

Special Equipment for Preventing Pressure Ulcers

Some patients or residents may need a special bed to help avoid problems associated with prolonged bed rest and immobility (Fig. 24-10). Several different types of specialty beds are available:

- An *airflow bed* supports the person on a fabric-covered layer of tiny ceramic beads (see Fig. 24-10A). The beads are kept constantly in movement by a current of air. The moving beads create a fluid-like effect, much like a waterbed but without the water, that helps to prevent pressure ulcers by relieving pressure on bony prominences. In addition, the circulating air keeps the person's skin dry. If the person soils the bed, some fluids will pass through the sheet and collect in the beads. The use of a bed

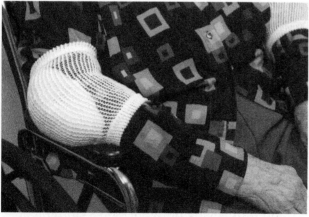

A

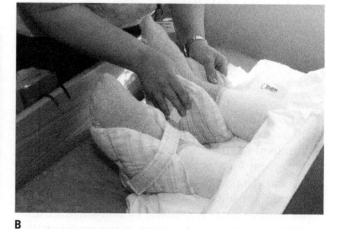

B

Figure 24-9
Pressure-reducing devices such as **(A)** elbow pads and **(B)** heel booties help to prevent the skin from rubbing against sheets and other surfaces.

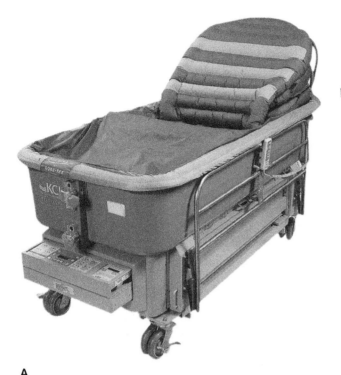

A

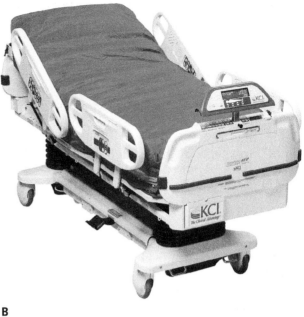

B

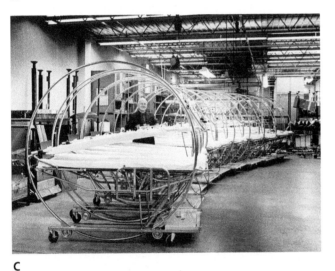

C

Figure 24-10

Specialty beds help to prevent problems related to prolonged bed rest and immobility. **(A)** The Fluidair Elite® airflow bed. **(B)** The TheraPulse®ATP™ alternating pressure bed. **(C)** A row of Circ-O-Lectric® beds. Pictured next to the row of Circ-O-Lectric® beds is Dr. Homer Stryker, the surgeon who designed the Circ-O-Lectric® bed. (*Photographs* **A** and **B** *courtesy of Kinetic Concepts Inc. [KCI], San Antonio, TX. Photograph* **C** *used with permission of Stryker Corporation.*)

protector helps to greatly reduce the amount of fluid that passes through the sheet into the beads. The beads are removed from the bed and decontaminated on a regular basis by a service technician. Airflow beds are particularly useful for critically ill patients with chronic watery diarrhea or weeping wounds.

- An *alternating pressure bed* supports the person on a series of compartments that fill with air and then deflate on a rotating basis (see Fig. 24-10B). The shifting areas of inflation shift the areas of pressure from place to place, helping to improve blood flow to the skin and underlying tissues and helping to

prevent pressure ulcers. These beds have protective covers, which can be wiped clean when soiled. The care of these beds is specific to type. If these beds are used in your facility, you will receive training in their care and use.

- A *Circ-O-Lectric®* bed (see Fig. 24-10C) helps to prevent pressure ulcers by making it easier to reposition people who may be difficult to reposition often, such as people with spinal injuries or severe burns. These beds allow a person to be turned from front to back without changing the alignment of his or her spine. A Circ-O-Lectric® bed is controlled electrically. Most facilities permit only nurses to operate these beds.

WOUNDS

A **wound** is an injury that results in a break in the skin (and usually the underlying tissues as well). Although this discussion focuses on wounds that occur as a result of surgery or trauma, pressure ulcers and burns (also discussed in this chapter) are technically considered "wounds" too.

Types of Wounds

An **intentional wound** is a wound that is the result of a planned surgical or medical intervention (Fig. 24-11). For example, a woman who has delivered a baby via cesarean section or a person who is recovering from open-heart surgery will have intentional wounds caused by their surgeries. Intentional wounds also occur when intravenous (IV) lines, percutaneous endoscopic gastrostomy (PEG) tubes, or other medical devices are inserted into the body through a "man-made" opening. Intentional wounds are usually created under controlled conditions. Precautions are taken to minimize the risk of

infection. The edges of the wound are usually clean and even, and held together with stitches (sutures) or staples.

An **unintentional wound** is an unexpected injury that usually results from some type of trauma. Falls, car accidents, and gun and knife violence can result in unintentional wounds (Fig. 24-12). Unintentional wounds can be *open*, which means that the surface of the skin is broken. The risk of infection is high with open wounds, because the open skin creates a portal of entry for microbes. In addition, the uneven wound edges and amount of tissue damage may make closing the wound difficult. A *closed* wound is one where the skin is not broken, but there is

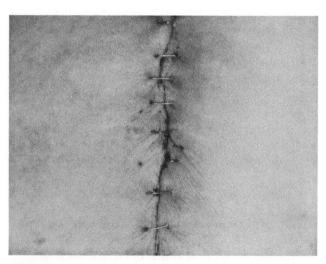

Figure 24-11
A surgical incision is an example of an intentional wound. Intentional wounds are usually created under controlled conditions, minimizing the risk of infection. The edges of the wound are usually brought together and secured with stitches or staples (shown here) to promote healing and minimize scarring. (Used with permission from Craven, R. F. [2007]. *Fundamentals of nursing: Human health and function* [5th ed., p. 1032]. Philadelphia: Lippincott Williams & Wilkins.)

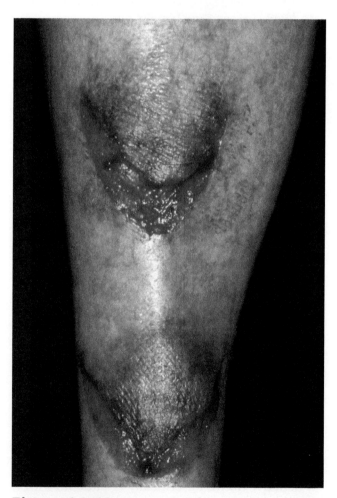

Figure 24-12
Cuts on the leg of an 80-year-old woman, who fell down the stairs. These cuts are open unintentional wounds. Open unintentional wounds carry a high risk of infection because they are often contaminated with dirt and microbes. The edges of the wound are often jagged, making it difficult to close the wound neatly. (© *Dr. P. Marazzi/Photo Researchers, Inc.*)

damage to the underlying tissues. The deep tissue damage associated with a closed wound can be considerable, even though the only signs of injury may be redness, swelling, or bruising of the overlying skin.

Wound Healing

The human body is quite efficient at healing wounds, especially when it is otherwise healthy. Having multiple, severe injuries; a chronic illness; or an impaired immune system can limit a person's ability to heal on his own. A person who is very young or very old may heal more slowly, or have a limited ability to heal. The same is true of a person who is malnourished.

For a wound to heal properly, there must be adequate blood flow to the injured area. This blood flow is responsible for the inflammation that is usually seen around an injury. Inflammation is characterized by redness, swelling, heat, and pain. It is a sign that the body is working to heal itself. Healing tissues also need good hydration and nutrition. Recall from Chapter 19 that adequate protein intake is especially important when the body is trying to rebuild injured tissues.

In the health care setting, we do many things to help support the wound healing process. Some of the measures taken by the health care team to support the wound healing process include closing the wound, inserting drains, and applying dressings. As a personal support worker, your duties related to wound care will vary, depending on your employer and the province or territory where you work. Usually, personal support workers are asked to assist the nurse with wound care. However, some facilities may train you to perform specific duties related to wound care on your own. As always, if you are asked to perform a task that is new to you, make sure that the task is covered by your job description and that you have received the training you will need to perform the skill properly. No matter where you work, the most important role you will play with regard to wound care is that of "observer." As a personal support worker, you will have the best opportunity to notice and report signs that might indicate that a wound is not healing properly or has become infected.

Wound closure

The wound must be closed so that the body's protective covering is once again intact. If a wound is kept clean but otherwise left alone, eventually the tissue will repair itself and the wound will close on its own. However, this can take a long time, it increases the risk of infection, and it often results in a scar. To speed this process up, minimize the risk of infection, and reduce the amount of scarring, the doctor may decide to close the wound using sutures or staples. The timing for, and approach to, wound closure varies depending on the situation:

- **First-intention wound healing.** In *first-intention wound healing,* open wounds are closed surgically with sutures or staples. Pulling the edges of the skin and underlying tissues together and holding them closed help speed up the healing process and minimize scarring.
- **Second-intention wound healing.** Wounds that are infected or are contaminated with dirt may be cleaned and rinsed and left open to heal from the inside out. This is called *second-intention wound healing.* Second-intention wound healing results in a wider, more noticeable scar after the wound has healed, but it prevents an unresolved infection from delaying the wound healing process.
- **Third-intention wound healing.** Sometimes it is necessary to leave a wound open, especially a traumatic wound, for a period of time to make sure that an infection is not going to occur. Then the wound edges are cleaned and closed with sutures or staples to speed the healing process. This is called *third-intention wound healing.*

Wound drains

As part of the healing process, some wounds will produce a lot of fluid, or drainage. A wound that is infected or bleeding will also often produce a lot of drainage. Fluid that is allowed to collect in a wound can promote infection, delaying the healing process. Therefore, wound drains are often used to allow blood and other fluids to flow out of the wound (Fig. 24-13).

Some drains allow fluid to collect in the wound dressing (the bandage covering the wound). Others are connected to a collection device. If a person you are caring for has a drain, take note of the characteristics of the drainage every time you check the dressing or the collection device. Is there more drainage than you expected? Does it have a foul odour that it did not have before? Has the appearance of the drainage changed? Report any unusual observations to the nurse.

When repositioning a person with a drain, take care not to pull on the drain tubing. Pulling on the drain tubing could pull the drain out of

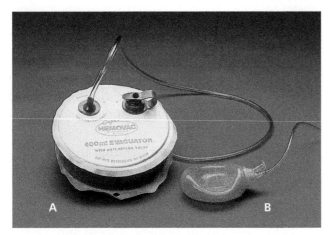

Figure 24-13
When drainage from a wound is significant, a drain may be placed. The drainage tube is placed in the wound and attached to a suction device, which draws the fluid out of the wound. Many types of drains are available. **(A)** A Hemovac drain. **(B)** A Jackson-Pratt or "grenade" drain. (Used with permission from Craven, R. F. [2009]. *Fundamentals of nursing: Human health and function* [6th ed., p. 1013]. Philadelphia: Lippincott Williams & Wilkins.)

the wound. The loss of the drain will allow fluid to collect in the wound until the doctor can replace the drain. Fluid in the wound puts the person at risk for infection.

Wound dressings

Sometimes dressings are applied to wounds to prevent microbes from gaining access to the body, to keep the wound dry during procedures such as bathing, or to absorb drainage from the wound. The type of dressing used depends on several factors, including:

- The type of wound
- The location of the wound
- The amount of drainage associated with the wound
- Whether or not the wound is infected
- Whether or not the wound must be kept dry
- How often the dressing must be changed

The doctor or the nurse determines which type of dressing is used.

Some dressings are made of a clear, plastic material (Fig. 24-14A). These dressings keep the wound clean and free from microbes and moisture, while allowing air to circulate freely. Some dressings are simply pieces of gauze held in place with tape (see Fig. 24-14B). Wounds that drain will have thick, absorbent dressings.

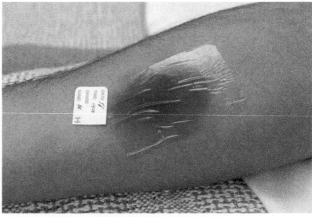

A

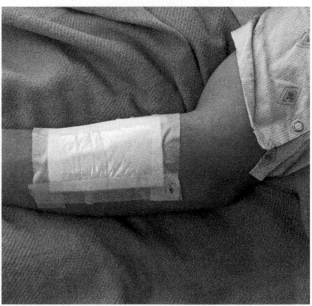

B

Figure 24-14
Various types of wound dressings and tapes are available. **(A)** Here, a wound is covered with a clear dressing that keeps moisture and microbes out of the wound, but allows air to reach the wound to promote healing. This type of dressing does not absorb drainage, but it does allow members of the health care team to look at the wound without removing the dressing. **(B)** This dressing is not waterproof, so it will need to be changed if it gets wet. The gauze prevents microbes from entering the wound, and it also absorbs drainage.

Many dressings are secured with tape. The type of tape used depends on the location of the wound and the needs of the person. For example, adhesive tape may irritate a person's skin, so a plastic or paper tape would be used instead.

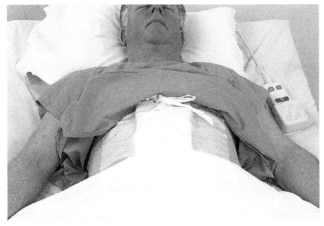

Figure 24-15
Montgomery ties can be used to secure a dressing that needs to be changed often. The adhesive is applied and then left in place. The ties secure the dressing and can be easily untied when a new dressing is needed. (© B. Proud.)

Elastic tape is stretchy and may be used when the wound is on a part of the body that must bend, such as the knee or elbow.

When a wound is draining heavily and the dressing must be changed often, a Montgomery tie may be used instead of tape. A Montgomery tie consists of a strip of adhesive that is attached to a cloth tie. The dressing is placed on the wound. Then, the adhesive strip of the Montgomery tie is applied to the person's skin alongside the dressing. Another Montgomery tie is placed in the same way on the other side of the dressing. Then the ties are tied together over the dressing, to hold it in place (Fig. 24-15). When it is time to change the dressing, the ties are untied, the dressing is replaced, and then the ties are retied. Because there is no need to remove the adhesive tape to change the dressing, Montgomery ties help to protect the person's skin from damage caused by the frequent removal and reapplication of tape.

You may be asked to assist the nurse with dressing changes. Procedure 24-1 explains how to help the nurse with a dressing change. Helping the nurse with a dressing change accomplishes two things. First, it minimizes the chance that the nurse's hands or other surfaces will become contaminated by the drainage on the soiled dressing. Second, it helps to ensure that the new dressing remains free of microbes that could contaminate the wound.

TELL THE NURSE

When caring for a person who has a wound, report the following observations immediately:

● The person complains of increased pain or discomfort

● There is increased redness, swelling, or warmth around the wound

● The person has a fever

● Drainage from the wound has changed in amount or appearance, or has developed a foul odour

● The dressing is excessively wet or soiled

● The drain tubing has pulled out or has become disconnected

BURNS

Burns are injuries to the skin and underlying tissues caused by contact with extreme heat (thermal burns), chemicals (chemical burns), or electricity (electrical burns). Burns can be minor, causing only slight redness and pain, or they can be very severe, extending down through the layers of the skin and possibly even involving the muscles and bones. Burns are classified according to the depth of the damage:

• *First-degree burns* cause injury to the outermost layer of the skin, the epidermis. Most sunburns are first-degree burns. Minor household accidents, such as touching a hot stove or leaving a heating pad that is too warm in place for too long, can also result in first-degree burns. The redness and pain usually goes away after a few days.

• *Second-degree burns* penetrate into the dermis of the skin. Second-degree burns are often associated with blisters. These burns are very painful and the loss of the epidermis increases the risk of infection.

• *Third-degree burns* involve the epidermis and dermis, the subcutaneous layer, and often the underlying muscles and bones as well (Fig. 24-16). People with third-degree burns need surgery and skin grafts to heal. Third-degree burns are associated with very high infection rates because the skin has been destroyed. In addition, the scarring that results from severe burns can cause severe disfigurement and contractures of the extremities.

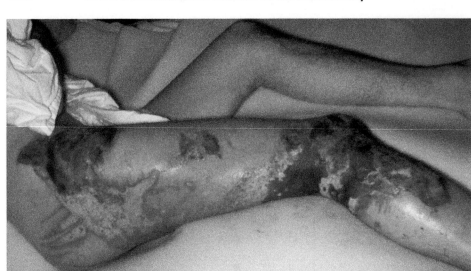

Figure 24-16
People with severe burns, such as the third-degree burns shown here, require special care to promote healing and prevent complications such as infection. (© *John Radcliffe Hospital/Photo Researchers, Inc.*)

People with second- and third-degree burns often require months or even years of rehabilitation, and they must have multiple surgical procedures. These people need very special care. Because of the risk of infection, they may be placed in reverse (protective) isolation. Caregivers must often wear sterile gloves and gowns when providing care, and bed linens may need to be sterilized before the bed is made, to reduce the chance of infection.

LESIONS

Lesion is a general term used to describe any break in the skin. Often you will see the term *lesion* used when discussing rashes or other skin disorders. Lesions often occur in groups, forming a **rash.** Rashes can be *localized* (limited to one area) or *systemic* (occurring all over the body).

Rashes are often caused by an infection, such as chickenpox or the measles. In this case, the skin itself is not infected, but it is showing signs of an infection inside of the body. Rashes may also be caused by contact with an irritant, such as poison ivy. In people with sensitive skin, contact with substances like bath soap or laundry detergent can cause a rash called *contact dermatitis.* **Dermatitis** is a general term for inflammation of the skin. **Eczema** is a type of chronic dermatitis that is usually accompanied by severe itching, scaling, and crusting of the surface of the skin.

Itching, burning, or redness of the skin accompanies many skin lesions. The redness of the skin that often accompanies these lesions is known as **erythema.** Dermatologists (doctors who specialize in knowledge of the skin) look at the characteristics of the lesions on the skin, as well as the location of the lesions and the person's other signs and symptoms, to find clues to their cause. There are many different types of skin lesions (Table 24-1):

- A **macule** is a small, flat, reddened lesion. Macules form the rash that is seen in measles.
- A **papule** is a small, raised, firm lesion. Papules can be easily felt by passing your fingers lightly over the affected area.
- A **vesicle** is a small, blister-like lesion that contains watery, clear fluid. Vesicles form the rash that is seen in chickenpox.
- A **pustule** is a vesicle that contains pus, a thick, yellowish fluid that is a sign of infection. Pustules are seen in acne.
- An **excoriation** is an abrasion, or a scraping away of the surface of the skin. Excoriations can be caused by trauma, chemicals, or burns (including friction burns from sliding a person's skin across a sheet). Urine or

Table 24-1 Types of Skin Lesions

LESION	DESCRIPTION
 Macule (© Custom Medical Stock Photo)	Small, flat, red lesions
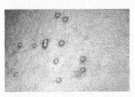 Papule (© Custom Medical Stock Photo)	Small, raised, firm bumps
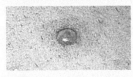 Vesicle	Small, fluid-filled, blister-like lesions
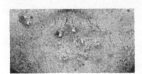 Pustule	Small, pus-filled, blister-like lesions
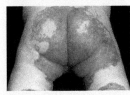 Excoriation (© Custom Medical Stock Photo)	Abrasion (wearing away of the surface of the skin)
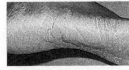 Fissure	A crack in the skin
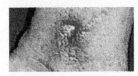 Ulcer	A crater-like open sore

feces, if left on the skin for too long, can cause a chemical excoriation.

- A **fissure** is a crack in the skin. Fissures can be caused by extreme dryness. Fungal infections, such as tinea pedis (athlete's foot), can also cause fissures.
- An **ulcer** is a shallow crater that is formed when the tissue dies. The dead tissue is shed, leaving a crater behind. Venous stasis ulcers, a common type of ulcer, develop as a result of poor blood flow through the veins in the legs.

Because skin lesions disrupt the skin's protective barrier, they place the person at increased risk for infection. Secondary bacterial infection of the skin is especially common when the lesion is itchy and the person scratches it excessively. *Secondary* means that the infection is occurring on top of the original problem. This is similar to what happens when you have a mosquito bite that you cannot stop scratching—eventually, you scratch it raw, it gets infected, and suddenly it takes much longer for the bite to heal than it would have if you had just left it alone.

When you are caring for a person with skin lesions, there are several things that you can do to increase the person's comfort and promote healing of the skin:

- Make sure that you are aware of any adjustments to the normal bathing and skin care routine that may be necessary. For example, you may need to use a special soap or lotion as part of the person's skin care. The nurse will be able to tell you about any necessary changes to the routine, or you can check the care plan.
- Help the person to choose clothing that does not rub or irritate the skin lesion.
- Discourage the person from scratching itchy or irritated skin. Although scratching may bring temporary relief, it causes additional skin injury and puts the person at risk for infection. Soft mitt restraints or gloves may be necessary to prevent a small child or confused adult from scratching the lesions.
- Observe the lesions for changes in colour, or for bleeding or drainage. Report any changes to the nurse immediately. Also note whether the lesions seem to be getting larger, or spreading to other parts of the body.

SUMMARY

- The integumentary system consists of the skin and its accessory structures (hair, nails, sweat glands, and sebaceous glands).
- As the body's most visible organ system, the integumentary system can provide clues to a person's overall health. Changes in a person's skin tone or the development of a rash may signal an internal problem, such as liver disease, a heart or lung problem, or an infection.
- The integumentary system has three major functions that help maintain the body's homeostasis.
  - The skin protects us from microbes, chemicals, and other agents that could harm the body.
  - The skin helps us to maintain our internal fluid balance.
  - The integumentary system plays a major role in temperature regulation. Narrowing and widening of the blood vessels in the skin helps our bodies to maintain or release heat, respectively. The sweat glands help to cool our bodies through evaporation. Hair on our scalps and bodies helps to keep us warm.
- Like all organ systems, the integumentary system changes as we age.
  - Changes that affect our appearance include wrinkles, grey hair, and age spots.
  - The skin becomes more fragile and more prone to injury with age. The number and output of the sebaceous glands decrease, making the skin dry. Circulation to the skin decreases.
  - The number and output of the sweat glands decrease. This change, along with the changes in the skin, makes it harder for the older person to adjust to changes in the environmental temperature.
  - The nails become tough and yellow, making them difficult to trim.
- Pressure ulcers are a major concern in the health care setting.
  - Pressure ulcers develop when soft tissues are squeezed between bone and a surface, such as a mattress or chair. The weight of the body disrupts the flow of oxygen-rich blood to the tissues, causing the tissues to die and leading to the formation of a pressure ulcer.
  - Immobility is the underlying cause of all pressure ulcers. Several factors, including old age, poor nutrition, and moisture trapped in the folds of the skin, can increase an immobile person's risk of developing a pressure ulcer.
- Warning signs of pressure ulcers include:
  - A reddened area that does not return to its normal colour after the pressure is relieved
  - A previously reddened area that is hot to the touch or painful
  - An area that is pale, white, or shiny
- Prevention of pressure ulcers is very important, because pressure ulcers are extremely painful, difficult to treat, and potentially fatal. The personal support worker does many things to prevent patients and residents from developing pressure ulcers, including repositioning, observing, providing good skin and perineal care, changing wet and soiled linens promptly, and encouraging exercise.
- A wound is a break in the skin. The underlying tissues are usually affected as well.
  - A wound can be intentional or unintentional.
  - A break in the skin puts the person at risk for infection. Therefore, the health care team does many things to help wounds to heal quickly and with minimal complications. Sutures, dressings, and drains are commonly used to help wounds heal.
  - Personal support workers are in an excellent position to notice and report signs and symptoms that suggest that the wound has become infected or is not healing well, such as a foul-smelling discharge or excessive drainage or bleeding.
- Burns are injuries caused by heat, chemicals, or electricity. People with burn wounds require special care because of the very high risk of infection.
- Lesions are breaks in the skin.
  - Many different types of skin lesions can form rashes.
    - The type of lesion is often a clue to the cause of the rash.
    - Rashes can be localized (limited to one area) or systemic (occurring all over the body).
  - Skin lesions can be caused by infections inside the body, infections of the skin itself, or irritation of the skin.
  - Personal support workers are often the first to notice an unusual lesion on a patient or resident.

PROCEDURE 24-1

Assisting the Nurse With a Dressing Change

WHY YOU DO IT   Helping the nurse with a dressing change minimizes the chance that the nurse's hands or other surfaces will become contaminated by the drainage on the soiled dressing. It also helps to ensure that the new dressing remains free of pathogens that could contaminate the wound.

Getting Ready WGKIEpS

1. Complete the "Getting Ready" steps.

Supplies

- gloves
- gown (if necessary)
- mask (if necessary)
- paper towels or a bed protector
- plastic bag
- tape or Montgomery ties
- dressing
- scissors

Procedure

2. Cover the over-bed table with paper towels or the bed protector. Place the dressing supplies on the over-bed table. Fold the top edges of the plastic bag down to make a cuff. Place the cuffed bag on the over-bed table.

3. Make sure that the bed is positioned at a comfortable working height (to promote good body mechanics) and that the wheels are locked. If the side rails are in use, lower the side rail on the working side of the bed. The side rail on the opposite side of the bed should remain up.

4. Help the person to a comfortable position that allows access to the wound.

5. Fanfold the top linens to the foot of the bed. Adjust the person's hospital gown or pajamas as necessary to expose the wound.

6. Put on the mask, gown, or both, if necessary. Put on the gloves.

7. The nurse will remove the old dressing. The nurse may ask you to take the old dressing and place it in the cuffed plastic bag. Be careful to keep the soiled side of the dressing out of the person's sight. Do not let the dressing touch the outside of the plastic bag.

8. Remove your gloves and dispose of them in a facility-approved waste container.

9. Wait while the nurse inspects the wound and measures it, if necessary.

10. Put on a clean pair of gloves.

11. Assist as the nurse applies a new dressing.

   a. Open the wrapper containing the dressing and hold it open so that the nurse can remove the dressing. Do not touch the dressing. Dispose of the wrapper in a facility-approved waste container.

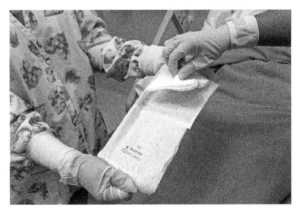

Step 11a Hold the wrapper open so that the nurse can remove the dressing.

   b. If the dressing will be secured with tape, cut four pieces of tape for securing the dressing. For a 4 × 4 dressing, each piece of tape should measure 20 centimetres long. Hang the tape from the edge of the over-bed table.

   c. If the nurse asks you to, use the tape strips to secure the dressing by placing one piece of tape along each side of

(continued)

the dressing. Center each piece of tape equally over the dressing and the person's skin.

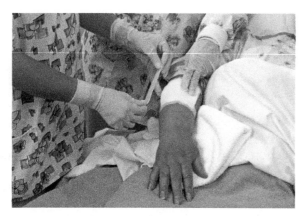

Step 11c The dressing is secured by placing one piece of tape along each side.

12. Remove your gloves (and gown and mask, if using) and dispose of them in a facility-approved waste container. Wash your hands.

13. Re-cover the wound with the hospital gown or pajamas. Help the person back into a comfortable position, straighten the bottom linens, and draw the top linens over the person.

14. Make sure that the bed is lowered to its lowest position and that the wheels are locked. If the side rails are in use, return the side rail to the raised position on the working side of the bed.

15. Dispose of disposable items in a facility-approved waste container. Clean equipment and return it to the storage area.

Finishing Up   CLSOWR

16. Complete the "Finishing Up" steps.

WHAT DID YOU LEARN?

Multiple Choice

Select the single best answer for each of the following questions.

1. Where are pressure ulcers most likely to form?
   a. On the heels, ankles, and toes
   b. On the elbows and shoulder blades
   c. On the spine
   d. All of the above

2. Why is it important to prevent pressure ulcers from forming?
   a. Pressure ulcers are disgusting to see
   b. People who have pressure ulcers require more care than people who do not, and this is expensive for the facility
   c. Pressure ulcers are difficult to treat and can lead to a person's death
   d. Pressure ulcers interfere with the skin's ability to make vitamin D

3. What is the underlying cause of all pressure ulcers?
   a. Continuous pressure applied to one area
   b. Poor nutrition
   c. Incontinence
   d. All of the above

4. Which of the following factors can increase a person's risk of getting a pressure ulcer?
   a. Advanced age
   b. Incontinence
   c. Poor nutrition
   d. All of the above

5. Mr. Underwood has developed a white, shiny area on his left hip about the size of a quarter. Yesterday, this same area was red and hot to the touch. If you were Mr. Underwood's personal support worker, what would be your biggest concern?
   a. That Mr. Underwood has the chickenpox
   b. That Mr. Underwood has a stage 1 pressure ulcer
   c. That Mr. Underwood's wound is not healing properly
   d. That Mr. Underwood has jaundice

6. You are caring for Mrs. Kling, a 93-year-old grandmother who has limited mobility following a stroke. What should you do to minimize Mrs. Kling's chances of developing a pressure ulcer?
   a. Dry Mrs. Kling's skin thoroughly after each bath
   b. Reposition Mrs. Kling regularly, according to the care plan
   c. Encourage Mrs. Kling to eat well
   d. All of the above

7. Which one of the following is an example of an intentional wound?
   a. A gunshot wound
   b. A surgical incision
   c. A lesion
   d. A burn

8. Why is it important to keep the skin healthy?
   a. The skin protects the body from microbes and helps to maintain the body's fluid balance
   b. The skin protects the body from sunburn
   c. It is easier to detect signs of disease in a person with healthy skin
   d. Keeping the skin healthy helps to prevent wrinkles in old age

Matching

Match each numbered item with its appropriate lettered description.

_____ 1. Macules

_____ 2. Melanin

_____ 3. Dermatitis

_____ 4. Vesicles

_____ 5. Erythema

_____ 6. Papules

_____ 7. Pustules

_____ 8. Excoriation

_____ 9. Fissure

_____10. Age spot

a. Redness of the skin that often accompanies rashes

b. Often seen on the backs of the hands; caused by melanin deposits

c. Cracks in the skin, such as those seen in athlete's foot

d. Abrasion or wearing away of the top layer of skin; caused by trauma, chemicals, or burns

e. Filled with pus, a thick yellow fluid associated with infection

f. Blister-like lesions that contain watery fluid, such as those seen in chickenpox

g. Flat, reddened lesions, such as those seen in measles

h. Firm, raised bumps

i. General term for inflammation of the skin

j. Gives the skin its colour

STOP and Think!

You have been assigned to help Mrs. Sills with her morning care. While you are helping Mrs. Sills to put on her socks, you accidentally scratch Mrs. Sills' ankle, causing her to bleed. What should you do? What are some steps you can take to avoid scratching a person's skin when you are providing care?

Richard is providing care to Mr. O'Meara, who has just been transferred to Willow Wood Care Center. Mr. O'Meara is confined to a wheelchair. While giving Mr. O'Meara a back massage as part of evening care, Richard notices a reddened area at the base of Mr. O'Meara's spine. What are the possible explanations for this finding? What should Richard do?

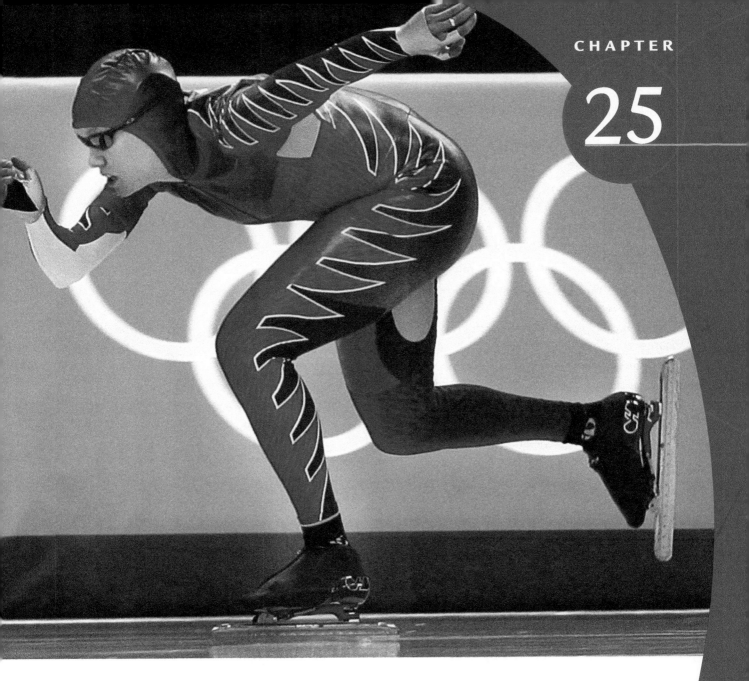

The Musculoskeletal System

WHAT WILL YOU LEARN?

Think about everything you have done so far today. Before you even left the house this morning, you did a number of different tasks requiring the services of your musculoskeletal system—getting out of bed, brushing your teeth, eating breakfast, and taking the dog for a walk or feeding the cat, just to name a few. Think about all of the individual movements that each of these small tasks requires, and you will get a sense of how very important the musculoskeletal system is to our daily functioning.

Photo: Cindy Klassen, from Winnipeg, Canada, powers around the oval in the ladies' 3000-metre speed skating competition to win an Olympic bronze medal at the Turin Winter Games. (AP Photo/Paul Chiasson, CP.)

The muscular system and the skeletal system work together to enable us to move. As you learned in Chapter 23, sometimes these two organ systems are referred to together as the *musculoskeletal system* because they work so closely together. In this chapter, you will learn about the structure and function of the musculoskeletal system, and about how it is affected by aging and illness. You will also learn about how personal support workers help residents and patients to maintain proper function of the musculoskeletal system. When you are finished with this chapter, you will be able to:

1. List the major parts of the musculoskeletal system.
2. List and describe the four types of bones found in the skeletal system.
3. Define terms used to describe joint movement.
4. List and describe the three types of muscles found in the muscular system.
5. Discuss the main functions of the musculoskeletal system.
6. Describe how normal aging processes affect the musculoskeletal system.
7. Describe some of the disorders that can affect the musculoskeletal system.
8. Define normal range of motion and describe methods used to maintain joint function in the health care setting.
9. Demonstrate how to help a person to perform range-of-motion exercises.
10. Discuss the use of heat and cold applications to promote a person's comfort.
11. Demonstrate how to safely use heat and cold applications in the health care setting.
12. Discuss rehabilitation measures that are commonly used in the health care setting that are specific to the musculoskeletal system.

Vocabulary

Skeleton	Tendons	Muscular dystrophy	Trapeze bar
Joints	Muscle tone	Fracture	Amputation
Range of motion	Atrophy	Reduction	Stump
Cartilage	Osteoporosis	Fixation	Phantom pain
Ligaments	Arthritis	Traction	

STRUCTURE OF THE MUSCULOSKELETAL SYSTEM

The musculoskeletal system consists of the skeletal system and the muscular system.

THE SKELETAL SYSTEM

The skeletal system consists of the bones. The 206 bones in the human body form a framework called the **skeleton** (Fig. 25-1). The skeleton gives structure and shape to the body, and protects key vital organs, such as the heart and the brain, from injury.

The bones of the skeleton vary in size and shape. Bones are classified according to their shape (Fig. 25-2):

- **Long bones.** When we think of a "bone," what we often picture is an example of a long bone. The long bones are found in the arms and the legs. Long bones consist of a shaft and two rounded ends.
- **Short bones.** Short bones are round or cube-shaped. Short bones are found in the wrists and ankles.
- **Flat bones** are relatively thin and may be curved. Examples of flat bones include the ribs and the bones that form the skull.
- **Irregular bones** are oddly shaped bones that are not flat. Irregular bones are found in the spinal column and face.

Bones must be strong enough to support and protect the body, yet light enough to allow us to move. Can you imagine how heavy a large bone like the bone in your thigh would be, if it were solid? Instead, bones have two layers. The

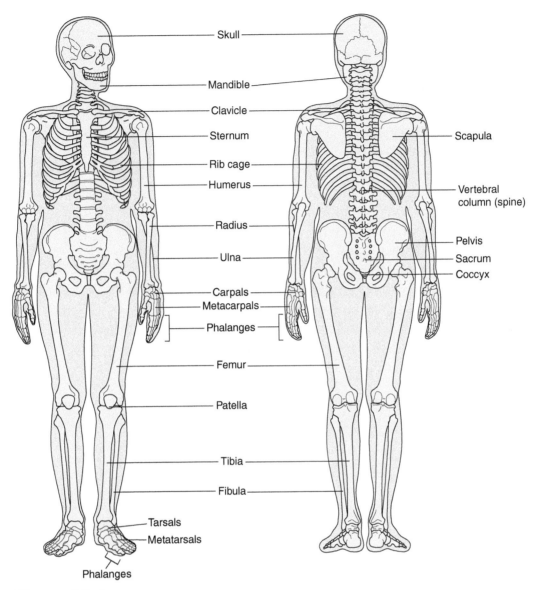

Figure 25-1
The human skeleton contains 206 bones. Some of the major bones are labelled here.

outside of the bone is hard and solid. The inside of the bone is sponge-like and airy. Thin strands of bone form a net-like structure, and the spaces in between the thin strands of bone are filled with bone marrow (Fig. 25-3). This combination of a solid, hard outside and a sponge-like inside results in bones that are very strong and able to resist a great amount of force, yet light-weight. The cells that form the bones are con-stantly broken down and replaced with new bone cells throughout a person's lifetime. A complex network of blood vessels supplies the bone cells with the oxygen and nutrients they need.

The areas where two bones join together are called **joints.** Joints allow us to move. The **range of motion** of a joint is the complete extent of

movement that the joint is normally capable of without causing pain. Joints can be classified according to the amount of movement they allow (Fig. 25-4):

- **Fixed joints** do not permit any movement at all. The joints between the bones of the skull are examples of fixed joints.
- **Slightly movable joints** allow for limited movement. Slightly movable joints are found between the vertebrae in the spine, and where the ribs attach to the sternum (breastbone). **Cartilage,** a tough, fibrous substance, fills in the space between the bones in the slightly movable joint. The car-tilage permits limited movement and acts as a "shock absorber" between the bones.

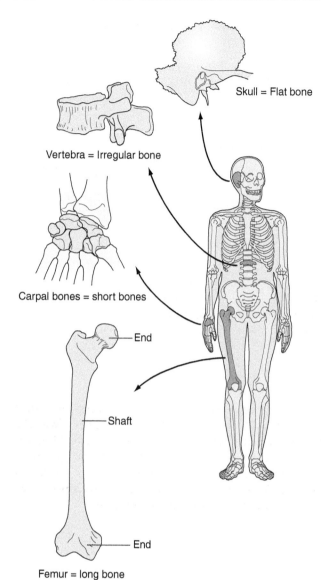

Skull = Flat bone

Vertebra = Irregular bone

Carpal bones = short bones

End

Shaft

End

Femur = long bone

Figure 25-2
Bones can be categorized by their shape. General types of bones include long bones, short bones, flat bones, and irregular bones.

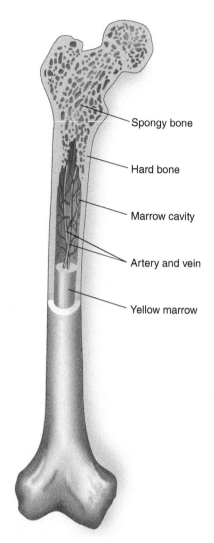

Spongy bone

Hard bone

Marrow cavity

Artery and vein

Yellow marrow

Figure 25-3
Bones have two layers, a solid outside and a net-like inside. As a result, bones are very strong, yet lightweight.

- **Freely movable joints** allow for a wide range of movement. Examples of freely movable joints include the knees, elbows, finger and toe joints, and hip joints. Some of the ways in which freely movable joints move are shown and defined in Table 25-1. The ends of the bones that form the freely movable joint are covered with cartilage, which provides a smooth surface for the other bones to move against. A capsule formed of connective tissue encloses the ends of the bones, forming a joint cavity. The lining of the capsule secretes a thick

fluid called *synovial fluid* into the joint cavity. The synovial fluid lubricates the joint, which helps the joint to move smoothly. **Ligaments,** which are very strong bands of fibrous tissue, cross over the joint capsule, attaching one bone to another and stabilizing the joint. If the ligament is torn or weak, the joint may be able to move too much in any one direction.

THE MUSCULAR SYSTEM

The muscular system consists of the muscles. As you learned in Chapter 23, there are three types of muscle tissue found in the body (see Chapter 23, Table 23-1). Of the three types, skeletal

A. Fixed joints (skull)

Sutures

B. Slightly movable joints (vertebrae)

Cartilage ("shock absorber")

C. Freely movable joints (knee)

Muscle

Tendon

Femur

Cartilage

Ligament

Fibula

Tibia

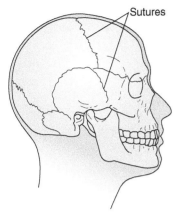
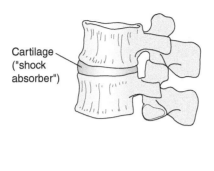
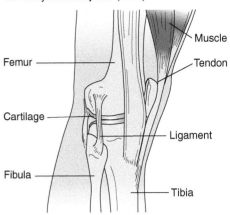

Figure 25-4

Joints are often categorized by the amount of motion they permit. **(A)** Fixed joints, such as the joints that join the bones of the skull, do not allow for any movement. **(B)** Slightly movable joints, such as those between the vertebrae in the spinal column, permit some movement. **(C)** Freely movable joints, such as the knee joints, allow for a wide range of movement.

muscle is the type of muscle tissue found in the musculoskeletal system. Skeletal muscle is said to be *striated*, because the muscle fibers make the muscles look like they have stripes. (*Striations* is another word for "stripes.")

There are almost 700 individual skeletal muscles in the body (Fig. 25-5). These muscles account for about 40% of your total body weight. Skeletal muscles vary in shape. Some are long, thick, and band-like. Others are flat or fan-like. Muscles are named according to their location, their shape, or their function.

The skeletal muscles are attached to the bones by bands of connective tissue called **tendons.** Occasionally, skeletal muscles are attached to other muscles by a broad, flat sheet of tendon called an *aponeurosis.*

FUNCTION OF THE MUSCULOSKELETAL SYSTEM

The musculoskeletal system has several vital functions.

PROTECTION

The bones of the skeletal system protect delicate internal organs. For example, the skull bones surround and protect the brain, and the rib cage surrounds and protects the lungs and heart.

SUPPORT

The bones of the skeleton form a framework that supports and gives shape to the body. **Muscle tone,** or the steady contraction of the skeletal muscles, helps us to maintain an upright posture, such as sitting or standing. The muscles of the back, neck, shoulders, and abdomen are responsible for maintaining posture.

MOVEMENT

Voluntary movement occurs when a skeletal muscle contracts (shortens) or relaxes (lengthens) across a freely movable joint. In freely movable joints, each skeletal muscle attaches to the bone in two places, the origin and the insertion. The origin and the insertion points are on opposite sides of the joint. So, when the muscle contracts, the muscle shortens and the origin and insertion points are drawn closer to each other, causing the part of the body to move (Fig. 25-6).

Skeletal muscles usually work in groups to provide body movement. For example, your biceps muscle is located on the front of your upper arm. When you contract your biceps muscle, your lower arm is drawn toward your body. When you are lifting a heavy object, the brachioradialis muscle, which is also located in your upper arm, also contracts, helping to stabilize the elbow and assisting the biceps muscle with lifting. When it is time to straighten the arm again, the biceps muscle relaxes and the triceps

Table 25-1   Words Used to Describe Movement

	WORD	DEFINITION
	Flexion	Bending of a joint
	Extension	Straightening of a joint
	Abduction	Moving a body part away from the midline of the body
	Adduction	Moving a body part toward the midline of the body
	Rotation	Twisting or turning of a joint
	Supination	Rotation of the palm so that it is facing up or forward
	Pronation	Rotation of the palm so that it is facing down or backward
	Eversion	Rotation of the sole of the foot outward
	Inversion	Rotation of the sole of the foot inward
	Dorsiflexion	Bending the foot upward at the ankle by pulling the toes toward the head
	Plantar flexion	Flexing the arch of the foot by pointing the toes downward

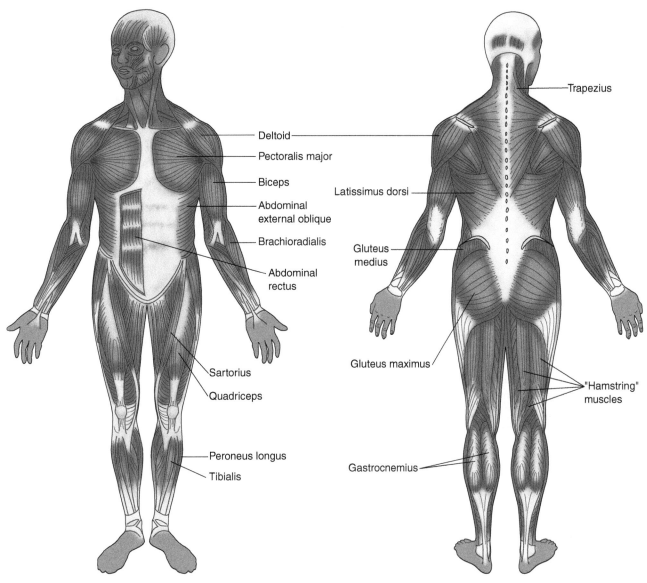

Figure 25-5
There are about 700 skeletal muscles in the body! Some of the more familiar ones are
labelled here.

muscle, located on the back of the upper arm, contracts, pulling the lower arm back into a straight position.

HEAT PRODUCTION

Contraction of the skeletal muscles produces heat and helps to maintain a constant body temperature. This is why we feel warmer when we move back and forth and stamp our feet while waiting outside on a cold day for a bus or train. The movement of the muscles produces heat, which makes us feel warmer. This is also why, when it is very cold, we may start to shiver. Shivering occurs when the skeletal muscles contract rapidly

in unison. The involuntary contractions help to increase the heat output of the muscles, raising the body temperature and making us feel warmer.

CALCIUM STORAGE

Calcium is an important mineral that is necessary for the proper functioning of skeletal and cardiac muscle. Calcium is also what makes the bone tissue hard and strong. Most of the calcium we need to function on a daily basis is obtained from calcium-rich foods and beverages, such as milk, cheese, yogurt, broccoli, leafy greens, tofu, and calcium-fortified orange juice. However, if we

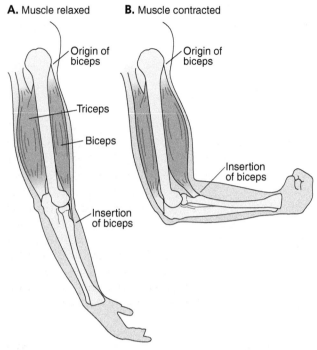

A. Muscle relaxed   **B.** Muscle contracted

Origin of biceps

Origin of biceps

Triceps

Biceps

Insertion of biceps

Insertion of biceps

Figure 25-6
The muscular and the skeletal systems work together to produce movement. The muscle attaches to the bone in two places, the origin and the insertion. **(A)** Shown here are the attachments of the biceps muscle, the muscle in your upper arm that bulges when you "make a muscle." **(B)** When you contract your biceps muscle, the origin and insertion points are drawn closer together. As the muscle shortens, it pulls on the bone, bringing your lower arm toward your body.

do not take in enough calcium through our diets, then calcium is released from the bones as it is needed. This is why it is important to obtain enough calcium through the diet, especially when a person is young.

Consuming enough calcium early on in life builds up the calcium stores in the bones. As we grow older, our intestines become less effective at absorbing the calcium that we eat, so calcium is released from the bones to keep the levels in our bloodstream constant. If the amount of calcium stored in the bones is not adequate, the bones become brittle and weak as the body draws on the calcium stored there and does not replace it. Consuming enough calcium while you are young is like putting money in the bank to use after you retire. If plenty has been stored away, then retirement can be quite comfortable. But if not enough has been put away, then you may not be able to do the things you want to do in retirement.

PRODUCTION OF BLOOD CELLS

In addition to storing calcium, the bones also function as a factory for the production of blood cells. There are many different types of blood cells, with many different functions. For example, some blood cells play a role in the immune response, and help us to fight off infection. Other blood cells carry oxygen to the tissues of the body. Blood cells form in red bone marrow, which is found in flat bones and the ends of the long bones. In young children, the shaft of the long bones also contains red bone marrow, but that red bone marrow is gradually replaced by yellow bone marrow as the person grows older. Yellow bone marrow is made up mostly of fatty tissue that can be used by the body for energy if necessary.

THE EFFECTS OF AGING ON THE MUSCULOSKELETAL SYSTEM

The normal processes of aging cause significant changes in the musculoskeletal system. It is the rare older person who does not have some degree of disability or discomfort related to the functioning of his or her musculoskeletal system! Aches, pains, and stiffness often accompany these changes. Occasionally, the person loses the ability to move one or more parts of his or her body. Age-related changes affecting the musculoskeletal system are the leading cause of disability in older adults.

It is now known that participating in regular physical exercise and eating properly are measures that can delay or decrease the effects of aging on the musculoskeletal system. Engaging in some form of weight-bearing exercise, such as brisk walking, aerobics, or moderate weight training, has been shown to have many positive effects, even in very old people (Fig. 25-7). Weight-bearing exercise helps to maintain bone strength by stimulating the body to store extra calcium in the bones. It improves blood flow, allowing more oxygen and nutrients to be carried to the tissues of the musculoskeletal system. Continued use of the muscles helps to retain strength. Flexibility of the joints is improved with regular exercise, which leads to fewer aches and pains.

People typically begin to experience age-related changes to the musculoskeletal system after the age of 40 years, although the onset of or a lack of physical activity are present, the loss of strong bone tissue occurs much more rapidly.

LOSS OF MUSCLE MASS

The number of muscle cells also starts to gradually decrease when a person is in his or her 40s, resulting in a decrease in the size and strength of each individual muscle. The loss of muscle size and strength is called muscle **atrophy** (Fig. 25-8). If a person is poorly nourished, is not physically active, or has a chronic medical condition, muscle atrophy progresses at a much faster rate. If you have ever had a broken bone that required a cast, you probably noticed that after the cast was removed, the affected limb was smaller and weaker than the other one. What you noticed was muscle atrophy as a result of not being able to use the muscle during the time that the limb was in the cast!

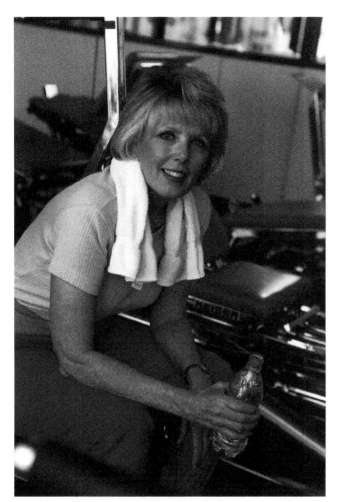

Figure 25-7
It is never too late to begin exercising! Regular exercise strengthens the muscles, helps to build bone mass, and lessens joint pain and stiffness.

these changes may be significantly delayed in people who exercise regularly and are relatively healthy. The normal age-related changes that affect the musculoskeletal system include loss of bone tissue, loss of muscle mass, and wear and tear on the joints.

LOSS OF BONE TISSUE

Aging decreases the body's ability to absorb calcium, a critical nutrient. When the body cannot get the amount of calcium it needs from the diet alone, it begins to draw on the calcium stored in the bones. Some people begin drawing on their calcium stores at a relatively young age, for example, when they are in their 40s. The continuous, gradual loss of calcium causes the bones to lose their strength and hardness, making them more fragile and prone to breaking. If other conditions, such as poor nutrition, poor circulation,

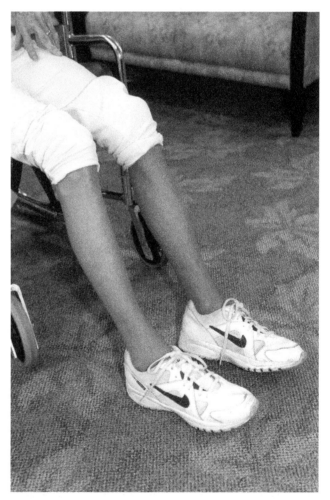

Figure 25-8
Muscle atrophy, or loss of muscle mass, is a normal age-related change. Immobility can make muscle atrophy much more severe.

Significant loss of muscle tissue can leave a person too weak to walk or carry out routine activities of daily living (ADLs). Loss of muscle tissue also affects the body's ability to produce heat. This is one reason why an elderly person might feel chilly in a room that a younger person would consider warm or even hot.

WEAR AND TEAR ON THE JOINTS

As we age, we lose the proteins that make the ligaments, tendons, and cartilage elastic and flexible, which can lead to stiffness and pain in the joints. The normal demands of daily life also cause a lot of wear and tear on the joints, which can, over time, lead to stiffness and pain. Overuse or injury of a joint, or being overweight, places extra strain on certain joints and will make the normal changes associated with aging more severe. Joint pain and stiffness can make simple activities, such as walking or getting out of a chair, difficult. Joint stiffness can also make a person more likely to fall.

DISORDERS OF THE MUSCULOSKELETAL SYSTEM

It is likely that many of the people in your care will have some degree of musculoskeletal disability, simply as a result of their age. You may also care for people who have musculoskeletal disability as a result of disease or trauma. Examples of diseases that affect the bones, joints, and muscles include osteoporosis, arthritis, and muscular dystrophy. Fractures (broken bones) are usually caused by trauma. Amputation (the loss of a limb) may be necessary because of trauma or complications of a disease, such as diabetes.

OSTEOPOROSIS

Osteoporosis is the excessive loss of bone tissue. Although everyone experiences some loss of bone tissue as a normal part of aging, people with osteoporosis lose excessive amounts of bone tissue, causing the bones to become crumbly and very fragile. The bones most commonly affected by osteoporosis are the bones of the spine, the pelvis, and the long bones in the arms and legs (Fig. 25-9).

Osteoporosis is most common in older women who have gone through menopause. This is because estrogen, a hormone that is present in the bodies of women who are still having menstrual periods, helps to prevent bone loss. However, when a woman's periods stop, her body stops producing estrogen, and this puts her more at risk for bone loss. Other risk factors for the development of osteoporosis include:

- White race
- "Small bones"
- Smoking
- Inactivity or immobility
- Diseases of the thyroid and adrenal glands
- A diet lacking in calcium, vitamin D (necessary for the absorption of calcium), and protein
- Certain drugs, such as steroids

Osteoporosis causes bones to break more easily, and physical activity becomes very difficult. Sometimes bones are so brittle that a person can break them just by bumping into a piece of furniture. Bones that have been fractured are difficult to repair and heal slowly. Crumbling of the bones of the spinal column causes the upper back to curve into the deformity known as a "dowager's hump" (see Fig. 25-9). These spinal column fractures are very painful and debilitating.

For people who have osteoporosis, some treatments are available. A drug that helps to slow the progression of osteoporosis has been developed. In addition, the use of calcium and vitamin D supplements can also help in the treatment of osteoporosis. Resistance training (lifting weights) slows the progression of the disease by helping to promote bone strength. However, as with most things, prevention is the best medicine! Osteoporosis can be prevented in many cases by exercising regularly and eating a diet rich in calcium, protein, and vitamin D, starting early in life.

When caring for a person with osteoporosis, remember to be gentle when helping the person with transfers. Encourage exercise by having the person take frequent walks with you. Carefully observe and document the types of foods and liquids the person eats and drinks, and encourage snacks that are high in calcium, such as milk, yogurt, ice cream, and cheese. Be especially observant of loss of function, swelling, or complaints of pain. These signs and symptoms may indicate a new fracture in a fragile bone.

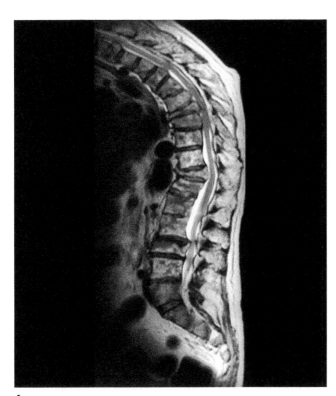

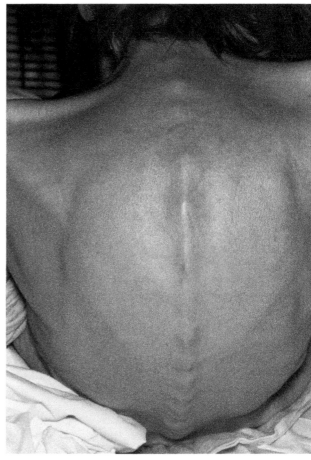

A

B

Figure 25-9

Osteoporosis. **(A)** A magnetic resonance imaging (MRI) scan of the spine of a 60-year-old patient with osteoporosis. This is a side view (the patient is standing, facing the left). The vertebrae (*brown*) enclose the spinal cord (*pink*). Some of the vertebrae (*orange*) have collapsed as a result of osteoporosis, causing the spine to curve. **(B)** This woman has a "dowager's hump" as a result of osteoporosis of the spine. The deformity occurs when the fragile bones of the spine crumble. (**A,** © *Zephyr/Photo Researchers, Inc.;* **B,** © *John Radcliffe Hospital/Photo Researchers, Inc.*)

ARTHRITIS

Arthritis is inflammation of the joints, usually associated with pain and stiffness. Arthritis is the most common disorder of the musculoskeletal system, affecting people of all ages. There are more than 20 different types of arthritis. Three of the most common types are osteoarthritis, rheumatoid arthritis, and gout.

Osteoarthritis

Osteoarthritis is the leading cause of physical disability among elderly people. In osteoarthritis, the cartilage that covers the ends of the bones wears away, making movement of the joint difficult and painful. Osteoarthritis appears to be the result of normal wear and tear on the joint, which

is why it is seen most often in elderly people. However, obesity, previous joint injury, or a family history of the disease may increase a person's risk of developing osteoarthritis earlier in life and more severely.

Osteoarthritis usually affects weight-bearing joints, such as the knees, hips, and joints of the spinal column. Osteoarthritis begins when the smooth cartilage on the ends of the bones becomes rough, due to normal use of the joint. The rough area then becomes inflamed, and bony deposits build up. These bony deposits rub against the cartilage, causing even more damage. This cycle repeats until the cartilage has been worn down to the point where bone is actually rubbing against bone as the joint moves. The joint becomes swollen, stiff, and very painful.

A person with osteoarthritis may take medications to decrease both the pain and swelling. Heat and cold applications, discussed later in this chapter, can also increase a person's level of comfort. Mild exercise that places the affected joints through their range of motion helps to diminish stiffness and maintain joint function. People who have very severe osteoarthritis may need surgery to replace the joint. Hips and knees are the joints most commonly replaced, but replacement of shoulder, elbow, wrist, and hand joints is also possible. Joint replacement surgery, also called total joint replacement, involves removing the ends of the bones in the affected joint and replacing them with parts made from metal and plastic (Fig. 25-10).

As a personal support worker, you may be responsible for caring for a person who is recovering from joint replacement surgery. People who have had a joint replaced are not allowed to bear weight on the affected joint for a period of time after the surgery, so you will need to help them with transfers. In addition, people who have had a hip joint replaced have several special care requirements during the recovery period:

- Following the surgery, the muscles and ligaments that normally hold the hip joint in place are weak, making it very easy for the head of the femur (the thigh bone) to dislocate, or pop out of joint. To prevent this from happening, the person's legs must be spread apart (abducted) when the person is in the supine or lateral position. Most people who have had hip replacement surgery will have a special wedge-shaped pillow, called an *abduction pillow,* which goes between the legs and attaches to each leg with Velcro™ fasteners (Fig. 25-11). The abduction pillow helps to keep the legs spread. If an abduction pillow is not available, a regular pillow can be used instead.

- When sitting, a person who has had hip replacement surgery must use a straight-backed chair. The person's hips must be flexed no more than 90 degrees, and his feet must rest flat on the floor. This is true when the person is using the toilet or commode, as well. A special device may be used to raise the height of the toilet seat to prevent

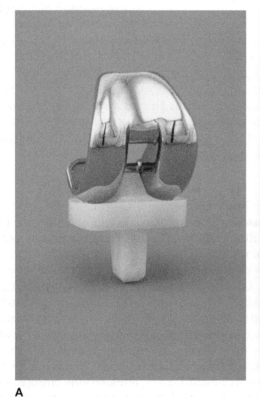
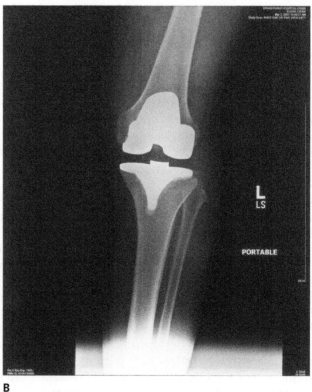

A　　　　　　　　　　　　**B**

Figure 25-10
In joint replacement surgery, a damaged joint is replaced with an artificial (prosthetic) joint.
(A) An artificial knee joint. **(B)** X-ray of an artificial knee joint in place. (**A,** © *SIU Bio Med/Custom Medical Stock Photo.*)

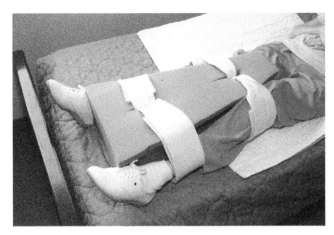

Figure 25-11
When a person is recovering from hip joint replacement surgery, an abduction pillow is used to help prevent the hip joint from becoming dislocated during the recovery period.

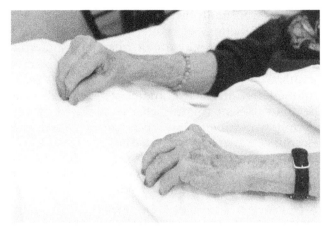

Figure 25-12
This woman has rheumatoid arthritis in the joints of her hands.

flexion in excess of 90 degrees when the person is using the toilet.

• A physical therapist will work with the person after surgery. If possible, you should be present while the therapist is working with the person. That way, you can see the specific ambulation and transfer techniques that are being used with your patient or resident.

As always, you should ask the nurse about any instructions or restrictions that are specific to your patient or resident.

Rheumatoid Arthritis

Rheumatoid arthritis is a crippling condition that can cause severe joint deformities (Fig. 25-12). Unlike osteoarthritis, rheumatoid arthritis affects people much younger in life, most often between the ages of 20 and 40 years. This disease is more common in women than in men.

Researchers believe that rheumatoid arthritis is an autoimmune disorder. In autoimmune disorders, the body's immune system begins to attack the body's own tissues. So, for example, in rheumatoid arthritis, the immune system attacks and destroys the cartilage that covers the ends of the bones. Scar tissue develops within the joints, causing them to become stiff and useless. For many months, a person's rheumatoid arthritis may seem to be under control, but then the person will experience an acute flare-up of the disease. During the acute phases of the disease, the person may experience pain, swelling, redness, and heat in the joints, as well as fever and general weakness. Bed rest may be necessary, and splints can help decrease joint deformity. The

gentle use of active and active-assistive range-of-motion exercises (discussed later in this chapter) helps to maintain joint mobility.

Gout

Gout is a type of arthritis that is caused by a disturbance in the body's metabolism. Uric acid is a waste product of metabolism that is usually eliminated from the body in the urine. If the body produces too much uric acid or the kidneys are unable to properly process the uric acid, the uric acid builds up in the body, forming crystals that are deposited within the joints. These uric acid crystals are extremely irritating to the tissues in the joint, and, as a result, the joint becomes inflamed and painful. While gout can affect any joint, the big toe is most commonly affected. Men past middle age are more commonly affected than women.

MUSCULAR DYSTROPHY

Muscular dystrophy is a general term for a group of disorders that cause the skeletal muscles to become more and more weak over time. These disorders are inherited. The types of muscular dystrophy vary according to the muscles that are affected, the age of the person typically affected, and the rate at which the disease progresses.

One type of muscular dystrophy is myasthenia gravis. In myasthenia gravis, the muscle's ability to respond to commands from the nervous system is affected. Therefore, the muscle cannot contract, and it becomes weak and atrophied. Duchenne's muscular dystrophy, another type of muscular dystrophy, usually affects children and causes death by the age of 20 years. The person dies because the muscles that allow him to breathe eventually become too weak to perform this vital function.

If one of your patients or residents has muscular dystrophy, the person will need assistance with range-of-motion exercises, walking, positioning, and ADLs. Eventually, when the disease begins to affect the muscles that control swallowing, you will also have to help the person with eating.

FRACTURES

A **fracture** is a broken bone. Fractures are usually caused by trauma, such as a fall or a car accident. However, some fractures are caused when a bone is put under constant and repeated stress. For example, you may have heard of a distance runner being diagnosed with a "stress fracture" in the small bones of the foot. Think about how many times a runner's foot pounds against the pavement, and the force behind each step, and you will understand how a stress fracture can occur!

Older people are especially at risk for fractures, because the bones become more fragile with age. Older people are also more likely to have diseases that put them at risk for fractures, such as osteoporosis or bone cancer. Weak, brittle bones can fracture easily, often from a seemingly minor fall or stumble. For example, hip fractures are quite common in older women who have fallen just a short distance, such as from a standing position to the floor or sidewalk. Not only do the bones of an older person fracture more easily, they take longer to heal and they may heal improperly. Delayed or improper healing may cause prolonged difficulty with mobility.

Types of Fractures

Fractures can occur in almost any bone in the body and are classified in the following manner (Fig. 25-13):

- **Closed fracture.** The bone is broken, but the broken ends do not protrude through the overlying skin.
- **Open (compound) fracture.** The bone is broken, and the sharp ends of the broken bone have broken through the skin. Because the skin is broken, open fractures carry a very high risk of infection.
- **Greenstick fracture.** Have you ever tried to snap a young, green twig? Unlike a dry, brown stick, a green twig will bend and splinter, but it will not break all the way through. In a greenstick fracture, the same thing occurs—the bone bends and splinters, but it does not break all the way through. Greenstick fractures occur most commonly in children because their bones are still quite flexible.
- **Impacted fracture.** The bone is broken all of the way through, and the broken ends of the bone are jammed into each other. These fractures are often seen in people who have jumped or fallen from a height, for example, off of a roof or ladder.

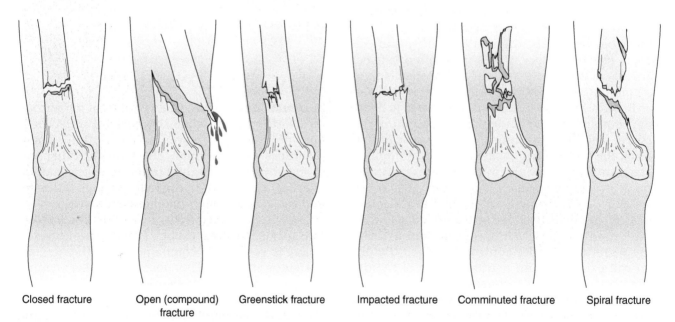

| Closed fracture | Open (compound) fracture | Greenstick fracture | Impacted fracture | Comminuted fracture | Spiral fracture |

Figure 25-13
There are many different types of fractures.

- **Comminuted fracture.** The bone is splintered into several little pieces. This type of fracture is common when a bone has been crushed under a great weight. The surrounding tissues, such as muscle and skin, may be seriously injured as well.
- **Spiral fracture.** The break circles around the bone in a winding fashion. Spiral fractures are common when the bone has been subjected to a twisting force.

Treatments for Fractures

Reduction and fixation

For a fractured bone to heal properly, the broken ends of the bone must be brought together (aligned) and then held in that position until the fracture heals. **Reduction** is the word used to describe the process of bringing the broken ends of the bone into alignment. **Fixation** is the word used to describe the process of holding the bone in one position until the fracture heals. There are many ways to accomplish reduction and fixation. The method used depends on the type and location of the fracture.

In a *closed reduction,* the doctor lines up the broken ends of the bone by simply pushing them back into place. In a closed reduction, it is not necessary to create a surgical incision to access the broken bone. Following a closed reduction, a cast (made of fiberglass or plaster of Paris) is applied to keep the bone in the proper alignment until healing occurs (Fig. 25-14A). First, a thin layer of cotton is placed on the skin to protect it. Then, the casting material is soaked in water and wrapped around the limb. As the casting material dries, it hardens, preventing movement of the broken bone. A cast is a method of *external fixation,* or fixation that is achieved without surgery. General guidelines for caring for a person with a cast are given in Guidelines Box 25-1.

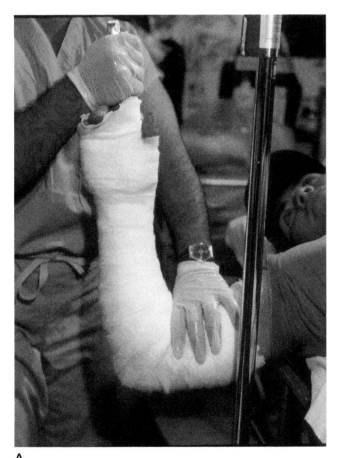

A

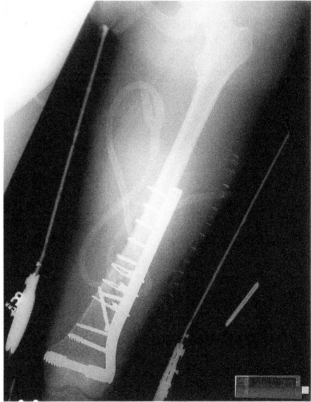

B

Figure 25-14

With any fracture, the broken ends of the bone need to be brought back together (reduction) and held in place (fixation). **(A)** Fixation can be accomplished externally, with a cast, or **(B)** it can be accomplished internally, with devices such as plates, screws, pins, or wires. (*A,* © L. Steinmark/ Custom Medical Stock Photo.)

Guidelines Box 25-1   Guidelines for Caring for a Person With a Cast

WHAT YOU DO	WHY YOU DO IT
Do not cover the cast or place it on a plastic-covered pillow until it has dried completely.	The casting material produces heat as it dries. Covering the cast can cause the person's skin underneath the cast to burn.
Do not touch the cast with your fingertips until it is totally dry. If you must handle the cast, use the palms of your hands.	Touching the cast can cause it to dent, creating pressure spots against the person's skin.
Keep the casted body part elevated on a pillow for several days.	Elevating the casted body part helps prevent and reduce swelling around the fracture site.
Because the skin underneath the cast can start to itch, the person may try to slide an object between the cast and the skin to scratch the itchy area. Advise the person that placing objects inside of the cast should be avoided.	Sliding an object between the cast and the skin may injure the skin, which puts the person at risk for infection.
Make sure the person's toes (or fingers, if the cast is on the arm) are pink, warm, and moving. Report any complaints of increased pain, numbness, or tingling. Report any observations of cyanosis, increased swelling, cold toes or fingers, increased drainage on the cast, or a foul odour immediately.	Cyanosis; increased swelling; increased pain, numbness, or tingling; or cold fingers or toes may indicate that swelling inside the cast is interfering with blood flow. If the tissues do not receive enough oxygen and nutrients, tissue death and skin breakdown may occur. Increased drainage or a foul odour may indicate infection.
Keep the cast clean and dry.	Plaster cast material becomes soft again when it becomes wet.
Do not allow the person to place pressure or weight on the cast unless he has been specifically instructed to do so.	Placing too much pressure or weight on the cast can cause the cast to break.

Sometimes it is necessary to surgically expose the bone to line up the broken ends of the bone. This is called an *open reduction*. Often, open reduction is followed by *internal fixation*. Internal fixation involves the use of metal plates, screws, rods, pins, or wires to hold the broken ends of the bone in place until the bone is healed (see Fig. 25-14B). You may see the notation "ORIF" on a person's chart. This means that the person has had surgery to achieve an "**O**pen **R**eduction, **I**nternal **F**ixation."

Traction

Some fractured bones cannot be repaired surgically for a period of time, especially if the person's overall medical condition is unstable. In these cases, traction is used to keep the broken ends of the bone in alignment until the fracture can be permanently repaired by surgery or casting. In **traction,** the ends of the bones are placed in the proper alignment and then weight is applied to exert a constant pull and keep the

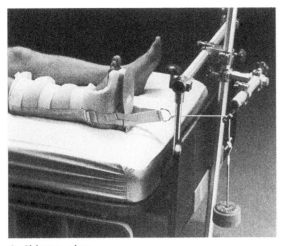

A. Skin traction

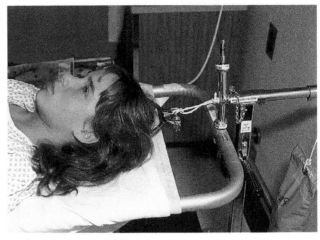

B. Skeletal traction

Figure 25-15

Traction is used to hold the broken ends of a bone in alignment until the fracture can be repaired permanently. **(A)** In skin traction, a device is attached to the person's skin, and weight is suspended from it. **(B)** In skeletal traction, pins are driven through the bone to support the weight. (**A,** *used with permission from Smeltzer, S. C., Bare, B. G., Hinkle, J. L., & Cheever, K. H. [2008].* Brunner & Suddarth's textbook of medical–surgical nursing *[11th ed., p. 2366]. Philadelphia: Lippincott Williams & Wilkins.* **B,** *used with permission from Rosdahl, C. B., & Kowalski, M. T. [2008].* Textbook of basic nursing *[9th ed.]. Philadelphia: Lippincott Williams & Wilkins.*)

bone in alignment. In skin traction, weight is suspended from a traction unit that is attached to the person's skin (Fig. 25-15A). In skeletal traction, weight is suspended from pins that are driven through the bone (see Fig. 25-15B). A **trapeze bar** may be attached to the overhead frame of the person's bed. The person grasps the trapeze bar to assist with movement.

A person in traction has several special care needs, many of which arise from the person's limited ability to move or change position:

- You may be asked to assist the person with range-of-motion exercises to work the unaffected joints and keep them limber.
- The person will have to use a fracture bedpan (see Chapter 20, Fig. 20-2B), which is easier to slide under the buttocks.
- Pressure ulcers are always a concern, so it is important to keep the person's skin clean and dry, and to monitor for signs of skin breakdown.
- Two people usually work together to change the bed linens, and the linens are changed from the top of the bed (working down), instead of from side to side. If you need to do this, the nurse will show you how.

When you are working with a person who is in traction, be very careful not to disturb or remove the weights attached to the traction unit. When you lower the person's bed height, check to make sure the weights are not resting on the floor. They must hang freely to apply the correct amount of tension to the affected limb.

AMPUTATIONS

The removal of all or part of an arm or a leg is called an **amputation.** For example, a person may lose just a toe, or the leg from the knee down, or the entire leg. Accidents are a common cause of amputation. For example, the body part may be severed from the body during the accident. Or, the body part may be so seriously damaged during the accident that the only treatment option is to surgically remove it.

Amputation may also be necessary as a result of disease. For example, some types of cancer are treated by amputation of the affected limb. Diseases that interfere with blood flow to all or part of an extremity can also eventually result in the need for amputation. For example, as you learned in Chapter 18, people with diabetes tend to have circulatory problems, and often, blood flow to their feet is poor. The poor blood flow to the feet is usually associated with poor sensation as well as an increased risk for infection. If a person with diabetes gets a foot infection, it may go

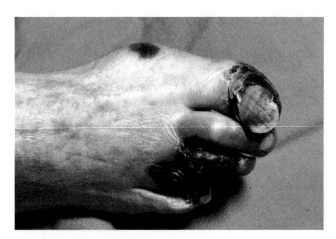

Figure 25-16
Impaired blood flow causes death of the tissues (gangrene). Once gangrene develops, the only treatment option may be amputation of the affected part. (© *M. English/Custom Medical Stock Photo.*)

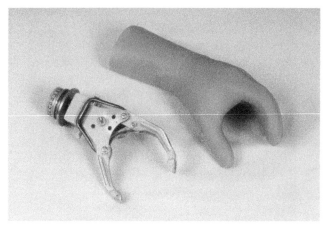

Figure 25-17
A prosthetic hand and its cover are shown here. Many times, it is hard to tell a false limb from a real one when the prosthesis is being worn. A prosthetic body part can help a person who has had an amputation regain function and mobility. (© *SIU Bio Med/Custom Medical Stock Photo.*)

unnoticed for a long time, and when it finally is noticed, it may be very difficult to treat. Eventually, death of the tissue (gangrene) occurs because the tissue is deprived of oxygen and nutrients (Fig. 25-16). Once gangrene develops, the only treatment option may be to remove the damaged part through amputation.

The loss of a body part, especially an arm or leg, is very emotionally traumatic for a person. The person's mobility, appearance, and sometimes even her ability to earn a living or enjoy a hobby she used to love can be affected by an amputation. For some people who have had a body part either partially or completely amputated, a prosthetic (false) part may allow the person to regain mobility, function, and a more normal appearance (Fig. 25-17).

For a prosthetic device to be fitted, the **stump,** or the end of the amputated limb that is left after surgery, must be cared for properly. Positioning is used to keep the muscles and tendons from shortening, and nearby joints are put through range-of-motion exercises to help maintain normal joint function and mobility. Wrapping the end of the stump with elastic bandages helps to shrink and shape the stump properly (Fig. 25-18). When assisting with caring for a person's stump, make sure to follow the nurse's or physical therapist's instructions exactly, as always. Finally, as you assist with the general care needs of your patient or resident, you will have numerous opportunities to observe the stump for any drainage, bleeding, or pain. These findings could be signs of poor tissue healing or

infection, and must be reported to the nurse immediately.

Many people experience what is known as **phantom pain,** or the feeling that the amputated body part is still present, after an amputation. Aching, itching, and other sensations are all types of phantom pain. The sensations are caused by the healing of the nerves that were cut when the body part was removed. Phantom pain usually goes away a short while after surgery, but some people report having these episodes for years afterward.

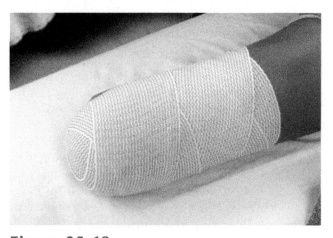

Figure 25-18
Wrapping the stump in bandages helps to shape it properly.

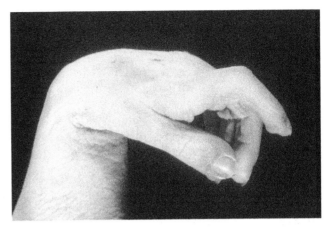

Figure 25-19

Contractures can occur when a joint is not exercised regularly. Use of the joint can be permanently lost.
(© *Siebert/Custom Medical Stock Photo.*)

GENERAL CARE MEASURES

As a personal support worker, you may be asked to assist a patient or resident with range-of-motion exercises, the application of heat or cold, or physical therapy. These techniques are used to prevent complications of immobility, relieve musculoskeletal discomfort, and maintain or restore musculoskeletal function.

RANGE-OF-MOTION EXERCISES

As you learned earlier, the range of motion of a joint is the complete extent of movement that the joint is normally capable of without causing pain. Normal activities—such as dressing, grooming, walking, and eating—usually put all of our joints through their complete range of motion several times throughout the day. However, some of the people you will be caring for will have conditions that prevent them from doing the activities that would normally exercise their joints and muscles.

As you know from this chapter and previous ones, immobility can have a serious impact on the musculoskeletal system. Muscle atrophy, loss of bone strength, and stiffness of the joints can quickly lead to permanent muscle weakness, brittle bones, and even contractures (Fig. 25-19). As a personal support worker, you will play a key role in preventing these complications by helping your patients or residents with range-of-motion exercises as ordered.

Range-of-motion exercises—movements that put each joint through its complete range of motion—are done to preserve joint and muscle function in a person who has limited use of his musculoskeletal system. Range-of-motion exercises are usually performed at least twice a day, often along with other personal care activities, such as bathing or dressing. The exercises can be done while the person is in bed or sitting down. Depending on the situation, range-of-motion exercises may be performed for only one, some, or all of the joints. Sometimes, the patient or resident will be able to perform the exercises on his own, and your role will be to provide guidance and encouragement. Other times, you will need to help the person to perform the exercises.

- In *active range-of-motion exercises*, the patient or resident performs the exercises independently, with verbal guidance from the personal support worker or nurse.

- In *passive range-of-motion exercises*, the personal support worker or nurse moves the patient's or resident's joints through the exercises, without active involvement on the part of the person. For example, a personal support worker might perform passive range-of-motion exercises for a person who is unconscious.

- In *active-assistive range-of-motion exercises*, the patient or resident performs the exercises with some hands-on assistance from the personal support worker or nurse. For example, a person may be able to lift his arm out to the side, but will need help from the personal support worker or nurse to complete the movement of bringing the arm up near the head.

Procedure 25-1 explains how to assist a patient or resident with passive range-of-motion exercises. Range-of-motion exercises can cause injury to the joints if they are not performed properly. Usually a physical therapist or nurse will evaluate the person and determine which joints should be exercised. When assisting a person with range-of-motion exercises, always follow the care plan (or the nurse's or physical therapist's instructions) exactly. This is important for two reasons:

1. There may be some exercises that the person is not allowed to do.
2. The physical therapist or nurse will most likely change the care plan as the person's condition either improves or worsens.

In addition to checking the care plan, you should make sure that helping the person with the ordered exercises is within your scope of practice. For example, in some facilities, personal support workers are not allowed to assist people with range-of-motion exercises involving the neck. General guidelines for assisting a person with range-of-motion exercises are given in Guidelines Box 25-2.

HEAT AND COLD APPLICATIONS

Disorders of the musculoskeletal system are usually painful. Pain can make it difficult for a person to relax, rest, or sleep. As a personal support worker, many of the things you do every day are related to promoting comfort and preventing pain. For example, ensuring that a person is in proper alignment when you reposition her helps to prevent pain. Personal support workers also play an important role in noticing and reporting pain. Many of the people you care for will be hesitant to complain about pain, even when the pain is severe or constant. Some people feel that their pain is just simply part of "growing old." Others are afraid that they will become addicted to pain medications. If you notice that a person seems to be in pain, report this to the nurse. There are many things that can be done to relieve pain, aside from the use of medications (or in addition to the use of medications). The nurse will work with the person and the other members of the health care team to find a way to lessen the person's pain.

Table 25-2	Uses of Heat and Cold Applications
HEAT	**COLD**
Reduces pain and swelling and promotes circulation to speed healing	Reduces pain and swelling
Relieves muscle spasms	Numbs sensation and controls bleeding
Provides warmth	Reduces fevers

As a personal support worker, you may be responsible for carrying out many of the tasks on the care plan related to relieving the person's pain. For example, back massage is especially beneficial when combined with pain medication. Also, many people with musculoskeletal pain can benefit from the application of heat or cold to an affected joint or muscle. The application of heat or cold can be used to reduce or prevent tissue swelling, promote healing, ease pain, and promote comfort. Heat and cold have opposite effects on the body, which are summarized in Table 25-2. Because the application of heat or cold can be dangerous, these treatments require a doctor's order, and in some facilities, the application of heat or cold may be outside of the personal support worker's scope of practice. However, even if you are not permitted to give these treatments, you will be involved with monitoring patients or residents who are receiving them.

Some people are at very high risk for injury from the application of heat or cold:

- **Older people, very young people, and chronically ill people.** The skin of people who are very old, very young, or chronically ill can be very fragile and sensitive.
- **People with very fair skin.** Fair skin tends to be more sensitive to temperature changes than darker skin.
- **People with impaired sensation.** People with impaired sensation, such as those who are paralyzed or who have diabetes, are at risk for injury because they are unable to detect whether an application is too hot or too cold.
- **People who are disoriented or taking pain medications.** People with impaired levels of consciousness are also at a higher risk for injury from heat or cold applications.

Guidelines Box 25-2   Guidelines for Assisting With Range-of-Motion Exercises

WHAT YOU DO	WHY YOU DO IT
Use good body mechanics.	Using good body mechanics saves energy and prevents muscle strain and injury.
Remove pillows and other positioning devices.	Pillows and positioning devices can prevent a person from achieving full range of motion of the joint.
Position the person so that each joint can be moved through all of the usual positions.	Positioning the person in a position that will allow each joint to be moved through all of its usual positions saves time (because the person will not have to be repositioned in between exercises) and helps to ensure that all of the exercises will be completed.
Move through the exercises in a systematic way (for example, from the head down).	Developing a routine helps to ensure that no exercise will be forgotten.
Unless instructed otherwise, perform the same exercise on each corresponding body part (for example, do the same thing for the right arm that you do for the left).	Exercising corresponding joints equally ensures that both sides of the body remain equally strong and flexible.
Support each joint as you exercise it.	Support reduces discomfort and strain on the joint.
Do not push a joint past its point of resistance.	Each joint has a limit to its range of motion. Attempting to exceed this limit can lead to joint pain and injury.
Watch the person's face for signs of pain or discomfort.	A person may not be able to tell you if what you are doing hurts. Therefore, it is important to watch the person's face for nonverbal cues, such as grimacing or wincing.
Avoid exercising a painful joint.	Exercising a painful joint can cause additional injury.
If you notice sudden, continuous contractions of the related muscles (spasticity), take a break or move the limb more slowly to allow the muscles to recover. Applying gentle pressure to the muscle can also relieve spasticity.	Spasticity is a sign that the muscles are working too hard. It may also indicate that the person is in pain, or that the joint's range of motion has been exceeded.
Expect the person's respiratory rate and heart rate to increase during the exercise. If these vital signs do not return to their normal resting rates after the activity ends, report this to the nurse immediately.	During activity, the tissues require more oxygen and nutrients, so the heart and lungs work harder to supply the tissues. However, once the activity ends, the heart rate and respiratory rate should return to normal because the tissues' demand for oxygen and nutrients will be less.
Encourage the person to help with the exercises as much as possible.	Active participation increases the person's sense of independence and improves function.

People with these risk factors for injury must be monitored especially carefully during the application of heat or cold.

Cold Applications

Cold applications are often used for people who have musculoskeletal injuries resulting from trauma, such as sprains and fractures. Cold applications are also frequently used on incisions following surgical procedures. The application of cold reduces pain and swelling and decreases bleeding. It does this by cooling the skin and underlying tissues, causing the blood vessels to constrict (narrow). Because the blood vessels are constricted, less blood is carried to the tissues, resulting in less bleeding and decreased tissue swelling. The numbing effect of the cold helps to reduce pain.

Cold applications can be either moist or dry (Fig. 25-20). In moist applications, moisture comes in direct contact with the skin. Moist applications allow the cold to penetrate the tissues more quickly and deeply. A cold compress, made by soaking a gauze pad, towel, or washcloth in cold water, wringing it out, and then applying it with pressure to the affected area, is an example of a moist application (see Fig. 25-20A). Procedure 25-2 explains how to give a moist cold application.

Dry applications prevent moisture from coming in direct contact with the skin. Dry applications are usually colder than moist applications. An ice bag is an example of a dry cold application (see Fig. 25-20B). Commercially prepared ice packs that are kept frozen until the time of use are available, or a dry cold application can be made by filling an ice bag with crushed ice and wrapping it in a towel or washcloth. Procedure 25-3 explains how to give a dry cold application.

When applied directly to a person's skin, cold can cause severe burns and blisters. Dry cold applications should be wrapped in a protective cloth to prevent the icy cold plastic from coming in direct contact with the person's skin. If a cold application is left in place for too long, prolonged constriction of the small blood vessels can keep oxygen and nutrients from reaching the skin, resulting in tissue death and skin breakdown. For this reason, cold applications should not be left in place for longer than 20 minutes. Make sure that you check the skin underneath the cold application every 10 minutes and stop the treatment immediately if you observe any evidence of a burn or blister. Pale skin, resulting from the constriction of the blood vessels, should return to its normal colour quickly after the cold application is removed. If it does not, or if you notice a burn or blister starting to develop, inform the nurse immediately. Also, if you have questions about how to apply the cold application or for how long, please ask the nurse for help.

Heat Applications

Although ice may be used initially after an injury or surgical procedure to reduce swelling and pain, heat may be used a day or so later to increase blood flow to the tissues to promote healing. In addition, heat may be used on joints that are painful and stiff as a result of arthritis. Heat relaxes the muscles, relieves pain, and promotes blood flow to the area. When heat is

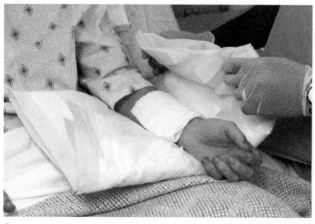

A

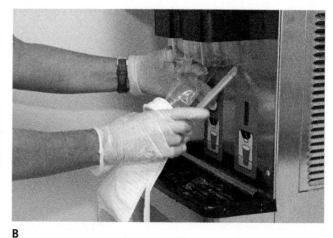

B

Figure 25-20
Cold applications are used to reduce pain and swelling. Cold applications may be either moist or dry. **(A)** A cold compress is a moist cold application. **(B)** An ice bag is a dry cold application.

applied to the skin, the blood vessels dilate (widen), allowing more blood to flow to the tissues. Increased blood flow speeds healing by bringing more oxygen, nutrients, and infection-fighting white blood cells to the area. The increased blood flow helps to reduce swelling by removing excess fluid from the tissues. In addition, heat relaxes the muscles and helps loosen stiff joints.

Like cold applications, heat applications can be either moist or dry (Fig. 25-21), and the applications may be either commercially prepared or homemade. Moist heat penetrates tissues more quickly and deeply than dry heat. Therefore, moist heat applications are used at a lower temperature to reduce the risk of burns. Examples of moist heat applications include warm compresses and hot water soaks (see Fig. 25-21A). Examples of dry heat applications include an electric heating pad or a hot water bottle wrapped in a towel. An Aquamatic pad (or K-pad) is a special type of electric heating pad (see Fig. 25-21B). The pad is connected to a heating unit that heats water to a preset temperature. The water circulates through the pad and then back into the heating device so that a constant temperature is maintained. A key is used to set the temperature, and then the key is removed, preventing anyone from accidentally turning the heat up or down. Procedure 25-4 describes how to apply a dry heat application using an Aquamatic pad.

Burns are the most common complication of heat applications. Some burns, especially on thin, delicate skin, can be very severe, resulting in blistering, tissue loss, and the need for skin grafting. It is common for a person to fall asleep with a heating pad in place and receive a burn from prolonged exposure to the heat. In addition to increasing the person's risk for burns, heat applications that are left in place for too long will eventually cause the blood vessels to constrict, putting the person at risk for tissue breakdown. For these reasons, heat applications should not be left in place for longer than 20 minutes. Make sure that you check the skin underneath the heat application every 5 minutes and stop the treatment immediately if you observe any evidence of burning. Warmth causes the skin to become pink or slightly reddened. Skin that is bright red or very pale could be burned. Report any observations that may indicate a burn to the nurse immediately, along with any complaints of pain, burning, or stinging.

REHABILITATION

Many of your patients or residents with musculoskeletal disorders will require physical, emotional, or vocational rehabilitation (or a combination of the three), as described in Chapter 23. Working to regain or maintain function, or learning to adjust to a loss of function,

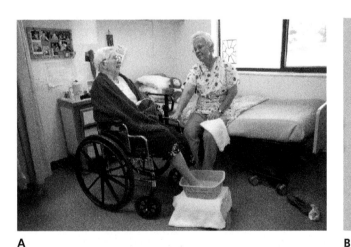
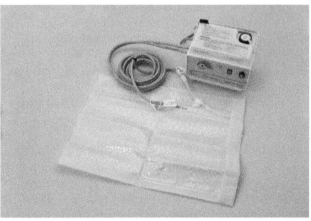

A

B

Figure 25-21
Heat applications are used to relax muscles, relieve pain, and promote blood flow to an area. Heat applications may be either moist or dry. **(A)** A warm soak is an example of a moist heat application. Soaks are done in either a wash basin (if the area to be soaked is small) or a tub (if the area to be soaked is large). **(B)** An Aquamatic pad is an example of a dry heat application. Water is heated in the heating unit. The heated water passes through the tubing and into a network of tubes inside the heating pad. The water never comes in contact with the person's skin.

can be a long, difficult, and painful process. It is very easy for patients or residents to become frustrated and discouraged. Your reassurance and encouragement are necessary to help keep your patients or residents focused. Be an active listener and an attentive observer. If you notice signs of skin breakdown or diminishing mobility, report these observations to the nurse. Make sure you are familiar with the supportive devices, assistive devices, and prosthetic devices used by your patients or residents so that you can assist them properly. Ask the physical therapist or nurse to explain any special procedures or rehabilitation techniques to you. As a personal support worker, there is much you can do to help your patients or residents as they work toward regaining maximum use of their musculoskeletal system.

SUMMARY

- The musculoskeletal system consists of the bones, skeletal muscles, and joints.
  - The primary function of the musculoskeletal system is movement.
    - Joints are the areas where two bones meet. Most movement occurs at freely movable joints.
    - The skeletal muscles attach to the bones. When the muscle contracts (shortens), it pulls against the bone, causing the body part to move.
  - Other functions of the musculoskeletal system include protection, support, heat production, calcium storage, and blood cell production.
- As we age, we lose bone tissue and muscle mass, and our joints begin to show the effects of a lifetime of wear and tear. Consuming a diet rich in calcium, vitamin D, and protein and exercising regularly throughout life can help to delay or decrease the effects of aging on the musculoskeletal system.
- Disorders of the musculoskeletal system can make mobility very difficult.
  - Osteoporosis is the excessive loss of bone tissue, resulting in bones that break very easily.
  - Arthritis is inflammation of the joints.
    - Osteoarthritis typically affects older people. In osteoarthritis, the cartilage that covers the ends of bones is worn away through normal use of the joint. Many people with osteoarthritis have joint replacement surgery to correct the condition.
    - Rheumatoid arthritis is a type of arthritis that affects younger people and can cause severe joint deformities. Rheumatoid arthritis is thought to be an autoimmune disorder, which means

  it is caused by a person's immune system attacking his or her own tissues.
    - Gout is a type of arthritis that results from the build up of uric acid in the joints.
  - Muscular dystrophy is a general term for a group of disorders that cause the skeletal muscles to become very weak over time. Muscular dystrophy is a genetic disorder, which means that it is inherited.
  - Fractures are broken bones.
    - Older people are especially at risk for fractures because of the normal loss of bone tissue that is a part of aging. Fractures may take longer to heal in an older person.
    - Fractures may be treated by casting or by surgical placement of plates, screws, pins, or wires. Traction may be necessary to hold the ends of the broken bone in alignment until the fracture can be permanently repaired.
  - Amputation is the removal of a limb or part of a limb.
    - Amputation may be necessary because of trauma or because of complications related to a medical condition, such as diabetes.
    - Proper care of the stump increases the likelihood that a person can be fitted with a prosthetic limb.
- Range-of-motion exercises, the application of heat or cold, and rehabilitation are measures taken to prevent complications of immobility, relieve musculoskeletal discomfort, and maintain or restore musculoskeletal function.
  - Range-of-motion exercises are used to preserve joint and muscle function in people who have conditions that limit their use of the musculoskeletal system.

Range-of-motion exercises are usually performed at least twice a day.

- Active range-of-motion exercises are performed by the patient or resident.
- Passive range-of-motion exercises are performed by the personal support worker or nurse on behalf of the patient or resident.
- Active-assistive range-of-motion exercises are performed by the patient or resident with some help from the personal support worker or nurse.

- Heat and cold applications can be beneficial for a person with disorders of the musculoskeletal system to help decrease pain and swelling and increase muscle relaxation and joint flexibility. Both heat and cold applications can cause severe injury to a person if they are used inappropriately.
- Rehabilitation is an essential part of the care needed by a person with a musculoskeletal disorder.

PROCEDURE   25-1

Assisting a Person With Passive Range-of-Motion Exercises

WHY YOU DO IT   Range-of-motion exercises help to keep the joints and muscles healthy in people who have a limited ability to move.

Getting Ready WORKIEDS

1. Complete the "Getting Ready" steps.

Supplies

- bath blanket

Procedure

2. Make sure that the bed is positioned at a comfortable working height (to promote good body mechanics) and that the wheels are locked. If the side rails are in use, lower the side rail on the working side of the bed. The side rail on the opposite side of the bed should remain up. Raise or lower the head of the bed to a horizontal or semi-Fowler's position.

3. Assist the person into the supine position.

4. Spread the bath blanket over the top linens (and the person). If the person is able, have him hold the bath blanket. If not, tuck the corners under his shoulders. Fanfold the top linens to the foot of the bed.

5. Perform each range-of-motion exercise in steps 6 through 13 according to the person's care plan, being careful to expose only the part of the body that is being exercised. Repeat each exercise three to five times, as written in the care plan.

6. If your facility permits, exercise the person's neck:

    a. Forward and backward flexion and extension (neck). Support the person's head by putting one hand under his chin and the other on the back of the head. Gently bring the head forward, as if to touch the chin to the chest, and then

bring it backward, chin pointing to the sky.

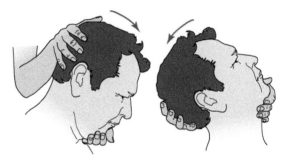

Step 6a Gently bring the head forward, then backward.

    b. Side-to-side flexion (neck). Support the person's head by putting one hand under his chin and the other near the opposite temple. Gently tilt the head toward the right shoulder and then toward the left.

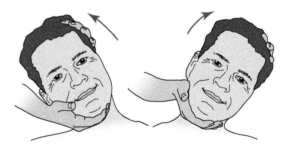

Step 6b Gently tilt the head toward the right shoulder, then the left.

    c. Rotation (neck). Support the person's head by putting one hand under his chin and the other on the back of the head. Gently move the head from side to side, as if the person were shaking his head "no."

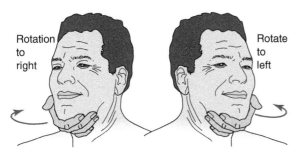

Step 6c Gently move the head from side to side.

7. Exercise the person's shoulder:

a. Forward flexion and extension (shoulder). Support the person's arm by putting one hand under his elbow and the other under his wrist. Keeping the person's arm straight with the palm facing down, lift the arm up so that it is alongside his ear and then return it to its original position.

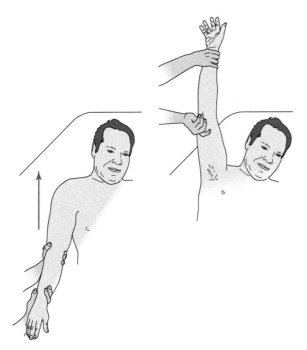

Step 7a Lift the arm up so that it is alongside the person's ear, then return it to its original position.

b. Abduction and adduction (shoulder). Support the person's arm by putting one hand under his elbow and the other under his wrist. Keeping the person's arm straight with the palm facing up, move his arm away from the side of his body and then return it to its original position.

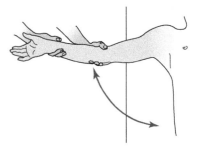

Step 7b Move the arm away from the person's side, then return it to its original position.

c. Horizontal abduction and adduction (shoulder). Support the person's arm by putting one hand under his elbow and the other under his wrist. Keeping the person's arm straight with the palm facing up, move his arm away from the side of his body. Gently bending the person's elbow, touch his hand to the opposite shoulder, then straighten the elbow and bring the arm back out to the side.

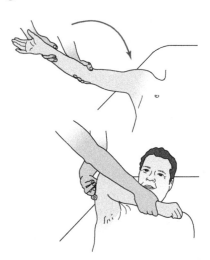

Step 7c Move the arm away from the person's side, then touch the person's hand to the opposite shoulder.

d. Rotation (shoulder). Support the person's arm by putting one hand under his elbow and the other under his wrist. Move the person's arm away from the side of his body and bend his arm at the elbow. Gently move the person's forearm up so that it forms a right angle with the mattress and then back down. This movement is similar to the motion a police officer makes when he or she is signaling someone to stop.

(continued)

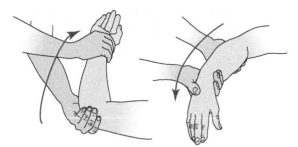

Step 7d Move the person's forearm up, then back down.

8. Exercise the person's elbow.

   a. Flexion and extension (elbow). Support the person's arm by putting one hand under his elbow and the other under his wrist. Starting with the person's arm straight and with the palm facing up, bend his elbow so that his hand moves toward his shoulder. Then, straighten out the elbow, returning the person's hand to its original position.

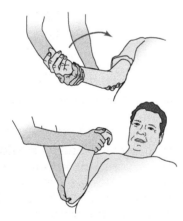

Step 8a Bend the arm so that the hand moves toward the shoulder, then return it to its original position.

   b. Pronation and supination (elbow). Support the person's arm by putting one hand under his elbow and the other under his wrist. Move the person's arm away from the side of his body and slightly bend his arm at the elbow. Gently move the person's forearm up so that it forms a right angle with the mattress. Gently turn the person's hand so that the palm is facing the end of the bed. Then turn the hand the other way so that the palm is facing the head of the bed.

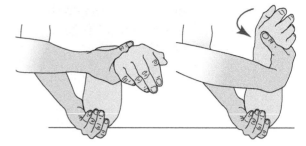

Step 8b Turn the hand so that the palm is facing the end of the bed, then turn the hand the other way so that the palm is facing the head of the bed.

9. Exercise the person's wrist.

   a. Flexion and extension (wrist). Support the person's wrist with one hand. Use the other hand to gently bend the person's hand down and then back.

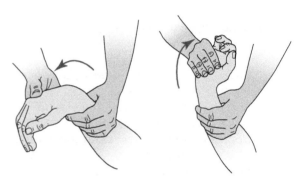

Step 9a Gently bend the person's hand down, then back.

   b. Radial and ulnar flexion (wrist). Support the person's wrist with one hand. Use the other hand to gently turn the person's hand toward his thumb. Then turn the hand the other way, toward the little finger.

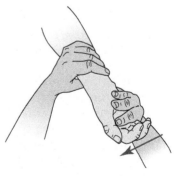

Step 9b Gently turn the person's hand one way, then the other.

10. Exercise the person's fingers and thumb.

a. Flexion and extension (fingers and thumb). Support the person's wrist with one hand. Using your other hand, flex the person's fingers to make a fist, tucking his thumb under the fingers. Then straighten each finger and the thumb, one by one.

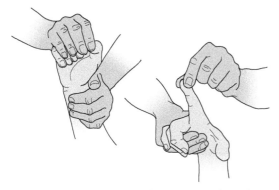

Step 10a Flex the person's fingers to make a fist, then straighten each finger and thumb, one by one.

b. Abduction and adduction (fingers and thumb). With one hand, hold the person's thumb and index finger together. With the other hand, move the middle finger away from the index finger. Then move the middle finger back toward the index finger and hold the middle finger, index finger, and thumb together. Next, move the ring finger away from the other two fingers and thumb, then move it back toward the group. Do the same with the little finger. Finally, reverse the process. Hold the little finger and the ring finger together and move the middle finger away and back. Complete with the index finger and thumb.

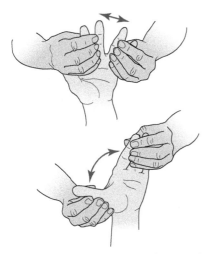

Step 10b Spread the fingers away from each other, then back together again.

c. Flexion and extension (thumb). Bend the person's thumb into his palm, then return it to its original position.

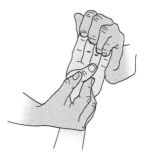

Step 10c Bend the thumb into the palm, then return it to its original position.

d. Opposition. Touch each fingertip to the thumb.

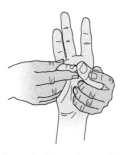

Step 10d Touch each fingertip to the thumb.

11. Exercise the person's hip and knee.

a. Forward flexion and extension (hip and knee). Support the person's leg by putting one hand under his knee and the other under his ankle. Gently bend the person's knee, moving it toward his head. Then straighten the person's knee and gently lower the leg to the bed.

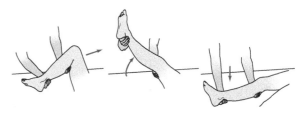

Step 11a Gently bend the knee, moving it toward the head. Then straighten the leg and lower it to the bed.

b. Abduction and adduction (hip). Support the person's leg by putting one hand under his knee and the other under his

(continued)

ankle. Keeping the person's leg straight, move his leg away from the side of his body and then return it to its original position.

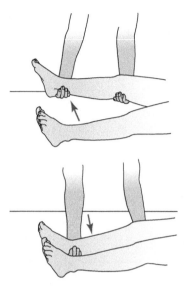

Step 11b Move the leg away from the person's side, then return it to its original position.

c. **Rotation (hip).** Support the person's leg by putting one hand under his knee and the other under his ankle. Keeping the person's leg straight, gently turn the leg inward and then outward.

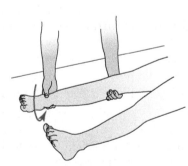

Step 11c Gently turn the leg inward, then outward.

12. Exercise the person's ankle and foot.
   a. **Dorsiflexion and plantar flexion (ankle and foot).** Support the person's ankle with one hand. Use the other hand to gently bend the person's foot up toward the head and then back.

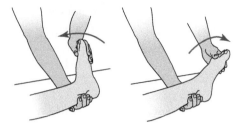

Step 12a Gently bend the foot toward the head, then back.

b. **Inversion and eversion (ankle and foot).** Support the person's ankle with one hand. Use the other hand to gently turn the inside of the foot inward and then outward.

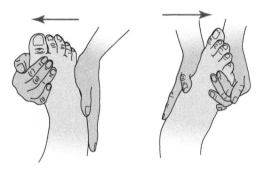

Step 12b Gently bend the foot inward, then outward.

13. Exercise the person's toes.
   a. **Flexion and extension (toes).** Put one hand under the person's foot. Put the other hand over the person's toes. Curl the toes downward and then straighten them.

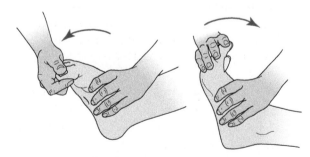

Step 13a Curl the toes downward, then straighten them.

b. **Abduction and adduction (toes).** Spread each toe the same way you spread each finger in step 10b.

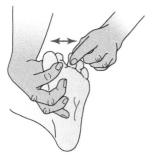

Step 13b Spread the toes away from each other, then back together again.

14. Straighten the bed linens and make sure the person is comfortable and in good body alignment. Draw the top linens over the person and remove the bath blanket.

15. If the side rails are in use, raise the side rail on the working side of the bed. Make sure that the bed is lowered to its lowest position and that the wheels are locked.

Finishing Up CLSOWR

16. Complete the "Finishing Up" steps.

PROCEDURE 25-2

Giving a Moist Cold Application

WHY YOU DO IT   Cold applications reduce pain and swelling and decrease bleeding.

Getting Ready WGKIEPS

1. Complete the "Getting Ready" steps.

Supplies

- bed protector
- compress (for example, 4 × 4 gauze pad or washcloth)
- rolled gauze or ties (optional)
- bath basin
- ice
- bath towel

Procedure

2. Put the ice in the bath basin and fill the basin with cold water at the sink.

3. Make sure that the bed is positioned at a comfortable working height (to promote good body mechanics) and that the wheels are locked.

4. Help the person to a comfortable position and expose only the area to be treated.

5. Position the bed protector as necessary to keep the bed linens dry.

6. Moisten the compress with the ice water as ordered. Wring out the compress and apply it to the treatment site.

7. Leave the compress in place for the designated amount of time, usually 15 to 20 minutes. The compress may be secured in place with ties or rolled gauze, or the patient or resident may assist by holding the compress in place.

   a. Keep the compress moistened with ice water.

   b. Check the skin beneath the compress every 10 minutes. If the skin appears pale or blue or if the person complains of numbness or a burning sensation, discontinue treatment immediately and notify the nurse.

   c. If you must leave the room, place the call light control within easy reach and ask the person to signal if he or she experiences numbness or burning.

8. When the treatment is complete, remove the compress and carefully dry the skin.

9. Remove the bed protector. Straighten the bed linens and make sure the person is comfortable and in good body alignment. Draw the top linens over the person.

10. Make sure that the bed is lowered to its lowest position and that the wheels are locked.

11. Gather the soiled linens and place them in the linen hamper. Dispose of disposable items in a facility-approved waste container. Clean equipment and return it to the storage area.

Finishing Up CLSOWR

12. Complete the "Finishing Up" steps.

PROCEDURE 25-3

Giving a Dry Cold Application

WHY YOU DO IT   Cold applications reduce pain and swelling and decrease bleeding.

Getting Ready WCKIEpS

1. Complete the "Getting Ready" steps.

Supplies

- paper towels
- rolled gauze or ties (optional)
- crushed ice
- ice bag
- towel

Procedure

2. Fill the ice bag with water, close it, and turn it upside down to check for leaks. Empty the bag.

3. Fill the bag one-half to two-thirds full with crushed ice. Do not overfill the ice bag. Squeeze the bag to force out excess air, and close the bag.

4. Dry the outside of the bag with the paper towels and wrap it in the towel.

5. Make sure that the bed is positioned at a comfortable working height (to promote good body mechanics) and that the wheels are locked.

6. Help the person to a comfortable position and expose only the area to be treated.

7. Apply the ice bag to the treatment site.

8. Leave the compress in place for the designated amount of time, usually 15 to 20 minutes. The compress may be secured in place with ties or rolled gauze, or the patient or resident may assist by holding the compress in place.

   a. Check the skin beneath the ice bag every 10 minutes. If the skin appears pale or blue or if the person complains of numbness or a burning sensation, discontinue treatment immediately and notify the nurse.

   b. Refill the bag with ice as necessary.

   c. If you must leave the room, place the call-light control within easy reach and ask the person to signal if he or she experiences numbness or burning.

9. When the treatment is complete, remove the ice bag.

10. Straighten the bed linens and make sure the person is comfortable and in good body alignment. Draw the top linens over the person.

11. Make sure that the bed is lowered to its lowest position and that the wheels are locked.

12. Gather the soiled linens and place them in the linen hamper. Dispose of disposable items in a facility-approved waste container. Clean equipment and return it to the storage area.

Finishing Up CLSOWR

13. Complete the "Finishing Up" steps.

PROCEDURE 25-4

Giving a Dry Heat Application With an Aquamatic Pad

WHY YOU DO IT   Heat applications relax the muscles, relieve pain, and promote blood flow to the area.

Getting Ready WGKIEPS

1. Complete the "Getting Ready" steps.

Supplies

- aquamatic pad
- heating unit
- distilled water
- cover
- ties or tape

Procedure

2. Check the pad for leaks. Make sure that the cord is not frayed and the plug is in good condition. Check the heating unit to be sure that it is filled with water. If you need to fill it, use distilled water. Tap water contains minerals that can corrode the unit.

3. Place the heating unit so that the tubing and pad are level with the heating unit at all times. Make sure that the tubing is free of kinks. Plug the cord into an outlet.

4. Allow the water to warm to the desired temperature, as specified by the nurse or the care plan. If the temperature is not preset, set the temperature with the key and then remove the key.

5. Place the pad in its cover.

6. Make sure that the bed is positioned at a comfortable working height (to promote good body mechanics) and that the wheels are locked.

7. Help the person to a comfortable position and expose only the area to be treated.

8. Apply the pad to the treatment site.

9. Leave the pad in place for the designated amount of time, usually 15 to 20 minutes.

The pad may be secured in place with ties or tape, or the patient or resident may assist by holding the pad in place. (Do not use pins to secure the pad. Pins can puncture the pad, causing it to leak.)

a. Check the skin beneath the pad every 5 minutes. If the skin appears red, swollen, or blistered or if the person complains of pain, numbness, or discomfort, discontinue treatment immediately and notify the nurse.

b. Refill the heating unit if the water level drops below the fill line.

c. If you must leave the room, place the call-light control within easy reach and ask the person to signal if he or she experiences numbness or burning.

10. When the treatment is complete, remove the pad.

11. Straighten the bed linens and make sure the person is comfortable and in good body alignment. Draw the top linens over the person.

12. Make sure that the bed is lowered to its lowest position and that the wheels are locked.

13. Gather the soiled linens and place them in the linen hamper. Dispose of disposable items in a facility-approved waste container. Clean equipment and return it to the storage area.

Finishing Up CLSOWR

14. Complete the "Finishing Up" steps.

WHAT DID YOU LEARN?

Multiple Choice

Select the single best answer for each of the following questions.

1. When a muscle atrophies, it:
   a. Becomes larger and stronger
   b. Becomes thinner and weaker
   c. Becomes stiffer
   d. Becomes more flexible

2. Which musculoskeletal disorder causes severe joint deformities and often affects younger people?
   a. Osteoarthritis
   b. Rheumatoid arthritis
   c. Multiple sclerosis
   d. Muscular dystrophy

3. What is the term for a fracture where the broken ends of the bone do not penetrate the skin?
   a. Impacted fracture
   b. Comminuted fracture
   c. Spiral fracture
   d. Closed fracture

4. Excessive loss of bone tissue is:
   a. Osteoarthritis
   b. Osteoporosis
   c. A normal effect of aging
   d. Gout

5. What does the skeletal system do?
   a. It acts as a storage site for calcium
   b. It works with the muscles to produce movement
   c. It produces blood cells
   d. All of the above

6. Ms. Vaughn broke her leg while skiing. Surgery is required to align the broken bone, and then the bone fragments are held together with metal plates and screws. What is the name of the procedure Ms. Vaughn has had?
   a. Open fracture, internal fixation
   b. Open reduction, internal fixation
   c. Open reduction, external fixation
   d. Traction

7. What does the muscular system do?
   a. It produces heat
   b. It helps to maintain posture
   c. It works with bones to produce movement
   d. All of the above

8. The purpose of cold applications is usually to:
   a. Prevent heat exhaustion
   b. Speed the flow of blood to an injured area
   c. Prevent swelling
   d. Prevent the formation of scar tissue

9. What is a heat application used for?
   a. To relieve muscle spasms
   b. To reduce pain
   c. To promote circulation and speed healing
   d. All of the above

10. Mr. Owen has severe osteoarthritis in his hips. You are caring for Mr. Owen following his hip replacement surgery. What do you need to remember?
    a. Mr. Owen's legs must always be kept together (adducted).
    b. When assisting Mr. Owen with range-of-motion exercises, make sure to flex the hips beyond 90 degrees to maintain flexibility in the joint.
    c. Mr. Owen should use an abduction pillow to keep his legs spread apart when he is in a supine or lateral position.
    d. Mr. Owen should be encouraged to get up and walk around within a day or two of the surgery.

11. Ms. Curtis has just had a cast put on her leg following a horseback riding accident. What should you remember when you are helping Ms. Curtis?
    a. Ms. Curtis's leg should not be elevated.
    b. You should check Ms. Curtis's toes frequently to make sure that the cast is not too tight.
    c. Ms. Curtis should be reminded that if the skin underneath the cast begins to itch, she can slide a tongue depressor inside the cast to scratch the itchy area.
    d. Ms. Curtis should be encouraged to get out of bed and take a shower as soon as the cast dries.

12. Mr. Jefferson has poorly controlled diabetes. He injured his toe, resulting in a severe infection. Now his toes are completely black as a result of gangrene. What is the most likely treatment for Mr. Jefferson's toe?
    a. Outside reduction, internal fixation (ORIF)
    b. Amputation of the toe
    c. Casting of the foot
    d. Application of heat

Matching

Match each numbered item with its appropriate lettered description.

F 1. Flexion/extension

C 2. Supination/pronation

D 3. Dorsiflexion/plantar flexion

E 4. Rotation

B 5. Abduction/adduction

A 6. Inversion/eversion

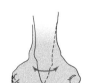
a.

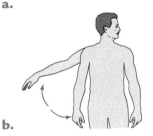
b.

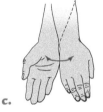
c.

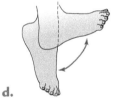
d.

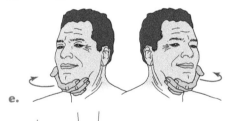
e.

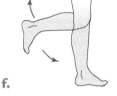
f.

STOP and Think!

You are assigned to care for Mr. Kuhlman. Mr. Kuhlman is 85 years old and fairly healthy, but he does have arthritis. One of your responsibilities is to assist Mr. Kuhlman to the dining room for meals. Today, while you are walking Mr. Kuhlman to breakfast, you notice that he is limping a bit and trying not to put weight on his left leg. You ask him if he is in pain, and he says, "I'm fine; it's just old age." What should you do?

You are caring for Mrs. Lasorda, who has crippling rheumatoid arthritis. She has many "good" days when she is able to manage her personal care and get around pretty well. This week, however, she is having a severe flare-up of her illness. What are some measures that you may be asked to do to help Mrs. Lasorda be more comfortable and prevent the loss of joint mobility?

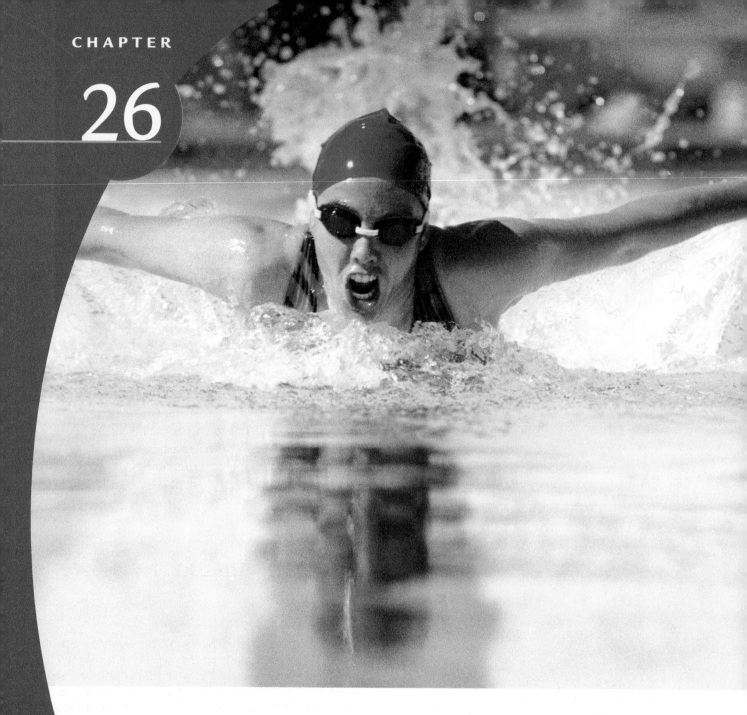

The Respiratory System

WHAT WILL YOU LEARN?

Have you ever heard the phrase, "It's as natural as breathing"? Breathing is certainly something that many of us take for granted, because we don't have to think about it. Air enters and leaves our lungs without any conscious effort on our part. With each breath, life-giving oxygen is delivered to the body, and carbon dioxide, a waste product of cellular

Photo: A swimmer comes up for air. Human beings need oxygen to live.

metabolism, is removed from the body. Breathing is the function of the respiratory system, the subject of this chapter. When you are finished with this chapter, you will be able to:

1. List and describe the main parts of the respiratory system.
2. Discuss the main functions of the respiratory system.
3. Describe how normal aging processes affect the respiratory system.
4. Describe some of the disorders that can affect the respiratory system.
5. Describe how oxygen therapy is used to assist a person with respiration.
6. Describe the guidelines that a personal support worker should follow when caring for patients or residents who are receiving oxygen therapy.
7. Discuss other methods used to help a person who is having trouble with respiration.

Vocabulary

Mucous membrane	Bronchioles	Asthma	Facemask
Mucus	Alveoli (alveolus)	Chronic obstructive	Nasopharyngeal
Nasal cavity	Gas exchange	pulmonary disease	airway
Pharyngitis	Pleura	(COPD)	Oropharyngeal
Pharynx	Diaphragm	Emphysema	airway
Larynx	Pneumonia	Chronic bronchitis	Mechanical
Laryngitis	Sputum	Pneumothorax	ventilation
Trachea	Hemoptysis	Hemothorax	Endotracheal tube
Bronchi (bronchus)	Pleurisy	Respiratory therapy	Tracheostomy
Lungs	Bronchitis	Flow metre	Suctioning
Respiration	Influenza	Nasal cannula	Hypoxic

STRUCTURE OF THE RESPIRATORY SYSTEM

The respiratory system consists of the lungs and a series of passages, collectively referred to as the *airway* (Fig. 26-1). You may hear people refer to the "upper respiratory tract" and the "lower respiratory tract." The upper respiratory tract consists of the structures located outside of the chest cavity (the nasal cavity, pharynx, and larynx). The lower respiratory tract consists of the structures located inside the chest cavity (the trachea, bronchi, bronchioles, and lungs).

AIRWAY

The purpose of the airway is to move air from the outside of the body to the lungs, and from the lungs to the outside of the body. The airway consists of a series of passages that become smaller in diameter as they approach the lungs. These passages are lined with a **mucous membrane,** a special type of epithelial tissue that lines many of the organ systems in the body. The surface of the membrane is kept moist by **mucus,** a slippery, sticky substance that is secreted by special cells.

Nasal Cavity

Air enters the body through the nostrils and passes into the **nasal cavity,** which is lined by a mucous membrane and coarse hairs. The coarse hairs and the mucous membrane help to trap dirt, dust, microbes, and other foreign particles, preventing these substances from entering the delicate lungs. The plentiful blood vessels in the mucous membrane transfer body heat to the air, warming it up to a comfortable temperature. In addition, the air picks up some of the moisture from the warm, moist nasal cavity. Warm, moist air is less likely than cold, dry air to damage the delicate lung tissue.

Pharynx

When you have a "sore throat," the part of your body that hurts is your pharynx. (You may have heard the term **pharyngitis,** which means inflammation of the pharynx, or a sore throat.) Both the nasal cavities and the oral cavity open into the **pharynx,** or throat region (see Fig. 26-1).

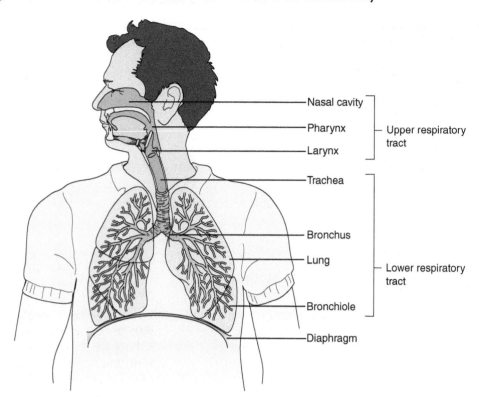

Nasal cavity ⎤
Pharynx   ⎬ Upper respiratory tract
Larynx   ⎦

Trachea   ⎤

Bronchus

Lung   ⎬ Lower respiratory tract

Bronchiole ⎦

Diaphragm

Figure 26-1
The respiratory system consists of the lungs and a series of passages collectively referred to as the "airway." The structures that form the airway include the nasal cavity, pharynx, larynx, trachea, bronchi, and bronchioles. Disorders of the respiratory tract are often said to affect either the "upper respiratory tract" or the "lower respiratory tract." The upper respiratory tract consists of those structures located outside the chest cavity, while the lower respiratory tract consists of those structures located inside the chest cavity.

This means that air passes through the pharynx on its way to the lungs, and food and fluids pass through the pharynx on their way to the stomach. This sharing of space is convenient when you have a stuffy nose, because it means that you have another way to get air into your body (that is, through your mouth). However, this sharing of space can also lead to complications, such as choking, which occurs when you try to breathe and swallow at the same time. The pharynx is divided into three sections: the nasopharynx (located right behind the nasal cavities), the oropharynx (located behind the mouth), and the laryngeal pharynx (located above the larynx).

Larynx

From the pharynx, air passes into the **larynx.** The opening of the larynx is covered by a flap of cartilage called the *epiglottis*, which snaps shut when you swallow, closing off the opening and preventing food from passing into the lower respiratory tract.

In addition to serving as part of the airway, the larynx is the organ responsible for speech. The larynx, often referred to as the "voice box," contains the vocal cords. When air flows over the vocal cords, it causes them to vibrate, producing sound. Humans and other animals make recognizable sounds by controlling the flow of air over the vocal cords. An inflammation of the larynx, or **laryngitis,** usually affects a person's ability to talk.

Trachea and Bronchi

The **trachea,** also called the "windpipe," is the passage that carries air from the larynx down into the chest toward the lungs. "C"-shaped rings of cartilage give the trachea its characteristic ridged appearance (see Fig. 26-1). These cartilage rings support the trachea and keep it open. At its lower end, the trachea divides into two separate passages called the **bronchi** (singular, **bronchus**). One bronchus goes to the right lung and the other goes to the left lung.

The mucous membrane lining of the trachea and bronchi contains millions of tiny hair-like structures called *cilia.* The cilia constantly move in a waving or beating fashion, moving mucus upward toward the pharynx so that it can be coughed up and removed from the respiratory tract along with any trapped particles or microbes.

LUNGS

The **lungs** are the main organs of **respiration,** the process the body uses to obtain oxygen from the environment and remove carbon dioxide (a waste gas) from the body. Once inside the lungs, the bronchi divide into smaller and smaller branches called **bronchioles** (Fig. 26-2). There are more than a million bronchioles in each lung! At the end of each bronchiole, there is a grape-like cluster of tiny air sacs called **alveoli** (singular, **alveolus**). Each alveolus is surrounded by a

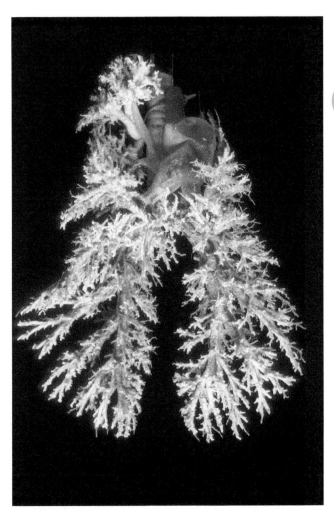

Figure 26-2
A resin cast of human lungs clearly shows the trachea, bronchi, and bronchioles. (© A. Siegel/Custom Medical Stock Photo.)

network of tiny blood vessels (Fig. 26-3). The transfer of oxygen into the blood, and carbon dioxide out of it, occurs in the alveoli. This process is called **gas exchange,** and it is described in more detail later in this chapter. The tissue of healthy lungs is elastic (stretchy) and sponge-like, because of all of the air-filled alveoli. The many blood vessels that surround the alveoli give healthy lung tissue its brilliant pink colour.

The lungs are divided into sections called *lobes.* The right lung has three lobes and the left lung has only two. The left lung is slightly smaller than the right lung because of the position of the heart in the chest cavity.

The lungs are located in the chest cavity. The inside of the chest cavity is lined with a membrane called the **pleura,** which also covers the outside of the lungs. Because the lungs almost fill the chest cavity, the pleura on the outside of the lungs almost touches the pleura on the inside of

the chest cavity. The pleura secretes a thin fluid that allows the lungs to slide easily against the chest cavity walls during the process of breathing.

FUNCTION OF THE RESPIRATORY SYSTEM

The main purpose of the respiratory system is respiration. Respiration is accomplished through the processes of ventilation and gas exchange.

VENTILATION

Ventilation is the mechanical process of moving air in and out of the lungs (breathing). Ventilation has two phases: inhalation and exhalation. The **diaphragm** is a strong, dome-shaped muscle that separates the chest cavity from the abdominal cavity (see Fig. 26-1). When we inhale, the diaphragm contracts, moving downward and making the chest cavity bigger. Air flows into the lungs, filling the alveoli and causing them to expand. When we exhale, the diaphragm relaxes, moving upward and pushing the air in the alveoli out of the lungs. Another group of muscles, called the *intercostal muscles,* helps with the respiratory effort as well. The intercostal muscles are located between the ribs.

The rate and depth of breathing is controlled mainly by the central nervous system, in the part of the brain called the *medulla.* Special cells, called *chemoreceptors,* are located in the medulla and in some of the major arteries. The chemoreceptors monitor the amount of carbon dioxide and oxygen in the blood and adjust the rate and depth of breathing as necessary. For example, if you are resting quietly, your body does not need as much oxygen and the amount of air inhaled and exhaled is minimal. But, if you are exercising, your body's need for oxygen is greatly increased, and ventilation increases as well. Although the brain ensures that breathing occurs automatically, the individual also has some control over breathing (for example, when you hold your breath while swimming).

GAS EXCHANGE

So, we now know how air moves in and out of the lungs. But just moving air in and out of the lungs is not enough. How does oxygen get from the air into the blood? How does the carbon dioxide in the blood get into the air we exhale? This is where the second phase of respiration, gas exchange, comes into play.

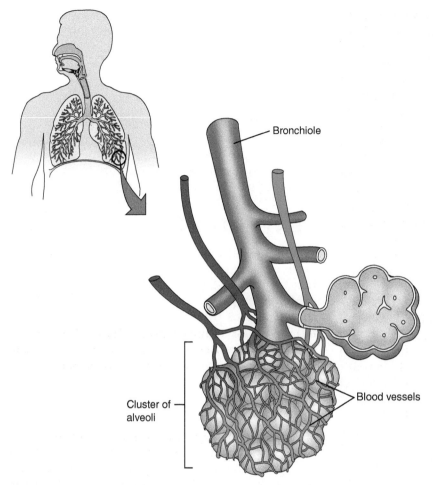

Figure 26-3
A cluster of air sacs, called alveoli, is found at the end of each bronchiole. The alveoli are surrounded by tiny blood vessels, which make gas exchange between the blood and the lungs possible.

Gas exchange occurs in the alveoli (Fig. 26-4). The walls of the alveoli are very thin—just one cell thick. Each alveolus is surrounded by a network of tiny blood vessels. The walls of the blood vessels are very thin too. As the blood passes through the blood vessels, it is brought very close to the air in the alveolus. Because the concentration of oxygen is greater in the air than it is in the blood, the oxygen in the air moves (diffuses) across the wall of the alveolus into the blood vessel, oxygenating the blood. At the same time, carbon dioxide moves from the blood (where it is more concentrated) into the alveolus, and is removed from the body when we exhale.

THE EFFECTS OF AGING ON THE RESPIRATORY SYSTEM

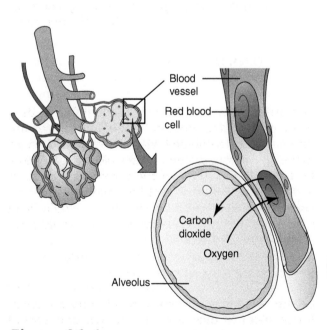

Figure 26-4
Gas exchange occurs in the alveoli. Oxygen moves from the alveolus into the blood vessel, and carbon dioxide moves from the blood vessel into the alveolus.

There is a good chance that many of the older people you will care for will have some type of respiratory problem. When the processes of aging are combined with chronic illness, immobility, or a lifetime of exposure to toxic chemicals (such as those in pollution and tobacco smoke), the respiratory system's ability to function properly is significantly reduced. For example, many people who are in their 60s, 70s, and 80s today began to smoke before anyone really knew about the harmful effects of tobacco smoke. In addition, many older people worked before regulations such as those resulting from the Canadian Centre for Occupational Health and Safety (CCOHS) were in place to keep them safe on the job. As a result, many were exposed to substances in the workplace that we now know are very harmful to the lungs, such as asbestos and coal dust.

When we inhale toxic substances (such as those in tobacco smoke and polluted air) day after day, the delicate membranes inside the lungs and airways become inflamed and stay that way. The chronic inflammation leads to scarring and may even cause changes that lead to cancer. In addition, chemicals in tobacco smoke paralyze the tiny cilia that line the trachea and bronchi. Recall that the purpose of the cilia is to sweep mucus upward, toward the pharynx, so that it can be eliminated from the respiratory tract. When the cilia are no longer able to perform this function because they have been paralyzed by tobacco smoke, the person must work harder to keep the airway and lungs clear of mucus. These attempts to keep the airway clear are what many of us know as a "smoker's cough." Fortunately, if a person is able to stop smoking, the cilia do regain their function and the tissues of the lungs will heal if the damage is not too severe.

Regular physical exercise and avoidance of tobacco smoke and other pollutants help to keep the respiratory system functioning properly well into old age (Fig. 26-5). However, as a person ages, there are two changes that are likely to occur to the respiratory system, even if the person is otherwise healthy. These changes include less efficient ventilation and an increased risk for respiratory tract infections.

LESS EFFICIENT VENTILATION

As you have learned in other chapters, loss of tissue elasticity and loss of muscle mass occur as a person ages. In the respiratory system, these changes result in less efficient ventilation. The very elastic lung tissue loses some of its ability to expand and bounce back as a person breathes, which reduces the amount of air that is taken in and let out with each breath. The diaphragm and intercostal muscles become weaker, which means

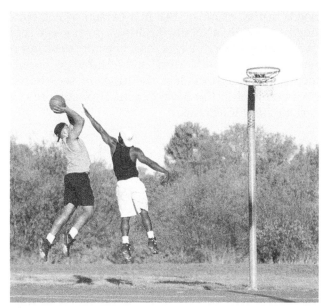

Figure 26-5
Exercise, especially when combined with avoidance of smoking and exposure to pollution, is a most effective way of keeping the respiratory system healthy for many years.

that the chest cavity may not expand as much with each breath, so the amount of air taken in will be smaller. However, in healthy older people who do not smoke, these changes do not usually cause any problems. Often, the person will not be aware of any change, except possibly during exercise, when oxygen demands are significantly increased.

INCREASED RISK OF RESPIRATORY INFECTIONS

The immune system becomes less efficient as a result of the aging process. This change in the immune system, combined with age-related changes to the respiratory system, makes older people more likely to get infections of the respiratory tract. In addition, a respiratory tract infection is likely to be more severe in an older person than it would be in a younger person. For example, what would have been a mild respiratory infection in a younger person can easily become a life-threatening respiratory infection in an elderly person.

Immobility also puts the older adult at higher risk for developing a severe respiratory infection. Many older people are less active because of changes in other body systems or because of chronic illness. In physically active people, the lungs are "exercised" along with the body, as they fully expand to meet the person's increased oxygen needs during exercise. But in a person who is confined to bed or a chair, the lungs do not get this "workout." A person who has become weak as a result of immobility may not be able to cough forcefully enough to clear the lungs of secretions. This can lead to the development of pneumonia, a serious lung infection.

DISORDERS OF THE RESPIRATORY SYSTEM

INFECTIONS

Pneumonia

Pneumonia is an inflammation of the lung tissue. It may be caused by infection with a virus or a bacterium. The infection causes the alveoli to fill with fluid and pus, which prevents air from entering the alveoli. As a result, gas exchange (the transfer of oxygen into the blood and carbon dioxide out of it) cannot occur.

Aspiration pneumonia occurs when foreign material (such as food, formula, saliva, or vomit) is inhaled into the lungs. The foreign material can damage the lung tissue, causing the alveoli to fill with fluid. The foreign material can also carry bacteria into the lungs, leading to bacterial pneumonia. Patients and residents who are receiving enteral nutrition (tube feedings) or who are unconscious are at increased risk for developing aspiration pneumonia because they are unable to protect their airway (by coughing or gagging).

Signs and symptoms of pneumonia include fever, pain when breathing, cyanosis (bluish skin as a result of decreased oxygen levels in the blood), and a productive cough. A productive cough is one in which a person coughs up sputum. **Sputum,** which is also known as "phlegm," consists of mucus and other respiratory secretions that are coughed up from the lungs, bronchi, and trachea. **Hemoptysis** is the coughing up of blood or blood-stained sputum (*hem* means "blood," and *-ptysis* means "to spit"). Hemoptysis may be seen in pneumonia, and can also occur with other respiratory disorders.

Pneumonia is usually diagnosed with a chest x-ray and treated with antibiotics. Knowledge about which microbe is causing the pneumonia will allow the doctor to prescribe the most effective antibiotic therapy. You may be asked to assist by collecting a sputum specimen for analysis. Guidelines for collecting sputum specimens are given in Guidelines Box 26-1.

Pleurisy is an inflammation of the pleura, the membrane that lines the chest cavity and covers the lungs. Pleurisy often accompanies lower respiratory tract infections such as pneumonia. The inflammation of the pleura causes pain during breathing as the layers of membrane rub against each other when the lungs expand and relax. Fluid may also collect in the space between the chest cavity and the lung. This build-up of fluid prevents the lungs from expanding fully. The doctor may need to insert a needle into the chest cavity to drain the fluid.

Bronchitis

Bronchitis is an inflammation of the bronchi. Like pneumonia, bronchitis can be caused by a viral or bacterial infection. Bronchitis may cause a dry, nonproductive cough that sounds like a "bark." Bacterial bronchitis is usually treated with antibiotics. Both bacterial and viral bronchitis can turn into pneumonia if the bronchial infection is not treated promptly.

Influenza

Influenza, commonly referred to as "the flu," is an acute respiratory infection caused by the influenza virus. You are probably already familiar with symptoms of the flu: sore throat, dry cough, stuffy nose, headache, body aches, weakness, and fever. Influenza is different from the "common cold," which can be caused by many different types of viruses and usually only affects the upper respiratory tract.

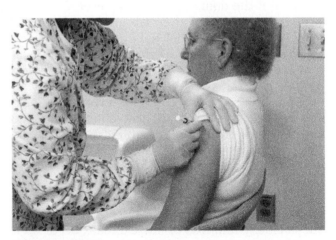

Figure 26-6

Flu shots are usually given to residents in the fall, before the start of flu season (November through April). Flu shots help to prevent infection with the influenza virus, which is very contagious and can cause serious complications in elderly people, very young children, and people with chronic illnesses.

Guidelines Box 26-1 Guidelines for Collecting a Sputum Specimen

WHAT YOU DO	WHY YOU DO IT
Explain to the person that the sputum for the specimen should be coughed up from deep down in the respiratory tract.	The sputum for analysis must come from the lungs, because that is where most of the infection-causing microbes are located. Explaining this to the person helps to ensure that he produces a specimen that will result in an accurate diagnosis. If you do not explain this to the person, he may just cough up saliva, which will not result in an accurate diagnosis.
Provide privacy.	Having to spit mucus into a cup can be embarrassing and unpleasant for some people.
Have the person rinse her mouth with water before coughing up the specimen.	Rinsing with plain water helps to remove microbes that are normally present in the mouth, resulting in a "cleaner" specimen.
Do not have the person rinse with mouthwash before coughing up the specimen.	The antiseptic effects of the mouthwash might actually kill the microbes in the sputum specimen that are responsible for the infection, which will result in inaccurate test results.
Have the person spit the specimen directly into a sterile specimen container and close the lid.	Having the person spit directly into the sterile specimen container reduces the risk of contaminating the specimen and results in more accurate test results.
Make sure that the specimen container is labelled properly and that the information is correct.	Labelling errors can result in misdiagnosis or the need to repeat the test.
Take the specimen container to the laboratory immediately after collecting the specimen or ask the nurse how to store it.	Allowing a specimen to sit around or storing it the incorrect way can result in the need to repeat the test.

The influenza virus is very contagious. Most people who get the flu will recover in about a week. However, elderly people, very young children, and people with chronic illnesses who get the flu are at risk for developing serious complications, such as an extremely severe form of pneumonia. Residents of long-term care facilities are especially at risk for getting and spreading influenza to other residents and to the staff. An annual "flu shot" for both staff members and residents is an effective way of preventing outbreaks of influenza in long-term care facilities (Fig. 26-6).

ASTHMA

Asthma is a condition that affects the bronchi and bronchioles. In people with asthma, triggers (such as cold weather, allergies, respiratory infections, stress, smoke, and exercise) cause the bronchi and bronchioles to constrict (become narrower). This makes breathing difficult, because air does not flow freely through the airways. An asthma attack can be very frightening for the person experiencing it, because the airways can narrow to the point that breathing becomes almost

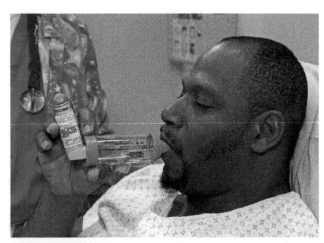

Figure 26-7
Asthma medications are often delivered through inhalers.
(© B. Proud.)

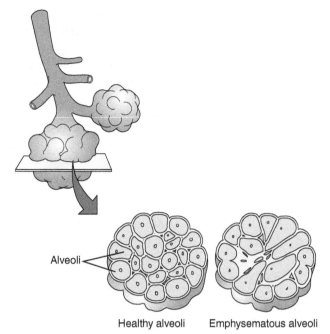

Figure 26-8
Emphysema occurs as a result of damage to the alveoli. The damage to the alveoli makes it difficult for the body to obtain oxygen and get rid of carbon dioxide. A healthy lung contains millions of tiny alveoli, where gas exchange takes place. In a person with emphysema, the walls of the alveoli break down, forming large areas where air can get trapped.

impossible. If one of your patients or residents is having trouble breathing or is making wheezing sounds, you should call the nurse immediately.

An acute asthma attack is usually treated with inhaled medications called bronchodilators (Fig. 26-7). Bronchodilators stop the muscle spasms responsible for the constriction of the airways. People with chronic asthma may need to take medication on a regular basis to prevent attacks from occurring. These medications may be given orally, or they may be inhaled.

CHRONIC OBSTRUCTIVE PULMONARY DISEASE

Chronic obstructive pulmonary disease (COPD) is a general term used to describe two related lung disorders: emphysema and chronic bronchitis. These disorders often occur together in the same person, which is why some health care professionals prefer the more general term, COPD. The leading cause of COPD is smoking.

Emphysema

Emphysema is a form of COPD that involves damage to the alveoli. As you learned earlier, the walls of the alveoli are very thin and delicate. When a toxin, such as tobacco smoke, is inhaled, it damages the thin walls of the alveoli. Over time, the damage causes the fragile walls of the alveoli to break. Eventually, instead of having millions of tiny alveoli where gas exchange can take place, the person has fewer, large, "merged" alveoli that are no longer effective for gas exchange (Fig. 26-8). Because the lung tissue is damaged, it is no longer "springy," and the air

gets trapped in the large, damaged alveoli. The trapped air cannot be exhaled and exchanged for new oxygen-rich air, which limits the amount of oxygen the lungs are able to supply to the body. In addition, excess fluid can collect in the damaged alveoli, creating an excellent place for infection-causing microbes to collect and multiply.

A person with emphysema has trouble getting a "proper breath." The person's breathing is shallow and rapid, and he may have to stop to catch his breath quite frequently when talking or engaging in any type of physical activity. As the person's emphysema gets worse, he will need supplemental oxygen just to carry out even the simplest activities of daily living (ADLs). If you are caring for a person with emphysema, you may notice that his chest is enlarged and rounded. This finding is referred to as "barrel chest" and is caused by years of having extra air trapped in the lung tissue, which causes the chest cavity to enlarge over time.

Chronic Bronchitis

The other form of COPD is chronic bronchitis. **Chronic bronchitis** is caused by long-term irritation of the bronchi and bronchioles, such as that caused by inhaling tobacco smoke. The irritation leads to the production of thick mucus, which blocks the airways. Because the air cannot pass freely through the bronchi and bronchioles, breathing is impaired. In addition, infection-causing microbes can collect in the mucus and multiply, leading to infection.

A person with chronic bronchitis has a nagging, productive cough. She may complain of a "tightness" in her chest, or difficulty breathing. She is likely to have frequent respiratory tract infections. Like a person with emphysema, a person with chronic bronchitis will eventually need oxygen therapy.

Helping Hands and a Caring Heart

FOCUS ON HUMANISTIC HEALTH CARE

People who have chronic conditions of the respiratory system, such as asthma or COPD, may be quite "needy." You may become frustrated with their frequent use of the call light control to ask for seemingly trivial things. Please stop for a moment and try to understand how frightening it would be to suddenly feel that you could not breathe! A person who is having an asthma attack or experiencing a flare-up of COPD feels that each breath might be his last. He might be afraid that in the event of another flare-up or attack, help will not arrive soon enough. Using the call light control frequently is the person's way of making sure that someone will actually come quickly if he calls. Instead of giving in to the desire to avoid a needy patient or resident, be patient and understanding of the underlying fears the person may have. Spend more time with the person, and get into the habit of stopping by to check on him, even when he has not called you. By addressing the person's underlying need for safety and security, you will be providing truly humanistic care.

CANCER

In Canada, cancers involving the lungs and airway are the most common cause of cancer-related death in both men and women. The types of cancers that affect the upper respiratory tract include tumours of the mouth, tongue, and vocal cords. Cancers of the lower respiratory tract can involve the lungs or the lining of the bronchi. People who smoke cigarettes are 10 times more likely to develop lung cancer than nonsmokers are. In addition, some cancers that begin in other body parts, such as the breast or intestines, commonly spread to the lungs.

You may care for a person who is having diagnostic tests done to determine whether or not she has cancer of the lungs or airway. It is important for you to remember that the person and her family members may be worried about both the diagnostic test itself and the results of the test. You may notice that your patient or resident seems quiet or distracted, or that she is having trouble concentrating on tasks. Or, you might come into the room and find the person crying. Sometimes worrying makes a person angry, short-tempered, or agitated. Family members may show similar behaviours as they worry about their loved one.

There are several different ways that the diagnosis of cancer can be made:

- **Radiologic studies,** such as chest x-rays, computed tomography (CT) scans, and magnetic resonance imaging (MRI) scans, allow the doctor to see the tumour without actually entering the body.
- **Bronchoscopy** involves using a special instrument to look inside the airway and obtain tissue or fluids for analysis. The bronchoscope is passed through the mouth and pharynx and into the person's airway (Fig. 26-9). The person may have some discomfort during the procedure, as well as a scratchy throat afterward.
- **Surgery** may be necessary to obtain tissue for analysis. Of all of the diagnostic methods, surgery carries the most risk for the person and is associated with the most discomfort.

You may also care for people who are in a health care facility because they are receiving treatment for cancer of the respiratory system. There are many different ways of treating cancer, which are discussed in detail in Chapter 37. Treatment of cancer of the mouth, tongue, or vocal cords may involve surgery to remove the cancer and possibly some of the surrounding tissues as well. This type of surgery often changes the person's appearance, in very noticeable ways. For many people, coping with the change in their appearance as well as the diagnosis of cancer is very difficult. Treatment of lung cancer may involve surgical removal of all or part of the lung. A person who has had lung surgery will usually have drains inserted in the chest cavity for several days after the procedure to remove blood and fluid and to help keep the lungs expanded properly (Fig. 26-10). Make sure you have been shown how to care for a person with chest tubes if caring for a surgical patient is included in your responsibilities.

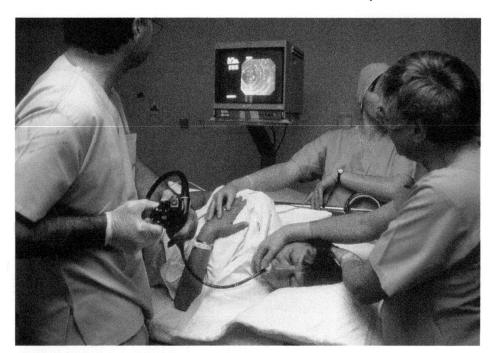

Figure 26-9
A doctor uses a flexible bronchoscope to examine a patient's airways. The bronchoscope is inserted in the patient's mouth, and an image of her trachea and lungs is displayed on the screen. (© *Antonia Reeve/Photo Researchers, Inc.*)

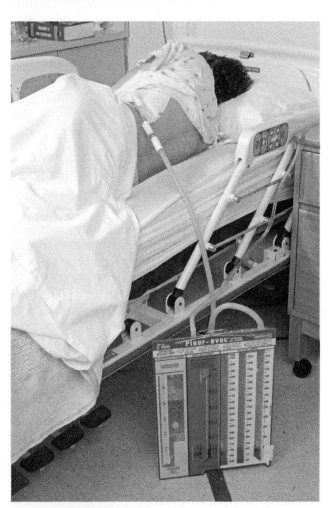

Figure 26-10
A chest tube drainage system is used to remove fluid (such as blood) or air that may build up in the chest cavity as a result of disease, injury, or surgery.

Helping Hands and a Caring Heart

FOCUS ON HUMANISTIC HEALTH CARE

When a person has a smoking-related illness, be careful not to be judgmental about the role the person's actions may have had in causing her disease. A person with a smoking-related illness, such as cancer or COPD, may choose to continue smoking, even though she knows doing so may significantly shorten her life. Smoking is very physically addictive and quitting can be extremely difficult, especially when the person is trying to cope with the stress of having a chronic or terminal condition. Each of your patients or residents must be allowed to make decisions concerning her own quality of life. For some people, this may mean not giving up smoking, even when it would seem to be the best thing to do.

PNEUMOTHORAX AND HEMOTHORAX

Pneumothorax and hemothorax are often complications of chest trauma. **Pneumothorax** occurs when air builds up in the space between the lungs and the chest wall. For example, a penetrating chest wound, such as a stab wound to the chest, can lead to pneumothorax because the stab wound is a "sucking" wound. That means that because of the pressure difference between the inside and the outside of the body, air is drawn into the chest cavity through the wound. The air in the chest cavity prevents the lungs from expanding fully and makes it hard for the person to breathe. Insertion of a chest tube to remove the air is usually necessary.

Hemothorax occurs when blood builds up in the space between the lungs and the chest wall. The bleeding can be caused by an injury to the chest or a rupture in the lung tissue. As with pneumothorax, the build-up prevents the lungs from fully expanding and breathing becomes difficult. Sometimes surgery is needed to stop the bleeding, and a chest tube is inserted to remove the blood.

RESPIRATORY THERAPY

Respiratory therapy is any treatment that is used to help a person achieve satisfactory respiration. Some of these treatments are relatively simple. For example, a humidifier may be used to add moisture to the air, helping to loosen secretions during a bout of bronchitis or pneumonia. Other treatments may be quite complex and involve the use of medications, such as oxygen, or mechanical ventilation.

Most health care facilities have a team of respiratory therapists who are specially trained to evaluate and treat problems of the respiratory system. The respiratory therapist listens to the person's breath sounds and looks at certain measurements to evaluate the person's respiratory function. For example, the respiratory therapist will measure the amount of air that is inhaled and exhaled, as well as the amount of oxygen in the person's blood. Next, the respiratory therapist helps to develop a treatment plan for the person. If you are caring for a patient or resident who is being cared for by a respiratory therapist, watch the therapist and ask questions about the types of treatments he is using. This knowledge will help you to better understand the specific needs of your patient or resident. The nurse or respiratory therapist can also alert you to signs or symptoms that you should watch for and report to the nurse immediately.

OXYGEN THERAPY

The air we breathe contains only about 20% oxygen. The rest is nitrogen. People with reduced lung function (for example, people with emphysema) may have trouble getting the oxygen their bodies need from inhaled air alone. For these people, the doctor might prescribe supplemental (extra) oxygen to increase the amount of oxygen

that they take in with each breath. The supplemental oxygen is pure, 100% oxygen.

Some people who are receiving supplemental oxygen will only need it for a short time. Others will need it for the rest of their lives. Oxygen can be given continuously, or it can be given on an as-needed basis. Some people only need supplemental oxygen when they are physically active.

Oxygen is considered a medication and requires a doctor's order to be used. The doctor determines the rate at which the oxygen should be delivered, and how it should be given. A nurse or respiratory therapist is responsible for setting up and adjusting the oxygen therapy. Many of the people you will care for will be receiving oxygen therapy. Therefore, you need to understand how oxygen is given and what precautions are necessary while oxygen is being used. Some provinces or territories and facilities do not allow personal support workers to adjust or assist with the administration of oxygen, but others do. Always make sure that you are familiar with your specific job responsibilities with regard to oxygen therapy. General guidelines for oxygen therapy are given in Guidelines Box 26-2. You should also review Chapter 9 for safety considerations related to oxygen therapy.

Oxygen is usually delivered to the patient or resident at a rate of 2 to 15 litres of oxygen per minute. The flow rate is set using a device called a **flow metre** (Fig. 26-11). Although you will not usually be responsible for adjusting the flow rate of oxygen, it is important for you to know what

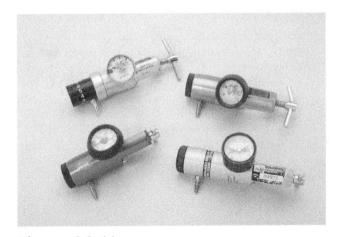

Figure 26-11

A flow metre controls the rate of oxygen flow to the patient or resident. Flow metres come in a variety of styles. You should learn how the flow metres used by your patients or residents work. This will allow you to check the flow metre to make sure that the person is receiving the ordered amount of oxygen.

Guidelines Box 26-2 Guidelines for Oxygen Therapy

WHAT YOU DO	WHY YOU DO IT
Avoid lighting matches or cigarette lighters in the person's room. Post a "No Smoking" sign, and remind the patient or resident and any visitors not to smoke when oxygen is in use.	Use of oxygen therapy can increase the oxygen content of linens and clothing in the immediate area. If burning ashes from a cigarette should happen to drop on the bed, a fire would be more likely to start and would burn much faster as a result of the added oxygen.
Make sure that any electrical equipment is in good working order, and that cords are not frayed. Use a battery-operated razor or a blade razor when shaving a person who is receiving supplemental oxygen.	Electrical equipment that is not properly maintained can be the source of a spark, which could start a fire.
Make sure that the tubing through which the oxygen is delivered is free of kinks, and that the person is not lying on it.	If the tubing is obstructed in any way, oxygen flow will be impaired and the person will not receive the correct amount.
Do not adjust the flow rate of oxygen.	Adjusting the flow rate of oxygen is out of the personal support worker's scope of practice. Receiving too much oxygen can be just as harmful to the patient or resident as receiving too little oxygen. The doctor decides how much oxygen the patient or resident should receive.
When you are caring for a person who is receiving supplemental oxygen, be aware of the ordered flow rate, and tell the nurse if the flow rate on the flow metre does not match the ordered flow rate.	The setting on the flow metre may get changed accidentally. Checking frequently to make sure that the ordered flow rate matches the flow rate on the person's medical chart helps to keep your patient or resident safe. Receiving too much oxygen can be just as harmful to the patient or resident as receiving too little oxygen.
When providing personal care, do not remove a person's facemask or nasal cannula, unless you are specifically told to do so by the nurse.	Removing the facemask or nasal cannula will deprive the person of the supplemental oxygen. Some people may not be able to tolerate a decrease in the amount of oxygen they are receiving, even for just a few minutes.
Make sure that the water level in the humidity bottle does not get too low.	Oxygen that is not humidified prior to delivery can be very drying to the mucous membrane lining of the person's nasal cavity and mouth. This dryness can be uncomfortable for the patient or resident.
Provide oral care frequently, as directed by the nurse.	Frequent oral care helps to relieve some of the dryness of the nose and mouth that occurs with supplemental oxygen therapy.
Watch for signs of skin irritation behind the person's ears, over his or her cheeks, or under his or her nose.	The pressure and friction from the tubing that holds the facemask or nasal cannula in place can cause skin breakdown.

flow rate was ordered. You should check the flow metre frequently when you are caring for a person who is receiving oxygen therapy to make sure that the flow rate is set properly. A patient or resident (or a visitor) might accidentally change the setting on the flow metre. If you notice that the setting on the flow metre does not match the amount of oxygen that has been ordered, notify the nurse immediately. Receiving too much oxygen is just as dangerous as receiving too little oxygen.

People who are receiving oxygen therapy may need to be monitored to make sure that enough oxygen is reaching the tissues. This monitoring may be constant for people who are critically ill. Other people will only require periodic monitoring. Monitoring of the oxygen content of the blood is done using a device called a *pulse oximetre*. The pulse oximetre is clipped to the person's fingertip or earlobe (Fig. 26-12). Infrared light is passed through the tissue to a sensor on the other side of the device. The amount of light that reaches the sensor is translated into a measurement of how much oxygen the blood is actually carrying. A normal reading is between 95% and 100%. Readings below 85% indicate that the person's tissues are not receiving enough oxygen. An alarm will usually sound if the person's blood oxygen level is too low.

Because oxygen therapy can be very drying to a person's mouth or nose, moisture is often added to the supplemental oxygen using a humidity bottle. The humidity bottle is filled with distilled water. The oxygen passes through the water before it is delivered to the patient or resident. This increases the water content of the oxygen, making it less drying to the person's nose and mouth. As the oxygen flows through the water in the humidity bottle, it creates bubbles. You should check the humidity bottle frequently for bubbles, which indicate that the oxygen is flowing freely. You should also check the water level often, to make sure that it does not drop too low. Your facility policy will specify how often the humidity bottle should be changed.

Sources of Supplemental Oxygen

Supplemental oxygen can be supplied through a wall-mounted delivery system, in a pressurized tank, or through an oxygen concentrator (Fig. 26-13).

Wall-mounted delivery systems

In many facilities, the oxygen is piped into the patient's or resident's room from a central location. A special valve and flow metre device is inserted into the wall to access the oxygen (see Fig. 26-13A). The nurse or respiratory therapist sets the flow metre so that the oxygen is administered to the person at the correct rate.

Pressurized tank

These tanks, which are placed in the patient's or resident's room, contain oxygen under pressure. Some of these tanks are small enough to be carried or wheeled around with the person (see Fig. 26-13B). The nurse or respiratory therapist sets the flow metre on the tank so that the oxygen is administered to the person at the correct rate.

A gauge tracks the amount of oxygen remaining in the tank. You should note when the dial shows that the supply of oxygen is getting low. If you notice that the tank is nearly empty, tell the nurse or respiratory therapist so that she can exchange the nearly empty tank for a full one.

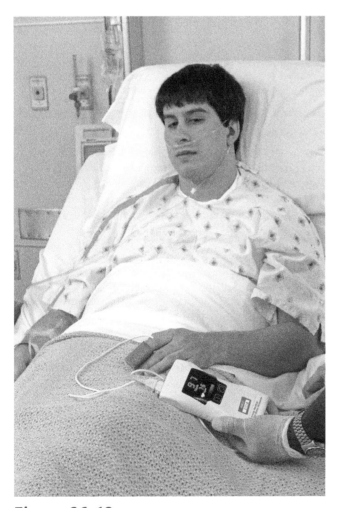

Figure 26-12
Pulse oximetry is used to monitor the amount of oxygen that is reaching a person's tissues.

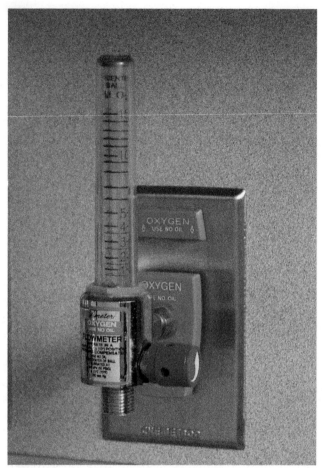

A. Wall-mounted delivery system

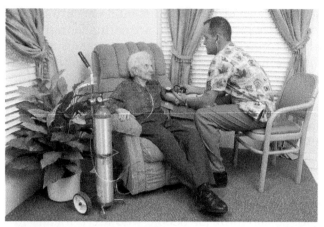

B. Pressurized tank

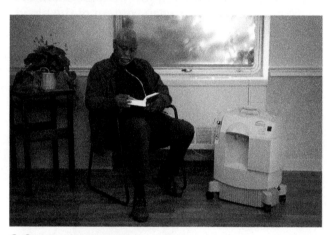

C. Oxygen concentrator

Figure 26-13

Supplemental oxygen can be supplied in various ways. **(A)** With a wall-mounted delivery system, the oxygen is piped into the person's room from a central location. A valve and flow metre device is inserted into the wall outlet to access the oxygen. **(B)** A pressurized tank of oxygen can go where the person goes. **(C)** An oxygen concentrator is often used in the home and long-term care settings, especially when the person only needs to use oxygen on an as-needed basis. Oxygen concentrators produce 100% oxygen by filtering the nitrogen out of room air.

Because the portable oxygen tanks are pressurized, they should be moved with caution. If the tank is accidentally knocked over and the valve at the top breaks, the escaping gas in the tank could propel the tank across the room with quite a bit of force. If the tank hits someone, it could cause a serious injury.

Oxygen concentrators

Oxygen concentrators are devices that take in air and filter out the nitrogen, leaving behind pure oxygen (see Fig. 26-13C). The oxygen is then delivered to the person at the rate that has been programmed into the unit. Because the delivery amount is preset, the person (or caregiver) only has to turn the switch to "ON" when oxygen is needed. These units run on electricity and are

often used in home and long-term care settings, especially if the person needs supplemental oxygen only once in a while.

Delivery of Supplemental Oxygen

A number of different devices are used to deliver oxygen to patients and residents. The type of delivery device used depends on several factors, including the amount of oxygen ordered, the condition being treated, and the overall physical condition of the patient or resident.

Nasal cannulas

A nasal cannula is the most common method of administering oxygen. A **nasal cannula** is two prongs of soft plastic tubing, which are inserted into the nostrils (Fig. 26-14A). The tubing to the

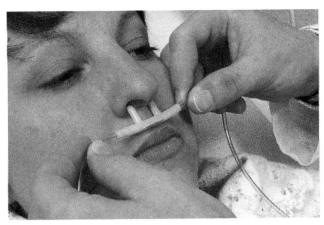

A. Nasal cannula

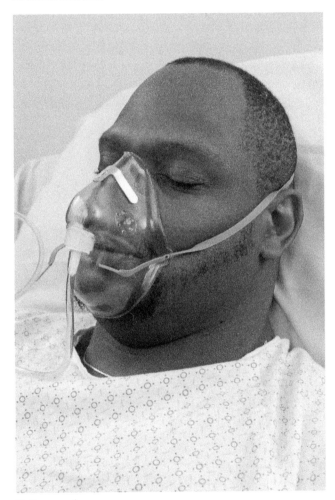

B. Facemask

Figure 26-14

Devices used for oxygen delivery. **(A)** A nasal cannula is a two-pronged device that is inserted into the nostrils to deliver oxygen to the patient or resident. A person who has a nasal cannula in place is able to eat, drink, and speak normally. **(B)** A facemask fits over the person's nose and mouth. A facemask may be used when a person requires a high level of supplemental oxygen. Facemasks come in a variety of styles.

cannula is connected to an oxygen source with a humidifier bottle and a flow metre. A nasal cannula is easy to apply, it does not interfere with eating or talking, and it is less likely to create a feeling of suffocation. However, the nasal cannula can dry out the mucous membranes in the nasal cavity if the oxygen is delivered at a high flow rate. The tubing can irritate the skin around the nostrils and cheeks and behind the ears. Finally, a nasal cannula may not be suitable for use in a critically ill patient, or in a person who breathes through his or her mouth, because the concentration of oxygen delivered may not be high enough.

Facemasks

Oxygen can also be delivered through a **facemask.** A facemask is made of soft, moulded plastic material that fits over the nose and mouth (see Fig. 26-14B). A facemask may be a simple device that just delivers the oxygen to the mouth and nose, or it may be quite complex, with attachments (such as bags that act as a holding place for extra oxygen). A facemask can deliver oxygen at a higher concentration than a nasal cannula can. In addition, a facemask is useful for a person who breathes through his or her mouth, instead of the nose. However, facemasks can make a person feel like he is suffocating (because they cover the person's nose and mouth), and they can interfere with the person's ability to eat, drink, and speak clearly. Sometimes a person is allowed to switch to a nasal cannula when it is time to eat or be shaved. Never remove a person's facemask without first asking the nurse. Removing the facemask, even briefly, can have serious consequences for the person.

Accessory devices

There are some other devices that are often used in combination with nasal cannula or facemask oxygen delivery systems (Fig. 26-15). Sometimes a person is unconscious or has been sedated to the point that the muscles that keep the upper airway open relax. The lower jaw falls open and the tongue falls backward into the throat, blocking the passage of air into the body.

To prevent this from happening, a nasopharyngeal airway (nasal trumpet) may be used. A **nasopharyngeal airway** is a soft rubber tube that is inserted into the person's nose (see Fig. 26-15A). It extends back toward the throat, providing an opening that air can flow through. Another commonly used airway device is the oropharyngeal airway. An **oropharyngeal airway** is a hard plastic device that is inserted into the

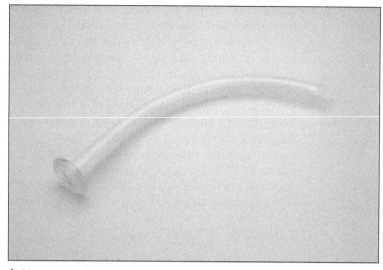
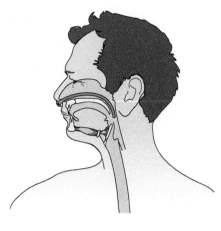

A. Nasopharyngeal airway

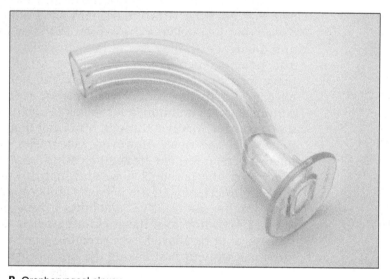
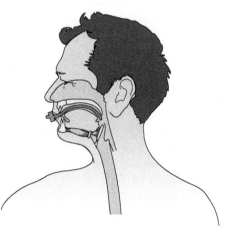

B. Oropharyngeal airway

Figure 26-15
An airway device may need to be used in a person who is unconscious or heavily sedated. The airway device keeps the airway open when the person cannot do this on his or her own. **(A)** A nasopharyngeal airway is inserted into the person's nose. **(B)** An oropharyngeal airway is inserted into the person's mouth.

person's mouth (see Fig. 26-15B). The oropharyngeal airway stops the tongue from falling back into the throat, keeping the airway open. The oropharyngeal airway is used only for a person who is either heavily sedated or unconscious, because it can cause gagging and choking in a conscious person.

MECHANICAL VENTILATION

In **mechanical ventilation,** a machine called a *ventilator* breathes for a person who cannot breathe on his own (Fig. 26-16). There are many

reasons that a person might need to be put on a ventilator. For example, a serious head injury, stroke, or drug overdose can affect the breathing control centers in the brain, which means that regular breathing will no longer occur automatically. In these situations, mechanical ventilation is needed. A spinal cord injury or a neurologic disorder can interfere with the nerve impulses that cause the diaphragm to contract and relax automatically, resulting in the need for mechanical ventilation. Other conditions that may result in a person needing mechanical ventilation include acute respiratory infections and heart

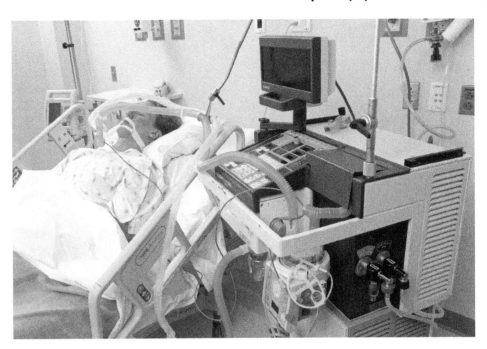

Figure 26-16
A mechanical ventilator performs the function of breathing for a person who cannot breathe on his own.

attacks. Mechanical ventilation is also often used both during and after surgery. Some people only need the ventilator for a short period of time, while others may need to be placed on a ventilator for the rest of their lives. Not all people who require mechanical ventilation are confined to bed. Some ventilators are portable (Fig. 26-17).

A ventilator works by forcing air into the person's lungs. The air is delivered through a tube that is inserted into the airway. Depending on the situation, an endotracheal tube or a tracheostomy tube may be used (Fig. 26-18).

Endotracheal Intubation

Many people who require mechanical ventilation for only a short time will have an endotracheal tube. The **endotracheal tube** is inserted into the person's nose or mouth. It extends to the trachea, where a balloon cuff on the end holds it in place and prevents secretions that drain from the mouth from entering the respiratory tract (see Fig. 26-18A). Being intubated with an endotracheal tube can be very uncomfortable and frightening for the patient or resident.

- Because the endotracheal tube travels through the larynx (voice box), a person who has an endotracheal tube in place is unable to talk, and will need to communicate using some other method, such as writing on a notepad. Imagine what it would be like to be dependent on a machine to breathe and unable to call out for help if you needed it. What would you do if the machine stopped?

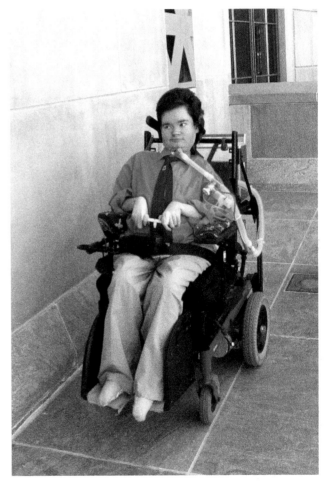

Figure 26-17
Portable ventilators allow some people with quadriplegia or other conditions that affect the muscles used for breathing to lead active lives. (*AP Photo/Jamie Martin.*)

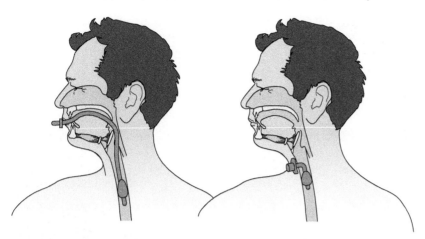

A. Endotracheal tube   **B.** Tracheostomy tube

Figure 26-18
Mechanical ventilation requires the use of an endotracheal tube or a tracheostomy tube. **(A)** An endotracheal tube is inserted into the person's nose or mouth and passed through the pharynx and larynx to the trachea. An inflatable balloon cuff at the end of the endotracheal tube holds it in place and helps to prevent secretions from passing into the lungs. **(B)** A tracheostomy tube is inserted into a surgically created opening in the neck called a tracheostomy.

This is something that a person on a ventilator might worry about. Making sure that the call light control is within easy reach and checking on the person frequently are things you can do to make an intubated person feel more secure.

- The endotracheal tube makes it impossible for the person to take food or fluids through the mouth. Frequent oral care can help to relieve some of the dryness and discomfort caused by having an endotracheal tube in place.
- Wrist restraints are often used for a person who is intubated, to keep the person from reaching up and removing the endotracheal tube from the airway. The tube is uncomfortable, and it is natural for a person to try and remove it. Although the wrist restraints may be necessary, they can add to the person's anxiety. As is always the case when restraints are being used, you will need to check on the person very frequently, and the restraints will need to be removed and reapplied at regular intervals.

Ensuring that a person with an endotracheal tube is as comfortable as possible and checking on the person frequently will help to relieve some of the person's worries and help him or her to feel safe.

Tracheostomy

If a person will need to be on a mechanical ventilator for more than a week or so, a tracheostomy is usually performed. A **tracheostomy** (often referred to as "a trach") is a surgically created opening in the neck that opens into the trachea. A short tube, called a tracheostomy or "trach" tube, is inserted into the opening and attached to the ventilator tubing (see Fig. 26-18B). The

tracheostomy tube is usually secured around the person's neck with ties or a special collar device (Fig. 26-19). If the tube is not secured, it could be coughed out very easily.

A tracheostomy tube is much more comfortable for the person than an endotracheal tube. The person is able to eat and drink normally. The tracheostomy and tubing require special care, which is performed by the nurse. You are responsible for making sure that the tubing stays connected at all times and for observing the person for any signs that she is having trouble breathing.

Depending on the situation, a tracheostomy may be permanent or temporary. For example, a

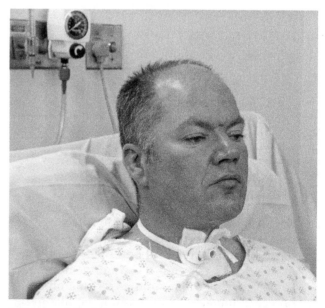

Figure 26-19
The tracheostomy tube is held in place with special ties or a collar.

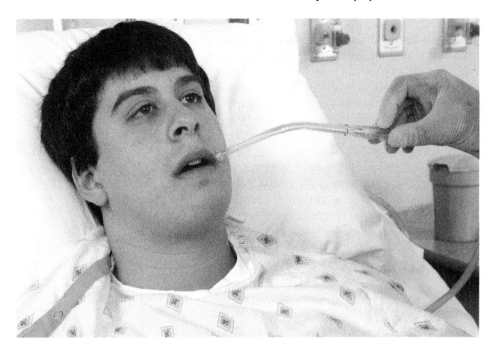

Figure 26-20
A Yankauer suction tip is used to remove secretions from the mouth and the back of the throat. You will be able to tell when a person needs to be suctioned. Always report this observation to the nurse so that he or she can perform the procedure.

person who requires mechanical ventilation for several weeks will have a temporary tracheostomy that will be allowed to heal once the person no longer needs to be on the mechanical ventilator. However, a person who is paralyzed and will need to be on a ventilator for the rest of his or her life will have a permanent tracheostomy. A person who has had his larynx removed as a result of cancer will also have a permanent tracheostomy. The person breathes, talks, sneezes, and coughs through the tracheostomy because the airway between the pharynx and the trachea is no longer complete.

SUCTIONING

People with respiratory disorders often need help removing secretions from the airway. Conditions such as pneumonia or chronic bronchitis can cause the production of large amounts of sputum, which builds up in the lungs and bronchi and makes it difficult to breathe. Other conditions interfere with a person's ability to cough up secretions. For example, a person who is in a coma or heavily sedated may not have an intact cough reflex. Therefore, the person does not cough and the secretions continue to build up. **Suctioning** is the process of removing fluid and mucus from a person's airway.

Suctioning is done using various types of suction catheters. The suction catheter is attached to tubing and a suction source, which works like a vacuum cleaner to remove the secretions from the airway. A Yankauer suction tip is

used to remove secretions that collect in the back of the throat (Fig. 26-20). The Yankauer tip is placed in the person's mouth, and suction is applied. A long, thin, flexible catheter is used when it is necessary to suction the airway in the lower respiratory system. This soft catheter can be passed through the nose or mouth, or down an endotracheal or tracheostomy tube.

Because suctioning removes air along with the bothersome secretions, a person can easily become **hypoxic** (that is, deficient of oxygen) during the suctioning procedure. Personal support workers are not responsible for suctioning patients and residents, but you will be responsible for letting the nurse know that suctioning may be needed, and for assisting during the procedure. Usually it is quite obvious when a person needs to have his airway suctioned. The person's breathing becomes noisy, and he may keep trying to cough up secretions, with little success.

GENERAL CARE MEASURES

Because there is little room for error when dealing with the respiratory system, many of the therapies that are used to help people with respiratory disorders can be carried out only by people who have received advanced training, such as nurses and respiratory therapists. However, many facilities and agencies offer additional training that will allow you to be more active in caring for people with special respiratory needs.

For example, you may work in a facility that provides specialized care for people who depend on mechanical ventilators to breathe. In this case, your scope of practice may be widened to include procedures that are not normally part of a personal support worker's responsibilities. Make sure that you have been adequately instructed in any special procedures that are required of you, and always be aware of what is and is not within your scope of practice, per your province/territory's or facility's policy. No matter where you work, there are several general care measures related to the respiratory system that are within every personal support worker's scope of practice.

OBSERVATION

A personal support worker's main responsibility in caring for any patient or resident with a respiratory problem is that of observation. Because you are the one who will spend the most time with your patients or residents, you will be the one who has the best opportunity to observe signs that a person may be having problems with ventilation or gas exchange. Some of your patients or residents who have chronic respiratory problems will always have difficulty breathing when they exert themselves. It is important for you to be able to recognize what is normal for each of your patients or residents, so that you can recognize changes if they occur. You should also be aware of a person's normal skin colour, so that you are able to recognize changes that may indicate that her tissues are not receiving enough oxygen.

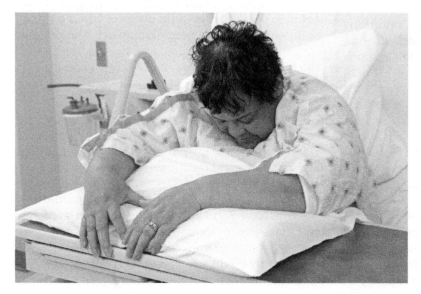

Figure 26-21
Certain positions make breathing easier for people with respiratory disorders. Many people find that leaning forward helps to make breathing easier.

PROMOTING COMFORT

There are many things that a personal support worker can do to help a person with respiratory problems feel more comfortable. Positioning the person in the Fowler's or semi-Fowler's position is often helpful. Some people are more comfortable when they assume a forward-leaning position using pillows on the over-bed table (Fig. 26-21). If the doctor has not placed any restrictions on the person's fluid intake, encourage the patient or resident to drink plenty of fluids. Fluids help to thin respiratory secretions so that they are easier to cough up. Providing frequent oral care will also help keep the person comfortable and will reduce the number of microbes that are present in the mouth.

SUMMARY

- "When you can't breathe, nothing else matters." (Canadian Lung Association)
  - The function of the respiratory system is to provide the body with oxygen and rid the body of carbon dioxide.
  - The respiratory system consists of the lungs and a group of structures known collectively as the *airway.* The airway consists of the nasal cavities, pharynx, larynx, trachea, bronchi, and bronchioles.
    - The upper respiratory tract consists of those structures located outside of the chest cavity (the nasal cavity, pharynx, and larynx).
    - The lower respiratory tract consists of those structures located inside of the chest cavity (the trachea, bronchi, bronchioles, and lungs).
- Respiration involves two processes: ventilation and gas exchange. If one or the other of these processes is impaired, respiration will not be effective.
  - Ventilation is the process of physically moving air in and out of the lungs (breathing). The diaphragm is the major muscle responsible for ventilation.
  - Gas exchange is the process of transferring oxygen from the air into the blood, and transferring carbon dioxide from the blood into the air. Gas exchange occurs in the alveoli.
- Like all organ systems, the respiratory system is affected by aging.
  - Loss of elasticity in the lung tissue and weakening of the muscles of respiration make breathing less efficient, because an older person is able to take in less air with each breath.

- The decreased ability of the immune system to fight infections may make an elderly person more likely to get pneumonia and other respiratory infections.
- Chronic illness, immobility, or a lifetime of exposure to pollution, chemicals, or tobacco smoke can make the effects of aging on the respiratory system much more noticeable. Regular physical exercise combined with healthy habits such as the avoidance of smoking helps to keep the respiratory system healthy throughout a person's lifetime.
- Disorders of the respiratory system can make breathing very difficult.
  - Infections can be caused by bacteria or viruses and include pneumonia, bronchitis, and influenza.
  - Asthma is a narrowing of the bronchioles in response to certain triggers, such as allergies, cold air, exercise, smoke, or stress. An asthma attack can be very frightening for the person experiencing it.
  - Chronic obstructive pulmonary disease (COPD) is a general term for two smoking-related disorders.
    - In emphysema, the alveoli are destroyed. Trapping of air in the lungs results. Breathing is difficult and gas exchange is impaired.
    - Chronic bronchitis affects the bronchi and bronchioles. Chronic bronchitis is associated with the production of excessive amounts of secretions.
  - Cancers of the lungs and airway are the most common cause of cancer-related deaths in both men and women in Canada. People who smoke are 10 times more likely to develop lung cancer than nonsmokers are.

- Respiratory therapy is used to help improve a person's processes of ventilation, gas exchange, or both.
  - Oxygen therapy is the administration of supplemental oxygen.
    - Oxygen is a medication and requires a doctor's order to be used.
    - Oxygen may be supplied by way of a wall-mounted system, an individual pressurized tank, or an oxygen concentrator.
    - Oxygen can be administered through a nasal cannula or facemask.
  - Mechanical ventilation is used for a person who cannot inhale and exhale on his own. A person who needs the assistance of a mechanical ventilator must be intubated with an endotracheal tube or a tracheostomy tube.
    - Suctioning is often necessary to remove excessive secretions from a person's respiratory tract.
- A personal support worker's responsibilities when caring for a person with a respiratory disorder are mainly observation and the promotion of comfort. A personal support worker also provides holistic care by helping the person to feel safe and secure. Not being able to breathe easily can be very frightening for the patient or resident.

WHAT DID YOU LEARN?

Multiple Choice

Select the single best answer for each of the following questions.

1. Who has to write the order for oxygen to be used?
   a. The nurse
   b. The respiratory therapist
   c. The doctor
   d. No order is necessary
2. The nurse asks you to obtain a sputum specimen from Mrs. Long, who has pneumonia. Which one of the following is correct to do when obtaining a sputum specimen?
   a. Have Mrs. Long rinse her mouth with mouthwash before producing the specimen.
   b. Have Mrs. Long cough the specimen into an emesis basin, and then transfer the specimen to the specimen container.
   c. Explain to Mrs. Long that the specimen must come from deep within her chest.
   d. Put the specimen container in the refrigerator after you have collected the sputum specimen and label the container with Mrs. Long's name and room number.
3. What colour is a healthy lung?
   a. Blue
   b. Grey
   c. White
   d. Pink
4. Where does gas exchange take place?
   a. In the alveoli
   b. In the bronchioles
   c. In the pleura
   d. In the nasal cavity
5. Which of the following is true about a person who has an endotracheal tube in place?
   a. The person is able to eat and drink normally.
   b. The person is able to talk normally.
   c. The person will need frequent oral care.
   d. The person is unconscious.
6. You have been assigned to care for Mr. Fenley, who has chronic obstructive pulmonary disease (COPD). He is on continuous oxygen by a nasal cannula at a rate of 4 litres per minute. One morning, you enter Mr. Fenley's room to do your morning checks, and you notice that the flow rate on the flow metre is set at 8 litres per minute. What should you do?
   a. Call the nurse immediately.
   b. Decrease the flow rate back to the prescribed 4 litres per minute.
   c. Tell Mr. Fenley that it is very dangerous for him to make adjustments to the flow metre on his own.
   d. Nothing. A patient or resident can adjust the flow rate of oxygen to meet his or her own needs.
7. One of your responsibilities is to assist Mr. Tang with shaving. Mr. Tang is receiving continuous oxygen via a nasal cannula.

What should you do when helping Mr. Tang to shave?

a. Remove the nasal cannula before you begin the procedure.

b. Use a battery-operated razor or a blade razor instead of an electrical razor.

c. Increase the flow of oxygen during the procedure.

d. Decrease the flow of oxygen during the procedure.

8. One of your newly admitted residents, Mr. Petersen, has emphysema. You are going to meet Mr. Petersen for the first time. Thinking back on what you learned during your personal support worker course about people with emphysema, which one of the following would you expect to be true of Mr. Petersen?

a. His breathing will probably be shallow and rapid.

b. He might need supplemental oxygen.

c. He may have to catch his breath frequently while talking.

d. All of the above

Matching

Match each numbered item with its appropriate lettered description.

_____ 1. Respiration

_____ 2. Lungs

_____ 3. Nasopharyngeal airway

_____ 4. Hemothorax

_____ 5. Pharynx

_____ 6. Trachea

_____ 7. Pneumothorax

_____ 8. Pleura

_____ 9. Hypoxic

_____ 10. Nasal cavity

a. Blood in the chest cavity

b. Also known as the "windpipe"; conducts air from the larynx to the bronchi

c. Membrane that covers the inside of the chest cavity and the outside of the lungs

d. Also known as the throat

e. A rubber tube that is inserted in a person's nose or mouth to keep the airway open

f. The process the body uses to obtain oxygen from the environment and remove carbon dioxide from the body

g. Primary organs of respiration

h. Space where air from the outside of the body is first warmed, humidified, and filtered

i. Air in the chest cavity

j. Deficient of oxygen

STOP and Think!

You have been assigned to care for Mrs. Nielsen, who has severe respiratory problems resulting from a long history of asthma. The light above Mrs. Nielsen's door is on, and you go to find out what she needs. When you enter the room, Mrs. Nielsen asks you if it is almost time for dinner and whether or not you think she will need to wear a sweater. You answer Mrs. Nielsen's questions, and then ask her if there is anything else she needs, because surely there must be! She says, "no," she just wanted to ask you those questions. Do you think that Mrs. Nielsen has needs she may not be telling you about? What might you do for Mrs. Nielsen?

Matthew is providing care for Mr. Thompson, who has smoked for more than 50 years. Mr. Thompson has advanced COPD, and requires a lot of assistance with nearly everything (including smoking, which he continues to do). One day, you and Matthew are leaving work together and you see all of the "smokers" outside having their cigarettes, shivering because it is the middle of winter. Matthew tells you that he thinks smoking is a disgusting habit, and that people who smoke are weak and lack willpower. How might Matthew's feelings about smoking affect his relationship with Mr. Thompson and other residents with smoking-related conditions?

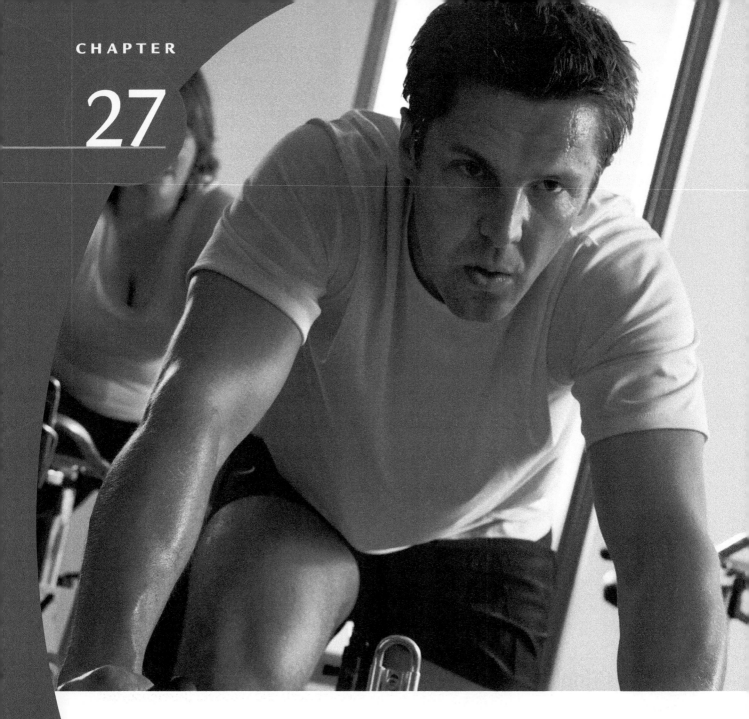

The Cardiovascular System

WHAT WILL YOU LEARN?

The heart and the other organs that make up the cardiovascular system are the subject of this chapter. It is likely that some of the people you will care for daily will have some sort of a cardiovascular problem. Not only will an understanding of how the cardiovascular system works help you to better serve your patients or residents, it will help you to

564

Photo: Exercising regularly is one way to keep your cardiovascular system healthy.

keep your own cardiovascular system healthy! When you are finished with this chapter, you will be able to:

1. List and describe the major parts of the cardiovascular system.
2. Discuss the major functions of the cardiovascular system.
3. Describe how aging affects the cardiovascular system.
4. Explain how exercise and a healthy lifestyle can lessen the effects of aging on the cardiovascular system.
5. Discuss various disorders that affect the cardiovascular system.
6. List diagnostic tests that are often used to diagnose disorders of the cardiovascular system.
7. Describe rehabilitation that may be necessary for a person who has a cardiovascular disorder.

Vocabulary

Plasma	Venules	Pulmonary circulation	Plaque
Erythrocytes	Lymph	Systemic circulation	Arteriosclerosis
Hemoglobin	Lymph node	Systole	Peripheral vascular
Leukocytes	Endocardium	Diastole	disease
Thrombocytes	Myocardium	Cardiac cycle	Coronary artery
Coagulation	Epicardium	Varicose veins	disease
Hemostasis	Pericardium	Anemia	Angina pectoris
Arteries	Atria	Leukemia	Myocardial infarction
Veins	Ventricles	Thrombi	Heart failure
Arterioles	Ischemia	Embolus	Conduction disorders
Capillary bed	Circulation	Atherosclerosis	Cardiac rehabilitation

STRUCTURE OF THE CARDIOVASCULAR SYSTEM

The cardiovascular system, also known as the *circulatory system*, is made up of the blood, the blood vessels, the lymphatic system, and the heart. *Cardio* means "heart," and *vascular* means "vessels."

BLOOD

Blood is the life-giving fluid of our bodies. The blood has two main components, the plasma and the blood cells (Fig. 27-1A).

Plasma

More than half of the total blood volume is plasma. **Plasma** is the liquid part of the blood (see Fig. 27-1B). Plasma is about 90% water. The other 10% is made up of substances that are dissolved in the water (such as glucose, amino acids, fats, and salts) and proteins. Important plasma proteins include albumin, fibrinogen,

and globulins. Albumin plays a role in moving fluid in and out of the bloodstream. Fibrinogen is used as part of the blood clotting process. Globulins help to fight infection.

Blood Cells

There are three main types of blood cells: red blood cells (erythrocytes), white blood cells (leukocytes), and platelets (thrombocytes).

Red blood cells (erythrocytes)

Red blood cells, or **erythrocytes,** carry oxygen. The name *erythrocyte* comes from *eryth-*, which means "red," and *cyt*, which means "cell." There are approximately 5 million red blood cells per cubic millimetre of blood! Red blood cells are made in the red bone marrow (see Chapter 25) and are continuously replaced as old ones wear out.

Red blood cells are tiny, disc-shaped cells that are thinner in the centre than at the edges (see Fig. 27-1A). The "dent" in the centre of the red blood cell contains a protein called **hemoglobin.** Oxygen molecules attach to the hemoglobin for transport to the tissues. When combined with

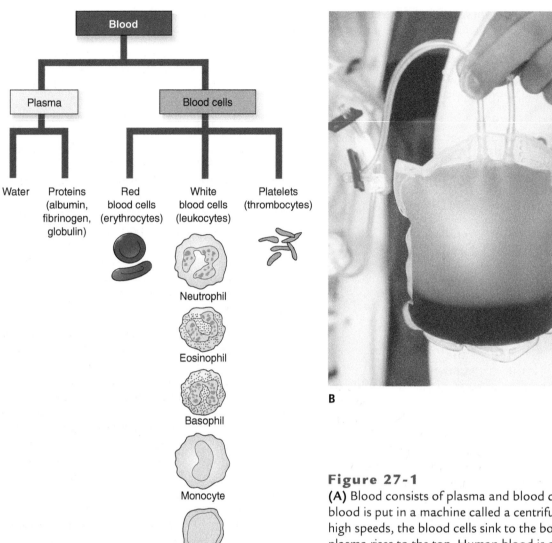

A

B

Figure 27-1

(A) Blood consists of plasma and blood cells. **(B)** When blood is put in a machine called a centrifuge and spun at high speeds, the blood cells sink to the bottom while the plasma rises to the top. Human blood is about 55% plasma. (*B, © Antonia Reeve/Photo Researchers, Inc.*)

oxygen, hemoglobin is bright red. This is what gives red blood cells their colour and name.

The hemoglobin molecule on each red blood cell can carry many oxygen molecules. The hemoglobin on red blood cells that have just received a full load of oxygen from the lungs is filled to capacity with oxygen, and therefore this blood is very bright red. As the blood circulates through the body, giving off oxygen and taking on carbon dioxide, the number of oxygen molecules on the hemoglobin molecule decreases, and the blood becomes darker red in colour.

White blood cells (leukocytes)

White blood cells, or **leukocytes,** fight infection. The name *leukocyte* comes from *leuk,* which means "white" and *cyt,* which means "cell."

The blood of a healthy person contains 5,000 to 10,000 white blood cells per cubic millimetre.

There are five different types of white blood cells (see Fig. 27-1A). Each type of white blood cell has a different function, related to fighting infection. Some destroy pathogens by surrounding them and "eating" them in a process called phagocytosis (see Chapter 7, Fig. 7-2). Others secrete substances that cause the pathogen to die. Still others make proteins called antibodies, which prevent us from getting some diseases twice.

White blood cells are formed in the red bone marrow and the lymphatic system (discussed later in this chapter). An infection causes white blood cell production to increase, sending more "troops" into the bloodstream to battle the invading pathogen.

Platelets (Thrombocytes)

Platelets, or **thrombocytes,** are responsible for clotting **(coagulation)** of the blood. When an injury occurs, the platelets stick together to form a temporary plug over the site of injury. They also release chemicals that react with the plasma protein fibrinogen, causing a more permanent clot (or scab) to develop. This process, known as **hemostasis,** stops the loss of blood from the circulatory system (*hem-* meaning "blood," *stasis* meaning "stop").

Platelets are not actually whole cells (see Fig. 27-1A). They are pinched-off pieces of larger cells that are formed in the red bone marrow. There are about 150,000 to 450,000 platelets per cubic millilitre of circulating blood.

BLOOD VESSELS

The blood vessels carry blood to and from all of the tissues in the body. The walls of the blood vessels have three layers (Fig. 27-2). The layer on the inside, the *tunica intima*, is a smooth lining that helps blood flow smoothly through the vessel. The middle layer, the *tunica media*, is formed of smooth muscle tissue. The smooth muscle in the tunica media is what allows the blood vessels to constrict or dilate according to the body's needs. Constriction (narrowing) of the vessels slows the flow of blood, while dilation (widening) of the vessels allows blood to flow more rapidly. The outer layer of the vessel wall, the *tunica externa*, is a tough protective layer of connective tissue.

Arteries carry blood away from the heart, and **veins** carry blood to the heart. Looking at Figure 27-2, you can see that there are two major differences between the walls of the arteries and the walls of the veins:

- The walls of the arteries contain more smooth muscle than those of the veins, because the arteries receive blood that is being pumped from the heart under great force and pressure. The smooth muscle in the walls of the arteries allows the arteries to handle the flow of blood from the heart.
- The tunica intima of the veins contains valves, which help blood to flow back to the heart. This is especially important in the arms and the legs, where blood would tend to flow away from the heart, due to the effects of gravity. The valves are assisted by contraction of nearby skeletal muscles. For example, when we walk, contraction of the leg muscles compresses the veins, pushing blood toward the heart.

Arteries carry blood away from the heart. As the arteries get farther away from the heart, they branch into a network, becoming smaller and smaller in diameter (Fig. 27-3A). The smallest arteries are called **arterioles.** Arterioles send off branches called *capillaries,* which form a network in the tissues called the **capillary bed** (Fig. 27-4). As blood passes through the capillary bed, the oxygen and nutrients in the blood pass into the tissues, and carbon dioxide and other waste materials from the tissues pass into the blood. This transfer of substances in and out of the blood is possible because the walls of the capillaries have only one thin layer, as opposed to the three layers in the walls of the arteries and veins. After the blood passes through the capillary bed, it starts its journey back to the heart by way of very tiny veins called **venules** (see Fig. 27-4). Venules drain into small veins, which become larger in diameter as they approach the heart (see Fig. 27-3B).

LYMPHATIC SYSTEM

The pressure of the circulating blood through the tiny capillaries forces some of the blood plasma to leak out into the surrounding tissues. Approximately 10% of the circulating plasma leaks out of the capillaries in this manner. The lymphatic system helps to return the fluid that leaks into the tissues to the bloodstream. The lymphatic system also produces some of the white blood cells that fight invading pathogens.

The lymphatic system is actually a one-way, open-ended circulatory system (Fig. 27-5). Lymph capillaries absorb excess fluid from the

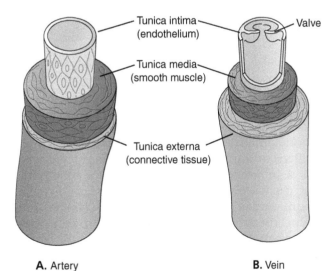

Tunica intima (endothelium)
Tunica media (smooth muscle)
Tunica externa (connective tissue)
Valve

A. Artery   **B.** Vein

Figure 27-2
The walls of the blood vessels have three layers. **(A)** An artery. **(B)** A vein.

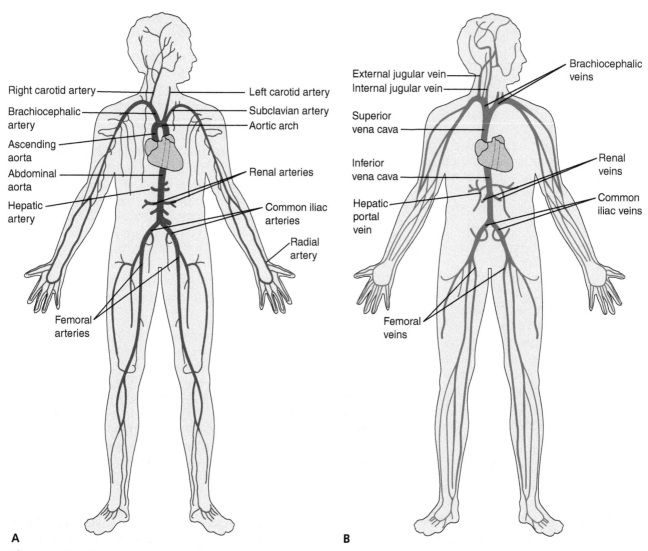

Figure 27-3
Blood vessels carry blood to every part of the body. **(A)** The major arteries of the body. Arteries carry blood away from the heart. Note how the arteries get smaller in diameter the farther away they get from the heart. **(B)** The major veins of the body. Veins carry blood back to the heart. Note how the veins get larger in diameter the closer they get to the heart.

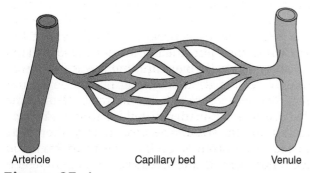

Figure 27-4
The capillary bed is where the transfer of substances between the blood and the tissues occurs.

surrounding tissues. (Once the fluid enters the lymph capillaries, it is called **lymph.**) The lymph capillaries join together to form larger vessels, called *lymphatics*. At certain points along the way, the lymph in the lymphatics passes through **lymph nodes,** masses of lymphatic tissue that "clean" the lymph by removing bacteria and other large particles. Eventually, all of the lymphatics empty into the large veins in the shoulder region, returning the fluid to the general circulation.

Other parts of the lymphatic system include the thymus gland, which is located in the chest. The thymus gland secretes a chemical that

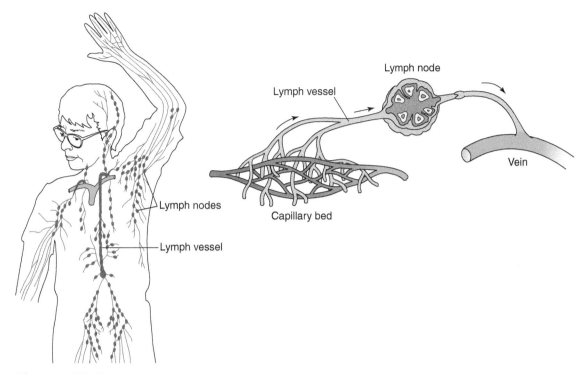

Lymph node

Lymph vessel

Vein

Lymph nodes

Capillary bed

Lymph vessel

Figure 27-5

The lymphatic system returns fluid to the bloodstream. It is a one-way system. Lymph capillaries, located in the capillary bed, absorb fluid from the surrounding tissues. The lymph capillaries join together to form larger lymph vessels (called lymphatics). Eventually, the lymphatics empty into the subclavian veins, large veins in the shoulder region. Lymph nodes, masses of lymphatic tissue located along the lymphatics, remove bacteria and other foreign particles from the lymph before the fluid is returned to the bloodstream.

stimulates the production of certain white blood cells (T cells) in the event of an infection. (Recall from Chapter 8 that T cells are the cells that the human immunodeficiency virus [HIV] virus attacks.) Another organ, the spleen, located in the abdomen, helps to filter blood and break down worn-out red blood cells. The spleen also acts as a reservoir where extra blood is stored. The body draws on this "extra" blood supply during times of massive blood loss, for example, following a major injury.

HEART

The heart is a hollow, muscular organ about the size of a fist that lies in the centre of the chest, tilted a bit toward the left, behind the sternum (breastbone). Like the walls of the arteries and veins, the walls of the heart are made of three layers of tissue. The **endocardium** is the smooth inner layer of the heart. The **myocardium,** the middle layer, is formed of cardiac muscle. Coordinated contraction and relaxation of the myocardium is what causes the heart to pump.

The **epicardium** is the smooth outermost layer of the heart. The epicardium forms part of the **pericardium,** a double-layered protective sac that surrounds the heart. A thin film of fluid between the epicardium and the outer layer of the pericardium allows the pericardial layers to slide smoothly against each other each time the heart pumps.

Atria and Ventricles

The hollow interior of the heart is divided into four chambers (Fig. 27-6). A thick wall of muscle, called the *septum,* separates the left side of the heart from the right side of the heart. *Valves,* flaps of tissue that help to ensure that blood flows only in one direction, separate the chambers on the top from the chambers on the bottom. The upper chambers are called the left atrium and right atrium, or the **atria.** The atria receive the blood that is being brought back to the heart from the body, and send it into the lower chambers of the heart, called the **ventricles.** When the ventricles contract, they send blood from the heart to other parts of the body. Because the ventricles must

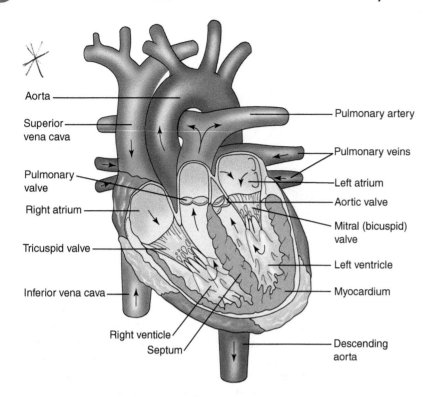

Aorta

Superior vena cava

Pulmonary valve

Right atrium

Tricuspid valve

Inferior vena cava

Right venticle

Septum

Pulmonary artery

Pulmonary veins

Left atrium

Aortic valve

Mitral (bicuspid) valve

Left ventricle

Myocardium

Descending aorta

Figure 27-6
The heart has four chambers. The atria receive blood that is being returned to the heart from the veins. Blood leaves the heart after passing through the ventricles.

send the blood much farther with each contraction, they are larger than the atria, and have thicker, more muscular walls.

Heart Valves

Blood can only flow through the heart in one direction. To keep blood flowing in the proper direction, the heart has four valves. Valves are flaps of tissue that snap shut after the blood passes through to prevent backflow.

- The tricuspid valve separates the right atrium from the right ventricle.
- The mitral (bicuspid) valve separates the left atrium from the left ventricle.
- The pulmonary valve is located where the pulmonary artery leaves the right ventricle.
- The aortic valve is located where the aorta leaves the left ventricle.

The four valves can be seen in Figure 27-6.

The valves that separate the upper and lower chambers of the heart may become diseased. For example, a type of infection called rheumatic fever can cause the valves to become thickened and scarred. Damaged valves are unable to create a seal when they close, which allows blood to backflow into the atria when the ventricles pump. This condition is called *valvular insufficiency*. A person with valvular insufficiency may need surgery to replace the defective valve.

Conduction System

The muscle cells that make up the myocardium are very specialized, so that they contract as a unit. This unified contraction is what allows the heart to work efficiently as a pump, moving blood continuously through the body. A small mass of special tissue in the heart, called the sinoatrial node (pacemaker), sets the pace for contraction by generating an electrical impulse. The electrical impulse travels through the myocardium via a special pathway called the conduction system. As it passes through, the electrical energy causes the cardiac muscle cells in the myocardium to contract. First the atria contract, there is a pause, and then the ventricles contract.

Coronary Circulation

Like all organs, the heart needs oxygen and nutrients. In fact, the heart's demand for oxygen and nutrients is very high because it works continuously, without rest. Think about it—the normal resting heart rate of an adult is 70 beats/min, or about 100,800 beats in a 24-hour period! The heart cannot stop to rest when it is tired; it has to continue pumping blood through the body. All of this hard work adds up to a very high, and constant, demand for oxygen and nutrients.

The coronary circulation meets this demand (Fig. 27-7). (*Coronary* is another word for "heart.")

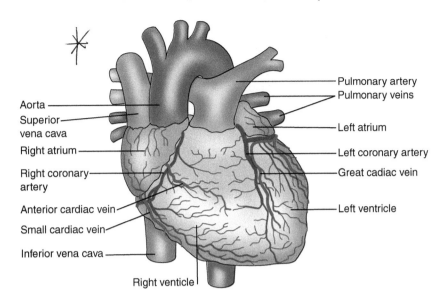

Figure 27-7
The heart has its own blood supply, called the coronary circulation.

Labels in figure:
Aorta
Superior vena cava
Right atrium
Right coronary artery
Anterior cardiac vein
Small cardiac vein
Inferior vena cava
Right venticle
Pulmonary artery
Pulmonary veins
Left atrium
Left coronary artery
Great cadiac vein
Left ventricle

Many people think that the cells of the heart just absorb oxygen from the blood that is passing through the chambers, but this is not the case. The tissues of the heart have their own special network of arteries and veins, just like all of the other organs in the body. Coronary arteries carry oxygen-rich blood into the heart tissue. Coronary veins remove carbon dioxide and other waste products. Any disruption in the flow of oxygen-rich blood to the tissues of the heart can cause **ischemia** (lack of oxygen to the tissues). Prolonged ischemia causes the tissue to die, resulting in permanent damage to the heart muscle.

FUNCTION OF THE CARDIOVASCULAR SYSTEM

The main function of the cardiovascular system is that of transport. However, the cardiovascular system also plays a role in regulating temperature and protecting the body from disease.

TRANSPORT

Bringing oxygen, nutrients, and other necessary substances (for example, hormones) to the cells and taking waste materials away from them is one of the most important functions of the cardiovascular system. Think of the cardiovascular system as a manufacturing company that serves customers across the nation. "Trucks" (red blood cells) are loaded up with merchandise at the "central warehouse" (the heart). The trucks set

out on a huge network of "highways" (the blood vessels) to deliver their goods. When they reach their destinations, the ordered merchandise is unloaded, and the empty crates are put back on the trucks to be returned to the warehouse.

Pulmonary and Systemic Circulation

While the blood is the vehicle that transports oxygen, nutrients, wastes, and other substances to their various destinations, the heart is the organ that powers the continuous movement of the blood (known as the **circulation**). The pattern of circulation actually involves two circuits: the pulmonary circulation and the systemic circulation (Fig. 27-8). The right side of the heart pumps blood to the lungs, where it picks up oxygen and releases carbon dioxide. This is the **pulmonary circulation** (*pulmonary* is another word for "lungs.") The left side of the heart pumps the newly oxygenated blood to the body. This is the **systemic circulation.**

The pattern of circulation goes like this (follow along on Figure 27-8):

Pulmonary circulation

- The largest veins in the body, the superior vena cava and the inferior vena cava, empty into the right atrium of the heart. The blood in these veins is returning from its journey to the tissues, so it has given up most of its oxygen and taken on a load of carbon dioxide.
- The right atrium pumps the oxygen-poor blood into the right ventricle.
- The right ventricle pumps the oxygen-poor blood into the pulmonary artery. The pulmonary artery branches into the right

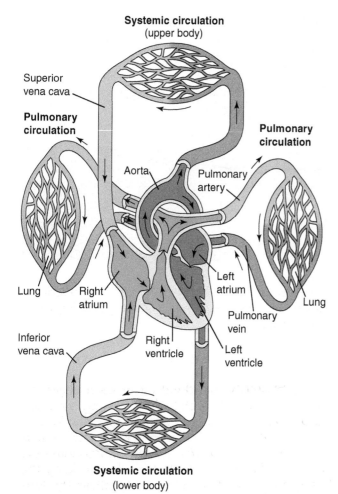

Figure 27-8
The pattern of circulation involves two circuits: the pulmonary circulation and the systemic circulation. In this diagram, *red* stands for oxygen-rich blood, and *blue* stands for oxygen-poor blood. Blood passes from the right ventricle into the pulmonary circulation. Once it is loaded up with oxygen, the blood returns to the left atrium, passes into the left ventricle, and is sent out to the rest of the body. This is the systemic circulation.

pulmonary artery, which goes to the right lung, and the left pulmonary artery, which goes to the left lung.

- Once in the lungs, the pulmonary arteries quickly branch into smaller arteries and arterioles to carry the oxygen-poor blood to the capillary beds surrounding the alveoli. As you remember from Chapter 26, gas exchange takes place in the alveoli. The oxygen in the alveolus moves into the blood, and the carbon dioxide in the blood moves into the alveolus, to be exhaled from the body.
- The blood, which now contains fresh oxygen, is carried by the network of venules, then

veins, to the pulmonary veins (right and left), which empty into the left atrium of the heart.

Systemic circulation

- The left atrium pumps the oxygen-rich blood into the left ventricle.
- The left ventricle pumps the oxygen-rich blood into the largest artery of the body, the aorta.
- The aorta branches very quickly into the coronary arteries to carry oxygen-rich blood to the heart muscle, and then into large branches of arteries that carry oxygen-rich blood to the rest of the body.
- The arteries branch into arterioles and then into capillaries, which join together to form a capillary bed. In the capillary bed, oxygen and nutrients move out of the blood and into the tissues, and carbon dioxide moves out of the tissues and into the blood.
- The blood, which now contains less oxygen, is carried by the network of venules, then veins, back to the right atrium, where the process begins again.

Cardiac Cycle

You may recall from Chapter 16 that the heart muscle contracts in two phases. During **systole,** or the active phase, the myocardium contracts, sending blood out of the heart. During **diastole,** or the resting phase, the myocardium relaxes, allowing the chambers to fill with blood. The atria are in systole when the ventricles are in diastole, and vice versa. The atria contract (atrial systole), sending the blood into the relaxed ventricles (ventricular diastole). Next, the atria relax (atrial diastole) while the ventricles contract (ventricular systole), sending the blood out to the body. This sequence is called the **cardiac cycle.**

The orderly sequence of systole and diastole is crucial for maximizing the amount of blood that is pumped throughout the body each time the heart contracts. During ventricular diastole, the ventricles are relaxed, which allows them to fill to capacity with blood. Without this rest period, the ventricles would never fill to capacity. Think about a plastic squirt bottle (the kind used at picnics to hold ketchup or mustard). If you fill the squirt bottle only partially with water, when you squeeze it, there is not enough force to push a large amount of water out. But, if you put as much water in the squirt bottle as it will hold and then squeeze, a small squeeze will cause a larger amount of water to squirt out with a lot more force. In other words, the heart is able to perform more efficiently when the ventricles are filled, because less force is required to send the maximum amount of blood out to the body.

As you may recall from Chapter 16, there are two distinct sounds that you will hear with your stethoscope when you are taking an apical pulse. The first sound, "lubb," is the sound of the tricuspid and mitral valves (the valves that separate the atria from the ventricles) snapping shut during ventricular systole. The second sound, "dupp," is the sound of the pulmonary and aortic valves closing during ventricular diastole. The two sounds heard together ("lubb–dupp") is what we know as a heartbeat.

REGULATION

Although transport is the cardiovascular system's major function, this system also plays a role in temperature regulation, as discussed in Chapter 24.

PROTECTION

The cardiovascular system helps to protect the body in two major ways. First, white blood cells, which play an important role in helping us to fight off disease, are circulated throughout the body in the blood. Second, when injury to the skin occurs, the blood has the ability to form a clot. The clot helps to protect us against excessive blood loss. It also helps to prevent microbes from gaining access to the body.

THE EFFECTS OF AGING ON THE CARDIOVASCULAR SYSTEM

Cardiovascular disorders are very common in Canada, especially among older people. Perhaps more than any other organ system, the cardiovascular system is affected by the choices we make in life. For example, smoking, poor dietary habits, and a lack of exercise can all contribute to cardiovascular disease later in life. In addition, common medical problems, such as diabetes, obesity, and hypertension (high blood pressure) can cause the cardiovascular system to age faster.

Many national organizations, such as the Heart and Stroke Foundation of Canada, provide information and education about "healthy heart

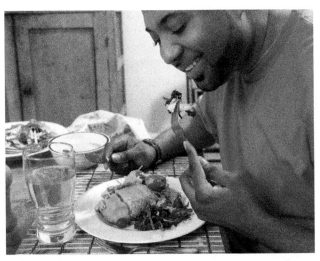

Figure 27-9
Regular exercise and a diet that is low in artery-clogging saturated fat are essential for maintaining a healthy heart throughout life.

living." By following the advice of these organizations, many people are able to maintain good cardiovascular function well into old age. The keys to cardiovascular health are exercise, a diet that is low in saturated (unhealthy) fats, and avoidance of smoking (Fig. 27-9). Exercise helps to keep the heart muscle strong and working efficiently. Eating a healthy diet helps to prevent atherosclerosis, a disease of the blood vessels that is discussed later in this chapter. Finally, chemicals in tobacco smoke cause the arterioles and capillaries to constrict, depriving tissues of vital blood flow. Smoking should be avoided because it has a very negative impact on the heart, which requires a healthy supply of oxygen and nutrients to function properly. In addition to preventing problems that affect the cardiovascular system directly, exercising, eating a healthy diet, and avoidance of tobacco smoke can help to prevent or control medical conditions that can contribute to cardiovascular disease, such as obesity, diabetes, and hypertension.

There are some changes to the cardiovascular system that will take place simply as a result of the aging process. In a healthy older person, these changes do not have a major impact on day-to-day life. However, when the processes of aging are combined with a chronic illness or a lifetime of unhealthy habits, the effect on cardiovascular function can be major. Age-related changes that occur include less efficient contraction of the heart, a loss of elasticity in the arteries and veins, and decreased numbers of blood cells.

LESS EFFICIENT CONTRACTION

Changes in the tissues of the heart, such as a loss of muscle tone and a loss of elasticity, affect the ability of the heart to contract forcefully, and it takes longer for the heart to complete the cycle of filling and emptying. A healthy older person might find that she tires faster while exercising, because the heart is not able to deliver oxygen and nutrients to the body as efficiently as it once was, in times of increased demand. Medical conditions, such as obesity or hypertension, place additional strain on the heart muscle and make the effects of normal aging on the heart worse. The heart of an older person who is ill may barely be able to meet the body's needs for oxygen and nutrients when the person is at rest.

DECREASED ELASTICITY OF THE ARTERIES AND VEINS

As we age, the walls of the blood vessels lose some of their elasticity. The loss of elasticity in the muscle layer of the arteries decreases the body's ability to control blood pressure and flow, because the arteries are not able to expand and "bounce back" as easily. This means that in an older person (especially one with cardiovascular disease), the arteries lose both the ability to dilate to allow for an increase in blood flow when needed, and the ability to constrict back to a smaller size afterward. The "stretch" is gone from the vessel. The effects of this age-related change are especially noticeable when an older person gets up quickly after lying down. The arteries do not constrict quickly enough to maintain adequate blood flow to the brain, and the person feels dizzy or lightheaded as a result. In other words, the person has orthostatic hypotension (see Chapter 16).

The loss of elasticity in the walls of the veins causes them to "stretch out," slowing the flow of blood back to the heart. The valves in the walls of the veins become less effective, which also slows the return of blood to the heart. Pooling of blood in the veins just underneath the skin can cause them to become swollen and "knotty" in appearance, a condition commonly known as **varicose veins.** Immobility and bed rest can make the effects of aging on the veins worse, because the large muscles of the legs are not working to help move the blood back toward the heart.

DECREASED NUMBERS OF BLOOD CELLS

The production of blood cells slows as a person ages. A decreased number of red blood cells affects the blood's ability to deliver oxygen to the tissues. A decreased number of white blood cells puts the older person at higher risk for developing infections, because the body's ability to fight them off is reduced.

DISORDERS OF THE CARDIOVASCULAR SYSTEM

Disorders of the cardiovascular system can involve the blood, the blood vessels, or the heart.

DISORDERS OF THE BLOOD

Blood disorders are often detected through laboratory analysis of the blood. Common blood disorders include anemia, leukemia, and clotting disorders.

Anemia

Anemia is a general term for a group of disorders affecting the red blood cells. Anemia decreases the blood's ability to transport oxygen to the cells. People who have anemia may become tired very easily. Their red blood cells simply are not able to transport the extra oxygen that is needed for exertion.

Anemia can result when the number of red blood cells is decreased, either because red blood cell production is impaired or the person is losing blood. For example, a disorder that affects the bone marrow, where blood cells are made, can cause a decrease in the number of circulating red blood cells, leading to anemia. Slow chronic blood loss (for example, from heavy menstrual periods or a stomach ulcer) can also cause anemia just by decreasing the amount of circulating blood.

Sometimes the number of red blood cells is adequate, but the red blood cells do not contain enough hemoglobin. Recall that hemoglobin is the molecule that binds with oxygen, so if the red blood cells lack hemoglobin, then they are unable to carry as much oxygen, resulting in anemia. The body needs iron to make hemoglobin. Therefore, people who have diets that are low in iron or certain B vitamins (which help the body to

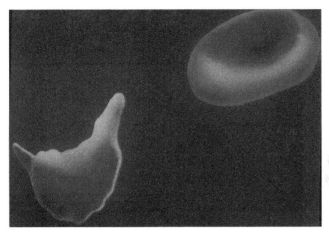

Figure 27-10

In sickle cell anemia, the red blood cells are abnormally shaped. Here, a sickled red blood cell is shown to the left of a normal red blood cell. (© *Roseman/Custom Medical Stock Photo.*)

absorb iron from the digestive tract) are at risk for anemia.

In disorders such as sickle cell anemia, red blood cells are produced, but they are abnormally shaped (Fig. 27-10). Because the cells lack the "dent" where the hemoglobin normally sits, they are unable to carry oxygen. Their abnormal shape also causes them to get stuck in the tiny capillaries, obstructing the flow of blood and causing pain, swelling, and fevers. Sickle cell anemia is an inherited disorder that is found mainly among people of African or Mediterranean heritage.

Leukemia

Leukemia is the excessive production of white blood cells. The white blood cells are abnormal in structure and they cannot perform their job of protecting the body from infection. Leukemia can be caused by cancer of the bone marrow or by cancer of the lymphatic tissue. Leukemia occurs in people of all ages, and can cause death if treatment is started too late or is not effective. People who have leukemia are at higher risk for developing infections. They may also have bleeding disorders, which can cause them to bruise very easily or bleed from their gums during oral care.

Bleeding Disorders

There are two types of bleeding disorders. Either the blood clots too much, or not enough.

In some people, the blood clots too easily. Clots can form in the small blood vessels, blocking

the flow of blood and depriving the tissues of oxygen and nutrients. The blood clots, called **thrombi,** can also break loose and travel to other parts of the body such as the brain, lungs, or heart. A blood clot that moves from one place to another is called an **embolus.** An embolus can be life-threatening. For example, the embolus may become stuck in the pulmonary artery, the artery that receives blood in need of oxygen from the heart. If blood cannot reach the lungs, then it cannot pick up the oxygen it needs for the rest of the body. People who have blood that clots too easily may need to take drugs called anticoagulants or "blood thinners" to help keep clots from forming where they are not needed.

Other people have the opposite problem—their blood does not form clots when it is supposed to (for example, after an injury). These people may lack fibrinogen, the protein in the blood plasma that assists with clotting. Or, they may have a low platelet count. (Recall that platelets are the blood cells that participate in clot formation.) For these people, even a small bump can cause a large bruise, while a more severe injury can result in a fatal hemorrhage.

DISORDERS OF THE BLOOD VESSELS

Atherosclerosis

Atherosclerosis is blocking of the arteries. Blood is unable to flow freely through the arteries because **plaque** (a fatty deposit) builds up on the inside of the vessel wall (Fig. 27-11). As a result, less oxygen and nutrients are delivered to the tissues of the body. In addition, plaque makes the normally smooth inner lining of the

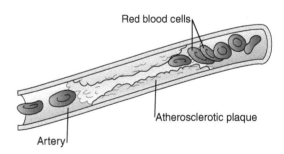

Figure 27-11

In atherosclerosis, fatty plaque builds up on the inside of the arteries, blocking the free flow of blood. This is particularly dangerous when the artery supplies a vital organ such as the heart, brain, or kidneys.

artery rough, which can cause blood clots to form. Sometimes the clots break off and become emboli. Finally, the plaque interferes with the elasticity of the arterial walls, making them brittle and prone to breaking (a condition called **arteriosclerosis**). This "hardening of the arteries" can lead to hemorrhages (bleeding) in the small vessels.

Depending on which arteries are affected, atherosclerosis can have serious consequences. The arteries that supply the brain, heart, kidneys, and legs are affected most often.

- Atherosclerosis of the arteries that supply the brain can cause a stroke. Strokes are discussed in detail in Chapter 28.
- Atherosclerosis of the arteries that supply the heart can cause myocardial infarction ("heart attack"). Myocardial infarction is discussed later in this chapter.
- Atherosclerosis of the arteries that supply the kidneys can cause renal failure, discussed in Chapter 32.
- Atherosclerosis of the arteries that supply the legs can cause **peripheral vascular disease.** In peripheral vascular disease, decreased blood flow to the leg muscles causes pain and cramping when the person walks. The pain and cramping, called *claudication,* occurs because the muscles are not receiving enough oxygen. In severe cases, the tissues in the leg die from lack of oxygen, and amputation may be necessary.

Although the exact cause of atherosclerosis is unknown, scientists now know that several factors contribute to the development of the disease. Diabetes, hypertension, and obesity are all medical conditions that have been associated with atherosclerosis. Heredity and stress may also play a role. Smoking, eating a diet high in cholesterol and saturated (unhealthy) fat, and a lack of physical activity can also increase a person's chances of developing atherosclerosis.

Venous Disorders

Loss of elasticity and decreased efficiency of the valves in the walls of the veins cause blood to "pool" in the legs, which can put the person at risk for several disorders:

- **Venous thrombosis.** In this disorder, blood clots form in the veins where the blood pools, because the blood is moving so slowly. These clots can block the vein, or they can become emboli. People with venous thrombosis are at risk for pulmonary embolism (an embolus that travels to the lung and blocks the pulmonary artery). Pulmonary embolism can be fatal.
- **Venous (stasis) ulcers.** As a result of pooling of the blood, plasma may leak into the tissues causing edema (swelling). The skin breaks down because of the poor circulation through the veins, resulting in sores that are slow to heal. These sores are called *venous ulcers* or *stasis ulcers.*

DISORDERS OF THE HEART

Heart disorders affect children as well as adults. Most heart disorders in children are *congenital,* which means that they were "present at birth." Congenital heart disorders occur when the fetus' heart does not form correctly. Many babies who are born with congenital heart disorders grow up to live long and healthy lives following surgery to correct the heart defect.

In adults, heart disorders have various causes. Conditions that are known to increase a person's risk of developing a heart disorder are called *cardiac risk factors.* Some of these risk factors can be changed, while others cannot. Risk factors that cannot be changed include the following:

- **Age.** The risk of developing a heart disorder increases with age.
- **Gender.** Men are at greater risk of developing heart disease at an earlier age than women. However, after a woman goes through menopause, her risk of developing heart disease is the same as a man's.
- **Heredity.** People who have parents or siblings with heart disease are more likely to develop heart disease themselves.
- **Body build.** Some people tend to put on weight in the abdomen or chest ("apples"), while others tend to carry it in the buttocks or thighs ("pears"). "Apple"-shaped people are more likely to develop heart disease than "pear"-shaped people.

Age, gender, heredity, and body build are risk factors that cannot be changed. However, there are many risk factors for heart disease that can be changed. These risk factors include:

- Smoking
- Physical inactivity
- Obesity
- A diet high in saturated fat and cholesterol
- Poorly controlled hypertension
- Poorly controlled diabetes

Common heart disorders in adults include coronary artery disease, heart failure, and heart block.

Coronary Artery Disease

Coronary artery disease occurs when the coronary arteries narrow as a result of atherosclerosis. Recall that the coronary arteries supply the heart muscle with blood containing oxygen and nutrients. Initially, the heart muscle may receive enough oxygen to work properly when the body is at rest, but it may be unable to meet the increased needs brought on by activity. Eventually, one or more of the coronary arteries may become so narrow that no blood gets through, causing areas of the heart muscle to die.

Coronary artery disease is treated in a number of ways. Medications are available that help to keep the arteries open, permitting maximum blood flow. Balloon angioplasty is a technique that involves the insertion of a catheter into the affected artery. A balloon on the end of the catheter is inflated, squeezing the plaque to the sides of the artery and creating a larger opening for blood to flow through. As an alternative to balloon angioplasty, springs may be placed in the artery to hold the narrowed portion open. Finally, surgery can be performed to bypass the blocked arteries and reestablish blood flow.

Conditions that are closely related to coronary artery disease include angina pectoris and myocardial infarction.

Angina pectoris

Angina pectoris is the classic chest pain that is felt as a result of the heart muscle being deprived of oxygen. Anginal pain varies among individuals. Some people describe it as a pain in the centre of the chest. Others experience pain that starts in the chest and extends to the arm or neck. A person who is experiencing angina may feel as though he is suffocating, and he may become very anxious.

Many people experience angina quite frequently and know what it is. These people often keep nitroglycerin pills on hand to relieve the pain when it occurs. Nitroglycerin relaxes the arteries, increasing the flow of blood. If you have been trained to help a person with her nitroglycerin, avoid handling the pills with your bare hands. The drug can be absorbed through the skin, which can cause a decrease in your blood pressure and a pounding headache.

Myocardial infarction

A **myocardial infarction** is a "heart attack." A myocardial infarction occurs when one or more of the coronary arteries becomes completely blocked, preventing blood from reaching the parts of the heart that are fed by the affected arteries (Fig. 27-12). The lack of blood (and vital

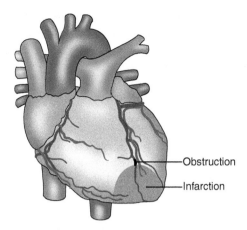

Figure 27-12

A heart attack occurs when one or more of the coronary arteries becomes blocked, preventing blood from reaching the myocardium. The lack of oxygen and nutrients causes the tissue that is supplied by the affected artery to die.

oxygen) causes the tissue to die. The dead tissue is called an *infarct*.

The severity of the myocardial infarction depends on the extent of the tissue damaged and the part of the heart affected. Although a myocardial infarction that affects the atria may not be life-threatening, one that severely damages the ventricles can reduce the heart's ability to pump blood to vital organs and cause death. Early recognition of the symptoms of a myocardial infarction (see Chapter 12) and early treatment can greatly increase a person's chances of surviving. Drugs that help to maintain a normal heartbeat and restore blood flow to the affected area can greatly improve the person's outcome.

Heart Failure

Heart failure occurs when the heart is unable to pump enough blood to meet the body's needs. Heart failure has many causes. For example, disorders that cause the ventricles to lose muscle tone and become large and flabby can cause heart failure. Heart failure can also occur as a result of a myocardial infarction that leaves the ventricles unable to function properly.

Heart failure can be either "right-sided" or "left-sided." Right-sided heart failure, also called *cor pulmonale,* causes blood to back up in the venous system because the right ventricle's ability to pump the blood into the pulmonary circulation is impaired. In a person with right-sided heart failure, the veins in the legs and abdomen become swollen, and fluid may leak into the tissues, causing significant edema and skin breakdown. Left-sided heart failure, also called *congestive heart failure,* causes the blood to back up in the lungs because the left ventricle's ability to pump the blood into the systemic circulation is impaired. The excess blood in the vessels of the lungs causes fluid to leak into the lung tissues, which causes congestion and makes breathing difficult.

For people with heart failure, medications may be used to help increase the heart's ability to pump more effectively and to pull excess fluid from the tissues. Many people with severe heart failure have their fluids restricted and their intake and output very carefully measured and monitored.

Conduction Disorders

Some conditions affect the pathway that the heart uses to transmit the electrical impulses that cause contraction. These disorders are called **conduction disorders.** Heart block is a common type of conduction disorder. Heart block can result from a myocardial infarction that damages the pathway, or it may occur as part of the normal aging process. A heart block causes the heart to slow down significantly, leading to dizziness or fainting episodes.

Heart block is usually treated with a pacemaker, an electrical device that stimulates the heart to contract. The pacemaker consists of a small, battery-operated device implanted under the skin below the collarbone and two wires that

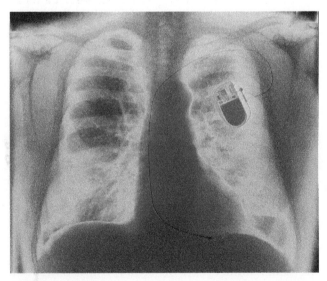

Figure 27-13

A pacemaker is a battery-operated device used to treat heart block. The pacemaker sends out an electrical signal that stimulates the heart to contract when the person's heart rate drops below a preprogrammed rate. In this photograph, you can see the pacemaker above the person's ribcage. A dark blue lead connects the pacemaker to the person's heart, which is the red area in the lower right of the photograph. (© *Salisbury District Hospital/Photo Researchers, Inc.*)

connect to the right side of the heart (Fig. 27-13). When the person's heart rate drops below a programmed rate, the battery-operated device sends a small electrical impulse through the wires that stimulates the heart muscle to contract.

TELL THE NURSE

The routine taking of vital signs, especially the pulse and blood pressure, is one of the best ways to detect abnormalities in the functioning of the cardiovascular system at an early stage. In addition, there are many signs and symptoms you may observe that could indicate that a patient or resident is having a cardiovascular problem. Report any of the following observations to the nurse immediately:

- Complaints of chest pain or pressure
- Laboured or difficult breathing
- A rapid or erratic pulse
- A slow, weak pulse
- A blood pressure reading that is either much higher or much lower than the person's usual reading
- Cyanosis of the face, lips, or fingers
- Decreased tolerance for usual exertion
- Red, painful, or swollen areas in the extremities, especially the calves of the legs
- Unusual swelling of the legs, especially if it is accompanied by red, shiny skin
- "Dusky" (blue or greyish) colouring of the legs, especially if it is accompanied by a diminished pulse and coldness of the skin

DIAGNOSIS OF CARDIOVASCULAR DISORDERS

Depending on where you work, you may be responsible for caring for people who are recovering from an acute cardiovascular disorder, such as a heart attack. Other people will be admitted to the hospital to have a procedure done to prevent a heart attack from occurring, such as balloon angioplasty. Often, people with cardiovascular disorders will have one or more tests done to help the doctor determine the extent of the problem, plan a course of treatment, and monitor the person after the treatment. Tests you may hear mentioned include the following:

- **Electrocardiography.** In electrocardiography, sensors are attached to the person's chest. These sensors pick up the electrical activity of the heart and record it on a piece of paper. The tracing is called an *electrocardiogram* (EKG). An EKG shows abnormalities in the conduction system of the heart. Some people have an EKG done while they are exercising. This is called a stress test (Fig. 27-14).
- **Echocardiography.** In echocardiography, sound waves are bounced against the body to produce an image. A computer translates the sound waves into an image. Echocardiography can provide the doctor with much helpful information, including the size and shape of the heart, its pumping strength,

and the location and extent of any damage to its tissues.
- **Doppler ultrasound.** In Doppler ultrasound, sound waves are used to check the blood flow in the large arteries and veins of the arms and legs.
- **Radiography.** Radiographs, commonly known as "x-rays," are often used in the diagnosis of cardiovascular disease. A chest x-ray can show enlargement of the ventricles. Sometimes, a special dye is injected into the veins and then an x-ray is taken. The dye allows the doctor to see any abnormalities in the vessels of the heart or other parts of the body.

CARDIAC REHABILITATION

Cardiac rehabilitation is often necessary for a person who has had a heart attack or has had heart surgery. **Cardiac rehabilitation** focuses on helping a person regain strength and adopt habits that will help the cardiovascular system become healthier. A person who is in cardiac rehabilitation will begin an exercise program under the guidance of a nurse or therapist who specializes in cardiac disorders. The exercise program is designed to strengthen the heart muscle and make it a more effective pump. As the person grows stronger, the therapist or nurse will work with the person to develop an exercise plan that will become a part of the person's daily routine. A dietitian will work with the person to teach him about dietary changes that are needed to help control obesity and blood cholesterol levels. Avoidance of unhealthy habits, such as smoking, may require the use of medications and supportive emotional therapy.

A person who has had a heart attack or heart surgery may not want to participate in cardiac rehabilitation. The person may be afraid that any type of activity will put too much stress on the heart. Or, the person may be depressed or in denial. When you are caring for a person who needs cardiac rehabilitation, use empathy and good communication skills to help reassure and comfort the person. Report your observations of any emotional difficulties to the nurse immediately.

Many people with cardiovascular disease benefit greatly from cardiac rehabilitation, especially if rehabilitation is started early. Cardiac rehabilitation gives people the energy and ability to pursue things that they enjoy doing, which improves quality of life.

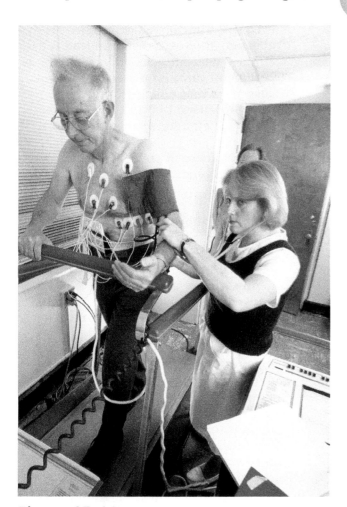

Figure 27-14
Electrocardiography is commonly used for diagnosis and monitoring of heart problems. This man is having a cardiac stress test. In a cardiac stress test, an electrocardiogram (ECG) is obtained while the person exercises. (© *Larry Mulvehill/Photo Researchers, Inc.*)

Summary

- The cardiovascular system, also known as the circulatory system, is made up of the blood, the blood vessels, the lymphatic system, and the heart.
    - Blood consists of plasma and blood cells (red blood cells, white blood cells, and platelets).
    - Arteries carry blood away from the heart, and veins carry blood to the heart. The transfer of substances into and out of the blood occurs in the capillary bed.
    - The lymphatic system is a one-way system that returns fluid that leaks into the tissues to the bloodstream.
    - The heart is the muscular organ that powers circulation.
        - The heart has four chambers. The atria receive blood from the body, and the ventricles send blood to the body.
        - The heart valves make sure that blood flows through the heart in the proper direction.
        - The heart's conduction system makes and conducts the electrical impulses that cause the heart to contract regularly.
        - The coronary circulation supplies the heart with oxygen and nutrients.
- The main function of the cardiovascular system is to transport oxygen, nutrients, and other substances *to* the tissues, and remove carbon dioxide and other wastes *from* the tissues.
    - The pattern of circulation involves two parallel circuits. The right side of the heart pumps blood into the lungs, where it picks up oxygen. The left side of the heart pumps the oxygenated blood to the rest of the body.
    - During systole, the heart contracts, sending blood out of the heart. During diastole, the heart relaxes, allowing the chambers to fill. The atria are in systole when the ventricles are in diastole, and vice versa.
- When the effects of aging are combined with a lifetime of unhealthy habits or a chronic disease, the effect on cardiovascular function can be major.
    - Exercising, eating a diet low in saturated fat and cholesterol, and avoiding tobacco smoke help to keep the cardiovascular system healthy. Controlling chronic diseases such as diabetes and hypertension is also important.
    - Risk factors for cardiovascular disease that cannot be changed include age, gender, heredity, and body build.
- Disorders of the cardiovascular system can affect the blood, the blood vessels, or the heart.
    - Disorders of the blood include anemia, leukemia, and bleeding disorders.
    - Disorders of the blood vessels include atherosclerosis, venous thrombosis, and venous (stasis) ulcers.
        - Atherosclerosis is blockage of the arteries. Depending on which arteries are affected, atherosclerosis can lead to strokes, heart attacks, kidney failure, or peripheral vascular disease.
        - Disorders that affect the veins are usually caused by widening of the veins, which allows blood to pool in the legs.
- Disorders of the heart include coronary artery disease, heart failure, and conduction disorders.
    - Coronary artery disease is caused by a narrowing of the arteries that supply the heart muscle with oxygen and nutrients.
        - Angina pectoris is chest pain that results from the heart muscle being deprived of oxygen.
        - A myocardial infarction occurs when the blood supply to the heart muscle is completely obstructed.
    - Heart failure results from the heart's inability to pump blood in sufficient amounts to supply the body.
    - Conduction disorders involve the electrical pathway in the heart. A person with a conduction disorder may have a pacemaker implanted to stimulate regular contraction of the heart.
- The goal of cardiac rehabilitation is to help a person with heart disease to regain strength and adopt habits that will improve the health of the cardiovascular system. An exercise plan and dietary and other lifestyle changes are part of cardiac rehabilitation.

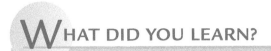

WHAT DID YOU LEARN?

Multiple Choice

Select the single best answer for each of the following questions.

1. The formation of artery-clogging plaque on the inside of the arteries is called:
   a. Atherosclerosis
   b. Arterioles
   c. Anemia
   d. Myocardial infarction

2. What is the function of the cardiovascular system?
   a. Transport of substances throughout the body
   b. Regulation of body temperature
   c. Protection of the body from blood loss and infection
   d. All of the above

3. Which circulation supplies the tissues of the heart with oxygen and nutrients?
   a. Pulmonary circulation
   b. Systemic circulation
   c. Coronary circulation
   d. Pericardial circulation

4. Which of the following is a risk factor for cardiovascular disease?
   a. Poorly controlled hypertension
   b. A diet high in cholesterol and saturated fats
   c. Lack of physical activity
   d. All of the above

Matching

Match each numbered item with its appropriate lettered description.

G 1. Red blood cells (erythrocytes)
D 2. White blood cells (leukocytes)
H 3. Ventricles
J 4. Veins
A 5. Atria
B 6. Arteries
C 7. Systole
i 8. Pulmonary circulation
E 9. Systemic circulation
F 10. Diastole

a. Upper chambers of the heart, which receive blood from the body
b. Vessels that carry blood away from the heart
c. Active phase of the cardiac cycle
d. Blood cells that help the body to fight infection
e. Circuit that sends newly oxygenated blood to the body
f. Resting phase of the cardiac cycle
g. Blood cells that contain hemoglobin and carry oxygen
h. Lower chambers of the heart, which pump blood to the body
i. Circuit that sends oxygen-poor blood to the lungs to pick up oxygen
j. Vessels that return blood to the heart

STOP and Think!

You are caring for Mr. Becker, a 74-year-old man with a history of heart disease. Mr. Becker keeps nitroglycerin in his bedside table to use when he has an angina attack. As you are assisting Mr. Becker back into his room from the dining room, he starts to complain of a tightness in his chest and seems to be having difficulty breathing. His lips also look a little blue. He asks you to help him with his nitroglycerin pill. What safety precaution needs to be taken while handling nitroglycerin? What else should you do?

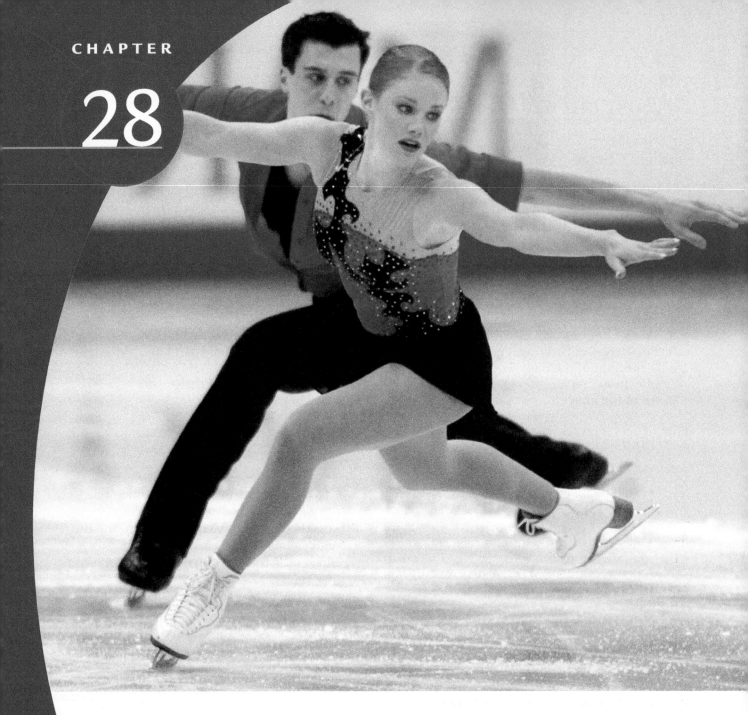

The Nervous System

WHAT WILL YOU LEARN?

The nervous system consists of the brain, the spinal cord, and the nerves. The nervous system receives information at a great rate, from both inside and outside the body. It then processes this information and issues instructions to other organ systems to carry out. "Command

Photo: The nervous system helps us to move with grace and coordination by directing the activity of the muscles. (AP Photo/Roberto Borea.)

central" of the human body, the nervous system, is the subject of this chapter. When you are finished with this chapter, you will be able to:

1. List and describe the structures that make up the two main divisions of the nervous system.
2. Discuss the main functions of the nervous system.
3. Describe how aging affects the nervous system.
4. Discuss various disorders that affect the nervous system.
5. List common diagnostic procedures that are used to help detect nervous system disorders.
6. Describe rehabilitation measures that a person with a nervous system disorder may need.

Vocabulary

Neuron	Central nervous system	Cerebrospinal fluid (CSF)	Stroke
Dendrites	(CNS)	Sensory nerves	Aphasia
Axon	Peripheral nervous	Motor nerves	Parkinson's disease
Synapse	system (PNS)	Transient ischemic	Epilepsy
Myelin	Meninges	attack (TIA)	Multiple sclerosis (MS)

STRUCTURE OF THE NERVOUS SYSTEM

Nervous tissue, which forms the organs of the nervous system, is made up of a special kind of cell, called a neuron. A **neuron** is a cell that can send and receive information. A neuron consists of dendrites, a cell body, and an axon (Fig. 28-1). **Dendrites** are short extensions from the cell body that *receive* information. The **axon** is a long extension from the cell body that *sends* information. An electrical signal, called a nerve impulse, enters the neuron at the dendrites. It passes through the cell body and travels down the axon, and then on to the dendrites of the next neuron in line. The movement of the nerve impulse is called *conduction.* The axon of one neuron does not actually connect with the dendrites of the next (see Fig. 28-1). Instead, chemicals called neurotransmitters carry the nerve impulse across the gap between the axon of one neuron and the dendrites of the next. This gap is called a **synapse.** The axons of some neurons are wrapped in **myelin,** a fatty, white substance that protects the axon. Myelin also helps to speed the conduction of nerve impulses along the axon.

The nervous system has two main divisions: the central nervous system and the peripheral nervous system (Fig. 28-2). The **central nervous system (CNS)** consists of the brain and spinal cord.

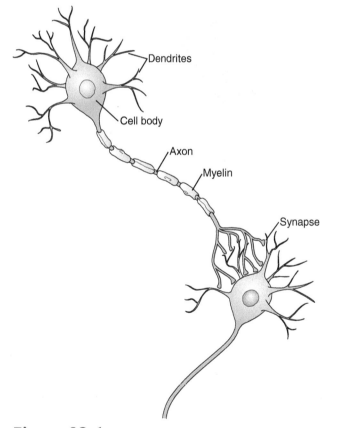

Figure 28-1

Neurons are special cells that have the ability to send and receive information.

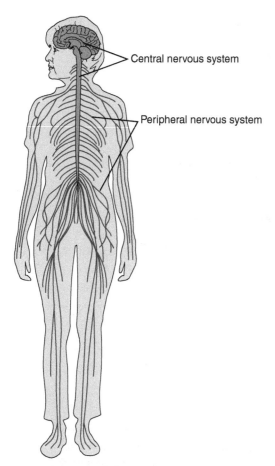
Central nervous system

Peripheral nervous system

Figure 28-2
The nervous system has two main divisions: the central nervous system and the peripheral nervous system. "Peripheral" means "along the edge" or "away from the centre."

The central nervous system receives information, processes it, and issues instructions. The **peripheral nervous system (PNS)** consists of the nerves outside of the brain and spinal cord. A nerve is simply a bundle of axons, wrapped in a connective tissue sheath. The peripheral nervous system receives information from the environment, and carries commands from the brain and spinal cord to the other organs of the body, such as the muscles.

THE CENTRAL NERVOUS SYSTEM

Because it is so vital to the body's functioning, the central nervous system is well protected by three layers of connective tissue, called **meninges,** and the bony skull and vertebrae (Fig. 28-3). The three meninges are, from the inside out:

- The *pia mater,* a thin delicate layer of tissue rich in blood vessels that is attached to the surface of the brain and spinal cord

- The *arachnoid mater,* the web-like middle layer
- The *dura mater,* a thick, tough outer layer that is attached to the inside of the skull and the vertebrae

The space between the pia mater and the arachnoid mater contains **cerebrospinal fluid (CSF),** a clear fluid that circulates around the brain and spinal cord and acts as an additional "shock absorber" to protect these structures.

The Brain

The brain, a large, soft mass of nervous tissue, is where information is processed and instructions are issued. The brain has four parts: the cerebrum, the diencephalon, the brainstem, and the cerebellum (see Fig. 28-3).

The cerebrum

The cerebrum is the largest part of the brain, with the characteristic "folds" that we always picture when we think of a brain (see Fig. 28-3). The cerebrum:

- Controls the voluntary movement of muscles
- Gives meaning to information received from the eyes, ears, nose, taste buds, and sensory receptors in the skin
- Allows us to speak, remember, think, and feel emotions

A deep groove divides the cerebrum into two hemispheres: the left hemisphere (or "left brain") and the right hemisphere (or "right brain"). The right and left hemispheres communicate with each other and are connected by a structure called the *corpus callosum.* The right side of the brain controls the left side of the body, and vice versa. So, an injury to the tissues in the left side of the brain may result in loss of function on the right side of the body.

The diencephalon

The diencephalon contains the thalamus and the hypothalamus (see Fig. 28-3). The thalamus sorts out the impulses that arrive via the spinal cord from other parts of the body and sends them to the correct part of the cerebrum. The hypothalamus controls body temperature, fluid balance, appetite, sleep cycles, and some of the emotions, and regulates the pituitary gland, a gland you will learn more about in Chapter 30.

The brainstem

The brainstem connects the spinal cord to the brain. It has three parts: the midbrain, the pons, and the medulla (see Fig. 28-3). The medulla

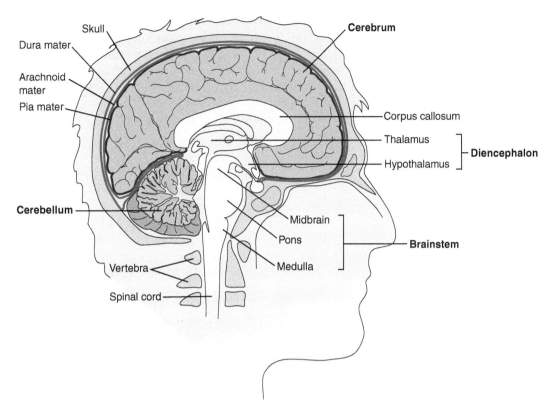

Figure 28-3

The brain and the spinal cord make up the central nervous system (CNS). The brain has four parts: the cerebrum, the diencephalon, the brainstem, and the cerebellum. Three layers of connective tissue, called the dura mater, the arachnoid mater, and the pia mater, help to cushion and protect the brain and spinal cord. Additional protection is provided by the bony skull and vertebrae.

contains the centres that control respiration, heartbeat, and blood pressure.

The cerebellum

The cerebellum helps to coordinate the brain's commands to the muscles so that the muscles move smoothly and in an orderly fashion. It also plays a role in balance.

The Spinal Cord

The spinal cord is a "cord" of nervous tissue that extends from the base of the brain downward, to a point approximately even with your bellybutton. The vertebrae (the bones that make up your spine) surround and protect the spinal cord.

The spinal cord is the main connection between the brain and the rest of the body. Pathways of nerve tissue in the spinal cord, also called *tracts*, carry messages to and from the brain. Ascending tracts carry information from the peripheral nervous system to the brain. Descending tracts carry information from the brain to the peripheral nervous system.

THE PERIPHERAL NERVOUS SYSTEM

The peripheral nervous system consists of the nerves, or the lines of communication between the central nervous system and the rest of the body. Every part of the body is innervated, or supplied, by nerves, which form a vast network throughout the body.

The nerves that form the peripheral nervous system are either sensory nerves or motor nerves. **Sensory nerves** carry information from the "outside in." In other words, the sensory nerves carry information from the internal organs and the outside world to the spinal cord and up into the brain so that the brain can analyze the information. **Motor nerves** carry information from the "inside out." In other words, the motor nerves carry commands from the brain down the spinal cord and out to the muscles and organs of the body. Motor nerves allow the brain to control voluntary muscle movement and the involuntary functions of the internal organs.

Thirty-one pairs of nerves, called spinal nerves, connect to the spinal cord. Each spinal nerve consists of one sensory nerve and one motor nerve. The spinal nerves that innervate the arms and the upper part of the body are located in the neck region, while the spinal nerves that innervate the legs and the lower part of the body are located in the back.

Some nerves are connected directly to the brain. These nerves are called cranial nerves. There are 12 pairs of cranial nerves.

FUNCTION OF THE NERVOUS SYSTEM

The nervous system receives, processes, and responds to information.

REGULATION OF THE INTERNAL ENVIRONMENT

By now, you are familiar with the concept of homeostasis, or balance. For the body to function well, a state of homeostasis must be maintained. The nervous system regulates what is going on within the body and makes adjustments as necessary to keep things within the range of normal. For example, control centres in the hypothalamus monitor the body temperature, and control centres in the medulla monitor heartbeat and respirations.

When the central nervous system detects an imbalance, a special part of the peripheral nervous system, called the autonomic system, is activated. The autonomic system has two lower divisions: the sympathetic nervous system and the parasympathetic nervous system. Generally speaking, the sympathetic nervous system speeds things up, and the parasympathetic nervous system slows them back down. Perhaps you have heard of the "fight or flight" response. When we are put in a dangerous situation, our heart rate and breathing increase, and the adrenal glands release adrenaline, a chemical that helps us to cope with stress. These changes allow us to run faster or be stronger in a fight, and they are caused by activation of the sympathetic nervous system. Once the danger has passed, the parasympathetic nervous system slows things back down.

INTERACTION WITH THE EXTERNAL ENVIRONMENT

The nervous system allows us to interact with the world around us. The special senses—touch, taste, smell, sight, and hearing—provide the brain with information about the outside world. The brain responds to this information. The ability to receive information about the outside world and respond to it not only makes life more pleasurable, it helps to protect us from harm. (The special senses are discussed in detail in Chapter 29.)

THE EFFECTS OF AGING ON THE NERVOUS SYSTEM

Neurons cannot divide and reproduce as other body cells do. That means that we keep the same 100 billion neurons our whole lives, give or take a few! Despite the fact that neurons are not replaced, they experience relatively little wear and tear over the course of a lifetime. Still, some structural changes occur as a result of aging, which can result in slowed conduction times and slight memory changes.

SLOWED CONDUCTION TIMES

You may notice that some of your elderly patients or residents are not as quick to react to things as they used to be. This is a normal age-related change that is caused by changes in the myelin sheath and the amount of neurotransmitters. As we age, the amount of myelin surrounding the axons decreases, reducing the speed of nerve conduction by approximately 10%. In addition, neurotransmitter imbalances can interfere with the ability of a nerve impulse to travel across a synapse, slowing conduction. These changes are a normal part of the aging process, and they occur gradually over time.

Slowed conduction times can increase an elderly person's risk for falling and other household accidents. For example, it will take an older person longer to regain his balance if he starts to fall, or to avoid an obstacle (such as a pet or small child) that suddenly darts into his path. For this reason, it is especially important to remember the general safety guidelines from Chapter 10 when caring for an older person. For example, when helping an older person to walk, you will want to make sure that the pathway is well lit and clear, that the person's clothes and shoes fit properly, and, if the person wears glasses, that she is wearing them.

MEMORY CHANGES

Memory and thought processes usually remain intact with normal aging. It may take an older person slightly longer to remember names, dates, or other information from the past, but given enough time, the person will eventually remember. Many older people experience a mild loss of memory for recent events, while still having excellent long-term memory. Engaging in activities that stimulate the mind (such as reading, traveling, working crossword puzzles, and doing crafts and other handiwork) throughout life helps to keep thought processes sharp and active well into old age (Fig. 28-4).

Dementia is a significant loss of mental capabilities. Dementia is a disorder, not a normal age-related change. If you work in a long-term care facility, it may seem to you that dementia is common, because dementia is a leading cause for admission to long-term care facilities. However, among the general population, the rate of dementia is much lower. Dementia is discussed in detail in Chapter 36.

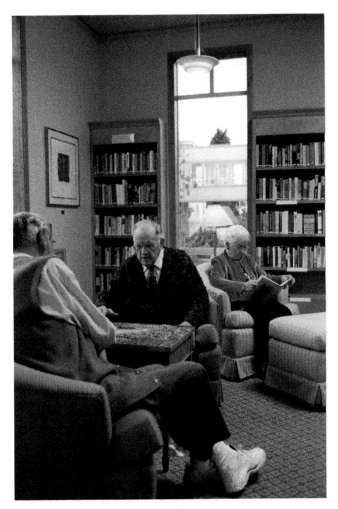

Figure 28-4
Use it or lose it! Studies have shown that actively exercising your mind throughout life helps to preserve mental function.

DISORDERS OF THE NERVOUS SYSTEM

There are many types of nervous system disorders. Some disorders affect a person's ability to control movement, or experience sensation. Other disorders may affect a person's ability to speak. Still other disorders affect a person's memory or behaviour. Disorders can be the result of a disease process, such as Parkinson's disease, or the result of an injury that damages the brain, spinal cord, or peripheral nerve pathways. Disorders of the nervous system are the most common causes of disability among elderly people. Approximately 50% of the disabilities seen in people older than 65 years are caused by a disorder of the nervous system.

TRANSIENT ISCHEMIC ATTACKS

Ischemia is decreased blood flow to the tissues. The tissue that is not getting enough blood is said to be *ischemic*. **Transient ischemic attacks (TIAs)** are temporary (transient) episodes of dysfunction that are caused by decreased blood flow (ischemia) to the brain. Any condition or situation that decreases blood flow to the brain can cause a TIA. For example, small blood clots can form in the heart or the arteries that supply the brain. These clots can break off and travel into the narrow arterioles of the brain, where they temporarily block the blood flow. Low blood pressure, certain medications, cigarette smoking, or standing up suddenly after lying down can also lead to a TIA.

Symptoms of a TIA vary according to the part of the brain affected by the decreased blood supply. Common symptoms may include dizziness, nausea, blurring or loss of vision, double vision, paralysis on one side of the body or face (with or without loss of sensation), or the inability to speak or swallow. The symptoms of a TIA may only last a few minutes, or they may last for several hours. The person usually recovers completely within 24 hours.

If you suspect that one of your patients or residents is having or has just had a TIA, please report this to the nurse immediately. TIAs are usually a warning that the person could have a stroke in the near future. A TIA may also be a sign of an underlying medical condition that needs to be addressed.

STROKE

A **stroke,** also known as a "brain attack" or cerebrovascular accident (CVA), occurs when blood flow to a part of the brain is completely blocked, causing the tissue to die. Unlike a TIA, a stroke causes permanent effects, because the obstruction of blood flow lasts long enough for the brain tissue to die or become damaged. Stroke is the third leading cause of death in people older than 65 years. Even if death does not occur, the person may be left with significant disabilities following a stroke. A very high number of the residents in long-term care facilities are survivors of a stroke.

A stroke can occur suddenly in a person who was previously healthy. Signs and symptoms vary, depending on the area of the brain that is affected. Personality changes, drooping of the eyelid or corner of the mouth, slurring of speech, paralysis, severe headache, and loss of consciousness can all be signs of a stroke. If you notice a difference in a patient's or resident's usual behaviour, appearance, or medical condition, you should report your observations to a nurse immediately (Fig. 28-5).

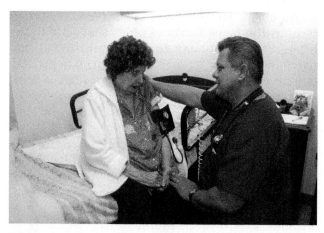

Figure 28-5
A severe headache, personality changes, slurring of speech, paralysis, or loss of consciousness may all signal the onset of a stroke.

 TELL THE NURSE

Signs and symptoms of stroke can vary. Observations that should be reported to the nurse immediately include the following:

- The person is unconscious or difficult to arouse from sleep
- The person suddenly seems confused or disoriented
- The person slurs his or her speech or is unable to speak clearly
- The person is drooling
- One of the person's eyelids or the corner of the mouth is drooping
- The person complains of the sudden onset of a severe headache
- The person complains of paralysis, tingling, or numbness of an arm or leg or the side of the face
- There is a change in the person's vital signs, especially the blood pressure or pulse

Causes of Stroke

The most common cause of a stroke is a blood clot that blocks the flow of blood to a part of the brain. Therefore, people who smoke, have atherosclerosis, or have poorly controlled hypertension or diabetes are at high risk for having a stroke. Another, less common, cause of a stroke is cerebral hemorrhage. A cerebral hemorrhage occurs when a small artery in the brain bursts. The bleeding into the surrounding brain tissue puts pressure on the delicate tissue, damaging it. A cerebral hemorrhage is more likely in people with chronic hypertension, arteriosclerosis ("hardening of the arteries"), or certain deformities of the blood vessels in the brain.

Effects of Stroke

The lasting effects of a stroke depend on the area of the brain that is affected and the amount of tissue that is damaged. For example, a stroke that affects the vital control centres of the brainstem will result in death, while a stroke that affects part of the cerebrum may result only in disability. The most common disabilities resulting from a stroke are hemiplegia and aphasia.

Hemiplegia, you will recall from Chapter 10, is paralysis on one side of the body. (Remember that the right side of the brain controls the left

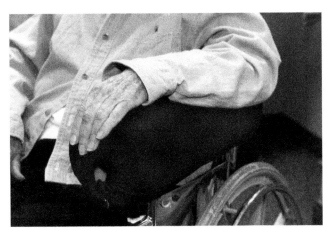

Figure 28-6
A person who has had a stroke may lose the ability to detect sensations on one side of the body. With these people, extra care must be taken to prevent pressure ulcers and other injuries, because the person will be unable to sense warnings of impending injury, such as pain, cold, or heat.

side of the body, and the left side of the brain controls the right side of the body—so a stroke that damages the right side of the brain will affect the left side of the body, and vice versa.) Depending on the amount of tissue damage, the hemiplegia may be mild or severe. A person with mild hemiplegia may have slight muscle weakness or shaking on the affected side, while a person with severe hemiplegia may not be able to move or feel any type of sensation at all on that side of the body. A person with severe hemiplegia who has lost sensation on one side of the body will need frequent repositioning to prevent pressure ulcers from forming (Fig. 28-6). Care must also be taken to prevent other injuries, such as burns, because the person will not have the ability to detect extreme heat, cold, or pain on the affected side.

Another common disability caused by a stroke is aphasia. **Aphasia** is a general term for a group of disorders that affect the ability of the person to communicate with others.

- *Expressive aphasia* is caused by damage to the motor centres of the brain that control the ability to speak or form sounds into meaningful words. A person with expressive aphasia may also have trouble swallowing, increasing her risk of choking.
- *Receptive aphasia* is caused by damage to the area of the brain that allows the person to understand words. The person can speak clearly, but he no longer knows the meaning of the words. For example, a person with

receptive aphasia may say "no" when he means "yes."

Treatment of Stroke

In the past, the treatment of stroke focused on stabilizing the person's medical condition and then using aggressive physical therapy to help retrain disabled muscles to perform simple tasks. However, now new treatments are available that can help to minimize the permanent damage caused by the stroke. For example, medications that dissolve blood clots are sometimes used to reestablish blood flow to the brain before permanent damage can occur. To work, these medications must be given very soon after the onset of the stroke.

Treatment immediately following a stroke depends on the severity of the damage to the brain, and on whether the person or family members want life-support measures to be taken. A person who has had a stroke may be very critically ill initially and need intensive care nursing. Respiratory support, oxygen, medications to support the heart rate and blood pressure, and continuous monitoring of vital signs may be necessary.

During this crisis period, the person's family members face uncertainty and difficult decisions. For example, they may need to decide whether or not to prolong life-support measures. If the person survives the stroke, family members may need to make some decisions about where the person will live in the future. For example, the person may need to move to a long-term care facility, or a home health care agency may need to be hired. During this difficult time, family members will appreciate a personal support worker who demonstrates empathy, patience, and understanding.

A person who suddenly experiences a stroke and regains consciousness only to find that she is paralyzed or unable to communicate can be totally devastated. Rehabilitation, which is started as soon as the person's medical condition stabilizes, can be physically and emotionally difficult. Depression, frustration, anger, and major behavioural and personality changes can be expected. As a personal support worker, you will be responsible for supporting the person both physically and emotionally during this difficult phase of his or her life.

PARKINSON'S DISEASE

As you learned earlier, neurotransmitters are chemicals that carry nerve impulses across the gap between the axon of one neuron and the dendrites of the next. There are many different types of neurotransmitters. In **Parkinson's disease,** one of these neurotransmitters, called *dopamine,* is not produced in sufficient amounts. Dopamine is necessary for proper functioning of the motor neurons. In a person with Parkinson's disease, the brain's instructions regarding muscle movement never reach the muscle, because of the lack of dopamine. Without enough dopamine, the impulse cannot be passed on to the next neuron in line. Because of this nervous system "short circuit," the brain loses its ability to properly control body movement.

Parkinson's disease is a progressive disease, which means that it gets worse with time. The average age for the onset of Parkinson's disease is 55 years. Men are affected more often than women. We do not know exactly what causes the neurons to stop producing dopamine, but some studies have linked this disorder to a history of metal poisoning, encephalitis (infection or inflammation of the brain tissues), or arteriosclerosis of the vessels of the brain.

Parkinson's disease usually starts with a faint tremor that gets worse over a long period of time. The tremor is most apparent when the person is resting and decreases when the person attempts purposeful movement. As the disorder progresses, muscles become weaker and rigid. The person may walk with a shuffling, leaning gait (Fig. 28-7), and it may be hard for the person to stop suddenly, once he has begun walking. A person with Parkinson's disease may speak very slowly, in a voice that does not vary in tone. The person may lose the ability to move the small muscles of the face that are responsible for facial expression, giving the face a "mask-like" appearance. Eventually, the person's ability to chew and swallow is affected, and drooling may occur.

Although a person with Parkinson's disease may have difficulty speaking, he will have no problem understanding what you are saying. Picture boards and asking simple questions that can be answered with a nod or shake of the head can help improve the person's ability to express himself.

EPILEPSY

Epilepsy is a disorder characterized by chronic seizure activity. Seizures are caused by interruptions of the normal electrical activity in the brain. A person with epilepsy experiences seizures periodically. The seizures may be grand mal seizures, which are characterized by generalized and violent

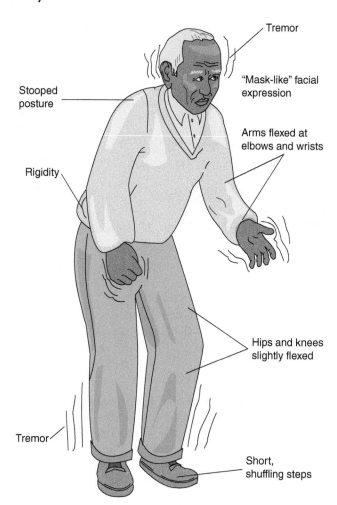

Figure 28-7
People with Parkinson's disease often develop a characteristic shuffling gait with a forward lean.

contraction and relaxation of the body's muscles, or they may be petit mal (absence) seizures, which can be very mild and hardly noticeable. Because the seizures often occur without any warning, a person with epilepsy may not be able to participate in certain activities, such as driving or swimming. Care for a person who is having a grand mal seizure is described in Chapter 12.

There are many possible causes of epilepsy. For example, a person may develop epilepsy following a head injury, brain infection, or stroke. A difficult delivery that results in the infant not getting enough oxygen during the birth process can also lead to epilepsy. Many times, the exact cause of a person's epilepsy is never determined.

Medications are available that help to reduce the frequency of seizures. For some people with epilepsy, these medications do not work, but for others, they are very successful. A person whose epilepsy can be well controlled with medications may have very few restrictions as far as activities are concerned.

MULTIPLE SCLEROSIS

It is thought that **multiple sclerosis (MS)** is an autoimmune disorder—the immune system attacks and destroys the myelin sheaths that protect the nerves, resulting in faulty transmission of nerve impulses. MS usually affects the nerves in the hands, feet, and eyes first, and then moves inward toward the central nervous system. Muscle weakness, tingling sensations, twitching of the eyes, and visual disturbances may be early signs of MS.

MS usually strikes people early in life, between the ages of 20 and 40 years. The disorder progresses at different rates, depending on the individual. Some people may have a period of remission (mild or no symptoms) followed by a relapse (the symptoms return and are much worse). In the late stages of the disease, the person may become totally paralyzed. At this time, there is no cure for MS, although some medications have been shown to slow the progression of the disease.

AMYOTROPHIC LATERAL SCLEROSIS (LOU GEHRIG'S DISEASE)

Amyotrophic lateral sclerosis (ALS), like MS, is a nervous system disorder that causes progressive muscle weakness. In ALS, the nerves that transmit impulses between the spinal cord and the muscles are totally destroyed. People in the late stages of the disease are totally paralyzed, yet their minds remain sharp. Death occurs when a person loses the ability to breathe and swallow.

ALS usually affects people later in life, between the ages of 40 and 60 years. Men are affected more often than women. Most people who have ALS die within 10 years of the diagnosis.

HEAD INJURIES

Head injuries leading to brain damage can be caused by falls, car and motorcycle accidents, bicycle accidents, and gunshot wounds to the head (Fig. 28-8). Brain damage can also occur from events that cause a person to stop breathing for a long period of time, such as near-drowning, drug overdose, or choking.

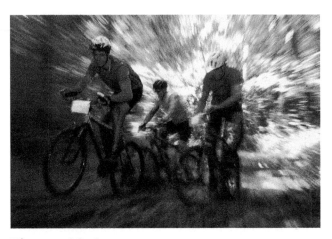

Figure 28-8
Taking standard safety precautions, such as wearing a helmet while riding a bike, can dramatically reduce the likelihood of a head injury should an accident occur.

Because neurons are not able to repair themselves or "grow back," traumatic injuries to the brain often result in physical disability, loss of mental function, or both. The type of disability will depend on the area and extent of the brain tissue damaged. Some people with head injuries will have paralysis similar to that seen in people who have had a stroke. Others will develop epilepsy, memory problems, or behavioural problems. Still others will be comatose and will need ventilator assistance to live. The type of care and rehabilitation that a person with a head injury needs is very individualized, according to the person's specific needs. Many of the younger people who live in long-term care facilities are there because of a head injury that resulted in severe disability.

SPINAL CORD INJURIES

Injuries to the spinal cord are usually caused by trauma, but they can also be caused by birth defects or tumours of the spine. Trauma can cause the vertebrae to break, and the sharp fragments of bone can cut the soft tissue of the spinal cord, causing damage. Permanent damage can also result from the swelling that occurs inside the spinal canal after an injury. Following an injury, the soft tissue of the spinal cord swells. The bones that surround the spinal cord do not "give." As a result, the spinal cord is squeezed, cutting off blood flow and resulting in tissue death from lack of oxygen.

The disability that results from a spinal cord injury depends on the severity of the injury and the level of the spine where the injury occurred.

Remember that the spinal cord is the line of communication between the brain and the rest of the body. If this line is broken at any point, then nerve impulses cannot travel beyond the break in the line. So, an injury to the spinal cord in the neck area can result in quadriplegia (paralysis from the neck down) because nerve impulses are not able to travel past the neck. An injury further down the spinal cord may result in paraplegia (paralysis from the waist down). The paralysis may be partial or complete, depending on the severity of the injury.

As with other types of disorders of the nervous system, the care and rehabilitation needed by a person with a spinal cord injury will depend on the severity and extent of the injury. A person with quadriplegia will usually need total assistance with his activities of daily living (ADLs), while a person with paraplegia may require little or no assistance following rehabilitation. For some people, the emotional effects of a spinal cord injury may be harder to overcome than the physical disabilities. Loss of control over one's body, and the accompanying loss of independence, can be very devastating. Some people may not be able to return to their jobs, which can cause financial problems. Others may never be able to enjoy a favorite hobby again. When you care for a person with a spinal cord injury, it is very important to encourage the person to do as much as possible for herself. Doing so helps the person to maintain a sense of independence.

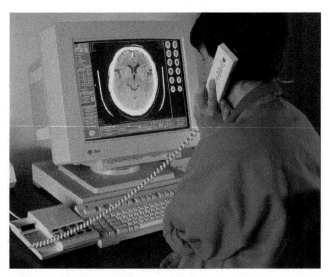

Figure 28-9
Imaging studies, such as computed tomography (CT) scans, allow doctors to see physical abnormalities of the brain, spinal cord, and surrounding bony structures. Here, a doctor looks at a CT scan of a patient's brain. (© *Simon Fraser/Photo Researchers, Inc.*)

DIAGNOSIS OF NEUROLOGIC DISORDERS

When a person is showing signs or symptoms that suggest a neurologic disorder, the doctor may order one of several diagnostic tests to help determine the exact cause of the person's signs and symptoms. Improved diagnostic tools have led to the earlier detection of many neurologic disorders. Diagnostic tests that are often ordered for people with signs and symptoms of a neurologic disorder include the following:

- **Imaging studies.** Tumours of the nervous system can occur in the brain, the spinal cord, or along the peripheral nerve tracts. Many of these tumours are not cancerous, but they may cause problems as they grow and press on healthy brain tissue or nerves. Imaging studies such as radiography ("x-rays"), computed tomography (CT),

and magnetic resonance imaging (MRI) are used to help locate tumours of the brain, spinal cord, or surrounding bony structures (Fig. 28-9). Imaging studies are also useful for detecting fractures of the skull or vertebrae. When used with special dyes (injected into a vein), imaging studies can help to reveal abnormalities in the blood vessels that supply the brain.

- **Electroencephalography.** An electroencephalogram (EEG) records the electrical activity of the brain (Fig. 28-10). EEGs are used to pinpoint seizure activity within the brain. Also, as you will recall from Chapter 22, a doctor can declare a person dead when there is a permanent loss of brain function. Therefore, when there is a possibility that someone is "brain dead" (for example, following a severe head injury), electroencephalography is used to monitor the person's brain activity. If there is no electrical activity for the period of time specified by the law (usually 24 hours or more), the person may be declared dead.

REHABILITATION

For people with neurologic disorders or injuries, rehabilitation is started as soon as possible after the person's medical condition stabilizes. One

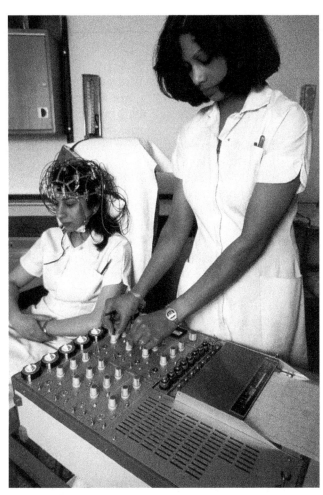

Figure 28-10
Electroencephalograms (EEGs) are used to monitor the electrical activity of the brain. (*Electro-* meaning "electric," *cephalo-* meaning "head," *-gram* meaning "tracing.") Here, a young woman is pictured having an EEG. The printout of her brain activity is visible in the lower right corner of the photograph. (© *Jerry Mason/Photo Researchers, Inc.*)

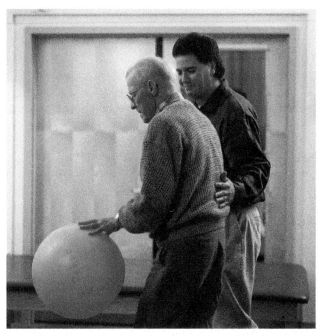

Figure 28-11
Learning about special equipment used by your patient or resident, as well as the rehabilitation techniques that the physical therapist is using with the person, can help you to provide better care.

very important aspect of the rehabilitation effort is the prevention of complications of immobility, such as contractures, muscle atrophy, and pressure ulcers. These complications can lead to failure of the rehabilitation effort and permanent disability. The use of splints, supportive devices, and assistive devices can help prevent complications and promote independence.

There are facilities that specialize in providing care and rehabilitation for people who are recovering from a brain or spinal cord injury. Perhaps working in a facility that specializes in helping people with neurologic disorders is a special

interest of yours. However, even if you do not work in a facility that is dedicated to helping people with neurologic disorders, you may still care for people who require restorative care as a result of a neurologic disorder or injury.

For a person with a neurologic disorder, rehabilitation can be a very long, frustrating experience. Although the brain has an incredible capacity for relearning basic functions, this process can be very slow. All successes, no matter how small, should be celebrated. As a personal support worker, you will be responsible for helping to prevent complications of immobility, and for reinforcing the rehabilitation efforts and techniques that are being used with your patient or resident (Fig. 28-11). Make sure you ask the nurse or physical therapist how to properly use any special equipment. Also make an effort to learn about any specific techniques that the patient or resident should be practicing. And above all else, be patient and empathetic with the person. Do not let the person's frustration and anger affect your ability to provide the best care possible. After all, how would you feel if you were suddenly put into a similar situation?

SUMMARY

- Neurons are the basic cell of the nervous system.
  - A neuron can send and receive information.
  - Information, in the form of a nerve impulse, enters the neuron at the dendrites, travels through the cell body and down the axon, and then across the synapse and onto the dendrites of the next neuron in line.
- The nervous system consists of the central nervous system (CNS) and the peripheral nervous system (PNS).
  - The central nervous system consists of the brain and the spinal cord. The central nervous system receives information, processes it, and issues commands. These delicate organs are protected by three layers of tissue (called meninges), the cerebrospinal fluid (CSF), and the bony skull and vertebrae.
    - The brain processes information and issues commands. The brain has four parts: the cerebrum, the diencephalon, the brainstem, and the cerebellum.
    - The spinal cord carries information to and from the brain.
  - The peripheral nervous system consists of the nerves. The nerves carry information to and from the central nervous system.
    - Sensory nerves carry information from the "outside in." Sensory nerves give the brain information about other organ systems or the outside world.
    - Motor nerves carry information from the "inside out." Motor nerves allow the brain to control the movement of muscles.
- The nervous system receives, processes, and responds to information.
  - The nervous system receives information from other organ systems and reacts to it, helping the body to maintain a state of homeostasis.
  - The nervous system allows us to experience the world around us. Without our nervous systems, we would not be able to enjoy the taste and smell of a ripe peach, a beautiful piece of music, the sight of a loved one, or the soft fur of a favourite pet. We would not be able to move, think, or create.
- The changes in the nervous system that result from normal aging are relatively few.
  - Older people are not as quick to react to things as younger people, which increases the older person's risk for falling and other household accidents.
  - Some older people find it harder to remember recent events, even though they remember events that happened long ago quite clearly. Extreme memory loss, such as that seen in people with dementia, is not a normal age-related change.
- Disorders of the nervous system can affect the brain, spinal cord, or nerves.
  - Transient ischemic attacks (TIAs) are caused by decreased blood flow to the brain. Once blood flow returns, the person's symptoms go away. Although the effects of a TIA are not lasting, a person who has had or is having a TIA needs medical attention because TIAs are often warnings that the person could have a stroke in the near future.
  - A stroke, also known as a cerebrovascular accident (CVA) or "brain attack," can be caused by a blood clot or hemorrhage that disrupts blood flow to the brain. The part of the brain that does not receive enough blood dies, due to lack of oxygen and nutrients. The effects of a stroke are permanent and can be mild or severe.
  - Parkinson's disease affects the brain's ability to conduct motor impulses to the muscles because of a lack of the neurotransmitter dopamine.
  - Epilepsy is a seizure disorder caused by abnormal electrical activity in the brain.
  - Multiple sclerosis (MS) is a nervous system disorder that affects the motor neurons, resulting in muscle weakness that gets worse over time.
  - Head injuries that result in brain damage and spinal cord injuries are the major reasons why younger people come to live in long-term care facilities or require the services of a home health care agency.
- Diagnostic procedures used to detect disorders of the nervous system include imaging studies—such as x-rays, computed tomography (CT) scans, and magnetic resonance imaging (MRI) scans—and electroencephalograms (EEGs).

● Rehabilitation can be a long, frustrating experience for the patient or resident, his or her family members, and the health care team. As a personal support worker, you will play an important role in helping people with disabilities caused by nervous system disorders or injuries to live the most satisfying lives possible.

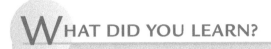

WHAT DID YOU LEARN?

Multiple Choice

Select the single best answer for each of the following questions.

1. Any condition that temporarily decreases blood flow to the brain can cause what to occur?
   a. A "senior moment"
   b. A transient ischemic attack (TIA)
   c. A heart attack
   d. A cerebral hemorrhage
2. Mrs. Romanelli has had a stroke and has a lot of trouble forming words. What term is used to describe Mrs. Romanelli's difficulty with language?
   a. Aphasia
   b. Dysphasia
   c. Paraplegia
   d. Hemiplegia
3. Mr. Owens had a stroke that left him paralyzed on the left side of his body. Which one of the following statements is true?
   a. The stroke occurred in the left side of Mr. Owens's brain.
   b. The stroke occurred in the right side of Mr. Owens's brain.
   c. The stroke affected Mr. Owens's brainstem.
   d. Mr. Owens has paraplegia.
4. What are the major goals of rehabilitation for a person who has a nervous system disorder or injury?
   a. To protect the person's self-esteem by not letting the person struggle with tasks he cannot do easily
   b. To get the person out of a wheelchair and back on his feet as soon as possible
   c. To prevent complications of immobility and help the person learn to do as much as possible for herself
   d. Because nervous system disorders and injuries often cause permanent damage, rehabilitation is of little use

5. Which of the following can increase a person's risk for a transient ischemic attack (TIA)?
   a. Low blood pressure
   b. Certain drugs
   c. Smoking
   d. All of the above
6. Which nervous system disorder is characterized by a lack of the neurotransmitter dopamine?
   a. Multiple sclerosis (MS)
   b. Epilepsy
   c. Parkinson's disease
   d. Dementia
7. What neurologic disorder is characterized by chronic seizure activity?
   a. Multiple sclerosis (MS)
   b. Epilepsy
   c. Parkinson's disease
   d. Stroke
8. What diagnostic test is used to monitor electrical activity of the brain?
   a. Electrocardiogram (ECG)
   b. Imaging studies, such as computed tomography (CT)
   c. Electroencephalogram (EEG)
   d. There is no test available to monitor the electrical activity of the brain
9. How does aging affect the nervous system?
   a. Older people usually become "senile" and forgetful.
   b. Older people lose the ability to form or understand words.
   c. Older people may take slightly longer to react to things.
   d. Aging does not affect the nervous system because old neurons are constantly replaced.

Matching

Match each numbered item with its appropriate lettered description.

__G__ 1. Meninges

__I__ 2. Cerebrospinal fluid (CSF)

__B__ 3. Central nervous system

__H__ 4. Peripheral nervous system

__A__ 5. Axon

__C__ 6. Myelin

__E__ 7. Dendrite

__D__ 8. Neuron

__F__ 9. Synapse

a. Sends a nervous impulse
b. Consists of the brain and spinal cord
c. Fatty white substance that speeds the conduction of nerve impulses
d. A cell that can send and receive information
e. Receives a nervous impulse
f. The gap between the axon of one neuron and the dendrites of the next
g. Three layers of connective tissue that protect the brain and spinal cord
h. Consists of the nerves
i. Clear fluid that cushions the brain and spinal cord

STOP and Think!

You have been caring for Mr. Elkins, a resident in the long-term care facility where you work, for about 6 months now. Normally, you and Mr. Elkins have quite a lively chat while you help him get ready for breakfast in the mornings. However, this morning, while you are helping Mr. Elkins with his morning care, you notice that he seems to be slurring his speech and saying things that don't really make sense. What do you think might be going on? What should you do?

Ken works in a facility that specializes in providing rehabilitation services to people with nervous system disorders. One of Ken's new residents is a 17-year-old named Mike, who was recently injured while "body surfing." After spending several weeks in the hospital, recovering from surgery to repair his fractured vertebrae and the pneumonia he developed when he aspirated sea water during the accident, Mike has come to the facility where Ken works. Because Mike broke his back during the accident and the spinal cord was damaged, there is a very good chance that Mike will be confined to a wheelchair for the rest of his life. Ken is not much older than Mike, and he has made a few attempts at friendly conversation, only to be snubbed every time. What might Mike be feeling that would make him act this way toward Ken? If you were Ken, how would you act going forward?

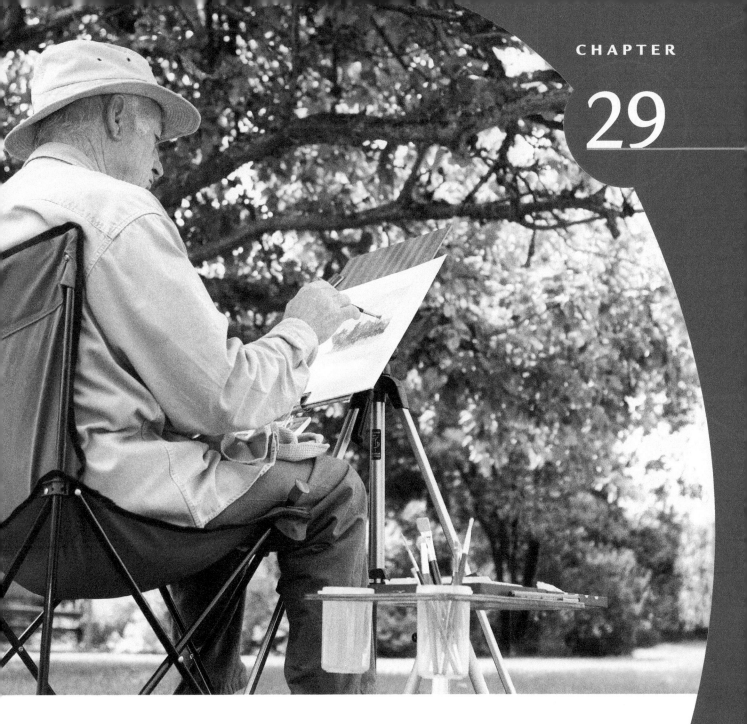

The Sensory System

WHAT WILL YOU LEARN?

We rely on our special senses—sight, hearing, taste, smell, and touch—to understand and interact with the world around us. Our sensory system allows us to experience the beauty and joy of the world we live in. It also helps to protect us from harm. Many of the people you will care for will have disorders or disabilities involving the sensory system. In this chapter, you will learn about how the sensory system works and about some of the disorders

Photo: Our sensory system allows us to experience and enjoy the world around us.

597

that can affect the sensory system. You will also learn how you can help to meet the needs of people who cannot see or hear well. When you are finished with this chapter, you will be able to:

1. Describe the main function of the sensory system.
2. List and define the two main divisions of the sensory system.
3. Understand the different types of pain that a patient or resident may experience.
4. Describe methods used to help control pain.
5. Describe how we experience taste and smell.
6. Discuss how aging affects a person's senses of taste and smell.
7. Describe how we experience sight.
8. Discuss the effects of aging on the eye.
9. List and describe disorders that can affect the eye.
10. Describe how to care for eyeglasses, contact lenses, and prosthetic (artificial) eyes.
11. Describe special considerations that are taken when caring for a blind person.
12. Describe how we experience sound.
13. Discuss the effects of aging on the ear.
14. List and describe disorders that can affect the ear.
15. Describe techniques for communicating with a hearing-impaired person.
16. Demonstrate proper technique for inserting and removing an in-the-ear hearing aid.

Vocabulary

Sensory receptors	Myopia	Diabetic retinopathy	Vertigo
Sense organs	Hyperopia	Macular degeneration	Tinnitus
Tactile receptors	Astigmatism	Braille	Conductive hearing
Referred (radiating)	Presbyopia	Cerumen	loss
pain	Conjunctivitis	Presbycusis	Otosclerosis
Acute pain	Cataract	Otitis media	Sensorineural hearing
Chronic pain	Glaucoma	Otitis externa	loss

STRUCTURE OF THE SENSORY SYSTEM

The sensory system is part of the nervous system. The sensory system consists of **sensory receptors,** specialized cells or groups of cells associated with a sensory nerve. The sensory receptor picks up information, called a *stimulus,* and translates it into a nerve impulse, which is then sent to the brain for interpretation, via the sensory nerve. Sensory receptors are found throughout the body. Some are found in the **sense organs,** which you probably can name already—the eyes, the ears, the nose, and the taste buds. Other sensory receptors are found throughout the skin, and even in the tissues of internal organs.

The sensory system is sometimes divided into two major parts. This division is based on the location of the sensory receptors. The first part is called *general sense.* The sensory receptors that are responsible for general sense are found everywhere throughout the body. The second part is called *special sense.* The sensory receptors that are responsible for special sense are located in the specific sense organs (the eyes, the ears, the nose, and the taste buds).

GENERAL SENSE

General sense is responsible for our sense of touch, position, and pain.

TOUCH

Our sense of touch allows us to feel textures (such as the plush velvet of a party dress or the hot sand between our toes at the beach) and the shapes of objects. The sense of touch is made possible

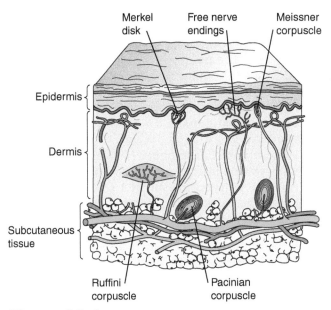

Figure 29-1

Tactile receptors and free nerve endings in the dermis of the skin allow us to feel things that come in contact with our bodies. There are four main types of tactile receptors: Ruffini corpuscles, Meissner corpuscles, Pacinian corpuscles, and Merkel disks.

by tactile receptors found in the skin (Fig. 29-1). (*Tactile* is another word for "touch.") The **tactile receptors** are stimulated when something comes in contact with the surface of the body and presses on them, causing them to change shape. Some areas of the skin have more tactile receptors than others, and are therefore more sensitive to touch. For example, the tips of the fingers and toes and the lips contain many tactile receptors and are more sensitive to touch than other parts of the body.

Some of the tactile receptors in the skin allow us to sense pressure, also known as *deep touch.* Intolerance to prolonged pressure is what makes us shift our position when we have been sitting in one position for a long time. A person who is unable to sense pressure (for example, a person who is paralyzed) does not become uncomfortable from being in one position for a long time. Therefore, the person is not motivated to change positions. What effect do you think this has on the person's risk for developing skin breakdown and pressure ulcers?

POSITION

Position receptors, found in the muscles, tendons, and joints, keep the brain informed about the position of various body parts in relation to each other. For example, you can tell if your leg is bent or straight without actually looking down to check its position. These same receptors also relay information to the brain about the degree of muscle contraction, especially when the muscle is contracting against resistance (for example, when you are lifting weights). Position sense provides us with muscle tone and the ability to move our muscles in a smooth, coordinated way.

PAIN

Pain is the body's distress signal. Pain tells us that we have been injured, that we have overworked a muscle group, that an organ is not working properly, or that we are ill.

Free nerve endings (dendrites) in the skin and the tissues of our internal organs allow us to detect pain. Your brain is usually pretty good at identifying what hurts when the cause of the pain is on the surface of your body (for example, when you burn your finger while removing a hot dish from the oven). But your brain may have more trouble pinpointing the exact location of pain that is coming from an internal organ. This results in the phenomenon known as **referred (radiating) pain.** For example, a person who is having a heart attack may complain of pain in the shoulder, neck, arm, or jaw. Gallbladder disease may cause pain in the back and shoulder on the person's right side. A back injury may cause pain to radiate down the leg and into a person's foot. Figure 29-2 shows how pain from certain internal organs can be referred to other areas of the body.

Many of the people you will care for will have some type of pain. There are two types of pain. **Acute pain** is sharp, sudden pain, such as that which occurs with an injury. Acute pain lasts a short period of time and decreases as the body's tissues repair themselves and heal. **Chronic pain** is widespread, constant pain that continues even after tissue healing has taken place. Chronic pain may be caused by conditions such as arthritis or certain cancers.

There are many factors that affect a person's response to pain. Culture and upbringing play a very large role in how people perceive and manage pain. For example, in some families, admitting to pain may be considered a sign of weakness. People who were raised in families that took a stoic approach to pain may feel that it is better to "work through" the pain than to complain about it or ask for relief. Other people, however, may come from families where family members discussed every little ache and pain loudly and in great detail. People with a background like this might not hesitate to discuss or ask for relief from their own pain. Other factors that can influence a person's response to

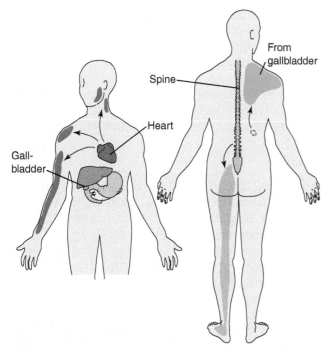

Figure 29-2

Pain may not always be felt at its exact source. Pain from the heart may be felt in the arm, shoulder, neck, or jaw (*red shading*). Pain from the gallbladder may be felt in the back and shoulder on the person's right side (*green shading*). A back injury can cause pain to radiate down the leg and into the foot (*yellow shading*).

pain include the person's age and past experience with pain, and the person's sense of responsibility toward others. For example, it is quite common for women with young children to ignore their own pain because they are so caught up in meeting the needs of their children.

As a personal support worker, you may be the first to notice that one of your patients or residents is in pain. Sometimes the person will tell you about his discomfort. Other times, your observation skills will tip you off. For example, facial expressions (such as grimacing or gritting the teeth) can be a clue that someone is uncomfortable. A person may try to avoid using a certain body part, or an area may be red and swollen. Profuse sweating or changes in the person's vital signs may also be signs that a person is in pain.

Once you determine that someone is in pain, you will need to get some details so that you can accurately report what the person is experiencing to the nurse. Pain is a totally subjective experience. Only the person feeling the pain can describe what she is feeling. The pain may feel sharp or dull. The person may describe it as "throbbing," or it may be more like a constant ache. If a person says that

she is in pain, ask her the following questions, and report the answers to the nurse:

- Where is the pain?
- How does the pain feel (for example, is it throbbing, aching, sharp, dull)?
- How long have you been feeling this pain?
- Does anything make the pain feel better (or worse)?
- How intense is the pain? (To help the person answer this question, you could ask her to rate the pain on a scale of 1 to 10, with 10 being the worst pain imaginable and 1 being slight discomfort.)

It is important for the nurse to know if a patient or resident is in pain. If the pain is new, the nurse will need to take steps to find out what is causing the pain. Even if the pain is familiar and the cause of it is known, there may still be something the nurse can do to help make the person more comfortable.

There are many ways of relieving and controlling pain. You have already learned about heat and cold applications, which are often used to treat musculoskeletal pain (see Chapter 25). Another common way of relieving pain is through the use of medication. Over-the-counter medications—such as aspirin, acetaminophen (Tylenol), and ibuprofen (Advil)—can be very effective for relieving mild to moderate pain. Severe pain, such as that which often accompanies traumatic injury, surgery, an acute illness, or some types of cancer, may only be controlled by the use of narcotics, such as morphine or meperidine (Demerol). People who need narcotics to control their pain should be encouraged to ask for the medication before the pain becomes too intense. Giving a small dose of a narcotic early on can help to stop the pain before it gets too bad. If left untreated, the pain will only get worse and a higher dose of the medication will be needed to relieve it. Many people hesitate to ask for pain medications because they have heard horror stories about people becoming addicted to painkillers. Although this can happen, it is rare.

Although giving heat and cold applications may be beyond your scope of practice, and most personal support workers are not permitted to give medications to patients and residents, there are many things that you can do to help a person who is experiencing pain and discomfort:

- Report any observations that suggest that a patient or resident is in pain, or any complaints that the person may have of pain, to a nurse promptly. Prompt and accurate reporting will help to ensure that measures are taken to make the person more comfortable, sooner.

- Help the person to relax. Anxiety causes the body to become tense, which increases pain. Simple care procedures, such as straightening the bed linens and positioning the person comfortably, can help the person to relax. Dim lights, a quiet environment, and a back massage can also be very comforting to a person who is in pain.

- Some people like to be distracted from their pain by listening to music, watching television, reading, or just talking.

Remember that each person's response to pain, and the methods that he is most comfortable using to address it, will vary.

TASTE AND SMELL

The sense organs of taste and smell are the taste buds and the roof of the nasal cavity, respectively. Special cells in these areas, called chemoreceptors, detect chemicals in the food we eat, the beverages we drink, and the air we breathe. The chemical signal is changed to an electric one and carried by sensory neurons to the brain, which tells us what we are tasting or smelling.

Taste buds cover the surface of the tongue. We have thousands of taste buds, and each taste bud consists of about 100 chemoreceptors, plus some supporting cells. The taste buds are bathed in fluid (either saliva or the liquids that we drink). The fluid contains dissolved chemicals, which stimulate the taste buds.

There are four basic tastes: sweet, salty, sour, and bitter. The taste buds that detect these four basic tastes are arranged in a particular pattern on the tongue. The "sweets" are found on the tip of the tongue. The "salties" are found on each side of the tongue, toward the front. The "sours" are located on each side of the tongue, toward the back. And the "bitters" are located across the back of the tongue.

The receptors that allow us to smell are located on the roof of the nasal cavity. Like the taste buds, these receptors are stimulated by chemicals that have been dissolved in fluid. However, in this case, the "fluid" is the moist mucous membrane lining of the nasal cavity. The sense of smell is easily fatigued, or worn out. This explains why an odour that is very strong at first becomes less noticeable over time.

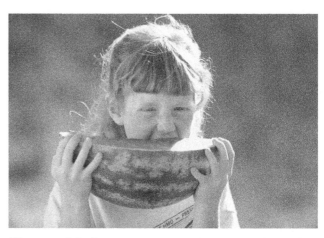

Figure 29-3
The senses of taste and smell are closely related. Eating a ripe piece of fruit is a treat for the tongue and the nose!

Together, taste and smell have a very powerful effect on the appetite (Fig. 29-3). Under normal circumstances, a person will not eat something that tastes or smells bad, even if he is hungry. But, how often have you found yourself eating too much of something just because it tastes or smells so good? Similarly, how often have you noticed that when you have a head cold and a stuffy nose, food seems to lose its appeal? This happens in large part because you can't smell the food!

As we get older, the number of chemoreceptors on the tongue and on the roof of the nasal cavity decreases. In addition, we produce less saliva, which makes it harder to dissolve the chemicals that stimulate the taste buds. As a result of these changes, the senses of taste and smell become less intense, leading to an overall decrease in appetite. To make up for a diminished sense of taste and smell, older people often season their food more heavily than younger people.

There are many dangers associated with a diminished ability to taste or smell. For example, an older person may not be able to tell that food has spoiled, and become ill from eating it. Or, he may not be able to detect the smell of smoke or a gas leak. It is surprising how much we rely on our senses of taste and smell to keep us safe.

SIGHT

Our sense of sight allows us to detect light, colour, and shape.

STRUCTURE OF THE EYE

The sense organ of sight is the eye. Each eye is protected by the bones of the skull, which form a protective cavity ("orbit," "eye socket") around the eye. Only the very front of the eyeball lacks the bony protection of the skull. To protect the front of the eye, we have eyelids that close and eyelashes and eyebrows that serve as "dust catchers" (Fig. 29-4A). Lacrimal glands, located above the eye in the orbit, form tears that help to keep the eye moist and free of dust and bacteria. Skeletal muscles located around the eyeball allow us to move our eyes.

It may be helpful to look at Figure 29-4B as we go through the internal structure of the eyeball. The eyeball itself is made up of three layers of tissue: the sclera, the choroid, and the retina:

- The *sclera* is the tough outer layer. The sclera is made of connective tissue. Although most of the sclera is white (hence the term, "white of the eye"), the front of the sclera, which is called the *cornea,* is clear. Light passes through the cornea to the inside of the eye.
- The *choroid* is the middle layer. This layer contains the blood vessels that supply the

A. External structure of the eye

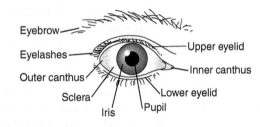

B. Internal structure of the eye

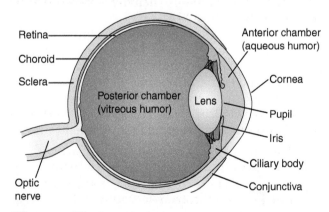

Figure 29-4
The eye. **(A)** External view of the eye. **(B)** Internal structures of the eye.

retina and other parts of the eye. At the front of the eye, the choroid also forms the ciliary body and the iris. The *ciliary body* is a muscular structure that attaches to the *lens,* a flexible, transparent, curved structure that adjusts to focus light rays onto the retina. The ciliary body changes the shape of the lens, allowing the eye to focus. The other structure formed by the choroid, the *iris,* is the coloured part of the eye. The iris is actually a round muscle with an opening in the center (the *pupil*). The iris controls the amount of light that enters the eye through the pupil.

- The *retina* is the innermost layer. The retina contains receptors, called *rods* and *cones,* which turn light into nerve impulses. The nerve impulses travel through the *optic nerve* to the brain for interpretation.

The eyeball also has two fluid-filled chambers (see Fig. 29-4B):

- The *anterior chamber* is located between the cornea and the lens. Special cells in the ciliary body secrete *aqueous humor,* a watery fluid that fills the anterior chamber. The aqueous humor passes through the anterior chamber and is reabsorbed back into the bloodstream.
- The *posterior chamber* is located between the lens and the retina. The posterior chamber is filled with *vitreous humor,* a jelly-like substance that gives the eyeball its shape.

FUNCTION OF THE EYE

Think about how a camera works. To take a picture, you need light and film. You also need a way of controlling the amount of light that enters the camera, and adjusting the distance between the camera lens and the film. If the amount of light entering the camera is not sufficient, or if the distance between the lens and the film is not correct, the resulting photograph will be out of focus.

The human eye works much like a camera:

- The retina is the "film."
- The iris and pupil control the amount of light that enters the eye. In bright sunlight, the iris constricts, making the pupil smaller so that less light is allowed into the inner part of the eye. In low light, the iris dilates, making the pupil bigger so that more light can enter the eye.
- The cornea and lens work to focus light rays onto the retina, resulting in a clear image.

First, the curve of the cornea focuses the light rays as they enter the eye. Next, the light rays pass through the lens, where the focus is refined (Fig. 29-5A). If the object the person is looking at is close, then the ciliary body contracts, causing the lens to become shorter and rounder. If the object is far away, then the ciliary body relaxes, causing the lens to become longer and flatter. The curved lens bends the light rays and brings them into focus on the retina, forming an image.

Clear, sharp vision is indeed a true gift. Many people need some help (in the form of corrective lenses, such as glasses or contact lenses) to see clearly. People who wear corrective lenses need help focusing the image properly on the retina. Some people need help focusing because of the shape of their eyeball. For example, the eyeball may be a little more oval than normal, causing the distance between the lens and the retina to be greater than usual. This results in nearsightedness, or **myopia** (Fig. 29-5B). People who are nearsighted are able to see fairly well close up, but they have trouble seeing images that are far away. This is because the distance between the person's lens and retina is longer than usual, which means that the image actually comes into focus before it hits the retina. This is a very common problem—20% of the people in Canada have some degree of nearsightedness!

Some people have the opposite problem, called farsightedness, or **hyperopia** (Fig. 29-5C). People who are farsighted are able to see objects in the distance fairly well, but they have trouble seeing objects that are close. In people who are farsighted, the eyeball is rounder than normal, causing the distance between the lens and the retina to be shorter than usual. Therefore, when the image hits the retina, it is not yet in focus.

Other people have trouble focusing on images properly because the cornea is not perfectly curved. This condition is called **astigmatism** (Fig. 29-5D). The irregular curve of the cornea bends the light rays in funny ways, which results in a blurred, distorted image.

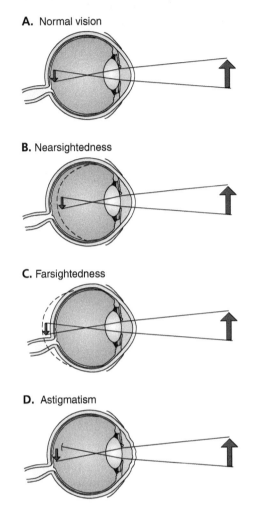

A. Normal vision

B. Nearsightedness

C. Farsightedness

D. Astigmatism

Figure 29-5
Many people need corrective lenses, such as glasses or contact lenses, to achieve clear vision. Three common problems that require the use of corrective lenses are nearsightedness (myopia), farsightedness (hyperopia), and astigmatism. **(A)** Normal vision. Light rays pass through the cornea and the lens and are focused on the retina. **(B)** Nearsightedness (myopia). The eyeball of a person who is nearsighted is more oval in shape than normal, which increases the distance between the lens and the retina. As a result, the image comes into focus before the retina. **(C)** Farsightedness (hyperopia). The eyeball of a person who is farsighted is more round in shape than normal, which decreases the distance between the lens and the retina. As a result, the image is not yet focused when it hits the retina. **(D)** Astigmatism. In astigmatism, the cornea is not perfectly curved. Some of the light rays that pass through the cornea are focused on the retina, but others are not, resulting in blurred vision.

THE EFFECTS OF AGING ON THE EYE

As we age, many changes occur in the eye that can affect vision:

- The number of receptors in the retina decreases, and the lens becomes more opaque (cloudy). As a result, images are not focused as sharply as in younger days, and colours may not be as bright.
- The iris becomes more rigid, which means that it takes longer for an older person's

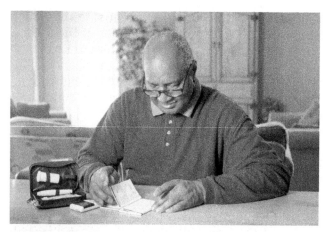

Figure 29-6
Presbyopia, which occurs when the lens becomes less elastic with age, is a common age-related change. People with presbyopia often need to use reading glasses to help them focus on things that are close.

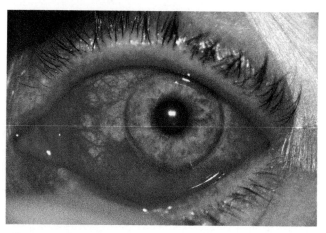

Figure 29-7
Conjunctivitis, or "pink eye," is a very contagious infection of the conjunctiva, the clear membrane that covers most of the surface of the eye and lines the inside of the eyelids. The affected eye is red, itchy, and teary, and there may be a sticky white or yellow discharge. (© *Science Photo Library/Photo Researchers, Inc.*)

eyes to adjust when she moves from a bright area to a dim one, or vice versa.

- The lens becomes less flexible, which affects the older person's ability to focus on objects that are close, a condition known as **presbyopia.** Presbyopia is why many people start using reading glasses in their 40s (Fig. 29-6).
- There is a decrease in tear production, which leads to dryness and irritation of the eyes. Many older people use lubricating eye drops to help keep the eyes moist and comfortable.

DISORDERS OF THE EYE

Conjunctivitis ("Pink Eye")

Conjunctivitis is an infection and inflammation of the conjunctiva, a clear membrane that lines the inside of the eyelids and covers most of the surface of the eye (see Fig. 29-4B). In conjunctivitis, the white of the eye appears red. The eye may itch or burn, and it tears excessively (Fig. 29-7). There may be a sticky white or yellow discharge.

There are many different causes of conjunctivitis. Microbes that cause colds and sinus infections can travel through the tear ducts and onto the surface of the eye, causing an infection. Or, microbes from an infection somewhere else in the body can be transferred into the eye when the person touches the infected area and then rubs his eyes. For example, methicillin-resistant *Staphylococcus aureus* (MRSA) and herpes virus can cause conjunctivitis in this way.

Conjunctivitis is highly contagious. Rubbing the eyes and then touching something transfers the microbes to that surface, where they can easily be picked up by someone else. All that person has to do is touch her own eyes, and she could find herself with her own case of conjunctivitis! Conjunctivitis is usually treated with eye drops or an eye ointment prescribed by a doctor.

Cataracts

Cataracts are very common in older people, but they can occur in younger people as well. It is thought that excessive exposure to sunlight increases a person's chances of developing cataracts. A **cataract** is the gradual yellowing and hardening of the lens of the eye. The lens becomes opaque and eventually prevents light from passing though to the retina. The person's vision becomes more and more cloudy as the cataract worsens (Fig. 29-8). It is like looking through a sheer curtain panel. When you look through one thickness of the sheer panel, your vision is only slightly cloudy. If you fold the panel to make a double thickness, your vision gets cloudier. And if you fold the panel again to make a triple thickness, your vision becomes cloudier still. This is what a person with a cataract experiences. Total blindness can result as a cataract becomes more opaque.

Many people with cataracts have surgery to remove the opaque lens and replace it with an artificial one. Improvements in equipment and surgical techniques have made this procedure

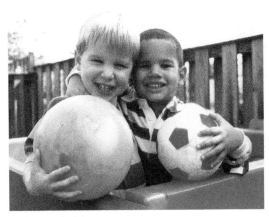

A. Normal vision

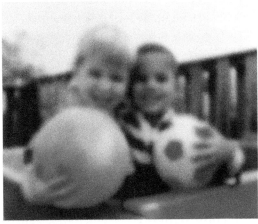

B. Cataract

Figure 29-8
Cataracts occur when the lens of the eye becomes yellow and hard over time, resulting in cloudy vision. This is what the world looks like to **(A)** a person with normal vision and **(B)** a person with cataracts. (*Courtesy of the National Eye Institute, National Institutes of Health.*)

simple and routine. Surgery is often performed on an outpatient basis using only a local anesthetic. The person usually can return home a few hours after the procedure. Cataract surgery enables people with cataracts to once again enjoy activities such as needlework and reading that would have been nearly impossible before.

Glaucoma

Glaucoma is a disorder of the eye that occurs when the pressure within the eye is increased to dangerous levels. This occurs when the aqueous humor in the anterior chamber is not reabsorbed into the bloodstream. As more and more aqueous humor is formed, it creates pressure, which builds up in the eye. The pressure squeezes the nerves and the blood vessels in the retina.

Eventually, the nerves are destroyed and vision is lost.

People who are older than 40 years and have a family history of glaucoma are at high risk for developing glaucoma themselves. Glaucoma also seems to be more common in people with dark irises (brown eyes), as opposed to light ones (blue or green eyes). The most common type of glaucoma occurs gradually, over a long period of time. However, in some people, the onset of glaucoma happens suddenly, and is accompanied by a great deal of pain. Both chronic and acute glaucoma can lead to blindness if left untreated.

Early detection and treatment of glaucoma can help to save the person's vision. This is why routine eye examinations are essential. If a person is found to have glaucoma, medicated eye drops are usually used to help control the pressure within the eye. Some people may need surgery if the eye drops are not effective.

Diabetic Retinopathy

Diabetic retinopathy is a complication of diabetes that can lead to blindness. In the early stages, the tiny blood vessels that supply the retina burst, leading to hemorrhages and damaging the retina. As the retina tries to heal, new blood vessels start to grow along the retina and in the vitreous humor. These new vessels are very fragile and they often burst as well, damaging the retina even more.

The number of cases of blindness caused by diabetic retinopathy in Canada is rapidly increasing. Early detection during an eye examination is essential for preserving the person's vision. Laser treatment is often necessary to help seal off hemorrhages in the retina.

Macular Degeneration

The macula is the small area in the middle of the retina where images are sharpest. In **macular degeneration,** deposits build up in the macula. The receptors in the area become damaged, and the person's ability to see is impaired. Factors that can increase a person's risk of developing macular degeneration are smoking, excessive exposure to sunlight, a diet high in cholesterol, and an inherited tendency for the disorder.

Blindness

Blindness has many different causes and takes many different forms. Many people are considered "legally blind" but have partial sight. Some people see nothing but darkness, but many others can see light, movement, shapes, and even colours, just not clearly enough to distinguish between them. Some people who are blind have been blind since birth and have never seen anything, while others may have lost their sight later in life. Most people who are blind adapt well and are very independent. People who have recently lost their sight, however, may be very frightened, especially of walking or moving around on their own.

Rehabilitation for a person who has recently lost his sight focuses on safety and the person's return to independence. Navigation skills are taught so that the blind person can be independent again. During rehabilitation, a blind person may learn to work with a companion animal that has been specially trained to guide the person as she walks (Fig. 29-9). The person may learn **Braille,** a system that uses letters made from combinations of raised dots (Fig. 29-10). The person runs her fingers over words written in Braille to read them. In addition, many books are available on tape for the person to listen to.

As a personal support worker, treating a person who is blind with respect and allowing the person to be as independent as possible are the best things you can do to help the rehabilitation effort. Learn the techniques that your patient or resident is being taught and reinforce them by

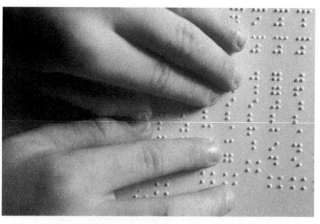

Figure 29-10
Braille uses a system of letters formed from raised dots to enable a blind person to read. (*Will & Deni McIntyre/Photo Researchers, Inc.*)

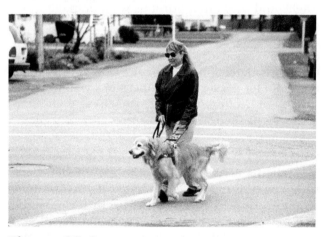

Figure 29-9
Many people who are blind have specially trained companion animals that help to keep them safe. For example, when preparing to cross a busy intersection, the blind person will listen to the traffic and tell the dog to move "forward" when she believes that the intersection is clear. If the dog judges that it is unsafe to move forward (for example, there is a car passing through the intersection that the person did not hear), the dog will refuse the command. This is called *intelligent disobedience*. Most companion animals require almost 2 years of training to learn how to do their jobs! (© *Peter Skinner/Photo Researchers, Inc.*)

helping the person to practice them continuously. Guidelines for caring for a person who is blind are given in Guidelines Box 29-1.

CARING FOR EYEGLASSES, CONTACT LENSES, AND PROSTHETIC EYES

Many of your patients or residents will wear glasses or contact lenses. Some may even have a prosthetic (artificial) eye. Most people are able to care for their own vision accessories, but others may need your help.

Eyeglasses

Eyeglasses are commonly used to correct vision. Some people wear eyeglasses only for reading or close work, while others may need to wear them all the time when they are awake. Always make sure that your patients or residents who need glasses wear them, especially if the person is confused or disoriented. Being unable to see clearly can make confusion and disorientation worse and adversely affect the person's quality of life.

Eyeglasses are very expensive to replace if broken or lost. As with all of your patients' or residents' personal belongings, you should be careful when handling a person's eyeglasses.

Clean eyeglasses with cloths or a special solution made specifically for that purpose, or with warm water (Fig. 29-11). If water or a special cleaning solution is used to clean the lenses, finish by drying them with a soft cloth or tissue. Paper towels or napkins may scratch the lenses and should not be used. When not in use, the person's

Guidelines Box 29-1	Guidelines for Caring for a Person Who Is Blind
WHAT YOU DO	*WHY YOU DO IT*
Speak in a normal tone of voice.	Unless the person is hearing impaired as well as blind, there is no need to raise your voice.
It is fine to use words such as "see," "look," and "watch." Be descriptive in the things you see around you. For example, tell the person that the sky is a beautiful shade of blue or that there are lovely yellow flowers blooming right outside the window.	There is no need to be self-conscious about your ability to see, as compared with the blind person's inability to see. Most people who are blind are comfortable with that fact. Many appreciate your ability to share what you see with them through your descriptions.
Ask the person about the extent of her blindness, and do not hesitate to ask the person what type of help she needs from you.	Asking the person about her blindness will help you to better care for the person. You might be surprised at what the person is able to do for herself, with little or no assistance from you!
When you enter the person's room, knock and tell the person who you are and why you are there. Similarly, when you leave, tell the person that you are leaving.	If you do not announce yourself when you enter the room, you could startle the person. Imagine how frightening it would be to hear someone walking around in your room and not know who they are or what they are doing! Similarly, if you do not tell the person that you are leaving, he may not be aware that you have left. How would you feel if you started talking to someone who was no longer in the room and were left to figure it out on your own that the other person had left?
Make sure you explain procedures completely and descriptively. Throughout the procedure, tell the person what type of equipment you are using, what you are doing, and what you are going to do next.	With all patients and residents, you should take care to explain procedures thoroughly. However, with a blind person, you may have to modify your approach a bit. For example, instead of just showing the person a piece of equipment, you will need to describe it to him, or let him touch it. Also, you should tell the person what is happening as it happens so that the person is not left wondering where you are in the procedure, or what is coming next.
Do not rearrange the furniture in the person's room, unless the person asks you to.	The person is used to moving around the room on her own. If you move the furniture, the person could injure herself by running into something that has been moved and is now in an unfamiliar location.
Leave the door either completely open or completely closed.	If the door is partially open, the person may feel for the door, think that it is all the way open, and walk into the edge of the door.

(continued)

Guidelines Box 29-1 Guidelines for Caring for a Person Who Is Blind (continued)

WHAT YOU DO	WHY YOU DO IT
When helping a blind person to walk, do not propel the person in front of you. Instead, let the person walk beside you and slightly behind you as she rests a hand on your elbow. Walk at a normal pace. Let the person know when you are about to turn a corner, or when a curb or step is approaching (and whether or not you will be stepping up or down).	In this way, you guide the person and reduce the risk of stumbles over unforeseen obstacles.

eyeglasses should be stored in their case within easy reach.

Contact Lenses

Contact lenses are also commonly worn to help make vision sharp. Contact lenses are made of moulded plastic and fit directly on the eyeball. Contacts may be soft or hard. How long they can be worn before taking them out depends on the type of lens. Some lenses are removed and cleaned daily, while others can be left in for several days at a time.

Contact lenses must be cared for carefully to prevent infection and irritation of the eyes (Fig. 29-12). Special cleaning and soaking solutions are used to clean and store the lenses. The types of solutions that are used vary according to the type of lens. Each lens is kept in its own case ("left" and "right") because the correction and size for the left and right eyes may be different. If one of your patients or residents wears contact lenses, make sure you are familiar with the proper technique for helping the person to care for them. Report any complaints of eye irritation or discharge to the nurse immediately.

Prosthetic Eyes

Sometimes a person's eye must be surgically removed, either because of injury or disease. A person who has had an eye removed may choose to wear a patch to cover the missing eye, or he may wear a prosthetic (artificial) eye. Prosthetic eyes are made of ceramic or plastic and are usually designed to be very close in appearance to

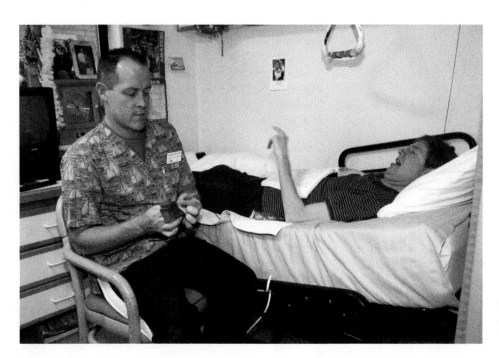

Figure 29-11
Take special care when handling a person's eyeglasses. They are expensive to replace.

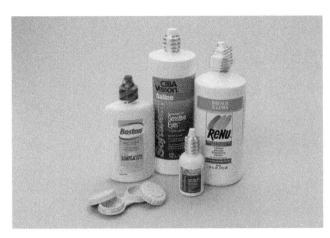

Figure 29-12
Contact lenses must be cleaned and stored properly to prevent infection and irritation of the eyes.

the person's own eye, in terms of colour and shape (Fig. 29-13). When the person's natural eye is removed, a supporting structure is often inserted into the empty socket and the tissues inside the eyelids (the conjunctiva) are closed over it. Many times, the muscles that move the eyeball are attached to the supporting structure. This allows the prosthetic eye, if the person chooses to wear one, to move with the other eye.

A prosthetic eye is usually a curved disc (not a ball) that fits underneath the person's eyelid. Some prosthetic eyes are removable and others are permanent. If your patient's or resident's prosthetic eye is removable, you may need to help him with cleaning and storing it. Like

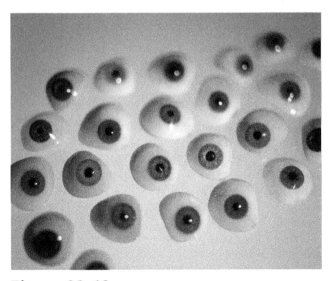

Figure 29-13
Artificial eyes are custom-made to look very similar to the person's other eye. (© *Lawrence Lawry/National Artificial Eye Service/Photo Researchers, Inc.*)

eyeglasses, a prosthetic eye is very expensive to replace and should be cared for carefully. Improper handling can cause scratches or nicks on the prosthetic eye that can injure or irritate the person's eyelids. Handling the prosthetic eye with dirty hands or not cleaning it properly can result in an infection. If one of your patients or residents wears a prosthetic eye, make sure you have been instructed in the proper way to care for it.

HEARING AND BALANCE

The sense organ of hearing and balance is the ear.

STRUCTURE OF THE EAR

The ear has three main sections: the outer ear, the middle ear, and the inner ear (Fig. 29-14).

The Outer Ear

The outer ear consists of the part of the ear that you can see (called the *pinna* or the *auricle*), plus a short canal called the *external auditory canal* (see Fig. 29-14). The shape of the pinna allows it to collect sound waves and direct them down the external auditory canal toward the *tympanic membrane* (also called the eardrum). The external auditory canal is lined with small hairs and special glands that secrete **cerumen** (ear wax). Cerumen helps to protect the ear canal by trapping dirt and other particles.

The Middle Ear

The middle ear consists of an air space containing three very small bones (called *ossicles*) and the opening of the *eustachian tube.* The eustachian tube connects the middle ear to the pharynx (throat) and serves to equalize the pressure in the middle ear. If you have ever gone up or down a mountain or flown in an airplane, then you have probably felt your eustachian tube at work. As you change altitudes, your ears feel funny and you yawn to open them. The yawn allows air to travel through the eustachian tube, making the air pressure in the middle ear equal to the air pressure outside of your body. Equalizing the air pressures prevents the tympanic membrane from rupturing.

The three small bones (ossicles) in the middle ear are connected to the tympanic membrane. These bones, individually called the *malleus,* the *incus,* and the *stapes,* form a tiny bridge between

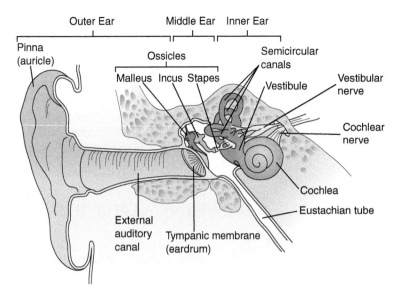

Figure 29-14
The ear.

the tympanic membrane and the inner ear (see Fig. 29-14).

The Inner Ear

The most complex part of the ear is the inner ear, which contains the receptors that make hearing and balance possible. The part of the inner ear that is responsible for hearing is called the *cochlea.* The cochlea looks like a snail's shell and is filled with fluid (see Fig. 29-14). Receptors for hearing are found within the cochlea.

The other part of the inner ear consists of two sac-like structures, called the *vestibule,* and three *semicircular canals* (see Fig. 29-14). Like the cochlea, the semicircular canals are filled with fluid. The vestibule and the semicircular canals, which are referred to together as the *vestibular apparatus,* help us to keep our balance.

FUNCTION OF THE EAR

Hearing

Sounds travel in the form of sound waves. Sound waves are captured by the pinna and sent down the external auditory canal. As the sound waves travel down the external auditory canal, they come in contact with the tympanic membrane, causing it to vibrate. The tympanic membrane vibrations are then passed to the first bone of the middle ear, the malleus, which sends the vibrations to the second bone, the incus, and then to the last bone, the stapes. The stapes rests against the oval window, a membrane at the opening of the cochlea. When the stapes vibrates, it causes the oval window to vibrate, sending the vibrations through the fluid inside the cochlea. The moving fluid stimulates

the receptors inside the cochlea, which then send nerve impulses via the cochlear nerve to the brain. The brain interprets these nerve impulses as sound.

Balance

When your body position changes, receptors in the vestibular apparatus are stimulated. These receptors then send nerve impulses via the vestibular nerve to the brain. These nerve impulses tell the brain what the body's position is, relative to the ground. Have you ever gotten sick on an amusement park ride, in a car, or on a boat? Motion sickness occurs when the messages your ears are sending to your brain about your body's position do not match the messages your eyes are sending to your brain about your body's position!

THE EFFECTS OF AGING ON THE EAR

Like other organs, the ear is prone to age-related changes. The tympanic membrane and ossicles become stiffer, and the number of sensory receptors decreases. As a result, many older people gradually lose the ability to hear high-pitched sounds. This type of hearing loss is called **presbycusis.**

A person with presbycusis has trouble telling the difference between similar-sounding high-pitched sounds like *th* and *s*, which can lead to frequent misunderstandings. Conversations can be difficult to follow, especially when many people are talking at once or there is a lot of background noise. As a result, an older person with presbycusis may start to avoid social situations, because she cannot hear well and is embarrassed to have to keep asking others to repeat themselves. Avoiding social gatherings can lead to a feeling of isolation and a decreased quality of life for the older person.

Many older people with presbycusis are mistakenly labeled "confused" or "disoriented" by family members, friends, or health care professionals. But think about it—how can a person answer a question correctly if she cannot hear it clearly in the first place? When speaking with an elderly person with presbycusis, it is helpful to speak slowly using a lower tone of voice. This may make it easier for the person to understand what you are saying.

DISORDERS OF THE EAR

Ear Infections

Otitis media is an infection of the middle ear that is common in young children. It occurs when fluid builds up in the middle ear. Bacteria from the throat find their way into the middle ear through the eustachian tube. Once there, they start to grow and multiply in the trapped fluid.

Otitis media is usually accompanied by ear pain, fever, and difficulty hearing. If untreated, otitis media can cause scarring of the tympanic membrane and a permanent loss of hearing. If the infection is bacterial, antibiotics are usually given to treat it. Children who have frequent middle ear infections may need to have "tubes put in their ears." During this surgical procedure, called a *myringotomy*, the doctor makes a small slit in the eardrum and inserts a tube to equalize the pressure and prevent the build up of fluid in the middle ear.

Another infection commonly seen in the ear involves the external auditory canal. **Otitis externa,** commonly referred to as "swimmer's ear," is an infection of the lining of the external auditory canal. Otitis externa is common in people who swim frequently or get the insides of their ears wet during showering or bathing. The ear becomes very painful to the touch. Antibiotic ear drops are usually needed to treat the infection.

Ménière's Disease

Ménière's disease, named after the French doctor who first described it, is a disease of the inner ear. Doctors do not know exactly what causes Ménière's disease. People with this disorder periodically experience episodes of dizziness (**vertigo**), ringing in the ear (**tinnitus**), temporary hearing loss, and a feeling of pressure or fullness in the ear. One or both ears may be affected, and with time, many people begin to experience permanent hearing loss in the affected ear or ears. There is usually no cure for this disorder.

Although Ménière's disease is not fatal, it can be very difficult to live with. Each attack can last between 2 and 4 hours, and is often accompanied by nausea, vomiting, or both. A person who is having an attack should lie down and keep his eyes fixed on an object that is not moving. This helps to reduce the nausea and lowers the risk of falling as a result of the dizziness. After a severe attack, the person may be very tired. A person with Ménière's disease may need to take more time when getting up from a sitting or lying position, to prevent an attack from occurring.

Deafness

Like blindness, deafness has many different causes and takes many different forms. Some people have been deaf since birth, while others may have lost their hearing gradually later in life. Deafness can be partial or complete. The two main types of deafness are conductive hearing loss and sensorineural hearing loss:

- **Conductive hearing loss** occurs when something prevents sound waves from reaching the receptors in the cochlea. For example, the external auditory canal may be blocked by built-up cerumen, or by a tumour. The tympanic membrane may be damaged and not vibrate well, or the ossicles might not move freely. **Otosclerosis** is a disorder that causes a change in the stapes, preventing it from moving properly. Often, surgical removal and replacement of the stapes with a wire prosthesis can help to restore some hearing in people with otosclerosis.
- **Sensorineural hearing loss** occurs when the receptors are unable to receive stimuli or transmit nerve impulses. Presbycusis, or age-related hearing loss, is sensorineural. However, there are many other causes of sensorineural hearing loss that are not necessarily the result of aging. For example, prolonged exposure to loud noise (especially industrial noise), recurrent ear infections, trauma to the ear, and some types of medications can all cause sensorineural hearing loss.

A person with hearing loss may work with a speech therapist to learn how to speak more clearly. In addition, many adaptive devices are available to help a person with hearing loss maintain his independence. For example, telephone devices for the deaf (TDD) systems can be used in combination with a standard phone to allow a hearing-impaired person to communicate using the telephone. Television shows are available with "closed captioning," a system that prints the words that are being spoken at the bottom of the screen so that the person can read them. The person's doorbell, alarm clock, telephone, and smoke alarms may flash instead of ring. Like a blind person, a deaf person may have a companion animal that is trained to act as the person's "ears."

Communicating with a person who is hearing impaired

When caring for a person with hearing loss, there are a few easy things you can do to ensure good communication:

- **Face the person when you are speaking to him or her.** Many people who lose their hearing gradually develop the ability to partially lip-read what people are saying to them. You should always face the person as you speak so that the person has a clear view of your mouth (Fig. 29-15). Avoid chewing gum or speaking fast. Doing so can hinder the person's ability to lip-read.
- **Use a notepad to write down important questions or directions so that the person can read them.** This helps to eliminate misunderstandings. If the person cannot read or reads in a language that is unfamiliar to you, a picture board (see Chapter 5, Fig. 5-4) may be quite helpful.

- **Make sure that the person fully understands what you said.** Some people, especially if the hearing loss is recent, hesitate to ask other people to repeat themselves. They may feel embarrassed by their hearing loss. When you are the "sender," you need to make sure that the person has gotten the message you were trying to send. If you are not sure that a person has understood what you have said to her, simply ask the person to repeat what you said back to you. For example, say, "If you could please repeat back to me what I said, I can make sure I told you everything I needed to." When the request is phrased in this way, the person feels as though she is helping you to do your job by repeating back the information. This helps to preserve the person's self-esteem and is a much better approach than just saying, "Now what did I say?"
- **Let the person know if you cannot understand what he is saying to you.** Many people with hearing impairments have difficulty speaking clearly. If you cannot understand what the person is saying to you, please do not pretend that you did to spare the person's feelings. The person may be trying to tell you something that is vitally important to his care or health. Tell the person that you did not understand and look for another way for him to get his message across. For example, you might offer him a notepad so that he can write down what he needs to tell you.
- **Consider learning sign language.** Many people who have significant hearing loss use sign language to communicate (Fig. 29-16).

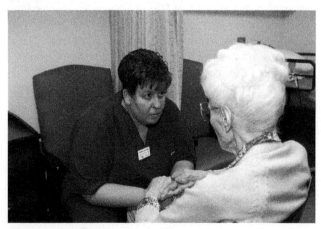

Figure 29-15
Always give a person who is hearing impaired an unobstructed view of your mouth. This will help the person to lip-read.

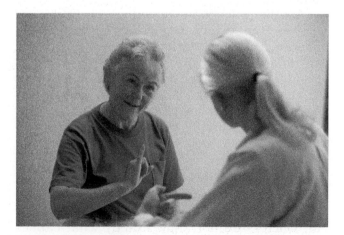

Figure 29-16
Some people who are deaf use sign language to communicate. (© Will & Deni McIntyre/Photo Researchers, Inc.)

Knowing how to communicate in this manner can be a very useful skill for a personal support worker to have.

Hearing aids

Many people who are hearing impaired use a hearing aid. A hearing aid is a battery-powered device that amplifies sound (makes it louder) before it enters the external auditory canal. There are many different styles of hearing aids (Fig. 29-17). Some styles fit entirely within the external auditory canal. Others attach behind the ear or to the person's eyeglasses. Others take the form of a small box that the person carries in his pocket.

Not all people with hearing loss can benefit from the use of a hearing aid. It depends on the type of hearing loss the person has. An otologist (ear specialist) evaluates the person's hearing deficit to determine whether a hearing aid will be useful, and to determine what type of hearing aid should be used.

Hearing aids amplify all sounds, not just the voice of the person who is speaking. Noises from the environment, such as traffic noise or background music in a restaurant, are also amplified. This can be distracting to a person wearing a hearing aid, and as a result, the person may choose to keep his hearing aid turned off most of the time.

Hearing aids are expensive and must be cared for carefully. General guidelines for caring for hearing aids are given in Guidelines Box 29-2. If one of your patients or residents uses a hearing aid, make sure that you know how to care for it and operate it. If a person who uses a hearing aid seems unable to hear you, make sure the hearing aid is turned on, and that the volume is turned up high enough. If the hearing aid still does not seem to be working, check the batteries to see if they need to be replaced and make sure the sound passageway is not blocked with cerumen. As with eyeglasses, it may be your responsibility to make sure that your patients or residents have their hearing aids in place because they may forget them or be physically unable to put them in and turn them on. Procedure 29-1 explains how to help a person to insert and remove an in-the-ear hearing aid.

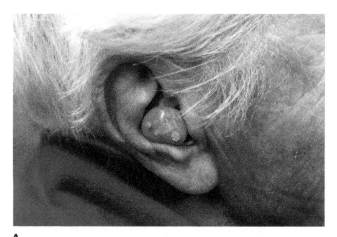

A

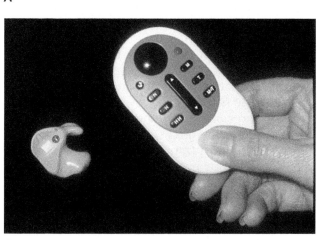

C

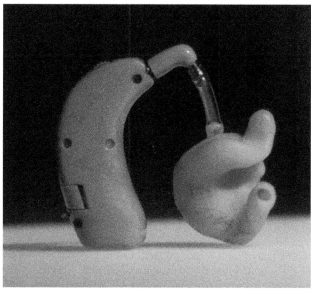

B

Figure 29-17
Hearing aids come in a variety of styles. **(A)** This type of hearing aid fits entirely inside the external auditory canal. **(B)** This type of hearing aid fits behind the person's ear. **(C)** This type of hearing aid is carried in a pocket. (*B, © Bishop/Custom Medical Stock Photo; C, © SPL/Custom Medical Stock Photo.*)

Guidelines Box 29-2 Guidelines for Caring for Hearing Aids

WHAT YOU DO	WHY YOU DO IT
Clean the hearing aid daily, according to the manufacturer's instructions.	If the hearing aid is not cleaned daily, the sound passages can become blocked with cerumen. The cerumen build-up can cause the hearing aid to stop working properly.
Make sure that the person has a spare set of batteries on hand at all times, and replace dead batteries immediately.	The hearing aid is battery operated and will not work if the batteries are dead. It is very inconvenient for a person who uses a hearing aid to be without it for any length of time.
Keep hearing aids away from heat and moisture.	Heat and moisture can damage the plastic ear mould.
Do not use hairspray or other hair care products on a person who wears a hearing aid while the hearing aid is in place.	The chemicals in many hair care products can damage the plastic ear mould.
Store hearing aids at room temperature when they are not being worn.	Hearing aids are delicate instruments. Exposure to very hot or very cold temperatures is not good for them.
Keep replacement batteries and small hearing aids away from children and pets.	These small objects can pose a choking hazard to children and pets. In addition, hearing aids are expensive to replace.

SUMMARY

- Our sensory system protects us from harm and lets us experience the world that we live in. The sensory system has two main divisions: general sense and special sense.
  - The receptors for general sense are spread throughout the body.
  - The receptors for special sense are located in special sense organs (the eyes, the ears, the nose, and the taste buds).
- General sense is responsible for our sense of touch, position, and pain.
  - Tactile receptors in our skin allow us to feel textures and the shapes of objects.
  - Position receptors in our muscles, tendons, and joints let us know where our body parts are in relation to each other.
  - Pain receptors (free nerve endings) in our skin and internal organs let us know when we are injured or ill.

- Pain can be referred, which means that the part of the body that hurts is not actually the part of the body that is injured. Referred pain is especially common when the pain is coming from an internal organ.
- Pain can be acute or chronic.
- The way a person responds to pain depends on several factors, including the person's culture and the person's previous experience with pain.
- As a personal support worker, one of the most important things you can do for your patients or residents is notice and report pain.
- There are many ways of controlling and relieving pain, including medications, massage, and heat and cold applications.

- Chemoreceptors in the taste buds and the roof of the nasal cavity give us our senses of taste and smell. Together, taste and smell play a very large role in stimulating the appetite. These senses also help to keep us safe by alerting us to signs of danger (such as spoiled food, a gas leak, or smoke from a fire).
- The eye is a complex organ that gives us our sense of sight.
  - Many people need corrective lenses (eyeglasses or contact lenses) to see clearly. Common problems with focusing include myopia (nearsightedness), hyperopia (farsightedness), and astigmatism.
  - Changes in the eye as a result of aging can lead to presbyopia (an inability to focus on objects that are close), cataracts, and dry eyes. In addition, older people need more time to adjust when moving from a brightly lit area to a dimly lit one, or vice versa.
  - Some eye disorders, such as glaucoma and diabetic retinopathy, can lead to permanent vision loss if they are not treated.
  - There are many different degrees of blindness.
    - Most people who are blind manage quite well on their own.
    - When caring for a person who is blind, you may have to make a few changes in the way you normally do things to make up for the person's inability to see.

- Always handle your patients' or residents' eyeglasses, contact lenses, and prosthetic (artificial) eyes with care. These items are expensive and difficult to replace. In addition, improper handling of contact lenses or prosthetic eyes can lead to infection of the eye.
- The ear is responsible for our senses of hearing and balance.
  - Sensory receptors for sound are located in the cochlea.
    - Presbycusis is age-related hearing loss caused by a gradual decrease in the number of sensory receptors for sound.
    - There are many different degrees of hearing loss. Hearing loss may be conductive or sensorineural in origin.
    - When talking to a person with hearing loss, be sure that the person can see your face, take care to speak clearly, and clarify information as necessary. Sometimes, it may be necessary to write information down or use a picture board to ensure complete understanding.
  - Sensory receptors for balance are located in the vestibular apparatus, which consists of the vestibule and the semicircular canals. These receptors tell the brain where the body is in relation to the ground.

PROCEDURE 29-1

Assisting a Person With an In-the-Ear Hearing Aid

WHY YOU DO IT   Being able to hear clearly makes communication easier and enhances the person's quality of life.

Inserting an In-the-Ear Hearing Aid

1. Complete the "Getting Ready" steps.

    WGKIEDS

2. Check the hearing aid to make sure the volume is down and the hearing aid is turned off.

3. Help the person to a comfortable position, with his head turned so that the ear needing the hearing aid is closest to you.

4. Inspect the ear canal for excessive cerumen (ear wax). If you see excessive wax build-up in the ear canal, gently wipe the ear canal with a warm, moist washcloth.

5. Gently insert the tapered end of the hearing aid into the external auditory canal. Gently rotate the hearing aid so that it fits into the curve of the ear. With one hand, push up and in. Use your other hand to pull gently down on the person's earlobe. The hearing aid should fit snugly but comfortably, flush with the ear.

6. Turn on the control switch. Adjust the volume by talking to the person as you increase the volume. Stop increasing the volume when the person can hear you.

7. Complete the "Finishing Up" steps.

    CLSOWR

Removing an In-the-Ear Hearing Aid

1. Complete the "Getting Ready" steps.

    WGKIEDS

2. Turn off the hearing aid.

3. Gently pull up on the person's ear. This will allow you to lift the hearing aid up and out of the person's ear.

4. Remove the batteries before storing the hearing aid in its case. Make sure the case is labeled with the person's name.

5. Complete the "Finishing Up" steps.

    CLSOWR

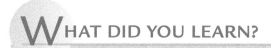

WHAT DID YOU LEARN?

Multiple Choice

Select the single best answer for each of the following questions.

1. Where are the sensory receptors that are responsible for "special sense" located?
   a. In the muscles, tendons, and joints
   b. In the eyes, ears, nose, and taste buds
   c. In the brain and spinal cord
   d. In all of the organs of the body

2. Mrs. Knight is having a heart attack. She complains to the nurse of pain in her arm and jaw. What type of pain is Mrs. Knight experiencing?
   a. Chronic pain
   b. Referred (radiating) pain
   c. Imagined pain
   d. Musculoskeletal pain

3. Which one of the following can be used to treat and control pain?
   a. Medications, such as aspirin and morphine
   b. Back massage
   c. Heat and cold applications
   d. All of the above

4. One of the residents in the facility where you work, Mr. Hepberg, is 85 years old and in fairly good overall health. Mr. Hepberg always says to you, "Don't ever get old, honey! When you get old, even the food doesn't taste good anymore." Why might Mr. Hepberg feel this way?
   a. The meals at the facility are very bland for dietetic reasons.
   b. Mr. Hepberg is depressed.
   c. As we get older, our sense of taste and smell decreases, making food less appealing.
   d. Mr. Hepberg has a head cold.

5. Which one of the following symptoms of conjunctivitis should be reported to the nurse?
   a. Itching and burning of the eye
   b. Redness of the eye
   c. A sticky white or yellow discharge from the eye
   d. All of the above

6. Jessica is assigned to take care of Mr. Golden, who has recently become blind. What should Jessica remember when caring for Mr. Golden?
   a. Jessica should greet Mr. Golden and state her name when she enters his room.
   b. Jessica can help Mr. Golden to feel more secure when walking by walking a step or two ahead of Mr. Golden and letting Mr. Golden rest his hand lightly on her elbow.
   c. During procedures, Jessica should explain each step of the procedure to Mr. Golden as she does it so that he knows what is happening.
   d. All of the above

7. Which one of the following is true about cataracts?
   a. Many elderly people develop cataracts, but young people can develop them too.
   b. Cataracts are very painful.
   c. There is no cure for cataracts.
   d. Cataracts are a complication of diabetes.

8. Michael is taking care of Miss Jordan, who has a hearing loss. Miss Jordan is wearing her hearing aid, but it does not seem to be working. What should Michael do first?
   a. He should raise his voice.
   b. He should make sure that the hearing aid is turned on, and that the volume is high enough.
   c. He should remove the hearing aid and replace its batteries.
   d. He should report the problem to the nurse immediately.

9. Mr. Campi, one of your elderly residents, is very hard of hearing. What should you remember when you are talking to Mr. Campi?
   a. You should sit or stand so that Mr. Campi has a clear view of your face, and you should avoid chewing gum or speaking quickly.
   b. If you think that Mr. Campi has not completely understood what you are saying, you should demand that he repeat it back to you so that you can correct his mistakes.
   c. If you do not understand what Mr. Campi has said, you should just let it pass. Letting him know that you did not understand might embarrass or frustrate him.
   d. There is no point in talking to Mr. Campi. He cannot hear you anyway. It is better to just write everything down.

Matching

Match each numbered item with its appropriate lettered description.

_C_ 1. Iris

_B_ 2. Cornea

_G_ 3. Lens

_A_ 4. Myopia

_E_ 5. Astigmatism

_H_ 6. Retina

_D_ 7. Hyperopia

_F_ 8. Pupil

_I_ 9. Vitreous humor

_J_ 10. Ciliary body

a. Nearsightedness

b. Clear portion of the sclera, through which light passes to the inside of the eye

c. A round muscle; the coloured portion of the eye

d. Farsightedness

e. A disorder of the cornea that results in blurred vision

f. The hole in the center of the iris

g. A flexible, transparent, curved structure that helps to focus images on the retina

h. Contains rods and cones, the sensory receptors responsible for vision

i. The jelly-like substance contained in the posterior chamber that helps to give the eyeball its shape

j. The muscle that allows the lens to either become shorter and rounder or longer and flatter

STOP and Think!

You work in an assisted-living facility and have known one of the residents, Mrs. Zinner, for almost 6 years now. Mrs. Zinner is in her 70s and enjoys very good health. In fact, her only disability seems to be related to macular degeneration, which is causing her to go blind. Mrs. Zinner's ability to see is now limited to being able to tell the difference between light and dark and make out the outlines of very large objects. What are some ways that you can help Mrs. Zinner adjust to her blindness physically? What are some things you can do that will help Mrs. Zinner adjust emotionally?

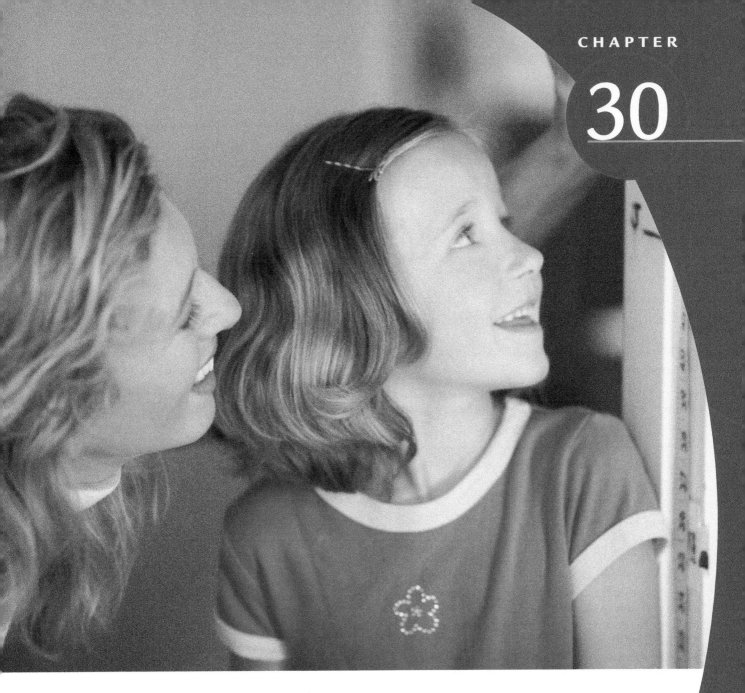

The Endocrine System

WHAT WILL YOU LEARN?

The endocrine system produces hormones, chemicals that act on cells to produce a response. The word "hormone" comes from the Greek word *hormaein*, "to set in motion." This is, in fact, exactly what hormones do—set things in motion. Sometimes, the effects of the hormone occur over a long period of time. For example, hormones allow us to grow to our adult height, and

Photo: Hormones, which are produced by the endocrine system, set processes in motion. For example, hormones are what cause us to grow! (©Elyse Lewin/Getty Images.)

they cause the physical changes that turn boys and girls into men and women. Other times, the effects of hormones are more immediate. Hormones with short-term effects help the body to maintain homeostasis (equilibrium). For example, insulin is a hormone that regulates blood sugar levels.

The hormones produced by the endocrine system control many of the body's functions. In this chapter, you will learn about the glands of the endocrine system, some of the hormones they produce, and how these hormones act to "set things in motion." You will also learn about some of the disorders that occur when the body produces too much or too little of a certain hormone. When you are finished with this chapter, you will be able to:

1. State the main function of the endocrine system.
2. List the glands that make up the endocrine system.
3. Describe the feedback mechanism that controls the endocrine system.
4. List the hormones produced by the different glands of the endocrine system.
5. Explain how the aging process affects the endocrine system.
6. Discuss various disorders that affect the endocrine system.
7. Discuss the special care needs of people who have endocrine system disorders.

Vocabulary

Hormones	Hyperthyroidism (Graves	Diabetes mellitus	Hyperglycemia
Goitre	disease)	Type 1 diabetes mellitus	Type 2 diabetes
Tetany	Hypothyroidism	Hypoglycemia	mellitus

STRUCTURE OF THE ENDOCRINE SYSTEM

A group of glands, called the endocrine glands, make up the endocrine system. Be careful not to confuse endocrine glands and exocrine glands! Endocrine glands produce hormones and release them directly into the bloodstream. Exocrine glands produce substances that are not hormones and release them into a hollow organ or onto a surface. Examples of exocrine glands include the salivary glands in the mouth, which produce saliva, and the sweat glands in the skin, which produce sweat. Exocrine glands are not part of the endocrine system.

The endocrine glands are located in specific places throughout the body (Fig. 30-1):

- The *pituitary gland* is about the size of a cherry and lies underneath the brain. It is connected by a stalk to the hypothalamus.
- The *pineal gland* is also located underneath the brain.
- The *thyroid gland* is located in the neck. It is butterfly-shaped, with two oval lobes located on either side of the larynx. The lobes are connected by a narrow band of tissue called the isthmus.

- The *parathyroid glands* are four tiny glands that are embedded in the back of the thyroid gland.
- The *thymus gland* is located in the upper part of the chest above the heart.
- The *adrenal glands* are located on top of the kidneys.
- The *pancreas* is located in the abdomen.
- The *sex glands (gonads)* are the ovaries in women and the testes in men. These glands are also considered part of the reproductive system and are discussed in detail in Chapter 33.

FUNCTION OF THE ENDOCRINE SYSTEM

The endocrine system controls many of the body's processes, such as growth and development, reproduction, and metabolism. It does this by producing **hormones,** chemicals that act on cells to produce a response. The hormones are released into the bloodstream, which means that they can affect cells far from the gland that produced them. The hormone travels in the blood until it reaches its target cell. Once there, it

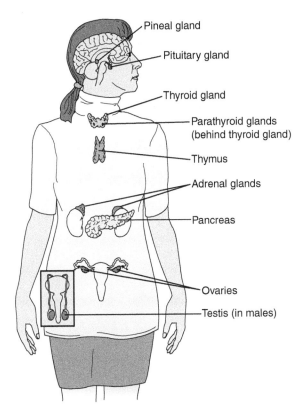

Figure 30-1
The endocrine system is made up of the endocrine glands, which are located throughout the body.

attaches to a special receptor in the cell wall. Just as turning a key in a lock causes a door to open, attaching a hormone to a receptor causes a specific reaction in the cell. Some hormones have receptors in all of the body's cells, while other hormones have receptors in only certain types of cells.

The release (secretion) of many hormones is regulated by a feedback system. In a feedback system, some change in the internal environment causes the gland to begin producing its hormone. The gland continues to produce the hormone until the amount of hormone (or some other related substance) reaches a certain level in the body. At that point, the gland stops producing the hormone. The feedback system works very much like a central heating unit in a house. The thermostat is pre-set to keep the temperature inside the house within a certain range. When the thermostat detects that the temperature has dropped below this pre-set range, the thermostat signals the furnace to turn on to heat the air. After the furnace creates heat and the temperature in the house rises to the desired range, the thermostat turns the furnace unit off.

In the rest of this section, we will explore the individual glands of the endocrine system, the hormones they secrete, and the effects of these hormones on the body.

PITUITARY GLAND

The pituitary gland, which is controlled by the hypothalamus, releases hormones that affect the function of other glands in the endocrine system. In this sense, the pituitary gland is like the "master gland." The pituitary gland has two parts: the posterior lobe and the anterior lobe.

Posterior Lobe Hormones

The posterior lobe of the pituitary gland stores and releases hormones that are produced by the hypothalamus. Two hormones are released by the posterior lobe (Fig. 30-2).

- *Antidiuretic hormone (ADH)* acts on the kidneys. ADH limits the amount of water that is lost from the body in the form of urine. When a person does not take in enough fluid or loses too much fluid through sweating, vomiting, or diarrhea, the hypothalamus detects a lower fluid level in the blood and signals the pituitary gland to release more ADH. The ADH causes the kidneys to save body fluid by decreasing the amount of urine produced. Similarly, when the hypothalamus detects that fluid levels are too high, it signals the pituitary gland to secrete less ADH. The lack of ADH causes the kidneys to produce more urine, eliminating the excess fluid from the body.
- *Oxytocin* is the hormone that causes labour to begin and is responsible for the let-down of milk in the breasts of a nursing mother.

Anterior Lobe Hormones

The anterior lobe of the pituitary gland makes and releases several different hormones (see Fig. 30-2).

- *Growth hormone* is what causes our bodies to get bigger and taller as we move from infancy into adulthood. Growth hormone is usually released in greater amounts during short periods of time, resulting in a child's "growth spurts." Although the output of growth hormone is highest during childhood, the anterior lobe continues to release growth hormone long after the growing phase of development is finished. Cells

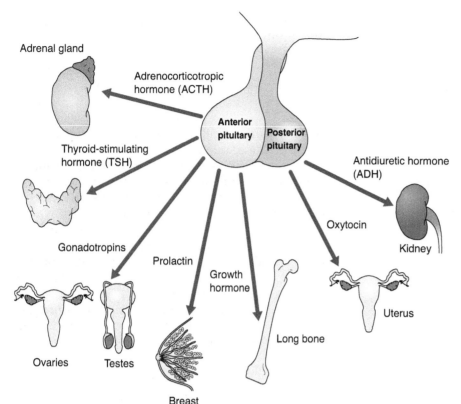

Figure 30-2
The pituitary gland, or "master gland," releases hormones that affect other glands in the endocrine system.

need to be replaced throughout a person's lifetime, and growth hormone is necessary for that to occur.

- *Thyroid-stimulating hormone (TSH)* stimulates the thyroid gland to produce thyroid hormones, which affect the rate of metabolism in the body's tissues.
- *Adrenocorticotropic hormone (ACTH)* stimulates the adrenal glands to produce their hormones, which help the body to deal with stress.
- *Prolactin* stimulates the milk glands of the breast to produce milk when a baby is born.
- *Gonadotropins* regulate the functioning of the *sex glands (gonads)* in both males and females. There are two gonadotropins: *follicle-stimulating hormone (FSH)* and *luteinizing hormone (LH)*. The action of the gonadotropins is discussed in more detail in Chapter 33.

PINEAL GLAND

The pineal gland secretes *melatonin,* which helps to regulate the body's sleep–awake cycles. The pineal gland is stimulated by light and darkness and secretes melatonin during the dark part of the day.

THYROID GLAND

The thyroid gland produces two hormones that help to regulate the body's metabolism, the main one being *thyroxine.* In addition, the thyroid gland produces *calcitonin,* a hormone that helps to regulate the amount of calcium in the bloodstream.

Thyroxine

The hormone thyroxine sets the rate of metabolism for the cells of the body. How quickly body cells and tissues use nutrients (especially protein) and produce energy is determined by the amount of thyroxine present in the bloodstream. If the thyroid gland releases more thyroxine, the metabolic rate of the cells increases, and if the thyroid gland releases less thyroxine, the metabolic rate of the cells decreases.

The thyroid gland needs iodine to produce thyroxine. Iodine is found naturally in fish and shellfish and is added to salt and other commercial products. When a person does not get enough iodine in her diet, the thyroid gland is not able to produce adequate amounts of thyroxine. The sensors in the hypothalamus and pituitary gland detect a decrease in the level of thyroxine in the bloodstream and release TSH to stimulate the

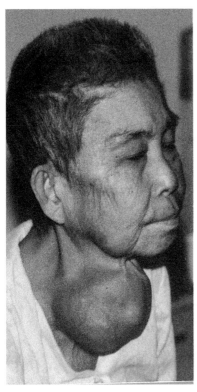

Figure 30-3
The swelling in this woman's neck is a goitre, or an enlarged thyroid gland. Goitre can be caused by a lack of iodine in the diet or by a tumour or disease that affects the thyroid gland's ability to produce thyroid hormone. (*From Rubin, R., & Strayer, D. S. [2008].* Rubin's Pathology: Clinicopathologic foundations of medicine *[5th ed., p. 942]. Philadelphia: Lippincott Williams & Wilkins.*)

thyroid gland to produce more. However, because the thyroid gland has no iodine, it cannot respond to the request for more thyroxine, and the cycle repeats itself. The constant stimulation of the thyroid gland causes it to enlarge. An enlargement of the thyroid gland is called a **goitre** (Fig. 30-3). Iodine deficiency is just one cause of goitre. Goitre can also occur when the thyroid gland does not produce enough hormone because of disease or tumours.

Calcitonin

Another important hormone produced by the thyroid gland is calcitonin. Calcitonin is one of the hormones that helps to maintain calcium levels in the bloodstream. As you learned in Chapter 25, calcium is important for proper functioning of the skeletal and cardiac muscle. Calcium helps transmit nerve impulses into and out of the muscle fibres, allowing for the smooth contraction and relaxation of the muscles. Too

little calcium makes the muscle fibres irritable and unable to relax after they contract, causing cramping. A condition called tetany (not to be confused with a tetanus infection) may result if the calcium level drops too low. **Tetany** is characterized by cramping of the skeletal muscles and an irregular heartbeat. Too much calcium in the bloodstream causes muscles to become weak and slow to respond.

Calcitonin lowers the amount of calcium in the bloodstream by allowing the calcium to be deposited in the bones and eliminated by the kidneys. For example, if a person drinks a lot of milk or takes calcium supplements, the level of calcium in the bloodstream increases as the calcium is absorbed from the intestines. The high calcium level in the blood stimulates the thyroid gland to produce calcitonin. Calcitonin transports the extra calcium to the bones. Any calcium that cannot be stored in the bones is excreted by the kidneys in the urine.

PARATHYROID GLANDS

The parathyroid glands produce *parathyroid hormone (PTH)*, which has the opposite effect of calcitonin. PTH causes calcium to be released from the bones into the bloodstream, increasing the amount of calcium in the bloodstream. In addition, PTH helps the kidneys to keep calcium, instead of excrete it in the urine. As you learned in Chapter 25, a calcium-rich diet is important to build up stores of calcium in the bones. PTH is what allows us to draw on these stores later in life, when our bodies become less efficient at absorbing the calcium that we eat. The actions of calcitonin and PTH balance each other and help to keep the levels of calcium in the bloodstream constant.

If the parathyroid glands are surgically removed or become damaged by disease, PTH is not produced in adequate amounts and the calcium levels may drop, causing tetany. Some tumours of the parathyroid gland can cause an overproduction of PTH that results in too much calcium being removed from the bones. The bones then become very fragile and fracture easily. Because the kidneys are responsible for excreting the excess calcium, kidney stones are likely to form.

THYMUS GLAND

The thymus gland secretes *thymosin*, a hormone that helps infection-fighting T cells to mature. An increase in the secretion of thymosin stimulates

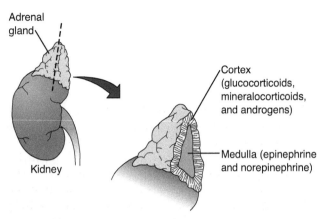

Figure 30-4
The adrenal gland consists of an inner part (the adrenal medulla) and an outer part (the adrenal cortex). Each part produces and secretes different hormones. Many of these hormones help us to deal with stressful situations.

the body to produce more T cells during an infection or illness.

ADRENAL GLANDS

Each adrenal gland has two separate parts: the *medulla*, or inner portion, and the *cortex*, or outer portion (Fig. 30-4). Each part secretes distinct hormones.

Medullary Hormones

The medulla of the adrenal glands secretes two hormones that are responsible for the "fight-or-flight" response of the body in emergency situations. Those hormones are *epinephrine* (also known as adrenaline) and *norepinephrine*. Epinephrine and norepinephrine help the heart and lungs deliver more oxygen and nutrients to the muscles, preparing the body to "stand up and fight or turn tail and run." A "side effect" of these hormones is the dry-mouthed, heart-pounding reaction that occurs when you are frightened!

Cortical Hormones

The outer portion of the adrenal glands secretes three main groups of hormones:

- *Glucocorticoids* play a role in the metabolism of fats and proteins, and help the body to maintain a reserve of glucose (sugar) that can be used in times of stress. They are also able to suppress the body's inflammatory response. For this reason, glucocorticoids

are often given in the form of medications for severe inflammatory disorders such as asthma, rheumatoid arthritis, or severe allergic reactions. Hydrocortisone is a common medication that is a glucocorticoid.
- *Mineralocorticoids* help to regulate the level of certain minerals in the body, particularly sodium and potassium. *Aldosterone* is the primary hormone in this group. Aldosterone helps the kidneys to reabsorb sodium and secrete potassium.
- *Androgens* are secreted in small amounts by the adrenal cortex. Androgens are converted by the body into the sex hormones *testosterone* (in men) and *estradiol* (in women).

PANCREAS

The pancreas is both an exocrine gland and an endocrine gland. It functions as an exocrine gland by producing and secreting enzymes into the small intestine that help to digest food. It functions as an endocrine gland by producing two hormones: *insulin* and *glucagon.*

Insulin

Special cells within the pancreas, called the *islets of Langerhans,* produce and secrete the hormone insulin. Insulin, which affects all of the body's cells, allows glucose (sugar) to be transported from the bloodstream into the individual cells, where it is used for energy. In this way, insulin lowers the blood glucose level.

When a person eats, food is digested and absorbed by the bloodstream in the form of glucose. The blood glucose levels determine how much insulin is released by the pancreas. After eating, a person's blood glucose is elevated, and the pancreas releases insulin. The insulin causes the glucose to move from the bloodstream into the cells, where it can be used for energy. Any extra glucose is converted to glycogen. Glycogen is stored in the liver for later use, or it is converted to fat and deposited in various places on the body.

Glucagon

Glucagon has the opposite effect of insulin. While insulin is responsible for lowering blood glucose levels, glucagon is responsible for raising them. When the glucose levels in the bloodstream drop, as they normally do when a person has not eaten for some time, the pancreas secretes glucagon. The glucagon stimulates the liver to release the glucose that has been stored as glycogen into the bloodstream, to supply the cells of the body with fuel for energy. Insulin and glucagon work together to keep the body's blood glucose levels stable.

SEX GLANDS

The sex glands (or gonads) secrete the hormones that result in the onset of puberty and that regulate reproduction. Because the ovaries and testes are also considered a part of the reproductive system, these glands are discussed in greater detail in Chapter 33.

THE EFFECTS OF AGING ON THE ENDOCRINE SYSTEM

The normal processes of aging decrease the amount of hormones produced and slow their secretion by the glands of the endocrine system. Many of the physical changes that are part of aging are directly related to the smaller amounts of hormone released. For example, decreases in growth hormone levels slow the rate at which the body's cells and tissues divide and replace themselves, and decreases in thyroid hormone levels slow the body's metabolism.

In women, menopause (the end of menstruation, which signals the end of a woman's ability to bear children) occurs as a result of decreased hormone production by the ovaries. In men, secretion of hormones by the testes decreases, affecting sexual drive and function.

DISORDERS OF THE ENDOCRINE SYSTEM

Disorders of the endocrine system occur when the body produces too much or too little of a certain hormone. Imbalances in hormone secretion can be caused by disorders of the hypothalamus, the pituitary gland, the specific endocrine gland responsible for the hormone, or as a result of poor nutrition. Corrective measures may be needed to restore the body's homeostasis and prevent the imbalances from causing health problems. There are many different types of endocrine disorders. Some of the ones you will be most likely to encounter in the health care setting are described here.

PITUITARY GLAND DISORDERS

Pituitary Dwarfism and Pituitary Gigantism

A deficiency in the amount of growth hormone secreted during the growing years results in a condition known as *pituitary dwarfism.* A person with pituitary dwarfism is much smaller than average, but still well proportioned. If the condition is diagnosed while the person is still a child, growth hormone may be given to help stimulate growth. Similarly, an excess in the amount of growth hormone secreted during the growing years results in a condition known as *pituitary gigantism* (Fig. 30-5). A person with pituitary gigantism is much larger than average, but still well proportioned.

Acromegaly

The secretion of too much growth hormone after a person has reached adulthood causes excessive

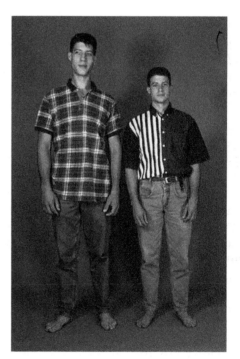

Figure 30-5
Pituitary gigantism occurs when the pituitary gland produces too much growth hormone during a person's growing years. These men are identical twins, but the man on the left is much taller than his average-sized brother because his body produced an excess amount of growth hormone. (*Photo courtesy of Gagel, R. F., & McCutcheon, I. E. [1999]. Images in clinical medicine.* New England Journal of Medicine (340), *524. Copyright © 2003, Massachusetts Medical Society.*)

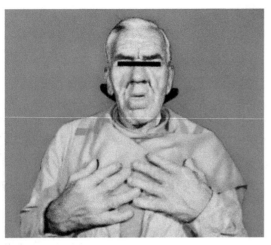

Figure 30-6
Secretion of too much growth hormone in an adult causes acromegaly, excessive growth of the bones of the hands, feet, and face.

growth of the bones of the hands, feet, and face. This condition is called *acromegaly* (Fig. 30-6). The person does not grow taller, but does have a disproportioned appearance, especially in the face and hands.

THYROID GLAND DISORDERS

Remember that the secretion of the thyroid hormones is controlled by the pituitary gland. Therefore, thyroid disorders can be caused by abnormalities of the pituitary gland or by abnormalities of the thyroid gland itself. Thyroid disorders can also result from nutrient deficiencies, such as a lack of iodine. A simple blood test can be used to detect imbalances in thyroid hormones. Once detected, these imbalances can usually be treated.

Hyperthyroidism

Hyperthyroidism (sometimes called **Graves disease**) is caused by the excessive secretion of thyroxine (*hyper* meaning "above"). In a person with hyperthyroidism, the metabolic rate of the body's cells is increased. Signs and symptoms of hyperthyroidism include increased hunger accompanied by weight loss, an irregular heartbeat, an inability to sleep, irritability, confusion, increased perspiration, and intolerance to heat. Hyperthyroidism may be treated by surgically removing part of the thyroid gland, or by destroying part of the gland with radiation.

Hypothyroidism

Hypothyroidism results when thyroxine secretion is too low (*hypo* meaning "below"). Some babies are born with hypothyroidism, which, if left untreated, can result in a condition known as *cretinism*. Because thyroxine's control of the body's metabolism is essential for growth and development, cretinism is characterized by a lack of physical growth and mental development. However, if the hypothyroidism is detected and treated soon after birth, cretinism is prevented and the child will go on to develop normally. Hypothyroidism is treated by administering thyroxine in the form of a pill.

Most cases of hypothyroidism develop later in life, as a result of a disorder of the hypothalamus, pituitary gland, or thyroid gland. In adults, hypothyroidism is more common among women and the elderly. Hypothyroidism causes signs and symptoms that are opposite those of hyperthyroidism. Signs and symptoms of hypothyroidism include fatigue, weakness, depression, anorexia, weight gain, constipation, and intolerance to cold. The administration of oral thyroxine helps to restore the body's metabolism to a normal rate and relieves the signs and symptoms of hypothyroidism.

ADRENAL GLAND DISORDERS

Two of the most common adrenal gland disorders, Addison's disease and Cushing's syndrome, result from imbalances of the adrenal cortical hormones.

Addison's Disease

In Addison's disease, the adrenal cortex is destroyed, resulting in low levels of the adrenal cortical hormones. Because the glucocorticoids play a role in protein metabolism, a person with Addison's disease develops muscle weakness and atrophy. Dark discolouration of the skin and disturbances in the body's salt and water balance are also seen. The person may have hypertension as a result of the Addison's disease. A person with Addison's disease may need assistance with walking and range-of-motion exercises.

Cushing's Syndrome

Cushing's syndrome results from excessive secretion of glucocorticoids. Cushing's syndrome can be caused by disorders of the pituitary gland that affect ACTH secretion or by disorders of the adrenal gland itself. Some people develop Cushing's syndrome after taking high doses of steroid

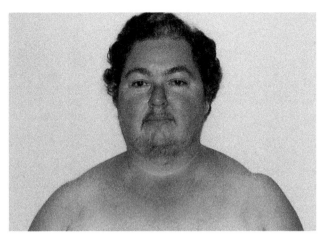

Figure 30-7
Cushing's syndrome results from excessive amounts of the adrenal cortical hormones. The excessive secretion of androgens, which are converted into sex hormones, is what caused this woman to develop facial hair. The accumulation of fat on the woman's back and face is the result of excess glucocorticoids. (*Reprinted with permission from Rubin, E., & Farber, J. L. [2005]. Pathology [4th ed., p. 1162]. Philadelphia: Lippincott Williams & Wilkins.*)

medications, such as hydrocortisone, for a long period of time. Because glucocorticoids help us to metabolize fat, people with Cushing's syndrome tend to develop pockets of fat in the abdomen, on the back, and in the face. Increased facial hair is also common (Fig. 30-7). A person with Cushing's syndrome will have high blood glucose levels because one of the effects of glucocorticoids is to decrease the use of glucose by the tissues. Easy bruising of the skin and muscle weakness are also seen.

DIABETES

Diabetes mellitus results when the pancreas is unable to produce enough insulin. Diabetes mellitus can occur in people of all ages and races, but people between the ages of 65 and 74 years and people of African descent are affected most often. Diabetes mellitus is the most common of all endocrine gland disorders and is the seventh leading cause of death among the elderly. There are two types of diabetes mellitus: type 1 and type 2.

Type 1 Diabetes Mellitus

Type 1 diabetes mellitus is less common but much more severe than type 2 diabetes mellitus. **Type 1 diabetes mellitus** is caused by destruction of the insulin-producing cells of the pancreas. Also called juvenile diabetes, type 1 diabetes mellitus is the form of diabetes that most often affects children. Most people who have type 1 diabetes are diagnosed while they are children or young adults.

Insulin

Because the pancreas is unable to produce adequate amounts of insulin, a person with type 1 diabetes mellitus must receive daily injections of insulin. The insulin is injected into the subcutaneous layer of the skin, where it is absorbed by the bloodstream. Several types of insulin are available. The types of insulin differ in the speed at which they start working and how long they last in the body. Some of your patients or residents will receive only one injection of insulin each day, while others may receive two or three. Insulin can also be delivered continuously by a pump device (Fig. 30-8).

Monitoring blood glucose levels

People who are receiving insulin injections need to have their blood glucose levels monitored closely. Too much insulin causes **hypoglycemia,** a dangerous drop in blood glucose levels. Hypoglycemia robs the brain of the glucose that is essential for it to function. Too little insulin results in **hyperglycemia,** or too much glucose in the bloodstream. If a person's blood glucose level increases too much, he can enter a state called diabetic coma. If not treated, diabetic coma can lead to death.

Many devices are available to monitor blood glucose levels, and new ones are constantly entering the market as new technology is developed. Most devices for monitoring blood glucose levels use a drop of blood obtained from the person's finger (Fig. 30-9). The "finger stick" method of monitoring blood glucose levels is painful for the person and can also expose the health care worker to bloodborne diseases. Make sure to wear gloves any time you are checking a person's glucose level using this method.

Many people with diabetes monitor their own glucose levels and have been taught to adjust their insulin intake as needed, but some residents or patients may need help with monitoring their blood glucose levels. Different facilities will have different policies about who is responsible for blood glucose monitoring. You may work in a facility that allows personal support workers to perform the glucose monitoring. Make sure that you have been adequately trained in how to use the equipment and record your findings. Be aware of which glucose levels need to be reported to the nurse immediately.

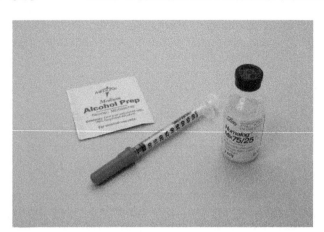

A

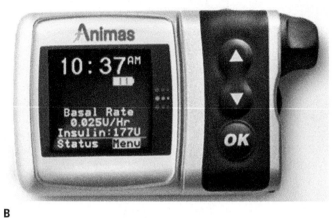

B

Figure 30-8

People with type 1 diabetes mellitus must inject insulin into their bodies daily. **(A)** A syringe is used to administer insulin at regular intervals throughout the day. **(B)** A portable insulin pump allows for the continuous infusion of insulin. (*B, courtesy of Animas Corporation, West Chester, PA.*)

Diet

It is very important for a person with diabetes to eat an adequate amount of nutritious food, especially if the person is taking insulin. In addition to regular meals, snacks are served to help regulate the person's blood glucose levels. A person with type 1 diabetes must eat a diet with specific amounts of carbohydrates, sugars, fats, and proteins to react with the amount of injected insulin. If a person does not eat at the recommended time after receiving her insulin, her blood glucose level can drop too low, resulting in a condition known as insulin shock. This is why it is important to serve meals and snacks at the scheduled time, especially when your patient or resident is taking insulin (Fig. 30-10). Also, if one of your patients or residents with diabetes refuses to eat or only

partially finishes his meal or snack, you should report this to the nurse immediately. Vomiting or being NPO (no food orally) for surgery or diagnostic testing can also affect a person's glucose levels.

Many people with diabetes understand how a balanced, nutritious diet can help them to manage their blood glucose levels and prevent complications from developing. However, some people may not follow their diet as closely as they should. For a person with diabetes, consuming too many sweets can result in hyperglycemia and lead to complications, both short term and long term. Some of your patients or residents, especially the older ones, may keep stashes of candy. If you

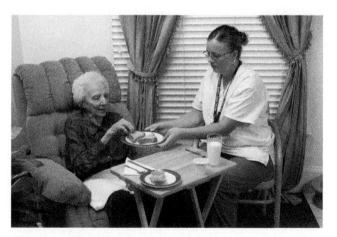

Figure 30-10

It is very important for a person with diabetes to eat regular, nutritionally sound meals and snacks. If one of your patients or residents with diabetes refuses to eat or only eats part of a meal or snack, report this to a nurse immediately.

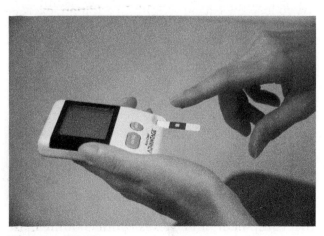

Figure 30-9

A glucometer is used to monitor blood glucose levels.

notice that a patient or resident is hoarding sweets, you should report this to the nurse.

Type 2 Diabetes

Type 2 diabetes mellitus, sometimes referred to as glucose intolerance, commonly occurs in overweight adults. In people with **type 2 diabetes mellitus,** the pancreas still produces some insulin, but the cells of the body are unable to respond to the insulin. This results in higher blood glucose levels because the body is unable to transport the glucose into the cells. Symptoms of type 2 diabetes mellitus may occur gradually and go undetected for a long time.

Type 2 diabetes is treated through diet, exercise, and the use of oral medications to increase the effectiveness of insulin. People with severe type 2 diabetes may need to be treated with insulin injections, especially during times of illness or stress. Controlling the diet may be quite difficult, especially for the person who enjoys sweets. When caring for a person with type 2 diabetes, be sure to watch closely the amounts and types of food the person eats, just as you would for a person with type 1 diabetes.

TELL THE NURSE

People with diabetes are very prone to developing both hyperglycemia (having too much sugar in the blood) and hypoglycemia (not having enough sugar in the blood). Hyperglycemia can be caused by eating too much food, not receiving enough insulin, being ill or under stress, being immobile or lacking exercise, or having diabetes mellitus that has not been diagnosed. Hypoglycemia can be caused by not having enough food, getting too much insulin, vomiting, or exercising more than usual.

Signs and symptoms of hyperglycemia and hypoglycemia are often very similar and should be reported to the nurse immediately. These signs include:

- Excessive hunger
- Excessive thirst

- Weakness, dizziness, or both
- Drowsiness and confusion
- Shaking and increased perspiration
- Rapid pulse and low blood pressure
- Headache
- Nausea and vomiting
- Slow, laboured respirations with sweet-smelling breath
- Frequent urination
- Convulsions
- Loss of consciousness

Complications of Diabetes

Many organ systems can be affected by uncontrolled diabetes mellitus of either type. Low insulin levels increase the release of lipids (fats) into the bloodstream. The lipids then build up in the linings of the arteries, damaging them. Atherosclerosis, high blood pressure, heart disease, kidney disease, and blindness (diabetic retinopathy; see Chapter 29) can result from the damaged blood vessels. In addition, peripheral nerve damage results from reduced blood flow to the neurons, causing diminished sensation in the arms and legs. Poor circulation to the feet and lower legs also increases the risk of infection and poor tissue healing in the event of injury.

Early detection of diabetes mellitus is essential for preventing complications. Once diabetes mellitus is diagnosed, there are many measures that can be taken to keep the disease under control and minimize the person's risk of developing complications. People who are overweight should try to lose the excess weight. In addition, exercising regularly, following the recommended diet closely, and taking prescribed medications correctly are also very important.

SUMMARY

- The endocrine system is made up of glands located in specific places throughout the body that produce hormones. Hormones are chemical messengers that allow the body to reproduce, grow, develop, metabolize energy, respond to stress and injury, and maintain homeostasis.
  - The pituitary gland is considered the master gland of the endocrine system because it secretes hormones that affect other

glands. The pituitary gland is controlled by the hypothalamus.

- The posterior lobe of the pituitary gland stores and releases antidiuretic hormone (ADH) and oxytocin.
- The anterior lobe of the pituitary gland produces and releases growth hormone, thyroid-stimulating hormone (TSH), adrenocorticotropic hormone (ACTH), prolactin, and the gonadotropins [luteinizing hormone (LH) and follicle-stimulating hormone (FSH)].
- The thyroid gland produces thyroxine, which helps to regulate metabolism, and calcitonin, which helps to maintain calcium levels in the bloodstream.
- The parathyroid glands secrete parathyroid hormone (PTH), which helps to move calcium from the bones into the bloodstream.
- The adrenal glands produce hormones that help us to deal with stress.
  - The adrenal medulla secretes epinephrine and norepinephrine, which play a role in the "fight or flight" response.
  - The adrenal cortex secretes glucocorticoids, mineralocorticoids, and androgens.
- The pancreas secretes insulin and glucagon, which play a role in regulating blood glucose (sugar) levels.
- Disorders of the endocrine system result from either too much hormone or too little hormone.

- Hypothyroidism (secretion of too little thyroid hormone) and hyperthyroidism (secretion of too much thyroid hormone) are common endocrine disorders. Thyroid hormone imbalances change the body's metabolic rate, causing many uncomfortable symptoms. Fortunately, hypothyroidism and hyperthyroidism can usually be treated.
- The most common of all endocrine disorders is diabetes mellitus.
  - There are two forms of diabetes mellitus.
    - Type 1 diabetes mellitus is the more severe form of diabetes. People with type 1 diabetes need daily insulin injections.
    - Type 2 diabetes mellitus is also called glucose intolerance because the cells and tissues of the body no longer respond to the action of insulin. Type 2 diabetes mellitus can usually be managed with diet, exercise, and oral medications.
- A person with diabetes mellitus is prone to hyperglycemia (blood glucose levels that are too high) and hypoglycemia (blood glucose levels that are too low). As a result, careful monitoring of the blood glucose level is necessary because both hyperglycemia and hypoglycemia can cause complications, some of which are life-threatening.
- A person with diabetes needs to eat regular, nutritionally balanced meals and snacks.

WHAT DID YOU LEARN?

Multiple Choice

Select the single best answer for each of the following questions.

1. Hormones are chemical messengers that allow the body to:
   a. Metabolize energy
   b. Grow
   c. Reproduce
   d. All of the above

2. Which endocrine disorder causes an increased metabolic rate, increased hunger, weight loss, an irregular heartbeat, an inability to sleep, irritability, and intolerance to heat?
   a. Hyperthyroidism
   b. Diabetes
   c. Acromegaly
   d. Pituitary gigantism

3. Mrs. Snow has type 1 diabetes mellitus. What special care considerations might a personal support worker who is caring for Mrs. Snow need to keep in mind?
   a. Mrs. Snow will be unable to tolerate cold, and therefore, will often need a sweater.
   b. Mrs. Snow will need to eat meals and snacks on a regular schedule.
   c. Mrs. Snow may grow tired very easily.
   d. Mrs. Snow is likely to be irritable.

4. Why must a person with type 1 diabetes mellitus receive regular doses of insulin?
   a. The cells of the body do not respond to the insulin produced by the pancreas.

(b.) The person's pancreas does not produce insulin on its own.

c. The person's pancreas produces too much glucagon.

d. People with type 1 diabetes do not need to take insulin; their disease can be controlled through diet, exercise, and oral medications.

5. Mr. Byron has type 2 diabetes mellitus. Although he knows that he should limit the amount of sweets that he eats, he has a real "sweet tooth" and often eats candy. In addition, he only monitors his blood glucose on days when he does not feel well. What complication is Mr. Byron at risk for developing if he does not make more of an effort to control his blood glucose levels?

a. Kidney failure

b. Blindness

c. Heart disease

(d.) All of the above

6. Mrs. Barney takes oral thyroxine to control her hypothyroidism. Without this medication, what sort of signs and symptoms do you think Mrs. Barney would have?

a. Loss of appetite, weight gain, and constipation

b. Frequent urination and excessive thirst

(c.) Fat deposits on her back, abdomen, and face

d. Excessive growth of the bones of the hands, feet, and face

Matching

Match each numbered item with its appropriate lettered description.

H 1. Parathyroid hormone (PTH)

B 2. Antidiuretic hormone (ADH)

C 3. Growth hormone

G 4. Thyroid-stimulating hormone (TSH)

E 5. Calcitonin

A 6. Adrenocorticotropic hormone (ACTH)

I 7. Thyroxine

J 8. Norepinephrine and epinephrine

F 9. Glucocorticoids

D 10. Insulin

a. Secreted by the adrenal cortex; helps the body to deal with stress

b. Secreted by the posterior pituitary gland; acts on the kidneys to limit the amount of water lost in the urine

c. Secreted by the anterior pituitary gland; causes our bodies to get bigger and taller

d. Secreted by the pancreas; helps the body to manage blood glucose levels

e. Secreted by the thyroid gland; lowers the amount of calcium in the bloodstream

f. Secreted by the anterior pituitary gland; stimulates the adrenal glands to produce their hormones

g. Secreted by the thyroid gland; sets the metabolic rate for the cells of the body

h. Secreted by the parathyroid glands; stimulates the release of calcium from the bones into the bloodstream

i. Secreted by the anterior pituitary gland; stimulates the thyroid glands to produce their hormones

j. Secreted by the adrenal medulla; participates in the "fight-or-flight" response

STOP and Think!

One of your residents, Mr. Singer, receives an insulin injection for his diabetes every morning. This morning, Mr. Singer had his injection and then ate most of his breakfast. About 30 minutes later, he vomited. Now Mr. Singer tells you that he feels shaky, and you can see that he is sweating. Why is it important for you to report these observations to the nurse immediately?

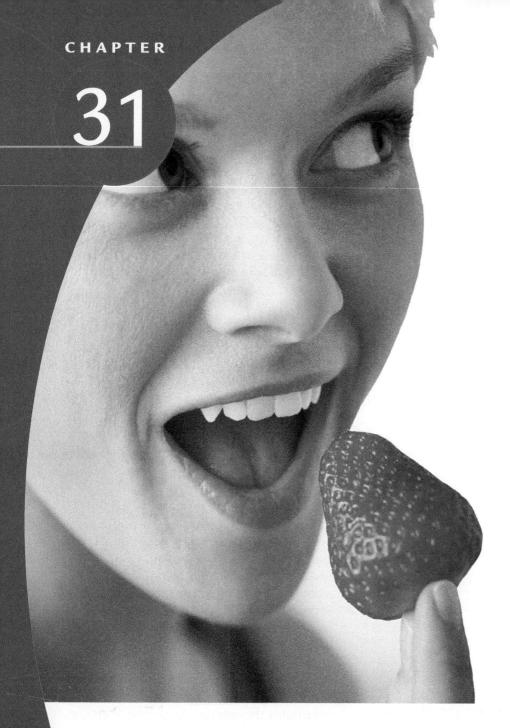

The Digestive System

WHAT WILL YOU LEARN?

Did you know that over the course of a lifetime, you will eat about 45,000 kg of food? As you already know from Chapters 19 and 20, it is your digestive system's job to process that food so that your body can use it, and to rid the body of the solid waste that is created as part of the food processing process. In this chapter, you will learn more about the

Photo: The digestive system processes the food that we eat.

individual organs of the digestive system and how they work. You will also learn about some common disorders of the digestive system. When you are finished with this chapter, you will be able to:

1. List the organs that are part of the digestive system.
2. Describe the function of the organs of the digestive system.
3. Discuss the effects of aging on the digestive system.
4. Discuss common digestive disorders and their symptoms.
5. Describe some of the tools used to diagnose digestive disorders.
6. Demonstrate how to provide routine stoma care.

Vocabulary

Esophagus	Salivary glands	Mechanical digestion	Ostomy
Stomach	Liver	Enzymes	Ileostomy
Esophageal (cardiac) sphincter	Bile	Chemical digestion	Colostomy
	Gallbladder	Villi	
Pyloric sphincter	Pancreas	Hernia	
Rugae	Mastication	Barium	

STRUCTURE OF THE DIGESTIVE SYSTEM

The digestive system, also known as the gastrointestinal system, is a long tube, or *tract*, consisting of the mouth, pharynx, esophagus, stomach, small intestine, and large intestine (Fig. 31-1). In addition, several accessory organs (appendages) along the way assist in the process of breaking down food so that our bodies can use it. These accessory organs include the teeth, tongue, salivary glands, liver, gallbladder, and pancreas.

THE DIGESTIVE TRACT

The walls of the "tube" that forms the digestive tract are made up of four layers of tissue (Fig. 31-2). The layers are basically the same throughout the digestive tract, although there is some variation from region to region. The four basic layers are the mucosa, the submucosa, the muscle layer, and the serosa:

- The *mucosa*, a mucous membrane, lines the digestive tract. The mucosa helps to trap disease-causing microbes. This is important because the digestive tract is open to the outside world at both ends (that is, the mouth and the anus). In addition to trapping microbes, the mucosa helps to protect the delicate tissues of the digestive tract from stomach acid, a very

harsh fluid produced by the stomach to help digest food.
- The *submucosa* contains blood vessels and nerves.
- The *muscle layer* contains smooth muscle. Recall from Chapter 23 that smooth muscle is not under voluntary control—it contracts and relaxes automatically. Peristalsis (contraction of the smooth muscle in the walls of the digestive tract) moves food through the system.
- The *serosa* is a tough outer layer of connective tissue.

Let's take a look now at the individual organs that form the digestive tract.

The Mouth, Pharynx, and Esophagus

Food begins its journey through the digestive tract at the mouth, or oral cavity. The mouth is lined with a mucous membrane and houses the teeth and tongue, accessory organs that assist with chewing and swallowing food. When you swallow, the epiglottis (a flap of cartilage that covers the opening to the larynx) snaps shut to prevent food from passing into the trachea. Instead, food moves into the pharynx (throat) and then into the esophagus.

The **esophagus**, a long narrow tube, serves mainly as a passageway for food to get from the pharynx to the stomach. The esophagus passes through the chest cavity, behind the heart (see Fig. 31-1). It enters the abdominal cavity at the

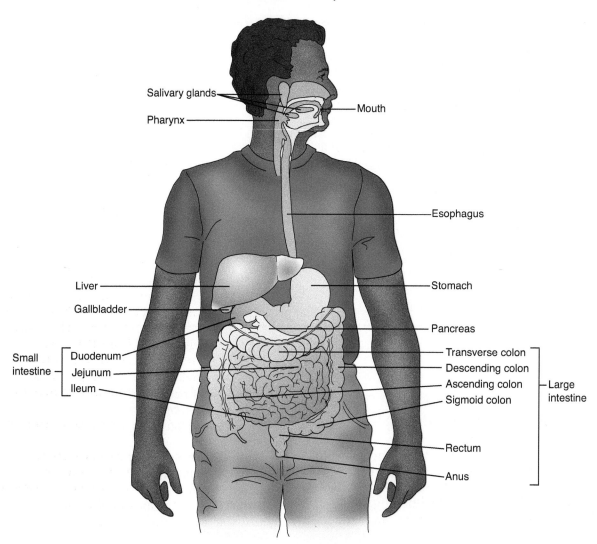

Figure 31-1
The digestive system breaks down food, absorbs nutrients, and gets rid of waste.

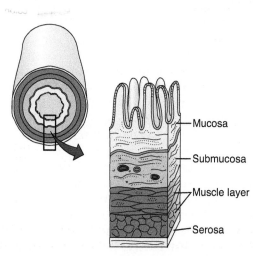

Figure 31-2
The walls of the digestive tract consist of four basic layers.

hiatus, an opening in the diaphragm (the large, flat muscle that separates the abdominal and chest cavities). After entering the abdominal cavity, the esophagus connects with the upper part of the stomach. The mucus secreted by the esophageal mucosa, as well as the action of the muscle layer, helps to move food downward and into the stomach.

The Stomach

The **stomach** is a hollow, muscular holding pouch for food. The stomach has three main regions (Fig. 31-3):

* The *fundus* is the upper region.
* The *body* is the main region. The esophagus enters the stomach here. The **esophageal (cardiac) sphincter,** a circle of muscular tissue, surrounds the place where the

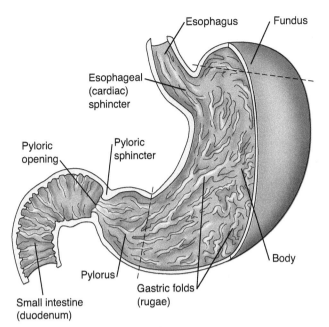

Figure 31-3
The stomach is a hollow holding pouch for food.

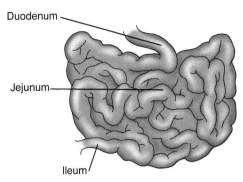

Figure 31-4
The small intestine has three regions: the duodenum, the jejunum, and the ileum.

esophagus enters the stomach and keeps food from going back up the esophagus after it has entered the stomach.

- The *pylorus* is the bottom region. Food leaves the stomach through the **pyloric sphincter,** a circle of muscular tissue that surrounds the place where the stomach empties into the small intestine. The pyloric sphincter helps to prevent food from returning to the stomach once it enters the small intestine.

As most of us have experienced after eating a large holiday dinner, the stomach is capable of stretching and holding a large amount of food. Folds of the mucosa, called **rugae,** flatten out as food enters the stomach, almost doubling the stomach's holding capacity.

The Small Intestine

The small intestine, which is about 610 centimetres long, is so named because its diameter is much smaller than that of the large intestine. The small intestine has three regions, called the *duodenum*, the *jejunum*, and the *ileum* (Fig. 31-4).

The Large Intestine

The large intestine (also called the *colon*) is about 140 centimetres long and is much larger in diameter than the small intestine. Like the small intestine, the large intestine has several distinct regions (Fig. 31-5):

- The *cecum* is like a waiting room for food that is leaving the small intestine through

the ileocecal valve and entering the large intestine. Food moves through the large intestine much more slowly than it moves through the small intestine. Therefore, incoming deliveries from the small intestine need a place to wait until the next segment of the large intestine, the ascending colon, is able to accept more food for processing.

- The *ascending colon* travels upward from the cecum.
- The *transverse colon* travels across.
- The *descending colon* travels down.
- The *sigmoid colon* is an S-shaped curve at the end of the descending colon.

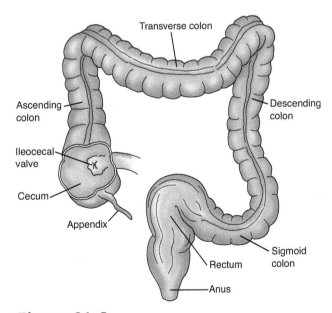

Figure 31-5
The large intestine has several regions: the cecum, the ascending colon, the transverse colon, the descending colon, the sigmoid colon, and the rectum. The appendix is a small pouch attached to the end of the cecum.

- The *rectum* is the last segment of the colon. The place where the rectum opens to the outside of the body is the *anus*.

The *appendix*, a tiny, closed pouch that dangles from the cecum, has no known function. Scientists think that in our ancient ancestors, the appendix may have played a role in digesting food, but that role has since been lost. Still, the appendix has a way of making its presence known. Inflammation or infection of the appendix causes *appendicitis*, a painful condition that is life-threatening if not treated. Treatment is surgical removal of the appendix.

THE ACCESSORY ORGANS

Several organs—the salivary glands, liver, gallbladder, and pancreas—play a role in digestion but are not actually part of the digestive tract (see Fig. 31-1).

- The **salivary glands** are located near the mouth. They produce and secrete saliva, a substance that helps with chewing and swallowing by moistening the food.
- The **liver** is a large organ located just underneath the diaphragm (see Fig. 31-1). The liver produces and secretes bile into the duodenum. **Bile** is a substance that helps with the digestion of fats. The liver also has several other important functions that are not related to digestion. For example, it produces clotting factors (chemicals that help our blood to clot) and it helps to clear our blood of toxins, such as alcohol and drugs.
- The **gallbladder,** a small pouch that is attached to the liver, stores bile produced by the liver that is not secreted directly into the duodenum.
- The **pancreas** is located behind the stomach, in the curve of the duodenum (see Fig. 31-1). The pancreas produces substances that aid in digestion and secretes them into the duodenum. The pancreas also produces insulin and glucagon, hormones that are secreted directly into the bloodstream. (Recall from Chapter 30 that insulin and glucagon regulate glucose levels in the blood.)

FUNCTION OF THE DIGESTIVE SYSTEM

The digestive system breaks down the food we eat into nutrients, which are then absorbed into the bloodstream for use by the body's cells. In addition, the digestive system removes unusable digested food from the body, in the form of feces.

DIGESTION

Digestion, or the breaking down of food into simple elements (nutrients), begins in the mouth. First, we physically break the food into smaller pieces by chewing it. Another word for chewing is **mastication.** This physical breaking up of the food, such as occurs when we chew, is called **mechanical digestion.** Next, chemical substances in our saliva start to work on the smaller pieces of food, breaking them down even more by breaking the bonds that hold the food molecules together. Substances that have the ability to break chemical bonds are called **enzymes.** The human body produces many different types of enzymes, each with a specific function. The process of breaking down food through the use of chemical substances such as enzymes is called **chemical digestion.**

After passing through the esophagus, the food we eat stays in the stomach for 3 to 4 hours, where digestion continues to take place. Special glands in the stomach lining produce hydrochloric acid (sometimes called "stomach acid") and enzymes. The stomach acid and enzymes act on the pieces of food to break them down even further. The peristaltic action of the stomach helps to mix the food with the acid and enzymes, creating a liquid substance called *chyme.*

The chyme passes into the duodenum, the first segment of the small intestine. Once in the duodenum, the chyme mixes with bile (secreted by the liver) and digestive enzymes secreted by the pancreas. These substances cause further breakdown of the food. From the duodenum, the chyme passes into the jejunum.

ABSORPTION

Once the chyme reaches the jejunum, absorption of nutrients begins. At this point, the food is fairly well digested. Now, it is time to start moving the nutrients from the digestive tract into the bloodstream. To reach the bloodstream, the nutrients pass through the mucosa and into the blood vessels in the next layer, the submucosa. The mucosa of the small intestine has millions of tiny finger-like structures called **villi** (Fig. 31-6). The villi increase the small intestine's ability to absorb nutrients by increasing the surface area of the mucosa.

Although most of the absorption of nutrients takes place in the small intestine, the large intestine also plays a role in absorption. Bacteria that live in the large intestine act on the chyme to

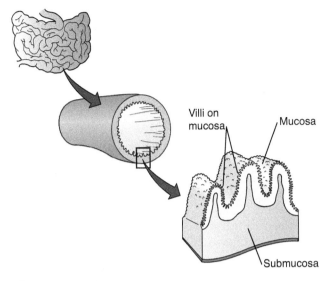

Figure 31-6
Villi are finger-like projections that increase the small intestine's ability to absorb nutrients.

produce vitamin K and some B vitamins, which are absorbed by the body. The action of these bacteria on the chyme can also produce gas as a by-product, especially when high-fibre foods such as beans, onions, and broccoli are part of the diet. As the chyme passes slowly through the large intestine, water is absorbed into the bloodstream. By the time the chyme reaches the end of the long intestine, all nutrients and most of the water have been removed, and the chyme has taken on the soft, moist, semi-solid consistency of normal feces.

EXCRETION

The feces (waste products of digestion) collect in the rectum, the last segment of the large intestine. The walls of the rectum gradually expand as the feces build up. At a certain point, the brain senses that the rectum is "full" and the urge to defecate (have a bowel movement) occurs.

EFFECTS OF AGING ON THE DIGESTIVE SYSTEM

Like all of the body's organ systems, the digestive system is affected by the process of aging.

LESS EFFICIENT CHEWING AND SWALLOWING

In older people, the production of saliva decreases, which may make chewing and swallowing more difficult. In addition, many older people have dental problems, such as missing or painful teeth. An older person may choke as a result of trying to swallow food that has not been chewed properly. Remember this when you are helping an older person to eat. Create a relaxed, social environment for eating and help the person to cut food up into small, easy-to-chew pieces. Also, report complaints of poorly fitting dentures, sores in the mouth or on the tongue, or a toothache to the nurse immediately.

LESS EFFICIENT DIGESTION

Food is most easily digested when it has been thoroughly chewed. Mechanical digestion increases the effectiveness of chemical digestion by making the pieces of food smaller. In an older person, the production of saliva, stomach acid, and digestive enzymes slows, making chemical digestion less efficient. Digestion is less efficient because not only are fewer chemicals available for chemical digestion, but the pieces of food that the chemicals must work on may be larger, due to inefficient chewing.

INCREASED RISK FOR CONSTIPATION

In an older person, the movement of food through the digestive tract may be slower. This can put the older person at risk for constipation. The chyme spends more time in the large intestine, which allows more water to be reabsorbed into the bloodstream. As a result, by the time the chyme reaches the end of the large intestine, almost all of the water has been removed and the resulting feces are hard, dry, and difficult to pass. Certain medications (such as prescription pain relievers) and immobility can also increase a person's risk for constipation. Measures that you can take to help your patients and residents avoid constipation were described in Chapter 20.

DISORDERS OF THE DIGESTIVE SYSTEM

Many of the people you will care for will have a digestive disorder of some sort, or will be recovering from one. Because the digestive system contains so many different organs, there are many different disorders that can occur. Four of the most common digestive disorders that you are likely to see in the health care setting are ulcers, hernias, gallbladder disorders, and cancer.

ULCERS

Ulcers (sores caused by wearing away of the protective mucosa that lines the digestive tract) can occur anywhere along the digestive tract. The most common sites are the stomach (*gastric ulcer*) and the duodenum (*duodenal ulcer*). Ulcers occur when the stomach produces too much hydrochloric acid. Factors such as smoking, frequent use of over-the-counter pain medications, and infection with a bacterium called *Helicobacter pylori* can increase a person's chances of developing ulcers. In severe cases, the ulcer may affect all of the layers of the stomach or duodenum wall, not just the mucosa. This condition, called a *penetrating ulcer*, is life-threatening.

A person with an ulcer may feel uncomfortably full or nauseous after eating. Stomach pain is common, especially within 3 hours of eating (or when the person does not eat). Most ulcers are chronic. The person will have periods of feeling well, interrupted by flare-ups of symptoms.

Most ulcers can be treated with medication. People with severe ulcers may need surgery.

HERNIAS

The abdominal cavity (the space in the body where most of the digestive organs are found) is bounded by muscular walls. The muscular walls of the abdominal cavity give structure to the body and help to keep the internal organs where they belong. A **hernia** occurs when an internal organ bulges through a weakness in the muscular wall of the abdominal cavity (Fig. 31-7). Sometimes the weakness occurs at the site of an old surgical incision. Other times, the muscle is just weak in certain areas. If there is a weak area in the muscular wall, and the person does something that requires a lot of physical effort (such as lifting a heavy object), a hernia may occur. Hernias can occur in a number of different places:

- *Inguinal hernias* and *femoral hernias* occur when a loop of intestine bulges through the abdominal wall in the groin area. Inguinal hernias are more common in men, and femoral hernias are more common in women. These types of hernias are repaired surgically.
- *Umbilical hernias* occur around the navel (belly button). If the umbilical hernia is very small, no treatment may be needed. However, surgery may be required to repair a larger umbilical hernia.
- *Hiatal hernias* occur when part of the stomach passes through the hiatus, the opening in the diaphragm that allows the esophagus to pass into the abdominal cavity. People with hiatal hernias often have heartburn because the stomach acid moves back up into the esophagus. A person with a hiatal hernia may find that eating small, frequent meals and sitting up for at least 2 hours after every meal helps to relieve the heartburn. Medication can also provide relief of symptoms. People with severe symptoms may need surgery to repair the hernia.

Complications occur if the muscle tightens around the trapped tissue, cutting off its blood supply. This situation, called a *strangulated hernia,* is a surgical emergency.

GALLBLADDER DISORDERS

Gallstones can form and block the flow of bile from the gallbladder into the duodenum (Fig. 31-8). This can lead to inflammation and infection of the gallbladder. A person with a gallbladder disorder has episodes of severe pain. The pain may stay in the upper abdominal region, or it may radiate to the back and shoulder on the person's right side. The person may also have indigestion, especially after eating foods that are high in fat. Because bile gives feces their characteristic brown color, in a person with a gallbladder disorder, the feces may be pale and "clay-colored" due to their low bile content. Remember also that bile helps the body to digest fat. Therefore, in a person with gallbladder disease, the feces may float because they contain a great deal of undigested fat.

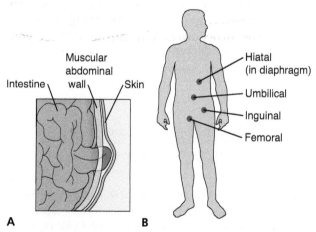

Figure 31-7

(A) A hernia occurs when an internal organ bulges through a weakness in the abdominal wall. **(B)** Hernias can occur in a number of different places.

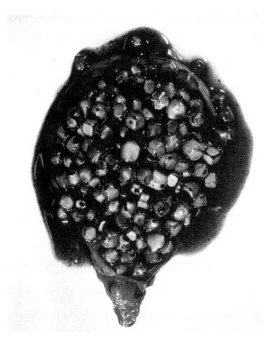

Figure 31-8
A gallbladder that has been removed and cut open to reveal the many gallstones inside. Gallstones can block the flow of bile into the duodenum, causing indigestion and severe pain. (*Rubin, R., & Stayer, D. S. [2008]. Rubin's Pathology: Clinicopathologic Foundations of Medicine [5th ed., p. 668]. Philadelphia: Lippincott Williams & Wilkins.*)

Medication or laser treatment may be used to dissolve the gallstones. In some cases, surgical removal of the gallbladder is needed.

CANCER

Any of the organs in the digestive system can be affected by cancer. The person's signs and symptoms will vary, depending on the location of the tumour. A person with cancer involving the digestive system may have one or more of the following signs and symptoms: loss of appetite, indigestion, pain, vomiting, constipation, changes in bowel movements, or blood in the feces (stool). Depending on the location and type of cancer, it may be treated with surgery, radiation, chemotherapy, or a combination of these.

DIAGNOSIS OF DIGESTIVE DISORDERS

Digestive complaints—such as heartburn, indigestion, nausea, vomiting, stomachache, gas, diarrhea, and constipation—are common. Often,

these symptoms are not a sign of anything serious. Sometimes, however, they may signal a serious disorder. Always report a new symptom, or a change in the person's symptoms, to the nurse immediately.

Sometimes, the doctor will order one or more tests to evaluate a person's symptoms. Some of these tests are simple, such as laboratory analysis of a stool sample. Others are more involved. Tests you may hear mentioned include the following:

- *Endoscopy* involves using a special instrument to look inside the digestive tract and obtain tissue or fluids for analysis. Endoscopy allows the doctor to look inside the digestive tract for tumours or other abnormal growths. The type of endoscope used depends on whether the instrument will be passed through the person's mouth (to view the upper digestive tract) or anus (to view the lower digestive tract).
- *Imaging studies*, such as x-rays, computed tomography (CT) scans, and magnetic resonance imaging (MRI) scans, allow the doctor to view the organs of the digestive system without actually entering the body. Sometimes, the person is asked to swallow barium or have a barium enema prior to the procedure. **Barium** is a liquid substance that coats the mucosa of the digestive tract and makes the organs appear on an x-ray (Fig. 31-9).

You may find yourself caring for a person who is about to have one of these diagnostic procedures. The person may have a special diet in the days leading up to the procedure, or be placed on NPO (no food orally) status. Sometimes, an enema is ordered to clean out the large intestine prior to the procedure. The nurse will let you know of any special care needs for a person who is having one of these procedures.

CARING FOR A PERSON WITH AN OSTOMY

As a personal support worker, you may care for people with ostomies. For example, a person with a tumour in the large intestine may have surgery to remove the diseased part of the intestine. Depending on the location of the tumour and the length of the segment of the intestine that had to be removed, the person may need an alternate way of eliminating feces from the

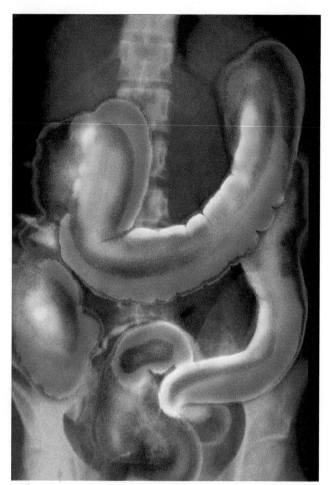

Figure 31-9

A person may be given a barium enema or asked to drink barium prior to having an x-ray taken. The barium helps to enhance the x-ray image. This is a false-color barium x-ray of a person's digestive tract. (© *BSIP/Custom Medical Stock Photo.*)

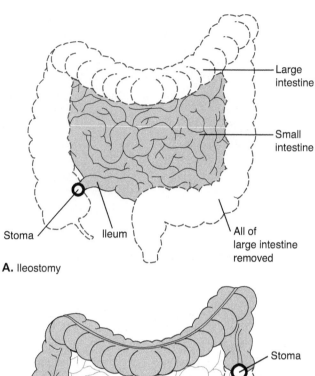

A. Ileostomy

B. Colostomy

Figure 31-10

Some of the people you will care for may have had surgery to remove all or part of the large intestine. Such a surgery may be necessary because of cancer, a bowel obstruction, or trauma. **(A)** Ileostomy. The entire large intestine is removed. A stoma is made in the abdominal wall, and the end of the small intestine (the ileum) is sewn into place. **(B)** Colostomy. Part of the large intestine is removed. A colostomy can be done at any point along the large intestine; here, a section of the descending colon was removed. A stoma is made in the abdominal wall, and the healthy end of the remaining large intestine is sewn into place.

body following the surgery. In this case, the person may have an **ostomy.** An artificial opening, called a stoma, is made in the abdominal wall and the remaining portion of the intestine is connected to it (Fig. 31-10). Feces pass through the stoma and into a pouch (called an *ostomy appliance*) that is worn over the stoma (Fig. 31-11).

- An **ileostomy** is created if the entire large intestine must be removed. The end of the small intestine (that is, the ileum) is attached to the abdominal wall. Because the chyme does not have the chance to travel through the large intestine (where water is reabsorbed), the person's feces are very liquid and may flow fairly continuously. For this reason, a person with an ileostomy is quite prone to dehydration.

- A **colostomy** is created if part of the large intestine is still present. After the diseased part of the large intestine is removed, the healthy end is attached to the abdominal wall. Among people with colostomies, the feces vary in consistency. If the portion of the intestine that was removed was near the

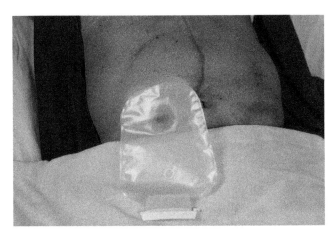

Figure 31-11
An ostomy appliance is worn over the stoma to collect the feces.

beginning of the large intestine, then the feces will be more liquid because the chyme will spend less time in the large intestine. On the other hand, if the portion of the intestine that was removed was near the end of the large intestine, then the feces will be more solid and formed.

Cancer is not the only reason a person might have to have an ostomy procedure. Bowel trauma and diseases such as diverticulitis (an inflammatory disease of the bowel) are other common reasons that ostomies are performed. Sometimes, a temporary ostomy is done to allow a portion of the bowel to "rest." Later, the ends of the bowel are sewn back together and normal bowel elimination resumes.

In some provinces or territories and facilities, helping patients or residents to care for an ostomy is within the personal support worker's scope of practice. Ostomies, like the people who have them, are very individual. Ostomies can be located in many different places on the abdomen. In addition, abdomens vary from person to person. For these reasons, the supplies used for ostomies vary greatly. Some ostomy appliances consist of a bag with an adhesive opening that adheres to the skin around the stoma. Other ostomy appliances have two pieces—a ring of flexible rubber that is applied to the skin around

the stoma, and a bag that is snapped on to the ring. Some appliances are used only once and then discarded, while others are emptied, cleaned, and used again. If you are permitted to provide ostomy care, make sure that you are familiar with the different types of ostomy appliances used in your facility and ask the nurse for help with any that are new to you.

No matter what type of ostomy appliance is used, certain principles of ostomy care remain the same for every patient or resident with an ostomy. Because the skin around the ostomy comes in contact with feces, it must be kept clean to prevent irritation. The ostomy appliance can be changed with the person sitting or standing in the bathroom, or while the person is in bed. If the ostomy appliance is being changed while the person is in bed, the person should either sit upright or lie flat. The procedure for providing routine stoma care is given in Procedure 31-1.

Helping Hands and a Caring Heart

FOCUS ON HUMANISTIC HEALTH CARE

For many people, having an ostomy is very difficult, emotionally. First, the person must cope with having an illness or injury serious enough to require major surgery. Second, many people consider elimination, especially bowel elimination, a very private activity. Having to wear a bag to collect feces on the outside of the body is very embarrassing for many people.

Especially in the beginning, it may be very hard for a person to accept the ostomy. If you are caring for someone who is getting used to the idea of having an ostomy, take the time to listen carefully if the person wants to talk about his fears or uncertainties. Be careful not to brush off the person's concerns with a comment such as "Oh, everything will be okay now; don't worry." Instead, put yourself in the person's shoes and think about how you would feel if you were in the same situation. Report the person's comments and questions to the nurse. Once the nurse knows that the person is having trouble adjusting to the ostomy, there are many things he or she can do to help the person adjust.

SUMMARY

- The digestive system consists of the digestive tract and several accessory organs.
  - The digestive tract consists of the mouth, pharynx, esophagus, stomach, small intestine, and large intestine.
    - The walls of the digestive tract are lined with a mucous membrane (called the mucosa).
    - The walls of the digestive tract contain smooth muscle, which contracts to help move food through the tube (peristalsis).
  - Accessory organs include the teeth, tongue, salivary glands, liver, gallbladder, and pancreas.
- The digestive system breaks down the food we eat into nutrients that can be used by the cells of the body. The digestive system also removes waste from the body in the form of feces.
  - Most digestion takes place in the mouth and stomach. There are two types of digestion: mechanical and chemical.
    - Mechanical digestion is the physical breaking down of food. Chewing is an example of mechanical digestion.
    - Chemical digestion is the breaking down of food through chemical means, such as digestive enzymes.
  - Most absorption takes place in the small and large intestines.
    - Most absorption of nutrients takes place in the jejunum and ileum, the last two segments of the small intestine.
    - Water is reabsorbed into the blood-stream as the chyme passes through the large intestine.
  - Feces are what are left after all of the nutrients and most of the water are removed from the chyme, during its passage through the small and large intestines. Feces collect in the rectum, the last segment of the large intestine, until the urge to defecate occurs.
- As a person gets older, he may have more trouble chewing and swallowing food. Digestion is less efficient. In addition, the older person may be at higher risk for becoming constipated.
- Common disorders of the digestive system include ulcers, hernias, gallbladder disorders, and cancer. Always report a new gastrointestinal complaint, or a change in a person's usual symptoms, to the nurse immediately.
- A person who is about to have a diagnostic procedure to evaluate her digestive system may have special care needs prior to the test. The nurse will let you know of any special instructions, which should be followed carefully.
- An ostomy is an alternate way of removing feces from the body.
  - For many people, having an ostomy is difficult, emotionally.
  - Proper care of the ostomy site is necessary to keep the skin clean and healthy.

Providing Routine Ostomy Care

WHY YOU DO IT Because the skin around the stoma comes in contact with feces, it must be kept clean to prevent irritation.

Getting Ready WORKTEPS

1. Complete the "Getting Ready" steps.

Supplies

- gloves
- paper towels
- bed protector
- toilet paper
- 4 × 4 gauze pad
- clean ostomy appliance
- clean ostomy belt (if one is used)
- skin barrier
- bedpan
- bedpan cover (or paper towels)
- wash basin
- soap (or other cleansing agent, per facility policy)
- adhesive remover (optional)
- deodorant for ostomy appliance (optional)
- washcloths
- towel

Procedure

2. Cover the over-bed table with paper towels. Place the ostomy supplies and clean linens on the over-bed table.

3. Make sure that the bed is positioned at a comfortable working height (to promote good body mechanics) and that the wheels are locked.

4. If the side rails are in use, lower the side rail on the working side of the bed. The side rail on the opposite side of the bed should remain up. If necessary, lower the head of the bed so that the bed is flat (as tolerated).

5. Fanfold the top linens to below the person's waist.

6. Position the bed protector on the bed alongside the person to keep the bed linens dry. Adjust the person's clothing as necessary to expose the person's stoma.

7. Put on the gloves.

8. Disconnect the ostomy appliance from the ostomy belt if one is used. Remove the belt. If the ostomy belt is soiled, dispose of it in a facility-approved waste container (if it is disposable), or place it in the linen hamper or linen bag (if it is not disposable).

9. Remove the ostomy appliance by holding the skin taut and gently pulling the appliance away, starting at the top. If the adhesive is making removal difficult, use warm water or the adhesive solvent to soften the adhesive. Place the ostomy appliance in the bedpan.

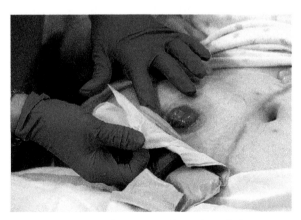

Step 9 Hold the skin taut and gently pull the ostomy appliance away.

(continued)

10. Gently wipe the stoma with toilet paper to remove any feces or drainage. Place the toilet paper in the bedpan. Cover the stoma with the gauze pad to absorb any drainage that may occur until the new appliance is in place.

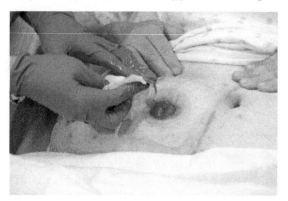

Step 10 Gently wipe the stoma with toilet tissue to remove drainage.

11. Cover the bedpan with the bedpan cover or paper towels. Take the bedpan to the bathroom. (If the side rails are in use, raise them before leaving the bedside.)

12. Note the color, amount, and quality of the feces before emptying the contents of the ostomy appliance and the bedpan into the toilet. (If anything unusual is observed, do not empty the ostomy appliance until a nurse has had a chance to look at its contents.)

13. Dispose of the ostomy appliance in a facility-approved waste container.

14. Remove your gloves and dispose of them in a facility-approved waste container. Wash your hands.

15. Fill the wash basin with warm water (43.3°C [110°F] to 46.1°C [115°F] on the bath thermometer). Return to the bedside. Place the basin on the over-bed table. If the side rails are in use, lower the side rail on the working side of the bed.

16. Put on a clean pair of gloves.

17. Form a mitt around your hand with one of the washcloths. Wet the mitt with warm, clean water and apply soap (or other cleansing agent, per facility policy). Remove the gauze pad from the stoma and dispose of it in a facility-approved waste container. Clean the skin around the stoma. Rinse and dry the skin around the stoma thoroughly.

18. Apply the skin barrier if needed, according to the manufacturer's directions.

19. Place the deodorant in the ostomy appliance if deodorant is used.

20. Put the clean ostomy belt on the person if an ostomy belt is used.

21. Make sure that the opening on the ostomy appliance is the correct size. Remove the adhesive backing on the ostomy appliance.

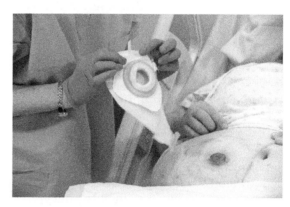

Step 21 Make sure the opening on the ostomy appliance is the correct size.

22. Center the appliance over the stoma, making sure that the drain or the end of the bag is pointed down. Gently press around the edges to seal the ostomy appliance to the skin.

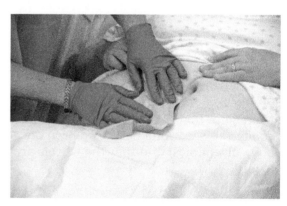

Step 22 Gently press the edges to seal the ostomy appliance to the skin.

23. Connect the ostomy appliance to the ostomy belt, if one is used.

24. Remove the bed protector.

25. Remove your gloves and dispose of them in a facility-approved waste container.

26. Adjust the person's clothing as necessary to cover the ostomy appliance. If the bedding is wet or soiled, change the bed linens. Help the person back into a comfortable position, straighten the bottom linens, and draw the top linens over the person. Raise the head of the bed, as the person requests.

27. If the side rails are in use, return the side rail to the raised position. Make sure that the bed is lowered to its lowest position and that the wheels are locked.

28. Gather the soiled linens and place them in the linen hamper or linen bag. Dispose of disposable items in a facility-approved waste container. Clean equipment and return it to the storage area.

Finishing Up CLSOWR

29. Complete the "Finishing Up" steps.

WHAT DID YOU LEARN?

Multiple Choice

Select the single best answer for each of the following questions.

1. Where does the process of digestion begin?
   a. In the stomach
   b. In the large intestine
   c. In the mouth
   d. In the esophagus
2. What is a hollow, muscular pouch for holding food?
   a. The appendix
   b. The gallbladder
   c. The duodenum
   d. The stomach
3. What is another term for the large intestine?
   a. Stomach
   b. Duodenum
   c. Colon
   d. Appendix
4. Where does most absorption of nutrients take place?
   a. In the jejunum and ileum of the small intestine
   b. In the rectum of the large intestine
   c. In the stomach
   d. In the liver
5. Where is most of the water absorbed from the chyme, resulting in the formation of formed, semi-moist feces?
   a. In the large intestine
   b. In the small intestine
   c. In the stomach
   d. In the gallbladder
6. Normal changes in the digestive system related to aging include:
   a. Less efficient chewing and swallowing
   b. Less efficient digestion
   c. Increased risk for constipation
   d. All of the above
7. Mr. Pak has an ileostomy, and you assist him with stoma care. What would you expect his feces to be like?
   a. Very liquid, continuously flowing
   b. Hard, dry, pellets
   c. Soft, brown, moist, and formed
   d. None of the above
8. What is the artificial opening for a colostomy called?
   a. A stoma
   b. A rectum
   c. An anus
   d. None of the above
9. You have been caring for Mrs. Zimmerman for several months. Mrs. Zimmerman has always had a "sensitive stomach." She often tells you that she is "queasy" or that something she ate "didn't agree with her." Although she always complains about the food at the facility, she usually cleans her plate. Today, however, you noticed that not only did Mrs. Zimmerman not eat her lunch, she has seemed particularly listless all afternoon. What should you do?
   a. Nothing; Mrs. Zimmerman always has "stomach issues"
   b. Record Mrs. Zimmerman's lack of appetite in her chart; the nurse will follow up later
   c. Report this change in Mrs. Zimmerman's behavior to the nurse immediately
   d. Wait and see if Mrs. Zimmerman has any appetite for dinner

STOP and Think!

Mr. Scott is a 42-year-old executive at an advertising agency who was recently diagnosed with colon cancer. Mr. Scott is married, with three young children. He is an avid golfer and swimmer. Following surgery to remove the cancer, Mr. Scott will have a colostomy. You are the personal support worker who will be caring for Mr. Scott in the hospital in the days following the surgery. Describe some of the emotions Mr. Scott may be feeling after the surgery, and how you would respond if Mr. Scott decided to share some of these feelings with you.

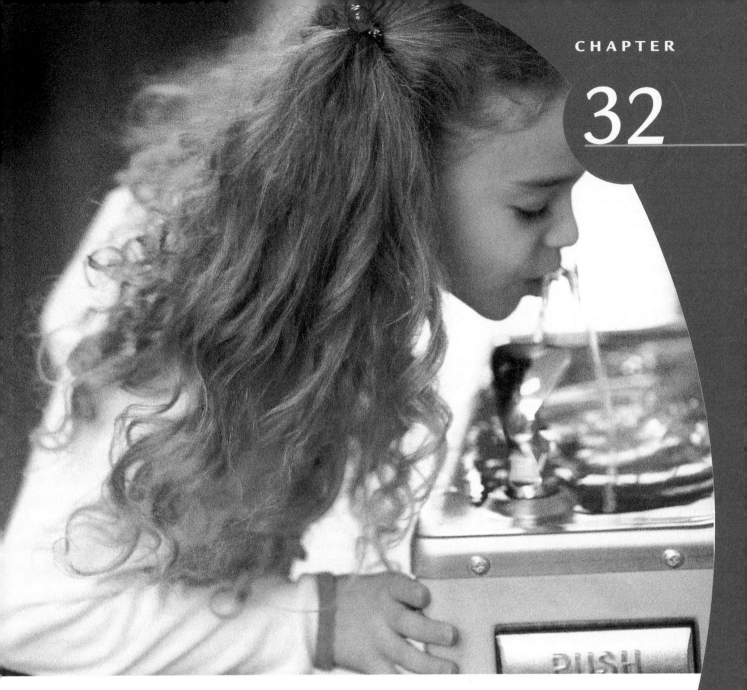

The Urinary System

WHAT WILL YOU LEARN?

As you learned in Chapter 20, the urinary system rids the body of waste products that have been filtered from the bloodstream, along with excess fluid, in the form of urine. In Chapter 20, you also learned how to assist patients and residents with urinary elimination. In this chapter, you will learn a little bit more about the organs that make up the urinary system and how they work. As a personal support worker, many of your daily responsibilities will allow you to observe changes in the functioning of a patient's or resident's urinary system that

Photo: Drinking plenty of fluids helps to keep the urinary system healthy.

647

could indicate a serious problem. This is why it is important for you to know about the effects of aging on the urinary system, and about some of the disorders that can affect this very important organ system. When you are finished with this chapter, you will be able to:

1. List the organs that make up the urinary system.
2. Describe the primary function of each organ of the urinary system.
3. Discuss the effects of aging on the urinary system.
4. Describe various disorders that can affect the urinary system.
5. Discuss the special care needs of people who have urinary system disorders.
6. List common diagnostic procedures that may be used to detect and diagnose urinary system disorders.

Vocabulary

Renal	Urine	Kidney stones (renal	Ureterostomy
Nephrons	Urethritis	calculi)	Urostomy
Glomerulus	Cystitis	Dialysis	
Filtrate	Pyelonephritis		

STRUCTURE OF THE URINARY SYSTEM

The urinary system consists of the kidneys, the ureters, the urinary bladder, and the urethra (Fig. 32-1).

THE KIDNEYS

We have two kidneys, which are like kidney beans in shape and color (only much larger!). The kidneys are located toward the back of the upper abdominal cavity, one on either side of the spinal column. The bottom of the rib cage and a layer of fat help to protect the kidneys.

Because the job of the kidneys is to filter the blood to remove waste products, the kidneys are supplied by two large arteries, called the left and right renal arteries. (**Renal** is a word meaning "related to, involving, or located in the region of the kidneys.") The renal arteries are branches of the aorta, the largest artery in the body. The blood flow through the renal arteries is so efficient that the kidneys are able to filter all of the body's blood every half-hour.

Inside each kidney are approximately 1 million tiny **nephrons,** the basic functional units of the kidney (Fig. 32-2). The nephrons are responsible for actually filtering the blood that passes through the kidney. Each nephron consists of a glomerulus and a series of tubules (see Fig. 32-2). The **glomerulus** is a capillary bed, enclosed

within a structure called *Bowman's capsule.* The blood entering the kidneys through the renal arteries is under great pressure. Once inside the kidneys, the blood passes through a series of arteries that get smaller and smaller, until it reaches the capillary bed of the glomerulus. The blood enters the glomerulus through a vessel called the afferent arteriole (*afferent* means "enter") (see Fig. 32-2). At this point, the blood is under a lot of pressure because the capillaries are very small. The walls of the capillaries in the glomerulus are semi-permeable, which means that they have tiny openings in them. Because the blood is under a lot of pressure, a lot of the liquid in the blood squeezes through the walls, taking the wastes and nutrients that are dissolved in it with it. This liquid, known as the **filtrate,** forms the basis of the urine. Next, two things happen (see Fig. 32-2B):

- The filtered blood leaves the glomerulus through the efferent arteriole (*efferent* means "exit"). It is returned to circulation through the renal veins, which empty into the inferior vena cava (the largest vein in the body).
- Meanwhile, the filtrate enters Bowman's capsule, and from there, flows into the tubules that make up the rest of the nephron. Small capillaries surround the tubules of the nephron. As the filtrate passes slowly through the tubules, these small capillaries reabsorb useful substances such as water, nutrients, and minerals from the filtrate. By

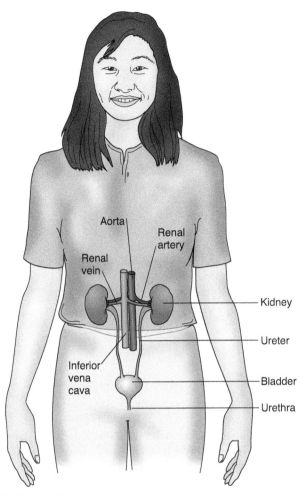

Figure 32-1
The urinary system consists of the kidneys, ureters, bladder, and urethra. Each kidney is supplied by a renal artery, which branches off of the aorta. After the kidneys filter the blood, the filtrate (urine) passes into the ureters and the blood passes into the renal veins, which empty into the inferior vena cava.

the time the filtrate reaches the end of the tubules, only excess fluid and waste substances remain. This is **urine.** The kidneys produce 160 to 180 litres of filtrate each day, but only about 1 to 1.5 litres are excreted from the body in the form of urine.

Urine from each nephron is emptied into a collecting area, called the *renal pelvis.* From the renal pelvis, the urine flows into the ureters.

THE URETERS

Two ureters, slender, muscular tubes approximately 25 to 32 centimetres long, carry urine from the kidneys to the bladder (see Fig. 32-1).

The ureters are wider at the top where they connect to the renal pelvis, but they quickly become very narrow. Where the two ureters enter the bladder, a small triangular fold of tissue called the *trigone* keeps urine from flowing back into the ureters after it has emptied into the bladder.

The ureters are lined with a mucous membrane, which helps to protect against infection. Smooth muscle in the walls of the ureters contracts rhythmically, moving urine away from the kidney and toward the urinary bladder. The peristaltic movements that help move urine through the ureters are similar to the peristaltic movements that help move food through the digestive tract.

THE BLADDER

The bladder is a hollow sac that is a holding place (reservoir) for urine. Urine is constantly produced by the kidneys and transported through the ureters to the bladder, where it is stored until urination occurs. The bladder is very small when empty but can become quite large as it fills with urine. Like the ureters, the inside of the bladder is lined with a mucous membrane. The walls of the bladder contain three layers of smooth muscle. When the walls of the bladder contract, urination occurs. Where the bladder and the urethra join (the *bladder outlet*), the internal sphincter (a ring of involuntary muscle) keeps the bladder closed while it fills.

THE URETHRA

The urethra is a tube that carries urine from the bladder to the outside of the body. The urethra begins at the bladder outlet, just below the internal sphincter, and ends at the external urinary opening (called the *urinary meatus* or *urethral orifice*). Below the internal sphincter, the external urethral sphincter, a ring of voluntary muscle, relaxes to allow urine to pass during urination.

Male and female urethras are very different in size and function (Fig. 32-3). In women, the urethra measures about 4 to 6 centimetres and is used only as a passageway for urine to leave the body. In men, the urethra measures about 15 to 20 centimetres and serves as a passageway for both urine and semen. In men, the urethra passes through the prostate gland soon after leaving the bladder outlet. The prostate gland produces seminal fluid, the fluid that, along with sperm cells, makes up semen.

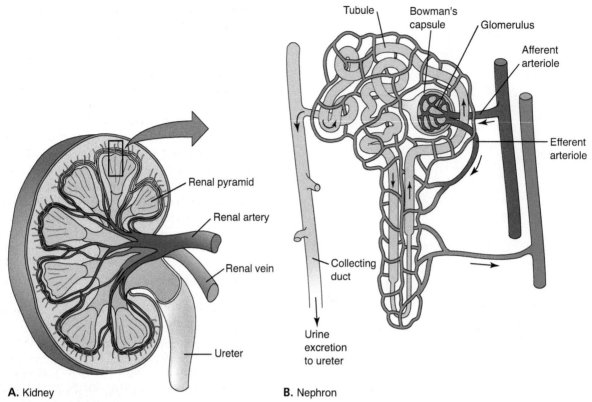

A. Kidney   **B.** Nephron

Figure 32-2
The kidney. **(A)** If you were to cut open the kidney and look at the tissue through a microscope, you would see nephrons, the functional units where filtration actually takes place. Each kidney contains about 1 million nephrons, arranged in a radiating pattern. **(B)** Each nephron consists of a glomerulus and a series of tubules. Blood (*red*) is filtered in the glomerulus, producing filtrate, the basis of urine (*yellow*). Filtered blood (*purple*) leaves the glomerulus through the efferent arteriole and is returned to the circulation through the renal veins.

FUNCTION OF THE URINARY SYSTEM

REMOVAL OF LIQUID WASTES

The main function of the urinary system is to filter the blood and remove waste products and excess fluid from the body. A moderately full bladder usually contains about 470 millilitres of urine. When about 200 to 300 millilitres of urine collect in the bladder, the internal sphincter opens and allows urine to flood the upper segment of the urethra. At this point, the urge to urinate occurs. The person voluntarily relaxes the external urethral sphincter and the muscles of the bladder contract, allowing urine to pass out of the body through the urethra. Although it is possible to delay urination for some time, the bladder continues to fill with urine and eventually, the bladder will empty itself automatically.

MAINTENANCE OF HOMEOSTASIS

The urinary system plays several important roles in maintaining the body's homeostasis:

- The urinary system helps to keep fluid levels within the body constant. As the filtrate passes through the tubules in the nephrons, water is reabsorbed as necessary to maintain the body's fluid balance. Too much fluid in the blood can lead to fluid overload, causing swelling in parts of the body. Too little fluid can lead to dehydration.
- The urinary system regulates the levels of essential minerals—such as potassium, calcium, and sodium—by either saving them or releasing them through urine.
- The urinary system regulates the acidity of the blood. The pH scale, which you might remember from chemistry class, is used to

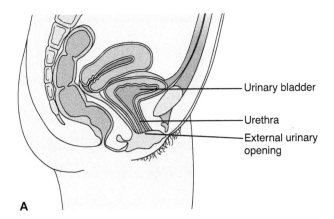

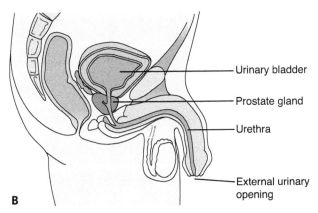

Figure 32-3
While a woman's urethra **(A)** is straight and only about 4 to 6 centimetres long, a man's urethra **(B)** is curved in an "S" shape and is about 15 to 20 centimetres long. Because of the differences in anatomy, women are more prone to urinary tract infections than men, but men are harder to catheterize than women.

rate the degree of acidity of a substance. Human blood is slightly above 7 on the scale, which ranges from 1 to 14. Anything above 7 is said to be basic, or alkaline. Anything below 7 is acidic. Our blood cannot be either too acidic or too basic. When there is even a slight change in the blood's pH, damage to the cells can occur. Acid is a normal by-product of cellular metabolism. So, to maintain the blood at a constant pH level, the kidneys excrete the excess acids produced by cellular metabolism.

THE EFFECTS OF AGING ON THE URINARY SYSTEM

The normal processes of aging affect the urinary system:

- **Less efficient filtration.** After a person reaches 40 years of age or so, the number of functioning nephrons in the kidneys starts to decrease, decreasing the kidneys' ability to filter waste products from the bloodstream.
- **Decreased muscle tone.** Loss of muscle tone as a result of aging can reduce bladder capacity and may contribute to stress incontinence. This type of urinary incontinence, which is most common in older women who have had children or are obese, can often be corrected with exercises or surgery.
- **Enlargement of the prostate gland (in men).** In older men, enlargement of the prostate gland is common. The enlargement may be benign (a normal effect of aging) or it may be due to cancer of the gland. As the prostate gland enlarges, it pushes against the urethra, causing it to narrow. Total emptying of the bladder of urine becomes difficult, and the man may experience episodes of overflow incontinence. As you recall from Chapter 20, overflow incontinence can occur when urine is retained in the bladder. Because the bladder does not empty completely when the man voids, it refills with urine quickly, and the urine simply overflows. As a result, the man may "dribble" urine in between visits to the bathroom. An enlarged prostate is treated with medications, surgery, or both.
- **Increased risk for urinary tract infections.** Older people are also more likely to get urinary tract infections. Incomplete emptying of the bladder can contribute to the development of infections, as can a decrease in immune system functioning.

Although it is important for everyone to drink plenty of water and other fluids, it is especially important for older people. Drinking plenty of fluids helps the kidneys to work properly, and regular urination flushes harmful bacteria from the bladder, helping to prevent urinary tract infections (Fig. 32-4).

DISORDERS OF THE URINARY SYSTEM

Illness or injury to any part of the urinary system affects the whole system, and, eventually, the whole body. Common disorders of the urinary system include infections, kidney stones, renal failure, and tumours.

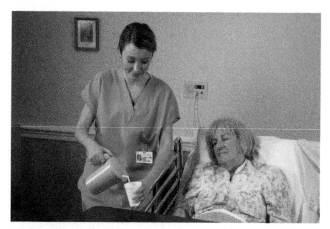

Figure 32-4
Encourage your patients or residents to drink plenty of fluids, unless a person has a medical condition that requires fluid restriction.

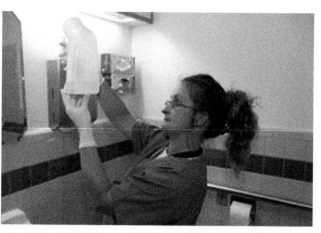

Figure 32-5
Urine that is cloudy, is an abnormal color, or has an abnormal odour may be a sign of a urinary tract infection. Always look at the urine before discarding it. If you notice anything unusual, get the nurse before discarding the urine.

INFECTIONS

Infections can affect any part of the urinary system:

- *Infection of the urethra* **(urethritis).** Urethritis is especially common in men, because the urethra is longer and curved. Microbes responsible for sexually transmitted diseases (STDs) such as gonorrhea, herpes, and chlamydia are common causes of urethritis in men. STDs are discussed in more detail in Chapter 33.
- *Infection of the bladder* **(cystitis).** Bladder infections are more common among women than men for two reasons. First, the urethral opening in women is located close to the anus. Because feces, which contain bacteria from the digestive tract, exit the body at the anus, this area is often contaminated with microbes that could cause a bladder infection. (This is why it is important to wipe from the front to the back when providing perineal care for a woman.) Second, a woman's urethra is short and straight, which means that once microbes gain access to the urinary tract, they do not have far to travel to infect the bladder.
- *Kidney infections* **(pyelonephritis).** If a bladder infection is not treated promptly with appropriate medications, the pathogens can travel up the ureters and infect the kidneys. A kidney infection can cause severe illness. If untreated, the infection might result in permanent damage to the nephrons.

In younger people, symptoms of urinary tract infections include urinary frequency, burning, and cramping. However, many older people do not have these symptoms. The personal support worker may be the first to notice a change in the appearance or odour of the urine or a change in a person's voiding habits that would indicate that a urinary tract infection may be present (Fig. 32-5).

KIDNEY STONES (RENAL CALCULI)

As you have learned, the main function of the kidney is to filter and remove waste products from the bloodstream. Many of these waste products are in the form of mineral salts, such as calcium salts and uric acid. If waste products become very concentrated, they can start to group together, forming tiny crystals that continue to grow in size as more of the mineral is deposited around them. These clumps of minerals are called **kidney stones (renal calculi)** (Fig. 32-6). Kidney stones are most common in middle-aged adults. Factors that may increase an older person's risk of developing kidney stones include immobility, not drinking enough fluids (which causes urine to be more concentrated with the waste salts), and infections of the urinary system.

Stones most often form in the collecting area (renal pelvis) of the kidney, but they can also form in the bladder. Kidney stones usually cause severe pain as they move downward through the ureter, and then through the urethra. The rough edges of the stone can damage the mucosal lining of the ureter or urethra, causing it to bleed, resulting in hematuria (blood in the urine).

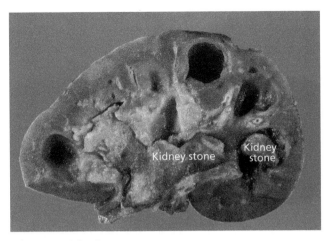

Figure 32-6
This is a kidney, cut open to reveal the kidney stones inside. Kidney stones can grow to be quite large, with sharp edges. They may cause obstruction of the ureters or urethra. Once the stone is passed, it is usually sent to the laboratory for analysis to determine which waste salt is causing the stones to form. (© Dr. E. Walker/Photo Researchers, Inc.)

A person with a kidney stone usually needs to drink plenty of fluids to help flush the stone through the urinary tract. Medication may be necessary to help control the pain. You may be asked to collect all of the person's urine after each voiding and strain it to retrieve the stone. To strain the urine, place a piece of filter paper or a 4 × 4 gauze pad in a graduate, and then pour the urine into the graduate (Fig. 32-7). The urine will pass through the filter paper or gauze pad, leaving any stones behind. It is important to retrieve the kidney stones because then they can be sent to the laboratory for chemical analysis. Once the doctor knows which waste salt is causing the stones to form, he may be able to prevent future stones from developing.

If a stone becomes lodged in the narrow ureter, it can block the flow of urine to the bladder. The urine builds up, placing pressure on the delicate nephrons of the kidney. In this case, the person will need to have the stone removed surgically. Often, the stones are removed using a procedure called *lithotripsy*. In lithotripsy, high-frequency sound waves are directed at the stone, causing it to break into smaller pieces that can then be passed through the urinary tract. Sometimes, a surgical incision needs to be made for stone removal.

KIDNEY (RENAL) FAILURE

Kidney (renal) failure is the inability of the kidneys to filter blood effectively. As a result of kidney failure, waste products and fluid build up in

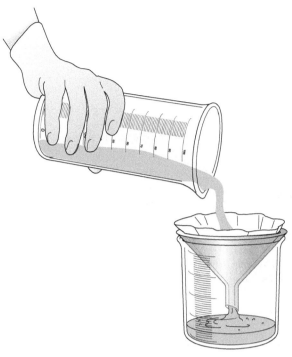

Figure 32-7
You may be asked to strain a person's urine to retrieve kidney stones. To strain urine, put a piece of filter paper or a 4 × 4 gauze pad in a graduate, and then pour the urine into the graduate. The urine will pass through the paper or gauze pad, leaving any stones behind. The stones are then transferred to a specimen container and sent to the laboratory for analysis.

the body, straining the heart and other organs. The person becomes very ill and can easily die if treatment is delayed.

Causes of Kidney Failure

Kidney failure can be either acute or chronic:

- Acute renal failure can result from a medical or surgical emergency that causes a decrease in the amount of blood flow through the kidneys. It can also be caused by poisoning, a severe infection, or a severe allergic reaction.
- Chronic renal failure results from a gradual loss of functioning nephrons. Because the kidneys lose their ability to function gradually, the person usually does not show signs of kidney failure until approximately 80% to 90% of kidney function is lost. The most common causes of chronic renal failure are hypertension and diabetes, chronic conditions that damage the blood vessels in the glomerulus. Other causes are related to chronic infections, blockage of

the urinary system by stones or growths, and cancer.

Signs of Kidney Failure

Signs of renal failure may include:

- Dehydration from excessive loss of fluid (usually early in acute renal failure because the kidneys cannot reabsorb filtrate back into the bloodstream)
- Swelling from the build-up of fluid in the tissues of the body (later in chronic renal failure when the kidneys are unable to eliminate excess fluid)
- Hypertension from fluid overload in the circulation
- Oliguria (scant amounts of urine, less than 400 millilitres in 24 hours), followed by anuria (the absence of urine)

Care of the Person With Kidney Failure

People with kidney failure often need to have dialysis. **Dialysis** does the job of the kidneys by removing waste products and fluids from the body. A person with acute renal failure may need dialysis treatment only for a short period of time, until kidney function returns. A person with chronic renal failure must remain on dialysis for the rest of her life, or until a donor kidney becomes available for transplant. There are two types of dialysis:

- In *hemodialysis,* the person's blood is drawn intravenously, passed through a machine with filters and solutions that clean the blood of waste, and then returned to the person's body through another vessel (Fig. 32-8A). A person who is receiving regular hemodialysis treatments will have surgery to create a *fistula* or *graft.* The fistula or graft provides access for the needles and tubing used during the dialysis treatment. Sometimes, this access is provided through a temporary device called a *shunt.*
- In *peritoneal dialysis,* solutions that absorb waste products are instilled (placed) into a person's abdominal cavity through a tube that has been surgically inserted for this purpose (see Fig. 32-8B). The solution remains in the abdominal cavity for a specified period of time so that waste products can be absorbed into the solution through

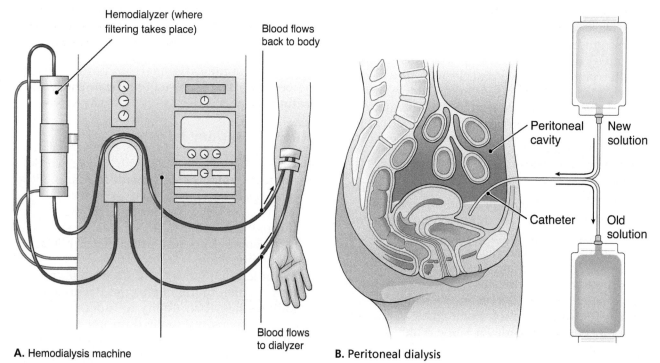

A. Hemodialysis machine   **B.** Peritoneal dialysis

Figure 32-8

Dialysis machines perform the job of the kidneys for people who have kidney failure.
(A) Hemodialysis. The dialysis machine receives blood drawn from an artery in the person's arm. The blood is filtered and then returned to the body. **(B)** Peritoneal dialysis. A special solution is placed in the person's abdominal cavity to absorb wastes, and then the solution is drained.

the membrane lining the abdominal cavity. The used solution is then drained into a collecting bag and is discarded according to facility policy.

Dialysis takes several hours and must be performed several times a week to keep the blood cleaned of waste products. Dialysis is performed by specially trained nurses. Most patients and residents who need dialysis travel to a health care center specifically designed to perform this service. Sometimes a patient or resident is too ill to be taken to a dialysis center, so nurses and technicians may bring portable equipment to the facility where you work. You may be asked to monitor vital signs quite frequently after your patient or resident has had a dialysis treatment. Guidelines for caring for a person with kidney failure are given in Guidelines Box 32-1.

TUMOURS

Tumours, which may or may not be malignant (cancerous), can affect all of the organs of the urinary system. Tumours can block the flow of urine

Guidelines Box 32-1	Guidelines for Caring for a Person With Kidney Failure
WHAT YOU DO	*WHY YOU DO IT*
Carefully measure the person's urine output and document the amounts accurately.	The doctor will use this information to monitor how well the person's kidneys are functioning.
Assist with obtaining urine samples as requested.	Testing the urine for waste products is another way of monitoring how well the person's kidneys are functioning.
Follow the person's care plan carefully with regard to food and fluid intake.	To reduce the amount of work the kidneys have to do, the person's fluid intake may be restricted and a special diet that is low in salt and protein may be ordered.
Monitor vital signs according to the person's care plan, and report any changes to the nurse immediately.	Changes in fluid balance, especially after dialysis, can significantly raise or lower a person's blood pressure.
When measuring the blood pressure of a person who receives hemodialysis treatments, avoid measuring the blood pressure in the arm in which the person's fistula, graft, or shunt is located.	Pressure can decrease blood flow through the fistula, graft, or shunt, which can lead to clots. Clots can make the fistula, graft, or shunt unusable for dialysis.
Provide frequent skin care.	Skin care helps prevent the skin irritation and itching that can be caused by kidney failure.
When assisting a person who receives peritoneal dialysis treatments with bathing or dressing, take care not to accidentally dislodge the tube used for peritoneal dialysis.	If the tube becomes dislodged, it will be necessary to reinsert it.
Provide care measures, such as frequent repositioning and range-of-motion exercises, to help prevent the complications of immobility.	People in kidney failure may be on bed rest, which can put them at risk for complications from immobility.

through the urinary system, resulting in kidney damage. Kidney damage may also result from tumours of the kidney that invade the healthy tissue, damaging the nephrons. Surgical removal of the affected kidney is usually necessary, but as long as the remaining kidney is functioning properly, it should be able to handle removal of waste and fluid.

Tumours of the bladder are common among people who have smoked cigarettes. The risk of bladder cancer increases with age, with older men twice as likely to develop bladder cancer as older women. Bladder tumours are usually malignant and may spread to other organs. Tumours may be treated with medication, radiation, or surgery, depending on the type of tumour and whether or not it has spread to other parts of the body. In some cases, it is necessary to remove the bladder, disrupting normal flow of urine out of the body. Because the urine needs a new pathway to leave the body, a *urinary diversion* is created. A surgeon can divert (redirect) the urine's flow out of the body in several ways:

- In a **ureterostomy,** the ureters are brought through the abdominal wall by way of small incisions, and sutured in place (Fig. 32-9A). The ureters then drain freely into an ostomy appliance designed to collect urine.
- In a **urostomy,** the ureters are attached to a small portion of the small intestine (usually the ileum) (see Fig. 32-9B). When the ileum is used, the person is said to have an *ileal conduit.* One end of the segment of intestine is sealed off, and the other end is brought through the abdominal wall and sutured into place to create a stoma. The urine then drains freely into an ostomy appliance designed to collect urine (see Fig. 32-9C).

Bladder cancer is a common reason for a person to have a ureterostomy or urostomy. However, injuries (for example, to the bladder or spinal cord) and birth defects (such as spina bifida) can also result in a person having a urinary diversion procedure done. Regardless of the reason for the procedure, good skin care around the ostomy site is

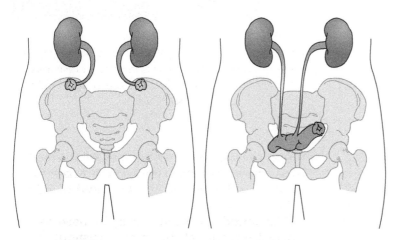

A. Ureterostomy   **B.** Urostomy (ileal conduit)

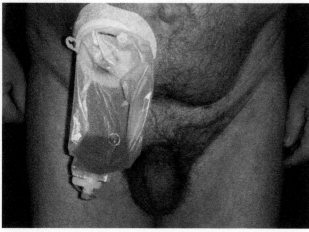

C

Figure 32-9
Urinary diversion procedures are necessary when part of the urinary system must be removed. **(A)** In a ureterostomy, the ureters are brought through the abdominal wall and sutured into place. **(B)** In a urostomy, the ureters are joined to a small segment of the small intestine, and then the intestine is brought to the surface of the body and sutured into place. **(C)** An ostomy pouch is worn to collect the urine, in both cases. The man shown here had a urostomy following removal of his bladder to treat cancer. (*C, © Dr. P. Marazzi/Photo Researchers, Inc.*)

essential. If urine is allowed to leak around the appliance, skin irritation and breakdown are very likely. The urostomy bags need to be emptied regularly and the urine may need to be measured and recorded. As always, the urine needs to be observed for any changes that might indicate infection or other urinary disorders.

TELL THE NURSE

Observations that may be a sign of a urinary system disorder and should be reported to the nurse immediately include:

- Complaints of sharp, sudden pain of the abdomen, side, or back

- Blood in the urine

- A significant increase or decrease in the amount of urine voided in a period of time

- Changes in a person's voiding habits, especially increased or decreased frequency, or a new onset of incontinence

- Pain or burning when urinating

- Urine that appears cloudy or has a strong ammonia smell

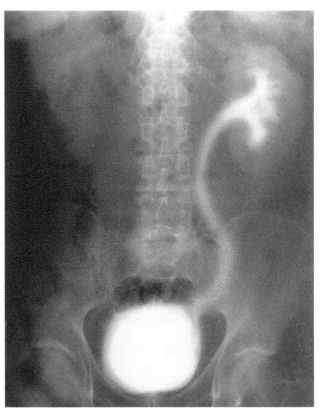

Figure 32-10
In intravenous pyelography (IVP), a type of radiographic (x-ray) procedure, a special dye is injected intravenously to allow visualization of the kidneys, ureter, and bladder. (© *Scott Camazine/Photo Researchers, Inc.*)

DIAGNOSIS OF URINARY DISORDERS

Observations that indicate problems affecting the urinary system are often nonspecific. For example, kidney stones or urinary tract infections can cause abdominal pain, a common symptom of many digestive disorders as well. Usually, additional testing is needed to find out what the real problem is. Many types of tests are used to diagnose disorders of the urinary system:

- **Urinalysis.** In urinalysis, the urine is examined under a microscope and by chemical means.
- **Imaging studies.** Computed tomography (CT) scans, magnetic resonance imaging (MRI) scans, and radiographs (x-rays) can allow a doctor to see tumours and other abnormalities of the urinary system.

With x-rays, a special dye may be injected into the veins before the x-ray is taken to highlight the kidneys, ureters, and bladder (Fig. 32-10).
- **Ultrasound.** Ultrasound may be used to detect tumours of the urinary system.
- **Cytoscopy and ureteroscopy.** A small, lighted scope is inserted through the urethra and used to view the inside of the bladder (cytoscopy) or ureters (ureteroscopy).

You may be asked to collect and measure urine for testing or to help prepare a patient or resident for other diagnostic tests or procedures. Make sure that you are informed about any specific procedures that you will be responsible for, such as keeping the person on NPO (no food orally) status, restricting or encouraging fluids, or straining urine.

SUMMARY

- The organs of the urinary system are the kidneys, the ureters, the urinary bladder, and the urethra.
  - The two kidneys filter the blood to remove waste products and excess fluid.
  - The ureters carry urine from the kidneys to the bladder.
  - The bladder is a holding place for urine.
  - The urethra carries urine from the bladder to the outside of the body.
- The main function of the urinary system is to remove waste products and excess fluid from the body. The urinary system also plays a key role in homeostasis by maintaining fluid balance and regulating the pH of the blood.
- Aging affects the urinary system just as it affects the other organ systems.
  - In an older person, loss of muscle tone affects the bladder's ability to hold urine and empty properly.

- Older men may experience difficulty voiding as a result of an enlarged prostate gland.
- An older person is more likely to develop urinary tract infections, because of decreased immune function and incomplete emptying of the bladder.
- As we age, the number of nephrons decreases, reducing the kidney's efficiency at filtering blood.
- Disorders of the urinary system include infections, kidney stones (renal calculi), kidney (renal) failure, and tumours.
  - As a personal support worker, you may be the first to notice signs and symptoms of a urinary problem that a patient or resident is having.
  - You may also be involved in helping a patient or resident to prepare for a diagnostic test used to evaluate the urinary system.

WHAT DID YOU LEARN?

Multiple Choice

Select the single best answer for each of the following questions.

1. Urine leaves the body through the:
   a. Nephrons
   b. Urethra
   c. Ureters
   d. Bladder
2. How does aging affect the urinary system?
   a. The number of nephrons is decreased, reducing the kidney's ability to filter blood efficiently
   b. The ability to empty the bladder completely is decreased
   c. Bladder capacity is decreased
   d. All of the above
3. How much urine does an average adult pass each day?
   a. 200 millilitres of urine per day
   b. 500 millilitres of urine per day
   c. 1 to 1.5 litres of urine per day
   d. 160 to 180 litres of urine per day

4. Why are urinary tract infections more common in women than in men?
   a. A woman's urethra is short, and the opening of the urethra is located close to the anus
   b. A woman's urethra is long and curved
   c. Women tend to be more careless with perineal care
   d. Women do not drink as much water as men
5. Which of the following might be a sign of a urinary tract infection?
   a. Pain or burning while urinating
   b. Extreme thirst
   c. Anuria (absence of urine)
   d. Kidney failure
6. Which procedure uses high-frequency sound waves to break up kidney stones?
   a. Lithotripsy
   b. Dialysis
   c. Filtration
   d. Urostomy

7. How is the male urethra different from the female urethra?
   a. It is longer
   b. It serves as a passageway for urine and for semen
   c. The opening is farther away from the anus
   d. All of the above
8. Mr. Loyd has a urostomy, which was done to treat his bladder cancer. What do you need to remember when caring for Mr. Loyd?
   a. He may develop kidney failure at any time
   b. He will require good skin care around the ostomy site to prevent skin irritation and breakdown
   c. He is more at risk for kidney stones
   d. He will not require any special care
9. Sally is caring for Mrs. Brady, who has been going to the bathroom more frequently than usual. Now, Mrs. Brady is complaining of a burning sensation when she urinates. Why is it important for Sally to report what she has observed to the nurse?
   a. Mrs. Brady may be in kidney failure
   b. Mrs. Brady may have a urinary tract infection
   c. The nurse will assign another personal support worker to help with Mrs. Brady's care
   d. It is not necessary for Sally to report these observations to the nurse

Matching

Match each numbered item with its appropriate lettered description.

E 1. Cystitis

D 2. Renal calculi

A 3. Pyelonephritis

C 4. Glomerulus

B 5. Urethritis

a. Infection of the kidneys
b. Capillary bed in the nephron; surrounded by Bowman's capsule
c. Infection of the urethra
d. Kidney stones
e. Infection of the bladder

STOP and Think!

Janice works in a hospital and is assigned to care for Mr. Roberts, who is in the hospital because of kidney stones. This morning, while helping Mr. Roberts with his A.M. care, she noticed that the urinal hanging on his side rail was full. Because Janice knows that Mr. Roberts was admitted for kidney stones, what extra steps will she take when she empties his urinal?

Kelly has been assigned to care for Mrs. Ralph, who has a urostomy. She is unfamiliar with this term and doesn't know what to expect. If you were on Kelly's team, what would you tell Kelly to expect? What things would you tell Kelly to look for in caring for Mrs. Ralph?

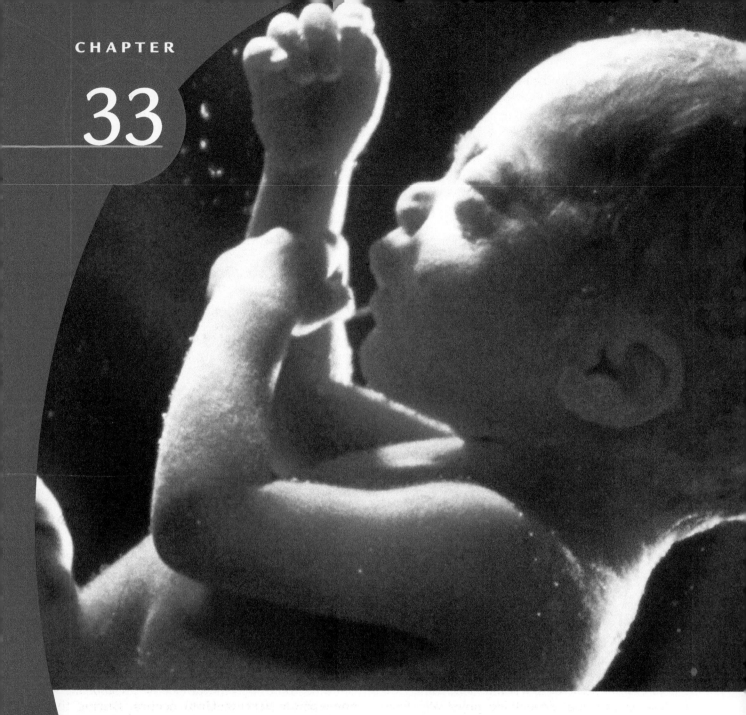

The Reproductive System

WHAT WILL YOU LEARN?

Of all of the systems that make up the human body, perhaps none is as fascinating and miraculous as the reproductive system. **Reproduction** is the process by which a living thing makes more living things like itself. Because all living things eventually die, the ability to reproduce is essential for the survival of any species. Without the ability to reproduce, the species would slowly die off and cease to exist.

Photo: A fetus develops from a single fertilized egg.
(© Petit Format/Photo Researchers, Inc.)

In this chapter, you will learn about the male and female reproductive systems, which are very different from each other. You will learn about their structure and function, the effects of aging on each, and common disorders that can affect each. In addition, you will learn about sexually transmitted infections (STIs), which can affect both men and women. When you are finished with this chapter, you will be able to:

1. Describe the main function of the reproductive system.
2. List the organs that make up the female reproductive system.
3. Discuss the normal function of the female reproductive system.
4. Explain the effects of aging on the female reproductive system.
5. Describe the disorders that may affect the female reproductive system.
6. List diagnostic tests commonly used to detect disorders of the female reproductive system.
7. List the organs that make up the male reproductive system.
8. Discuss the normal function of the male reproductive system.
9. Explain the effects of aging on the male reproductive system.
10. Describe the disorders that may affect the male reproductive system.
11. List diagnostic tests commonly used to detect disorders of the male reproductive system.
12. Discuss STIs that may affect the male or female reproductive systems.
13. Discuss ways to prevent STIs.

Vocabulary

Reproduction	Ovulation	Infertility	Impotence (erectile
Sex cell (gamete)	Lactation	Postmenopausal	dysfunction)
Sperm cell	Menstrual period	bleeding	Sexually transmitted
Egg (ovum, ova)	Amenorrhea	Mastectomy	infection (STI)
Conception	Dysmenorrhea	Hysterectomy	Pelvic inflammatory
(fertilization)	Menorrhagia	Ejaculation	disease (PID)

Has anyone ever told you that you have "your mother's eyes" or "the family nose"? Do you look very much like your brothers or sisters, or not much like them at all? Each of us receives our genes, the bundles of DNA that determine how we develop and what we look like physically, from our parents. Your mother gave you half of your genes and your father gave you the other half, to make a full set. This is why you may look a lot like either one of your parents, or like a blend of the two. Or why you may look very much like one of your siblings, and not much like another one. It all depends on the combination of genes that you received.

Each species has a set number of genes, or chromosomes. For example, human beings have 46 chromosomes. This means that to keep the number of chromosomes the same from generation to generation, the father contributes 23 chromosomes and the mother contributes 23 chromosomes. The special cells contributed by each parent that contain half of the normal number of

chromosomes are called **sex cells (gametes).** The male sex cell is called a **sperm cell.** The female sex cell is called an **egg (ovum; ova,** plural). When the sperm joins the egg, forming a cell that contains the complete number of chromosomes, **conception (fertilization)** occurs. During the 9 months leading up to the birth of a baby, the single original cell that formed at conception copies itself over and over again, forming all of the baby's tissues and organs.

One of the main functions of the reproductive system in both males and females is to produce and transport sex cells. However, unlike other organ systems in the body, the organs that make up the reproductive system are very different in men and women. The male reproductive system is designed to produce sperm and deposit it inside the female's body. The female reproductive system is designed to produce eggs, receive sperm cells, contain and nourish a developing baby, give birth, and provide nourishment after the baby's birth by producing breast milk. Because of the physical and functional differences between the male and female reproductive systems, we will look at each system separately in the sections that follow.

THE FEMALE REPRODUCTIVE SYSTEM

STRUCTURE OF THE FEMALE REPRODUCTIVE SYSTEM

The organs and structures of the female reproductive system are located both inside and outside of the body. The internal organs are the ovaries, fallopian tubes, uterus, and vagina (Fig. 33-1A). The outer structures are the labia, the clitoris, and the vaginal opening (see Fig. 33-1B). These outer structures are sometimes referred to collectively as the *vulva*. In addition, the breasts (mammary glands) are considered accessory organs of the female reproductive system, because they play a role in nourishing a newborn baby.

The Ovaries

The ovaries are two small, almond-shaped organs located deep inside the abdomen on either side of the uterus (see Fig. 33-1A). The ovaries store the ova, or eggs. When a baby girl is born, her ovaries contain all of the eggs that she will ever have. The stored eggs are kept in a "holding pattern" until they are needed. Once a girl passes through puberty and reaches reproductive age, she begins to ovulate. **Ovulation** is the release of a ripe, mature egg from the ovaries each month.

The Fallopian Tubes

The fallopian tubes, also called *uterine tubes* or *oviducts*, are slender tubes about 10.2 to 12.7 centimetres long that transport the egg from the ovary to the uterus. After leaving the ovary, the egg moves through the fluid in the abdomen to the entrance of the nearest fallopian tube. The open ends of the fallopian tubes nearest the ovaries have small, fringe-like projections called *fimbriae* (see Fig. 33-1A). The fimbriae beat in a wave-like motion, helping to move the egg into the tube.

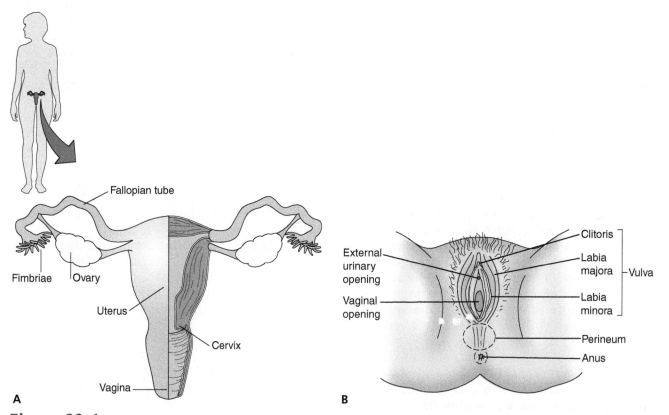

A

B

Figure 33-1

The female reproductive system. **(A)** Internal structures include the ovaries, fallopian tubes, uterus, and vagina. **(B)** External structures, collectively known as "the vulva," include the vaginal opening, labia, and clitoris.

Once in the fallopian tube, the egg moves toward the uterus, helped along by the peristaltic contractions of the smooth muscle layer in the walls of the fallopian tube and the tiny, hair-like cilia on the lining of the fallopian tube. Like the cilia in the airways of the lungs, the cilia in the fallopian tubes move gently back and forth, creating a sweeping motion that helps to move the egg along the length of the tube. Conception, if it occurs, occurs in the fallopian tubes.

The Uterus

The uterus, sometimes referred to as the *womb,* is a hollow, pear-shaped organ (see Fig. 33-1). The uterus has three sections:

- The *fundus* is the upper, rounded portion of the uterus.
- The *body* is the mid-portion of the uterus.
- The *cervix* is the lower, narrow portion of the uterus. Normally, the cervix is closed, except for a very tiny opening. This opening, which is no larger than a pinpoint, allows sperm to enter the uterus, and menstrual blood to pass out of it. When a woman is about to give birth, the cervix dilates (opens), becoming as large as 10 centimetres in diameter. Dilation of the cervix creates an opening wide enough for the baby to pass through into the vagina.

The walls of the uterus are made of thick, smooth muscle tissue. The muscular walls of the uterus expand to accommodate a growing baby and then contract during labour to push the baby out. The inner cavity of the uterus is shaped like a capital "T" and is lined with tissue called *endometrium.*

The Vagina

The vagina is a muscular tube about 7 centimetres long that connects the uterus to the outside of the body (see Fig. 33-1A). The vagina is the receiving organ for sperm. It also serves as the birth canal, through which a baby passes during birth. The mucous membrane lining of the vagina helps to lubricate the vagina during sexual intercourse and protect the body from infection. It contains many folds, which allow the vagina to expand enough to allow a baby to pass through.

The Vulva

The vulva consists of the vaginal opening, the labia, and the clitoris (see Fig. 31-B).

- The vaginal opening, also called the *vaginal orifice,* is where the vagina opens to the outside of the body. The vaginal opening is located between the external urinary opening (the urinary meatus or urethral orifice) and the anus. The area between the vaginal opening and the anus is often called the *perineum.* However, the term *perineum* can also be used to describe the entire external genital area of both men and women.
- The labia, or "lips," are folds of tissue that surround the vaginal opening. The many folds of the external female reproductive system can create difficulties with hygiene, especially if a woman is injured, ill, or otherwise unable to provide for her own cleanliness needs. Perineal care and hygiene assistance is discussed in Chapter 17.
- The clitoris is located at the upper folds of the internal labia. This tissue, which is very sensitive to touch, helps to initiate a woman's sexual arousal.

The Breasts (Mammary Glands)

In women, the breasts are considered accessory organs of the reproductive system because they play a role in nourishing the newborn. Although the female breasts develop during puberty, they do not become functional until the end of pregnancy. The breasts are made up of lobes, or sections, that contain glandular tissue and fat (Fig. 33-2). When it is stimulated by the hormone prolactin (which is secreted by the pituitary gland at the end of pregnancy), the glandular tissue of the breasts produces milk, a process known as **lactation.** In response to an infant's suckling, the glandular tissue contracts, sending the milk through the ducts to the nipple.

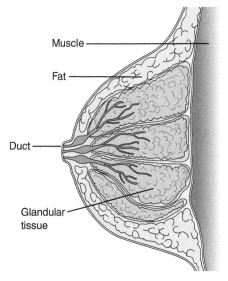

Muscle

Fat

Duct

Glandular tissue

Figure 33-2
The breasts consist of glandular tissue and fat.

FUNCTION OF THE FEMALE REPRODUCTIVE SYSTEM

Each month during a woman's reproductive years (from puberty to menopause), her body prepares itself to become pregnant. If pregnancy does not occur, the woman has a menstrual period and the cycle begins again.

The cycle begins when the pituitary gland releases follicle-stimulating hormone (FSH), a hormone that causes about 20 eggs in the ovaries to begin to grow and mature (Fig. 33-3). Each egg grows within its own "shell," called a *follicle.* FSH also stimulates the follicles to produce estrogen, another hormone. As the estrogen level increases, it "turns off" FSH production. This feedback mechanism limits the number of follicles that mature each month. One egg-containing follicle continues to grow and mature, and the others die off.

When the egg has matured, luteinizing hormone (LH), another hormone released by the pituitary gland, causes the follicle to burst, releasing the egg from the ovary (ovulation) (see Fig. 33-3). Following ovulation, the empty follicle becomes known as the *corpus luteum.* The corpus luteum continues to produce estrogen, and it also begins to produce progesterone. Estrogen and progesterone cause the uterus to begin to prepare itself to receive a fertilized egg.

In response to estrogen and progesterone, the lining of the uterus (the endometrium) thickens, creating a soft, nourishing environment for a fertilized egg, should one arrive (see Fig. 33-3). Estrogen and progesterone allow the fertilized egg to attach itself to the endometrium (a process called *implantation*). Once the fertilized egg implants, it begins to divide, forming the cells and tissues that will eventually become a new human being. If fertilization does not occur, the egg passes into the uterus, where it usually dissolves. The levels of hormones decrease, causing the endometrial lining to break down and pass through the vagina as the **menstrual period.**

This cycle of hormone secretion and egg development occurs in a regular pattern throughout a woman's reproductive years. The average cycle from the first day of one menstrual period until the start of another one is 28 days, but the cycle can be as short as 22 days or as long as 45 days.

THE EFFECTS OF AGING ON THE FEMALE REPRODUCTIVE SYSTEM

Unlike the age-related changes that affect other organ systems, the age-related changes that affect the female reproductive system are usually very noticeable.

Increased Difficulty Becoming Pregnant

Many women in their late 30s and early 40s have difficulty becoming pregnant. This is because each month, the number of healthy eggs remaining in a woman's ovaries decreases. (Remember that at birth, a female's ovaries contain all of the eggs that she will ever have.) Becoming pregnant is often still possible at this age, just more difficult. Fertility treatments, such as the use of drugs to cause more eggs to ripen each month or in-vitro fertilization (IVF), are often very helpful for women in this age group who wish to become pregnant.

Decreased Sex Hormone Production

As a woman ages, her body produces lower amounts of sex hormones, especially estrogen and progesterone. Eventually, this decreased

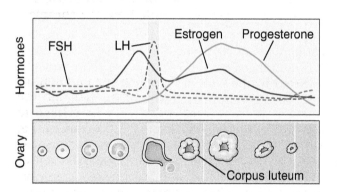
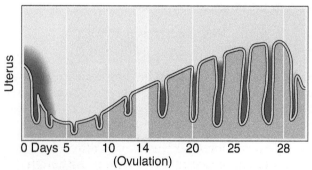

Figure 33-3

Each month during a woman's reproductive years, her body prepares itself for pregnancy. In response to hormones, an egg develops and is released, and the lining of the uterus prepares itself to receive the fertilized egg, should fertilization occur. If fertilization does not occur, the egg and the lining of the uterus are shed during the woman's menstrual period, and the cycle begins again.

hormone production results in *menopause,* the complete ending of a woman's menstrual cycles. Menopause occurs in most women sometime between the ages of 45 and 55 years and is caused by the loss of ovary function due to age. After the onset of menopause, the reproductive organs do not function and shrink to the size they were before puberty. Menopause can cause many bothersome symptoms, including "hot flashes," irritability, a loss of energy, and an inability to sleep. Decreased production of estrogen and progesterone, which are "feminizing" hormones, may also cause some women to develop facial hair and a coarse ("scratchy") voice. Some women experience vaginal dryness and irritation and may need to use a lubricant during sexual intercourse.

Many women who have gone through menopause choose to replace the hormones their bodies no longer produce by taking estrogen and progesterone orally. This is called hormone replacement therapy (HRT). HRT helps to minimize some of the more annoying "side effects" of menopause, such as hot flashes. In addition, some research shows that taking estrogen and progesterone after menopause can help keep bones strong and prevent heart disease and some types of dementia. However, other research indicates that HRT may increase a woman's chances of developing certain types of cancer. Each woman must work with her health care provider to determine whether HRT is right for her, given her unique situation and health history.

DISORDERS OF THE FEMALE REPRODUCTIVE SYSTEM

Many types of disorders can affect the female reproductive system. For example, many factors, such as hormone imbalances, can cause a woman to have problems with her menstrual cycle. Cysts (fluid-filled sacs) and noncancerous tumours can interfere with the functioning of the reproductive system, or cause pain or excessive bleeding. Finally, cancer can occur in almost any organ of the female reproductive system.

Menstrual Disorders

A woman may have problems with her menstrual cycle, such as irregular periods, excessive pain, or excessive bleeding. Common disorders associated with the menstrual cycle include the following:

- **Amenorrhea** is the absence of menstrual flow. Primary amenorrhea occurs when a girl has not begun to menstruate by the age of 16 years. Abnormalities in the reproductive organs, a hormone disorder, or malnutrition may be the cause. Secondary amenorrhea is the absence of menstrual flow in a woman who has had previous menstrual periods. Secondary amenorrhea can result from hormone imbalances or tumours, and is usually the first sign of pregnancy.
- **Dysmenorrhea** is painful menstruation. Many women experience cramps in the lower abdomen during menstrual periods, but for some women the pain is severe enough to interfere with daily activities. Extremely painful periods that prevent a woman from doing what she normally does should be brought to the attention of a health care provider.
- **Menorrhagia** is excessive bleeding during a menstrual period, either in terms of the amount of blood lost or the number of days that bleeding lasts. Hormonal disturbances, infections, and growths inside the uterus can cause menorrhagia. Excessive bleeding for an extended period of time can cause a woman to become anemic from the chronic blood loss.

Infertility

Infertility is the inability to become pregnant or to carry a pregnancy to full term. Although the cause of a couple's infertility may be related to the man's inability to produce the amount of sperm needed to fertilize the egg, in many cases, it is related to a problem with the woman's reproductive system. Hormone imbalances, deformities of the reproductive organs, or scar tissue can lead to infertility.

Cysts and Noncancerous Growths or Tumours

Many organs in the female reproductive system can be affected by cysts or other noncancerous growths. Although these cysts and growths are not cancerous, they can still cause problems.

- *Cysts* can form on the ovaries after ovulation, causing intense pain. Although not malignant, ovarian cysts may need to be surgically removed if they occur frequently and are painful. Cysts may also form in the lubricating glands located inside the vagina, creating a painful, infected lump that may have to be surgically drained.
- *Fibroids (myomas)* sometimes form in the muscle wall of the uterus. Fibroids can

cause problems during pregnancy if they are large enough to crowd a developing baby inside the uterus. They may also cause severe menorrhagia if they grow toward the inside of the uterine cavity.

Cancer

Cancers affecting the female reproductive system include cervical cancer, endometrial cancer, ovarian cancer, and breast cancer.

- *Cervical cancer* (cancer of the cervix, the lower region of the uterus) is more common among women between the ages of 30 and 50 years and can be caused by a sexually transmitted viral infection. Other factors that can increase a woman's risk of developing cervical cancer include having sexual intercourse at an early age and having multiple sexual partners. If diagnosed early enough, cervical cancer can be effectively treated without putting a woman's ability to have children at risk.
- *Endometrial cancer* (cancer of the lining of the uterus) is the most common type of cancer that affects the female reproductive tract. It is most common in women after menopause. The first sign of this type of cancer is **postmenopausal bleeding,** uterine bleeding that occurs after a woman has completed menopause. Postmenopausal bleeding can also result from hormone imbalances.
- *Ovarian cancer* (cancer of the ovary) most commonly occurs in women between the ages of 40 and 65 years. Ovarian cancer is a leading cause of cancer death for women. This cancer is associated with a high rate of death because it grows quickly and spreads easily to other organs. Early diagnosis and treatment can improve a woman's chances of survival.
- *Breast cancer* is the most commonly occurring cancer in women. Breast cancer can develop in women with relatives with breast cancer, especially a mother or sister. But it can also develop in women who have no family history of the disease. Women are encouraged to get into the habit of examining their breasts at the same time each month. During the breast self-examination (BSE), the woman looks and feels for any changes in the breast tissue (Fig. 33-4). The monthly BSE can help a woman to become familiar with the way her breast tissue normally looks and feels. This knowledge may allow her to recognize lumps or other

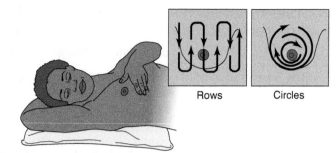

A. Feeling for abnormalities

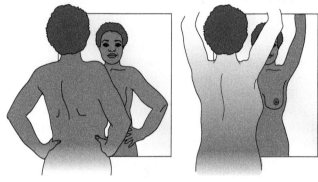

B. Looking for abnormalities

Figure 33-4
Women are encouraged to examine their breasts monthly, so that they become familiar with the way their breast tissue normally looks and feels. A breast self-examination (BSE) involves **(A)** feeling the breasts for abnormalities and then **(B)** looking at the breasts for abnormalities. There are many different ways to do a BSE. For example, the BSE can be performed while lying down or standing up, and the fingers can be moved across the breast in circles or in rows. The important thing is to do the BSE the same way each time, at the same time each month, and to report any unusual findings to a health care provider immediately.

problems that need to be reported to the nurse or doctor for further evaluation. Many breast lumps are not cancer, but the only way to be sure is to have them checked. Early detection and new treatment methods for breast cancer allow many women to be completely cured of this disease.

TELL THE NURSE

Your duties will include assisting your female patients or residents with their personal hygiene and toileting needs. Because of this, you may be the first to observe signs of a problem involving the reproductive organs. In addition, a female patient or resident may tell you about a problem that she is experiencing. Report any of the following observations or complaints to the nurse immediately:

- The woman has an unusual vaginal discharge

- The woman has vaginal bleeding, but she has already gone through menopause

- The woman has very heavy vaginal bleeding during her menstrual period

- The woman has pain or cramping in her lower abdomen

- The woman reports itching or burning around the vulva

- The skin around the vulva is inflamed or irritated

- There are changes in skin coloring, sores that do not heal, lumps, unusual swelling, or thickened areas around the vulva

- There is a lump or thickened area in the breast

- There is a discharge from the nipples or puckering of the skin of the breasts

COMMON DIAGNOSTIC PROCEDURES

As a personal support worker, you may need to help prepare a female patient or resident for a procedure used to diagnose problems with the reproductive system. Many women are hesitant or embarrassed to discuss problems involving the reproductive organs. You must be especially careful to help maintain a woman's modesty and privacy when she is being prepared for a diagnostic procedure involving the reproductive system. Make sure that the privacy curtains and the door are closed, and keep sensitive body parts (such as the breasts or vulva) covered as much as possible. Also be aware that your patient or resident may be fearful or anxious about the test results. Be careful not to give advice or tell the person what you would do if you were in her situation. Instead, listen, give competent and compassionate care, and report your observations to the nurse.

Routine physical examinations are very effective for detecting disorders of the female reproductive system while they are in the early stages and easier to treat. In addition to routine physical examinations, several diagnostic procedures are used to screen for female reproductive disorders:

- **Pap test.** A Pap test (named after the doctor who invented the test, George Papanicolaou) is routinely performed to detect changes in the cervix that may indicate early cervical cancer. The doctor uses a swab to gather a sample of cells from the cervix, and then the cells are examined under a microscope to make sure they are healthy.

- **Biopsy.** In a biopsy, a tissue sample is obtained and examined under a microscope for cancerous cells. A biopsy may be used to detect endometrial, cervical, or breast cancer.

- **Dilation and curettage (D&C).** A D&C is a surgical procedure. The cervix is dilated (made wider) and tissue is curetted (scraped) from the inside of the cervix and the uterus. This tissue is then examined to determine the cause of abnormal bleeding.

- **Imaging studies.** Radiographic imaging studies can allow a doctor to see tumours or scar tissue that may be blocking the fallopian tubes, a common cause of infertility.

- **Ultrasonography.** During an ultrasound study, sound waves are "bounced off" an organ and then translated into a three-dimensional image. Ultrasound can reveal tumours or cysts on the ovaries and in other structures of the female reproductive tract. Ultrasound can also be used to check breast cysts. In addition, ultrasound is used when a woman is pregnant to check on the fetus and make sure that it is developing properly (Fig. 33-5).

- **Mammography.** A mammogram is an x-ray of breast tissue (Fig. 33-6). Mammography can detect breast lumps at a very early stage, before they become large enough to be seen or felt. For this reason, many doctors recommend that women receive routine mammograms, in addition to performing monthly BSEs.

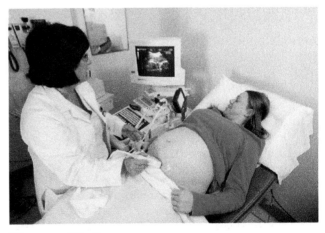

Figure 33-5
Ultrasound, a common diagnostic procedure, is used to view a developing baby inside the uterus. It can also be used to detect tumours or cysts on reproductive structures.

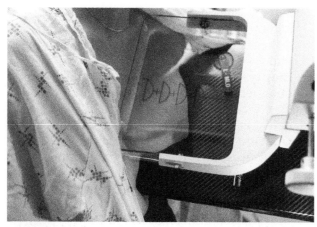

Figure 33-6
Mammograms can detect early forms of breast cancer. Many doctors recommend that women 40 years and older have a mammogram done annually.

COMMON SURGICAL PROCEDURES

Many of your patients or residents may be preparing for, or recovering from, surgery involving the reproductive organs. Common surgical procedures involving the female reproductive system include mastectomy and hysterectomy.

Mastectomy

A **mastectomy** (surgical removal of a breast) may be performed on a woman who has been diagnosed with certain types of breast cancer. For some women with breast cancer, the cancer can be treated by removing only the cancerous lump and some of the surrounding tissue. This procedure is called a *lumpectomy*. But for many women, the entire breast must be removed to treat the cancer effectively. When this is the case, many women choose to follow the mastectomy with reconstructive surgery. A new breast is created either by inserting a prosthesis (implant) under the skin and muscle, or by grafting tissue from another part of the body. For many women, removal of a breast is very difficult to handle emotionally. This means that in addition to healing physically from the procedure, the woman will need to heal emotionally.

Hysterectomy

A **hysterectomy** (surgical removal of the uterus) may be used to treat uterine cancer, excessive bleeding, or other disorders of the female reproductive tract. When a hysterectomy is performed

through an incision in the abdomen, it is called a *total abdominal hysterectomy (TAH)*. When it is performed through the vagina by cutting around the cervix, it is called a *total vaginal hysterectomy (TVH)*. The woman's fallopian tubes and ovaries may or may not be removed, depending on the reason for the surgery.

THE MALE REPRODUCTIVE SYSTEM

STRUCTURE OF THE MALE REPRODUCTIVE SYSTEM

The organs and structures of the male reproductive system include the testicles (testes), the epididymis, the vas deferens, and the penis (Fig. 33-7). Accessory organs include the seminal vesicles and prostate gland, which play a role in producing semen (the fluid that carries sperm cells out of the body).

The Testicles (Testes)

The testicles are two walnut-like organs located in the *scrotum*, a loose, bag-like sac of skin that is suspended outside of the body, between the thighs. The testicles have two important functions: they secrete testosterone, the hormone that is responsible for the development of male secondary sex characteristics and for the proper functioning of the male reproductive system, and they produce sperm cells. The testicles are located outside of a man's body because the temperature necessary for the proper development of sperm is lower than the temperature inside the body.

The Epididymis

After the sperm cells leave the testes, they move into the epididymis, a series of coiled tubes where the sperm cells mature and gain the ability to "swim." A sperm cell's ability to swim comes from its flagellum, a whip-like "tail" (Fig. 33-8). The whip-like motion of the flagellum moves the sperm cell forward, allowing it to "swim" through the female reproductive tract in search of an egg to fertilize. The sperm cell is the only human body cell that has a flagellum.

The Vas Deferens

From the epididymis, the sperm cell moves into the vas deferens, a passageway that transports the sperm cell to the urethra (see Fig. 33-7). While

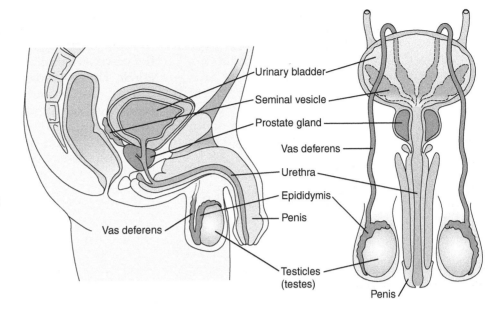

Figure 33-7
The male reproductive system consists of the testicles (testes), the epididymis, the vas deferens, and the penis. Accessory organs include the seminal vesicles and prostate gland.

in the vas deferens, the sperm cells are mixed with the secretions from the seminal vesicles and the prostate gland. These secretions, which nourish and protect the sperm cells, form the fluid portion of semen. In the prostate gland, the vas deferens joins with the urethra, which is the final passageway through which the sperm cells leave the man's body.

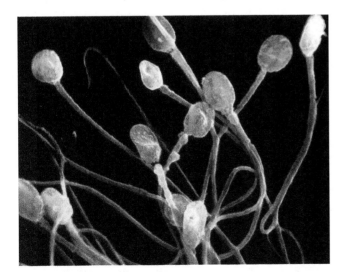

Figure 33-8
Each sperm cell has a whip-like "tail," called a flagellum, that allows it to move. The ability to move is important for sperm cells. After leaving the man's body, the sperm cells need to travel through the woman's vagina, into the uterus, and then into the fallopian tubes to meet the egg. (*CNRI/Photo Researchers, Inc.*)

The Penis

The male urethra, described in Chapter 32, is contained in the penis. Semen leaves the man's body by way of the external urinary opening, which is located at the tip of the *glans penis,* the enlarged portion at the end of the penis. If a male has not been circumcised, a loose fold of skin called the *foreskin* covers the glans penis.

The urethra is surrounded by "spongy" tissue. Stimulation by the nervous system causes this spongy tissue to fill with blood. This, in turn, causes the penis to become hard and erect. When erect, the penis can be inserted into a woman's vagina, allowing sperm cells to be deposited into the woman's reproductive tract.

FUNCTION OF THE MALE REPRODUCTIVE SYSTEM

The function of the male reproductive system is to produce and nourish male sex cells (sperm), and to deposit these cells inside the female's body so that fertilization can occur. The mature female reproductive system usually produces only one egg each month. In contrast, the mature male reproductive system produces sperm cells constantly. Many millions of sperm cells are needed to fertilize one egg because so many sperm cells die during their journey through the woman's reproductive tract. After puberty, sperm cells are produced in the testicles in response to the release of FSH by the pituitary gland. The pituitary gland also secretes interstitial cell-stimulating hormone (ICSH), which stimulates the testicles to produce testosterone. Testosterone is needed for the continued development and growth of the sperm cells.

Sperm cells are deposited in the female reproductive tract through the process of **ejaculation.** During sexual intercourse, stimulation of the erect penis causes the forceful release of semen from the body. Ejaculation is how sperm cells leave the man's body and enter the woman's vagina so that the process of fertilization and reproduction can begin.

THE EFFECTS OF AGING ON THE MALE REPRODUCTIVE SYSTEM

As they get older, many men find that the frequency and duration of their erections decreases. Many men also develop enlargement of the prostate gland.

Decreased Frequency and Duration of Erections

Beginning at around the age of 20 years, production of testosterone and sperm begins to gradually decline. A man can remain fertile until late in life, even as late as 80 years of age, but most men find that as they get older, erections occur less frequently and last for shorter periods of time. This is a result of decreased production of testosterone. The ability to have and maintain an erection is also affected by the effects of aging on the cardiovascular system, which can result in decreased blood flow to the penis. Finally, medications taken for hypertension and other common disorders can also affect sexual abilities.

Enlargement of the Prostate Gland

As a man ages, the prostate gland tends to enlarge. Because the prostate gland surrounds the urethra, this enlargement can make urination difficult. Prostate problems associated with aging are discussed in Chapter 32.

DISORDERS OF THE MALE REPRODUCTIVE SYSTEM

Common disorders of the male reproductive system include impotence (erectile dysfunction) and cancer.

Impotence (Erectile Dysfunction)

Impotence (erectile dysfunction) is the inability to achieve or maintain an erection long enough to engage in sexual activity. A patient or resident may experience erectile dysfunction for several reasons. Lowered levels of male hormones, circulatory problems that restrict blood flow to the penis, medications, or emotional disturbances can all affect a man's ability to have an erection, either temporarily or permanently. In many cultures, the ability to have an erection and father children is often considered a mark of "manliness." Because of this, many men who have erectile dysfunction are embarrassed to tell a health care provider about this problem. However, once the cause has been discovered, many effective methods of treatment can allow a man to remain sexually active throughout his life span.

Cancer

Cancers affecting the male reproductive system include testicular cancer, prostate cancer, and penile cancer. In addition, men may get breast cancer, although this cancer is much less common in men than in women.

- *Testicular cancer* usually affects young to middle-aged adult men and can easily spread to other parts of the body through the lymphatic system before it is detected. Men of all ages are encouraged to examine their testicles regularly (Fig. 33-9). Testicular self-examination (TSE) can help detect lumps and other abnormalities at an early stage. Early detection and treatment of cancer leads to a better survival outcome.
- *Prostate cancer.* Cancer of the prostate gland most commonly occurs in men older than 50 years. Rectal examination, during which a doctor inserts a finger into the man's rectum to feel for enlargement of the gland, can lead to early detection. A blood test can also be used to screen for prostate cancer. Prostate cancer typically grows slowly and has a good cure rate with early detection.
- *Penile cancer.* Occasionally, lesions that appear on the penis may be cancerous. As always, it is important for you to report any changes in the skin of patients or residents, no matter what part of the body they appear on.

TELL THE NURSE

A conscientious personal support worker always observes a patient or resident for changes that indicate that something is "not quite right" and reports those observations to the nurse immediately. Listed below are

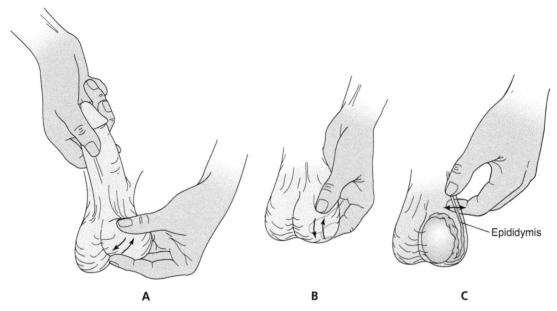

Figure 33-9
Men are encouraged to examine their testicles monthly. This is an effective and easy way to detect testicular cancer. To perform a testicular self-examination (TSE), first roll each testicle from side to side between the thumb and middle finger to feel for any lumps or abnormalities **(A)**. Then repeat the procedure, except this time, roll the testicle between the fingers in an up-and-down direction **(B)**. Finally, feel along the epididymis, the cord-like structure on the top and back of the testicle **(C)**.

some observations that may indicate disorders of the male reproductive system. Report any of the following observations or complaints to the nurse immediately:

- The man has an unusual discharge from the penis, especially if it contains blood or other discolored secretions

- The man has pain or burning when urinating

- There is a lump or thickened area in the testes

- There are changes in the skin surrounding the scrotum or penis

- There is reddened or irritated skin in the genital area

- The man complains of pain or aching in the scrotum or rectal area

one of these tests, or for one of the following tests:

- *Bloodwork.* A blood sample can be used to determine hormone levels (for example, in a man with erectile dysfunction). A blood sample can also be analyzed for prostate-specific antigen (PSA), a substance that is found in the blood of men with prostate problems.
- *Biopsy.* A biopsy may be necessary to test tissue for the presence of cancer in the prostate gland or the testes.

As always, be sensitive to how your patient or resident might be feeling. The person may be afraid of finding out that he has cancer, or worried that problems with sexual functioning will be permanent.

COMMON DIAGNOSTIC PROCEDURES

Many of the diagnostic procedures that are used to detect disorders of the urinary system (see Chapter 32) are also used to detect disorders of the male reproductive system. You may care for a male patient or resident who is scheduled for

SEXUALLY TRANSMITTED INFECTIONS

A **sexually transmitted infection (STI)** is an infection that is most often transmitted by sexual contact. These infections, also known as *sexually* *transmitted diseases (STDs)* or *venereal diseases,* can be caused by bacteria or viruses. The pathogens are transmitted through semen and vaginal secretions. Infection of the organs of the reproductive system is most common, although the mucous membranes of the eyes, mouth, or anus may also become infected following contact with infected semen or vaginal secretions. Some STIs, such as acquired immunodeficiency syndrome (AIDS), involve the entire body.

TYPES OF SEXUALLY TRANSMITTED INFECTIONS

There are many different types of STIs. Some of the most common include the following.

- *Herpes simplex* is a viral infection. There are two forms of herpes simplex. Herpes simplex type I causes the common "cold sore" or "fever blister" on the lip. Herpes simplex type II, or genital herpes, causes painful blisters to form around the vaginal opening and perineum (in women) or the external urinary opening (in men) (Fig. 33-10). There is no cure for genital herpes and the blisters may return over and over again throughout the lifetime of the person who is infected.
- *Gonorrhea* is a bacterial infection. In men, the bacterium that causes gonorrhea infects the urethra. The man may experience a burning sensation during urination and notice a

greenish discharge from the urethra, or he may have no symptoms at all. Women who are infected with the bacterium that causes gonorrhea also may not have any symptoms. Because the infection may not be detected and treated for some time, the bacterium can travel to the fallopian tubes and into the abdominal cavity, resulting in a condition called **pelvic inflammatory disease (PID).** PID often results in severe pain and scar tissue that can lead to infertility. If detected, gonorrhea can be treated with antibiotics.

- *Chlamydia,* the most commonly occurring STI, is caused by a type of bacteria. Like gonorrhea, chlamydia often is not associated with any noticeable symptoms. Chlamydia can cause infertility in both men and women and is treated with an antibiotic.
- *Genital (venereal) warts* are caused by a virus. In men infected with the virus, small, wart-like growths may occur inside the urethra. In women, the warts may be seen around the vaginal opening, inside the vagina, or on the cervix. Infection with genital warts increases a woman's risk of developing cervical cancer. Treatment may involve removal of the growths with a laser.
- *Syphilis* is a bacterial infection. The signs and symptoms of syphilis occur in three stages. During the first stage, a painless lesion is seen on the genitals. This lesion heals, and 2 to 4 weeks later, the person

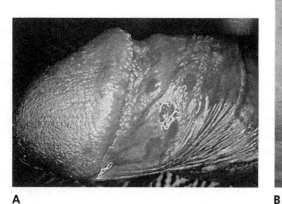
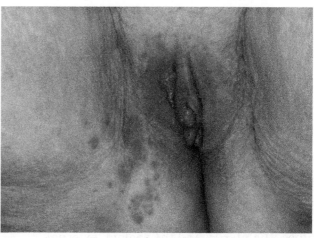

A   **B**

Figure 33-10
Genital herpes is a viral infection that causes blisters to form **(A)** on the penis (in men) and **(B)** on the vulva (in women). There is no cure for genital herpes. The sexual partner of a person with genital herpes is at risk for infection even when blisters are not seen, if a condom is not used. (**A,** *used with permission from Goodheart, H. P. [2003]. Goodheart's photoguide of common skin disorders. Diagnosis and management [2nd ed., p. 284]. **B,** © Dr. P. Marrazi/Photo Researchers, Inc.*)

develops a skin rash and a fever. This is the second stage. If not detected and treated, the infection becomes latent. This means that the pathogen that is causing the infection is still in the person's body, but it is not active. As many as 20 or more years later, the pathogen can become active again, resulting in the third stage. The third stage usually involves damage to the cardiovascular and nervous systems, which can result in confusion, dementia, and paralysis.

- *AIDS* is caused by human immunodeficiency virus (HIV). The virus can be transmitted in semen, vaginal secretions, or blood. To date, there is no cure for AIDS, and many people with AIDS die as a result of the disease. AIDS is discussed in detail in Chapters 8 and 38.

PREVENTION OF SEXUALLY TRANSMITTED INFECTIONS

People who begin having sexual relations at a young age (for example, in their early teens) and people who have many sexual partners are at increased risk for getting an STI. Women are also at greater risk than men for STIs. Although some STIs can be effectively treated and cured with antibiotics, the best treatment still remains prevention. The following methods are useful in the prevention of STIs.

- When having sexual relations, use a barrier, such as a condom. Condoms help to prevent the transmission of infected secretions from one person to another. Some contraceptive creams, when used with a condom, help to increase the condom's effectiveness against both pregnancy and STIs.
- If someone has signs or symptoms of an STI, they should not have sexual relations until treatment has been sought. Remember that both partners must be treated. If they are not both treated, then reinfection can occur. After the course of treatment has been completed, it is important for both partners to return to the health care provider for a follow-up examination to ensure that treatment was successful.

Knowing about STIs can help to keep a person safe and healthy. In addition, this knowledge will help you to care for your patients or residents. Even if you work in a health care setting where you care mostly for elderly people, information about STIs is still useful. Some of the residents of long-term care facilities may continue to be sexually active and can still get an STI if they have relations with an infected partner. Also, symptoms of the third stage of syphilis may not appear until late in a person's life. To provide quality care to the people who depend on you for assistance, you need to be aware of the many different types of disorders that require the services of the health care industry.

SUMMARY

- Reproduction is the process by which a living thing makes more living things like itself. Although in both men and women, the reproductive system produces the cells and hormones that are necessary to create a new life, the organs that make up the reproductive system are very different in men and women.
- The female reproductive system consists of internal structures (the ovaries, the fallopian tubes, the uterus, and the vagina), external structures (the labia, the clitoris, and the vaginal opening, referred to collectively as the vulva), and the accessory organs (the breasts).
  - The female reproductive system is designed to produce eggs, receive sperm cells, contain and nourish a developing baby, give birth, and provide nourishment after the baby's birth by producing breast milk.
- Each month during a woman's reproductive years (from puberty to menopause), her body prepares itself to become pregnant. If pregnancy does not occur, the woman has a menstrual period and the cycle begins again.
- Aging affects the female reproductive system by causing a decline in the amount of hormones produced and the number of eggs that mature.
- Many disorders may affect a woman's reproductive system throughout her lifetime, including menstrual disorders, cancer, infertility, and infections.
- The male reproductive system consists of the testicles (testes), the epididymis, the vas

deferens, and the penis. Accessory organs include the seminal vesicles and prostate gland, which play a role in producing semen (the fluid that carries sperm cells out of the body). Sperm cells leave the body through the urethra.

- The male reproductive system is designed to produce sperm and deposit it inside the female's body.
- After puberty, the male reproductive system produces sperm cells continuously. Sperm cells are produced in the testes and mature in the epididymis. From the epididymis, they pass through the vas deferens and urethra to reach the outside of the body. Before leaving the body, the sperm cells are mixed with secretions from the seminal vesicles and the prostate gland, forming semen.
- As they get older, many men find that the frequency and duration of their erections decreases. Many men also develop enlargement of the prostate gland.

- Disorders of the male reproductive system include impotence (erectile dysfunction), cancer, and infection.
- Sexually transmitted infections (STIs) are infections of the reproductive system that are commonly transmitted by sexual contact.
  - Some STIs do not cause signs or symptoms. Because they may not be diagnosed for a long time, the infected person can spread the infection to his or her sexual partners without knowing it. In addition, the untreated infection can damage the passageways that carry the sperm or eggs, causing infertility.
  - Common STIs include herpes simplex, gonorrhea, chlamydia, genital (venereal) warts, syphilis, and AIDS. Although some STIs can be treated, there is no known cure for herpes simplex or AIDS.
  - The best treatment for STIs is prevention. The risk of getting an STI can be lowered by using a barrier (such as a condom) when engaging in sexual activity and avoiding sexual activity with infected partners.

WHAT DID YOU LEARN?

Multiple Choice

Select the single best answer for each of the following questions.

1. What occurs when a male sex cell joins the female sex cell, forming a cell that contains the complete number of chromosomes?
   a. Ovulation
   b. Menstruation
   c. Menopause
   d. Conception (fertilization)
2. Which one of the following is a sexually transmitted infection (STI)?
   a. Breast cancer
   b. Herpes simplex
   c. Hepatitis A
   d. Tuberculosis (TB)

3. Which sexually transmitted infection (STI) is caused by a bacterium and may cause a man to have a burning sensation during urination and a greenish discharge from the urethra?
   a. Gonorrhea
   b. Syphilis
   c. Pelvic inflammatory disease (PID)
   d. Acquired immunodeficiency syndrome (AIDS)
4. Where does conception (fertilization) usually occur?
   a. In the uterus
   b. In the vagina
   c. In the fallopian tube
   d. In the vas deferens

Matching

Match each numbered item with its appropriate lettered description.

c 1. Sperm
e 2. Estrogen and progesterone
f 3. Amenorrhea
h 4. Egg (ovum)
a 5. Hysterectomy
g 6. Menopause
b 7. Menorrhagia
d 8. Mastectomy
j 9. Impotence (erectile dysfunction)
i 10. Infertility

a. Surgical removal of the uterus
b. Excessive menstrual bleeding
c. Male sex cell
d. Surgical removal of the breast
e. Female sex hormones
f. Absence of menstruation
g. The complete ending of a woman's menstrual cycles
h. Female sex cell
i. Inability to become pregnant or to carry a pregnancy to full term
j. Inability to achieve an erection

STOP and Think!

You work in a busy health clinic that provides services for people with sexually transmitted infections (STIs). One day, one of your friends confides in you that she is afraid she might have an STI. Based on your knowledge of these infections, what advice can you offer your friend?

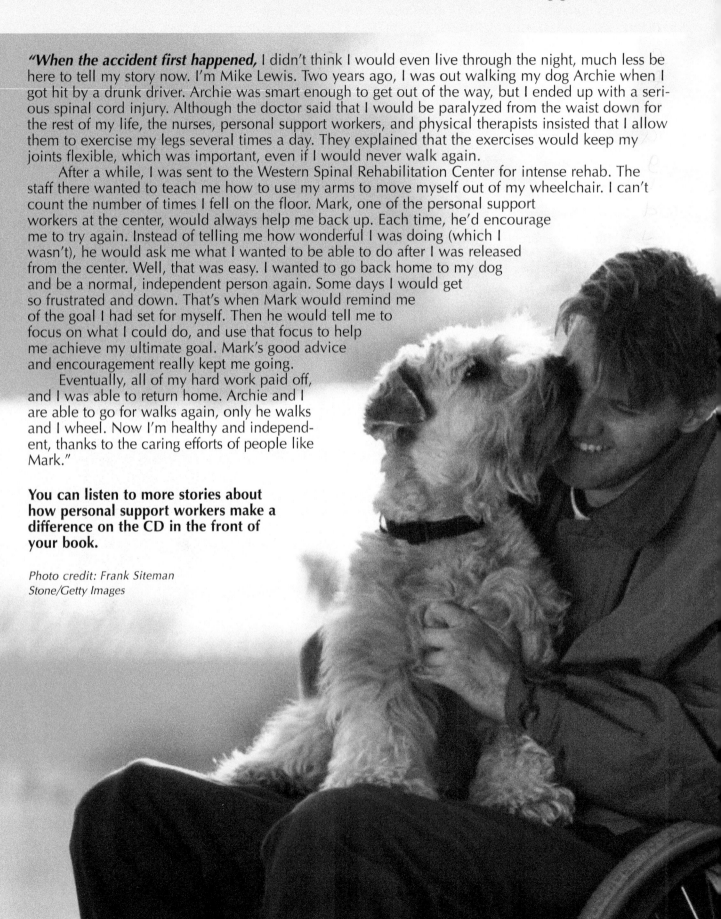

Personal Support Workers Make a Difference!

"When the accident first happened, I didn't think I would even live through the night, much less be here to tell my story now. I'm Mike Lewis. Two years ago, I was out walking my dog Archie when I got hit by a drunk driver. Archie was smart enough to get out of the way, but I ended up with a serious spinal cord injury. Although the doctor said that I would be paralyzed from the waist down for the rest of my life, the nurses, personal support workers, and physical therapists insisted that I allow them to exercise my legs several times a day. They explained that the exercises would keep my joints flexible, which was important, even if I would never walk again.

After a while, I was sent to the Western Spinal Rehabilitation Center for intense rehab. The staff there wanted to teach me how to use my arms to move myself out of my wheelchair. I can't count the number of times I fell on the floor. Mark, one of the personal support workers at the center, would always help me back up. Each time, he'd encourage me to try again. Instead of telling me how wonderful I was doing (which I wasn't), he would ask me what I wanted to be able to do after I was released from the center. Well, that was easy. I wanted to go back home to my dog and be a normal, independent person again. Some days I would get so frustrated and down. That's when Mark would remind me of the goal I had set for myself. Then he would tell me to focus on what I could do, and use that focus to help me achieve my ultimate goal. Mark's good advice and encouragement really kept me going.

Eventually, all of my hard work paid off, and I was able to return home. Archie and I are able to go for walks again, only he walks and I wheel. Now I'm healthy and independent, thanks to the caring efforts of people like Mark."

You can listen to more stories about how personal support workers make a difference on the CD in the front of your book.

Photo credit: Frank Siteman
Stone/Getty Images

SPECIAL CARE CONCERNS

34 Caring for People With Developmental
Disabilities
35 Caring for People With Mental Illness
36 Caring for People With Dementia
37 Caring for People With Cancer
38 Caring for People With HIV/AIDS

Because personal support workers are employed in so many different health care settings, you may be involved with the care of patients, residents, or clients who have developmental disabilities, mental illness, dementia, cancer, or HIV/AIDS. Along with the normal assistance needed for feeding, bathing, and toileting, these groups have other unique needs. The purpose of this unit is to introduce you to these groups and help you to recognize, and assist with meeting, their special needs.

Photo: An athlete competes in the Special Olympics.
(© Lawrence Migdale/Photo Researchers, Inc.)

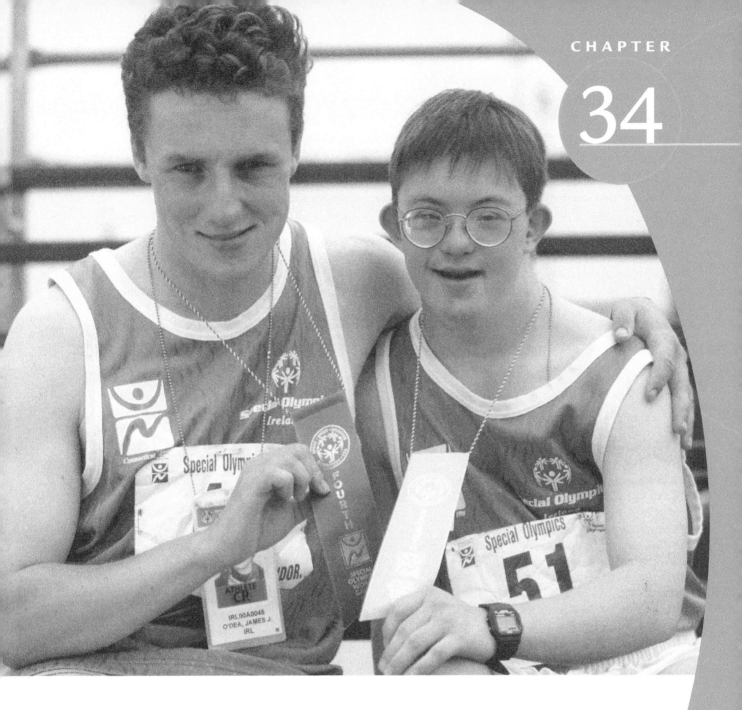

Caring for People With Developmental Disabilities

WHAT WILL YOU LEARN?

In this chapter, you will learn about caring for people with developmental disabilities. Permanent disabilities that affect a person before adulthood are called developmental disabilities because they interfere with normal physical or mental development.

Photo: Participating in events such as the Special Olympics provides physical as well as emotional benefits for people with developmental disabilities. (Richard Hutchings/Photo Researchers, Inc.)

679

As a personal support worker, you will be primarily responsible for providing the assistance that people with developmental disabilities need to meet their physical and emotional needs on a daily basis. When you are finished with this chapter, you will be able to:

1. Define the term developmental disabilities and discuss various causes.
2. List common developmental disabilities and describe characteristics of each one.
3. Describe the special needs of people with developmental disabilities.
4. Discuss physical problems that people with developmental disabilities may have.
5. Discuss types of rehabilitation that may be used to help people with developmental disabilities.

Vocabulary

Developmental disability	Down syndrome	Fragile X syndrome	Spina bifida
Congenital	Autism	Fetal alcohol	Hydrocephalus
Mental retardation	Cerebral palsy	syndrome	

WHAT IS A DEVELOPMENTAL DISABILITY?

A **developmental disability** is a permanent disability that affects a person before he reaches adulthood (that is, before 18 to 22 years of age) and interferes with the person's ability to achieve developmental milestones. A developmental disability may be **congenital** (something a child is born with) or acquired (occurring after birth, as a result of trauma or illness). Common causes of developmental disabilities are shown in Box 34-1. A developmental disability may affect mental function, physical function, or both. Developmental disabilities vary in severity. Some people with developmental disabilities are very independent, while others require total care.

SPECIAL NEEDS OF PEOPLE WITH DEVELOPMENTAL DISABILITIES

People with developmental disabilities have the same physical and emotional needs as everyone else. For example, they need good nutrition, plenty of exercise, and the sense of well-being that comes from feeling loved and cared for. However, many people with disabilities have additional special needs.

SPECIAL EDUCATION

Many children with developmental disabilities go to public school alongside friends and classmates who have no disabilities. This is called *mainstreaming*. Mainstreaming benefits children with developmental disabilities by making them feel less isolated. Children with disabilities who are "mainstreamed" have higher self-esteem and better social skills, because they have the opportunity to interact with other children who are not disabled (Fig. 34-1). Mainstreaming also benefits children who are not disabled by making them aware that people with disabilities are just like they are, except that they need extra help to do certain things.

BOX 34-1	**Common Causes of Developmental Disabilities**

Congenital (present at birth)
Genetic (inherited) disorders
Consumption of alcohol, drugs, or other toxic
  substances during pregnancy
Infections during pregnancy, such as German
  measles (rubella) or human immunodeficiency
  virus (HIV)
Poor nutrition during pregnancy
Conditions that deprive the baby of oxygen

Acquired (occurring after birth)
Birth trauma
Head injury
Near-drowning
Poisoning

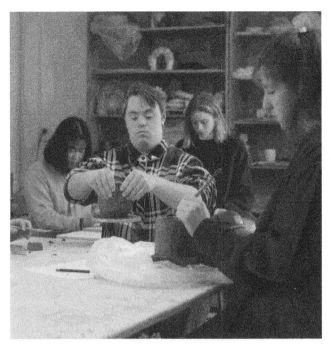

Figure 34-1
"Mainstreaming" benefits everyone. Here, a teenager with Down syndrome participates in a pottery class at his high school. (*Richard Hutchings/Photo Researchers, Inc.*)

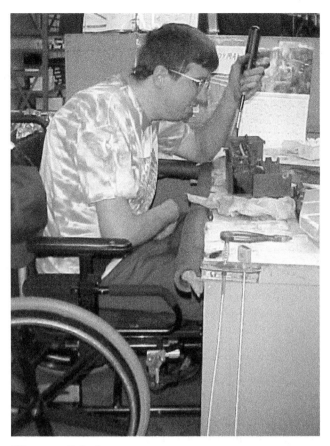

Figure 34-2
Vocational training helps to prepare people with disabilities for the workforce. (*Courtesy of the Wood County Board of Mental Retardation and Developmental Disabilities, Bowling Green, OH.*)

Children with developmental disabilities may also take part in special educational programs. Special educational programs are focused on the individual's needs and cover a wide range of topics, such as self-care skills (for example, eating or dressing), life skills (for example, counting money), and social skills (for example, understanding appropriate behaviour and "limits"). Vocational training focuses on teaching work skills that help people with disabilities become less dependent on others for their care (Fig. 34-2).

PROTECTION OF RIGHTS

Government agencies and organizations help protect the rights of people with developmental disabilities. This ensures that people who have disabilities are treated the same as those without disabilities, by guaranteeing people with disabilities access to public education, employment, and public places such as parks, restaurants, and transportation. The Canadian Mental Health Association is a national charitable organization that promotes the rights of people with mental disabilities.

EMOTIONAL AND SOCIAL NEEDS

Reassurance, love, and acceptance are vital for everyone's well-being, and especially for those who have disabilities that can make them appear or feel "different." Similarly, all people, even those with disabilities, have the need to interact with other people and participate in activities that they find enjoyable. One notable way in which people with developmental disabilities can fulfill their emotional and social needs is through events like the Special Olympics. The Special Olympics is a sporting event established to promote the physical and emotional health of people with developmental disabilities. The participants are matched for their competitions according to their level of physical and mental ability. The athletes compete against their own personal best performance. The Special Olympics emphasizes the joy that comes with physical activity, recognizing each athlete as a winner. Participating in events such as the Special

Olympics benefits athletes with disabilities emotionally as well as physically.

TYPES OF DEVELOPMENTAL DISABILITIES

MENTAL RETARDATION

A person with **mental retardation** has below-average intellectual functioning and problems with adaptive skills. *Intellectual functioning* is the ability to reason, think, and understand. *Adaptive skills* are skills needed to live and work, such as communication skills, social skills, and self-care skills. A mentally retarded person has an intelligence quotient (IQ) score of less than 70 points and limited adaptive skills in two or more areas.

Mental retardation can be caused by abnormalities in the brain that are present at birth. It can also be caused by problems that interfere with oxygen getting to the brain before, during, or after birth. The severity of mental retardation, like that of other disabilities, varies:

- **Mild mental retardation.** Most people with mental retardation fall into this category. Mild mental retardation may go unnoticed until a child begins school and starts having trouble with reading or solving math problems. With special education, a person with mild mental retardation is usually able to achieve a third- to sixth-grade learning level and master the skills needed for socially appropriate behaviour. Vocational (job) training is useful.
- **Moderate mental retardation.** People with moderate mental retardation have delays in both motor (manual) skills and speech development. With special education, a person with moderate mental retardation is usually able to learn self-care skills, communication skills, and safety habits. However, academically, she will probably not progress beyond a second-grade learning level. The person may also have trouble learning socially appropriate behaviour.
- **Severe mental retardation.** With special education, people with severe mental retardation are able to learn some communication and basic self-care skills, such as how to feed themselves. A person with severe mental retardation can usually learn to walk, if he does not have other physical disabilities.

- **Profound mental retardation.** *Profound* means "deep." People with profound mental retardation have minimal function in all developmental areas, physical and mental. These people need complete assistance with their activities of daily living (ADLs), and constant supervision to provide for their safety.

One of the great rewards that you will experience as a personal support worker is the satisfaction of helping a person with mental retardation to feel loved, and allowing her to express love back to you (Fig. 34-3). Many people with mental retardation need guidance with "appropriate" methods of displaying their love and affection to other people. In the same manner that a child learns that hugging a kitty too hard will lead to being scratched, people with mental retardation may need gentle reminders that a hug may sometimes be too tight and that not everyone appreciates physical affection.

Adults with mental retardation may function mentally at the level of a 7- or 8-year-old, with child-like curiosity and innocence. However, they are adults and will experience the same hormonal changes and sexual drives as everyone else. Because the person may not understand what is happening, these physical drives may be very confusing. Education and guidance from caregivers is very important to help a person with mental retardation learn about appropriate touch and sexual behaviour. In addition, caregivers must protect the person from sexual abuse. Because people with mental retardation tend to

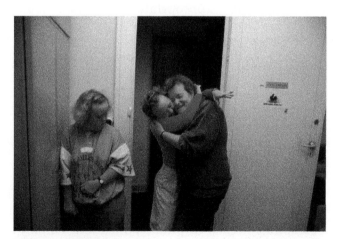

Figure 34-3

One of the great rewards that you will have as a personal support worker is the satisfaction of helping a person with mental retardation to feel loved, and allowing him to express love back to you. (© *Stephanie Maze/CORBIS.*)

be very trusting, and because they are not able to understand what is happening to them, they are often targets of sexual abuse. As a personal support worker, you must be especially observant for signs of sexual abuse when caring for a person with mental retardation. Any observations you make or suspicions that you have should be reported to the nurse immediately.

DOWN SYNDROME

Down syndrome is a developmental disability that is the result of a genetic disorder. Normally, each of our body's cells contains 23 pairs of chromosomes, for a total of 46. A person with Down syndrome has one extra chromosome. Down syndrome is the most common chromosome-related disorder, affecting 1 in every 1000 children born. Although the exact cause of Down syndrome is unknown, studies have shown that babies with Down syndrome are born more often to women who have children later in life.

People with Down syndrome have some degree of mental retardation and muscle weakness. In addition, they have certain characteristic physical features (Fig. 34-4):

- Eyelid folds that give the eyes an almond-shaped appearance
- A large tongue in a small mouth
- Square hands with short, stubby fingers
- A small, wide nose and small ears
- Short stature and a wide, short neck

Many people with Down syndrome are also born with heart defects that require corrective

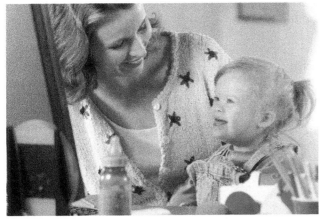

Figure 34-4
Certain physical characteristics are typical of Down syndrome, such as almond-shaped eyes. (© *LWA-Dann Tardif/CORBIS.*)

surgery or medication. Frequent respiratory tract infections are also common among people with Down syndrome, due to muscle weakness (which affects the muscles used for breathing) and a compromised immune system.

Many people with Down syndrome live independently and hold down jobs. Children with Down syndrome are usually raised in their own homes with their families. Once a person with Down syndrome reaches adulthood, the person may continue to live with family members, or he may choose to move to a group home. Group homes allow a person with Down syndrome to live independently within a supervised and supportive environment.

AUTISM

A person with **autism** has extreme difficulty communicating and relating to other people and surroundings. Although the specific cause of autism is unknown, experts suspect a genetic link. Like Down syndrome, autism affects about 1 in every 1000 children born. Boys are affected more often than girls.

Autism affects a person's reasoning skills, language skills, ability to socialize, ability to perform self-care activities, and response to touch and pain. A person with autism may seem very withdrawn, like he is in his "own world" (*auto* means "self"). The person may have lengthy or extreme tantrums, or show aggressive or violent behaviour that can result in self-injury. Other disorders, such as mental retardation and seizure disorders, may accompany autism. However, many people with autism have average or above-average intelligence. Therapy focusing on communication and social skills can be very useful for a person with autism.

CEREBRAL PALSY

Cerebral palsy is caused by damage to the cerebrum, the part of the brain involved with motor control. Cerebral palsy has many possible causes, including physical brain deformity and conditions that interfere with the flow of oxygen to the baby's brain before, during, or shortly after birth. Babies who are born prematurely or have a low birth weight are at higher risk for cerebral palsy. Accidents in early childhood can also cause cerebral palsy. For example, head trauma that causes swelling or bleeding in the brain and events that interfere with the flow of oxygen to the brain (such as choking, near-drowning, or

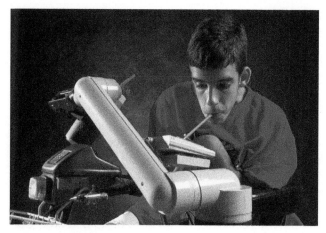

Figure 34-5
Cerebral palsy affects a person's motor function. Here, a child with cerebral palsy is using a pencil held in his mouth to operate a computer. (© *Richard T. Nowitz/Photo Researchers, Inc.*)

poisoning) can all cause this disability. The degree of disability depends on the extent of the damage to the brain.

The cerebrum plays a role in motor activity. This is why cerebral palsy typically affects the person's ability to voluntarily move parts of her body. Cerebral palsy can affect body movements in two different ways. One type of cerebral palsy causes spasms and shortening of the muscles. The affected joints may develop contractures. If the hands and arms are affected, the person may be unable to perform self-care skills such as feeding, bathing, or dressing. If the feet and legs are affected, the person may be unable to walk (Fig. 34-5). The second type of cerebral palsy causes involuntary movements of the arms, legs, and upper body. Facial and tongue muscles may also be involved, making the person appear to be chewing constantly. Varying degrees of mental retardation may also accompany the physical disabilities associated with cerebral palsy.

FRAGILE X SYNDROME

Fragile X syndrome is an inherited type of mental retardation caused by a defect in the X chromosome. Fragile X syndrome is more common and usually more severe in boys, as compared with girls. People who have fragile X syndrome are usually moderately to severely mentally retarded and may have physical characteristics such as large, cupped ears; a slim build; wide-set, somewhat squinting eyes; and velvet-like skin. They usually have delayed speech and communication skills. They may be hyperactive, and prone to

"mood swings." Autism may also accompany fragile X syndrome.

Special education helps people with fragile X syndrome learn self-care and behaviour skills. A calm, structured environment that keeps distractions and disturbances to a minimum is useful when caring for a person with fragile X syndrome. Unfortunately, because the syndrome has only recently been identified as a developmental disorder, more research is still needed to determine the most effective methods of caring for people with this disability.

FETAL ALCOHOL SYNDROME

Fetal alcohol syndrome is a combination of physical and mental problems that affect a child whose mother consumed alcohol during pregnancy. The degree of disability seems to depend on the amount of alcohol the mother drank during her pregnancy, as well as on how frequently she drank. Babies born with fetal alcohol syndrome are usually smaller than normal and have mental retardation, behavioural problems, learning difficulties, and facial deformities. Although the disabilities caused by fetal alcohol syndrome are permanent, special education and therapy can help to maximize the person's abilities.

SPINA BIFIDA

Spina bifida is a congenital defect of the spinal column. Normally, the vertebrae enclose the spinal cord, protecting it from harm. In a person with spina bifida, the vertebrae do not close properly during development, leaving the spinal cord exposed. As with other developmental disabilities, spina bifida varies in severity. Some people with spina bifida have only a slight bone deformity that is not even visible on the outside of the body, except for possibly a dimple or tuft of hair on the back. Other people have more severe deformities that result in the meninges, the spinal cord, or both bulging through a large opening on the back. The person may just have weakness in the legs, or she may be totally paralyzed below the waist (Fig. 34-6). Problems with bowel and bladder control are common. Sometimes, people with spina bifida also have mental retardation.

HYDROCEPHALUS

Hydrocephalus, sometimes called "water on the brain," results from a build up of cerebrospinal fluid (CSF). Recall from Chapter 28 that the

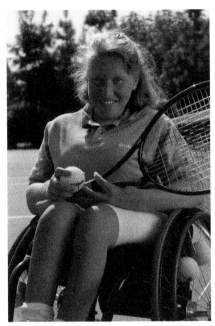

Figure 34-6
Spina bifida occurs when the vertebrae do not close properly during development. People with spina bifida have varying degrees of weakness or paralysis from the waist down, depending on the severity of the defect. (© *Jim Sugar/ CORBIS.*)

ventricles of the brain constantly produce CSF, which circulates around the brain and spinal cord. Normally, the CSF is reabsorbed into the bloodstream after it circulates through the central nervous system (CNS). In hydrocephalus, either too much CSF is produced, or the CSF cannot drain properly. Eventually, the fluid builds up, placing pressure on the delicate tissues of the brain and putting the person at risk for permanent brain damage.

Many cases of hydrocephalus are congenital. For example, babies with spina bifida often have hydrocephalus as well. When hydrocephalus occurs in a child younger than 2 years, the child's head often enlarges, because the bones of the skull have not yet fused together (Fig. 34-7A). Hydrocephalus may also occur later in life, as a result of a tumour, head trauma, or infection. Whether the hydrocephalus is congenital or acquired, it is often treated by surgically inserting a tube (called a *shunt*) that allows the fluid to drain from the brain to another part of the person's body (see Fig. 34-7B).

CARING FOR A PERSON WITH A DEVELOPMENTAL DISABILITY

During your career as a personal support worker, you may have many opportunities to care for people with developmental disabilities, in many different types of health care settings:

- **Hospitals.** If you work in a hospital, you may care for a person with a developmental disability while he is receiving treatment for an acute health problem, such as a heart problem, a respiratory tract infection, a nutritional deficiency, or seizures.
- **Home health care agencies.** Many parents who have children with disabilities choose to

Figure 34-7
Hydrocephalus results from a build up of cerebrospinal fluid (CSF). **(A)** In children younger than 2 years, the accumulation of cerebrospinal fluid can cause the head to grow larger because the bones of the skull have not yet fused together. **(B)** To prevent additional brain damage from occurring, a shunt is inserted to drain the cerebrospinal fluid. (*A*, © *Southern Illinois University/Photo Researchers, Inc.*)

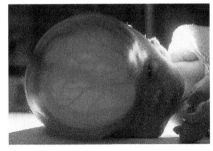

A

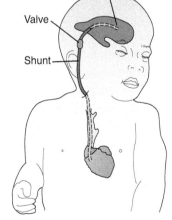

Catheter tip in venticle

Valve

Shunt

B

raise them at home, with their brothers and sisters. The parents of a child with severe disabilities may need the assistance of a home support worker to provide the best care to the child at home.

- **Day care centers.** Some day care centers specialize in the care of people with developmental disabilities. Clients may be children with developmental disabilities or adults with developmental disabilities who live at home with their parents. These facilities provide care for the person while family members go to work. These facilities usually provide educational services and social activities for their clients.
- **Long-term care facilities.** People with developmental disabilities become residents of long-term care facilities for many reasons. A young person may become a resident of a long-term care facility because her disabilities are simply too difficult or too numerous for the family to manage at home. Older people with disabilities often become residents of long-term care facilities because their parents or other caregivers die or become too old to physically care for them. If you work in a long-term care facility, be aware that the adjustment of having to leave home—where the person felt comfortable and safe—and move into a health care facility can be incredibly traumatic for a person with developmental disabilities, just as for any other resident or patient. These new residents may feel angry, isolated, or deserted, and will need your compassion and understanding to help them become comfortable in their new surroundings. It is important that you understand the frustrations that may accompany a change like this for a developmentally disabled person so that you avoid taking actions personally.

The degree to which a person is disabled varies greatly from person to person. Some physical disabilities are very mild and may only cause minor muscle weakness and coordination problems. Others are more severe and may leave the person without any control over her muscles at all. The severity of mental disabilities also varies from person to person. People with mild mental retardation are able to function independently, holding down jobs and raising families with minimal support from others. Severely mentally disabled people, however, require constant care and supervision just to keep them safe.

Helping Hands and a Caring Heart
FOCUS ON HUMANISTIC HEALTH CARE

When working with a person who has a developmental disability, the care that you provide must be specific to the person's abilities and disabilities. Learn as much as you can about each person in your care. Focusing on each person's abilities, whether developmentally disabled or not, will help you to provide the standard of care that each of your patients or residents needs from you.

COMMUNICATING WITH A PERSON WITH A DEVELOPMENTAL DISABILITY

Many people with developmental disabilities have difficulty communicating with other people. Some are unable to speak or to learn language skills due to a lack of motor skills, mental capabilities, or both. Vision or hearing problems can also make communication difficult. However, many people with developmental disabilities find other ways of communicating. For example, they may rely heavily on nonverbal communication techniques, such as facial expressions, nods, and body language. When caring for a person with a developmental disability:

- Ask family members what communication techniques work best with the person. Family members are often glad to share with you what they have learned about which communication methods work best.
- If the person has a mental disability, use simple words and short phrases. This allows the person to comprehend ideas or tasks, one at a time.
- Perhaps the most useful communication method is that of a touch, a smile, or a kind word, all of which transmit the message of your care and compassion for the person (Fig. 34-8).

Because many people with severe developmental disabilities have difficulty communicating, they may be unable to tell you if they are experiencing pain or discomfort. Learn to watch for small, subtle changes in your patients or residents, such as changes in behaviour, eating habits, or sleeping habits. Changes like these may be a sign that the person is ill. Because you will most likely be the member of the health care

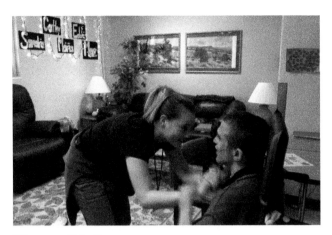

Figure 34-8
Good communication skills are especially important when working with people with developmental disabilities. (*Sacramento Bee/Jose Luis Villegas.*)

team who spends the most time with the person, you will likely be the first to notice that "something is not quite right." Always be sure to report your observations to the nurse.

TELL THE NURSE

A person with a developmental disability may not be able to tell you when something is wrong. Use your observation skills and be sure to report any of the following to the nurse immediately:

- There is a change in the person's vital signs, especially body temperature or pulse rhythm
- There is a change in the person's appetite
- There is a change in the person's level of activity
- There is a change in the person's physical abilities (for example, a person who usually has no trouble walking starts having falls)
- There is a change in the person's level of mental functioning (for example, the person seems confused or disoriented)
- There is a change in the person's behaviour (for example, a normally gentle person becomes aggressive)
- The person complains of pain or discomfort
- The person's skin is red or swollen in areas
- The person shows signs of physical or mental abuse

MEETING THE PHYSICAL NEEDS OF A PERSON WITH A DEVELOPMENTAL DISABILITY

A person with a developmental disability has the same physical needs as everyone else. Because of the person's disability, however, he may need some help in meeting those needs. As always, you will need to consider the specific needs of each person. Personal support workers often are involved with assisting people with disabilities with their ADLs, and with activities related to rehabilitation.

Assisting the Person With Activities of Daily Living

Depending on the severity and type of disability, the person may need assistance with ADLs. Some types of disability, such as cerebral palsy, can cause muscle weakness on one or both sides of the body, making dressing and grooming difficult. The short fingers of a person with Down syndrome may make it hard for the person to manage buttons or zippers on clothing. Assistive devices, many of which you have learned about in previous chapters, allow many people with physical disabilities to manage their ADLs independently or with minimal assistance. A person with mental disabilities may simply need supervision and reminders (for example, about which step comes next) to complete his ADLs. As with any patient or resident, helping a person achieve the greatest possible level of independence is the best type of assistance that you can give.

Assisting With Rehabilitation

Physical therapy or respiratory therapy may be needed to help the person maintain levels of function or to treat accompanying illnesses. For example, a person who has physical limitations may need assistance with passive range-of-motion exercises to keep the affected parts of her body functional. As a personal support worker, you may play a very important role in helping the person with physical rehabilitation.

SUMMARY

- Permanent disabilities that affect a person before she becomes an adult are called *developmental disabilities* because they interfere with that person's normal physical or mental development.
  - Developmental disabilities can be due to congenital abnormalities, traumatic injury, infection, disease, deprivation of oxygen or nutrition, or the result of poisoning or drug use.
  - Developmental disabilities can affect a person physically or mentally.
  - The severity of the disability varies greatly with each individual.
  - Special education, assistive devices, and rehabilitation can help a person with a developmental disability maximize his abilities and become more independent.
- Many developmentally disabled people have special needs.
  - Educational opportunities designed specifically for people with developmental disabilities help teach self-care, communication, and social and vocational skills.
  - Government legislation, and organizations such as the Canadian Mental Health Association help to protect the rights of people with disabilities.
  - The Special Olympics was established to promote the physical and emotional health of people with developmental disabilities.
- There are many different types of developmental disabilities. The degree to which a person's abilities are affected varies considerably, even among people who have the same type of disability.
  - Mental retardation affects a person's general intellectual functioning. A person with mental retardation has an IQ score of less than 70 and limited adaptive skills in two or more areas.
  - Down syndrome is a developmental disability that is the result of having an extra chromosome. People with Down syndrome

have some degree of mental retardation as well as certain physical characteristics.
  - Autism is a congenital disorder. People with autism have extreme difficulty communicating with and relating to other people and their surroundings.
  - Cerebral palsy affects the motor region of the brain (the cerebrum) and causes varying degrees of paralysis in the body. Some people with cerebral palsy also have some degree of mental retardation.
  - Fragile X syndrome is an inherited type of mental retardation that is more common in boys.
  - Fetal alcohol syndrome is a combination of physical and mental abnormalities that affect a child whose mother consumed alcohol during pregnancy.
  - Spina bifida is a defect of the spinal column that can cause paralysis of the lower extremities.
  - Hydrocephalus occurs when the ventricles of the brain produce too much cerebrospinal fluid (CSF), or when the fluid is not able to drain properly. Hydrocephalus can result in brain damage.
- Personal support workers care for people with developmental disabilities in a variety of health care settings.
  - Because people with developmental disabilities may have trouble communicating with others, personal support workers often must rely on their observation skills to tell when something is wrong.
  - Personal support workers often must provide some or complete assistance with activities of daily living (ADLs). However, many people with developmental disabilities are able to manage their ADLs quite independently by using assistive devices.
  - Personal support workers are often very involved in assisting people with developmental disabilities with tasks related to rehabilitation.

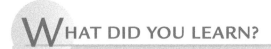

WHAT DID YOU LEARN?

Multiple Choice

Select the single best answer for each of the following questions.

1. Which one of the following statements about mental retardation is correct?
   a. It affects the motor region of the brain
   b. It can occur before, during, or after birth
   c. It is always severe
   d. None of the above

2. What physical characteristics does a person with Down syndrome have?
   a. Large, cupped ears; a slim build; wide-set, somewhat squinting eyes; and velvet-like skin
   b. Almond-shaped eyes, square hands with short fingers, large tongue in a small mouth
   c. A large head
   d. Facial deformities and small stature

3. What do researchers think is a cause of autism?
   a. Genetics
   b. Oxygen deprivation at birth
   c. Drugs
   d. Trauma at birth

4. Cerebral palsy can be caused by:
   a. Infection during pregnancy
   b. A lack of oxygen to the brain
   c. An extra chromosome
   d. Alcohol intake during pregnancy.

5. A person with autism may have:
   a. An extra chromosome
   b. Hearing and vision problems
   c. Problems with social relations
   d. Muscle weakness

6. A person with Down syndrome always has some degree of:
   a. Mental retardation
   b. Spastic movements
   c. Cerebral palsy
   d. Autism

7. Which one of the following statements about fetal alcohol syndrome is correct?
   a. It occurs when a woman smokes during pregnancy
   b. A newborn with fetal alcohol syndrome is larger than normal
   c. It occurs when a woman drinks alcohol during pregnancy
   d. It is caused by oxygen deprivation at birth

8. What is spina bifida?
   a. A seizure disorder
   b. A defect of the spinal column
   c. A shunt
   d. Another name for fragile X syndrome

9. What is common in a person with spina bifida?
   a. Autism
   b. Bowel and bladder incontinence
   c. Drooling
   d. Seizures

10. Hydrocephalus occurs when:
    a. Cerebrospinal fluid (CSF) collects in the brain
    b. The person has a seizure
    c. A person is born with an extra chromosome
    d. A person has nerve damage

STOP and Think!

Today a new resident has been admitted to the long-term care facility where you work. Mr. Theodore has severe cerebral palsy. He is an only child. His parents, who are in their 80s, are experiencing health problems of their own and are no longer able to provide the physical care that Mr. Theodore needs. Mr. Theodore is very upset. He is crying, and he keeps asking why his family doesn't want him anymore. What can you do in the coming days and weeks to help Mr. Theodore make the adjustment to his new home?

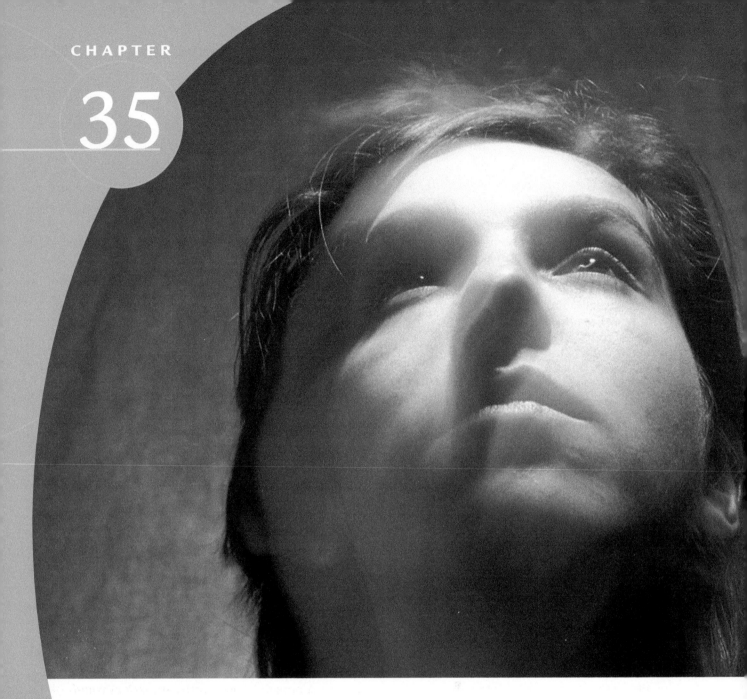

Caring for People With Mental Illness

WHAT WILL YOU LEARN?

A **mental illness** is a disorder that affects a person's mind, causing the person to act in unusual ways, experience emotional difficulties, or both. (*Mental* means "mind.")

Photo: Mental illnesses are disorders that affect the mind and emotions.
(© Piko/Photo Researchers, Inc.)

In many societies and cultures, mental illness is viewed as something shameful. A mentally ill person's odd behaviour may be frightening to those who do not understand it. In addition, movies, television, and books have contributed to the popular image of mentally ill people as crazy, violent, and out of control. Although some people who are mentally ill may behave in violent or dangerous ways, most do not. There are many different types of mental illness, and mental illness varies in severity from person to person.

As a personal support worker, you will care for many people with different types and degrees of mental illness. You may find the idea of caring for a mentally ill person frightening. Learning about common mental illnesses can help you to overcome this fear. In this chapter, you will learn about several common mental illnesses, and how they affect the people who suffer from them. When you are finished with this chapter, you will be able to:

1. Define the term *mental illness*.
2. Describe some of the qualities that define good mental health.
3. Discuss methods that people use to cope with stress effectively.
4. List possible causes of mental illness.
5. Discuss the different treatments that are available for people with mental illness.
6. Describe common mental illnesses that you may encounter in the health care setting.
7. Discuss special concerns related to the health care setting and aging that may affect a person's mental health.
8. Describe the responsibilities of the personal support worker when caring for mentally ill patients and residents.

Vocabulary

Mental illness	Suicide	Depression	Anorexia nervosa
Stress	Anxiety	Bipolar disorder	Bulimia nervosa
Coping mechanisms	Panic disorder	(manic depression)	
Defense mechanisms	Obsessive-compulsive	Schizophrenia	
Psychiatrist	disorder	Delusions	
Psychologist	Phobia	Hallucinations	

MENTAL HEALTH

To better understand mental illness, it is often useful to start by understanding mental health. Simply put, mental health is the absence of mental illness. One of the main qualities of mental health is a state of emotional balance. In Unit 5, you learned how physical health is related to the body's ability to make adjustments to maintain a state of physical balance, or homeostasis. Similarly, mental health is characterized by a person's ability to make adjustments to maintain a state of emotional balance.

Stress, which results from any change from the normal routine, affects a person's ability to maintain a state of balance. Changes that affect us physically, such as illness or disability, cause physical stress. Life events, such as getting married, getting divorced, starting a new job, having

a baby, or losing a loved one cause a great deal of mental stress. For most of us, stress is a constant in our lives. Even day-to-day activities, such as reading the newspaper, raising children, or performing our jobs, are sources of stress (Fig. 35-1). Stress that is not managed properly can affect a person's physical health, as well as his mental health. For example, not being able to manage stress can put a person at risk for cardiovascular problems, such as a heart attack, and digestive disorders, such as ulcers.

Each person has a limit to the amount of stress that she can effectively deal with at any given time. Fatigue, illness, and everyday stress sometimes affect our ability to cope well with change. Many times, stress does not come from a single source. For example, a person may be able to cope fairly well with one type of stress, such as the loss of a job. But when other stresses, such as a sick child,

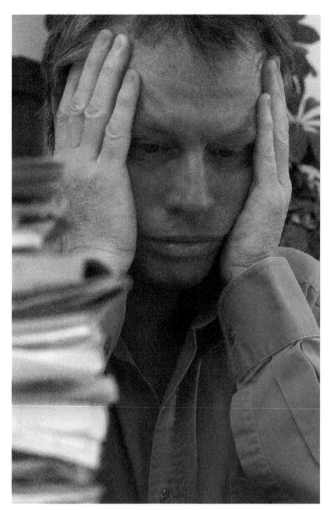

Figure 35-1
Stress is a constant in most people's lives. Work, family, and world events are common sources of stress.
(© Jean-Paul Chassenet/Photo Researchers, Inc.)

are added, the person may reach his "breaking point." When this happens, the person may cry, sleep excessively, be unable to sleep, have difficulty concentrating, or feel depressed for a time. Most people with good mental health are able to eventually overcome these feelings and regain their emotional balance (Fig. 35-2). People who are mentally ill cannot cope effectively with stress and may become unable to work, care for their children, make simple decisions, think clearly, or even provide their own self-care. A mentally ill person may need medication, counselling, or support groups to help regain emotional balance.

COPING MECHANISMS

What do you do when you start to feel overwhelmed or "stressed out"? Maybe you exercise, practice a hobby, get together with friends, meditate or pray, or just find a quiet place to relax (Fig. 35-3). Over time, many people come to know what they can do to make themselves feel better when they start to feel overwhelmed by life's pressures. These conscious and deliberate ways of dealing with stress are called **coping mechanisms.**

Many people rely on positive coping mechanisms, such as exercise, prayer and meditation, getting together with friends, or engaging in a hobby. Other people rely on less effective coping mechanisms. These people seek short-term relief through behaviours such as nail biting, pacing, overeating or not eating enough, smoking, or abusing drugs or alcohol (Fig. 35-4). Initially, these behaviours may help the person to reduce stress.

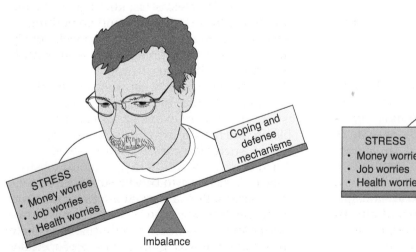
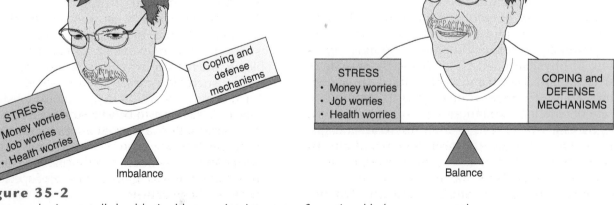

Figure 35-2
A person who is mentally healthy is able to maintain a state of emotional balance on most days. Stress can drag us down, causing the scale to tip out of balance, but a person who is mentally healthy is able to adjust to the stress and return to a state of emotional balance.

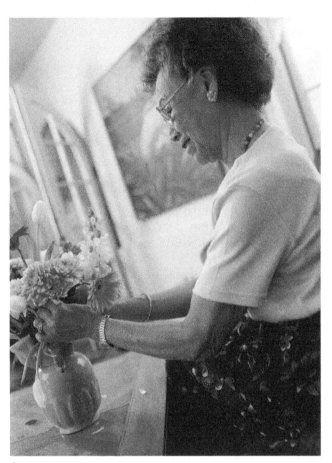

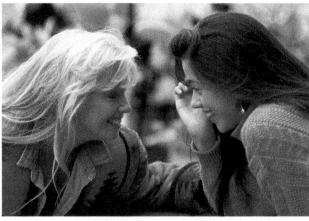

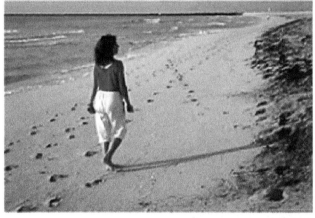

Figure 35-3
Our physical and mental health depends on our ability to manage everyday stress. Enjoying a hobby **(A)**, laughing with friends **(B)**, and taking a long walk **(C)** are just some of many positive approaches people take to relieve stress! (**B,** © Christopher Briscoe/Photo Researchers, Inc.; **C,** © Jeff Greenberg/Photo Researchers, Inc.)

But over time, they place the person at risk for serious physical problems, mental problems, or both.

DEFENSE MECHANISMS

As you know, our bodies are "programmed" to try and return to a state of balance. Therefore, when a person is under stress, the mind may try to return the person to a state of emotional balance by using defense mechanisms. **Defense mechanisms** are methods of dealing with stress that "just happen." Usually the person is not even aware that he is using them. Defense mechanisms help to protect us from emotionally traumatic events. The behaviours associated with defense mechanisms occur when the mind attempts to restore or maintain emotional balance in response to stress. Common defense mechanisms include the following:

- *Compensation* means to make up for a loss by "filling in" or "substituting" something else. For example, a person who feels lonely may eat too much. This person is substituting food for affection.
- *Conversion* means "to change." For example, a person who is depressed (an emotional problem) may develop a stomachache (a physical problem), and then use the physical problem as a reason to avoid participating in an activity.
- *Denial* is refusing to believe something that is true, especially if the truth is unpleasant. For example, a person who has been diagnosed with cancer may truly believe that the doctor has made the wrong diagnosis, and that she does not have cancer.
- *Displacement* is shifting an emotion from one person to another who is less threatening. For

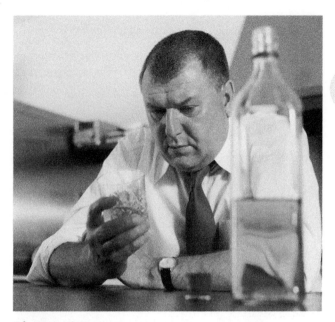

Figure 35-4
Many people drink alcohol excessively, use illegal ("street") drugs, or abuse legally prescribed drugs to deal with stress. This is called substance abuse. Although substance abuse may provide short-term relief from the pressures of daily life, in the long run it is not an effective coping mechanism.

example, a resident who is angry with her daughter for moving her to a long-term care facility—and who is afraid of expressing this anger because she fears the daughter will abandon her—may take her anger out on the personal support worker instead.

- *Projection* is blaming someone else for your own uncomfortable or unacceptable actions or feelings. For example, a resident may accuse a personal support worker of breaking a vase when in fact, the resident actually broke the treasured vase herself.
- *Rationalization* is making excuses or creating acceptable reasons for poor behaviours or actions. For instance, a student who does not study for a test and then fails it may tell herself that the reason she failed is because the teacher is "too hard."
- *Regression* means to turn back to a former or earlier state. For example, many older children who experience stress as a result of being hospitalized begin demonstrating behaviours from when they were younger, such as thumb-sucking or bedwetting.
- *Repression (suppression)* is the refusal to remember or think about a frightening or painful memory. A person may repress

memories of an automobile accident or childhood abuse.

CAUSES AND TREATMENT OF MENTAL ILLNESS

There are many different types of mental illness, and many different causes. Some types of mental illness run in families (that is, they are inherited). Others result from chemical imbalances in the brain. In Chapter 28, you learned about chemicals called *neurotransmitters*. An imbalance in these chemicals can lead to some forms of mental illness. Finally, some mental illnesses may be caused by a person's environment. For example, a person who is abused by a family member may develop ineffective coping or defense mechanisms that lead to mental illness.

Fortunately, many mental illnesses, just like many physical illnesses, can be successfully managed with medications, psychiatric counselling, or both. The word *psychiatric* comes from the Greek words *psyche* (the soul) and *iatreia* (healing). A **psychiatrist** is a medical doctor trained in diagnosing and treating mental illness. A psychiatrist is allowed to prescribe medications. A **psychologist,** while not a medical doctor, has education and training that allows him to provide counselling services to help people with mental illness. A psychologist is not allowed to prescribe medications. Depending on the person's situation, he may need the services of a psychiatrist, a psychologist, or both. With treatment, many people with mental illnesses are able to lead happy, productive lives. Because many people with mental illnesses are at risk for committing **suicide** (taking their own lives, intentionally and voluntarily), diagnosis and treatment of mental illness are very important.

Treatment for mental illness has changed dramatically over the past 50 years. In the past, mentally ill people were usually sent to special hospitals ("mental institutions"), where they were given large doses of medications to keep them quiet and sedated. Techniques such as electroshock therapy (passing electricity through the brain to cause a seizure) and lobotomy (surgical removal of part of the brain) were used frequently, often with little success. Now we know more about why mental illnesses occur and how they should be treated. For example, now that we know that moods and behaviours can be affected by chemical imbalances, we have developed new medications that help to restore the brain's chemical balance. Rather than simply sedating the person into submission, these new medications help the person to act and think more "normally." And electro-shock therapy, while still used in some cases, is used much more effectively.

TYPES OF MENTAL ILLNESS

Some of the more common mental illnesses include anxiety disorders, depression, bipolar disorder (manic depression), schizophrenia, and eating disorders. In this chapter, we will give you only a brief overview of these disorders. As you care for patients or residents who suffer from these mental illnesses (or others not discussed here), make an effort to learn more about their conditions. For example, you might ask the nurse if she can explain the person's condition to you more fully. The nurse may also be able to recommend articles or books for you to read to learn more about the person's condition. Increasing your knowledge about your patients' or residents' specific conditions allows you to better understand and care for them.

ANXIETY DISORDERS

Anxiety is a feeling of uneasiness, dread, apprehension, or worry. Anxiety is a normal feeling that we have in response to situations that are threatening to our body, lifestyle, values, or loved ones. A certain level of anxiety is normal and may actually lead us to do something positive about a bad or potentially dangerous situation. But too much anxiety or prolonged periods of anxiety can make it hard for us to function or cope with everyday situations. Feelings of anxiety can cause many physical signs and symptoms, such as sleeplessness, restlessness, fatigue, changes in appetite, or an increased heart rate and blood pressure. It is also common for an anxious person to be irritable and to have difficulty thinking clearly.

Although we all have periods of increased anxiety, some people have periods of anxiety that continue to build until they can no longer function. Anxiety is a typical symptom in many common mental illnesses. However, in some mental illnesses, overwhelming anxiety is the key feature of the disorder. These mental illnesses are grouped under the general term *anxiety disorders*. Common anxiety disorders include panic disorder, obsessive-compulsive disorder, and phobias.

Panic Disorder

Panic is a sudden, overpowering fright. A person with a **panic disorder** has terrifying episodes or "panic attacks," during which she experiences sudden increases in anxiety and feelings of intense fear. A person who is having a "panic attack" usually also has physical signs and symptoms, such as chest or abdominal pain, a rapid heartbeat, shortness of breath, and dizziness (Fig. 35-5). These symptoms may be similar to those of a heart attack or other severe physical illness. Panic attacks can be brief, or they may last for some time. Some people will experience these attacks rarely, while others will have them quite often. It is important to remember that even though the physical symptoms may not be a sign of a serious physical condition, they are no less real and frightening to the person who is experiencing them.

Obsessive-Compulsive Disorder

Obsessive-compulsive disorder is an anxiety disorder that causes a person to suffer intensely from recurrent unwanted thoughts (*obsessions*). The obsessions are usually associated with rituals that the person cannot control (*compulsions*). The rituals may include actions such as handwashing, counting, or checking that are repeated over and over again in hopes that the obsessive thoughts will go away. Not performing the rituals

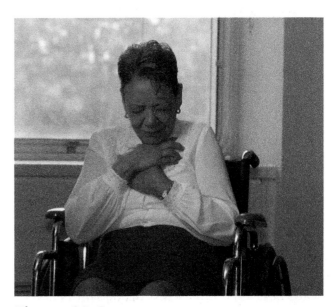

Figure 35-5
People with panic disorder suffer from "panic attacks," which are characterized by feelings of intense fear and anxiety, accompanied by physical signs and symptoms such as chest pain and a rapid heartbeat.

increases a person's level of anxiety. When it is severe, obsessive-compulsive disorder takes over the person's life. The person becomes unable to perform the tasks that are associated with normal daily activities because of his obsessions and compulsions.

Phobias

A **phobia** is an excessive, abnormal fear of an object or situation. Phobias can be incredibly disabling for the person affected by them. The person will do anything to avoid the thing she is afraid of, to the point where she may be unable to do something as simple as leaving the house. There are three main groups of phobias:

- *Simple phobias* are the most common type. A person with a simple phobia is abnormally afraid of a specific thing (for example, dogs, cats, insects, heights, water, or flying in an airplane).
- *Social phobias* involve a fear of being humiliated or embarrassed in front of other people. Social phobias may be related to feelings of inferiority and low self-esteem and may cause a person to drop out of school, avoid making friends, or remain unemployed.
- *Agoraphobia* is the fear of having a panic attack in a place from which there is no easy escape, or in a place where help is not available. For example, a person may be intensely afraid of having a panic attack in an elevator or on a crowded bus.

DEPRESSION

Depression is a feeling of excessive sadness or hopelessness. Many events in life, such as the loss of a loved one, can cause temporary feelings of intense sadness and hopelessness. In a person with good mental health, the painful emotions of an event-related depression (such as the loss of a loved one) go away over time. Sometimes, short-term treatment with medication or counselling may be needed to help the person through the crisis.

Some people, however, experience intense feelings of sadness and hopelessness that do not go away, even with time. These feelings may or may not be brought on by a sad event, such as the death of a loved one. When depression is severe and persistent, it is called *clinical depression.*

Clinical depression is one of the most common mental illnesses. It affects more than 1 million Canadians each year. Some research indicates that a family history of clinical depression

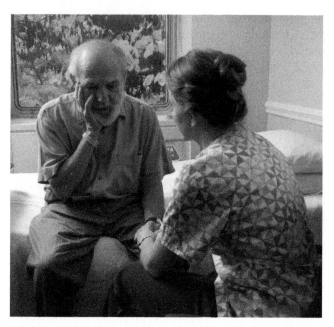

Figure 35-6
Depression is common among older people. If you think that one of your patients or residents is depressed, you should report your suspicions to the nurse.

increases a person's risk of developing this mental illness. Women seem to experience clinical depression about twice as often as men do. Clinical depression is also the most frequently treated mental illness among elderly people (Fig. 35-6).

Several factors can lead to the development of clinical depression, including:

- Chemical imbalances in the brain
- Low self-esteem and poor coping skills
- Hormonal changes, such as those that affect women during pregnancy, menstruation, childbirth, and menopause
- Medications

A person who is depressed loses interest in activities that she usually finds pleasurable or fulfilling, such as eating, working, socializing with friends, and pursuing hobbies. The person may feel sad or anxious, and she may cry frequently. Many people who are depressed have problems sleeping. The person may sleep too much, or not enough. The person may be restless or irritable. Instead of being grateful when someone tries to help, the person may become angry and defensive. The person may have feelings of guilt and worthlessness and struggle with thoughts of death or suicide. Physical complaints (for example, of pain or a digestive disorder) are also common among people who are depressed.

Prompt treatment is needed to help a clinically depressed person return to an enjoyable, productive life.

The incidence of depression increases with age. Unfortunately, elderly people are less likely to seek treatment for this disorder. Many older people who are depressed feel that their depression is just part of getting older and must be accepted. However, this is not the case. If you will be working with older patients or residents, pay attention to changes in their behaviours or moods that may indicate clinical depression. By reporting these observations to the nurse, you play an important role in helping to ensure that the person receives treatment that will help him feel better.

BIPOLAR DISORDER (MANIC DEPRESSION)

Bipolar disorder (manic depression) is a mental health disorder that causes mood swings. Periods of excessive happiness and excitement that may cause the person to engage in impulsive or reckless behaviour (*mania*) are followed by periods of excessive sadness and hopelessness (*depression*). Experts believe that bipolar disorder is caused by chemical imbalances in the brain that affect a person's moods.

A person with bipolar disorder may have mood swings several times a day, or less frequently, with days or even weeks passing between episodes. Between mood swings, a person with bipolar disorder may have periods of "normal" mood. Bipolar disorder can be difficult to recognize and properly diagnose.

SCHIZOPHRENIA

Schizophrenia is a very disabling form of mental illness. It tends to run in families and may have a genetic basis. As with other mental illnesses, schizophrenia may be mild or severe. A person with severe schizophrenia that is untreated may be a danger to himself, or to others.

A person with schizophrenia has trouble determining what is real and what is imaginary. He may suffer from **delusions,** or false ideas. For example, the person may believe that he is someone famous or that someone is spying on him or trying to take his belongings. He may also experience **hallucinations,** or episodes where he sees, feels, hears, smells, or tastes something that does not really exist. For example, the person may hear voices in his head telling him to perform a certain act. The person's thinking and speech become disordered. He may switch from one topic to another during a conversation, or make up new words or patterns of speech. As a result of these symptoms, the person may say or do very strange things, making it hard for him to function normally in social situations. A schizophrenic person's behaviour is often frightening and confusing to others.

EATING DISORDERS

There are many different types of eating disorders. Two of the most commonly known types are anorexia nervosa and bulimia nervosa. No matter what the type, all eating disorders involve serious (and potentially fatal) changes in eating behaviour, such as reducing the amount of food eaten to almost nothing, or severe overeating. Eating disorders cause many physical problems, including kidney failure and serious heart problems that can lead to death. Like people with other mental illnesses, people with eating disorders cannot voluntarily control their impulses, and they need treatment to help them learn to eat normally again.

Eating disorders usually start during adolescence or early adulthood. Women are at higher risk than men for developing an eating disorder. Many people who suffer from depression or anxiety disorders also suffer from eating disorders.

Anorexia Nervosa

People with **anorexia nervosa** see themselves as very overweight, even though they are excessively thin (Fig. 35-7). Anorexia (loss of appetite) is a key feature of this disorder. The person simply does not eat enough food. She will skip meals, take tiny portions at meal times, or make excuses for why she cannot eat. She may only allow herself to eat small amounts of very "safe" low-calorie foods. Many people with anorexia nervosa exercise excessively, in addition to severely reducing their food intake.

Bulimia Nervosa

A person with **bulimia nervosa** regularly eats huge amounts of food (*binging*) and then induces vomiting or uses laxatives to rid the body of the food before it is digested (*purging*). A person with bulimia nervosa often is of normal weight for her age and height. However, like a person who suffers from anorexia nervosa, a person with bulimia nervosa is extremely focused on her body weight and shape, and believes that she is excessively overweight.

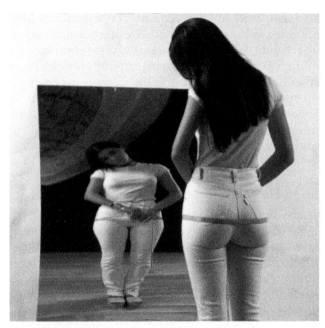

Figure 35-7
A person with anorexia nervosa has an intense and irrational fear of being overweight. Without treatment, many people with anorexia nervosa die. (© *Oscar Burriel/Photo Researchers, Inc.*)

CARING FOR A PERSON WITH MENTAL ILLNESS

You may choose to work in a facility that specializes in the care of people with mental illnesses. Treatment facilities for people with mental health disorders differ in purpose. Some facilities care for mentally ill people who cannot function on their own and need assistance with activities of daily living (ADLs) and safety. These facilities provide a form of long-term care specifically for people with mental illnesses. Other facilities specialize in acute care services. These facilities provide care to a person who is experiencing a mental crisis that may result in attempted suicide, drug overdose, or danger to others. After the crisis phase has passed, the person may be able to return home and receive treatment on an outpatient basis. Outpatient mental health clinics see people on a regular basis and offer services such as counselling, medication, and support groups. They may even help the person to obtain education, job training, or employment.

Even if you do not choose to work in a facility that specializes in the care of people with mental illnesses, it is likely that some of the patients or residents at the facility where you work will have

or develop mental illnesses. The additional stress of illness or injury that brings a person to a health care facility could become the person's "breaking point," causing a mild mental illness to worsen. Remember all the new challenges that your patients or residents face when they enter a health care facility. They may have fears of being disabled or disfigured from illness or injury. The people you care for have been separated from loved ones and are now in unfamiliar surroundings. A lengthy illness can mean the loss of a job and income. Many people will have worries related to their current and future health. Any of these additional emotional stresses can push a person toward mental illness if he has poor or ineffective coping mechanisms.

Many of the people cared for in health care facilities are elderly with mental health problems. Most elderly people have successfully lived through many struggles and stresses during their lives and have developed excellent abilities to cope. However, some of the unique losses and challenges that an elderly person faces may overwhelm the person emotionally and promote mental illness (Fig. 35-8). For example:

- Elderly people face the loss of spouses, friends, and sometimes even adult children. Often, an elderly person has to face the death of several loved ones within a short period of time.
- Elderly people face retirement. Although many people view retiring from a job as an event to be celebrated, some people miss the structure, routine, and sense of identity that their jobs gave them. Retirement also means that a person's income becomes fixed, which can lead to money worries.
- Elderly people face the loss of physical abilities and independence, either as a result of illness or the normal process of aging. As a result, many elderly people feel that they are a burden to their families. Others fear the need to move to a long-term care facility, because of the associated loss of independence.

LISTENING AND OBSERVING

Listening and observation skills are very important when you care for a person with mental illness. In some cases, your observations may lead to the diagnosis of a mental illness in one of your patients or residents. As noted earlier, the diagnosis and treatment of mental illness is very important. Not only might the person be suffering needlessly, she

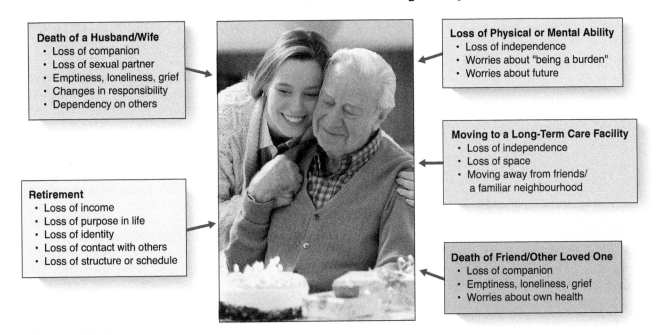

Death of a Husband/Wife
- Loss of companion
- Loss of sexual partner
- Emptiness, loneliness, grief
- Changes in responsibility
- Dependency on others

Loss of Physical or Mental Ability
- Loss of independence
- Worries about "being a burden"
- Worries about future

Retirement
- Loss of income
- Loss of purpose in life
- Loss of identity
- Loss of contact with others
- Loss of structure or schedule

Moving to a Long-Term Care Facility
- Loss of independence
- Loss of space
- Moving away from friends/
  a familiar neighbourhood

Death of Friend/Other Loved One
- Loss of companion
- Emptiness, loneliness, grief
- Worries about own health

Figure 35-8
As we age, we face very challenging life events. These additional stresses can put an elderly person at risk for clinical depression and other mental illnesses.

may be at high risk for committing suicide. The rate of suicide increases as a person ages and is highest among elderly white men, especially those who have lost their wives. Nearly 25% of all people who commit suicide are 65 years of age or older. As a personal support worker, you may hear a person speak of "ending it all," or the person may wonder aloud "if anyone would miss me if I were gone." Take comments like these seriously and tell the nurse immediately.

Sometimes a physical problem can cause a person to appear to be mentally ill. This is especially common in older people. Nervous system disorders, kidney disorders, and the effects of other chronic illnesses such as hypertension and diabetes may cause a person to seem depressed or anxious. The symptoms that accompany hypothyroidism and anemia are often mistaken for clinical depression. Early signs of dementia (see Chapter 36) can also be very similar to some types of mental illnesses. Infections, dehydration, and the side effects of many medications can also affect an elderly person's behaviour. When you notice a change in a patient's or resident's behaviour or mental status and report this change to the nurse, you are taking the first step toward making sure the person gets the help he needs. The health care team will work to determine the cause of the person's change in behaviour, which will lead to prompt treatment. Never assume that your elderly patient or resident is just "entering his second childhood" or becoming senile. The

person may have a serious mental or physical problem that needs to be treated.

If you work in a facility that specializes in caring for mentally ill people, special methods of recording and reporting may be used. Know what is expected of you and how to report and record according to facility policy. When reporting and recording subjective information about patients and residents with mental illnesses, be very careful to use the person's own words, and avoid adding your own opinions or judgments. This is especially important when caring for a person with mental illness because certain phrases or words may have special meaning for the person. To accurately gauge the person's mental status, the health care team will need to know exactly what the person said.

TELL THE NURSE

There are many signs and symptoms of mental illness. Sometimes a physical problem or a medication will make a person show signs of mental illness. As a personal support worker, you must know what types of behaviours and moods are "normal" for each patient or resident who is in your care. Watch for the subtle signs that something is not quite right and make sure to tell the nurse immediately if you notice any of the following in your patients or residents:

- Changes in appetite, such as eating too much, or not eating enough

- Changes in sleep patterns, such as sleeping too much, or not being able to sleep
- Restlessness, pacing, or unusual "handling" of objects such as bed linens
- An inability to concentrate
- Crying for long periods of time or crying frequently
- Loss of interest in daily activities that were previously enjoyed
- An inability to focus during a conversation, or an unwillingness to make conversation
- Fatigue or irritability
- Expressions of feelings of hopelessness or helplessness

ASSISTING WITH ACTIVITIES OF DAILY LIVING

Mental illness may affect a person's ability to eat, sleep, rest, or manage routine grooming and hygiene. People with mental illnesses will need different levels of assistance with their ADLs, depending on the severity of their disorders. As always, help to promote the person's independence by allowing the person to provide as much of his self-care as possible. Because some mental illnesses affect a person's ability to think through the steps of routine care, you may need to gently remind the person of what step comes next. For instance, you may need to say, "Okay, you're all dressed now . . . you just need to brush your teeth before we take our walk."

SUMMARY

- One of the main qualities of mental health is a state of emotional balance.
  - Life causes stress, which can threaten our ability to maintain emotional balance.
  - People who are mentally healthy are able to manage stress effectively. People who are mentally ill have trouble effectively coping with stress.
  - Coping mechanisms and defense mechanisms help us to deal with stress.
    - Coping mechanisms are actions that a person does deliberately to manage stress, such as going to an exercise class or engaging in a hobby.
    - Defense mechanisms occur when the mind attempts to restore or maintain emotional balance in response to stress. Defense mechanisms often occur automatically, without conscious effort.
- A mental illness is a disorder that affects a person's mind, causing the person to act in unusual ways, experience emotional difficulties, or both.
  - Mental illnesses may be temporary or permanent, and of varying severity.
  - Mental illnesses may be caused by genetics, chemical imbalances in the brain, or a person's environment.
  - Mental illnesses are typically treated using a combination of medication and psychiatric therapy.
  - Mental illness places a person at risk for committing suicide. Therefore, diagnosis

and treatment of mental illness is extremely important.
- Common mental illnesses include anxiety disorders, depression, bipolar disorder (manic depression), schizophrenia, and eating disorders.
  - Anxiety disorders are characterized by overwhelming feelings of uneasiness, dread, apprehension, or worry. Specific anxiety disorders include panic disorder, obsessive-compulsive disorder, and phobias.
  - Clinical depression is characterized by feelings of excessive sadness and hopelessness that do not go away with time.
  - Bipolar disorder (manic depression) is a mental illness that causes mood swings. The person's mood varies between periods of mania (extreme highs) and depression (extreme lows).
  - Schizophrenia is a mental illness that causes a person to have trouble determining what is real and what is imaginary. The person may have delusions and hallucinations.
  - Eating disorders such as anorexia nervosa and bulimia nervosa are characterized by serious (and potentially fatal) changes in eating behaviour, such as reducing the amount of food eaten to almost nothing, or severe overeating.
- Personal support workers care for people with varying degrees of mental illness in all types of health care settings.

- The additional stress of illness or injury that brings a person to a health care facility may trigger the onset of mental illness, or make an existing mental illness worse.
- The unique losses and challenges that face the elderly may trigger a mental illness. For example, clinical depression is very common among elderly people.
- By using their observation and listening skills, personal support workers are able to give the health care team important information about subtle changes in a person's behaviour or mood. These observations help to ensure that the person receives prompt treatment.
- Learning more about specific mental illnesses and special ways of caring for people with these illnesses enables the personal support worker to provide better care to affected patients and residents.

WHAT DID YOU LEARN?

Multiple Choice

Select the single best answer for each of the following questions.

1. Which physical sign or symptom can be caused by anxiety?
   a. Sleeplessness
   b. Fatigue
   c. Increased heart rate and blood pressure
   d. All of the above
2. What is depression?
   a. An overwhelming feeling of uneasiness, dread, apprehension, or worry
   b. An overwhelming feeling of sadness and hopelessness
   c. A sudden, overpowering fright
   d. Recurrent, unwanted thoughts
3. One of your residents insists that she is the Blessed Virgin Mary. What is your resident experiencing?
   a. A manic episode
   b. An hallucination
   c. A delusion
   d. A religious vision
4. You are caring for a resident who has schizophrenia. You know that when you are recording or reporting subjective information about this resident, you should:
   a. Report or record what the resident has said, using his own exact words
   b. Report or record your interpretation of what the resident has said, since the resident often says things that do not make much sense
   c. Report or record your own opinion about what the resident has said, in addition to reporting or recording the subjective information in the resident's own words
   d. Avoid reporting or recording any subjective information about this resident at all

5. One of your elderly residents, Mrs. Sigfried, has been acting strangely the past few days. She is refusing to eat, and she insists on sleeping all of the time. Why is it important for you to report your observations to the nurse immediately?
   a. Refusing to eat and extreme sleepiness are signs that death is approaching
   b. Mrs. Sigfried's change in behaviour could be caused by a physical or mental problem, and sharing your observations with the nurse will help Mrs. Sigfried to get the help she needs, sooner
   c. Mrs. Sigfried is in violation of facility policy
   d. Mrs. Siegfried is a danger to the other residents
6. One of your residents tells you that he hears voices inside his head, telling him to contact aliens on another planet. What is this resident experiencing?
   a. The effects of doing too many drugs in the 1970s
   b. Hallucinations
   c. Delusions
   d. Mania
7. Which one of the following is a negative way to manage stress?
   a. Smoking in moderation
   b. Taking an exercise class
   c. Taking a bubble bath
   d. Getting together with friends

Matching

Match each numbered item with its appropriate lettered description.

_E_ **1.** Panic disorder

_B_ **2.** Phobia

_D_ **3.** Obsessive-compulsive disorder

_C_ **4.** Schizophrenia

_G_ **5.** Bipolar disorder (manic depression)

_F_ **6.** Anorexia nervosa

_A_ **7.** Bulimia nervosa

a. An eating disorder characterized by eating excessive amounts of food, and then vomiting it up or taking laxatives to remove the food from the body before it can be digested

b. An anxiety disorder characterized by an extreme, abnormal fear of an object or situation

c. A mental illness characterized by an inability to tell what is real from what is imaginary

d. An anxiety disorder characterized by recurrent unwanted thoughts and rituals that the person cannot control

e. An anxiety disorder characterized by sudden increases in anxiety, often accompanied by physical signs and symptoms such as a rapid heartbeat and chest pain

f. An eating disorder characterized by an extremely reduced food intake

g. A mental illness characterized by mood swings, from extreme highs to extreme lows

STOP and Think!

Think about an elderly person whom you know well. What major life events has this person experienced in recent years? How did these events affect the person? What coping mechanisms did the person use to deal with the stress caused by these life events?

You work in a hospital. One patient on your floor is a 36-year-old woman named Anne who is receiving treatment and evaluation following her second failed suicide attempt. In your opinion, Anne has everything anyone could possibly want—a loving husband, two young children, and a comfortable lifestyle. You are finding it hard to understand why Anne wants to kill herself, and as a result, you are having a hard time feeling empathetic toward her. What are you forgetting?

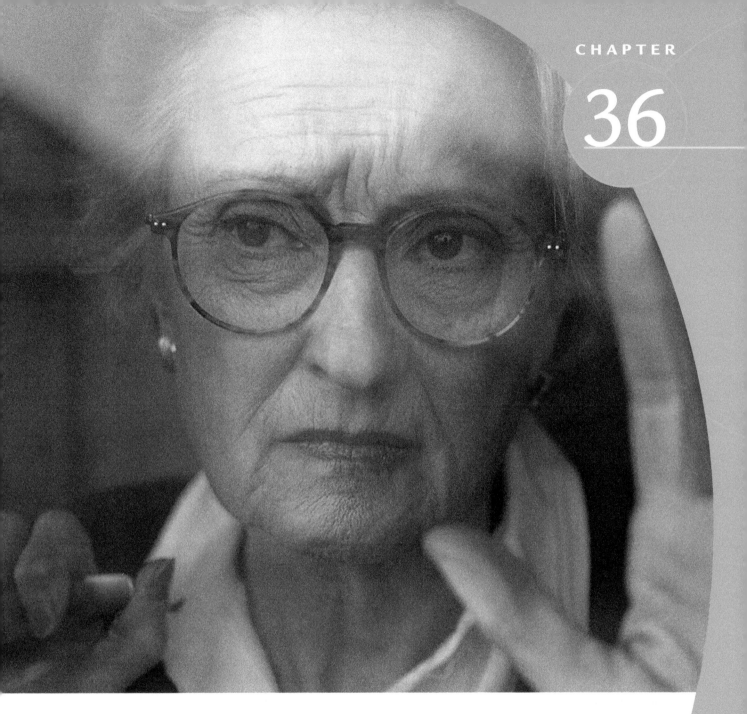

Caring for People With Dementia

WHAT WILL YOU LEARN?

Can you imagine what it would be like to know that there is something terribly wrong with your ability to remember or to think? For example, you are out to lunch with friends and when the check comes, you can't remember how to figure out the tip. Or you leave your house to go to the grocery store, a place you have been many times before, and you can't remember

Photo: Dementia robs a person of her identity and sense of self.
(© Benelux Press/Index Stock Imagery.)

how to get home. Or you can't remember the middle name of the person you have been married to for the past 40 years. For a person with dementia, a frightening experience like this is often the first sign that something is wrong. Dementia, which is caused by changes in the brain tissue, affects a person's ability to remember and think. As the disorder progresses, the person loses the ability to perform even the most basic tasks related to self-care. Dementia is devastating, both for the person who has it and for his or her family members.

More than 50% of the residents in long-term care facilities are there because they have dementia and are no longer able to care for themselves. In this chapter, you will learn about some of the types of dementia, and about the special care needs of people with dementia. When you are finished with this chapter, you will be able to:

1. Explain the difference between dementia and delirium.
2. Describe two major types and causes of dementia.
3. List and describe the stages of Alzheimer's disease, a common form of dementia.
4. Describe behaviours that are common in people with dementia.
5. Describe strategies for managing difficult behaviours in people with dementia.
6. Describe special considerations that the personal support worker must keep in mind while helping a person with dementia with activities of daily living (ADLs), such as bathing, eating, and toileting.
7. Describe special care measures that are taken to help maintain quality of life for a person with dementia.
8. Describe the effects of caring for a person with dementia on the caregiver, and strategies for coping.

Vocabulary

Dementia	Vascular (multi-infarct)	Catastrophic	Validation therapy
Delirium	dementia	reaction	Reminiscence
Alzheimer's disease	Perseveration	Sundowning	therapy

WHAT IS DEMENTIA?

Dementia is the permanent and progressive loss of the ability to think and remember, caused by damage to the brain tissue (Fig. 36-1). A person with dementia experiences the following:

- Problems with memory, especially short-term memory
- Difficulty putting thoughts together and understanding concepts
- Problems with judgment (the person is not able to make good decisions)
- Disorientation (the person is not oriented to person, place, or time)
- An inability to manage activities of daily living (ADLs)

In the early stages of dementia, the person is aware that his memory is lacking, and may take action to make up for, or cover, the memory loss. Disorientation becomes more evident as the disease progresses. The person may develop problems with language, and may act "out of character" or in socially inappropriate ways. The person loses the ability to recognize others and, eventually, the ability to remember his own identity. In the final stage of the disease, the person dies.

Dementia must not be confused with **delirium,** which is a temporary state of confusion. Delirium is a symptom of an underlying disorder, such as an infection. It may also be a side effect of medication. Once the underlying disorder is treated or the medication is stopped, the delirium goes away. In some cases, the person may die if the underlying cause of the delirium is not identified and treated.

TELL THE NURSE

As a personal support worker, you may be the first to notice changes in a resident's behaviour that may suggest delirium. If you notice any of the following in a person who is normally alert and oriented, report your observations to a nurse immediately:

- The person is hallucinating (seeing or hearing something that you know cannot possibly

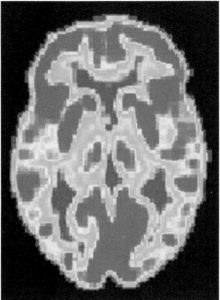
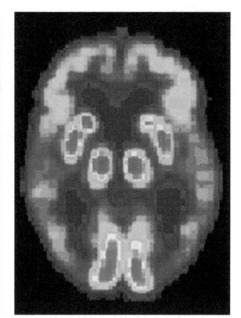

Figure 36-1
Dementia is the permanent and progressive loss of the ability to think and remember.
(A) Brain scan of a healthy person. **(B)** Brain scan of a person with Alzheimer's disease, the most common type of dementia. The blue areas indicate areas where brain activity is lost. (*Alzheimer's Disease Education Referral Center, a service of the National Institute on Aging.*)

A   B

be true, such as mice crawling all over the bed)

- The person does not recognize someone familiar, or mistakes a stranger for a family member or close friend

- The person is very restless, especially at night

- The person seems confused

- The person talks frequently about events from the past, but cannot remember events that occurred recently (such as a meal eaten 2 hours ago)

- The person gets lost and wanders the halls aimlessly, even though the person knows his or her way around the facility

TYPES OF DEMENTIA

There are many different types of dementia (Table 36-1). In a person with advanced dementia, it is usually hard to tell exactly what type of dementia the person has, because people with all types of dementia show similar behaviours and have similar disabilities in the late stages of the disease. In many cases, the type of dementia is not known for sure until after the person dies and an autopsy is done. Two of the most common types of dementia are Alzheimer's disease and vascular (multi-infarct) dementia.

ALZHEIMER'S DISEASE

Alzheimer's disease is the most common type of dementia, accounting for more than 50% of cases of dementia. Approximately 500,000 people in Canada have Alzheimer's disease. If no cure is found, it is estimated that around 1 to 1.3 million people will have the disease or a related dementia in 25 years.

Alzheimer's disease occurs in 10% of people older than 65 years, and nearly 50% of people older than 85 years. However, people as young as 40 years may also get the disease. Alzheimer's disease is the fourth most common cause of death, after heart disease, cancer, and stroke. However, a person can live anywhere from 3 to 20 years or more after the disease is diagnosed.

Alzheimer's disease is named after Alois Alzheimer (1864–1915), a German doctor who discovered the disease in 1906. One of Dr. Alzheimer's patients, a 51-year-old woman, died after showing unusual mental changes and behaviours. To learn why these changes occurred, Dr. Alzheimer performed an autopsy on her brain. He found that certain areas of her brain seemed soft and shrunken. In addition, he saw abnormal deposits of protein, especially in the parts of the brain that function in memory. He called these abnormal deposits *plaques* and *tangles* (Fig. 36-2).

Although we do not know exactly what causes Alzheimer's disease, researchers have a number of theories. One of the leading theories is that Alzheimer's disease can be caused by an

Table 36-1   Causes of Dementia

CAUSE	SOURCE OF DAMAGE TO BRAIN TISSUE	COURSE OF DISEASE
Alzheimer's disease	Plaques and tangles (abnormal protein deposits in brain)	Slow, steady decline; death occurs 3 to 20 or more years after diagnosis
Vascular (multi-infarct) dementia	Lack of blood flow to brain results in tissue death	Variable
Pick's disease	Atrophy (shrinking) of the neurons in the brain	Relatively rapid decline; death occurs within 4 years of diagnosis
Creutzfeldt-Jakob disease ("mad cow disease")	Viral infection of brain tissue	Rapid decline; death occurs within 2 years of diagnosis
Huntington's chorea	Genetic defect	Slow, steady decline; death occurs (on average) 25 years after diagnosis
Parkinson's disease*	Neurotransmitter (dopamine) deficiency	Slow, steady decline
AIDS dementia (HIV encephalopathy)	AIDS-related infections and tumours	Onset variable, but may be abrupt; decline is rapid
Syphilitic dementia	Infection with the bacterium *Treponema pallidum* (tertiary syphilis)	Onset occurs many years after the initial infection; decline is slow

*Only about 20% of people with Parkinson's disease develop dementia, and then only during the later stages of the disease.

abnormality in a person's genes. The abnormal gene causes the body to start producing the abnormal protein that forms plaques and tangles. The plaques and tangles interfere with the way that nerves inside of the brain communicate with each other. Another theory is that exposure to toxins, such as aluminum and mercury, may play a role in the development of Alzheimer's disease.

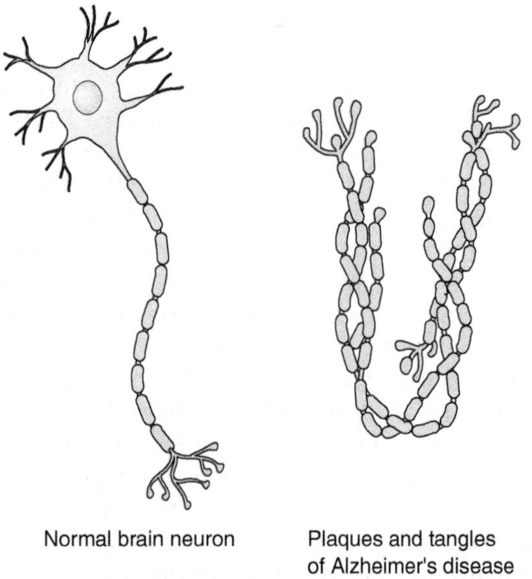

Normal brain neuron   Plaques and tangles of Alzheimer's disease

Figure 36-2
Protein deposits, called plaques and tangles, are found in the brains of people with Alzheimer's disease.

A person with Alzheimer's disease passes through three major stages (Box 36-1). Most people with Alzheimer's disease are cared for by family members during the early stages of the disease. However, as the disease progresses, many people with Alzheimer's disease must move to a long-term care facility because they become very difficult to care for. The person needs more and more assistance with basic activities, such as bathing and toileting. In addition, the disease can cause the person to behave in disruptive or annoying ways, which can place a great deal of emotional stress on the caregiver. The emotional pain suffered by a person with Alzheimer's disease, as well as her family members, is immeasurable (Fig. 36-3).

VASCULAR (MULTI-INFARCT) DEMENTIA

Damage to the blood vessels that supply the brain can affect the delivery of oxygen to the brain tissue, and may contribute to the onset of vascular (multi-infarct) dementia. In **vascular (multi-infarct) dementia,** mental functions are lost because multiple areas of the brain tissue die due to lack of adequate oxygen and nutrients. (An *infarction* is death of tissue due to lack of oxygen and nutrients.) Vascular dementia is thought to be the cause of dementia in approximately 20% to 25% of people with dementia.

Stages of Alzheimer's Disease

Mild Alzheimer's Disease

● The earliest sign of the disease is minor forgetfulness. For example, the person may forget where she has placed common objects, such as the car keys.

● Later, the person begins to have trouble doing complex tasks, especially in social settings or at work. Other people begin to notice that the person is having trouble with routine daily tasks, such as planning meals or managing money.

● The person's confusion increases, and she becomes less aware of current events.

● Because the person is aware of these changes, she may have feelings of fear, shame, anxiety, and depression. The person may avoid social activities. The person is at increased risk for suicide.

Moderate Alzheimer's Disease

● The person becomes disoriented to time and place.

● She needs help with dressing, but can usually manage eating and toileting without help. The person begins to forget the names of familiar people, such as a spouse or other family members.

● The person's personality may change, and she may begin to behave differently, often in challenging ways.

● The person eventually loses the ability to manage bathing and toileting independently, and she may become incontinent of urine and feces.

Advanced Alzheimer's Disease

● In the final stage of dementia, the person loses the ability to walk and sit independently. She is no longer able to speak, swallow, or smile. The person becomes totally incontinent of urine and feces.

● The person dies.

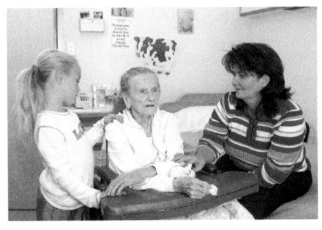

Figure 36-3
The emotional pain suffered by a person with dementia, as well as his or her family members, is immeasurable.

- Obesity
- Smoking
- High blood cholesterol levels

Symptoms may appear suddenly and they may vary from person to person, depending on which areas of the brain are affected. Like Alzheimer's disease, vascular dementia is irreversible and incurable. Keeping the person's blood pressure, blood glucose, and blood cholesterol levels within normal limits can help to slow the progression of the dementia.

BEHAVIOURS ASSOCIATED WITH DEMENTIA

People with dementia often show a wide range of behaviours, especially as the dementia progresses. Some of these behaviours can be dangerous for the person, such as the tendency to wander. Others are not dangerous, but they can be very annoying to caregivers or other residents. Many of these behaviours occur because of changes in the brain caused by the disease. When you are caring for a person with dementia, you will come to know the behaviours that are "normal" for that person. A change in a person's "normal" behaviour is a cause for concern. As the dementia progresses, the person loses the ability to communicate effectively. A change in the person's behaviour may be a sign that the person is trying to tell you something. For example, the person may have an acute physical problem, such as a bladder infection, pain, dehydration, or constipation.

Vascular dementia most often affects people between the ages of 55 and 75 years, most commonly occurring in people who are about 70 years old. It is more common in men than in women. Conditions that put a person at risk for developing vascular dementia include:

- A history of myocardial infarction (heart attack)
- Hypertension (high blood pressure)
- Diabetes mellitus
- Peripheral vascular disease
- Transient ischemic attacks (TIAs)

TYPES OF BEHAVIOURS

Common behaviours in people with dementia include the following.

Wandering

People with dementia may stray away from home. When this occurs, it is very dangerous because the person is confused and disoriented. The person might get lost, walk into the path of an oncoming car, or drown in a body of water, such as a lake or river. Depending on the weather and climate, the person may not be dressed appropriately to be outside. For example, if it is raining or cold, the person may not have a coat.

Because this tendency to wander cannot be stopped, many long-term care facilities have developed ways to allow residents to wander safely. Many facilities have outside courtyards with high fencing, which allow the resident to wander outside while still keeping her within the safe environment of the facility (Fig. 36-4). A resident who tends to wander may also wear a bracelet or an anklet that will set off an alarm if the resident tries to leave the facility through a doorway that leads to an unsafe area. When the alarm sounds, staff members are alerted and can guide the person back to safety.

Pacing

A person with dementia may pace back and forth. Often, the person is pacing because he has a physical need that is not being met. For example, the person may be hungry or need to use the bathroom. A person might also pace in response to a noisy, overstimulating environment, or because he is feeling scared or lost. If one of your residents is pacing, try to figure out what is causing the behaviour, and take steps to relieve the cause of the behaviour. Sometimes there is nothing to do but to let the person pace. In this case, you might take the person to a safe place (for example, a fenced-in garden) and walk alongside him until the behaviour has run its course.

Repetition

A person with dementia may do the same thing over and over again. This is called **perseveration.** For example, the person might repeat the same phrase or question constantly. Or she might constantly move a piece of cloth around on a coffee table, as if dusting. Although these behaviours are usually not physically harmful to the person, they can be a sign that the person is bored. These behaviours can also be annoying to caregivers and other residents. Distracting the person by offering to take her for a walk, or by getting her involved in an activity such as looking through a magazine, may help to break the cycle.

Rummaging

A person with dementia may go through drawers or closets, searching for an item that he is never able to find. If you notice that a resident is rummaging, ask the person what he is trying to find, and offer help in finding it. If the person tends to rummage through other residents' belongings or every single drawer in his own dresser, it may be necessary to make certain areas "off-limits" by locking them. You can then show the person a special drawer or a box filled with small personal items that he can rummage through.

Delusions and Hallucinations

A person with dementia may think that she is someone she is not, such as the Queen of England. Thoughts like these are called *delusions.* If one of your residents is delusional, do not try to correct the person. This will only upset her, because she honestly does believe that she is the Queen of England. It would be like someone telling you that you are not who you think you are! Instead, just try to redirect the conversation. For example, you might say, "Tell me about your day" or "Would you like to take a walk now?"

Hallucinations are also common in people with dementia. A *hallucination* is seeing, hearing,

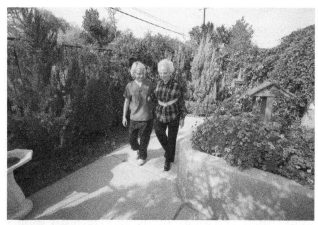

Figure 36-4
Wandering and pacing are two very common behaviours in people with dementia. Many long-term care facilities that specialize in the care of people with dementia have enclosed areas outdoors where people can wander and pace safely.

tasting, or smelling something that is not really there. For example, a person with dementia may tell you that there is a cat in the hallway or insects on the bed. If a person is hallucinating, reassure the person. For example, you might tell the person that you will ask the cat to leave, or go through the motion of sweeping the bugs off the bed. Then, gently redirect the person's attention.

Agitation

People with dementia often become very upset and excited. When a person with dementia is agitated, he may pace, shout, or strike out at caregivers or other residents. Remember that people with dementia often lose the ability to communicate effectively with others, so they express themselves through behaviour (Fig. 36-5). Many things can cause agitation, including pain or an infection, an unmet physical need (for example, hunger, a full bladder, or lack of sleep), or a noisy environment.

Catastrophic Reactions

A person with dementia may overreact to something that would cause a healthy person minimal or no stress. This is called a **catastrophic**

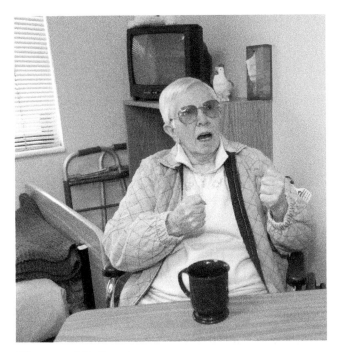

Figure 36-5
People with dementia often lose the ability to communicate effectively with others, so they express themselves through behaviour. Agitation is often a sign that a physical or emotional need is not being met.

reaction. For example, a person with dementia may become very agitated or begin to scream or sob loudly when you try to give him a bath. Catastrophic reactions often occur when the person feels threatened. For example, the person may feel that his privacy is being threatened when you attempt to give him a bath. Feeling overwhelmed can also cause a person to have a catastrophic reaction. For example, a ringing telephone in a room where the television is on and people are talking might be too much for a person with dementia to handle.

Sundowning

Sundowning is the worsening of a person's behavioural symptoms in the late afternoon and evening, as the sun goes down. For example, the person may become more agitated, restless, and confused in the evening hours, and may have trouble getting to sleep.

No one knows for sure exactly why sundowning behaviour occurs. Some people think that it might be brought on by fatigue, especially if the person frequently wanders, paces, or engages in other repetitive behaviour of a physical nature. Helping to ensure periods of quiet and rest during the day might help to reduce fatigue, in turn reducing sundowning. Another theory is that sundowning occurs because the person cannot see as well in the evening hours, when the sun starts to go down. Not being able to see well can increase the person's confusion and agitation. Turning on lights earlier in the evening may help to prevent or reduce sundowning behaviour.

Inappropriate Sexual Behaviours

A person with dementia may attempt to get into bed with a resident who is not her spouse. Sometimes the person will begin to masturbate or undress in a public area, such as the dining room. These behaviours occur because the person is disoriented to person, place, and time.

You must take measures to stop inappropriate sexual behaviours, especially if the person is making unwelcome sexual advances toward another person. Gently, but firmly, lead the person back to her room and redirect the person's attention by introducing another activity. Although a resident of a long-term care facility must be allowed to fulfill her sexual needs with another consenting resident, another resident with dementia is not able to give that consent. Therefore, you have a responsibility to protect all of the residents of the facility from unwelcome sexual advances.

BOX 36-2 **Situations That Can Cause Dementia-Related Behaviours**

- The person is in a room that is too large or too small.
- The person is in a room that is overstimulating (cluttered, noisy, or decorated with fabrics and wallpapers with "busy" patterns).
- The person is in a place that is new or unfamiliar (for example, the person is hospitalized for treatment of an acute problem).
- The person is being asked to do something that is too complicated, has too many steps, or is unfamiliar.
- The person is trying to express a physical or emotional need.

MANAGING DIFFICULT BEHAVIOURS

Many of the behaviours demonstrated by people with dementia can be difficult to deal with on an ongoing basis. Try to remember that the person with dementia does not want to act this way and cannot help it. He is not behaving this way to be difficult or annoying. Often, there is some physical or emotional reason for the behaviour (Box 36-2).

In many cases, finding the underlying cause of the behaviour and addressing it causes the behaviour to stop, providing relief to you and the person. Also, remember, in a person with dementia, a change in the person's behaviour might be the first and only sign of a medical problem. For example, a problem such as a urinary tract infection can cause a person with dementia who is normally pleasant and calm to become agitated and strike out at a caregiver. Therefore, it is important to try and determine the cause of the behaviour, rather than just accepting it as a normal part of the person's disease process.

When caring for a person with dementia who is demonstrating a particular behaviour, you must use your observation skills to try and answer the following questions:

- **What** is the behaviour? Describe the behaviour in as much detail as possible.
- **Whom** is the behaviour associated with? For example, does the person act this way only in the presence of certain people?
- **When** does the behaviour occur?
- **Where** does the behaviour occur?

Having answers to these questions can help you to answer the biggest question of all: "Why is the behaviour happening?" Once you have a few ideas about what is causing the behaviour, you can try doing different things to see if the person's behaviour improves. For example, if you suspect that the person is acting a certain way because she is hungry or needs to use the bathroom, you can try offering a snack or taking the person to the restroom. If you observe that the room is noisy and there is a lot of activity, you might try taking the person to a quieter place. If you suspect that the person is behaving in a certain way because he has a medical problem or is in pain, report your suspicions to the nurse so that the nurse can investigate further. Knowing your resident is the key to stopping (and sometimes preventing) difficult behaviours.

The way that you interact with a person with dementia can also affect the person's behaviour. Many years ago, caregivers used a technique called *reality orientation* with people with dementia. Reality orientation was based on the idea that it is important to bring the person back to the "here and now" by constantly orienting the person to time, place, people, and things. If the person was given enough information to stay on track, then he could be brought back to the present. We now know that although reality orientation is useful for people who are experiencing temporary confusion that is reversible and treatable (that is, delirium), it is not an effective technique to use with a person who has dementia. People with dementia often cannot remember what they have been told just a few minutes earlier. Because of this, attempting to orient the person to reality can embarrass the person and increase her irritation and agitation.

Now, caregivers use a technique called **validation therapy** with people with dementia (Table 36-2). Validation therapy stresses the importance of acknowledging the person's reality. Rather than correcting the person, you attempt to distract the person and redirect the conversation whenever possible. For example, you might change the course of the conversation by encouraging the person to talk about things from her past. Pay special attention to the words, phrases, and body language that the person uses, so that you can better understand what the person is trying to communicate. What the person is saying may seem like nonsense to you, but there may be important meaning behind the words. Validation therapy protects the feelings of the person with dementia. It also helps the caregiver to understand what the person with dementia is experiencing.

Table 36-2   Reality Orientation Versus Validation Therapy

EXAMPLE	REALITY ORIENTATION APPROACH	VALIDATION THERAPY APPROACH
Mrs. Rivera is trying to leave the facility. She is very agitated. She keeps repeating that she needs to go home to take care of her mother.	Personal support worker: "Don't you remember? Your mother died 20 years ago. You are staying here with us." Mrs. Rivera's agitation increases. She may continue to insist on going home, or begin to grieve her mother's death.	Personal support worker: "You want to go home to see your mother. Aren't mothers wonderful? Here, sit down and tell me about your mother." Mrs. Rivera is diverted from wanting to go home. She happily sits down with the personal support worker to discuss mothers.
Dr. Carroll, a retired family doctor, believes that he needs to leave the facility and go to the hospital to deliver babies and make rounds on his patients.	Personal support worker: "I'm sorry. Don't you remember that you are retired? You live here in the nursing home with us now. We can't let you leave because you might get lost or hurt." Dr. Carroll becomes agitated because what the personal support worker is saying does not match his current reality.	Personal support worker (leading Dr. Carroll to the nurse's station): "I bet we can find you a nurse who would love to have you make rounds with her and see the patients here." Dr. Carroll is diverted while still thinking that he has some value as a doctor.

CARING FOR A PERSON WITH DEMENTIA

As a person's dementia progresses, he will need more and more help with all activities of daily living (ADLs). In addition to physical needs, the person will have emotional needs that must be met as well. General guidelines for caring for a person with dementia are given in Guidelines Box 36-1.

MEETING THE PHYSICAL NEEDS OF A PERSON WITH DEMENTIA

For a person with dementia, everyday activities such as bathing, dressing, eating, and using the bathroom can be challenging. The person cannot remember how to do these things, and as a result, may become frustrated. Sometimes the person will resist doing what you need her to do.

When you are helping a person with dementia with her ADLs, there are several general things you can do to make the task go more smoothly:

- **Speak clearly, in a calm tone of voice.** Also, consider gently resting one of your hands on the person's arm or hand. Many people with dementia respond positively to touch (Fig. 36-6).
- **Remind the person at each step what she needs to do next.** The person may be able to complete tasks such as dressing, shaving, or brushing the teeth with your guidance.

Allowing a person to complete tasks independently for as long as possible is important for the person's self-esteem.

- **Use hand gestures in addition to spoken instructions.** For example, if you are trying to get the person to sit down at the table and eat, pat the seat of the chair as you ask the person to come sit down.
- **Plan for the procedure in advance.** "Getting ready" steps are always important, but especially so when you are caring for a person with dementia. Many routine procedures, such as bathing, are very stressful for a person with dementia. Being prepared and having everything you need before you begin a procedure will allow you to accomplish the task as quickly as

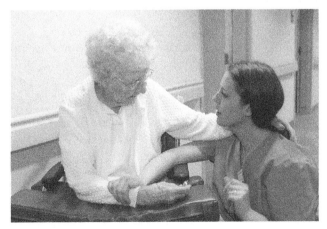

Figure 36-6
Many people with dementia respond well to touch.

Guidelines Box 36-1 Guidelines for Caring for a Person With Dementia

WHAT YOU DO	WHY YOU DO IT
Maintain a calm, structured environment.	A person with dementia can become overwhelmed very easily. When the person becomes overwhelmed, difficult or dangerous behaviours such as wandering, agitation, or a catastrophic reaction are likely to increase.
Approach the person with dementia slowly, announcing yourself before touching him.	Many people with dementia also have hearing problems, vision problems, or both. If you approach quickly without warning, you may startle the person, triggering a catastrophic reaction.
Avoid arguing or disagreeing with the person.	A person with dementia exists in a different reality from the rest of the world. Trying to force the person with dementia to understand or acknowledge anything other than her own reality will increase the person's agitation.
When asking a person with dementia to do something, use short words and short sentences. Avoid negatively worded instructions (such as, "Don't put that there!"). Avoid instructions that require the person to remember more than one action at a time.	Because a person with dementia has problems with short-term memory, he will not be able to remember or process long words and sentences. A positively worded command ("Please put that here") is easier to understand than a negative one. Failing at a task increases the person's frustration. When you give the person instructions in a way that she can understand, you increase the person's chances of successfully completing the task.
Give a person with dementia enough time to respond to questions and directions.	It may take the person a while to think of the word or words he needs to answer your question, or the actions he must take to follow your directions. Feeling rushed can cause the person to become agitated or upset.
"Listen" to the person by paying attention to body language. Make good use of your observation skills.	As a person's dementia gets worse, she loses the ability to communicate effectively. Often, body language and behaviours become the person's main way of expressing herself.
When managing difficult behaviours, be aware that solutions that work today may not work tomorrow. Be creative, and do not give up.	Dementia is a progressive disease. Therefore, the person's abilities, disabilities, and needs change over time, and your approaches to managing difficult behaviours may also need to change.
Help the person with dementia to feel secure and loved by showing affection (kind words, a gentle touch) and smiling.	Like all people, people with dementia have emotional needs that must be met.

Guidelines Box 36-1	Guidelines for Caring for a Person With Dementia (continued)
WHAT YOU DO	**WHY YOU DO IT**
Allow the person with dementia to do as much as he can for himself, for as long as possible.	This is important for maintaining the person's dignity and self-esteem. No one likes to feel helpless or useless.
Help the person to maintain independence for as long as possible by using visual cues to orient the person to place and time. For example, place a large-faced clock in the person's room, decorate for the holidays, and post names and other reminder signs in prominent, meaningful places. (For example, if a person keeps trying to walk out the front door, apply a big, red and white "stop" sign to the inside of the door.)	Using visual cues can help the person to maintain his independence longer, which is important for the person's self-esteem.
Help the person to exercise her mind by getting the person involved in activities that relate to the person's former interests and experiences.	Participating in activities helps to prevent boredom and increases the person's sense of purpose and accomplishment.
Protect the person from physical injury.	People with dementia often become clumsy as a result of their disease, which increases their risk of falling. In addition, they lose the ability to make good decisions related to their well-being. For example, a person with dementia might walk in front of an oncoming car, leave the house without a coat in the middle of a snowstorm, or drink the contents of a bottle found under the sink.
Maintain the person's hygiene and good grooming habits.	This is important for the person's health as well as for her self-esteem.
Be as tolerant as possible of the person.	The person's behaviours are a result of his dementia, and are beyond the person's control. The person is not purposely trying to frustrate or annoy you.
When you become tired and frustrated, take time out, be good to yourself, and share your feelings with the nurse. Know that these emotions and thoughts are normal.	Caring for a person with dementia is emotionally draining and physically difficult. If you do not take measures to protect your own mental health, you run the risk of "burn-out." In addition, you place the resident at risk for abuse, should you lose your temper.

possible, which can help to reduce the amount of stress the person feels.

- **Keep to a regular schedule.** A person with dementia responds best to a very structured environment. To a person with

dementia, the world is very confusing. Structuring the person's world as much as possible, by following an established routine, can reduce the person's confusion and fear.

Assisting With Bathing

Bath time can be a frightening time for a person with dementia. The person may not remember what a bath or shower is, or why he needs to take one. The sound of running water, the bright lights, and the shiny surfaces in the tub room can be upsetting. Being naked makes the person feel exposed and vulnerable. The person may be very afraid of falling.

As a result, the person may become agitated when you tell him that it is "time to take a bath." If this is the case, try to avoid the word "bath." Instead, say "Let's go freshen up" or "It's time for an activity you will enjoy." If the person seems very agitated, you might try singing to the person. Singing can have a very calming effect on people with dementia.

Bath time will generally go more smoothly if you prepare the tub room in advance. Make sure that the room is warm, and fill the tub ahead of time so that the person does not become frightened by the sound of the running water. Put a folded towel on the shower chair for comfort. Allow the person to wear his robe as long as possible, and consider draping a bath blanket or towel over the person's shoulders while he is bathing (Fig. 36-7). The bath blanket or towel will make the person feel less exposed and it will also provide some warmth. Hand the person a washcloth and let the person assist as much as possible.

Assisting With Dressing

Many people with dementia have trouble selecting an outfit to wear. They often want to wear the same clothes every day. Limiting the number of outfits the person has to choose from and asking family members to purchase several identical outfits for the person can help to solve these problems.

For a person with dementia, putting on and fastening clothing can also be difficult. To help make dressing less frustrating for the person, select articles of clothing that are simple, rather than complex. For example, a shirt that pulls over the head is easier to manage than a shirt that buttons up the front. Pants with elastic waistbands are easier to manage than pants with zippers and buttons.

Assisting With Eating

You might find that it is difficult to get a person with dementia to focus on eating at meal times. The person may forget why she is at the table, or become distracted by others at the table. A quiet setting and limited food choices can help. Many times, the person will not recognize eating utensils, or she will forget how to use them. You may have to remind the person how to eat by placing your hand over the person's hand. Together, you bring the fork or spoon with the bite of food to the person's mouth (Fig. 36-8). Make sure that the person is swallowing the food after chewing it. People with dementia often have a tendency to chew and then pack the food in the cheeks, increasing the risk of choking. If the person cannot focus long enough to eat a proper meal, try offering the person "finger foods" such as sandwiches, cut-up vegetables or fruit, or a stuffed baked potato. A plastic cup with a lid and a straw or a spout can help to ensure that the person drinks enough fluids.

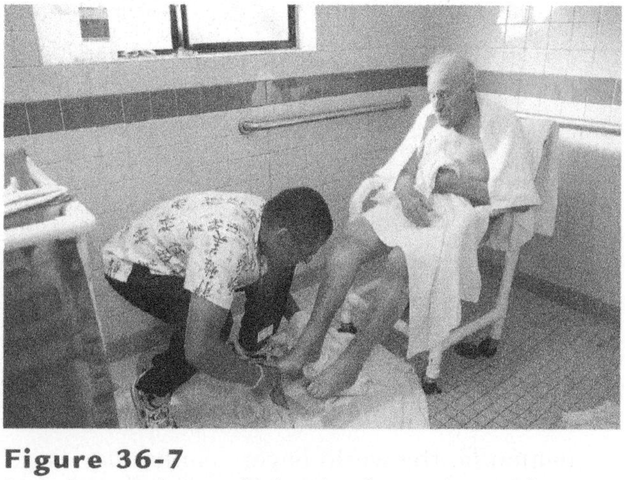

Figure 36-7
Bath time can be very frightening for a person with dementia. Making every effort to maintain the person's modesty is important.

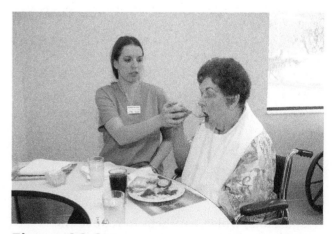

Figure 36-8
You may have to remind a person with dementia how to eat.

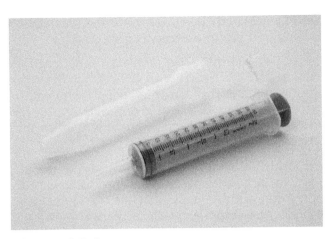

Figure 36-9
A feeding syringe is sometimes used instead of a spoon to feed people in the advanced stages of dementia.

People in the advanced stages of dementia eventually lose the ability to eat independently. When we eat, the tongue pushes the food to the back of the throat so that we can swallow it. People with advanced dementia often "forget" how to do this. Most of the food placed in the mouth of a person with advanced dementia just comes right back out again. Because a person with advanced dementia loses the ability to use his tongue to move food to the back of the throat, sometimes a special syringe with a nozzle-shaped tip is used for feeding instead of a spoon (Fig. 36-9). The food is semi-liquid and the syringe is used to place the food farther back in the mouth so that the person can swallow it more easily. The food is given slowly in small amounts to prevent choking. Using a feeding syringe may allow the person with advanced dementia to continue taking food by mouth for a longer period of time, instead of through a feeding tube. Feeding tubes can be very uncomfortable. Some facilities consider this feeding technique to be outside the personal support worker's scope of practice, so before using a syringe to feed a person, check with the nurse.

Assisting With Elimination

Elimination can present many problems for the person with dementia. The person may forget where the bathroom is, or fail to recognize the toilet. Sometimes, the person will have an accident because he is unable to move the necessary clothing out of the way fast enough. Taking the person to the bathroom on a regular schedule (for example, every 2 hours) can help, as can helping the person to select clothing with fasteners that are easy

to manage. If a person suddenly seems to be having a lot of accidents, report this to the nurse. The person may have a medical problem, such as a urinary tract infection, that needs to be addressed.

MEETING THE EMOTIONAL NEEDS OF A PERSON WITH DEMENTIA

Helping a person with dementia to meet his emotional needs is just as important as helping the person to meet his physical needs. Just like everyone else, a person with dementia needs to feel loved and needed. Several approaches are taken to help meet the emotional needs of a person with dementia.

Reminiscence Therapy

To *reminisce* means to remember. In **reminiscence therapy,** the person with dementia is encouraged to remember and share experiences from his past with others (Fig. 36-10). For example, if a person with dementia insists that she needs to go see her mother (who has been dead for years), you might say, "What does your mother look like?" or "Tell me about a favourite food that your mother used to make when you were growing up." Talking about

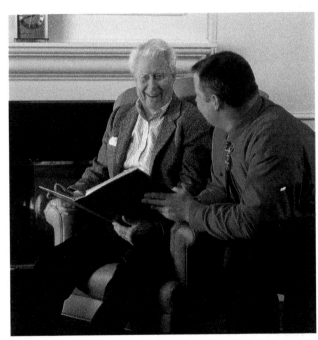

Figure 36-10
Reminiscence therapy increases a person's self-esteem and happiness by encouraging him to remember the past. (*Courtesy of Copper Ridge.*)

the past diverts the person's attention and increases her self-esteem. Reminiscence therapy can be used in a "one-on-one" setting, or in a group setting. When done in a group setting, reminiscence therapy gives the person a chance to socialize with other residents.

Activity Therapy

People with dementia, like all people, need to exercise their minds. Even though a person with dementia is confused, he still can become bored. In fact, boredom may be an underlying cause of some difficult behaviours, such as wandering or rummaging. Activities are so important to a resident's well-being that many facilities display a large calendar with daily planned activities on the wall (Fig. 36-11A). Engaging in activities helps the person to feel useful and gives him a sense of purpose and accomplishment.

Activities may be planned for a group of residents, or just for one resident (see Fig. 36-11B). There are many different types of activities that a person with dementia can enjoy:

- Creative activities (flower arranging, painting, baking)
- Intellectual activities (looking at a book of photographs, reading the newspaper aloud together, attending a play)
- Social activities (hosting a tea party, going on a picnic)

- Physical activities (taking a walk, participating in a group exercise class)

When planning an activity, take care to choose one that relates to the former interests and abilities of the person or people who will be participating in it. For a group activity, assign tasks according to each resident's abilities and interests. For example:

Debra, a personal support worker, works in a facility that specializes in providing care to people with dementia. Debra is responsible for planning one special activity a week for a group of residents. This week, she decides that she, Mr. Pitt, Mrs. Winger, and Mrs. Kemp will make fruit smoothies and then share them with some of the other residents. Debra knows that both Mrs. Winger and Mrs. Kemp used to enjoy baking for their families, so she asks Mrs. Winger to peel the bananas and Mrs. Kemp to measure the orange juice. Mr. Pitt worked for years as a bartender, so once all of the ingredients are in the blender, Debra asks Mr. Pitt to turn the blender on, and then to help her pour the drinks into cups to serve to the other residents.

Debra's activity was successful because she considered the special interests and talents of each of the residents who would be participating

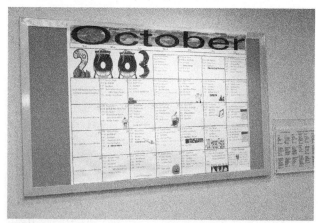

A

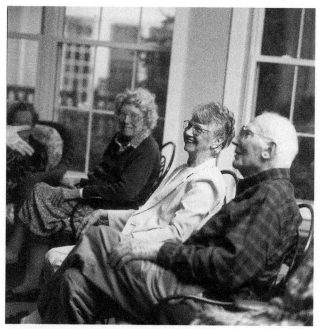

B

Figure 36-11
Activity therapy is an important part of caring for people with dementia. **(A)** Many facilities keep a large calendar so that residents can see the activities that are planned for each day. **(B)** Activities can be planned for an individual or for a group of residents. (**B,** *courtesy of Copper Ridge.*)

in it. Planning the activity in advance, gathering all necessary supplies, and having a back-up plan "just in case" are other things that a personal support worker can do to help ensure success when planning an activity for residents.

Music Therapy

Music can be very beneficial for people with dementia. Research has shown that when we listen to music we enjoy, our heart and respiratory rates slow, and our blood pressure becomes lower. In this way, music can calm an agitated person. Holiday music, religious music, or music from a certain time period (for example, 1940s big band music) may be particularly appealing to residents with dementia.

Pet Therapy

Spending time with companion animals, such as dogs and cats, can have many benefits for people with dementia (Fig. 36-12). The facility may participate in a visiting pet program, in which volunteers bring specially selected animals to the facility for a few hours each week to share with the residents. Or the facility may have a pet cat or dog that lives in the unit. A person with dementia may benefit from pet therapy in many different ways. The person may get pleasure simply by watching the animal. Some people may like to stroke the animal's fur, or sit with the animal in their laps. This can be very calming. Other people will benefit from pet therapy by remembering and talking about pets they had in the past.

EFFECTS ON THE CAREGIVER OF CARING FOR THE PERSON WITH DEMENTIA

Caring for people with dementia is very important work. The difference you make in the life of the person with dementia, as well as those of her family members, is significant. However, caring for a person with dementia can take its toll on you, physically and emotionally.

- A person with dementia is prone to outbursts of anger, and can become agitated very easily. Therefore, it is likely that on any given day, you may be cursed at, spit on, slapped, hit, scratched, or pinched. Because you will most likely develop a fondness for the

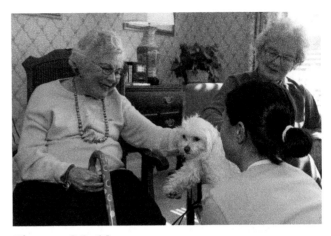

Figure 36-12
Pet therapy can improve the quality of life for many residents with dementia.

residents in your care, it can be very difficult when a resident has a "bad day" and that affection is not returned!

- Many of the behaviours of people with dementia can be very annoying, because they are repetitious. It is not always easy to figure out what you can do to make the behaviour stop, and until a solution is found, the behaviour can really try your patience.
- Caring for a person is hard physical work. As the dementia progresses, the person becomes completely dependent. Exhaustion and fatigue can put you on edge, making it difficult for you to keep your emotions in check.

If you feel yourself becoming overwhelmed by your responsibilities or a particular situation, take a deep breath and remind yourself that a person with dementia cannot be held responsible for her actions. If you still feel angry, make sure that the person is safe and walk away. Ask a co-worker or the nurse for help with the person. Sometimes you may need to ask to be assigned to another resident for a while. If your frustration or anger moves you to the point of actually causing a resident physical harm, you will lose your job (as well as all chances of future employment in the health care field). You may even be punished by a court of law for abuse. Remember, a member of the health care team is particularly at risk for becoming abusive when the resident is "difficult" or hard to manage, and the relationship is a long-term relationship. When you become tired and frustrated, take time out, be good to yourself, and share your feelings with the nurse. To provide the best care to your residents, you need to care for yourself.

SUMMARY

- Dementia is the permanent and progressive loss of the ability to think and remember, caused by damage to the brain tissue.
  - There are several types and causes of dementia. Two of the most common types are Alzheimer's disease and vascular (multi-infarct) dementia. Currently, there is no cure for dementia.
  - Dementia must not be confused with delirium, which is confusion in a person who is normally alert and oriented. Delirium goes away when the underlying cause is treated.
- A person with dementia often shows a wide range of behaviours, especially as the dementia progresses.
  - A change in a person's behaviour is often a sign that the person has a physical or emotional need that is not being met.
  - Personal support workers use their observation skills to try and figure out the underlying cause of the person's behaviour. If the cause can be determined,

then actions can be taken to stop the behaviour.
- The way that you interact with a person with dementia can affect the person's behaviour. Try to understand what is "real" for the person with dementia, and do not try to correct the person. This technique of communicating is called *validation therapy.*
- A person with dementia has physical and emotional needs that must be met.
  - As the person's dementia gets worse, he needs more and more help with activities such as eating, bathing, dressing, and toileting.
  - Reminiscence therapy, activity therapy, music therapy, and pet therapy are used to help meet the emotional needs of the person with dementia.
  - Caring for a person with dementia is very demanding, yet very important, work. Dementia is a terrible disease that is devastating both to the person who has it, as well as his family members.

WHAT DID YOU LEARN?

Multiple Choice

Select the single best answer for each of the following questions.

1. Which one of the following is experienced by a person with dementia?
   a. Problems with memory, especially short-term memory
   b. Confusion and disorientation
   c. An inability to manage activities of daily living (ADLs)
   d. All of the above
2. When caring for a person with dementia, it is helpful to:
   a. Be understanding and see the person's behaviours as part of the disease
   b. Take the same approach with every resident
   c. Correct the person to bring him or her back to the "here and now"
   d. Avoid acknowledging your own feelings
3. When communicating with a person with dementia, what is the best approach to take?
   a. Speak loudly and quickly to get the person's attention

   b. Speak clearly, in a calm tone of voice
   c. Avoid touching the person or using hand gestures
   d. Avoid talking about the past
4. Which statement about validation therapy is true?
   a. Validation therapy stresses the importance of bringing the person with dementia back to the "here and now."
   b. Validation therapy is based on the belief that people with dementia are able to return to the present, if given enough information to do so.
   c. Validation therapy stresses the importance of acknowledging the person's reality.
   d. Validation therapy encourages the caregiver to correct the person, to help the person to stay on track.
5. A person with dementia may show which one of the following behaviours?

a. Pacing and wandering
b. Hallucinations
c. Agitation
d. All of the above

6. Which statement about reality orientation is true?
   a. Reality orientation helps a person with dementia to remember the past, which might be less painful than thinking about the "here and now."
   b. Reality orientation suggests that when we interact with someone with dementia, we pay special attention to the words, phrases, and statements that the person uses to understand what the person is trying to express.
   c. Reality orientation ties past memories to the present and helps bring the person back to the current time.
   d. Reality orientation is useful for people who are temporarily confused but not permanently impaired.

7. What is sundowning?
   a. Increased confusion, restlessness, and insecurity that occurs late in the day, as it becomes darker outside
   b. Aimless wandering after dark
   c. Worry and increased suspicion
   d. Crying inconsolably for a long time

8. Mr. Greene, one of the residents in your care, has Alzheimer's disease. For the past hour, Mr. Greene has been folding and unfolding a piece of paper, and he is showing no signs of stopping. What should you do?

   a. Let him keep doing it; perseveration is a normal behaviour in a person with dementia.
   b. Try to distract Mr. Greene by starting a new activity with him, such as reading the newspaper together or going for a walk.
   c. Tell the nurse; she will be able to give Mr. Greene a sedative to make the behaviour stop.
   d. Tell Mr. Greene firmly that the behaviour is unacceptable and it must stop, immediately.

9. What is a catastrophic reaction?
   a. A response to a situation that is more extreme than would normally be expected
   b. An abnormal protein deposit that is found in the brains of people with Alzheimer's disease
   c. The belief that you are someone you are not (for example, the Queen of England)
   d. The reaction family members have on learning that a loved one has Alzheimer's disease

10. When helping a person with dementia with her activities of daily living (ADLs), such as bathing, eating, and dressing, what should you remember?
    a. Keep to an established routine as much as possible
    b. Prepare for the procedure ahead of time
    c. Many ADLs are very frightening or frustrating for the person with dementia
    d. All of the above

STOP and Think!

You work in the dementia unit of a long-term care facility. Mrs. Darden, one of the residents you are responsible for, needs a great deal of help with all of her activities of daily living (ADLs). Lately, Mrs. Darden has started having a catastrophic reaction every time you help her to bathe. What are some things you could do to make bathing easier and less frightening for Mrs. Darden?

You work in a long-term care facility. One day, you go to the room of one of your residents, Mrs. Craven, to answer her call light. When you enter the room, Mrs. Craven cries out to you in a frightened voice, "Get them out of here! Get them out of here now!" You don't know what she is talking about—you don't see anybody or anything

in the room. You ask Mrs. Craven to explain what she means, and she tells you that there are spiders crawling all over the walls. Normally, Mrs. Craven is alert and oriented, but today, she definitely seems "out of it." What do you think is wrong with Mrs. Craven? What should you do?

Mrs. Rowan has Alzheimer's disease. You have cared for Mrs. Rowan for a long time and know pretty much what to expect from her in terms of behaviour. Although she does tend to pace and to rummage quite frequently, she is usually calm and pleasant. Today in the dining room, however, when you are trying to help Mrs. Rowan eat lunch, she becomes angry and strikes out at you. What might be the explanation for this behaviour?

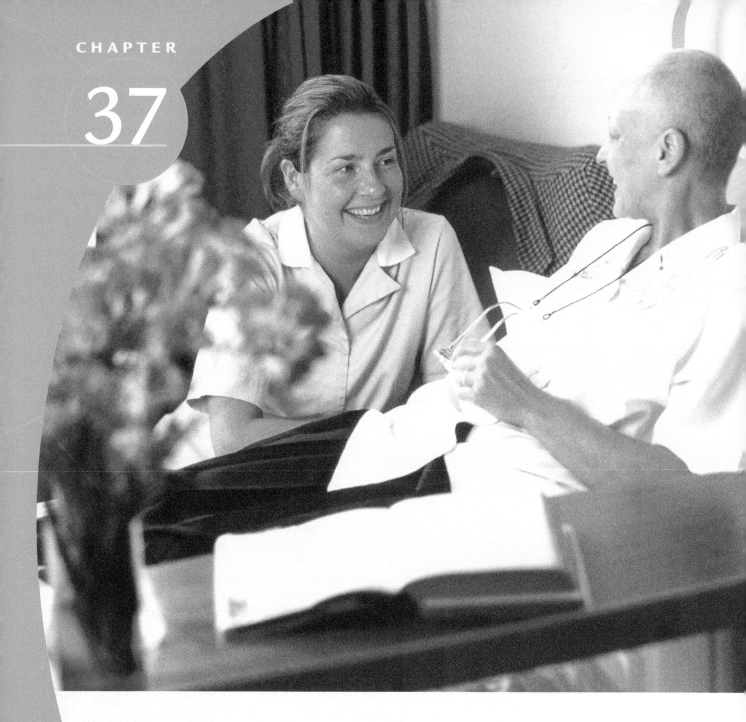

Caring for People With Cancer

What WILL YOU LEARN?

Cancer is the second leading cause of death in the Canada. Only heart disease kills more people in this country each year. However, it is important to remember that many people who are diagnosed with cancer survive it, especially when the cancer is diagnosed and

Photo: A personal support worker talks with a patient who is receiving chemotherapy to treat cancer. A common side effect of chemotherapy is hair loss.
(© Colin Cuthbert/Photo Researchers, Inc.)

treated early. As a personal support worker, you will play an important role in making sure that changes in a patient or resident that might be early signs of cancer are reported to the nurse promptly. In addition, you will care for people who have already been diagnosed with cancer and are receiving treatment for it, or who are waiting to find out if they have cancer. In this chapter, you will learn more about cancer, how it is diagnosed, and how it is treated. You will also learn about the special physical and emotional needs of people with cancer. When you are finished with this chapter, you will be able to:

1. Describe the difference between benign and malignant tumours.
2. List the common causes of cancer.
3. Describe the warning signs of cancer.
4. List some common types of cancer.
5. Describe how early detection and treatment affect the outcome of a cancer diagnosis.
6. List and explain the types of treatment used for people with cancer.
7. Describe some of the side effects of cancer treatment, and discuss how a personal support worker can help a person who is experiencing these side effects feel more comfortable.
8. Discuss how cancer affects a person emotionally.

Vocabulary

Tumour	Metastasis	Chemotherapy	Stomatitis
Benign	Biopsy	Radiation therapy	Prognosis
Malignant			

WHAT IS CANCER?

The word *cancer* comes from the Greek word *karkinos,* or "crab." Indeed, cancers are "crab-like," with a central body and arms that reach out into the surrounding tissues (Fig. 37-1). The central body is a mass of abnormal cells, called a tumour. A **tumour** is simply an abnormal growth of tissue. Not all tumours are necessarily cancer.

Tumours that are not cancerous are called benign. (*Benign* means "kind.") A **benign** tumour is made up of abnormal cells that tend to stay

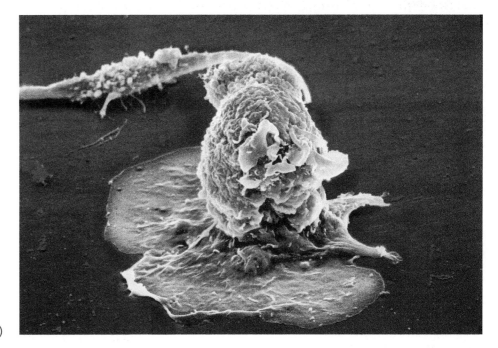

Figure 37-1
Cancerous tumours have the ability to send crab-like arms of cancerous cells into the surrounding tissue. This is a scanning electron micrograph (SEM) of a breast cancer cell. Colour has been added to the photograph to make the cancer cell stand out. (© *Biophoto Associates/Photo Researchers, Inc.*)

together, without spreading into surrounding tissues. In addition, benign tumours tend to grow slowly, because their cells do not divide rapidly. Many benign tumours are easily treated, because they are slow growing and their cells tend to stay together. However, an untreated benign tumour can enlarge and press on vital organs, which can cause serious problems (or even death), depending on the organs that are affected.

Cancerous tumours are called malignant. (*Malignant* means "evil.") A **malignant** tumour is made up of abnormal cells that do not function properly. Malignant cells divide rapidly and invade nearby healthy tissue. Malignant cells can also travel through the bloodstream to other parts of the body, where they "take root" and start a new cancerous tumour. The process by which cancer cells spread from their original location in the body to a new location (which may be quite distant from the first) is called **metastasis** (Fig. 37-2). Death from cancer almost always results from metastasis. The cancer simply takes over the body.

TYPES OF CANCER

It is estimated that 200 different types of cancer can affect the human body. All organ systems can be affected by cancer. Some cancers are very rare, while others are quite common. Common cancers that you may have heard of include skin cancer, lung cancer, breast cancer, brain cancer, colon cancer, ovarian cancer, prostate cancer, leukemia, and lymphoma. Cancer can occur at any age, but 67% of cancer deaths occur in people older than 65 years. The most common cancers seen in elderly people are breast, lung, prostate, and colon cancers.

CAUSES OF CANCER

There has been much research into what causes cancer and why some people get cancer and others do not. At present, the exact cause of cancer is still unknown. Currently, researchers believe that whether or not a person develops cancer may be related to a combination of many factors, including:

- **Inheritance.** Some cancers seem to "run in families." For example, a woman with a mother or sister who has had breast cancer is more likely to develop breast cancer herself. This suggests that genetics may play a role in whether or not a person develops cancer.
- **Environmental factors.** What we are exposed to on a daily basis also seems to play a role in the development of cancer. For example, a person who smokes or spends a

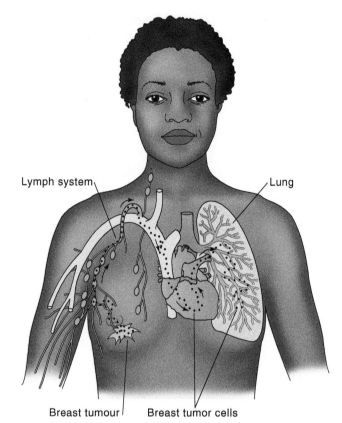

Figure 37-2
Metastasis is the process by which malignant cells spread to other parts of the body, or metastasize. A common example of metastasis is when a woman with breast cancer also develops lung cancer. First, the malignant cells of the breast tissue gain access to the lymphatic system, which empties into the bloodstream. The malignant cells are pumped, along with the blood, through the right side of the heart. Some of the malignant cells are deposited in the tiny blood vessels in the lungs, where they begin to multiply and grow, forming a new tumour.

lot of time around people who smoke is more likely to develop lung cancer than a person who is not exposed to tobacco smoke. Some people work in jobs or live in places that expose them to cancer-causing agents (*carcinogens*), such as radiation, asbestos, chemicals, and pollution.
- **Lifestyle.** Factors such as a person's diet and the amount of time he or she spends exercising have been shown to play a role in the person's risk for developing cancer. For example, diets that contain lots of fruit and vegetables are known to lower a person's risk for many cancers, while diets that are high in fat increase a person's risk for some cancers. Similarly, exercising on a regular basis can lower a person's risk for developing cancer, while not exercising can increase the person's cancer risk.

The Canadian Cancer Society (CCS) reports that approximately one third of the deaths caused by cancer in Canada are the result of smoking, and another third are related to dietary habits. Eating a healthy diet, exercising, and avoiding smoking and job-related carcinogens are important steps that people can take to lower their risk of developing cancer.

DETECTION OF CANCER

Early detection of cancer can lead to early treatment, which greatly improves a person's chances of surviving the disease. Many cancers are caught in their early stages when a person notices signs and symptoms and reports them to a health care provider. For example, a person may feel an odd lump, or notice blood in the stool. Other cancers are caught in their early stages through routine physical examinations and screening tests.

WARNING SIGNS OF CANCER

Our bodies are good at letting us know when something is not quite right. A person who has cancer may experience one or more of the following early warning signs. These warning signs can be remembered by thinking of the word *CAUTIONS*:

Change in bowel or bladder habits. A person with colon cancer may have diarrhea or constipation, or he may notice that the stool has become smaller in diameter.

A person with bladder or kidney cancer may have urinary frequency and urgency.

A sore that does not heal. Small, scaly patches on the skin that bleed or do not heal may be a sign of skin cancer. A sore in the mouth that does not heal can indicate oral cancer.

Unusual bleeding or discharge. Blood in the stool is often the first sign of colon cancer. Similarly, blood in the urine is usually the first sign of bladder or kidney cancer. Postmenopausal bleeding (bleeding after menopause) may be a sign of uterine cancer.

Thickenings or lumps. Enlargement of the lymph nodes or glands (such as the thyroid gland) can be an early sign of cancer. Breast and testicular cancers may also present as a lump.

Indigestion or difficulty in swallowing. Cancers of the digestive system, including those of the esophagus, stomach, pancreas, and biliary system, may cause indigestion, heartburn, or difficulty swallowing.

Obvious change in a wart or mole. Moles or other skin lesions that change in shape, size, or colour should be reported (Fig. 37-3).

Nagging or persistent cough or hoarseness. Cancers of the respiratory tract, including lung cancer and laryngeal cancer, may cause a cough that does not go away or a hoarse (rough) voice.

Sudden, unexplained weight loss. Loss of a significant amount of weight (for example, about 22 kg) without trying may be an early sign of cancer.

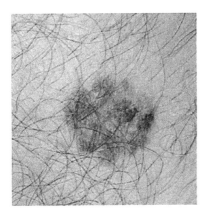 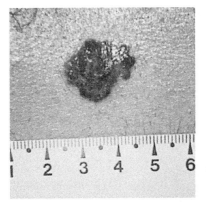 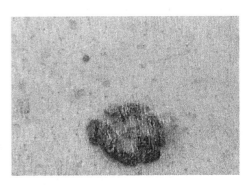

Figure 37-3

Moles that change in appearance or bleed, have jagged borders, display two or more colours (for example, brown, black, pink, grey, or white), or are larger than a pencil eraser may be malignant melanoma. Malignant melanoma is the most lethal type of skin cancer, accounting for 4% of deaths from cancer overall. (*Photographs courtesy of Goodheart, H. P. [2003]. Goodheart's photoguide of common skin disorders: Diagnosis and management [pp. 325, 354]. Philadelphia: Lippincott Williams & Wilkins.*)

Unfortunately, many people recognize these early warning signs of cancer but put off making an appointment with a health care provider because they are embarrassed or scared. As a personal support worker, you may be the first to notice that a patient or resident has an early warning sign of cancer. Reporting your concerns to the nurse immediately can lead to early detection and treatment. Early detection and treatment play a very important role in preventing deaths due to cancer.

ROUTINE PHYSICAL EXAMINATIONS AND SCREENING TESTS

Many cancers are detected during routine physical examinations, or by screening tests that are done on a regular basis. Examples of screening tests include mammograms (used to detect breast cancer), Pap smears (used to detect cervical cancer), and fecal occult blood tests (used to detect colon cancer). These tests can help to detect cancer long before the person develops noticeable signs or symptoms of the disease. The early detection of cancer allows the tumour to be removed before it has time to spread (metastasize) to nearby tissues or other organs.

If physical examination or screening tests reveal that a person might have cancer, the doctor may order additional studies or exploratory surgery (surgery that is performed when a person is thought to have a significant medical problem but the doctors do not know the extent of the problem or what is causing it). As a personal support worker, you may need to help prepare a patient or resident for surgery or other diagnostic tests that will be performed to determine if cancer is present. Examples of additional studies that may be ordered for a person who might have cancer include the following (Fig. 37-4):

- *Imaging studies,* such as x-rays, computed tomography (CT) scans, and magnetic resonance imaging (MRI) scans, allow the doctor to see the tumour without actually entering the body (see Fig. 37-4A).
- *Endoscopic studies* involve using a special lighted instrument to look inside the body

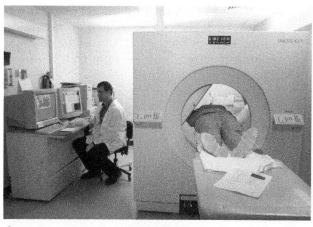

A

B

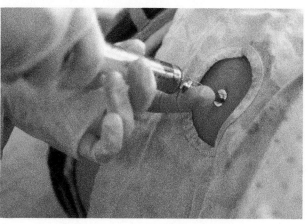

C

Figure 37-4
As a personal support worker, you may need to help prepare a patient or resident for studies that are done to diagnose cancer. **(A)** Radiologic imaging studies, such as magnetic resonance imaging (MRI) scans, allow the doctor to see the tumour without actually entering the person's body. **(B)** Endoscopic studies, such as colonoscopy, involve passing a lighted instrument through an opening in the body to view the inside of a structure. **(C)** In a needle biopsy, cells are removed from the body so that they can be examined under a microscope for abnormalities. Here, a surgeon is performing a needle biopsy to check for breast cancer. (*A,* © R. Gould/Custom Medical Stock Photo; *B,* © Antonia Reeve/Photo Researchers, Inc.; *C,* © Daiwei/Custom Medical Stock Photo.)

and obtain tissue or fluids for analysis (see Fig. 37-4B). Examples of endoscopic studies that you read about in Unit 5 include bronchoscopy (when a scope is passed into the lungs through the mouth), gastroscopy (when a scope is passed into the stomach through the mouth), and colonoscopy (when a scope is passed into the large intestine through the anus).

- **Biopsy** is the surgical removal of cells or a small piece of tissue for microscopic examination (see Fig. 37-4C). Biopsy is done to determine if cells are cancerous, and to determine exactly what type of cancer is present.

TREATMENT OF CANCER

There are three main approaches to treating cancer (Fig. 37-5). The approach used depends on the type of cancer and the extent to which the cancer has spread to other tissues and organs. Treatment methods may be used alone or in combination with each other, depending on the type and extent of the cancer.

- **Surgery** involves cutting away the tumour and surrounding tissue to remove the cancer and stop the spread of the disease (see Fig. 37-5A). Many cancer surgeries change the person's physical appearance significantly. For example, a woman with breast cancer may lose one or both breasts. A person with bone cancer may lose all or part of an arm or leg. A person with colon cancer may need to use an ostomy appliance for the rest of his life. Although it is a relief to have the cancer gone, the person must still deal emotionally with the change in his or her appearance.
- **Chemotherapy** involves the use of medications (chemical agents) to destroy the cancer cells (see Fig. 37-5B). There are many different chemotherapy drugs available now, each for specific types of cancer. Chemotherapy is often used in combination with surgery to help destroy any malignant cells that the surgery may not have removed completely. Alopecia (the loss of hair) may accompany chemotherapy. Chemotherapy works by killing cells that divide rapidly,

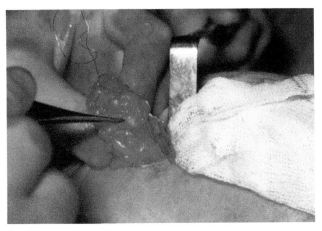

A

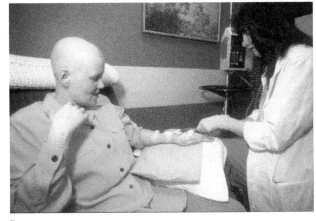

B

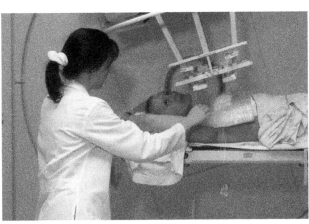

C

Figure 37-5
The three main approaches to treating cancer are **(A)** surgery, **(B)** chemotherapy, and **(C)** radiation therapy. Doctors may choose to use these methods alone or in combination, depending on the type and extent of the cancer. (*A,* © *St. Bartholomew's Hospital/Photo Researchers, Inc.; B and C,* © *Bradford/Custom Medical Stock Photo.*)

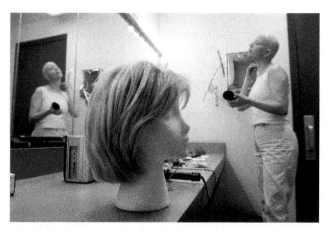

Figure 37-6
Hair loss (alopecia) is a common side effect of cancer chemotherapy. Many people who have lost their hair temporarily as a result of chemotherapy find that wearing a wig, hat, or scarf helps them to feel more confident about their appearance. (© *AP Photo/Eric Gay*)

such as cancer cells. Unfortunately, some types of normal cells in the body also divide rapidly, such as the cells in the hair follicles. This is why people who are receiving chemotherapy often lose their hair. Many people, especially women, may be very self-conscious about their hair loss. These people may find that wearing a wig, hat, or scarf helps them to feel more confident about their appearance (Fig. 37-6).

- **Radiation therapy** involves the use of powerful x-ray beams to destroy the cancer cells (see Fig. 37-5C). The beams are directed at the tumour to destroy the cells. Sometimes tiny pellets that contain radiation are placed inside the tumour so that the cells are destroyed from the inside. This is a common method of treating prostate cancer—radioactive pellets are placed inside the prostate gland with a needle-like instrument to destroy the cancerous cells.

Surgery, chemotherapy, and radiation may be either *curative* or *palliative*. When a treatment is performed with the goal of curing the person of cancer by completely removing the cancerous cells from the body, the treatment is said to be *curative*. However, sometimes the cancer cannot be cured. When this is the case, the goal of treatment is to make the person as comfortable as possible until death occurs. This sort of treatment is referred to as *palliative* (see Chapter 21, Fig. 21-9). Examples of palliative cancer treatments include surgery to bypass an obstruction

caused by a tumour and chemotherapy or radiation to shrink a large tumour that is pressing on an organ and causing pain.

Helping Hands and a Caring Heart

FOCUS ON HUMANISTIC HEALTH CARE

A person who has cancer may need to decide among several different treatment options. Sometimes, the person will have to decide whether she even wants to go ahead with treatment. Some people may choose to have every type of treatment available. Others may choose to skip treatment, even if it means a chance for longer survival. You must always remember that each patient or resident has the right to choose. The reasons behind treatment choices are unique and specific for each individual person. Although one choice may be right for one person, a different choice will be the right one for another. To truly provide humanistic care to a person with cancer, you must respect the person's decisions and choices concerning treatment. You do not have to necessarily agree with your patients' or residents' choices, but you must respect what they have decided to do. Use your listening skills to show the person that you care. Allow the person to verbalize his fears and feelings without adding your own opinion as to whether you think the person is doing the right thing or not. When you respect the decisions of the people you provide care for and support them emotionally, you demonstrate true compassion and caring.

CARING FOR A PERSON WITH CANCER

Many of us know someone who has had cancer. In fact, the experience of losing someone to cancer, or of witnessing someone's recovery from cancer, may be what inspired you to become a personal support worker in the first place. Like all patients and residents, those with cancer have special physical and emotional needs that must be met.

MEETING THE PHYSICAL NEEDS OF A PERSON WITH CANCER

People with cancer have special physical needs that are directly related to the cancer, the treatment, or both. Cancer can be very painful. The pain may be temporary, related to surgery or radiation treatment. Or it may be chronic, related to the cancer itself. In addition, many of the treatments used for cancer have unpleasant side effects. As a personal support worker, you will play an important role in helping your patients or residents who have cancer to manage their pain and deal with the unpleasant side effects of treatment.

Managing Pain

Pain control is an essential part of the treatment for a person with cancer. Advanced cancerous tumours often cause severe pain that can only be relieved by the regular use of strong pain medications. Report any observations that suggest that a patient or resident is in pain, or any complaints that the person may have of pain, to a nurse promptly. (See Chapter 29 for a complete discussion of pain, and the personal support worker's role in detecting it and helping to control it.) As a personal support worker, you will also need to be aware of and look for side effects of pain medication, such as constipation. The discomfort from the constipation alone may be as bad as the tumour pain. Recall what you learned in Chapter 20 about the measures you can take to help prevent your patients or residents from becoming constipated. And if one of your patients or residents does become constipated, please report this to the nurse immediately.

Managing Side Effects of Treatment

The treatments used for cancer, especially chemotherapy and radiation therapy, may have severe side effects:

- **Digestive problems.** Nausea, vomiting, anorexia (loss of appetite), and diarrhea are common with chemotherapy and radiation treatments. Patients or residents who are having digestive problems as a result of cancer treatment will appreciate frequent mouth care. In addition, you can offer ice chips to prevent the person from becoming dehydrated. Many people are able to tolerate ice chips when nothing else will stay down. If a person is able to tolerate some foods or liquids and has an appetite for something special, try to accommodate the person's request.
- **Skin problems.** People who are receiving radiation therapy may develop irritation and burning where the skin is exposed to the treatment rays. Skin breakdown can be prevented with gentle, thorough skin care.
- **Mouth problems.** People who are having chemotherapy may develop **stomatitis** (inflammation of the mouth). Sores in the mouth may be very painful and cause

discomfort during eating. Offering the person drinks that are blended with ice, ice cream, yogurt, and fruit may be very soothing and provide much-needed nutrition at the same time. Frequent, gentle oral care is necessary to prevent infection. A special mouthwash or spray may be used to numb the inside of the person's mouth before providing oral care.

- **Fatigue.** People who are receiving cancer treatment may be very tired, all of the time. Mild exercise combined with periods of rest is necessary to maintain muscle strength.
- **Increased risk for infection.** Some cancer treatments temporarily interfere with the body's ability to fight off infections. People who are having these treatments will be at high risk for getting contagious illnesses, such as colds or the flu. In addition, if they do get a cold or the flu, it could turn into something more serious, such as pneumonia. For this reason, you must be very careful to protect patients or residents with lowered immunity from contact with other people who have a contagious illness.

TELL THE NURSE

When caring for a person who has cancer, be sure to report any of the following observations to the nurse immediately:

- The person has severe nausea, vomiting, or both
- The person has pain or sores in the mouth
- The person's skin is red or irritated in areas
- The person has an unusual discharge or bleeding from the vagina, urethra, or rectum
- The person complains of pain, or shows body language that suggests he is in pain
- The person has diarrhea or is constipated
- The person has redness, swelling, or pain around an intravenous (IV) or venous access site
- The person has a fever or other signs of infection

MEETING THE EMOTIONAL NEEDS OF A PERSON WITH CANCER

A person who is awaiting test results or who has just been diagnosed with cancer will have many emotional needs. The word *cancer* is very frightening to many people, because the disease is so often associated with death. However, a diagnosis of cancer is not necessarily a "death sentence." Many types of cancer can be successfully treated. Still, many people are very anxious about their prognosis, especially right after the cancer is diagnosed. A **prognosis** is the doctor's prediction of the course of a disease, and his estimation of the person's chances of recovering from it.

A person who has cancer may have many other fears as well. For example, the person may fear the side effects of treatment. Or he may worry about how his body will look during treatment or following surgery. The person may be afraid of experiencing a great deal of pain as a result of the cancer or treatment. The person may worry that even if the cancer is treated successfully now, it may return later in life.

If one of your patients or residents has been diagnosed with cancer, be sure to check in on the person as often as you check in on your other patients or residents. Spend time with the person. Many personal support workers are uncomfortable with the subject of cancer, and as a result may avoid a person with cancer without even being aware that they are doing so. You might be afraid that you "won't know what to say." Remember, caring for a person with cancer does not require you to say anything—the person will be comforted just by the fact that you are there and willing to listen.

Often, people with cancer find comfort in their spiritual beliefs and practices. The person may request visits from clergy members. Time spent praying, reading religious texts, meditating, or listening to spiritual music may be comforting to the person. Provide privacy for the person during these times, and make sure you relay any requests for clergy visits to the nurse so that the appropriate calls can be made, according to facility policy.

Summary

- A tumour, or mass of abnormal cells, may be *malignant* (cancerous) or *benign* (not cancerous). The cells that make up malignant tumours divide rapidly and spread into nearby tissues. They can also enter the bloodstream and spread to distant organs, a process called *metastasis.*
- Early detection of cancer can lead to early treatment, which greatly improves a person's chances of surviving the disease.
  - The nature of your duties as a personal support worker will put you in an ideal position to observe changes in a patient or resident that may be early warning signs of cancer.
  - Many cancers are detected at an early stage through routine physical examinations or screening tests. If the doctor suspects cancer, he or she might recommend follow-up tests (such as radiologic studies, endoscopic studies, or biopsy).
- The three main approaches to treating cancer are surgery, chemotherapy, and radiation therapy.
  - These approaches may be used alone or in combination, depending on the type of cancer and whether it has spread.
  - Treatment may be curative or palliative. The goal of curative treatment is to rid the body of the disease. The goal of palliative treatment is to keep the person comfortable when the disease cannot be cured.

- Cancer treatment can be associated with unpleasant side effects, including hair loss (alopecia), nausea, vomiting, diarrhea, loss of appetite (anorexia), mouth sores (stomatitis), skin breakdown, lowered immunity, and fatigue.
- A person with cancer often faces many treatment choices, including the choice of not having treatment at all. It is important to respect the person's choice, even if you do not agree with it.
- A patient or resident with cancer requires humanistic care, just as any other patient or resident does. Personal support workers must take steps to prevent their own discomfort with the subject of cancer from compromising their ability to care for their patients or residents with the disease.
  - A person with cancer has many physical needs that are directly related to the cancer, or to its treatment. Personal support workers play an important role in helping the person with cancer to manage pain and deal with unpleasant side effects of cancer therapy.
  - A person with cancer will need assistance to meet emotional and spiritual needs as well. Often, the best thing a personal support worker can do is listen if the person wants to talk, or spend quiet time with the person if he or she does not want to talk.

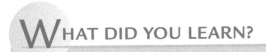

WHAT DID YOU LEARN?

Multiple Choice

Select the single best answer for each of the following questions.

1. Which one of the following statements best describes a malignant (cancerous) tumour?
   a. It consists of abnormal cells that divide rapidly and are capable of spreading to nearby tissues and distant organs.
   b. It consists of abnormal cells that divide slowly and tend to stay together.
   c. All tumours are malignant.
   d. All malignant tumours are fatal.

2. Which of the following factors plays a role in whether or not a person develops cancer?
   a. Inheritance (genes)
   b. Lifestyle choices, such as diet and exercise
   c. Environment
   d. All of the above

3. Mrs. Worthington is receiving chemotherapy following surgery to remove a malignant tumour. Following each treatment, she is nauseous and often vomits. What could you do to help Mrs. Worthington feel better?
   a. Offer her strong pain medications
   b. Offer her ice chips, and sit with her and hold her hand
   c. Enter her room only when necessary to avoid disturbing her
   d. Serve her meal tray as usual, in hopes that the smell of the food will increase her appetite

Matching

Match each numbered item with its appropriate lettered description.

__C__ 1. Alopecia

__E__ 2. Stomatitis

__A__ 3. Biopsy

__F__ 4. Metastasis

__B__ 5. Palliative

__G__ 6. Tumour

__D__ 7. Prognosis

a. Surgical removal of cells or tissue for examination under a microscope
b. Treatment done with the goal of reducing pain and discomfort, not curing the disease
c. Loss of hair
d. The doctor's prediction of the course of a person's disease, and the person's chance of recovering from it
e. Inflammation of the mouth
f. The spread of malignant cells to other parts of the body
g. Abnormal growth of tissue

STOP and Think!

You are caring for Mr. Lukens, a resident who was recently diagnosed with cancer. The doctors have presented Mr. Lukens and his family with a number of different treatment options, and for the past few days, Mr. Lukens has been weighing the pros and cons of each. In addition, he is still trying to adjust to the diagnosis he has just been given, and what it means for his future. One morning, while you are making Mr. Lukens' bed, he starts to talk to you about his father, who died of cancer after going through several months of agonizing treatments. He tells you that he is scared that he, too, will go through the treatments and in the end, all of his suffering might be for nothing. "Maybe it would just be easier to give up now and die peacefully," he says. How would you react to what Mr. Lukens is telling you? Is there anything you can do or say that might help Mr. Lukens with the difficult choices he needs to make?

CHAPTER

38

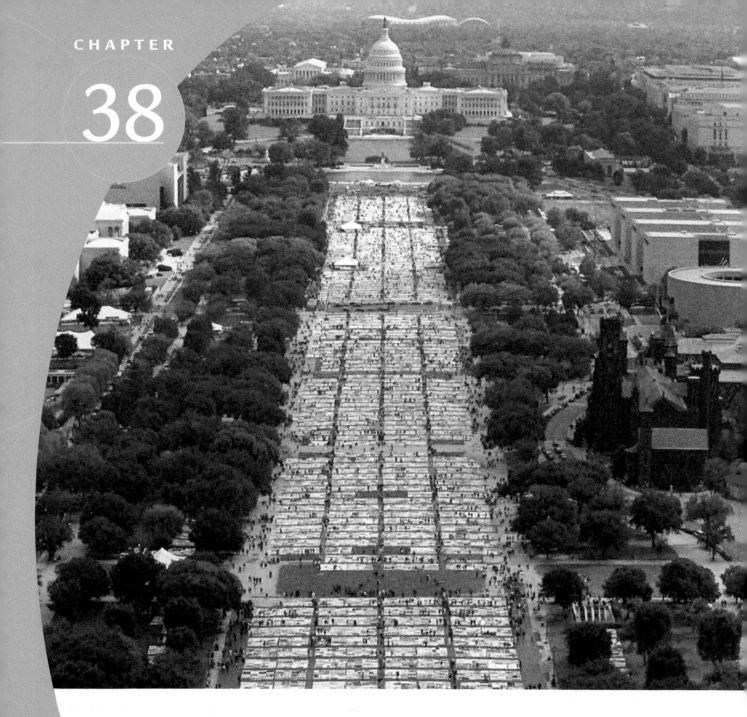

Caring for People With HIV/AIDS

WHAT WILL YOU LEARN?

In Chapter 8, you learned how human immunodeficiency virus (HIV), the virus that causes acquired immunodeficiency syndrome (AIDS), is transmitted. You also learned about measures you can take to protect yourself from HIV infection in the workplace, and about

Photo: The AIDS memorial quilt on display in Washington, D.C. The quilt contains more than 44,000 panels. Each panel memorializes a person who died from AIDS. (AP Photo/Ron Edmonds.)

730

how HIV takes over the body's immune system, eventually leading to the condition known as AIDS. In this chapter, you will learn more about AIDS, and how it affects the people who have it, physically and emotionally. When you are finished with this chapter, you will be able to:

1. Describe how HIV/AIDS affects a person physically.
2. Discuss who is at risk for HIV infection and AIDS.
3. Discuss legal concerns related to caring for people with HIV/AIDS.
4. Describe how HIV/AIDS affects a person emotionally.
5. Recognize the importance of the personal support worker's responsibility to provide for the physical and emotional needs of the person with HIV/AIDS.

Vocabulary

HIV-positive

WHAT IS AIDS?

A person who is infected with HIV is said to be **HIV-positive,** because he or she has tested positive on the blood test for HIV antibodies. HIV invades a person's white blood cells. In doing so, the virus destroys the cells that are responsible for protecting the body. As HIV takes over the body's immune system, the infected person begins to have more and more health problems, such as severe infections and aggressive cancers. Most HIV-positive people eventually develop AIDS, an advanced stage of HIV infection. AIDS is said to occur when the person's battered immune system is no longer able to fight off infections and malignancies. People with AIDS do not die from the virus that has infected their bodies. Rather, they die from infections and malignancies that the body is no longer able to fight.

Most people who become infected with HIV experience a brief, flu-like illness about 2 to 4 weeks after they are first exposed to the virus. During this brief illness, the person may have a fever, swollen lymph nodes, a sore throat, a rash, or any combination of these signs and symptoms. These signs and symptoms eventually go away, and may be forgotten. In many cases, if the person is tested for the virus within the next 3 to 6 months, the test will not be positive, even though the person is infected with the virus. A person can be infected with HIV for many years before developing AIDS, or he may never develop AIDS. The amount of time that it takes before AIDS develops and death occurs varies greatly from person to person. For example, in children and people in poor health, HIV infection is likely to progress to AIDS more

quickly. As HIV infection progresses, the person is likely to experience:

- Loss of appetite, nausea, vomiting, or diarrhea
- Weight loss
- Fever (with or without night sweats)
- Pain or difficulty swallowing (dysphagia)
- Fatigue
- Swollen lymph nodes in the neck, armpits, and groin
- A cough or recurrent episodes of pneumonia
- Sores or white patches in the mouth
- Bruises or dark bumps on the skin that do not heal (Kaposi's sarcoma; Fig. 38-1)
- Forgetfulness and confusion
- Dementia

To date, there is no cure for HIV/AIDS, although medications have been developed that can delay the onset of AIDS in HIV-positive people. These medications can cost more than $10,000 per year and are not always successful. In addition, they often have severe and disabling side effects, such as headache, dizziness, nausea, diarrhea, fever, skin rash, severe anemia, and extreme fatigue. Currently, no medication can kill HIV or offer a complete cure for AIDS.

TELL THE NURSE

When caring for a person with HIV/AIDS, it is very important for you to immediately report any of the following observations to the nurse:

- The person has a fever
- The person has sores or white patches in the mouth

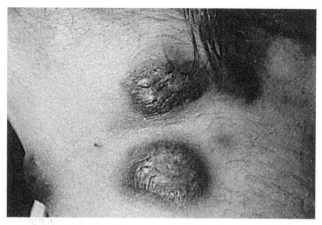

Figure 38-1

As a result of their weakened immune systems, people with AIDS often develop malignancies, such as Kaposi's sarcoma. The lesions of Kaposi's sarcoma are often seen on the skin and mucous membranes of people with advanced HIV infection (AIDS). (*Photograph courtesy of Goodheart, H. P. [2003]. Goodheart's photoguide of common skin disorders: Diagnosis and management [p. 374]. Philadelphia: Lippincott Williams & Wilkins.*)

- The person has diarrhea, nausea, or vomiting
- The person is coughing
- The person has a skin rash or bruises
- The person's mental status has changed (for example, he or she has become confused or disoriented)
- The person seems depressed or talks of suicide
- The person is bleeding from any body opening

WHO IS AT RISK FOR HIV/AIDS?

Although the first cases of HIV/AIDS were reported in homosexual men, we now know that *anyone* can get AIDS—young, old, homosexual, heterosexual, male, or female. In Chapter 8, you learned that HIV is transmitted from one person to another through body fluids, such as blood, semen, and vaginal secretions. Exposure to HIV can also occur either before or during birth, or through breast milk. Behaviours and situations that increase a person's risk for becoming infected with HIV include the following:

- **Having unprotected sex.** Unprotected sexual intercourse, both homosexual and heterosexual, is the most common method of HIV transmission.

- **Sharing of needles.** Sharing of needles among people who abuse intravenous drugs is the second most common method of transmission.

- **Receiving tissue transplants or transfusions of blood or blood products.** Before 1985, people who received blood transfusions may have been exposed to HIV. This method of transmission is less common now in developed nations with more advanced health care systems, because donated blood is screened for the virus. However, some developing countries still do not screen their blood supplies.

A GLOBAL HEALTH CRISIS

Today, HIV/AIDS is considered a global health crisis. The rate of infection continues to increase around the world, and there is no cure for this devastating disease. In the United States, the Centers for Disease Control and Prevention (CDC) reports that more than 90 million people worldwide are HIV-positive or already have AIDS. In 2005 alone, approximately 5 million new infections were reported. AIDS awareness programs, which teach people about AIDS and how to lower their risk of becoming infected with HIV, have helped to lower the rate of infection in developed countries, such as Canada, the United States, and many European nations (Fig. 38-2). For example, in Canada, the federal government, through the Public Health Agency of Canada, has identified eight key population groups who are at

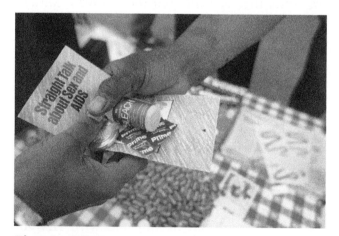

Figure 38-2

AIDS awareness programs provide information about HIV infection and AIDS to the general public. These programs provide free advice about the disease, how it can be prevented, and where a person can go to get tested for HIV. (*© Allen Russell/Index Stock Imagery.*)

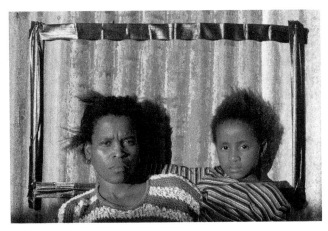

Figure 38-3
AIDS is a global health crisis. Some developing countries report HIV infection in as many as 70% of adults. This woman, who lives in Africa, discovered that she was HIV-positive when her daughter was born HIV-positive. Developing nations are hit hardest by the AIDS epidemic because they lack money for education and health care. (© *Gideon Mendel/CORBIS.*)

especially high risk for HIV/AIDS. Through federal initiative programs, the government is committed to developing specific approaches to lower the risk for HIV/AIDS among members of these groups. People who live in developed countries also often have better access to health care if they do become infected with HIV.

But in developing nations, such as India and many countries in Africa and Southeast Asia, the rate of HIV infection is increasing, and the number of people dying from AIDS is doubling and even tripling (Fig. 38-3). In these countries, access to health care services and information about the prevention of HIV infection may be extremely limited, especially to women. Women in these countries often have a low social or economic status. As a result, they may not be able to insist on safe sex practices, or afford treatment. These women may become pregnant without knowing that they are HIV-positive. Even if they do know that they are infected with HIV, they may not be able to afford treatments to reduce the chance that the virus will be transmitted to their unborn children during pregnancy. As a result, more and more babies in developing nations are being born with HIV.

PROTECTION OF RIGHTS

In many cultures, being HIV-positive or having AIDS is considered shameful. As a result, a person who is HIV-positive or who has AIDS may experience discrimination and poor treatment by others. There are many factors that contribute to the negative attitude many people have toward those who are HIV-positive or have AIDS:

- Because HIV infection is associated with many behaviours that people can control (such as whether or not they practice safe sex), some people may feel that the person with HIV/AIDS "has only himself to blame."
- Many of the behaviours associated with HIV infection are behaviours that many people do not approve of for moral or religious reasons (such as abusing street drugs or being homosexual).
- Many people lack information about how HIV is transmitted, and as a result, fear becoming infected with HIV through casual contact with an infected person.

Because a person with HIV/AIDS is at risk for discrimination, many provinces and territories have laws designed specifically to protect the rights of people with HIV/AIDS. These laws ensure the person's right to employment, education, privacy, and health care. It would be difficult to detail all of the laws here, because they vary from province to province and they change frequently, as lawmakers write and introduce new laws. However, as an example, in most provinces, people with HIV/AIDS are protected under the Canadian Human Rights law.

As with all of your patients or residents, protecting the person's privacy and right to confidentiality is very important. This is especially true when a person has a condition, such as HIV/AIDS, that could cause him to experience discrimination. For example, if a person is known to be HIV-positive, he may have trouble getting a job, or renting an apartment. Although laws are in place to protect the person from discrimination, discrimination can still occur.

As a personal support worker, you are responsible for maintaining absolute confidentiality about a person's HIV status. You need to know the HIV status of a person to whom you are providing care. However—no one else needs to know. Know your facility's or agency's policies related to keeping health information private, and follow these policies carefully at all times, with all patients and residents.

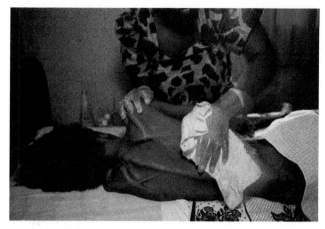

Figure 38-4
Toward the end of their lives, most people with AIDS require almost complete assistance with activities of daily living (ADLs). As a result, many seek care from home health care or hospice agencies, or in long-term care facilities. (© *Joel Steffenheim/CORBIS.*)

CARING FOR A PERSON WITH AIDS

People with HIV/AIDS often require the services of the health care industry throughout the course of their illness. In many communities, organizations exist for the sole purpose of serving people with AIDS. These organizations can help the person with transportation, housing, employment, mental health counselling, financial aid, and medical services. As the disease progresses, the person may be hospitalized several times for the treatment of severe infections and other problems. In the advanced stage of AIDS, pain and weakness cause the person to become almost completely dependent on others for assistance with activities of daily living (ADLs) (Fig. 38-4). As a result, the person may need the services of a home health care agency, or she may need to move to a long-term care facility. Most people with AIDS also eventually require the service of hospice agencies.

MEETING THE PHYSICAL NEEDS OF A PERSON WITH AIDS

A person with AIDS becomes more dependent on others for basic physical care as the disease progresses. Fatigue and disability will make it difficult for the person to perform basic activities, such as those related to personal hygiene and grooming. As a result, you will need to help the person with any ADLs that he can no longer manage. As always, encourage the person to do as much for himself as possible, for as long as possible. Special considerations with regard to physical care for the person with AIDS include the following:

- People with AIDS often develop painful sores on the inside of the mouth. These sores can make eating difficult, putting the person at risk for poor nutrition. In addition, people with AIDS often suffer from chronic diarrhea, which puts them at risk for dehydration. As a result, you may be required to measure and record intake and output. You should also offer the person fluids, as ordered.
- As a result of sores on the inside of the mouth, oral hygiene can be painful for a person with AIDS. A special mouthwash or spray to numb the inside of the person's mouth may be used before providing oral care. Rashes and other skin disorders may require the use of special cleansing agents, special bathing techniques, or both.
- Because people with AIDS are at high risk for opportunistic infections, you will need to ask visitors who have colds or other contagious illnesses to delay their visit until after they have recovered from their illnesses. In addition, the person with AIDS needs to avoid other potential sources of infection, such as undercooked meat and eggs. Always practice proper infection control measures, especially good handwashing. Avoid coming to work if you have a contagious illness. This is important with all patients and residents, but especially so when you are caring for people with weak immune systems.

As you already know, your job responsibilities place you at risk for contacting body fluids that are known to transmit HIV and other blood-borne pathogens. For this reason, you must use standard precautions (see Chapter 7) with every patient or resident, not just those who are known to be infected with HIV (Fig. 38-5). Remember that a person can be infected with HIV and not know it. You may find it frightening to provide physical care for a person who is known to have a communicable, potentially fatal illness. Know that with the proper and consistent use of standard precautions, your risk of exposure to HIV and other bloodborne pathogens in the workplace is actually quite low.

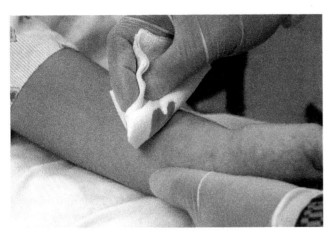

Figure 38-5
Practicing standard precautions is essential with all patients and residents, not just those who are known to have an illness caused by a bloodborne pathogen (such as AIDS).

MEETING THE EMOTIONAL NEEDS OF A PERSON WITH AIDS

People with HIV/AIDS can face a great deal of emotional stress. Because of increasing levels of stress, people with HIV/AIDS may lose their ability to cope. As a result, clinical depression and an increased risk for suicide are very common among people with HIV/AIDS. Sources of emotional stress include the following:

- Fear, shame, or disapproval can cause friends and even family members to abandon a person when they find out that she is HIV-positive. They may avoid the person because they fear that they, too, could get the disease from casual contact or conversation. Or they may just be ashamed to know a person with HIV/AIDS. Can you imagine how you would feel if your friends or family members could not give you emotional support when you needed it most?
- People with HIV/AIDS may lose their jobs as a result of their disease. Health care and the medications used to slow the progression of HIV are very expensive, and the loss of employment usually means the loss of health care benefits. For these reasons, the person with HIV/AIDS may have many worries about money.
- A person with HIV/AIDS may suffer from a lot of guilt, especially if the cause of infection was due to risky behaviour. For example, a man who finds out that he is

HIV-positive must face the fact that he may have transmitted a deadly disease to his sexual partner.

- A person with HIV/AIDS may have many fears related to his declining health and how this will affect his ability to care for himself. The person may also have fears about pain related to the disease, or about death itself.

Providing emotional care for the person with HIV/AIDS is an essential responsibility of the personal support worker. When caring for a person with HIV/AIDS, you can use touch to comfort the person, spend time listening and talking, or share a simple hug (Fig. 38-6). None of these activities will transmit the virus to you. Many times, the only human touch a person with HIV/AIDS will experience will come from the person providing care within the health care setting. How would you feel if people were afraid to touch you? Would you feel dirty, unloved, and alone? Instead of being afraid to care for people with HIV/AIDS, learn how to protect yourself from infection and practice what you have learned consistently.

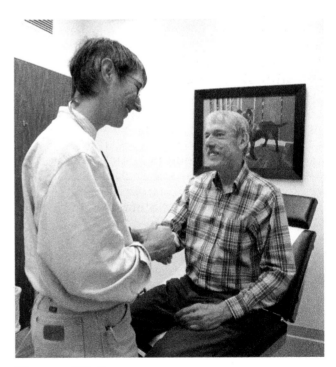

Figure 38-6
HIV cannot be transmitted from one person to another through touching or hugging. Lack of human touch can make a person feel unloved and alone. When caring for a person with HIV/AIDS, try not to let fear get in the way of your ability to provide compassionate care. (*AP Photo/ Paul Sakuma.*)

Helping Hands and a Caring Heart

FOCUS ON HUMANISTIC HEALTH CARE

Remember that it does not really matter how a person became infected with HIV. Even if you do not approve of the person's lifestyle, you must not let your personal beliefs affect the care that you give the person. Instead of focusing on *how* the person got HIV, focus on *who* the person is. What does she enjoy about life? Whom does she admire? Try to remember that a person is defined by a lot more than just her HIV status. A patient or resident with HIV/AIDS needs your care and support, perhaps more than anything else she has ever needed before. Your ability to provide supportive and compassionate care to your patients or residents with HIV/AIDS will make a significant difference in their quality of life.

SUMMARY

- Acquired immunodeficiency syndrome (AIDS) is caused by infection with the human immunodeficiency virus (HIV). HIV invades the body's immune system, leaving it unable to do its job. As a result, the person eventually dies from infections or cancers that take over the body.
  - A person who has tested positive for having antibodies to HIV in his or her blood is said to be *HIV-positive.*
  - Most HIV-positive people eventually develop AIDS, an advanced stage of HIV infection. A person who is infected with HIV may live for many years before AIDS develops. AIDS is a terminal illness.
- HIV/AIDS is a global health crisis. Since it was first identified in the early 1980s, HIV/AIDS has spread rapidly, killing a large number of people throughout the world in a short period of time.
  - In developed countries, such as the United States, Canada, and England, rates of HIV infection and death from AIDS are decreasing due to the efforts of AIDS-awareness programs and the availability of funding for research and health care.
  - Rates of HIV infection and death from AIDS continue to soar in developing countries, such as India and many nations in Africa and Southeast Asia, where money and access to health care and education about HIV infection are limited.
- Anyone can get HIV/AIDS, regardless of race, gender, sexual orientation, or age.
  - Behaviours that increase a person's risk of becoming infected with HIV include having unprotected sexual intercourse and using dirty needles to inject street drugs.
  - The virus can also be transmitted through tissue transplants or transfusions of blood or blood products, and from a mother to a child during birth or through breast milk.
- A person with HIV/AIDS may experience discrimination and poor treatment by others. It is important for the personal support worker to keep information about a person's HIV status, or any other medical condition, private and confidential.
- People with HIV/AIDS often require the services of the health care industry throughout the course of their illness.
  - Infections that cause pneumonia, diarrhea, and malignancies such as Kaposi's sarcoma are common in people who are infected with HIV, causing them to be hospitalized repeatedly.
  - As the disease progresses, the person becomes unable to care for himself, and he may need the services of a home health care agency or long-term care facility.
  - In the final months of their lives, people with AIDS may require the services of a hospice agency.
- In addition to providing physical care, the personal support worker plays an important role in providing emotional care to the person with HIV/AIDS.
  - With the proper and consistent use of standard precautions, your risk of exposure to HIV and other bloodborne pathogens in the workplace is actually quite low.
  - Human touch is a very effective way of comforting a person and communicating care and concern. You cannot get HIV/AIDS from holding a person's hand or giving a person a hug.
  - Remember that it is not important how a person became infected with HIV. Try not to let your personal beliefs or fears get in the way of your ability to provide compassionate, competent care.

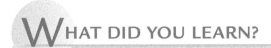

WHAT DID YOU LEARN?

Multiple Choice

Select the single best answer for each of the following questions.

1. When should a personal support worker use standard precautions?
   a. When a person who is HIV-positive develops AIDS
   b. When a person is HIV-positive or has AIDS
   c. When caring for a patient or resident who is homosexual
   d. When caring for any patient or resident and contact with blood or body fluids is possible

2. Which one of the following statements about HIV infection and AIDS is true?
   a. Anyone can become infected with HIV, regardless of age, gender, sexual orientation, or race.
   b. The only people who become infected with HIV and get AIDS are drug abusers and homosexuals.
   c. HIV infection and AIDS are not a problem among the elderly.
   d. AIDS usually develops soon after a person is first exposed to HIV.

3. When caring for a person with HIV/AIDS, which one of the following observations should be reported to the nurse?
   a. The person has diarrhea
   b. The person seems depressed
   c. The person seems disoriented
   d. All of the above

4. Why is it especially important for personal support workers to keep information about a person's HIV status private and confidential?
   a. AIDS is a shameful disease and should not be discussed in public.
   b. There are laws to protect the rights of HIV-positive people and people with AIDS, including their right to privacy and confidentiality of medical information.
   c. Personal support workers have a responsibility to make sure that everyone who might come in contact with the person knows the person's HIV status, so that others can protect themselves.
   d. AIDS is a global health crisis.

5. Which one of the following physical problems is a person with AIDS at risk for?
   a. Alopecia (loss of hair), due to the medications used to slow the progression of HIV to AIDS
   b. Dehydration, due to chronic diarrhea
   c. Blindness, due to nerve damage as a result of HIV infection
   d. Heart failure, due to myocardial infarction

STOP and Think!

You work in a hospital. One of the patients you will be caring for today, Camilla, is a 34-year-old woman who has been admitted for the treatment of AIDS-related pneumonia. Although Camilla has been admitted to the hospital for AIDS-related infections and complications several times in the past, you have never had her as a patient because you are a relatively new employee. In fact, you have never cared for any patient with AIDS. Frankly, you are a little bit nervous about meeting Camilla and about providing hands-on physical care to a person who is known to be HIV-positive. What will be your approach to Camilla and your responsibilities as a personal support worker?

Personal Support Workers Make a Difference!

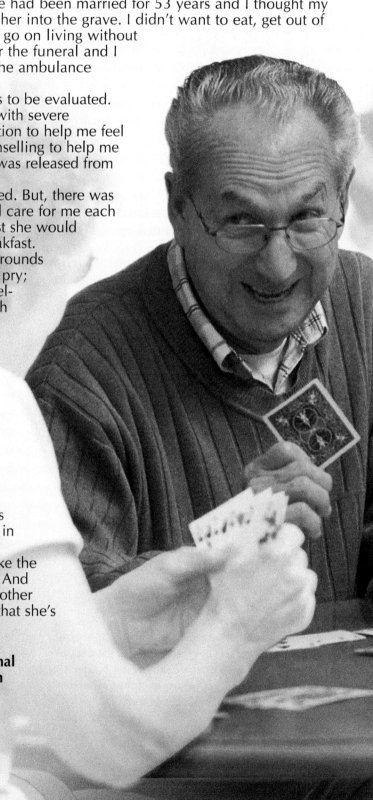

"I am Clarence Wright and I live in the Sunny Shores Nursing Facility. I came here about a year ago after my dear wife, Callie, passed away. We had been married for 53 years and I thought my heart was broken forever the day they lowered her into the grave. I didn't want to eat, get out of bed, or even take a bath; heck, I didn't want to go on living without her! A good friend visited me a week or so after the funeral and I guess I frightened him so much that he called the ambulance for me.

I went to the hospital and stayed a few days to be evaluated. There, a mental health specialist diagnosed me with severe depression. The doctor prescribed some medication to help me feel more 'normal' and arranged for me to have counselling to help me come to terms with losing Callie. Shortly after I was released from the hospital, I decided to move to Sunny Shores.

After moving here, I was still pretty depressed. But, there was this really nice woman named Celia who helped care for me each day. She was my personal support worker. At first she would help me get dressed and shaved and out for breakfast. Then she would ask me to go walk around the grounds with her. We didn't talk much at first. She didn't pry; instead, we just walked quietly. After I started feeling like talking, she let me talk about my life with Callie, and would sit and look at pictures of her with me. One day I broke down and just cried like a baby and Celia just sat quietly with me and held my hand. That day, I knew I would be able to make it.

Yes, I still get sad when I think of Callie's death. But I've learned to make use of what I have left of my life. I help Celia out with some of the residents who aren't as fortunate as I am. I read to one fellow who is blind and we have some of the most wonderful conversations. Also, a group of us meet every Thursday night to play cards. I have regained the feeling that my life has meaning and I know that Celia had a major part in that. Medicine is great for helping people with depression, but no medicine ever created can take the place of knowing that a person cares about you. And Celia shows that she cares about me and all the other residents down this hall. We love her and think that she's our angel in disguise."

You can listen to more stories about how personal support workers make a difference on the CD in the front of your book.

Photo credit: Jupiterimages Corporation

ACUTE CARE

39 Caring for Surgical Patients
40 Caring for Mothers and Newborns
41 Caring for Pediatric Patients

The acute care setting can be an exciting place to work. If you choose to work in an acute care setting, such as a hospital, you will have the opportunity to meet and care for many different people. In this unit, you will learn about how to care for three special groups of patients who often receive treatment in hospitals: surgical patients; women who are about to deliver, or have just delivered, babies; and children.

Photo: The acute care setting offers the opportunity to work with many different types of patients. Here, a personal support worker helps a woman in labour.

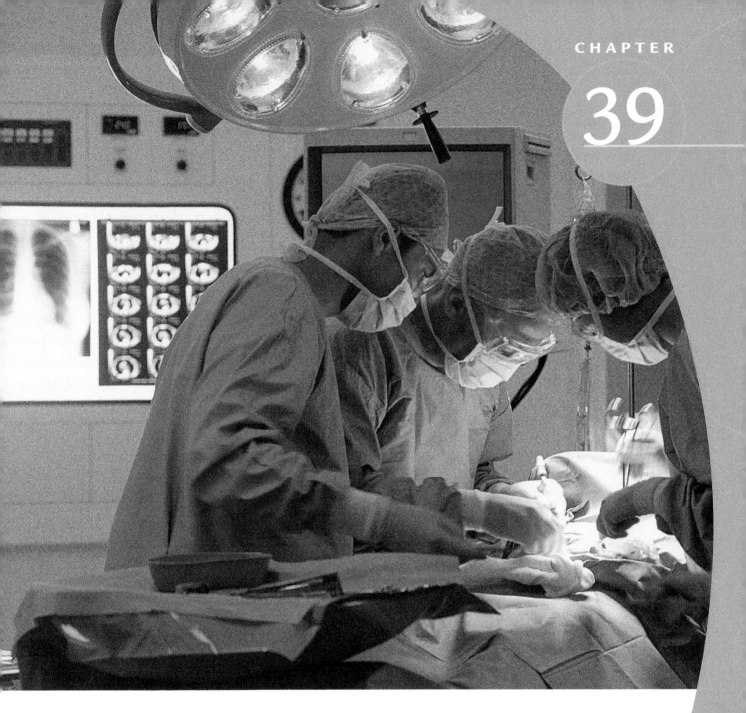

Caring for Surgical Patients

WHAT WILL YOU LEARN?

Surgery is a branch of medicine that involves treating diseases and disorders by entering the body and physically removing or repairing damaged organs or tissues. Advances in surgical tools and techniques have made many surgeries safer and have opened up treatment options for many diseases and disorders that were considered fatal in the past. Surgeries that once made headlines, such as kidney transplants, are now done fairly routinely.

Photo: A surgical team performs an operation.

741

The longer a person lives, the greater the chance the person will need surgery sometime during her lifetime, simply because the person will have more of a chance to develop a disease or disorder that is treated surgically. As a personal support worker, you may have many opportunities to help prepare people for surgery and care for them afterward. When you are finished with this chapter, you will be able to:

1. Discuss the various reasons surgery is done.
2. Define the term *anaesthesia* and describe the three main types of anaesthesia.
3. Describe changes in the health care field that affect the care of the surgical patient.
4. Understand the fears and concerns that a person who is about to have surgery may have, and describe actions the personal support worker can take to help relieve some of these worries.
5. Describe what needs to be done to physically prepare a person for surgery, and explain the personal support worker's role in these preparations.
6. Describe potential complications of surgery, and the measures taken to prevent them.
7. Discuss observations that are important to report to the nurse when caring for a patient who is recovering from surgery.
8. Demonstrate the proper way to apply anti-embolism (TED) stockings.

Vocabulary

Exploratory surgery	General anaesthesia	Post-operative phase	Atelectasis
Definitive surgery	Regional anaesthesia	Peri-operative period	Thrombophlebitis
Elective	Local anaesthesia	Pre-operative teaching	Pulmonary embolism
Urgent	Pre-operative phase	Post-anaesthesia care	Sequential compression
Emergent	Intra-operative phase	unit (PACU)	device (SCD)

A person may need surgery for many different reasons. **Exploratory surgery** may be performed when a person has a significant medical problem but the doctors do not know how bad the problem is or exactly what is causing it. For example, doctors might want to do exploratory surgery following an accident when the extent of the damage to the person's internal organs is unknown, or when cancer is suspected but cannot be confirmed by other means. Often, the problem is discovered and solved during the same surgery. **Definitive surgery** is performed when the person's medical problem is known and the best way to address it is through surgery. For example, surgeries are performed to repair organ defects or injuries, as in a hernia repair or surgical repair of a fractured bone. Surgeries are also performed to remove diseased body parts, as when the cancerous part of the colon is removed as treatment for colon cancer.

Surgeries may be elective, urgent, or emergent. Surgeries are performed on an **elective** basis when the procedure is planned for and scheduled ahead of time. An example of an elective procedure would be cataract surgery or a plastic surgery procedure, such as a face-lift. **Urgent** surgeries are planned and scheduled ahead of time, but usually an effort is made to schedule the procedure as soon as possible to prevent the person's condition from getting worse. Examples of urgent procedures would include a mastectomy (in a person with breast cancer) or cardiac bypass surgery (in a person with coronary artery disease). An **emergent** surgery is one that must be performed immediately to prevent the person from dying or becoming disabled. Emergent surgeries are unplanned and unscheduled and are usually the result of an acute illness or injury, such as a ruptured appendix.

Most surgical procedures are done under anaesthesia. Anaesthesia prevents the person from feeling pain during the surgery, and is accomplished through the use of medications. Depending on the situation, the doctor may choose to use a general anaesthetic, a regional anaesthetic, or a local anaesthetic:

- **General anaesthesia** causes a loss of consciousness. Usually, a combination of inhaled medications (in the form of a gas) and injected medications are given to cause general anaesthesia. The person is "put to sleep" for the duration of the surgical procedure. When the procedure is completed, the medications are stopped and the person "wakes up." The person will be sleepy for several hours after the procedure and may experience some nausea or vomiting during the recovery period.

- **Regional anaesthesia** causes a loss of sensation in part, but not all, of the body. The person remains conscious throughout the procedure. A sedative may be given in addition to the anaesthetic to help the person relax. The anaesthetic is injected near a nerve pathway, causing the part of the body beyond the injection site to become numb. After surgery, the sensation returns gradually. The person may experience temporary paralysis and weakness of the anaesthetized body part until the anaesthetic has completely worn off. An example of regional anaesthesia is "an epidural block," which numbs the body from the waist down and is often given to women during childbirth.

- **Local anaesthesia** causes a loss of sensation in only a very small part of the body (the surgical site). As with regional anaesthesia, the medication is injected near a nerve pathway, the person remains conscious throughout the procedure, and a sedative may be given to help the person relax. The surgical site remains without sensation until the local anaesthetic wears off. Eye surgeries, breast biopsies, and hernia repairs are examples of surgeries that are often performed under local anaesthesia.

In the past, people who were having a planned surgical procedure were admitted to the hospital the day before the scheduled surgery. The tests required prior to surgery were done, the surgical site was shaved and cleaned, the person and his family members were told what to expect during and after the surgery, and the person was given a sleeping pill to ensure a restful night's sleep. Following the surgery, the person usually stayed in the hospital for several days to recover under the watchful eyes of the hospital staff.

Now, changes in health care have led to changes in the lengths of hospital stays. People are discharged from the hospital "quicker and sicker." For the surgical patient who is having elective or urgent surgery, this means that most of the tasks that used to be done in the hospital the day before surgery are now done in the surgeon's office or on an outpatient basis in the days leading up to the surgery. The person remains home until the morning of surgery and goes to the hospital or surgical center an hour or two before the surgery is scheduled. Hair is removed from the surgical site and the skin is cleaned in the operating room or in a preparation area next to the operating room just prior to the procedure. After the surgery, the person is often discharged from the hospital within a few hours to recover at home, in an extended care facility, or in a long-term care facility. Even though surgery is performed in a hospital or surgical center, these changes mean that as a personal support worker, you can expect to care for people who are either preparing for surgery or recovering from it, no matter where you work.

There are three phases of care for the person having surgery (Fig. 39-1). These phases are:

- The **pre-operative phase,** or before surgery
- The **intra-operative phase,** or during surgery
- The **post-operative phase,** or after surgery

The term **peri-operative period** is used to describe all three phases of the surgical process as a whole.

CARE OF THE PRE-OPERATIVE PATIENT

The pre-operative phase begins when the person is first informed about the need for surgery, and ends when the person actually enters the operating room. The pre-operative period can be as long as several weeks (for an elective, scheduled procedure) or as short as a few minutes (for an emergent procedure). During the pre-operative period, the person who is having surgery is prepared both emotionally and physically for the procedure.

EMOTIONAL PREPARATION

A person facing surgery usually has many fears, concerns, and worries. For example, the person may be afraid of not waking up from the anaesthesia, dying as a result of the surgery, or experiencing pain during or after the procedure. He may worry that the doctor will make a mistake and remove the wrong organ or limb. If the person is

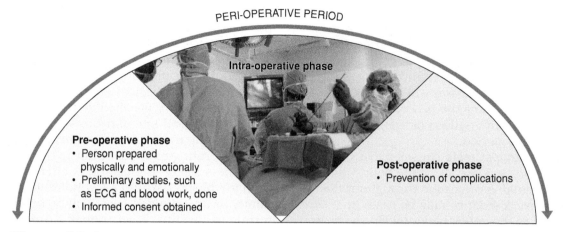

Figure 39-1

There are three phases of care for the person having surgery. As a personal support worker, you will provide care during the pre-operative and post-operative phases.

having exploratory surgery, the person may be worried about what the doctor will find (for example, a malignant tumor). Many people worry about how long it will take to recover from the surgery, and what this will mean in terms of time missed from work and lost income needed to support a family.

To help reduce a person's anxiety about the upcoming surgery, the health care team spends time talking with the person and his family members about the procedure, its benefits and possible risks, and what can be expected during the post-operative recovery period. These conversations, which occur during the pre-operative phase, are commonly called **pre-operative teaching.** Pre-operative teaching begins with the doctor's explanation of why he or she feels the procedure is the best treatment option for the person. The doctor tells the person what complications can occur as a result of the procedure, what will actually occur during the procedure, and what other treatment options, if any, are available (Fig. 39-2).

The doctor must explain these things in a way that is understandable to the person, so that the person can make an informed decision about whether he wants to have the surgery. To go ahead with the procedure, informed consent must be given by the person and documented in the person's medical record. If the person is not able to make an informed decision on his own, informed consent must be obtained from the person's family members. The nurse is responsible for making sure that informed consent has been obtained and that the person signs a form giving permission for the procedure to take place (Fig. 39-3). As a personal support worker, you

will not be responsible for either explaining the procedure to the person or obtaining the person's signed consent for it.

Once informed consent for the procedure is obtained, the nurse continues the pre-operative teaching by explaining what will need to be done both before and after the surgery. The nurse explains the pre-operative procedures that are done to physically prepare the person for surgery, as well as the purpose of any medications or tests that are required during the pre-operative period. The nurse also explains what will happen during the post-operative period, and teaches the person how to do any exercises that may be necessary to prevent complications following the surgery.

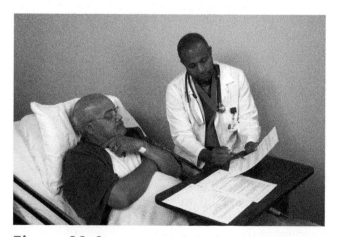

Figure 39-2

During the pre-operative period, the doctor tells the person why he or she feels surgery is the best treatment option, explains the surgical procedure and any associated risks to the person, and obtains informed consent to perform the surgery.

Davis Hospital and Medical Center

Acknowledgement of Informed Consent for Procedures / Invasive Procedures

1. My treating Physician,_____, has explained my medical condition to my satisfaction and I have had an opportunity to have my questions answered.

2. My proposed treatment, its purpose, risks and alternatives, have been explained to me. I accept this treatment in hopes of obtaining the desired beneficial result of such care.

3. I recognize that, during the procedure(s), unforeseen conditions may require additional or different procedures than those explained. I request that my physician(s) and associates perform those procedures as, in their professional judgment, are desirable.

4. I agree to observation by medical personnel in training during my procedure in order to advance medical education.

Check all that apply:

❑   I agree to the administration of anesthesia or intravenous sedation.

❑   I agree to the administration of intravenous therapy to include blood products, chemotherapy, or antibiotics as ordered by my physician.

❑   I understand that any tissues removed from my body may be examined and then disposed of by hospital personnel.

❑   I agree to the presence of a medical product representative, as required and requested by the physician, for consultation purposes only.

❑   I agree to photography/video, during the procedure for the purposes of advancing medical education.

❑   As a <u>cardiac patient,</u> I acknowledge that the risks of no on-site surgical back-up have been explained to me by my physician.

❑   As a <u>cardiac patient,</u> I agree to be transferred to another facility in the event that surgical intervention becomes necessary.

❑   I understand that the procedure that is being done to me results in <u>sterilization</u>. I understand that the word "sterility" means that I may forever and irrevocably be unable to conceive or bear children, and in giving my consent to the operation have in mind the possibility, (probability) of such a result.

❑   I certify that I have had nothing to eat or drink, including water, since_____AM / PM.

❑   I have been given patient information sheets on_____and have had my questions answered.

Proposed Medical Procedure (in layman's terms) _____

_____

_____

_____   _____

Patient's Signature   Signature Witnessed By:

_____

Signature of Next of Kin or Legal Guardian

Time_____   Date_____

Figure 39-3

A signed informed consent form is necessary before any surgical procedure can be done. By signing the informed consent form, the person indicates that he or she understands what is going to be done, why it is being done, and what the possible risks are. (*Courtesy of Davis Hospital and Medical Center, Layton, Utah.*)

Although as a personal support worker you will not participate directly in pre-operative teaching, you will still play a very important supporting role. You will reinforce what the nurse has told the person, and keep the nurse informed of any questions the person may ask you about the procedure. Anxiety can make the person forget to ask important questions when the doctor or nurse is explaining the surgery. Often, the person will remember questions she wanted to ask later, when the doctor or nurse is no longer in the room. The person may ask you the questions instead. If the question is about an aspect of pre-operative or post-operative care that you are directly involved with, such as the reason for the NPO (no food or water by mouth) status prior to the procedure or the purpose of taking vital signs frequently after the procedure, you can answer the question yourself. But if you do not know the answer to the person's question, or if the question is about the surgical procedure itself, please tell the nurse immediately that the person has a question. The nurse will see to it that the person's question is answered.

Helping Hands and a Caring Heart

FOCUS ON HUMANISTIC HEALTH CARE

It is very easy to tell a person that a procedure is "minor" or "just routine." Many surgical procedures are, indeed, relatively low risk, and considered "routine" by health care professionals who see these procedures done every day. But no matter how simple or low-risk a surgical procedure is, there is nothing minor or routine about it to the person who is having it! Recognizing the person's fears, listening to his questions and concerns, and taking action to get those questions or concerns addressed are all very important things that you can do to help a person to prepare emotionally for the upcoming surgery.

PHYSICAL PREPARATION

Several things are done to physically prepare the person for surgery.

In the Days Leading Up to the Surgery

Typically, a person who is having surgery will need to have several tests done before the surgery to assess her level of health. Tests to assess the functioning of the person's cardiovascular, respiratory, and urinary systems are typically done. In addition, the doctor may request blood work.

The Evening Before Surgery

A person who is scheduled for surgery will usually be on NPO status for 6 to 8 hours before surgery (Fig. 39-4). This is necessary to ensure that the person's stomach is empty during and after the procedure. It is common for a person who has had general anaesthesia to vomit as the anaesthesia is given or starts to wear off. Vomiting while in a semi-conscious state puts the person at risk for aspiration (the inhalation of foreign material into the lungs). Aspiration puts the person at risk for developing pneumonia. Going into the procedure with an empty stomach helps to reduce the risk of aspiration and pneumonia.

You will need to tell the person, as well as any visitors, that NPO means that the person may not have anything by mouth, including water, ice, gum, and mints. It can be difficult for a person who is on NPO status to be around other people who are eating and drinking. For this reason, it may be helpful to show visitors to an area outside of the person's room where they can enjoy their snacks and beverages, away from the person who is on NPO status. Remember to remove the water pitcher and the drinking glass from the bedside table. Frequent mouth care helps to keep the person on NPO status comfortable. The person is usually allowed to brush her own teeth as long as no water is swallowed.

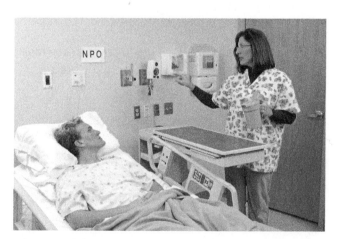

Figure 39-4

Many people will not be allowed to have anything by mouth for 6 to 8 hours before the surgery. When a person is on NPO status, the water pitcher and drinking glass are removed from the person's room.

The Morning of Surgery

Many things are done the day of surgery to prepare the patient. You should arrange your schedule as necessary, allowing enough time to help the person get ready for surgery. This is especially important if you work in a long-term care facility or for a home health care agency, to ensure that the person arrives at the hospital or surgical center at the appointed time. The nurse will tell you what you need to do to help to prepare the person for surgery. Tasks that you may be involved with include the following:

- **Administering an enema or vaginal douche.** A cleansing enema is given before many procedures to empty the bowel. For example, an enema may be given if the person is scheduled for intestinal surgery, to prevent feces from contaminating the abdominal cavity during the surgery. If a woman is having a vaginal procedure, the doctor may order vaginal irrigation (a douche) prior to the surgery to clean the vagina. When vaginal irrigation is ordered, a special solution is placed in the vagina and then allowed to drain out.
- **Bathing.** You may need to help the person to bathe and wash his hair prior to the surgery. Bathing and shampooing reduces the number of microbes on the skin. In some cases, the doctor may order a special antimicrobial soap to be used.
- **Grooming.** Makeup, including nail polish, is not permitted during surgery. Prosthetic devices, glasses, contact lenses, hearing aids, dentures, wigs, jewelry, and hair ornaments may also be removed prior to the surgery. Although the person may want or need to wear some of these items up until the very last minute, you should let the person know about these restrictions and encourage him to leave all but the most necessary items at home.
- **Dressing.** If the person will be going to the hospital or surgical center the day of the surgery, have him wear clothing that is loose and comfortable. This will make changing into a hospital gown before the procedure easier, and it will also ensure that when the person goes home, the clothing will fit over any bulky dressings or casts that may have been applied during the procedure.

Immediately Before the Surgery

Outpatients

Once the person arrives at the hospital or surgical center, she will go to a preparation area next to the operating room. The person will be shown to a private area and asked to undress and put on a clean hospital gown and surgical cap.

A nurse will check that all paperwork has been properly completed, and will answer any questions that the person has. The person will then be asked to void, and may be given an antiemetic medication (to prevent nausea) and a sedative (to help relieve anxiety). After these medications have been given, the side rails must remain up on the bed or stretcher and the person must not get up without assistance, because the sedative may make the person drowsy and weak (Fig. 39-5). Make sure the call light control is within easy reach, and that the person is comfortable and warm.

If the surgery will be performed under general anaesthesia, the person's glasses or contact lenses, hearing aids, dentures, prosthetic devices, jewelry, and hair ornaments may be removed at this time. If the surgery will be performed under regional or local anaesthesia, the doctor may request that the person wear hearing aids or dentures during the surgery, to make communication easier. Items that are removed from the person are documented and given to the person's family or placed in the facility safe.

The surgical site may be prepared at this time, or this may be done in the operating room. The surgical site is the area of the body that will be operated on. Preparation of the surgical site may or may not involve removal of body hair. If hair removal is ordered, an electric clipper with a

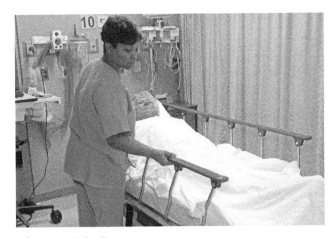

Figure 39-5

Last-minute preparations for surgery take place in the preparation area next to the operating room. Once medications have been given to prevent nausea and reduce anxiety, the person must remain in bed with the side rails up to reduce the risk of falling.

disposable head will most likely be used. If one of your duties is to perform pre-operative hair removal, make sure you have been instructed in the proper technique.

Last, a pre-operative checklist is completed (Fig. 39-6). The checklist is used to confirm that all pre-operative tests and procedures have been completed. The personal support worker is often responsible for completing and recording many of the tasks on the checklist.

Inpatients

If the person was admitted to the hospital prior to the surgery, the tasks that are completed immediately before the surgery may be completed in the person's room, before taking her to the operating room. In addition, you may need to help your patient from the bed onto the stretcher when it is time to go to the operating room. Let the person's family members know where they can wait while the person is in surgery. Some

---

1. Patient's name: _____ Date: _____ Height: _____ Weight: _____
   Identification band present: _____
2. Informed consent signed: _____ Special permits signed: _____
3. Surgical site: _____ (Ex: Sterilization)
4. History & physical examination report present: _____ Date: _____
5. Laboratory records present: _____
   CBC: _____ Hgb: _____ Urinalysis: _____ Hct: _____

6. | Item | Present | Removed |
   |---|---|---|
   | a. Natural teeth | | |
   | Dentures; upper, lower, partial | _____ | _____ |
   | Bridge, fixed; crown | _____ | _____ |
   | b. Contact lenses | _____ | _____ |
   | c. Other prostheses—type: _____ | _____ | _____ |
   | d. Jewelry: | | |
   | Wedding band (taped/tied) | _____ | _____ |
   | Rings | _____ | _____ |
   | Earrings: pierced, clip-on | _____ | _____ |
   | Neck chains | _____ | _____ |
   | Any other body piercings | _____ | _____ |
   | e. Make-up | _____ | _____ |
   | Nail polish | _____ | _____ |

7. Clothing
a. Clean patient gown	_____	_____
b. Cap	_____	_____
c. Sanitary pad, etc.	_____	_____

8. Family instructed where to wait? _____
9. Valuables secured? _____
10. Blood available? _____ Ordered? _____ Where? _____
11. Preanesthetic medication given: _____
    Type: _____ Time: _____
12. Voided: _____ Amount: _____ Time: _____ Catheter: _____
    Mouth care given: _____
13. Vital signs: Temperature: _____ Pulse: _____ Resp: _____ Blood Pressure: _____
14. Special problems/precautions: (Allergies, deafness, *etc.*): _____
15. Area of skin preparation: _____
16. _____ Date: _____ Time: _____
    Signature: Nurse releasing patient

Figure 39-6

A pre-operative checklist documents that all of the tasks that must be completed during the pre-operative period have been completed. The pre-operative checklist goes in the person's medical record and must be completed before the person goes into surgery.

facilities have surgical waiting rooms, while others allow the family to wait in the person's room. Please remember that family members are often anxious and nervous about the surgery. Refer any questions family members may have about the procedure or the person's condition to the nurse.

CARE OF THE POST-OPERATIVE PATIENT

Immediately after surgery, the person is taken to the **post-anaesthesia care unit (PACU),** also known as the recovery room (Fig. 39-7). While in the PACU, the person is closely monitored by the health care team to make sure that he is recovering without complications from the surgery or the anaesthesia. The person is usually groggy, but can be awakened. Once awake, the person will usually be oriented to person and place. The person will remain in the PACU until his condition is stable. While in the PACU, the person usually receives supplemental oxygen. Suctioning is also available, in case the person vomits or has secretions that interfere with respiration.

While the person is in surgery, you will most likely be responsible for preparing the person's room for his arrival post-operatively (Fig. 39-8). The bed linens are usually changed and a surgical bed is prepared (see Chapter 15). The bed is raised to make transferring the person from the stretcher to the bed easier. Furniture is moved, if necessary, to ensure a clear pathway for the

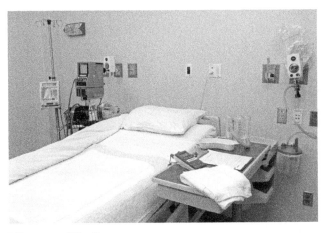

Figure 39-8
The personal support worker prepares the person's room for her return while the person is in surgery. The linens are changed and a surgical bed is made. The bed is raised to a height that will make transferring the person from the stretcher to the bed easier. The equipment that may be needed during the post-operative period is gathered and placed in the room. Before the occupant of this room arrives, the over-bed table will need to be moved out of the way to ensure a clear pathway from the door to the bed.

stretcher. Finally, items that may be needed at the time of the person's arrival are gathered and placed in the room. Items that may be needed include:

- Equipment for taking vital signs and a flow sheet for recording the vital signs
- An intravenous (IV) pole
- A towel and washcloth
- An emesis basin
- A bed protector
- Suction to connect to drainage devices
- Supplemental oxygen
- Pillows or other positioning aids to elevate the extremities
- Warmed blankets

When the person is returned to his room, you will need to assist in transferring the person from the stretcher to the bed. The nurse assesses the person's overall condition, checks for blood on the dressing and for the presence of drains and catheters, and adjusts the IV flow rate. While the nurse is doing this, you may be asked to take the person's vital signs. Vital signs are taken as ordered and recorded on the flow sheet. Post-operatively, routine vital sign measurements, including temperature, are usually taken every 15 minutes for the first hour, every 30 minutes for the next 1 to 2 hours, every hour for the next

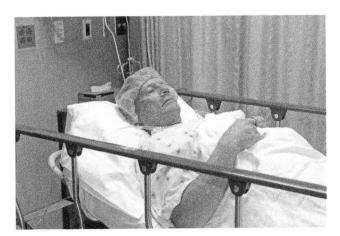

Figure 39-7
Following surgery, the person is taken to a post-anaesthesia care unit (PACU), also known as a recovery room. The person remains here and is monitored closely until the anaesthesia has worn off.

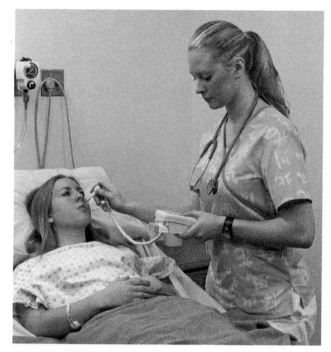

Figure 39-9
Vital signs are taken frequently during the immediate postoperative period because a change in vital signs could signal a complication of the surgery or the anaesthesia.

4 hours, and then every 4 hours as ordered (Fig. 39-9). As always, any changes in vital signs must be reported to the nurse immediately. In a person who is recovering from surgery, a change in a vital sign could be the first sign that the person is developing a post-operative complication.

The person may need to be positioned in a particular way post-operatively. For example, if the person is recovering from an anesthetic that was injected into the spinal canal, she may need to remain in the supine position for a period of time. Children may be positioned laterally or in the Sims' position to help prevent aspiration in the event of vomiting. If the person had surgery on an arm or leg, the arm or leg is usually elevated on a pillow or folded blanket to help prevent swelling and pain. Make sure you check with the nurse for any specific instructions or restrictions regarding the person's position. In all cases, the person should be positioned comfortably and in a way that will prevent stress on the surgical incision.

In the hours and days that follow surgery, the health care team focuses on preventing complications and assisting the person with routine tasks, such as grooming and elimination, as necessary. As a personal support worker, you will play a large role in helping the person to make a good recovery.

PREVENTING COMPLICATIONS

People who have had surgery are at risk for developing complications, especially related to breathing and circulation. In addition, the surgical site may become infected or the wound may not stay closed. As a personal support worker, there are several things that you will do to prevent complications from developing. Also, if one of your patients develops a complication from surgery, you may be the first one to notice. Reporting your observations to the nurse promptly helps to ensure that action will be taken quickly to prevent the person's condition from getting worse.

Respiratory Complications

The combined effects of general anaesthesia, the medications given to relieve post-operative pain, and a painful incision make it difficult for a person who is recovering from surgery to clear the lungs and airways of fluid and mucus. The person is drowsy from the anaesthesia and pain medication, and it hurts to cough! If the person also has a chronic respiratory disorder, such as asthma or chronic obstructive pulmonary disease (COPD), or if the person smokes, then her risk of developing a respiratory complication increases even more.

Common respiratory complications of surgery include pneumonia (fluid fills the alveoli) and **atelectasis** (the alveoli collapse). Both atelectasis and pneumonia make it difficult for oxygen to pass into the blood, and carbon dioxide to pass out of it.

To prevent fluid and mucus from collecting in the person's lungs, you may need to assist the person with frequent repositioning and with performing respiratory exercises. Commonly used respiratory exercises include coughing and deep breathing, and incentive spirometry (Fig. 39-10).

- **Coughing and deep breathing.** The person is helped into a comfortable position and then instructed to take a few deep breaths and cough forcefully. If the person has had abdominal or chest surgery, you may need to support the incision site with a small pillow or folded towel while the person coughs (see Fig. 39-10A). Supporting the incision site helps to minimize pain.
- **Incentive spirometry.** The person forcefully inhales through a special device called an incentive spirometer (see Fig. 39-10B). The device consists of a tube and a chamber that contains balls. The goal is for the person to inhale hard enough through the tube to raise the balls in the chamber.

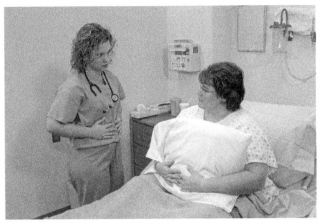
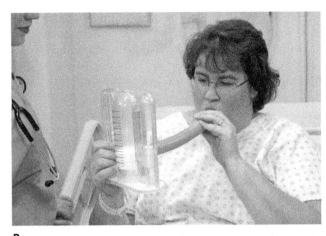

A   B

Figure 39-10
Respiratory exercises may be ordered during the post-operative period to prevent the person from developing respiratory complications such as pneumonia and atelectasis. **(A)** Coughing and deep breathing exercises. The person takes a few deep breaths and then coughs forcefully. **(B)** Incentive spirometry. The person inhales through an incentive spirometer with the goal of causing the balls to rise in the chamber.

If your patient has orders to perform respiratory exercises, these exercises will need to be done every few hours, or as directed. Elevating the head of the bed while the person is supine will also make it easier for the person to breathe.

Cardiovascular Complications

Anesthetic agents, pain medications, and general immobility after surgery can cause the body's circulation to slow down, leading to pooling of blood in the legs. When blood flow slows and blood pools, a thrombus, or blood clot, may form. Surgical patients who are elderly or have a history of circulatory problems are at the most risk for developing thrombi. Certain conditions (such as fractures of the femur, or thigh bone) and certain surgeries (such as joint replacement surgery) also carry a high risk of thrombus formation.

A thrombus in one of the veins of the legs causes inflammation and pain, a condition known as **thrombophlebitis.** Sometimes the blood clot will break loose and travel through the bloodstream. This puts the person at great risk. A blood clot that breaks loose and moves through the bloodstream is known as an *embolus.* The embolus can travel to the brain and get stuck in one of the blood vessels there, causing a stroke. Or, the embolus can travel to the pulmonary artery, the artery that carries blood from the heart to the lungs so that it can receive oxygen. Blocking of the pulmonary artery by an embolus is called a **pulmonary embolism** and it is often

fatal. Restlessness and shortness of breath may be signs of pulmonary embolism and should be reported to the nurse immediately.

A number of different measures are taken to lower the person's risk of cardiovascular complications.

Sequential compression device

A **sequential compression device (SCD)** is a device that is applied to the calves to help prevent pooling of blood in the lower legs (Fig. 39-11).

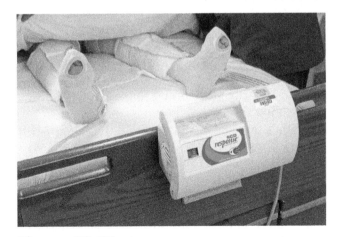

Figure 39-11
A sequential compression device (SCD) helps to prevent pooling of blood in the lower extremities. The plastic sleeves around the person's lower legs contain multiple chambers, which alternately inflate and deflate, pushing blood through the veins.

Disposable plastic sleeves are wrapped around the person's lower legs. The sleeves, which have several different compartments, are connected to an air pump via tubing. Air is pumped into the first compartment (the one closest to the foot) to inflate it. Then the next compartment inflates, then the next, helping to move the blood from the lower legs toward the heart. When the top-most compartment has been inflated, all the compartments deflate and the cycle begins again at the bottom. The inflating and deflating action massages the veins, pushing the blood through the veins and back to the heart. Many of your patients will return from the PACU with SCDs in place.

Anti-embolism stockings

Anti-embolism (TED) stockings are made of a tight-fitting elastic fabric. The stockings, which may be knee-high or thigh-high, are specially fitted for the person by the nurse or the physical therapist. The elastic fabric applies pressure, compressing the veins and helping to return blood to the heart. This helps to prevent pooling of blood in the legs.

Anti-embolism stockings may be applied before surgery, or ordered afterward. If the stockings are allowed to be removed at night, they should be reapplied before the person gets out of bed for the day. Once the person stands up, gravity increases blood flow to the veins in the lower legs, causing the veins to widen and the blood to pool. Procedure 39-1 describes how to apply anti-embolism stockings.

Leg exercises

The doctor may also order leg exercises for the person following surgery, to help reduce the risk of embolism. If the person is weak or unconscious, you may need to help her with these exercises (Fig. 39-12). The person usually must do these exercises every 1 to 2 hours while he or she is awake.

The exercises are done while the person is in the supine position. One leg is exercised at a time. The person rotates the ankle, flexes and points the foot, flexes and extends the knee, and finishes by raising the leg off the bed and lowering it again. Each movement is repeated five times, and then the movements are repeated with the other leg, unless the person had leg surgery. In this case, the exercises might only be done on the "well" leg. A doctor's order is required to exercise the leg that was operated on. Always check with the nurse to see if there are any specific instructions for your patient.

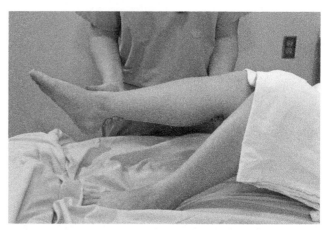

Figure 39-12
If your patient is weak or unconscious, you may have to help him or her to perform leg exercises. Leg exercises help to prevent blood from pooling in the veins of the legs.

TELL THE NURSE

During the post-operative period, you may be the first person to notice signs of a post-operative complication. Report any of the following observations to the nurse immediately:

- There is an increased amount of bright red drainage (blood) on the person's wound dressing or in the drainage device

- There is a significant change in the person's vital signs (blood pressure, pulse, respirations, temperature)

- The person is having trouble breathing, or is making wheezing or gurgling sounds

- The person is restless, confused, or disoriented

- The person's lips or nailbeds are very pale or have a bluish tinge

- The person's skin is cool and clammy

- The person complains of increased pain, tingling, or numbness of an extremity with a cast or bandage

- The person complains of pain or swelling at the IV site, or the IV is not dripping

- The person complains of abdominal pain, nausea, or vomiting

ASSISTING WITH POSITIONING

During the post-operative period, most people will need assistance with repositioning themselves every 1 to 2 hours. Frequent repositioning is necessary for the person's comfort. In addition, it helps to prevent the post-operative complications of pneumonia and embolism. Depending on where the incision is, moving may be very painful for the person. Use a lift sheet to help reposition the person, and move him gently and slowly.

ASSISTING WITH NUTRITION

A person who is recovering from surgery usually needs intravenous (IV) therapy until she is able to take fluids orally and is no longer nauseated. If the person has had surgery involving the digestive system, she may have a nasogastric tube. The nasogastric tube is connected to suction to keep the stomach empty. These patients may need to remain on IV fluids for several days.

Once the person is able to take fluids orally and is no longer nauseated, she will usually be started on a clear liquid diet. The diet is progressed as the person's condition improves. From a clear liquid diet, the person usually progresses to a full liquid diet and then gradually to a regular diet. Good hydration and a proper diet help with the healing process.

ASSISTING WITH ELIMINATION

Following surgery, the person may have difficulties related to elimination. Some people may need to use a bedpan or a urinal after surgery. The person's NPO status, pain medications, and immobility can lead to constipation. A full bladder can increase pain from an abdominal incision, making voiding difficult. As a result, some people may need to be catheterized. Other patients will return from surgery with an indwelling urinary catheter already in place. Your responsibilities will include reporting the person's first voiding after surgery. Often, you will also need to measure and record the person's intake and output (I&O) for a period of time following surgery as well.

ASSISTING WITH HYGIENE

People who are recovering from surgery may need help with personal hygiene. Assisting with frequent oral care, helping the person to wash his face and hands, and changing soiled gowns promptly are all things you can do to help promote comfort. Many people will not be able to take a bath or a shower for a few days following surgery, because the incision cannot get wet. These people will need your help in the form of either partial or complete bed baths.

ASSISTING WITH WALKING (AMBULATION)

Early and frequent ambulation is helpful in preventing many of the complications that can result from surgery. Many times, a person who has had surgery is able to get out of bed within a few hours of returning to his room. Because the person will be weak and unsteady, he will need your help when ambulating. Allow the person time to sit on the edge of the bed ("dangle") before getting out of bed. If the person complains of feeling dizzy or lightheaded while he is dangling, help the person to lie back down and call the nurse. Otherwise, check the person's pulse and blood pressure and then help the person to stand. Usually, you and the person will walk only a short distance to begin with. As the person's strength returns, you can go for longer walks.

SUMMARY

- Surgery is a branch of medicine that involves treating diseases and disorders by removing or repairing damaged organs or tissues.
  - Surgery may be exploratory or definitive. It may be elective, urgent, or emergent.
  - Surgery is performed under anaesthesia. A general, regional, or local anesthetic may be used.
  - Because many surgeries are now done on an outpatient basis, you may be responsible for helping a person to prepare and recover from surgery, even if you do not work in a hospital or other acute care setting.
- There are three phases of care for a person who is having surgery. The term *perioperative period* is used to describe all three phases of the surgical process as a whole.
- During the pre-operative period, the patient is prepared emotionally and physically for the procedure.

- People who are about to have surgery often have many fears and concerns. Pre-operative teaching helps to relieve some of the person's fears. By listening to your patients and promptly relaying any questions they may have to the nurse, you can make an important contribution to the pre-operative teaching process.
- A pre-operative checklist is completed to verify that the tasks needed to prepare the person physically for surgery have been accomplished, and that informed consent has been obtained.

- During the intra-operative period, surgery is performed.

- During the post-operative period, the nursing team's efforts focus on preventing complications and helping the person to recover.

- Coughing and deep breathing exercises, along with incentive spirometry, may help to reduce the person's risk of developing respiratory complications, such as pneumonia and atelectasis.
- Application of sequential compression devices (SCDs) or anti-embolism (TED) stockings may help to prevent cardiovascular complications, such as thrombophlebitis or embolism. Leg exercises and frequent ambulation are also helpful.
- In addition to performing tasks related to preventing complications, personal support workers may need to assist surgical patients with activities of daily living (ADLs), such as bathing and elimination, during the post-operative period.

PROCEDURE **39-1**

Applying Anti-embolism (TED) Stockings

WHY YOU DO IT   Use of anti-embolism (TED) stockings as ordered helps to prevent the formation of blood clots in the lower legs.

Getting Ready

1. Complete the "Getting Ready" steps.

Supplies

- anti-embolism (TED) stockings in the correct size

Procedure

2. Make sure that the bed is positioned at a comfortable working height (to promote good body mechanics) and that the wheels are locked. If the side rails are in use, lower the side rail on the working side of the bed. The side rail on the opposite side of the bed should remain up.

3. Help the person into the supine position.

4. Fanfold the top linens to the foot of the bed. Adjust the person's hospital gown or pajama bottoms as necessary to expose one leg at a time.

5. Turn the stocking inside out down to the heel.

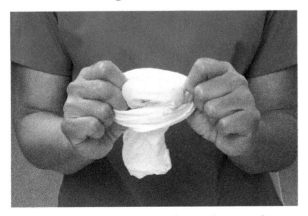

Step 5 Turn the stocking inside out down to the heel.

6. Slip the foot of the stocking over the person's toes, foot, and heel. The stocking has an opening in the toe area, which allows the health care team to assess the person's toes to make sure they are receiving enough blood. Depending on the manufacturer, this opening may be on the top or on the bottom of the stocking.

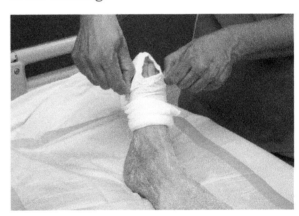

Step 6 Slip the foot of the stocking over the person's toes, foot, and heel.

7. Grasp the top of the stocking and pull it up the person's leg. The stocking will turn itself right-side out as you pull it up the person's leg.

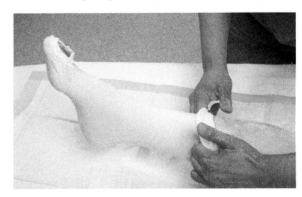

Step 7 Grasp the top of the stocking and pull it up the person's leg.

(continued)

8. Check to make sure that the stocking is not twisted and that it fits snugly against the person's leg, with no wrinkles. Also make sure that the stocking fits smoothly over the heel and that the opening in the toe area is correctly located in the toe region.

9. Cover that leg, expose the other leg, and repeat steps 5 through 8.

10. Help the person back into a comfortable position, straighten the bottom linens, and draw the top linens over the person. Raise the head of the bed as the person requests. Make sure that the bed is lowered to its lowest position and that the wheels are locked.

Finishing Up   CLSOWR

11. Complete the "Finishing Up" steps.

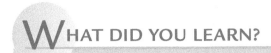

WHAT DID YOU LEARN?

Multiple Choice

Select the single best answer for each of the following questions.

1. Mrs. Jones is recovering from surgery. How often will she need assistance with repositioning?
   a. Every shift
   b. Every 1 to 2 hours
   c. Every 3 to 4 hours
   d. Every 15 minutes

2. Which one of the following patients is at high risk for an embolism?
   a. Mr. Smith, who is 75 years old and has just had cardiac bypass surgery
   b. Mrs. Greene, who is 60 years old and has just had a hip joint replaced
   c. Ms. Kirkpatrick, who is 40 years old and has just had surgery to repair a fractured leg
   d. All of the above

3. Which one of the following may be a sign of pulmonary embolism?
   a. Fever
   b. Fatigue
   c. Profuse sweating
   d. Restlessness and shortness of breath

4. The nurse asks you to help Mr. Huang in Room 340 with coughing and deep breathing exercises. What is the purpose of these exercises?
   a. To help Mr. Huang build up his strength following the surgery
   b. To lower Mr. Huang's risk of pulmonary embolism
   c. To lower Mr. Huang's risk of pneumonia or atelectasis
   d. All of the above

5. Why might emergent surgery be necessary?
   a. The person has been in a car accident and is bleeding internally
   b. The person needs to have a cataract removed
   c. The person needs to have a hip joint replaced
   d. The person needs to have a tumour in the breast removed

6. During which type of anaesthesia is the person unconscious?
   a. Regional anaesthesia
   b. Local anaesthesia
   c. General anaesthesia
   d. All of the above

7. Which one of the following activities takes place before surgery?
   a. Frequent ambulation
   b. Completion of the pre-operative checklist
   c. Performance of coughing and deep breathing exercises
   d. Careful monitoring in the post-anaesthesia care unit (PACU)

8. Why must a person who is having surgery avoid taking food or fluids by mouth for 6 to 8 hours before the surgery?
   a. If the person vomits as a result of the anaesthesia, he or she could be at risk for aspiration
   b. An empty stomach is necessary to prevent infection of the abdominal cavity
   c. The anaesthesia is more effective if the person's stomach is empty
   d. An empty stomach helps to prevent problems with elimination after the surgery

STOP and Think!

You are a personal support worker in an assisted-living facility. One of your residents, Mrs. Wight, is scheduled to have a surgical procedure done on an outpatient basis at the local hospital. Mrs. Wight is a very stylish woman who takes a lot of pride in her appearance. Her nails are always done, she always accessorizes her outfits, and she always makes sure to apply a fresh coat of lipstick before leaving her room. Mrs. Wight knows that she is not permitted to wear makeup during the surgery, but when you arrive in her room to help her get ready the day of the surgery, you find that she is looking like her usual self—nails done, jewelry on, lipstick applied. What would you do, and why?

You work as a personal support worker in a hospital. One of your patients, Mr. Newman, is scheduled for exploratory surgery to determine whether a tumor in his brain is cancerous. Mr. Newman is married, with three children ranging in age from 8 to 14 years. He has a very large extended family, many of whom have been staying at the hospital day and night since Mr. Newman was admitted. How might Mr. Newman and his family members be feeling right now? Is there anything you could do to help them?

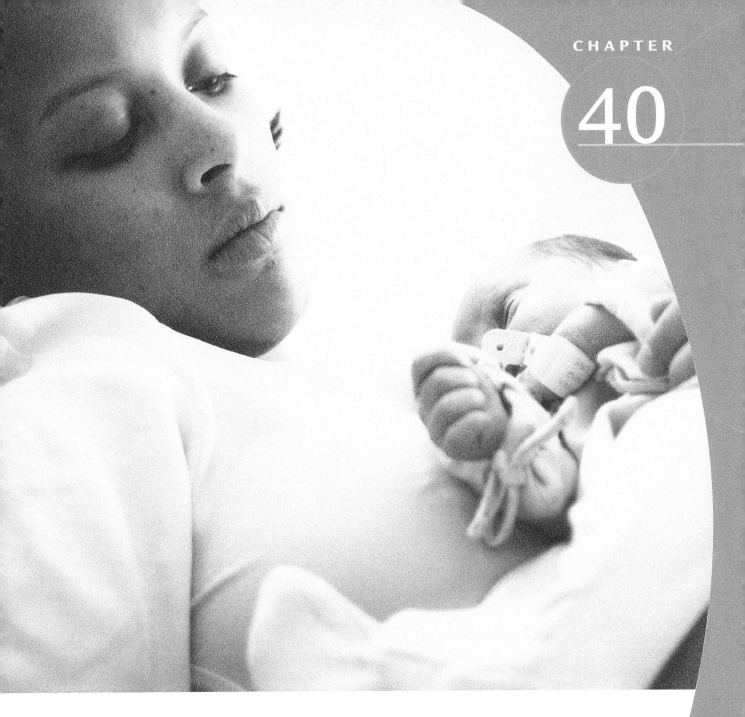

Caring for Mothers and Newborns

WHAT WILL YOU LEARN?

In this chapter, you will learn how to care for a newborn baby. You will also learn about the care required by the mother in the months leading up to the birth, during the birth, and following the birth. Although many provinces or territories and health care facilities do not allow personal support workers to participate in the care of an expectant mother

Photo: Few events are met with as much excitement as the birth of a baby.
(© Laurent/Ravonison/Photo Researchers, Inc.)

or a newborn, others do. You may work in a hospital, providing care for mothers and newborns before, during, and after delivery. Or you may be employed by a home health care agency that provides home care to expectant and new mothers and their newborns. When you are finished with this chapter, you will be able to:

1. Describe physical changes that occur in the female reproductive system during pregnancy.
2. List reasons that an expectant mother may need home care or hospitalization during her pregnancy.
3. Describe the two ways of delivering a baby.
4. Describe the personal support worker's responsibilities when caring for a new mother.
5. List observations you might make while caring for a new mother that should be reported to the nurse immediately.
6. Discuss important security and safety issues related to caring for a newborn.
7. Explain how to care for the umbilical cord stump.
8. Explain how to care for a baby boy who has been circumcised.
9. Explain how to bottle-feed a baby.
10. Explain how to bathe a baby.

Vocabulary

Antepartum (prenatal) period	Pre-eclampsia/ eclampsia	Vernix	Sitz bath
Placenta	Labour	Bonding period	Colostrum
Prenatal care	Cesarean section	Postpartum period	Umbilical cord
Pre-term labour	Epidural block	Lochia	
		Episiotomy	

THE ANTEPARTUM (PRENATAL) PERIOD

When a woman is pregnant, the period of time from conception until the baby is born is called the **antepartum (prenatal) period.** (The prefixes *ante-* and *pre-* both mean "before," and the roots *partum* and *natal* both mean "birth.") The antepartum period lasts approximately 9 months and is divided into three trimesters of 3 months each.

PHYSICAL CHANGES IN PREGNANCY

Very soon after conception, the pregnant woman's body undergoes dramatic changes that allow for the growth and development of the new life she carries inside. The changes are the result of hormones secreted by the woman's pituitary gland and the **placenta,** the structure that develops from the inside lining of the uterus during pregnancy and participates in the exchange of gas and nutrients between the mother and the developing baby (called a *fetus*). Prolactin, a

hormone secreted by the pituitary gland, causes the woman's breasts to enlarge and prepare for the production of milk to nourish the baby after birth. The uterus enlarges to make room for the growing fetus. More blood is formed to manage the extra demand created by the fetus's need for oxygen and nutrients. The extra blood also helps to remove the extra waste products created by the fetus.

These physical changes can result in many "signs and symptoms" of pregnancy. For example, changes in hormone levels may be responsible for the morning sickness that many women have during the first trimester of pregnancy. In a pregnancy that is progressing normally, certain "signs and symptoms" are expected at certain times (Fig. 40-1).

ROUTINE PRENATAL CARE

Prenatal care, or the health care given to a woman in the months leading up to the birth of her baby, helps to ensure the health of both the mother and the fetus during the pregnancy. Routine prenatal care involves screening tests and regular check-ups. The woman is also given

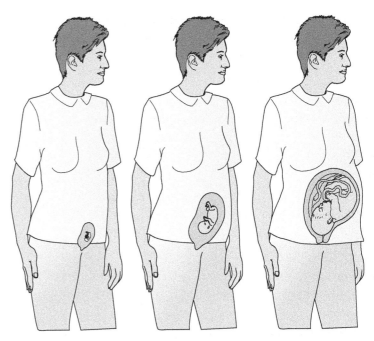

First trimester
- First missed menstrual period
- Morning sickness
- Swollen, tender breasts

Second trimester
- Visibly enlarged uterus
- Weight gain
- Breast enlargement
- Will feel baby move

Third trimester
- Indigestion and shortness of breath (caused by enlarged uterus pressing on stomach and lungs)
- Difficulty sleeping
- Swollen ankles

Figure 40-1
The antepartum period is divided into three trimesters. In a pregnancy that is progressing normally, certain signs and symptoms are expected at certain times.

advice about how to care for herself and her developing fetus:

- **Nutrition.** A pregnant woman should eat a healthy diet, containing a variety of nutritious foods. Because a pregnant woman must meet her own body's nutritional needs, plus those of the developing fetus, her nutritional needs are increased. For example, because she has an increased need for calcium, a pregnant woman should consume three to four servings of dairy foods each day (versus two to three servings for a woman who is not pregnant). Most doctors also suggest that pregnant women take a special prenatal vitamin supplement daily to ensure that their nutritional needs are met.

- **Avoidance of toxins.** A pregnant woman should avoid smoking, drinking alcohol, or taking any medications that have not been specifically approved by her doctor. Many of these substances are known to harm the growth and development of the fetus.

- **Exercise.** Moderate exercise throughout pregnancy has been shown to have benefits for both the mother and the fetus. If a woman is interested in either starting an exercise program or continuing one during her pregnancy, the health care team will provide information about how to safely do this.

Helping Hands and a Caring Heart

FOCUS ON HUMANISTIC HEALTH CARE

When caring for a pregnant woman, be aware that the woman's feelings may differ from what you consider "normal." Some women have mixed emotions when they find out that they are pregnant. The pregnancy may be unplanned, or another child may cause financial hardship for the family. Sometimes there are health concerns associated with the pregnancy. All of these are reasons that an expectant mother may not behave in a "typical" way. It is important to respect your patient's feelings, even if they differ from what yours would be in a similar situation. Also, avoid being judgmental about a woman's marital situation or other lifestyle choices. Remember that not all pregnant women have (or necessarily want) husbands.

COMPLICATIONS DURING PREGNANCY

Prenatal care helps to prevent complications from developing during the pregnancy. It also helps to detect complications at an early stage, should any develop. If a complication develops, the pregnant woman may be hospitalized or placed on partial or complete bed rest at home for the rest of her pregnancy to help protect her own health, as well as that of the fetus. Examples of complications that can develop during pregnancy include **pre-term labour** (labour begins too early, before the fetus can survive on its own) and **pre-eclampsia/ eclampsia** (the woman develops dangerously high blood pressure). Some pregnancies are "high risk" right from the start—for example, the woman has had trouble carrying a baby to term in the past, she is carrying more than one baby, or she has a chronic health condition, such as diabetes. These women may also be hospitalized or put on bed rest at some point during their pregnancies.

A pregnant woman who is having, or is at risk for, complications may be hospitalized for weeks or even months prior to the birth of the baby. Depending on the situation, she may be permitted to stay at home, but with extreme limitations on activity. In this case, she will often need the services of a home support worker.

MEETING THE PREGNANT WOMAN'S PHYSICAL NEEDS

A personal support worker who is caring for a pregnant woman in the hospital or home health care setting may have the following responsibilities:

- **Measuring and recording vital signs.** Any change in the woman's vital signs must be reported to the nurse immediately.
- **Obtaining urine samples.** Depending on the situation, the woman may need to provide urine samples on a regular basis. The urine is tested for glucose and protein. You may be responsible for obtaining these samples.
- **Helping with personal care.** Many women who are on bed rest are allowed to get up to go to the bathroom, but they will need assistance with bathing in bed and grooming. If the woman is not allowed to get out of bed at all, then she will also need assistance with toileting.

Make sure you follow all instructions that are given to you regarding the woman's care, and ask the nurse for help if you are unsure about how to complete any of your assigned duties.

TELL THE NURSE

Complications during a pregnancy can endanger the life of the mother and the baby if they are not reported promptly. When caring for a pregnant woman, report the following observations to the nurse immediately:

- There is a change in the woman's vital signs (especially an elevated blood pressure or body temperature)
- The woman complains of a headache or of seeing "spots" or "bright flashes" in front of her eyes
- The woman faints or is dizzy
- The woman has nausea, vomiting, or diarrhea
- The woman complains of abdominal pain
- The woman is experiencing uterine contractions that are frequent or severe and are not relieved by resting
- The woman has vaginal bleeding or there is fluid leaking from the vagina

MEETING THE PREGNANT WOMAN'S EMOTIONAL NEEDS

Pregnancy can be a time of great joy and anticipation. It can also be a time of great stress, especially if complications develop that jeopardize the mother's health and that of the baby.

A pregnant woman who is experiencing complications and has been placed on partial or complete bed rest prior to the birth of her child may have many emotional needs. The woman may feel lonely and bored—imagine what it would be like to be stuck in the same bed, in the same room, for weeks, or even months. Making pleasant conversation as you complete your duties can help to ease the woman's loneliness. The woman may also have lots of worries. She may be worried about her own health, as well as that of her unborn child. She may worry about children she already has, and how they are being cared for in her absence. She may worry about how she will pay her bills during the time that she cannot work. Taking the time to listen to the woman's concerns, and reporting these concerns to the nurse, is important (Fig. 40-2).

Sometimes pregnancy does not end with the birth of a healthy baby. Many pregnancies result

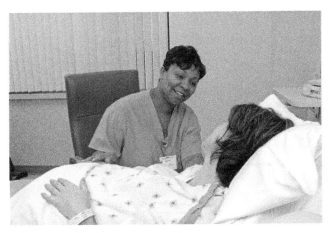

Figure 40-2
A pregnant woman who is having complications is likely to be lonely, bored, scared, or all three. Making yourself available to listen is part of providing humanistic care.

in miscarriage. Some babies are born too early to survive on their own, and die. Some babies are stillborn (born dead). The loss of a child is an emotional time for the family. Loss affects each person differently. Be respectful of the family's feelings. Acknowledge the loss, and simply say "I'm sorry."

LABOUR AND DELIVERY

LABOUR

When it is time for a baby to be born, the mother's pituitary gland releases oxytocin, a hormone that stimulates the uterus to contract. The contractions of the uterus squeeze the baby downward, forcing his head against the cervix so

that it opens, or *dilates*. This process is known as **labour.** The length of time a woman is in labour varies greatly from person to person. Some women have very short labours, while other labours may last as long as 36 hours or so. When caring for a woman who is in labour, your responsibilities will be defined by facility policy. In many cases, your only responsibility will be to measure and record vital signs and other observations. However, some facilities or birth centers provide additional training, which will allow you to perform more specialized tasks when assisting a woman who is in labour.

DELIVERY

A woman may deliver (give birth to) the baby vaginally or by cesarean section (Fig. 40-3). Delivery of the baby through the vagina (a vaginal delivery) is usually preferred, unless there are complications. A **cesarean section** (delivery of the baby through a surgical incision made in the mother's abdomen) is done when a vaginal delivery is not possible or safe for the mother or the baby. For example, many doctors choose to do a cesarean section when labour has gone on for too long, when the baby is not positioned correctly for a vaginal delivery, or when the mother has a serious health problem (such as heart disease) that would make a prolonged labour dangerous. Because a cesarean section is a surgical procedure, the recovery time following a cesarean delivery is generally longer than the recovery time following a vaginal delivery.

Women who give birth vaginally may choose to deliver with or without pain medications. Many

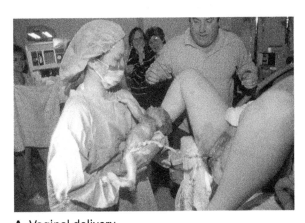

A. Vaginal delivery

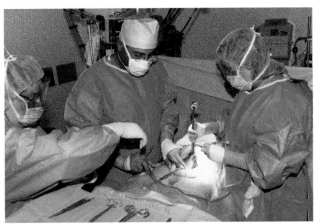

B. Cesarean delivery

Figure 40-3
A baby may be delivered (**A**) vaginally or (**B**) by cesarean section. (*A,* © *B. Proud*)

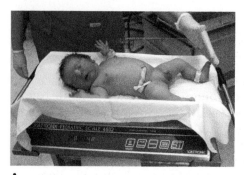
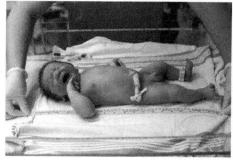

A   B

Figure 40-4
The baby is **(A)** weighed and **(B)** measured.

women choose to have an **epidural block,** anesthesia given through a catheter that is placed in the spinal canal. The catheter is placed in the lower back, so that the anesthetic affects only the pelvis and legs. This allows the woman to be awake and participate fully in the birth of her child, while numbing the pain of labour.

Woman who give birth by cesarean section are having major abdominal surgery, and therefore require an anesthetic of some sort. The woman may be given an epidural block, or in some cases, general anesthesia. An incision is then made in the woman's abdomen, and the baby is lifted out of the uterus. After delivery, the incision is closed and the mother is recovered in the same manner as with any other type of operation (see Chapter 39).

IMMEDIATELY FOLLOWING DELIVERY

Immediately following the birth of the baby, if the baby is breathing well and otherwise stable, she may be handed directly to her mother for a few moments. Then, the baby is weighed and measured and evaluated by the nurse or doctor (Fig. 40-4). The baby's footprints are taken, and identification bracelets are applied to her wrists and ankles. Because it takes a while for a newborn's body to adjust to life outside of the mother's body, the baby may be placed for a short period of time in a special bed to help keep her warm. A temperature monitor may be taped to the baby's skin, or you may need to measure the baby's axillary temperature as often as ordered or until the baby's temperature has stabilized. Once the baby's temperature has stabilized, she is given a bath to remove the **vernix,** a protective, cheese-like substance that is present on the skin of newborns. Finally, the baby is wrapped snugly in a blanket; a soft, stretchy cap is put on the baby's head to prevent heat loss;

and the baby is placed in the waiting arms of her mother.

The first hour or two immediately following delivery is important for mother–infant bonding. This **bonding period** helps to develop the emotional and physical attachment between the mother and the infant. It is important to remember the importance of the bonding process for the father also (Fig. 40-5).

THE POSTPARTUM PERIOD

During the **postpartum period** (the 6-week period of time following the birth), you may be involved in the care of both the new mother and the new baby.

CARE OF THE MOTHER

Birth is a stressful, difficult activity affecting the entire body. After delivery, the mother will likely be tired, hungry, and thirsty. She may want to

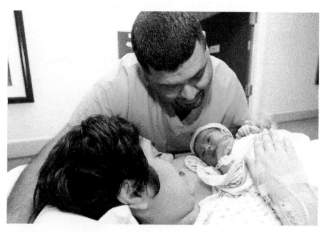

Figure 40-5
The first 1 to 2 hours following birth is a critical time for parents to bond with their newborn, and vice versa.

sleep, especially if the labour was long and difficult. She may only want privacy, to cuddle and get to know her new baby.

When you are caring for a woman who has just delivered a baby, you will have several general responsibilities related to her care, including:

- **Taking vital signs as ordered.** You will need to take the woman's vital signs as often as ordered. As always, any change in vital signs should be reported immediately.
- **Assisting with transferring and walking.** If the woman has had an epidural block, she may be unsteady on her feet for some time after delivery, and she will need help with transferring and walking.
- **Assisting with toileting.** Assist the new mother to the bathroom, or provide a bedpan if needed. Measure and record the amount of urine voided. Many women experience swelling after delivery and may not be able to void. If this is the case with your patient, tell the nurse. The woman may need to be catheterized.
- **Observing.** A complication that develops during the immediate postpartum period can become life-threatening very quickly. Being observant can make the difference between life and death for the new mother.

TELL THE NURSE

When caring for a woman who has just given birth, report any of the following observations to the nurse immediately:

- There is an increased amount of vaginal bleeding
- There is a change in the woman's vital signs, especially an increase in pulse rate and a decrease in blood pressure, or an increase in temperature
- The woman complains of dizziness or excessive thirst
- The woman has trouble breathing or complains of pain in the chest
- A woman who has had an epidural block complains of increased numbness in her legs and pelvic region, or a headache
- The woman is having trouble urinating or is unable to urinate

You may also have additional responsibilities, as described in the sections that follow.

Managing Vaginal Discharge

Following delivery, the mother will have vaginal discharge, called **lochia:**

- *Rubra lochia.* Initially, the discharge is bright red and is called *rubra lochia* (*rubra* means "red"). The woman will wear special sanitary napkins to collect this flow, which may last for 2 to 3 days. If she is recovering from a cesarean section or is on bed rest for other reasons, you may have to assist her with changing these napkins. Note the amount and colour of the discharge and report your observations to the nurse. Remember that vaginal secretions should be handled according to standard precautions. Always wear gloves anytime you might come into contact with soiled sanitary napkins, bed linens, or bed protectors.
- *Lochia serosa* follows for approximately 3 to 10 days longer. Serosa is pink- or brown-tinged fluid. Any large clots are abnormal and should be reported immediately.
- *Lochia alba* follows for another week or two and is mostly creamy white to yellowish in colour (*alba* means "white").

Assisting With Perineal Care

If the woman delivered her baby vaginally, she may have perineal tears, caused by the baby's head as it exited the birth canal. Sometimes, doctors perform an episiotomy to prevent the perineum from tearing so much. An **episiotomy** is an incision made in the perineum to enlarge the vaginal opening, making delivery of the baby's head easier. If the perineum was torn during the delivery, or if an episiotomy was done, the perineum will be sore and tender for several days and the new mother may find sitting uncomfortable.

Ice may be applied to the perineum for a period of time immediately following delivery to help prevent swelling. Afterward, the use of Sitz baths may help ease the discomfort. A **Sitz bath** is a hot water soak for the perineal area. The basin, which usually fits over the toilet seat, is filled with hot water [40.5°C to 43.4°C (105°F to 110°F)] and the woman sits in it for the prescribed amount of time. Be sure to follow the nursing care plan; the maximum amount of time allowed is 20 minutes. After the Sitz bath, help the woman to stand up. She may be dizzy because the hot water causes the blood vessels to dilate. Depending on facility policy, new mothers may also be instructed to cleanse the perineal area after each trip to the bathroom by spraying warm water over the area using a small plastic sprayer. Increased pain, swelling, or drainage from the episiotomy site could indicate an infection and should be reported to the nurse immediately.

Assisting With Breastfeeding

Many women choose to breastfeed their babies. Immediately following delivery of the baby, the new mother's breasts produce **colostrum,** a thin yellowish fluid that contains extra calories and protein, as well as important antibodies. Colostrum is usually secreted for 2 to 3 days after birth and is then replaced by the mother's breast milk. Breastfeeding requires the mother to take in extra calories and fluids. Therefore, you should offer the mother fresh water frequently, as directed by the nurse.

The woman's breasts may become swollen and painful when the milk comes in. Frequent nursing of the infant will help to ease the discomfort, which usually only lasts for a couple of days. The appearance of a painful lump, reddened areas, or an elevated temperature could indicate a breast infection and should be reported to the nurse immediately.

If a woman chooses to breastfeed her baby, the nurse will teach her how. You may need to help the new mother get in a comfortable position, especially if she has had a cesarean section or an episiotomy. Help her to first wash her hands and then gently clean the nipple of the breast with warm water. Next, hand the mother the baby. There are several different ways to hold a baby during breastfeeding. With time, the mother will usually find the way of holding the baby that works best for her. Have the mother stroke the baby's cheek with her nipple to stimulate the baby's rooting reflex. The baby will turn his head toward the breast and open his mouth. The mother needs to place all of the nipple and part of the *areola* (the coloured portion of the breast surrounding the nipple) into the baby's mouth. She may need to use her finger to help keep her breast from blocking the baby's nose while he nurses (Fig. 40-6). As the baby sucks on the breast, the mother may experience cramping pains in her lower abdomen. This is normal. After the baby has finished feeding from the first breast, the mother inserts her finger gently into his mouth to break the suction before removing him from the breast. After burping the baby, the process is repeated with the other breast.

After the baby has finished nursing, have the mother clean her breasts with warm water. Soap should not be used, because it can cause dryness or irritation of the nipples. Some women use special creams or ointments when they first start

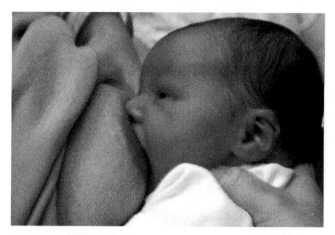

Figure 40-6
When breastfeeding, the mother may need to use a finger to hold the breast away from the baby's nose. Note that the baby's mouth covers both the nipple and the areola.

breastfeeding to help keep the nipples from cracking and becoming sore. Some women find that a supportive nursing bra is more comfortable than a regular bra, while others do not.

CARE OF THE BABY

A newborn is considered a neonate for the first 28 days of his or her life. You may help to care for a neonate in the hospital or birth center, or in the home as a home support worker. You may also find yourself caring for older babies, especially if you work in the home health care setting or in the pediatrics unit of a hospital.

TELL THE NURSE

A baby can become very sick very quickly. When caring for an infant, report any of the following observations to the nurse immediately:

- The baby appears weak or "floppy"
- The baby is pale
- The baby cries, and nothing you try makes him stop
- The baby's temperature is abnormal (either high or low)
- The baby's heart rate is abnormal (either fast or slow)
- The baby is breathing rapidly and shallowly
- The baby cannot be wakened

- The baby has a rash
- The baby will not eat
- The baby's eyes are red or discoloured
- The baby has vomited

Taking Vital Signs

You may be responsible for taking vital signs on the newborn infant. If the baby is in the room with the mother, make sure you explain what you are going to do before beginning.

- A newborn's temperature may be measured either by the axillary or tympanic method (Fig. 40-7). Rectal temperatures are not routinely taken on newborns. The range of normal is 36.6°C to 37°C (97.6°F to 98.6°F).
- A newborn's apical pulse is taken for a full minute by listening (auscultating) with a stethoscope over the heart. The normal heart rate in a newborn is 110 to 160 beats/min. A newborn's respirations are also counted for a full minute by watching the abdomen rise and fall. The normal respiratory rate in a newborn is 30 to 60 breaths/min. Vital signs taken on a crying baby are not going to be accurate, so it is best to measure the baby's pulse and respirations while the baby is sleeping, if possible.
- A newborn's blood pressure is measured in the baby's arm using a cuff specifically sized according to the baby's weight (Fig. 40-8). Most facilities use electronic blood pressure devices for taking a newborn's blood

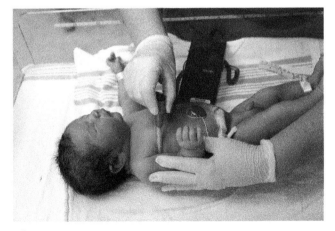

Figure 40-7
A newborn's temperature is measured using either the axillary or tympanic method. The axillary method is shown here.

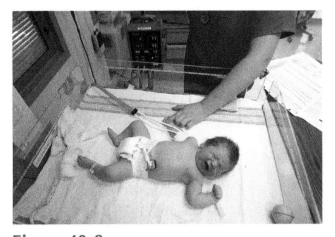

Figure 40-8
A newborn's blood pressure may be measured manually or using an electronic measuring device. Here, an electronic measuring device is being used. Note the very small cuff, which is sized according to the baby's weight.

pressure. These devices inflate the cuff and measure the blood pressure automatically. The range of normal for a newborn is 50 to 80 mm Hg systolic, 30 to 50 mm Hg diastolic.

Ensuring Security

If you work in the postpartum unit of a hospital or in a birthing center, there will be many policies and procedures in place to ensure the security of the newborn (Fig. 40-9). These security measures are taken to prevent newborns from being kidnapped from the facility by people posing as relatives or health care workers. Always follow the security procedures in place at your facility. These procedures usually require visitors to sign in. The baby is brought from, and returned to, the nursery by a member of the health care team. A member of the health care team must also accompany the baby if a family member wishes to take him to another part of the hospital. Finally, the identification bands on the baby's wrist and ankle are always checked against the parent's identification band before the baby is handed to the parent. The identification bands cannot be removed until after the baby goes home with his parents.

Caring for the Umbilical Cord Stump

The **umbilical cord** supplies the growing fetus with nutrients and oxygen, and removes waste. When the baby is born, the umbilical cord is clamped and cut. Eventually, the "stump" (the part of the cord that remains) dries up and falls off, leaving behind the navel (or belly button).

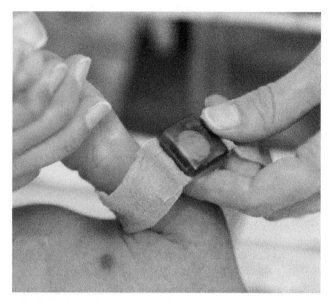

Figure 40-9
Protecting the security of the newborn is very important. Many facilities attach a sensor device to the newborn's wrist (shown here) or umbilical cord stump (see Figure 40-10). If someone tries to remove the baby from the nursery, the device sounds an alarm.

Until the stump dries up and falls off, it must be cared for properly to prevent infection (Fig. 40-10). At each diaper change, rub an alcohol swab over the entire stump. The purpose of this is to clean and to dry the stump. Fold the diaper down in front so that it does not cover the stump. If the stump or surrounding area is red, bleeding, or has any drainage, tell the nurse. The baby should not

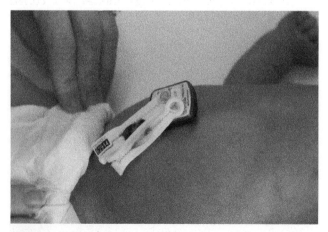

Figure 40-10
Proper care of the umbilical cord stump is necessary to prevent infection. At each diaper change, the umbilical cord stump is wiped with an alcohol swab to promote drying, and the diaper is folded down so that it does not cover the stump. The stump will dry up and fall off in about 10 days.

be given a complete bath (in a bath basin) until the umbilical cord stump has dried up and fallen off. This usually occurs within about 10 days of the birth.

Providing Circumcision Care

Circumcision is the surgical removal of the foreskin from the head of the penis. Many studies have been done regarding the long-term benefits and risks associated with circumcision. To date, whether to circumcise remains largely a matter of parental choice. Circumcision is also a rite of the Jewish religion.

The circumcision is done using local anesthetic. The procedure can be performed at the hospital before the baby is discharged home, or it may be done at the doctor's office. Following circumcision, the penis should be kept clean and dry. A petrolatum dressing may be applied to keep the penis from sticking to the diaper. Triple antibiotic ointment may also be applied, as an added precaution against infection. Be sure to follow any specific instructions that are given to you regarding care of the circumcision.

The baby's penis will be red and sore (Fig. 40-11). If you notice bleeding, drainage, or odour when you are changing the baby's diaper, tell the nurse. The circumcision should heal within 10 to 14 days. After the circumcision has healed, the baby can be given a complete bath in a bath basin.

Feeding

Babies who are not being breastfed are fed with a bottle. The bottle may contain the mother's breast milk, or a prepared formula. Infants who are younger than 1 year should not be fed cow's

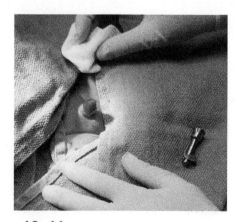

Figure 40-11
Following circumcision, the penis will be red and sore, but there should not be any bleeding, discharge, or odour. Report any of these observations to the nurse immediately.

milk. Cow's milk can cause the baby to develop food allergies. In addition, it does not contain many of the nutrients that are essential for the baby's growth.

Many commercial formula preparations are available. Some formulas come prepared and

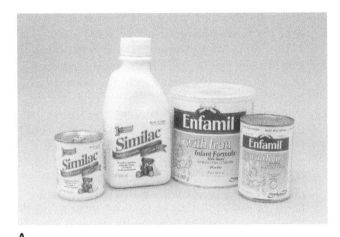

A

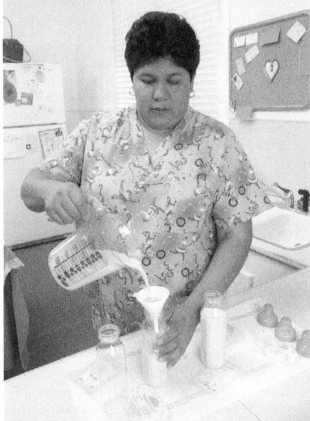

B

Figure 40-12
Babies who are not breastfed are bottle fed. **(A)** Many types of prepared formulas for bottle feeding are available. **(B)** When preparing bottles, always be sure to mix the formula according to the label instructions, if the formula is not "ready-to-feed."

ready to feed to the baby, while others are in the form of a powder or a concentrated liquid that must be mixed with water prior to feeding (Fig. 40-12A). Make sure you follow the label instructions carefully when preparing infant formula, so that the prepared formula is neither too strong nor too weak. Often, several bottles are prepared at once and stored in the refrigerator (see Fig. 40-12B). Before preparing the bottles, wash your hands.

Prepared bottles that have been stored in the refrigerator will need to be brought to room temperature before feeding the baby. To warm the bottle, place the prepared bottle in a container of warm water. Check the temperature of the bottle by shaking a few drops of the formula on to your wrist before feeding the baby. Never use a microwave oven to warm the bottle. Microwaving can cause the formula inside the bottle to become very hot in some spots, while remaining cool in others. When you test the formula on your wrist, the "hot spots" might go undetected. The hot formula will then burn the baby's mouth when she swallows it.

Hold the baby upright while feeding her (Fig. 40-13). Never prop the bottle up during feeding, or lay the baby down to take the bottle. After every few ounces of formula, stop feeding the baby so that she can burp. Burping gets rid of the excess air that is swallowed during feeding. The baby can be burped in several ways (Fig. 40-14). Hold the baby upright on your knee, or place the baby over your shoulder, and gently rub or pat her back. Be patient—some infants burp easily, while others may need more time.

Bottles, nipples, and rings should be cleaned in the dishwasher. They can also be washed by hand in hot, soapy water and rinsed well. Bottles do not need to be boiled for sterility, unless the

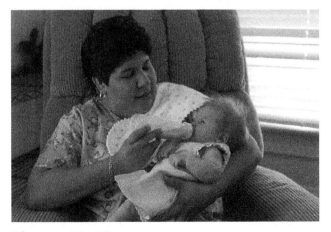

Figure 40-13
Always hold a baby upright to feed her.

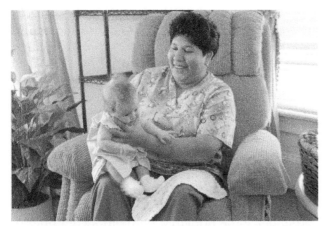

A

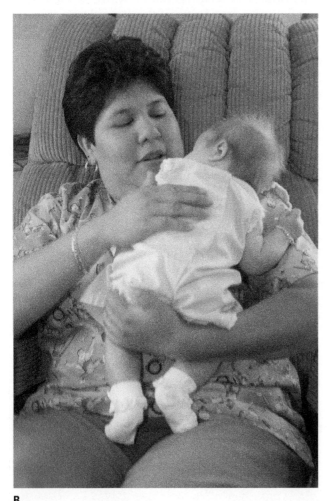

B

Figure 40-14
To burp the baby, **(A)** hold her upright on your knee, or **(B)** place her over your shoulder.

doctor specifies that this should be done. In a hospital setting, disposable bottles are usually used.

Diapering

Infants are diapered, using disposable or cloth diapers. To prevent diaper rash and skin break-

down, change the baby's diaper every time the baby has a bowel movement or urinates. An infant usually urinates 6 to 10 times each day. The frequency of bowel movements depends on whether the baby is fed breast milk or formula. To change a diaper:

1. Wash your hands and gather your supplies. It is important to gather all of your supplies first because you must never leave a baby alone, even for a moment. Even very small infants can easily roll off the changing table or other surface, leading to serious injury.
2. Put on the gloves, and remove the soiled diaper. Clean the perineal area, wiping from front to back if the baby is a girl. The perineal area can be cleansed with baby wipes (soft disposable wet cloths that contain a cleansing agent) or with a warm, wet washcloth. A mild baby soap may be used in addition to a warm, wet washcloth if the baby had a bowel movement. Be sure to rinse and dry the area thoroughly. Apply diaper rash ointment or a light dusting of cornstarch powder, if used.
3. Position the clean diaper, fastening it with the provided tabs (or diaper pins, if you are using a cloth diaper). Place the baby in an infant carrier or some other secure place.
4. Dispose of the soiled diaper in an appropriate waste container. Before placing a cloth diaper that is soiled with stool in the diaper pail, rinse it in cool water to prevent the stool from drying in the diaper.
5. Remove your gloves and wash your hands.

Bathing

A newborn infant is given a complete bath at birth. Once the umbilical cord stump has fallen off and the circumcision has healed (if the baby was circumcised), the baby may be given a complete bath in a bath basin on a routine basis. Until that time, partial baths (sponge baths) are given as needed.

To bathe a baby in a bath basin:

1. Wash your hands and gather all of your supplies. It is important to gather all of your supplies first because you must never leave a baby alone in a bath.
2. Fill the bath basin with only 2.5 to 5 centimetres of warm water. Check the water temperature with a bath thermometer before putting the baby in the bath basin (Fig. 40-15A). The temperature should be between 37.8°C to 40.5°C (100°F and 105°F).

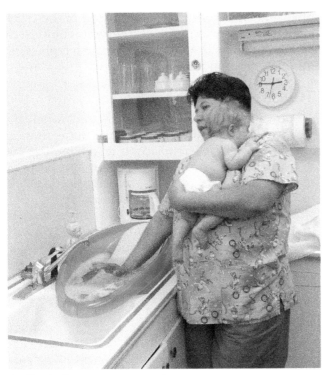

A. Check the water temperature.

Figure 40-15
Bathing a baby. **(A)** The bath basin is only filled to a depth of 2.5 to 5 centimetres. Always check the temperature of the bath water before you put the baby in it. **(B)** Wash the baby's hair first. **(C)** Then wash the baby's body.

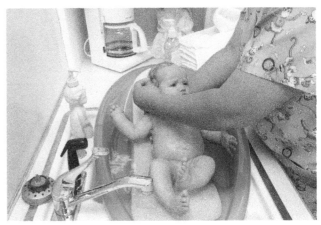

B. Wash the baby's hair.

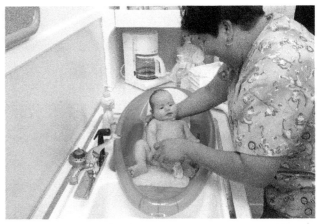

C. Wash the baby's body.

3. Place the baby in the bath basin. Lather the baby's hair with a baby shampoo and rinse well (see Fig. 40-15B). Next, use a washcloth and soap formulated for infant skin. Wash the baby's face first. Then move on to the rest of the body, making sure to rinse all soap from the skin (see Fig. 40-15C). Keep a firm grip on the baby at all times and work quickly to avoid chilling the baby.
4. After the bath, dry the baby thoroughly. Baby lotion may be applied as desired.

Putting a Baby Down to Sleep

A baby should be placed on his back or side to sleep. Research has shown that positioning babies on their backs or sides is safer than positioning them on their stomachs (Fig. 40-16). When placing a baby on his side to sleep, roll a receiving blanket or towel and tuck it securely next to the baby's back. This will help the baby to stay in the side-lying position. Remove all fluffy blankets, pillows, and toys from the sleeping area. These items pose a suffocation risk

(the baby may get tangled in them and not be able to breathe). Instead of using blankets, place the baby in a blanket sleeper to keep him warm.

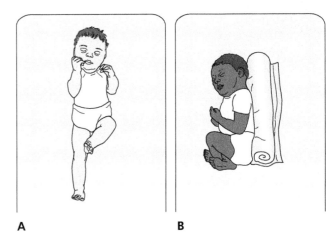

A   B

Figure 40-16
A baby is placed on his back or side to sleep, never on his stomach. **(A)** Positioning on the back. **(B)** Positioning on the side. Note the rolled receiving blanket bolstering the baby's back.

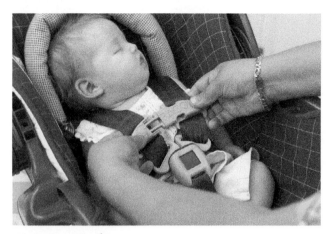

Figure 40-17
A baby may also sleep in her carrier. Always make sure to secure the baby in the carrier.

A baby can also be placed in an infant carrier to sleep. After putting the baby in the carrier, make sure that the carrier straps are properly secured (Fig. 40-17). Place the carrier on a low, level surface (such as the floor) so that it does not tip. Make sure that the carrier is out of the reach of pets or other small children who could accidentally knock the carrier over. Never place an infant carrier on a table or counter.

Transporting a Baby

A baby's first ride in a car seat occurs when the parents leave the hospital or birthing center. In all provinces and territories, it is against the law to transport a baby in a car without first properly securing her in a car seat. You may need to help the parents install the car seat correctly, and show them how to place the baby in it. Written instructions for installation are provided with the car seat packaging. Instructions for installation can also be found on many manufacturers' websites.

An infant car seat is placed in the back seat. The baby faces the back of the car, not the front. This is safer in the event of an accident. An infant car seat is required until the child reaches the age of 1 year and weighs more than 44 kilograms. The use of car seats for older babies and children is discussed in Chapter 41.

SUMMARY

- Personal support workers often are involved in the care of pregnant women, women who are in labour or have just given birth, and newborns.
  - Complications during pregnancy can require a woman to be on complete or partial bed rest, either at home or in the hospital, for weeks or even months before delivery. When this occurs, the personal support worker is usually responsible for measuring and recording vital signs and assisting with personal care for the expectant mother. In addition, the personal support worker provides companionship and emotional support.
  - When assisting a woman who is in labour, the personal support worker is usually only responsible for measuring and recording vital signs and other observations, unless he or she has received advanced training from the facility.
  - Following the delivery of the baby, the personal support worker cares for both the new mother and the baby. The immediate post-delivery period is a critical time physically for both the mother and the infant.

  The personal support worker plays an important role during this time by reporting any unusual observations or vital sign measurements to the nurse promptly.
- During the postpartum period, the personal support worker helps the new mother recover from the birth. The personal support worker may also assist the new mother with breastfeeding her baby.
- A personal support worker may care for a baby in the hospital, birthing center, or home setting.
  - Neonates require special care.
    - The umbilical cord stump is wiped with an alcohol swab after each diaper change to prevent infection. The umbilical cord stump falls off after about 10 days.
    - If a baby boy has been circumcised, the circumcision will also require special care for about the first 2 weeks.
    - The neonate should not be submerged in bath water until the umbilical cord stump (and circumcision, if applicable) have completely healed, approximately 10 to 14 days.

- Personal support workers also assist with feeding, diapering, and bathing babies.
- Following procedures and policies designed to keep the infant safe and secure is very important.
  - Procedures and policies related to security in the postpartum units of facilities such as hospitals and birthing centers are designed to prevent babies from being kidnapped.
- When bathing or diapering a baby, never leave the baby alone, not even for a minute.
- Babies are placed on their backs or sides to sleep, never their stomachs.
- A baby must never be taken anywhere in a car without first placing him or her in a car seat. The car seat must be properly installed, and the baby must be properly positioned in it and strapped in.

WHAT DID YOU LEARN?

Multiple Choice

Select the single best answer for each of the following questions.

1. Mrs. Gutierrez had an episiotomy during the birth of her son. What might the personal support worker do to help relieve the soreness and tenderness at the episiotomy site?
   a. Apply triple antibiotic ointment to the perineum
   b. Give Mrs. Gutierrez a bed bath
   c. Assist Mrs. Gutierrez with a Sitz bath
   d. Avoid washing the area until the episiotomy has healed
2. What is the period of time after delivery during which the parents and the new baby develop an emotional and physical attachment called?
   a. The epidural period
   b. The prenatal period
   c. The bonding period
   d. The antepartum period
3. You are caring for Ms. Bergen, who just had a baby. Which one of the following observations should you report immediately to the nurse?
   a. Ms. Bergen has what you think is an abnormal amount of vaginal discharge
   b. Ms. Bergen's pulse rate is elevated
   c. Ms. Bergen's blood pressure is low
   d. All of the above
4. Mrs. Ling has just delivered a daughter by cesarean section. You are helping her to breastfeed her baby, and she complains of cramping in her lower abdomen while the baby nurses. What is this a sign of?
   a. Mrs. Ling may be hemorrhaging
   b. The baby is kicking her in the stomach
   c. Cramping in the abdomen is a normal response during breastfeeding
   d. Mrs. Ling is not holding the baby correctly for breastfeeding

5. What position should an infant be placed in to sleep?
   a. On his back
   b. On his stomach
   c. On his side
   d. Either on his back or on his side
6. Which one of the following observations would be a cause for alarm when caring for a baby?
   a. The baby is pale
   b. The baby cries all the time, no matter what you do
   c. The baby will not eat
   d. All of the above
7. Mr. and Mrs. Saccamundi are going home from the hospital today with their new baby. How should the car seat be placed?
   a. In the front seat, facing the back of the car
   b. In the back seat, facing the back of the car
   c. In the back seat, facing the front of the car
   d. It makes no difference, as long as the baby is secure
8. You are checking vital signs on a newborn. Which one of the following measurements would you report to the nurse immediately?
   a. Heart rate 80 beats/min, respiratory rate 20 breaths/min
   b. Heart rate 160 beats/min, respiratory rate 34 breaths/min
   c. Heart rate 152 beats/min, respiratory rate 58 breaths/min
   d. None of the above

Matching

Match each numbered item with its appropriate lettered description.

_____ **1.** Lochia.

_____ **2.** Colostrum.

_____ **3.** Vernix.

a. Whitish, cheese-like protective coating on the skin of newborns

b. Vaginal discharge following the birth of a baby

c. Thin, yellowish fluid produced by the breasts before the milk comes in; rich in calories, protein, and antibodies

STOP and Think!

You work in the newborn nursery at your local hospital. The other personal support worker who works in the nursery with you, Shelly, has just left to take a baby to his mother for his noon feeding. You are attending to the other babies, when a pleasant-looking woman approaches and asks to see the new Sitko baby. She explains that she is the baby's grandmother, and she has just arrived from out of town to visit her son, daughter-in-law, and new grandchild. How would you respond to this request?

Donna is a home support worker who has been assigned to care for Mrs. Upchurch and her new baby, David. David was born very prematurely and spent several months in the hospital, but now the doctors have allowed him to come home. David still has numerous problems related to his premature birth, but coming home is a big milestone. Donna cannot help but notice that Mrs. Upchurch does not seem to be as thrilled about David's homecoming as Donna herself would be. Mrs. Upchurch seems very high-strung and almost frightened of the baby. In addition, she cries frequently. Why might Mrs. Upchurch be feeling this way? If you were Donna, how would you behave around Mrs. Upchurch?

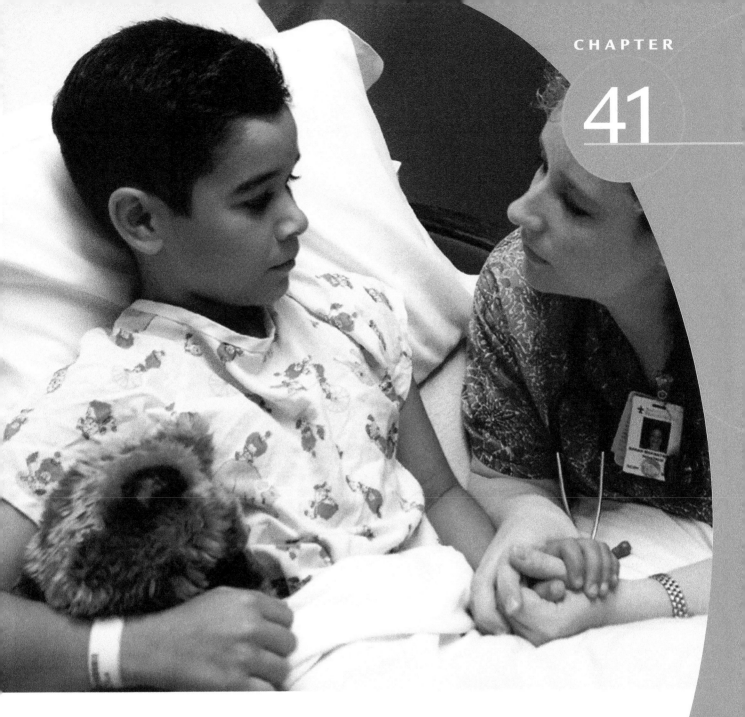

Caring for Pediatric Patients

WHAT WILL YOU LEARN?

Children receive health care in many different types of health care settings. For example, children who have acute illnesses or injuries are often cared for in a hospital setting. Children who need regular therapy or medical treatment for congenital or chronic health conditions may receive this care in a hospital, clinic, or home health care setting. Other children are residents of long-term care facilities because of developmental disabilities, injuries, or illnesses.

Photo: Children who have acute illnesses or injuries are often cared for in a hospital setting.

Although many of the procedures used to provide physical care to a child are very similar to those used with adults, it is very important to remember that children are not simply "little adults." In this chapter, you will learn about the unique physical and emotional needs of children of different ages. You will also learn about your role in reporting suspected cases of child abuse. When you have finished with this chapter, you will be able to:

1. Discuss the specific physical needs that children in health care settings have, according to their ages and abilities.
2. Understand how the stages of development affect the emotional needs of children in health care settings.
3. Describe measures that the personal support worker can use to assist a child in a health care setting.
4. List safety considerations that are specific for a child's age and developmental level.
5. Discuss signs of child abuse and the personal support worker's role in reporting suspected abuse.

Vocabulary

Failure to thrive	Magical thinking	Shaken baby	Munchausen syndrome
Regress	Egocentric	syndrome	by proxy

In Chapter 6, you learned about the stages of growth and development that we all pass through as we live our lives. Childhood is a time of rapid growth and development. A child's physical and emotional needs change constantly as he grows. Although only a few years separate a 3-year-old from an 8-year-old, there is a huge difference between these two age groups in terms of growth and development. A child's ability to understand and cooperate with the health care team depends on his particular stage of development. While a 3-year-old will need to be cuddled and sung to for comfort during a treatment or procedure, an 8-year-old will need answers to specific questions before he will feel comfortable. For example, an 8-year-old might ask *"What exactly is going to happen?" "What are you going to use to do that?" "Can I see it/touch it/hold it?"* and *"How will it feel?"* An understanding of the basic stages of growth and development will better prepare you to provide the type of care that each child requires.

In Chapter 6, you also learned how illness, injury, or disability affects people and their needs. You learned that although providing physical assistance to a person in a health care setting is an important responsibility of the personal support worker, recognizing and providing for the person's emotional needs is just as important. Think about what a frightening place a health care setting must be to a child. A child, especially a very young child, does not understand illness and pain. She has been taken from the comfort of her home and is now surrounded by people she does not know. Her room may be filled with strange, frightening machines, and "getting better" might mean having to have painful treatments first.

Think also about the effect a child's illness has on the family as a whole. Family members will worry that the child is suffering or uncomfortable. If the child's injury or illness is severe or acute, family members may wonder whether the child will survive the event, and if he does, what effects the illness or injury will have on his future growth and development. Sometimes, a child's illness requires one family member to travel to a distant health care facility to be with the child, while the rest of the family stays at home. When this is the case, the family member who is away may worry about the rest of the family at home, and how they are managing on their own. Families may worry about how they will pay for the health care that the child is receiving. The other children in the family may feel "left out" while most of the family's attention is being focused on the child who is sick or injured. Or they may feel guilty that they are healthy while their brother or sister is sick. Including the child's family members in his or her care whenever possible is one thing you can do to help the family cope with a child's illness (Fig. 41-1). The family members will feel like they are actively doing something to help the child, and the child will be happier being cared for by familiar people.

When working with children and families, remember that families come in all different shapes and sizes. Many families are "traditional," in the sense that they consist of two parents and one or more children. However, many families

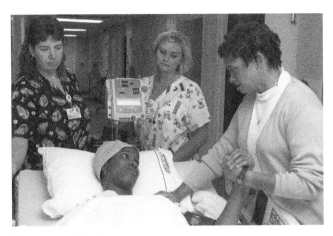

Figure 41-1
A child's illness can be very stressful for the family.

consist of only one parent and the children. Or, the children may be raised by grandparents, guardians, foster parents, or other caregivers. Regardless of the family structure, the effects of a child's illness on the people who care about the child are the same.

CARING FOR INFANTS

Infancy is the period of time from a child's birth to his first birthday. Infants grow and develop very rapidly during the first year of life. They progress from being totally helpless—unable to roll over, sit up, or move about without help—to being able to crawl, walk, and feed themselves small pieces of food by the time they reach the age of 1 year.

MEETING THE INFANT'S PHYSICAL NEEDS

An infant is totally dependent on her caregiver to help her meet her most basic physical needs. The procedures for feeding, diapering, bathing, and positioning a newborn that you learned in Chapter 40 apply for older infants as well. In addition, you may be responsible for monitoring food and fluid intake and output, and for monitoring the infant's temperature:

- **Monitoring food and fluid intake and output.** An infant who is ill or unable to drink or eat properly can quickly become dehydrated. An infant who is receiving adequate food and fluid will urinate regularly and have regular bowel movements. Since it is not possible to know exactly how much breast milk a nursing infant is taking at each feeding, keeping track of the number of wet diapers or weighing the wet diapers may be necessary to ensure that the baby is not dehydrated. Observing and recording the number, consistency, and amount of bowel movements may also be one of your responsibilities.

- **Monitoring body temperature.** An infant, especially one who is ill or very young, must be kept warm. A very small infant can be wrapped securely in a blanket. An older, more mobile infant can be clothed in snuggly one-piece pajamas if the weather is cold. A change in body temperature (either above or below the normal range) is cause for concern and should be reported immediately.

Because an infant's medical condition can change very quickly, you must report any unusual signs or symptoms (see Chapter 40) to the nurse immediately.

MEETING THE INFANT'S EMOTIONAL NEEDS

Aside from being clean, warm, and fed, an infant's greatest need is to feel secure. Infants need to be spoken to or sung to softly (Fig. 41-2). They need to be rocked gently, touched, and held. Human contact is essential for an infant to develop physically and emotionally. Many studies have shown that infants, even those who are well cared for physically, fail to grow and develop both physically and emotionally if they are not held and talked to. This is called **failure to thrive.**

To help meet an infant's emotional needs, you must take the time to touch, cuddle, stroke, and talk soothingly to him. Encourage family members to hold the baby, if the baby's condition allows. The nurse can show family members how to hold the baby without disturbing medical devices, such as monitors and tubes. Provide music and infant-appropriate toys. If possible, position the infant's bed so that he can watch activity out a window or through a doorway.

MEETING THE INFANT'S NEED FOR SAFETY

Safety and the prevention of accidents are essential for children of all ages, but especially for the youngest. As helpless as they may seem, infants can wriggle, roll, and twist themselves into dangerous situations very quickly.

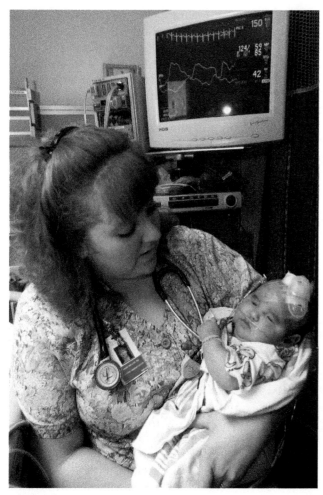

Figure 41-2
The infant's greatest emotional need is to feel safe and secure. Infants need to be held, cuddled, rocked, and spoken or sung to.

- Never leave an infant on a surface unattended, even for a moment. Even very young infants can easily roll off of a bed, changing table, or examination table. An infant who falls to the floor could receive severe or fatal head injuries. If you are changing diapers, taking vital signs, or bathing an infant, keep one hand on the child at all times to prevent a fall.
- As the infant grows and is placed in an infant carrier, swing, or high chair, make sure that safety straps are securely fastened both across the infant's waist and between his legs to prevent him from falling out of, or sliding down in, the carrier, swing, or chair.
- Always secure the infant in a car seat when traveling in a car or other vehicle. An infant car seat is placed in the back seat. The baby faces the back of the car, not the front.

- An infant explores her world by placing everything she can get her hands on in her mouth. Make sure that toys are age-appropriate and that they have no small, removable parts that the infant could choke on. Clean the toys by washing them frequently in warm, soapy water and rinsing them thoroughly. As the infant learns to crawl and move about, make sure that the floor or play area is free of small objects or plants that the infant could place in her mouth.
- Keep plastic bags and balloons away from infants. A young infant could roll over and become tangled in a plastic bag. An older infant could put the bag over his head. The infant is unable to breathe through the plastic, and suffocates. Balloons are also a suffocation risk. The infant may put the balloon (or a piece of a broken balloon) in his mouth. When the infant inhales, the rubber balloon gets sucked into the airway, blocking air flow and leading to suffocation.
- Do not leave an infant unattended, even for a moment, in water of any depth. Babies who can stand up have drowned in a mop bucket!
- Make sure that electrical cords and window blind cords are out of the reach of the infant. The infant could become tangled in the cord and strangle himself. Or, he could put the electrical cord in his mouth, which could result in electrocution.

These are just a few of the many safety concerns that you must be aware of when caring for very small children. A primary rule of thumb is that if a child can reach an object, he will grab it and try to put it in his mouth. Child-proofing everything, whether in the home or the health care setting, is critical for the safety of the infant.

CARING FOR TODDLERS

A toddler is a child between the ages of 1 and 3 years. Toddlers are mobile, curious, and independent. They explore everything. Toddlers can feed themselves, and are busy learning how to communicate, how to use the potty, and how to dress themselves. Because of their new independence, toddlers may not cooperate with the efforts of health care workers.

Toddlers who need health care services are also likely to be very frightened. It is common for a child of this age to **regress,** or return to an earlier stage of development. For instance, a child who has been potty trained for some time may suddenly start wetting her pants, or she may ask for a bottle or pacifier after being previously weaned from these items. While frustrating, especially for the child's caregivers, regression is just a normal way for a young child to cope with stress. A toddler is still too young to talk about her fears or even understand what exactly she is afraid of, so she just returns to an earlier, more comfortable stage of development temporarily until the stress passes. When caring for a toddler, it is important to recognize regression for what it is and ignore it. For example, rather than scolding a potty-trained child who has had an accident and telling her to "stop acting like a baby," clean her up and comfort her, without drawing a lot of attention to the accident.

MEETING THE TODDLER'S PHYSICAL NEEDS

A toddler will need your help to meet many of his physical needs. Ask the toddler's regular caregiver how much help the child usually needs with eating, toileting, and dressing. Find out what words the child uses for urination and bowel movements. It is important for you to allow the toddler to remain as independent as possible. One way to do this is to offer choices that are realistic. For example, instead of asking the child what he wants to wear, limit his choices to those that are actually possible ("Do you want to wear your red pajamas, or your blue ones?").

Because a toddler's physical growth slows during this stage, his appetite may also be small. Being scared can also affect the toddler's appetite. Ask the child's caregiver what he likes to eat and drink. Many children in this age group have very clear, and very limited, food preferences. Most toddlers enjoy finger foods such as crackers, fruit cut into small pieces, and dry cereal. They can drink from a cup and may enjoy a variety of juices and milk. Toddlers are usually on an "eat and run" type of dietary schedule and need to have small amounts of food provided throughout the day. You may be responsible for monitoring and recording the toddler's food and fluid intake. If the toddler's fluid intake is low, try offering foods such as popsicles, ice cream, or gelatin. These foods count toward the fluid intake and may be more enticing than a cup of water.

Older toddlers who sleep in a regular bed at home may be offered a small adjustable bed in the health care facility if their condition allows. However, a toddler who is at risk for falling out of bed may need a crib with side rails and a top

cover. The use of restraints is common among children in this age group, because toddlers are simply too young to understand that intravenous lines, drains, catheters, and other medical devices are a necessary part of their treatment and should not be pulled out. If restraints are being used, be sure to check on the toddler very frequently (at least every 10 minutes). The best alternative to using a restraint is to keep the toddler occupied by offering distracting activities and toys, and by having someone stay with the toddler at all times.

MEETING THE TODDLER'S EMOTIONAL NEEDS

Most toddlers are afraid of strangers and prefer to be with their usual caregivers. Remember that you are a stranger to the toddler. Speak softly and get down on the toddler's level when you are talking with him. That way you will not appear quite so tall and scary. Many toddlers are more cooperative during procedures if they are allowed to sit in their usual caregiver's lap. They also like to touch any equipment that is being used in the procedure (Fig. 41-3). Allow the child to handle your stethoscope and blood pressure cuff before attempting to measure vital signs.

Toddlers love to play with brightly coloured toys such as blocks, simple puzzles, and stuffed toys. They also love to clap, move, and sing along with children's songs. Because their attention spans are very short, toddlers become bored and fretful very quickly. Make sure that the toddler

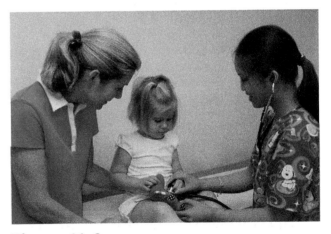

Figure 41-3
Most toddlers enjoy handling the equipment that will be used in a procedure. Procedures will usually go more smoothly if it is possible for the toddler's usual caretaker to be present.

has access to activities that can help keep him entertained. Toddlers also may need to nap in the middle of the day, especially if they are sick or injured. Provide quiet time, soothing music, and a comforting touch to help the child fall asleep.

MEETING THE TODDLER'S NEED FOR SAFETY

Toddlers are sometimes referred to as "tornadoes in training pants" because of their boundless energy, mobility, and natural curiosity. They learn to open locked doors quickly and can wander away from the facility or home. They run, climb, and reach for things without any thought to safety. They love to explore cabinets and will taste the contents of any containers they find there. As a result, accidental poisonings are very common among this age group. Toddlers must be observed at all times to help prevent accidents, and safety locks on doors, cabinets, and drawers are essential.

When a child reaches 1 year of age and 9 kilograms in weight, she moves from an infant car seat to a toddler car seat. Toddler car seats, like infant car seats, are placed in the back seat of the car. However, the toddler sits facing forward. As with infants, it is illegal in all provinces and territories to transport a toddler in a car without first properly securing him in a car seat.

CARING FOR PRESCHOOLERS

Preschoolers are children between the ages of 3 and 5 years. Like toddlers, preschoolers are very physically active and love to run, jump, ride on toys, and swing. Because the preschooler enjoys being physically active, being confined to bed or indoors because of an injury or illness can lead to boredom. Art supplies, games, movies, and television can be good entertainment for a child of this age (Fig. 41-4). Preschoolers also love to have stories read to them, and many are learning to read simple books on their own.

MEETING THE PRESCHOOLER'S PHYSICAL NEEDS

At this age, a child has developed most of his or her self-care skills. A healthy preschooler can dress himself, go to the bathroom unassisted,

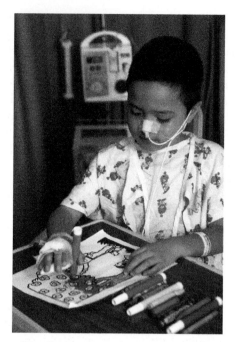

Figure 41-4
Art projects, books, games, movies, and television can be good entertainment for the preschooler who is injured or ill.

and brush his own teeth. However, a sick or injured preschooler may need help with these daily tasks.

Most preschoolers are picky eaters and eat only a small variety of foods, in small amounts. You may find it frustrating when your attempts to get a preschooler to eat nutritious foods fail. A preschooler who is not feeling well is even less likely to have an appetite for foods that are "good for her." Offering a variety of nutritious foods in small amounts throughout the day is often more effective than insisting that the preschooler eat regular meals.

You may be required to help hold or restrain a preschooler during a procedure. Make sure you plan ahead and have been shown how to hold a child gently but securely, so that the procedure can be performed as efficiently as possible. A frightened child can be very strong, and he may kick, pinch, hit, or bite to get away. You will have to protect both the child and yourself from injury in this situation.

MEETING THE PRESCHOOLER'S EMOTIONAL NEEDS

Preschoolers have vivid imaginations and enjoy pretend play. As a result, preschoolers may have a lot of anxiety about being in a health care facility. A young preschooler may fear that a procedure will involve "cutting off" body parts or other drastic measures. An older preschooler has begun to understand the concept of death and may think that the hospital is "where people go to die." Because children of this age have learned to understand that discipline or punishment is the consequence of bad behaviour, they may think that the reason they have to have a painful treatment or stay in bed is because they were "bad."

"Magical thinking" is a thought process that is common among preschoolers. Preschoolers believe that if they wish for something hard enough, it will happen. As a result, a preschooler may think that because she wished for something bad to happen to a parent or a sibling, her current medical condition is punishment for having those bad thoughts. Or she may think that her bad thoughts actually made something bad happen (for example, if several members of a family are now hospitalized because of an accident or fire).

Preschoolers need their questions answered simply and honestly. They are very interested in whether a procedure will "hurt." If the procedure will cause discomfort, be truthful and describe what the procedure will feel like in words that the child can understand. For example, you might tell the child that the procedure will "pinch," "squeeze," or "pull." Not being honest about the procedure and what it will feel like will destroy the child's ability to trust you and the other members of the health care team.

Using a stuffed animal or doll to demonstrate the procedure helps the child to understand what is expected of her and will help to relieve the child's fears. For example, you could use a doll to demonstrate how you do range-of-motion exercises. Similarly, the preschooler will enjoy being able to listen to her own heart through the stethoscope, or seeing a demonstration of how the blood pressure cuff "squeezes her arm to check her muscles."

MEETING THE PRESCHOOLER'S NEEDS FOR SAFETY

A preschooler is beginning to learn the difference between right and wrong behaviour. As a result, he is more able to "follow the rules of safety," if these rules are explained to him in a way that he understands. Some preschoolers are still likely to place items in their mouths and are therefore at risk for choking. As in younger children, balloons pose a choking risk and should be used with caution. Scissors used for crafts projects should be

blunt-tipped, and markers, crayons, glue, and other art supplies should be nontoxic and approved for use for children between the ages of 3 and 5 years.

The toddler car seat is used until the child weighs 18 kilograms. At that point, the child will have outgrown the toddler car seat and will need a booster seat. The booster seat raises the child up so that the lap and shoulder belts in the car fit properly. The booster seat is placed in the back seat of the car, facing forward. As with younger children, it is illegal to drive with a child in the car who is not properly restrained.

CARING FOR SCHOOL-AGE CHILDREN

School-age children are children between the ages of 5 and 12 years. School-age children are developing many interests outside of their own families. They are learning to socialize and spend a lot of time playing with their friends. They enjoy physical activities, such as riding bicycles, swimming, skating, skiing, and climbing. Unfortunately, these activities often result in injury and the need for health care. "Fitting in" socially is very important to the school-age child, and children who are physically or mentally disabled may be excluded from play or teased by their peers.

Caring for a child of this age in a health care setting involves answering lots of questions. School-age children are typically very cooperative if their questions are answered in a manner that they can understand. These children like to be included as active participants in their own care and are very good at following directions.

MEETING THE SCHOOL-AGE CHILD'S PHYSICAL NEEDS

School-age children are very independent and are quite proud that they no longer have to rely on anyone else for self-care, although they do need to be reminded that the purpose of a bath or shower is to clean their bodies. If a child is not able to bathe, dress, or go to the bathroom by himself as a result of injury or illness, he will need the assistance of others, and this is likely to make him very unhappy. Allow the child to do as much as he is able to by himself. Sometimes, taking the approach that the child is helping you because you simply cannot do the task without his assistance is helpful.

When caring for a school-age child, you must check on her frequently. Although the child may be badly injured and in pain, she may not pay attention to your directions to call for help if she needs to get out of bed. She will want to do it herself. A reward system for following the rules may be necessary. For example, you might tell the child that if she uses the call light control to ask for your assistance each time she needs to get out of bed, then you will allow her to choose a small treat or privilege. Rewards and praise work very well for children of this age.

MEETING THE SCHOOL-AGE CHILD'S EMOTIONAL NEEDS

School-age children expect to receive direct, simple answers to their questions. If a school-age child asks you a question that you cannot answer, be sure to relay the question to the nurse, so that she can answer it for the child. Never make promises or assurances about a school-age child's condition or treatment that are not certain. Children of this age are usually aware of when they are being told the truth, and when they are not. A school-age child usually has developed a strong moral conscience and feels very strongly about what is right and what is wrong.

A school-age child will enjoy reading, doing arts and crafts projects, playing video games, and talking with caregivers. If possible, allow the child to accompany you throughout the health care facility in a wheelchair for company, or take her to a common area where there may be other children her age to socialize or play games with. For a child of this age who is confined due to accident or illness, staying in touch with friends is a huge emotional boost. Phone calls, visits (if possible), and cards from friends and classmates are thoroughly enjoyed (Fig. 41-5). Make sure you help the child to place cards and notes safely on a table or bulletin board so they can be looked at often.

MEETING THE SCHOOL-AGE CHILD'S NEED FOR SAFETY

The school-age child is less vulnerable to certain dangers than younger children are. For example, school-age children know not to drink poisonous liquids or stick objects into an electrical socket. However, their curiosity and habit of pushing their physical abilities to the limit bring new dangers. School-age children are often interested in fire. They may dart into the path of oncoming traffic on bicycles and skateboards or when

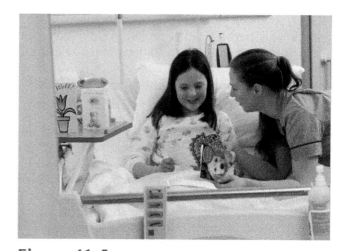

Figure 41-5
School-age children who must be confined to bed due to injury or illness will miss socializing with their friends. Greeting cards, phone calls, and visits from peers are thoroughly enjoyed. (© *Chris Whitehead/Photodisc Red/ Getty Images.*)

chasing a ball. They climb trees and buildings, and then fall. Burns, broken bones, and head injuries are the reason many children in this age group require hospitalization and rehabilitation.

When transporting a school-age child in a car, use a booster seat until the car's lap and shoulder restraints fit the child properly. This usually occurs when the child reaches a height of 1.4 metres, and a weight of about 36 kilograms. Children should continue to ride in the back seat until the age of 12 years.

CARING FOR ADOLESCENTS

Adolescents are children between the ages of 12 and 17 years. Adolescence is a time of tremendous growth and development. We enter adolescence as children and exit as young adults. During adolescence, logical thinking skills develop. Adolescents have the ability to understand possibilities and make judgments. As a result, it is essential that children of this age be included in plans and decisions regarding their medical care.

MEETING THE ADOLESCENT'S PHYSICAL NEEDS

Allow the child to be as independent as possible with his daily care. An adolescent may hesitate to ask for help or for pain medication if he is trying to seem "tough," mature, or grown up. He may act angry or aloof when in reality he is really just frightened. Adolescence is a difficult time of life to require health care. The physical changes that occur during adolescence can make adolescents self-conscious about their bodies. As a result, they are often very embarrassed by care or treatments that expose their bodies to others. Remember this when caring for an adolescent, and make a special effort to provide privacy. Also be aware that an adolescent girl may need your assistance with obtaining or changing sanitary napkins or tampons, if she is too ill to manage this task on her own. Be sensitive to the embarrassment she may feel at having to ask for your help.

To help adolescents meet their nutritional needs, offer the types of foods that they like to eat. A teenager may totally refuse the types of meals served in a health care facility, but will eat pizza, milkshakes, or other nutritional alternatives. Because of the increased need for extra calories during periods of growth spurts, an adolescent may need nutritious snacks in between meals. Peanut butter and crackers, cheese, fruit, yogurt, and ice cream are good nutritious alternatives to chips and soda and should be readily available for the teenager if her dietary orders allow.

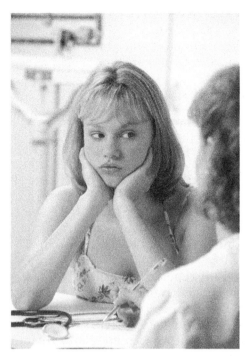

Figure 41-6
Adolescents need to be included in plans and decisions regarding their medical care. It is important to listen to what the adolescent is telling you. Avoid lecturing her on morals or proper behaviour.

MEETING THE ADOLESCENT'S EMOTIONAL NEEDS

Psychologically, the period of adolescence is stormy. Adolescents are **egocentric,** meaning that they think of themselves as being at the center of the world and often overestimate their importance to others. They begin to question the moral teachings of authority figures and parents. As a result, experimentation with alcohol, drugs, and sex may occur during this stage.

Adolescents are torn between wanting to be treated as grown-ups and being afraid to make their own decisions. They need adults to respect their individuality. When caring for an adolescent, listen to what she is saying. Try not to lecture her on morals or proper behaviour. Include the adolescent in discussions and decisions regarding her care and treatment. Adolescents need to feel that their opinions count (Fig. 41-6).

Many adolescents require care in a health care facility because of complications related to mental illnesses, such as depression, attempted suicide, or eating disorders. Others may have had accidents related to drug or alcohol abuse. An adolescent girl may need health care as a result of a pregnancy, which may not be planned or wanted. Sexually transmitted infections (STIs) are common among this age group. All of these situations require tact and sensitivity on the part of caregivers. Be very observant for any changes in the adolescent's emotional behaviour or mood and report anything unusual to the nurse immediately.

MEETING THE ADOLESCENT'S NEED FOR SAFETY

In the health care setting, most adolescents are fairly safe. However, an adolescent who has a history of abusing drugs or other substances may try to obtain pain medication that is not needed. Depressed adolescents will need to be observed closely for suicide attempts or other types of self-injury. Make sure that the adolescent knows you are available if he needs assistance, and answer the call light promptly.

CHILD ABUSE

Children, like the elderly, are often targets of abuse.

FORMS OF ABUSE

Like elder abuse, child abuse can be physical, psychological (emotional), or sexual in nature.

Physical Abuse

Neglect is a common form of physical abuse in children. The child's caregiver simply fails to provide for the child's basic physical needs. For example, the child may be malnourished from lack of nutritious food, dirty from lack of proper hygiene, or ill from a lack of medical care.

Physical abuse can also take the form of striking, biting, slapping, shaking, or handling a child roughly. Violently shaking an infant or toddler can cause the child's brain to hit the inside of his skull repeatedly, leading to severe brain damage or death. This is called **shaken baby syndrome.** Shaken baby syndrome is most often seen in children younger than 1 year. About 25% of children with shaken baby syndrome die, and the rest suffer from permanent disabilities. Many cases of shaken baby syndrome occur accidentally, when a frustrated caregiver shakes a child to get him to stop crying. Because of the risk of head injury, it is never acceptable to shake an infant or toddler.

In **Munchausen syndrome by proxy,** another form of physical abuse seen in children, the child's caregiver (usually the mother) deliberately does things to make the child appear ill. For example, the caregiver may feed the child soap or other substances to make her vomit. Or she might smother the child for a period of time to deprive her of oxygen, leading to neurological symptoms. Often, the child is forced to have painful diagnostic procedures or surgery as health care providers try to discover the cause of the child's strange signs and symptoms. Munchausen syndrome by proxy is often difficult to detect and to prove, because nearly constant observation is needed to determine the cause of the child's health problems. In some cases, it becomes necessary to hide a camera in the child's hospital room to observe what happens when the caregiver is alone with the child.

Psychological (Emotional) Abuse

A caregiver can inflict psychological (emotional) abuse on a child in many ways. A caregiver might make a child fearful by threatening him with physical harm or abandonment. Or he might say cruel things to the child, such as "You're no good," "You're stupid," or "I wish you had never been born." Isolating a child by preventing him from seeing friends or other family members (an act called *involuntary seclusion*) is another form of psychological abuse. Involuntary seclusion can involve keeping a child in a room alone with the door closed. In extreme cases, it may involve locking a child in a closet or attic for years. Children who are the victims of psychological abuse can struggle for the rest of their lives with emotional pain, depression, thoughts of suicide, and lack of self-esteem.

Sexual Abuse

Sexual abuse occurs when a parent or caregiver:

- Touches or fondles a child's sexual organs
- Shows his or her sexual organs to a child, or asks the child to touch or otherwise stimulate them
- Forces a child to have sexual intercourse with him or her (rape)
- Forces a child to engage in a sexual act and then films or photographs it (pornography)
- Forces a child to engage in a sexual act for money, often with many different people (prostitution)

When a stranger sexually abuses a child, it is called *sexual assault*.

RISK FACTORS FOR CHILD ABUSE

Child abuse can occur in all levels of society and in all ethnic groups. However, there are certain situations that seem to increase the risk that abuse will occur. Risk factors for child abuse include the following:

- Caregivers who are very stressed by situations such as unemployment, depression, marital or relationship problems, substance abuse, or health problems of their own
- Caregivers who are very young, lack parenting skills, or lack knowledge about the normal behaviours and developmental stages of children
- Caregivers who have no family or social support and feel "trapped" by their parenting responsibilities
- Children who are "difficult" to care for, such as those who cry frequently, do not sleep well, are hyperactive or aggressive, wet the bed, or have physical or mental disabilities

ROLE OF THE PERSONAL SUPPORT WORKER IN REPORTING ABUSE

As a personal support worker, you may suspect that one of your pediatric patients is being abused (Box 41-1). You may see physical signs that suggest abuse, or the child's behaviour or play-acting may raise your suspicions. In some cases, the child might tell you something that makes you suspicious. Make sure to listen carefully to what the child is telling you. Report the child's words exactly as you heard them. Be very careful not to influence the child's ideas or "put words in her mouth." In the event of an abuse investigation, a young child may repeat what she has been told, rather than describe what actually happened. If you are suspicious about something a child has told you, do not question the child further yourself. Report your suspicions to the nurse and allow a person who has experience and training in detecting child abuse to continue the questioning.

It may be difficult to work with parents or caregivers if you suspect that they have abused their child. You may feel angry toward the parents or caregivers, or disgusted by their behaviour. Remember that it is not your place to pass judgment on a parent or caregiver. Your responsibility is to simply report your suspicions, and to let the agencies that handle abuse reports determine if abuse has occurred and, if so, who did it. The agencies will also determine how the child will be protected going forward. Your top priority is to meet the child's physical and emotional needs as best you can while the child is in your care. If you feel that your emotions about a particular situation may affect your ability to provide care, talk with your supervisor and ask for help or to be assigned to another area.

BOX 41-1	Signs of Child Abuse

- Unclean or unsafe living conditions, as evidenced by rotting food, unchanged sheets, or a lack of heat or water services
- Poor personal hygiene, as evidenced by an unclean body, clothes, or both; uncombed hair; skin irritation (from wearing urine-soaked undergarments for long periods of time); dried stool on buttocks; or a lack of oral hygiene
- Loss of weight or dehydration
- Multiple, unexplained fractures or bruises in various stages of healing; explanations of injuries that are not consistent with the location of the injury
- Burn marks (for example, from cigarettes or stove burners) or scalds (for example, from having a hand or foot held in hot water)
- Abrasions from ropes or other bindings
- Patches of missing hair
- Vaginal bleeding or discharge; urinary tract infection; or pain, itching, redness, or bruising around the genitals or anus
- Excessive sexual curiosity or play
- Sleeping problems or nightmares
- An anxious, fearful, or withdrawn demeanor, especially in the presence of the abuser
- Uncontrolled medical conditions (possibly the result of a lack of prescribed medication or treatment)
- A history of requiring health care for similar injuries

SUMMARY

- Children receive health care in many different types of health care settings, for many different reasons. To provide humanistic care for children, you must first understand that children are not simply "little adults." An understanding of the basic stages of growth and development will better prepare you to provide the type of care that each child requires.
- Pediatric patients range in age from newborn through 17 years.

- Infants are children younger than 1 year. Infants are totally dependent on others for their physical care. Their greatest emotional need is to feel secure and to develop trust.
- A toddler is a child between the ages of 1 and 3 years. Toddlers may have a fear of strangers that could affect their response to health care providers. In addition, they commonly regress to an earlier stage of development in response to the stress of being in a health care setting.

- Preschoolers are children between the ages of 3 and 5 years. Preschoolers have vivid imaginations and enjoy pretend play. Preschoolers may indulge in magical thinking. The preschooler's questions must be answered simply and honestly.
- School-age children are children between the ages of 5 and 12 years. School-age children like to be included as active participants in their own care and are very good at following directions. However, they may resist asking for help when they need it.
- Adolescents are children between the ages of 12 and 17 years. Adolescents have a great need for privacy, and for control over what is happening to them.
- Children are frequently the helpless victims of many types of abuse. All members of the health care team are legally obligated to report any type of suspected abuse.
  - Physical abuse can take the form of neglect or deliberate injury.
  - Psychological (emotional) abuse can involve threatening a child, saying demeaning or cruel things to a child, or isolating the child from others.
  - Sexual abuse occurs when an adult touches a child inappropriately or forces the child to perform sexual acts.

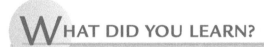

WHAT DID YOU LEARN?

Multiple Choice

Select the single best answer for each of the following questions.

1. A pediatric patient is most likely to cooperate with the health care team when:
   a. Members of the health care team treat him like a "little adult"
   b. Members of the health care team recognize the child's particular stage of development and provide age-appropriate care
   c. Members of the health care team always give the child what he wants
   d. The child is restrained
2. To help determine whether a breast-fed infant is receiving an adequate amount of milk, the personal support worker may need to:
   a. Supplement the breastfeeding with extra formula
   b. Monitor the baby's intravenous (IV) line
   c. Have the mother pump her breasts and measure the amount of milk she produces
   d. Weigh the infant's wet diapers
3. A behaviour that could indicate regression in a toddler might be:
   a. Asking for a bottle or pacifier
   b. Becoming potty trained
   c. Feeding herself
   d. Fearing strangers
4. Which one of the following is an example of magical thinking?
   a. Believing in Santa Claus
   b. Fearing strangers
   c. Thinking that an accident occurred because you were mad at your sister
   d. Pretending to be a princess

Matching

Match each numbered item with its appropriate lettered description.

_____ **1.** Infant

_____ **2.** Toddler

_____ **3.** Preschooler

_____ **4.** School-age child

_____ **5.** Adolescent

a. This child has developed a very strong moral conscience and will expect truthful answers to his many questions.

b. This child may be very self-conscious and become embarrassed if she is exposed during a medical procedure.

c. This child needs to be touched, cuddled, stroked, and spoken to soothingly to thrive.

d. This child has a vivid imagination and may fear monsters under the bed and doctors who will "cut off" body parts.

e. This child is at the highest risk for accidental poisoning.

STOP and Think!

You are the personal support worker on a pediatric floor of a hospital. One of your small patients, Sarah, is 5. As you walk into her room, you notice that she is playing with a doll and a teddy bear. As you listen, you hear her talking to the toys. Sarah is pretending that the bear is asking the doll to touch him between the legs. When the doll refuses, the bear becomes very angry and demands that the doll touch him. What is happening in this room? What should be your response?

You are caring for a 2-year-old child who has a fractured arm. You notice that the mother seems very fearful of talking about what happened and her version of the story changes frequently. As you are helping to bathe the child you notice small burn marks on his buttocks and some bruises on his back. What do you report and to whom?

Personal Support Workers Make a Difference!

"My husband, Fred, and I are both in our early 70s and enjoying Fred's retirement. We are active and travel to many places. My husband has had arthritis in his knees for a long time and has managed pretty well with it, but a few months ago, the arthritis in his right knee really started giving him trouble. It was so bad, Fred started skipping our weekly golf outings, something he has always enjoyed. When Fred spoke to our doctor about his knee, Dr. Bowen suggested that Fred have a joint replacement so he could continue to be active without so much pain.

One of the first people we met when we went to the hospital the morning of Fred's surgery was a personal support worker named Patrick. Patrick took us up to Fred's room and then got Fred ready for the surgery. He took his vital signs, and got him into a hospital gown. The surgery went well and Fred was back in his room before lunch time, still snoring from the pain medication he had been given. Patrick was there as well, taking his vital signs fairly frequently. Patrick explained that this was normal procedure for a person who had just been through surgery.

Early that afternoon, Patrick took Fred's pulse and blood pressure, but instead of writing them down, he took them again. When I asked Patrick about his puzzled expression, he reassured me that it was probably nothing, but that he had noticed something that he wanted the nurse to take a look at. Well, come to find out, Fred had had a minor heart attack after the surgery, and Patrick had noticed an irregularity in Fred's pulse rhythm. Because he had noticed it and reported the change to the nurse, the doctors were able to start treating Fred's heart soon enough to prevent any permanent damage from occurring.

Now, 8 months later, we're back on the golf course and Fred's swing is as bad as it always was! Fred has started taking a medication to regulate his heart rate, but he feels great and we're loving life. Thank goodness for Patrick and his attention to detail!"

You can listen to more stories about how personal support workers make a difference on the CD in the front of your book.

Photo credit: Digital Vision/Getty Images

8

HOME HEALTH CARE

42 Introduction to Home Health Care
43 Safety and Infection Control in the Home Health Care Setting

Home health care—skilled care that is given to a person in his or her home—is a rapidly growing part of the health care industry. In Canada, the number of home care clients has increased almost 100% between 1995 and 2006. It is estimated that 1 million Canadians have used home care services, and that number is expected to keep growing each year (Canadian Home Care Association). The purpose of this unit is to introduce you to the home health care setting.

Photo: Home support workers care for clients in their homes. (© John Henley/CORBIS.)

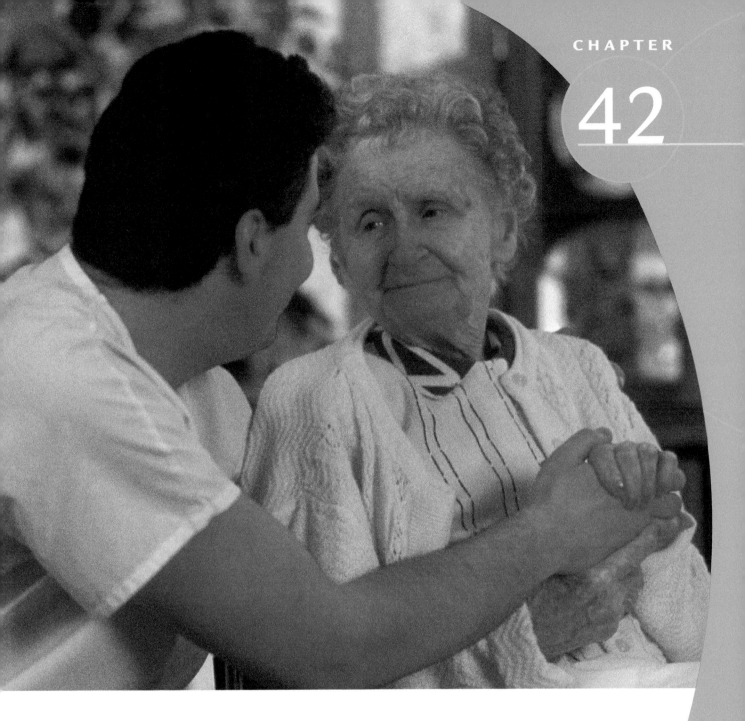

Introduction to Home Health Care

WHAT WILL YOU LEARN?

Many personal support workers choose to work in home health care. A personal support worker who works in home health care is often called a **home support worker.** Perhaps becoming a home support worker is something you have thought about. The basic skills and concepts that you have learned will apply no matter where you decide to work. But some aspects of providing care to a person in his or her own home are unique. In this chapter, you will

Photo: A home support worker interacts with a client.
(© Frank Siteman/Index Stock Imagery.)

learn why a person might need the services of a home health care agency, and how these services are paid for. You will also learn about some of the key responsibilities you would have, if you decided to work in the home health care setting. Finally, we will discuss the personal qualities that a person must have to succeed as a home support worker. When you are finished with this chapter, you will be able to:

1. Describe why a person might need home health care.
2. Discuss how home health care is paid for.
3. Describe how the home health care team works together to provide client care.
4. Describe the major duties of a home support worker.
5. List personal qualities that a home support worker must have to be successful.

Vocabulary

Home support worker	Respite care Homebound	Case manager Nurse's bag	Abandonment

WHAT IS HOME HEALTH CARE?

If you were ill, where would you rather be? In your own home, surrounded by the people, pets, and things that you love? Or in a hospital or long-term care facility? Given a choice, most people would prefer to stay in the comfort of their own homes when they are sick. Home health care, also known as *home care*, makes it possible for people who are not critically ill to receive health care in the comfort of their own homes. A person who is receiving the services of a home health care agency is called a *client*, instead of a "patient" or a "resident." There are many reasons why a person might become a client of a home health care agency:

- **The person may have just been discharged from the hospital following an acute illness or injury.** The care provided in a hospital is costly, and the number of beds in the hospital is limited. For these reasons, a person may be discharged from the hospital as soon as she is out of danger, but before she is fully recovered. In this situation, a home support worker may be needed to help care for the person at home until she has made a full recovery.
- **The person may have a chronic illness or disability that makes it hard for him to manage some tasks independently.** For example, a person who is paralyzed might need a home support worker to help him get out of bed and ready for work each morning.

- **The person may have an illness, such as dementia, that makes it dangerous for the person to be left alone in the house.** In this case, a home support worker might come to the home on a regular basis to provide care and companionship for the person and to relieve the primary caregiver. Care that allows the primary caregiver to rest or leave the house for a short period of time is called **respite care** (Fig. 42-1). Being able to "take a break" and leave the house is critical for managing the stress that can be caused by providing constant care for a family member who is ill.
- **The person may be terminally ill.** Hospice care is often provided in the person's home. A home support worker who works for a hospice agency will receive special training in providing end-of-life care.

PAYING FOR HOME HEALTH CARE

Home health care is paid for in many different ways. A client may pay for home health care entirely from his own income or savings. Or, he might have insurance coverage that covers all or part of the costs. Insurance coverage is provided by private insurance companies and by government agencies.

Insurance companies and government agencies often have strict rules regarding what type of care is covered, and under what circumstances. For example, many times the client must

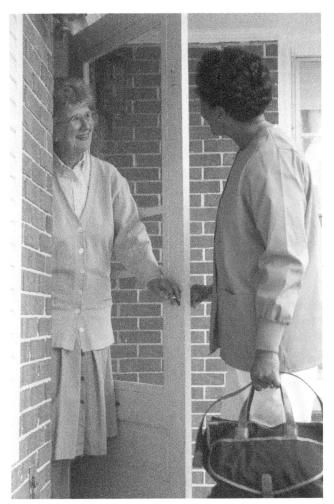

Figure 42-1
Part of a home support worker's duties may be to provide respite care. Respite care allows the family member who has primary responsibility for caring for the client to have time to herself. (© *Sally Moskol/Index Stock Imagery*.)

payment for home care services and to determine the frequency and length of future visits.

THE HEALTH CARE TEAM

Just as in any other health care setting, health care that is provided in the home is provided by a health care team. The health care team consists of the client, the client's family members, the home support worker, a nurse, a doctor, a case manager, and other specialists (such as a physical therapist or social worker). As always, the client is the focus of the health care team's efforts, and the goal of the health care team is to provide holistic care. Each team member provides a specific aspect of care for the client. For example, the home support worker may be responsible for monitoring vital signs and helping the client with routine activities of daily living (ADLs), while the nurse may be responsible for giving medications or providing wound care (Fig. 42-2). The health care team provides care in the home as directed by the client's care plan. The care plan is a set of instructions for the client's care, created by the case manager with input from all members of the health care team. The **case manager,** usually a registered nurse, is responsible for overseeing all of the client's care, from admission through discharge.

The home support worker is a very important member of the health care team. Because the home support worker is often scheduled to

be completely homebound before the insurance company will pay for the costs of home care. **Homebound** means that the person is unable to leave the house without a lot of help from another person. Insurance companies and government agencies may also control the length of each visit and the number of visits a person may have each week. For example, a client who needs minimal assistance with bathing may be allowed three visits per week, while a client who cannot get out of bed and is at risk for developing pressure ulcers may be allowed two visits each day. One client may be allowed a 1-hour visit, while another client is allowed a 2-hour visit. Proper documentation (recording) of the care provided to the client during each visit is necessary to justify continued

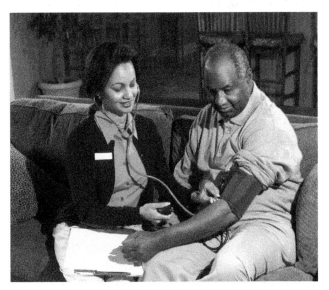

Figure 42-2
Home support workers are often responsible for monitoring the vital signs of their clients.

visit the client on a frequent, routine basis, he has the best chance to observe changes that could indicate a change in the client's health. In addition, the client may feel most comfortable with the home support worker, and as a result, may tell him things she might not tell other members of the health care team. By communicating his observations to the rest of the health care team, the home support worker becomes the "eyes and ears" of the members of the team who do not see the client as frequently. For this reason, communicating with the case manager and other members of the health care team is an essential part of the home support worker's responsibilities.

In the hospital and long-term care settings, team members often have the chance to communicate face-to-face, because everyone is together in the same building. This is not true in the home health care setting. Team members travel to the client's home according to their own individual schedules. As a result, they may rarely see one another. In the home health care setting, most communication among team members takes place through documentation. As always, you must accurately document the care you provide on the appropriate paperwork, including the date, time, and duration of the visit. Proper documentation is necessary to ensure that all members of the home health care team are kept "in-the-know."

TELL THE NURSE

As a home support worker, you will play an important role in reporting changes in a client's medical condition that could indicate a serious problem. Your agency will have written guidelines about observations that should be reported. Make sure you are familiar with these guidelines, and if you are ever in doubt about whether an observation should be immediately reported to the case manager, choose to err on the side of safety and report it. Make sure you report any of the following observations to the case manager immediately:

- One or more of the client's vital signs is above or below the standards set by the agency

- The client has a fever or other signs of infection

- There is a change in the client's mental alertness or orientation

- The client has signs of skin breakdown or pressure sores

- The client has signs or symptoms that could indicate a medical emergency

- You suspect that the client is being abused (physically, sexually, or psychologically)

- There are unsafe or unsanitary conditions in the home

RESPONSIBILITIES OF THE HOME SUPPORT WORKER

The home support worker usually assists clients with tasks related to personal care, such as bathing, grooming, and repositioning. Depending on the client's needs, the home support worker may also be assigned light housekeeping duties, such as cleaning, preparing meals, and doing laundry. The home support worker's responsibilities are clearly outlined in the client's care plan. You must follow the care plan exactly. Any changes to the care plan must first be approved by the case manager.

As noted earlier, it is very important for you to keep accurate records of the care that you provide and the observations that you make. Proper documentation of the care that you provide helps to ensure that the client's insurance will continue to pay for the services. In addition, good documentation is necessary to ensure that all of the members of the health care team are kept informed of the client's status. Each home health care agency has specific policies related to documentation. Your supervisor will review these policies with you.

In addition to documenting the care that you provide to the client, you may be required to keep a daily record of your activities. For example, you might be asked to keep a *time and travel log*, which details how much time you spent at each client's house, how much time you spent traveling between houses, and your mileage for the day. Always record information in a timely manner. If you must wait until the end of the day to record something, keep accurate notes so that the information you record will be accurate.

You will provide care for many different clients. Some of your clients may have limited income and live in very small homes or apartments. Others may be quite wealthy and live in large homes with many modern conveniences. Some homes will be very clean, while others will not live up to your personal standards. Each home, and each family, is different. Remember that you are a guest in the client's home. You must be careful not to allow your opinions about how a person lives to affect the care that you provide. If you feel that something about a client's home environment puts the client at risk for injury (such as extremely dirty conditions, an abusive relationship with a family member, or a potential fire hazard), report your concerns to the case manager.

PERSONAL CARE

As a home support worker, many of your responsibilities will be related to helping your clients with activities such as bathing, eating, getting dressed, exercising, toileting, repositioning, and transferring (Fig. 42-3). As always, the amount of help you will need to provide will vary from client to client, and you should encourage the client to do as much as possible for himself.

The skills you will use to assist with personal care are the same no matter where you work. However, in the home setting, some of the equipment may be different. Medical equipment, such as shower chairs, bedside commodes, or adjustable beds, can be purchased or rented from a medical supply store for use in the home, but this can be expensive. Many clients will not be able to afford this expense. Therefore, many times you must be resourceful and use items that are readily available in the home. For example, if the person's bed is not adjustable, you can use extra pillows or a back rest to position the person in the Fowler's position. A sturdy webbed or plastic lawn chair may substitute for a shower chair (Fig. 42-4). However, as with the use of any type of equipment, safety is a top priority. If you think that a client is at risk for injury because he or she does not have a certain piece of medical equipment, ask the case manager for advice. The case manager may be able to work with outside resources to get the equipment the client needs at low cost, or no cost.

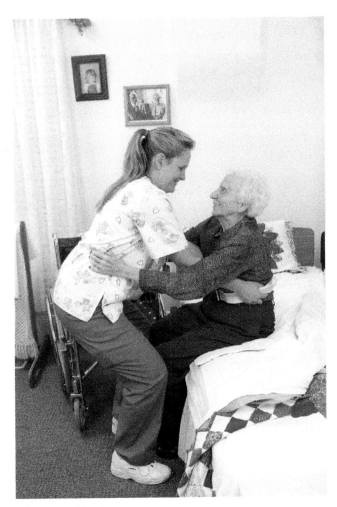

Figure 42-3
Home support workers assist with all types of personal care. Here, a home support worker helps a client to transfer out of bed.

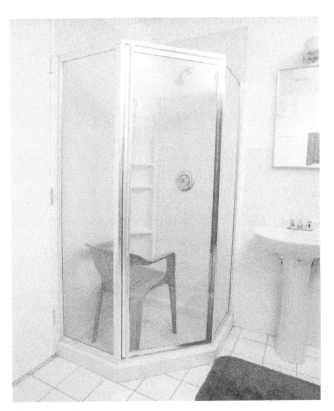

Figure 42-4
Sometimes common household items can be used in place of expensive medical equipment. Here, a plastic lawn chair is used as a shower chair.

HOMEMAKING

Depending on the client's needs, part of your responsibilities as a home support worker may include preparing and serving meals, cleaning, and doing laundry. Homemaking duties are outlined on the client's care plan. You will document the homemaking duties that you perform on a *homemaker flow sheet,* according to your agency's policies. The homemaker flow sheet becomes part of the client's medical record. As always, you must accurately document your work.

Meal Preparation

Preparing meals is a duty frequently assigned to the home support worker (Fig. 42-5). Some training programs require home support workers who will be preparing and serving food to take a food handler's course. Because requirements may differ from province to province it is important for you to know your agency's policies and to check with the personal support worker's registry in the province or territory where you work.

When preparing a meal, consider the special needs and individual preferences of the client. The meal should be nutritious. If the person is on a special diet, such as a restricted-sodium diet, then you must make sure that the meal you prepare

meets the diet's requirements. For some clients, you will have to cut the food into very small pieces or puree it in a blender before serving it.

Serve the meal or snack at the time specified in the care plan. As always, make an effort to make meal time as pleasant as possible. Present the meal in an attractive way, and sit down and talk with the person as she is eating. The amount of assistance with eating that your client will need will vary. For example, some clients will be able to feed themselves if you assist with opening cartons or peeling a piece of fruit. Others will need more help. Involve the person in the process of eating by allowing her to do as much as she can for herself.

Housekeeping

Many times, the home support worker is also responsible for providing some cleaning services (Fig. 42-6). These tasks may be done on a weekly basis, or as scheduled on the care plan.

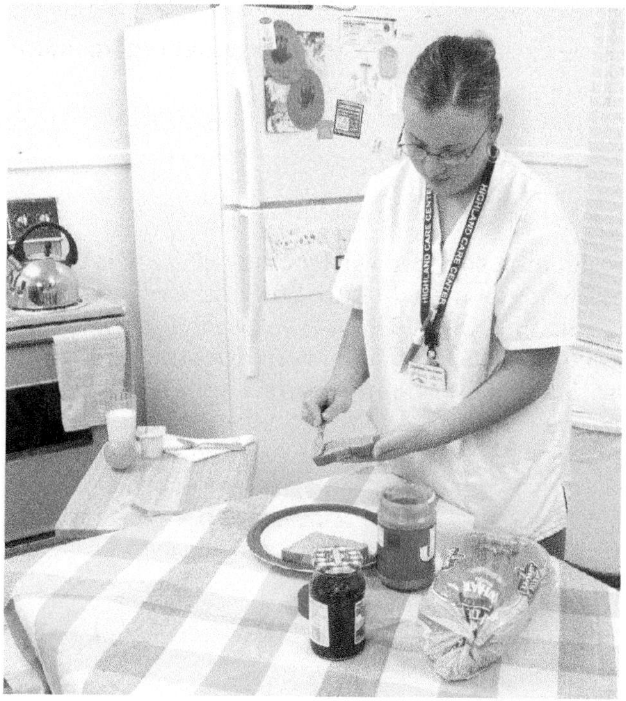

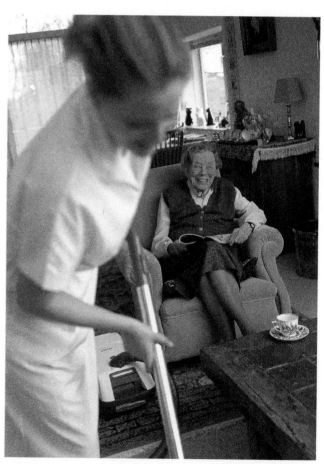

Figure 42-5
Meal preparation is often part of the home support worker's routine duties.

Figure 42-6
Light housekeeping might also be part of the home support worker's responsibilities. (© *Benelux Press/Index Stock Imagery.*)

Depending on the client's needs, you may be responsible for:

- Dusting
- Vacuuming carpets
- Mopping floors
- Disinfecting kitchen and bathroom surfaces
- Changing the client's bed linens
- Washing and drying the client's bed linens and clothing

When providing housekeeping services, care for the client's home as if it were your own. Be careful not to damage decorative items on tables and shelves. Pay attention to details. For example, when vacuuming a room, be thorough. Don't just vacuum the center of the room—make sure the edges and baseboards are clean too. When using cleaning solutions, make sure that the product you are using is approved for use on the surface you are cleaning, to avoid causing permanent damage (Fig. 42-7). It is important to be respectful of the client's home and its contents. When you show respect for a client's home and personal belongings, you are letting the person know that you truly care for him or her.

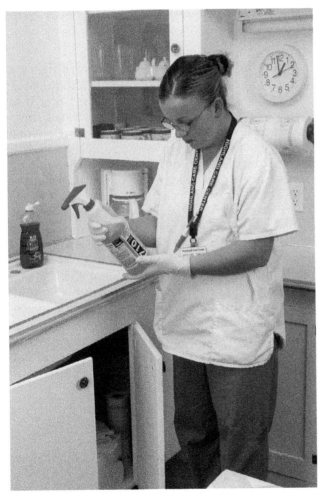

Figure 42-7
When using cleaning solutions, make sure the product you are using is approved for use on the surface you are cleaning. Cleaning solutions should always be kept in properly labelled containers.

QUALITIES OF THE SUCCESSFUL HOME SUPPORT WORKER

So maybe you are thinking that you would like to work in the home health setting. Of course, just as in any health care setting, a strong work ethic is important. For example, being honest, compassionate, courteous, conscientious, and reliable will serve you well, no matter where you work. However, the people who make the best home support workers also have other qualities that help them to succeed in the home health care setting. The most successful home support workers:

- Enjoy working independently and are self-motivated
- Are organized and able to manage their time well
- Are reliable
- Are able to set professional boundaries

Let's look at each of these qualities in more detail.

ABILITY TO WORK INDEPENDENTLY

As a home support worker, you will be working in a client's home without direct supervision most of the time. If you like a lot of feedback and guidance as you complete your assignments, then working in the home health care setting might not be right for you. To work in the home health care setting, you need to be very comfortable with your own caregiving and problem-solving skills. You also need to be self-motivated. No one will be there to help you, or to tell you what to do next.

ABILITY TO BE ORGANIZED AND MANAGE TIME

Because you will be working independently, you will be responsible for making sure that you complete your assigned duties as scheduled. You will be given a list of the clients you must care for each day, and you will be told the length of each client visit. However, it will be up to you to determine how to best provide the required care, complete the necessary documentation, and travel between clients during the workday. You must work efficiently and safely.

Organization is one key to working efficiently and safely. When preparing to visit a client's home, gather all of the supplies you will need before you enter the person's home. Having the necessary supplies on hand allows you to work more efficiently, because you will not have to interrupt care to search for something you need. Some supplies and equipment may be kept at the client's home in a designated place (Fig. 42-8). Others, you will have to carry with you to each client's home in your **nurse's bag** (Fig. 42-9). For example, some of the things you might carry in your nurse's bag include:

- Forms needed for documentation, and a pen
- Personal protective equipment (PPE)
- Equipment used for taking vital signs
- Supplies for cleaning your equipment
- Alcohol-based hand rub

The nurse's bag has many compartments, which makes it easy for you to organize and find your supplies and equipment. Keeping each item in a special place makes it easy for you to see if you need to restock your nurse's bag. It also makes it easy for you to check that you have everything you need before you leave for the day. Organizing the paperwork needed for documentation in the order of your visits for the day is also very helpful.

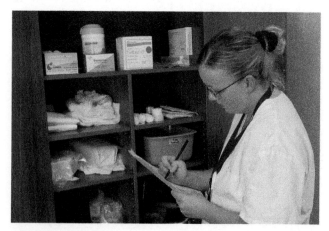

Figure 42-8
Some of the supplies and equipment you will need to care for your client will be kept in a special place in the client's home. Here, a home support worker is checking to see if any of the supplies are getting low.

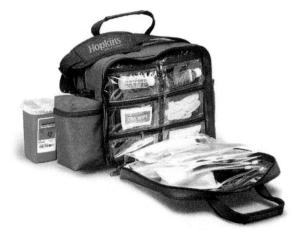

Figure 42-9
A nurse's bag is used to carry supplies that will be used with every client, such as equipment for taking vital signs and personal protective equipment. The many compartments help you to keep the bag organized and clean. (*Courtesy of Hopkins Medical Products, Baltimore, MD/ (800)835-1995, www.hmponline.com.*)

Planning is the other key to working efficiently and safely. If possible, you should plan your day so that you visit clients in an order that allows for the most efficient use of travel time. For example, it would not be the best use of your time to spend all day traveling back and forth across town, when you could see all of your clients on the east side in the morning and all of your clients on the west side in the afternoon. When planning your day's work, map out your client's addresses and try to limit your travel time as much as possible. However, keep in mind that your clients' preferences and needs must also be taken into account when arranging care schedules. For example, a client with paraplegia may need your help to get ready for work in the morning, while another client with diabetes might need you at his house at a certain time to prepare and serve lunch. It takes planning to make sure that your clients' needs are met while minimizing your travel time between homes.

RELIABILITY

Clients who receive home care depend on the home support worker to arrive and provide the appropriate care. For example, how would you feel if you depended on someone to help you get out of bed, shower, and get ready for work in the morning, and that person did not come to help you when she said she would come? Failing to keep appointments is not only inconsiderate, it can cause the client harm. For example, if you are responsible for preparing lunch for a client with diabetes, then you must do that at the scheduled time, or else the person is at risk for an adverse insulin reaction due to low blood glucose levels. Being reliable is a critical quality for a home support worker to have.

The term **abandonment** means to withdraw one's support or help from another person, in spite of duty or responsibility. A home support worker who fails to show up at a client's home to provide scheduled care is guilty of abandonment (Fig. 42-10). Similarly, a home support worker who leaves a client's home without completing the scheduled tasks may also be guilty of abandonment. As with any job, there may be situations beyond your control that will cause you to

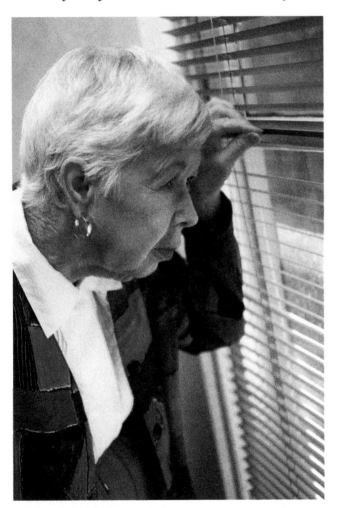

Figure 42-10
Your clients depend on you to arrive and provide the appropriate care, as scheduled. Leaving a client alone and without proper assistance is called *abandonment*.

be unable to keep your appointments. If you are running late, it is your responsibility to notify the home health care agency. You must also try to contact the clients who are expecting you and let them know that you will be late. If you are unable to report to work at all, you must notify the home health care agency so that another home support worker can be sent to care for your scheduled clients. Also make sure you notify your agency if a personal emergency arises during your work-day that would make it necessary for you to leave before completing your scheduled visits and care duties. Follow your agency's policies regarding situations of this nature so that the care needed by your clients is provided without delay.

ABILITY TO SET PROFESSIONAL BOUNDARIES

Many of your clients and their family members will come to regard you as a friend, or maybe even part of the family. You may also become close to clients and their family members. As a result, the line between your professional life and your personal life might become blurry. To succeed as a home support worker, you must be able to maintain a professional relationship with both clients and their family members at all times. Although it may be tempting to "drop in" on a client, or to go to the client's home after working hours to visit socially, this is not appropriate. Also, you should refuse any gift (including gifts of food or money) that may be offered to you by a client or family member. Your employer will have very specific policies regarding personal relationships between health care professionals and clients, and the acceptance of gifts. Make sure that you always follow these policies, and if you are in doubt about any type of relationship or gift, ask your supervisor for clarification.

Professional boundaries are also necessary to prevent clients or their family members from taking advantage of you. You will have a helping relationship with the client and family members that can easily be taken advantage of in many different ways. For example, a family member might ask you to provide care that has not been listed in the care plan. If you ever have any question about whether or not it is acceptable to perform additional duties or "favors" for a client or family member, make sure you ask your supervisor first.

SUMMARY

- Home health care is skilled care that is given to a person in his or her home.
  - People of all ages, and with all types of illnesses and disabilities, use the services of home health care agencies. Home care may be needed for a short time to help a person recover from an acute illness or injury, or it may be needed for the rest of the person's life.
  - Home health care can be paid for privately by the client, by insurance, or by government. Proper documentation of the care that you provide helps to ensure that the client's insurance will continue to pay for the services. The information that you record is also used to plan the client's future care.
  - Home health care is provided by a health care team. At minimum, the home health care team consists of a client, the client's family members, the home support worker, a nurse, a doctor, and a case manager. Other specialists may be included as well, depending on the client's needs.
    - The home support worker is the "eyes and ears" of the health care team. Most communication with other health care team members takes place through recording.
    - The home support worker's major responsibilities include tasks related to personal care and light housekeeping.
- To succeed as a home support worker, a person must have several qualities.
  - The home support worker must be resourceful. All of the standard equipment that is available in other health care settings may not be available in a person's home.
  - The home support worker must be able to work independently, without a lot of supervision or help from others.
  - The home support worker must be organized, with good time management skills.
  - The home support worker must be reliable. Leaving a client alone and without proper assistance is called *abandonment.*
  - The home support worker must have the ability to set appropriate professional boundaries with the client and family.

WHAT DID YOU LEARN?

Multiple Choice

Select the single best answer for each of the following questions.

1. Which one of the following is a routine responsibility of a home support worker?
   a. Providing respite care for the wife of a client with dementia
   b. Picking up a client's prescription at the drugstore
   c. Grocery shopping for the family
   d. Washing the windows of the home
2. One of your clients is turning 90 next week, and his family has invited you to attend his birthday party. What should you do?
   a. Accept the invitation, and take a card or a gift to the party
   b. Decline the invitation, but give the client a card or gift during your next scheduled visit
   c. Decline the invitation after thanking the family for inviting you
   d. Accept the invitation, but avoid bringing a card or a gift to the party
3. You are scheduled to work today, but the weather is beautiful and your best friend is begging you to take the day off and go to the beach with her. What should you do?
   a. Ask your friend if she would be willing to go with you in the afternoon. You will take care of all of your scheduled clients in the morning, and then you will be free to go.
   b. Call the case manager on your way to the beach and tell her that you will not be able to visit your clients today. This will allow

the case manager to find another home support worker to cover for you.

c. Tell your friend that you are sorry, but you cannot go to the beach today.

d. Call each of the clients who you are scheduled to visit and ask them if it would be okay if you came tomorrow instead.

4. Why is documentation a very important responsibility of the home support worker?

a. Documentation is the main way that the members of the home health care team communicate with one another about the care given to the client and the client's condition, and the home support worker has the most frequent contact with the client.

b. Documentation provides information that is used to determine if a client is recovering, or getting worse.

c. Documentation of all care provided is needed to justify continued payment for home care services.

d. All of the above

5. Peggy is a home support worker. Today, while Peggy is helping a client, her son's teacher calls Peggy on her cell phone to tell her that her son has had an accident on the playground, and he needs to be picked up. What should Peggy do?

a. Tell the client that she has a family emergency and she has to leave

b. Tell the teacher that she will be there to pick up her son after her shift ends, in another 2 hours

c. Call her supervisor and ask if there is another home support worker who could cover for her while she goes to pick up her son at school

d. Take the client in the car with her to pick up her son

6. Elizabeth has been caring for Mrs. Robinson for several months and has become friendly with her bachelor son, Richard. One day, Richard asks Elizabeth out for a cup of coffee after she is finished working. What should Elizabeth do?

a. Decline Richard's invitation because dating family members of clients is against the home health care agency's policy

b. Accept Richard's invitation—after all, she is single and she likes to date

c. Ask Mrs. Robinson if it is all right if she dates her son

d. Ask Richard if he would be willing to go for a cup of coffee on a day when she is not scheduled to work

Matching

Match each numbered item with its appropriate lettered description.

B **1.** Case manager

E **2.** Care plan

F **3.** Respite care

A **4.** Hospice care

C **5.** Time and travel log

D **6.** Homemaker flow sheet

a. End-of-life care provided to a person who is terminally ill

b. Member of the health care team responsible for overseeing a client's care, from admission through discharge

c. Form the home support worker uses to record how much time he spent at each client's house, how much time he spent traveling between houses, and his mileage for the day

d. Form used to document housework that is done

e. A set of instructions for the client's care

f. Care that allows the primary caregiver to rest or leave the house for a short period of time

STOP and Think!

You are thinking about becoming a home support worker, and you decide to talk to your friend Darlene, who has worked in both the long-term care setting and as a home support worker. What do you think Darlene will tell you is different about working in the home health care setting? What will she tell you is the same?

You work for the Home-Aid Home Health Care Agency, which is located in a city called Evergreen. You have received your assignments for the day and are trying to plan your day's work. Look at the assignment list and the map of Evergreen below, and decide how you will organize your day. You know that it will take you 15 minutes to travel between each client's home.

CLIENT	ASSIGNMENT	LENGTH OF VISIT	ADDRESS
Mr. Diaz, a 93-year-old man who is confined to bed	Assist client with toileting and repositioning	45 minutes, twice daily	13th & Chestnut
Miss Louise, an 84-year-old woman who is blind and has diabetes	Assist client with eating snack, change bed linens	45 minutes	7th & Spruce
Ms. Lindgren, a 65-year-old woman with advanced dementia	Assist client with activities of daily living (ADLs) and provide respite care for client's daughter	3 hours	16th & Walnut
Ms. Chang, a 26-year-old woman with paraplegia	Assist client with morning care and breakfast so that she can leave for work by 8:30 A.M.	90 minutes	14th & Arch

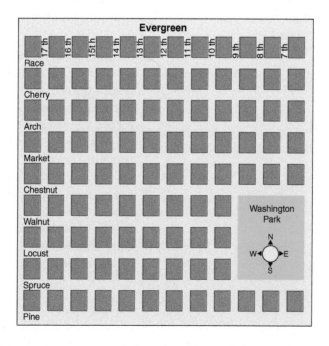

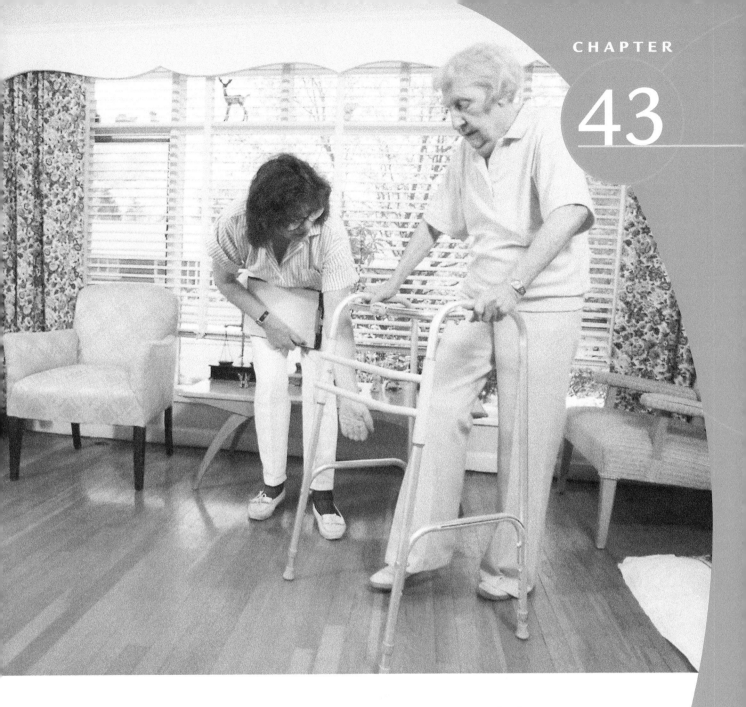

Safety and Infection Control in the Home Health Care Setting

WHAT WILL YOU LEARN?

Keeping yourself and your clients safe, from both physical hazards and infection, is a priority in the home health care setting, just as it is in other health care settings. As a home support worker, you must be aware of unsafe situations that could put your client at

Photo: A home support worker checks to make sure a client is comfortable using her walker. This is just one of many ways that home support workers help to keep their clients safe.

803

risk for injury in his own home. In addition, working as a home support worker poses unique risks to your safety and well-being. In this chapter, you will learn how to adapt the principles of safety and infection control that you learned earlier to meet the unique needs of the home health care setting. When you are finished with this chapter, you will be able to:

1. List safety concerns that are unique to the home health care environment.
2. Understand ways that home support workers can spread infection.
3. Identify ways to reduce the spread of infection within the home.
4. Identify ways to properly prepare and store food.
5. Describe measures that the home support worker can take to protect herself from personal harm while carrying out her duties.

Vocabulary

Bag technique

WORKPLACE SAFETY

Many of us consider our homes places of safety and security. However, the home environment can actually be quite dangerous. As a home support worker, you need to be aware of conditions in the home that put the client at risk. You also need to know how to react in the event of an emergency.

ACCIDENTS AND MEDICAL EMERGENCIES

Health care settings, such as long-term care facilities and hospitals, are built with safety in mind. The hallways are wide and well lit; there are no throw rugs to trip over; and the bathrooms come equipped with handrails and other safety devices. A person's private home is a different story, however. Many factors in the home can put a person at risk for falling, especially if the person has limited mobility or poor eyesight:

- Many homes are old, with worn carpets or uneven floors.
- Hallways, rooms, and staircases might be dimly lit, or not lit at all.
- The bathroom may be small, or not located in a place that is easy for a person with poor mobility to reach.
- The home may be filled with a lifetime of collected objects and furniture, which can lead to crowding and clutter.
- Many people have pets, which can run underfoot.

Remember from Chapter 10 that falling is the most common type of accident that occurs in the health care setting, and the number one cause of accidental death among elderly people.

Fire is also a concern in the home:

- The wiring in the house may be old.
- Outlets may be overloaded. Overload can be caused by plugging too many cords into a single outlet, or by using extension cords.
- Electrical cords may be covered by carpet. This is a fire hazard as well as a tripping hazard.
- The family may rely on a space heater to provide heat. Space heaters can be dangerous if they are not used properly.
- Many people do not have functioning smoke detectors in their homes.

Guidelines for helping to maintain a safe home environment are given in Guidelines Box 43-1. It is not your responsibility to change the client's home to ensure safe conditions. However, your observations about the overall safety of the home are important and should be reported to the case manager. For example, based on your observations, the case manager might decide that the client needs better lighting and a smoke detector installed in the hallway, handrails installed on the staircase, and grab bars installed in the bathroom. The client may also need assistive devices, such as an elevated toilet seat or a bedside commode (to make toileting easier) or a side rail (for help with getting into and out of bed). The case manager will arrange for the necessary modifications and equipment. Your job is to make the case manager aware of the client's needs.

Guidelines Box 43-1 Guidelines for Maintaining a Safe Home Environment

WHAT YOU DO	WHY YOU DO IT
Make sure that the furniture is arranged to allow for wide walkways. Chairs and small tables should be placed around the edges of the room, rather than in the center.	A cluttered, narrow walkway increases a person's risk of tripping and falling.
Remove any clutter or obstacles from indoor and outdoor walkways and steps. Provide adequate lighting.	Proper lighting enhances the ability to see, which helps to prevent falls. Removing obstacles and clutter that a person could trip over helps to prevent falls as well.
Place a small lamp and a telephone on the person's bedside table.	Having these items close at hand can help to prevent falls. If the phone rings, the person can answer it without getting out of bed. If the person needs to get out of bed in the middle of the night, he can turn on the light first. The ability to see helps to prevent falls.
Install night-lights as needed.	Some people may hesitate to turn on the light when they get up in the middle of the night. Night-lights can help the person to see the route to the bathroom or kitchen without turning on the lights in the room or hallway. The ability to see helps to prevent falls.
Avoid running cords across walkways. Instead, move the furniture so that the electrical cords for lamps and other appliances are close to the outlet.	A person could trip over a cord that is stretched across a room or walkway.
In wintry climates, make arrangements for snow and ice to be removed from outdoor walkways and steps.	A person could easily slip and fall on icy or snowy walkways and steps.
Clean up spills on the bathroom or kitchen floor promptly.	Tile or linoleum floors become very slippery when wet, increasing the person's risk of falling.
Use a no-slip rubber bath mat on the floor of the bathtub.	A no-slip rubber bath mat helps to provide traction, reducing the person's risk of falling while getting into or out of the bathtub.
Provide a bath bench or a shower chair for the person to use while showering.	An unsteady person will be more stable and at less risk for falling if he can sit down during the shower.
Be aware of potential fire hazards (for example, frayed wires and overloaded outlets) and report these immediately.	A house fire can have tragic consequences, especially when the people who live in the home are relatively unable to help themselves should a fire break out.

(continued)

Guidelines Box 43-1	Guidelines for Maintaining a Safe Home Environment (continued)
WHAT YOU DO	**WHY YOU DO IT**
Keep chemicals, cleaning solutions, and other poisonous substances in a locked storage area.	Poor eyesight, confusion, or a decreased sense of taste or smell can cause an elderly person to eat or drink something that will cause her harm. Children are also at risk for accidental poisonings because they are curious.
Program emergency telephone numbers into the telephone (for example, for the person's doctor, a family member, and emergency services), or keep a written list next to the telephone.	Having emergency phone numbers handy will make it easier for the person to call for help in the event of an emergency.

It is quite possible that despite your efforts to maintain a safe home environment, an accident, fire, or medical emergency will occur. For example, you may arrive at the home to find that your client has fallen and hurt himself. You may smell smoke or gas when you enter the client's home. The client may have a medical emergency, such as a heart attack or stroke, while you are there, or she may choke on food. Remember what you learned in Chapters 9 and 12 about reacting to fire and medical emergencies. Remain calm, and use good judgment. Call the fire department or activate the emergency medical services (EMS) system by calling "911" or the emergency telephone number specified by your agency. Then provide appropriate care until help arrives. After the situation has been resolved, you will need to report and record according to your agency's policy. For example, if an accident occurred while you were working, most agencies will require you to complete an incident (occurrence) report (see Chapter 10, Fig. 10-3).

ABUSIVE SITUATIONS

In Chapter 4, you learned about abuse. Abuse can be physical, psychological (emotional), or sexual. Anyone can be a target for abuse. Families are complex, and many things go on "behind closed doors." As a home support worker, you may witness some of these things. For example, one of the family members may be the target of abuse, either by another family member or a friend of the family. A disabled or elderly person is more likely to be abused in the privacy of his or her own home because the abuser may feel

that the abuse will go undiscovered. Children are also often targets of abuse.

As a home support worker, you may find yourself in a situation where you suspect that one of your clients is being abused (see Chapter 4, Box 4-1). Laws require that any health care worker who suspects the abuse of a child or elderly person must report his or her suspicions to the proper authorities. Your agency will have specific policies regarding the chain of reporting. It is not your responsibility to investigate whether or not abuse has actually occurred, or who has caused it. The agencies that handle abuse reports will proceed through the proper channels. Your responsibility is to simply report your suspicions.

If a family situation turns violent while you are in the client's home, and you feel unsafe, you should leave the home after doing your best to make sure that the client is also safe. Activate the EMS system by calling "911" or the emergency telephone number specified by your agency if you feel that someone in the house is in immediate danger, and then report the situation to the case manager.

INFECTION CONTROL

Just as in any other health care setting, infection control is a top priority. Many of the people you will care for as a home support worker will have risk factors for infection. Your clients will be sick, recovering from surgery, elderly, or have a chronic illness or conditions that will increase their risk of getting an infectious disease. One of your major responsibilities is to protect the people you care for from infection.

As a home support worker, you will visit several clients' homes each day. Improper or careless use of infection control methods can result in pathogens being carried from the home of one client to the home of another one. You can transmit pathogens on your hands, clothes, or equipment. By maintaining a sanitary environment and using standard precautions, you can protect your clients and yourself from communicable disease.

MAINTAINING A SANITARY ENVIRONMENT

No matter where you work, you will do many things to help maintain a sanitary work environment (see Chapter 7, Guidelines Box 7-1). When working in a client's home, you will have additional responsibilities related to maintaining a sanitary environment and preventing the spread of infection.

Using Proper Bag Technique

Bag technique is a procedure that is used to keep your nurse's bag free from contamination. Using proper bag technique helps to prevent the transmission of microbes from one client's home to another client's home. To practice proper bag technique:

1. When you arrive at the client's home, place your nurse's bag on a clean surface, such as the kitchen table, after laying down a newspaper, plastic bag, or other clean barrier object (Fig. 43-1). Placing a barrier between your nurse's bag and the surface helps to prevent contamination of the nurse's bag.
2. After washing your hands, remove the equipment you will need from your nurse's bag.
3. After you use the equipment, clean it and disinfect it according to agency policy and return it to its proper location in your nurse's bag (Fig. 43-2). Equipment that is used with all clients, such as your stethoscope, is not to be transported to another client's home until it has been properly cleaned and disinfected. Equipment that has been cleaned and disinfected is stored in the "clean" area of the nurse's bag.
4. Some items that are used for a client's care must be returned to the agency for proper cleaning and disinfection before they are used again. You may also be required to transport specimens, such as urine or sputum samples, to the agency or laboratory.

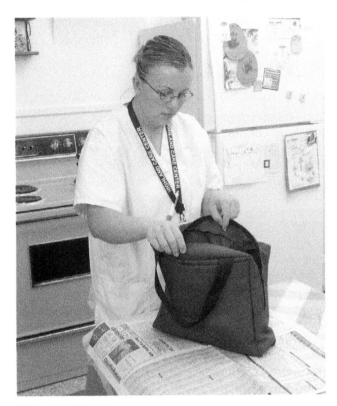

Figure 43-1
The nurse's bag is placed on a barrier, such as a clean sheet of newspaper, to help prevent the bag from becoming contaminated.

Dirty equipment and specimens are considered contaminated and are stored in the "dirty" area of the nurse's bag. (If equipment is too large to fit in the nurse's bag, then it can be stored in the "dirty" area of your car

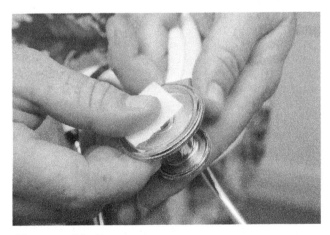

Figure 43-2
Equipment that is used for each client, such as equipment for measuring vital signs, is cleaned after each use and before placing it back in the nurse's bag. Alcohol wipes are usually used to clean the ear pieces, bell, and diaphragm of a stethoscope.

trunk, which may be divided in a way similar to the way the nurse's bag is divided.)

Cleaning Equipment and Household Surfaces

You will use many pieces of equipment as you care for your clients. Some of this equipment will be kept in the client's home, such as a bedside commode or equipment used for bathing. As always, this equipment must be properly cleaned and disinfected after each use. A commercial disinfectant solution or a solution of bleach and water mixed 1:10 (1 cup of bleach to 10 cups of water) may be used, according to your agency's policy. Use gloves when cleaning any equipment.

Many of your duties as a home support worker will be related to keeping areas clean where food is prepared or personal care is given. A disinfectant solution is used to clean floors, kitchen counters, bathroom fixtures (including the toilet, bathtub, sink, and counters), and surfaces that are frequently touched by many people (such as doorknobs, telephone receivers, and refrigerator handles). These areas should be cleaned according to agency policy to decrease the spread of pathogens in the home. When cleaning floors and other household surfaces, remember the following:

- Empty dirty mop water into the toilet, *not* into sinks where food will be prepared.
- Disinfect mop heads and sponges after use by soaking them in a 1:10 bleach and water solution.
- Clean up blood or body fluid spills immediately. Wearing gloves, use paper towels to soak up as much fluid as possible. Place the soiled towels in a plastic bag and seal it. Then place that plastic bag in a second plastic bag. Seal the second bag, write "biohazard" on the outside of it, and dispose of it according to your agency's policies. Then clean the area where the spill occurred with a disinfectant solution.
- Pregnant women and people who have weak immune systems should not clean litter boxes, bird cages, or other pet-related items. Cat feces, bird droppings, and other animal wastes can contain microbes that can cause harm to a developing fetus, or to a person with a weak immune system.

Handling Food Properly

You may be responsible for preparing meals for clients. Before preparing any food, always wash your hands using proper handwashing tech-

nique, and make sure that the surface where you will be preparing the food is clean. When preparing foods, remember to:

- Take note of expiration dates on packaged foods
- Avoid using eggs that are cracked
- Thoroughly wash and dry fresh fruits and vegetables before serving them
- Wash your hands after handling raw meat or poultry, and before touching anything else
- Wash cutting boards, utensils, and dishes used to prepare raw meat or poultry in hot, soapy water immediately after use
- Cook meat and poultry thoroughly, according to the safe food handling labels that are attached to all grocery store meat packages
- Use a clean spoon each time if you must taste the food to check for seasonings

Raw or cooked food that is not stored properly can easily spoil and cause food poisoning. Leftovers should be placed in appropriate sealed containers, labelled with the date and contents, and refrigerated (Fig. 43-3). Food in the refrigerator should be inspected and disposed of before it is outdated or spoiled. The refrigerator itself should be cleaned with hot, soapy water periodically.

After each use, clean kitchen counters and stovetops with a disinfectant solution. If the house has a dishwasher, rinse the dishes and utensils and place them in the dishwasher. When the dishwasher is full, run it using the hot water cycle and dishwasher detergent. Items that are not "dishwasher safe" should be washed by hand using hot, soapy water. If possible, allow these items to air dry in a rack. Otherwise, use a clean dishtowel or paper towels to dry them. If no dishwasher is available, the dishes and utensils will need to be washed by hand and dried. Be sure to wear gloves when washing dishes.

Assisting Clients With Personal Hygiene

Helping your clients to maintain good personal hygiene is essential to maintaining a sanitary environment. Bathing, washing hair, brushing teeth, and wearing clean clothing are all grooming practices that help prevent the spread of infection. Change the client's bed linens frequently, and encourage the client to wear clean clothing each day. (As always, soiled bed linens and clothing should be changed immediately.) Wash soiled linens and clothing in the washing machine, using the warmest water temperature

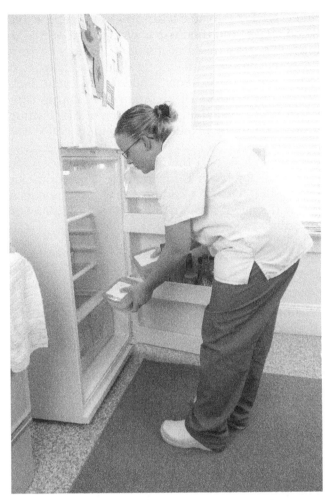

Figure 43-3
Leftovers should be placed in appropriate sealed containers, labelled (contents and date), and stored in the refrigerator.

available. Use a lengthy wash cycle and laundry soap. Add bleach if fabrics are colorfast. Dry the laundry on the high heat setting in a dryer. If a dryer is unavailable, hang laundry in the sun to dry.

TELL THE NURSE !

As a home support worker, you will have the unique opportunity to observe the home for conditions and situations that may increase a client's risk of spreading or getting an infection. You must be very diligent about observing your client for signs or symptoms of a developing infection. You must also be aware of practices of the client or family members that may spread an infection. Report any of the following observations to the case manager immediately:

● The client has signs of an infection, such as fever, pain, reddened skin, coughing, a thick nasal discharge, vomiting, or diarrhea

● A family member has signs of infection, especially if the client is at high risk for catching a communicable infection (because of a weakened immune system)

● Members of the household have poor sanitation practices (for example, there is spoiled food, accumulated trash, or soiled linens lying around the house)

● The house lacks running water or toilet facilities

USING STANDARD PRECAUTIONS

Maintaining a sanitary workplace is one important way to limit the spread of pathogens. In addition, you must always use standard precautions when providing client care. Standard precautions, covered in detail in Chapter 7, are used to reduce your risk of getting a communicable disease from a client. Proper use of standard precautions also helps to prevent the transmission of an infection to family members or other clients.

Handwashing

Handwashing is the single most important method of preventing the spread of infection in any type of health care setting (see Chapter 7). Always wash your hands:

• When you first arrive at a client's home
• Whenever your hands become visibly soiled with blood or other body fluids or substances
• Whenever you remove your gloves
• After each task or procedure that you perform

Wash your hands with soap and warm water, using the technique you learned in Chapter 7 (Fig. 43-4; see also Procedure 7-1). If paper towels are not available, use a *clean* cloth towel to dry your hands.

If handwashing facilities are not available or are inadequate, and your hands are not visibly soiled with dirt, blood, or other body fluids or substances, you can use an alcohol-based hand rub to decontaminate your hands (Fig. 43-5). If your hands are visibly soiled, then you should seek proper handwashing facilities as soon as possible.

Using Personal Protective Equipment

As in other health care settings, gloves, gowns, masks, and goggles are worn as necessary to control the spread of pathogens. Your agency is required by the Canadian Centre for Occupational Health and Safety (CCOHS) to provide you

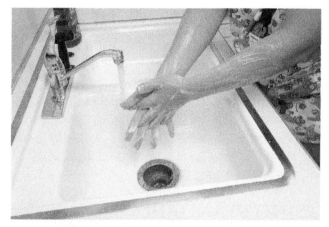

Figure 43-4
Handwashing is the single most important method of preventing the spread of infection, no matter where you work. Here, a home support worker washes her hands at the kitchen sink.

with adequate personal protective equipment (PPE). You may carry PPE in your nurse's bag, or store it on site, depending on the situation. It is your responsibility to make sure that you have the PPE that you need before you leave for work, and to use the PPE consistently, conscientiously, and correctly (see Chapter 7). Eye protection that is not disposable must be cleaned and disinfected after each use.

Disposing of Sharps

Many clients will use needles, lancets, or other sharp instruments or devices on a routine basis. For example, a client who has diabetes may rou-

tinely prick his finger with a lancet to check his blood sugar, and then use a syringe and needle to inject his daily doses of insulin. Clients who routinely use needles and lancets should be instructed to dispose of these items properly to prevent accidental needlesticks. If a commercial sharps container is not available, one can be made by cutting a small slit in the plastic lid of an empty coffee can or in the side of a heavy plastic bottle. When it is two-thirds full, seal the container with wide tape and write "biohazard" on the side. The container should be disposed of according to the guidelines set by the client's waste management company or according to agency policy.

PERSONAL SAFETY

As a home support worker, you will use standard methods to keep yourself safe on the job. For example, you will use proper body mechanics to minimize your risk of physical injury when lifting or transferring clients, and you will use standard precautions to protect yourself from infection. But some aspects of the home support worker's job pose unique safety risks. Instead of working in one building, you will be required to travel from one client's home to another. This puts you at increased risk for traffic accidents, flat tires, and other hazards of driving. In addition, some of your clients may live in unsafe neighborhoods, which could put you at risk for being attacked. Protecting yourself while traveling to and from your clients' homes is a top priority. Here are

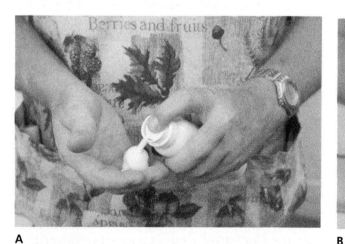

A

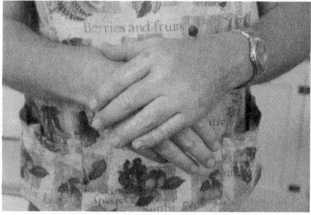

B

Figure 43-5
An alcohol-based hand rub can be used for routine hand decontamination. Alcohol-based hand rubs are easy to use. **(A)** Apply the recommended amount of product to one of your palms. **(B)** Rub your hands together, covering your hands and fingers (front and back) with the product. Keep rubbing your hands together until your skin is dry.

some things you can do to keep yourself safe while traveling between clients' homes:

- Keep your car in good repair, and always start out with a full tank of fuel.
- Choose the safest route of travel. Avoid driving or walking through unknown areas and alleys.
- Take a defensive driving course.
- Keep an emergency kit in the trunk of your car. Include flares, a blanket, a shovel, food, drinking water, a flashlight and batteries, jumper cables, and a tire jack.
- Be aware of the dangers of driving in ice and snow. When the weather is bad, be prepared with snow tires, a bag of sand or kitty litter (for weight and traction), antifreeze, and windshield washer fluid.
- Always keep your car doors locked and stay alert for strangers who may wish to cause you harm.
- Leave excessive amounts of cash and expensive personal items (such as jewelry or electronics) at home. Do not leave items in plain view on the car seat. Instead, take them with you or put them in the trunk or under the seat before leaving the car. Always lock your car.

- Visit clients who live in unsafe neighborhoods during the day, preferably during the morning hours. Or, speak with the case manager about arranging an escort to help ensure your safety.
- Park your car in a safe, well-lighted area as close to the client's home as possible.
- Choose the safest walking route to reach the home. When walking between your car and the client's home, be aware of other people, strange animals, and your surroundings in general.
- Wear a name badge identifying yourself as a home support worker according to your agency policy. If you are attacked, let the attacker know that you do not carry syringes, needles, or medication.
- Consider taking a self-defense course. If you are attacked, use your bag, arms, and hands to protect your face, neck, and throat. Kick the attacker with your legs. Use your car keys to slash the attacker's face. Scream or yell loudly to attract attention.
- Make sure that someone else (your case manager, a friend, or family member) knows your planned schedule. Follow your schedule and check in with the office frequently.
- Carry a fully charged cell phone with you at all times.

SUMMARY

- Home support workers are responsible for protecting themselves and those in their care from physical harm and infection.
- The home environment poses many safety risks. Home support workers are responsible for noting dangerous situations in the home and reporting their observations to the case manager, and for knowing how to react should an emergency occur.
  - Worn carpets or uneven floors, poor lighting, and clutter increase a person's risk of falling, especially if the person has poor mobility or eyesight.
  - Fire is always a risk in the home.
  - Abuse can take place in the home.
- Infection control is a priority in the home health care setting, just as it is in any other health care setting. The home support worker helps to prevent the spread of infection by maintaining a sanitary environment and using standard precautions.

- Using proper bag technique helps to prevent the spread of microbes from one client's home to another client's home.
- Disinfecting household surfaces, especially those where food is prepared or personal care is given, is essential to maintaining a sanitary environment.
- Handling and storing food properly is important for preventing food poisoning and other illnesses.
- Practicing good personal hygiene, and helping clients to do the same, is an important part of infection control.
- Home support workers must be concerned with keeping themselves safe while traveling between clients' houses. Keeping your car in good repair, being prepared for roadside and weather emergencies, using common sense, and being aware of your surroundings are important safety measures to take when traveling.

WHAT DID YOU LEARN?

Multiple Choice

Select the single best answer for each of the following questions.

1. You have just entered a client's home and are preparing to wash your hands at the kitchen sink, when you notice that there is no soap. How else could you accomplish the task of decontaminating your hands?
   a. Wipe your hands with moisturizing hand lotion and a tissue
   b. Use an alcohol-based hand rub
   c. Run your hands under hot water and dry them with a dishtowel
   d. Skip washing your hands at this time because you have just arrived in the home, and you have not done anything yet

2. Where are laboratory specimens stored for transport?
   a. In the "dirty" section of the nurse's bag
   b. In the "clean" section of the nurse's bag
   c. In the home support worker's uniform pocket
   d. In a cooler on the front seat of the car

3. You have just finished mopping a client's kitchen floor. Where do you dispose of the dirty water?
   a. Out the back door
   b. Down the kitchen sink
   c. Down the toilet
   d. Down the bathroom sink

4. You arrive at a client's home and find the client tied down in bed. The client's daughter tells you that her mother keeps falling out of bed, so she has tied her to the bed for her own protection. What should you do about this situation?
   a. Ignore it. The client's daughter obviously knows what is best for her mother.
   b. Report your observations to the case manager immediately.
   c. Call the police.
   d. Untie the client and tell the daughter that she is guilty of abusing her mother.

5. You are caring for Mrs. DiTomo, who has advanced emphysema. Suddenly, Mr. DiTomo, who also has health problems, complains of chest pain and slumps to the floor. What should you do first?
   a. Call the case manager.
   b. Dial "911" to activate the emergency medical services (EMS) system.
   c. Call the DiTomos' daughter and ask her to come over right away.
   d. Leave for your next assignment. You owe it to your next client to be on time, and caring for Mr. DiTomo is not your responsibility.

6. Which one of the following observations about a client's home should be reported to the client's case manager?
   a. The client has all of the most modern kitchen appliances
   b. The client has newspapers and magazines stacked 3 metres high lining both sides of a hallway
   c. The client has a large collection of dishes, which she stores in a sideboard in the dining room
   d. The client has very poor taste in decorating

CHAPTER 43 Safety and Infection Control in the Home Health Care Setting 813

STOP and Think!

Janis has been assigned a new client, Mrs. Peterson. Mrs. Peterson is a widow who lives alone in a small home on a limited income. She is recovering from a stroke, so her ability to get around independently is limited. Janis is expected to assist Mrs. Peterson with her activities of daily living (ADLs) and to do some light housekeeping. When Janis arrives at Mrs. Peterson's home for her first visit, she notices the garbage cans outside of the house are overflowing, and there are a lot of flies. On entering the kitchen she notices the kitchen sink is full of dirty dishes, there are dirty dishes all over the counter, and there is a strange odour coming from the refrigerator. After Janis finishes helping Mrs. Peterson to bathe and she has cleaned up the bathroom, she starts to wonder what to do about Mrs. Peterson's breakfast. Mrs. Peterson needs breakfast, but the kitchen is too filthy to do any cooking. In addition, Janis only has another half hour before she must leave for her next appointment. If you were Janis, what would you do?

You have been assigned to provide home health care for Mrs. Abrams. Mrs. Abrams is pregnant with her third child and on complete bed rest because of pregnancy-related complications. During your visits, you are assigned to help Mrs. Abrams with personal care, as well as look after her twin 2-year-old boys, Sammy and Alex. When you arrive at the Abrams' home today, you learn that both Sammy and Alex have had diarrhea and have been vomiting since the middle of the previous night, as the result of a virus. You really do not want to take this virus home to your own kids, or get it yourself. Nor do you want Mrs. Abrams to get it, since being sick will only make her more uncomfortable than she already is. And you definitely do not want the client you will be visiting next, Mrs. Jefferson, to get it. Mrs. Jefferson has been receiving chemotherapy as part of her treatment for cancer and as a result, her immune system is weak. What measures will you take to try to contain the virus and prevent anyone else from getting it?

Personal Support Workers Make a Difference!

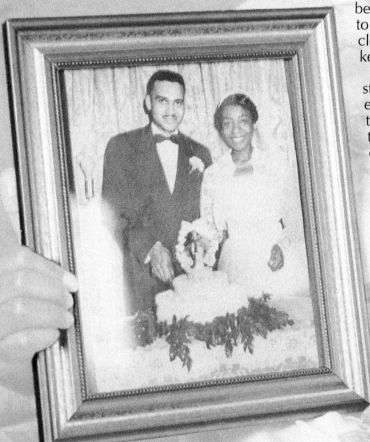

"I'm Sally Richards, and my husband Carl had a severe stroke about 4 months ago. The stroke left him totally paralyzed on his right side and I was afraid that I would have to place him in a nursing home. Carl was a big man, and I just wouldn't have been able to lift him and care for him properly by myself.

The social worker at the hospital suggested that we use the services of a local home health care agency. The agency sent a nurse to our home to evaluate our needs even before Carl came home from the hospital. When we got home, a hospital bed, wheelchair, and specialized bathroom equipment had already been delivered and set up for his arrival. That day, we also met Angie, our home support worker.

The home health nurse explained that in addition to helping with Carl's personal care, Angie would be responsible for handling some housekeeping duties. I must admit that this caused me some concern. I have always taken great pride in making sure that my home was as neat as a pin. I figured that I would have to go back and re-do everything Angie did to my own standards.

Well, that Angie really surprised me! She was always personally clean and neat, and she took great care to avoid bringing germs from other clients' homes into ours. She gave Carl the best care anyone could ask for. And, I hate to admit it, but I think my bathroom was cleaner after she finished with it than I ever kept it!

Carl lived for 3 months after his first stroke. He then had another one that ended his life, but I feel very comforted that I was able to have him at home for those last months. Angie really made a difference in our lives."

You can listen to more stories about how personal support workers make a difference on the CD in the front of your book.

Photo credit: Photodisc Red /Getty Images

Glossary

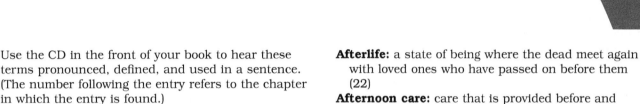

Use the CD in the front of your book to hear these terms pronounced, defined, and used in a sentence. (The number following the entry refers to the chapter in which the entry is found.)

A

Abandonment: the act of withdrawing support or help from another person, in spite of duty or responsibility (42)

Absorption: transfer of nutrients from the digestive tract into the bloodstream (19)

Abuse: intentional act that causes harm to another person (4)

Acceptance: one of the stages of grief; the person comes to terms with the reality of his or her own impending death, and is finally at peace with this knowledge (21)

Acquired immunodeficiency syndrome (AIDS): a disease caused by human immunodeficiency virus (HIV), a bloodborne virus that attacks the body's immune system; death usually results when the body becomes unable to recognize and fight off infections (8)

Activities of daily living (ADLs): routine tasks of daily life, such as bathing, eating, and grooming (17)

Acute illness: an illness with a rapid onset and a relatively short recovery time, usually unexpected (6)

Acute pain: sharp, sudden pain (29)

ADLs: see *activities of daily living*

Admission: official entry of a person into a health care setting (14)

Admission sheet: form that is completed when a person is admitted to a health care setting; gathers standard information about the person such as the person's name, address, date of birth, age, Social Security number, gender, and employment information, emergency notification information, and advance directive information (14)

Advance directive: a document that allows a person to make his wishes regarding health care known to family members and health care workers, in case the time comes when he is no longer able to make those wishes known himself; examples include living wills and durable powers of attorney for health care (21)

Aerobic: an adjective used to describe bacteria that need oxygen in order to live (compare with *anaerobic*) (7)

Afterlife: a state of being where the dead meet again with loved ones who have passed on before them (22)

Afternoon care: care that is provided before and after lunch and dinner (17)

Against medical advice (AMA): term used to describe a person's actions when a person leaves a health care facility without a doctor's order (14)

AIDS: see *acquired immunodeficiency syndrome*

Airborne pathogen: pathogens that can be transmitted through the air (8)

Airborne precautions: used when caring for people infected with pathogens that can be transmitted through the air; include placing the patient or resident in a private room with the door closed, wearing a mask when caring for the person, and minimizing the amount of time the person spends out of his or her private room (7)

Alignment: good posture; the "A" in the ABCs of good body mechanics (9)

Alopecia: baldness, loss of hair (18)

Alveoli (singular, *alveolus*): grape-like clusters of tiny air sacs in the lungs, where gas exchange takes place (26)

Alzheimer's disease: the most common type of dementia; characterized by the permanent and progressive loss of the ability to think and remember caused by damage to the brain (36)

Ambulate: to walk (11)

Amenorrhea: absence of menstrual flow (33)

Amino acids: molecules that are the building blocks of the body's cells; found in proteins (19)

Amputation: the surgical removal of all or part of an extremity (25)

Anaerobic: an adjective used to describe bacteria that can survive without oxygen (compare with *aerobic*) (7)

Anaphylactic shock: shock caused by a serious allergic reaction to a medication, bee sting, or certain foods (12)

Anatomy: the study of what body parts look like, where they are located, how big they are, and how they connect to other body parts (23)

Anemia: a general term for a group of disorders that affect the ability of the red blood cells to carry oxygen to the cells and tissues of the body (27)

Anger: one of the stages of grief; the person realizes that she is actually going to die as a result of her illness and has feelings of rage, which may be directed toward herself or others (21)

Angina pectoris: the classic chest pain that is felt as a result of the heart muscle being deprived of oxygen (27)

Anorexia: loss of appetite (19)

Anorexia nervosa: an eating disorder characterized by an intense fear of gaining weight or becoming obese; people with this disorder cannot maintain a healthy body weight because they engage in activities such as extreme dieting, excessive exercising, or both (35)

Antepartum (prenatal) period: the period of time from conception until the baby is born (40)

Antibodies: specialized proteins produced by the immune system that help our bodies to fight off specific microbes, preventing infection (7)

Antiperspirant: a grooming product that contains ingredients to stop or slow the production of sweat (17)

Antisepsis: practices that kill microbes or stop them from growing; one of the techniques of medical asepsis (compare with *sanitization, disinfection,* and *sterilization*) (7)

Anuria: the state of voiding less than 100 mL of urine over the course of 24 hours (20)

Anxiety: feeling of uneasiness, dread, apprehension, or worry (35)

Aphasia: a general term for a group of disorders that affect a person's ability to communicate with others; may be expressive (an inability to form words) or receptive (an inability to understand words); often occurs following a stroke (28)

Appetite: the desire for food (compare with *anorexia*) (19)

Arteries: vessels that carry blood away from the heart (27)

Arterioles: the smallest arteries (27)

Arteriosclerosis: "hardening of the arteries"; occurs when atherosclerotic plaque interferes with the elasticity of the arterial walls, making them brittle and prone to breaking (27)

Arthritis: inflammation of joints, usually associated with pain and stiffness (25)

Aspiration: the accidental inhalation of foreign material (such as food, liquids, vomitus) into the airway (12)

Assault: threatening or attempting to touch a person without the person's consent (4)

Assisted-living facility: type of long-term care facility that provides residents with limited assistance with tasks such as medication administration, transportation, meals, and housekeeping (1)

Assistive devices: devices that make certain tasks (such as walking, eating, or dressing) easier for a person with a disability (23)

Asthma: a condition that affects the bronchi and bronchioles of the lungs; triggers (such as cold weather, allergies, respiratory infections, stress, smoke, and exercise) cause the bronchi and bronchioles to become narrower, making breathing difficult (26)

Astigmatism: an inability to focus images properly because the cornea of the eye is not perfectly curved (29)

Atelectasis: collapse of the alveoli of the lungs; a common respiratory complication following surgery (39)

Atherosclerosis: blocking of the arteries, caused by the build up of fatty deposits called plaque on the inside of the vessel wall (27)

Atria (singular, *atrium*): the upper chambers of the heart (27)

Atrophy: the loss of muscle size and strength (25)

Attitude: the side of ourselves that we display to the world, communicating outwardly how we feel about things (3)

Autism: a developmental disability characterized by extreme difficulty communicating and relating to other people and surroundings (34)

Autonomy: an ethical principle that requires health care workers to respect a person's rights and personal preferences (4)

Autopsy: examination of a person's organs and tissues after the person has died, done to confirm or identify the cause of the person's death (22)

Axon: a long extension from the body of a neuron that *sends* information to other neurons (compare with *dendrites*) (28)

B

Bag technique: an infection control procedure used in the home health care setting to keep the nurse's bag free from contamination (43)

Balance: stability produced by the even distribution of weight; the "B" in the ABCs of good body mechanics (9)

Bargaining: one of the stages of grief; the person wants to "make a deal" with someone he or she feels has control over his or her fate, such as God or a health care provider (21)

Barium: a substance that coats the mucosa of the digestive tract, making the organs appear sharper and brighter on radiologic studies (x-rays) (31)

Basic life support (BLS): basic emergency care techniques, such as rescue breathing and cardiopulmonary resuscitation (CPR) (12)

Bath blanket: a lightweight cotton blanket used to cover a person during a bed bath or linen change to help provide modesty and warmth (15)

Battery: touching a person without his or her consent (4)

Bed board: a piece of wood that is placed under the mattress to provide extra support; helps to keep the person's body properly aligned by preventing the mattress from sagging (15)

Bed cradle: a metal frame that is placed between the bottom and top sheets to keep the top sheet, the blanket, and the bedspread away from the person's feet; used when pressure on the person's feet could result in pain or skin breakdown (15)

Bedpan: a device used for elimination when a person is unable to get out of bed; women use a bedpan for both urination and bowel movements; men use a bedpan for bowel movements only (20)

Bed protector: a square of quilted absorbent fabric backed with waterproof material that measures approximately 91 cm × 91 cm; used to prevent soiling of the bottom linens; sometimes called an *incontinence pad* or a *soaker pad* (15)

Bedside commode: a device used for elimination when a person is able to get out of bed, but unable to walk to the bathroom; it consists of a chair-like frame with a toilet seat and a removable collection bucket (20)

Bell: the small, rounded surface on a stethoscope that is used to pick up faint sounds; commonly used to listen to the apical pulse in infants and small children (16)

Beneficence: an ethical principle that requires health care workers to do good for those in their care by preventing harm and promoting the health and welfare of the person above all else (4)

Benign: adjective used to describe a noncancerous tumour (that is, a tumour that does not progress or invade other tissues) (compare with *malignant*) (37)

Bile: a substance produced by the liver that helps with the digestion of fats (31)

Biological death: occurs when the tissues of the brain and heart die from lack of oxygen; biological death is not reversible (compare with *clinical death*) (12)

Biopsy: a diagnostic procedure that involves obtaining a tissue sample and examining it under a microscope for cancerous cells (37)

Bipolar disorder (manic depression): a mental health disorder characterized by mood swings; people with this disorder experience excessively "high" or happy periods, followed by excessively "low" or depressed periods (35)

Bisexual: a person who is sexually attracted to members of both sexes (6)

Bloodborne pathogen: a disease-producing microbe that is transmitted to another person through blood or other body fluids (8)

Blood pressure: the force that the blood exerts against the arterial walls; one of the vital signs (16)

BLS: see *basic life support*

Body alignment: positioning of the body so that the spine is not twisted or crooked (11)

Body fluids: liquid or semi-liquid substances produced by the body, such as blood, urine, feces, vomitus, saliva, drainage from wounds, sweat, semen, vaginal secretions, tears, cerebrospinal fluid, amniotic fluid, and breast milk (8)

Body mechanics: the efficient and safe use of the body (9)

Body temperature: how hot the body is; one of the vital signs (16)

Bonding period: the first hour or two immediately following delivery of a baby, during which emotional and physical attachments between the parents and the infant develop (40)

Bony prominences: parts of the body where there is very little fat between the bone and the skin, such as the ankles, heels, hips, and elbows (24)

Bradycardia: a heart rate that is slower than normal (less than 60 beats/min in an adult) (16)

Bradypnea: a respiratory rate that is lower than normal (less than 10 breaths/min in an adult) (16)

Braille: a system that uses letters made from combinations of raised dots that allows a blind person to read (29)

Bronchi (singular, *bronchus*): passageways that carry air from the trachea ("windpipe") to the lungs, one bronchus goes to the right lung and the other goes to the left (26)

Bronchioles: the smallest branches of the bronchi (26)

Bronchitis: inflammation of the bronchi (26)

Bulimia nervosa: an eating disorder characterized by an intense fear of gaining weight or becoming obese; people with this disorder cannot maintain a healthy body weight because they engage in activities such as binging (eating large amounts of food in one sitting) and purging (vomiting the food back up) (35)

C

Call light system: a system that allows a patient or resident to call for help; usually consists of a call light control, a light in the hall, and a panel of lights at the nurses' station or some other central location (13)

Calories: the unit of measure used to describe the energy content of food (19)

Canada Health Act: federal legislation that outlines the types of health care services that are insured; includes five principles that each province and territory must adhere to in order to qualify for federal subsidy (1)

Canada Privacy Act: this law, which took effect in 1983, protects the privacy rights of Canadians by establishing ground rules for how organizations may use, collect, or disclose personal information (4)

Canadian Centre for Occupational Health and Safety (CCOHS): a Canadian federal government agency that serves to support the vision of eliminating all Canadian work-related illnesses and injuries (8)

Canadian Human Rights Law: states that it is against the law for an employer to ask a candidate questions related to these subjects at any time during the hiring process (3)

Capillary bed: the network of tiny vessels in the tissues where the oxygen and nutrients in the blood pass into the tissues, and carbon dioxide and other waste materials from the tissues pass into the blood (27)

Cardiac arrest: the condition that is said to occur when the heart stops beating (12)

Cardiac cycle: the pumping action of the heart in an organized pattern (all of the events associated with one heart beat) (27)

Cardiac rehabilitation: therapy that helps a person regain strength and adopt habits that will help the cardiovascular system become healthier (27)

Cardiogenic shock: shock that occurs when the heart is unable to pump enough blood throughout the body to meet the tissues' need for oxygen (12)

Cardiopulmonary resuscitation (CPR): a technique used to sustain breathing and circulation for a person who has gone into respiratory or cardiac arrest (12)

Care plan: a specific plan of care for each patient or resident developed by the nursing team (5)

Carrier: a person who is infected with a virus but never develops symptoms of the disease; the virus lives in the person's body and can be transmitted to another person (8)

Cartilage: a tough, fibrous substance found in joints and other parts of the body; in slightly movable joints, the cartilage acts as a "shock absorber"; in freely movable joints, the cartilage provides a smooth surface for the bones of the joint to move against (25)

Case manager: in the home health care setting, the member of the health care team who is responsible for overseeing the client's total care, from admission through discharge (42)

Cataract: the gradual yellowing and hardening of the lens of the eye (29)

Catastrophic reaction: an extreme reaction to a situation that would normally cause minimal or no stress; often seen in people with dementia (36)

Catheter: a tube that is inserted into the body for the purpose of administering or removing fluids (20)

Catheter care: thorough cleaning of the perineal area (especially around the urethra) and the catheter tubing that extends outside of the body, to prevent infection (20)

CCOHS Bloodborne Pathogens Standard: standards created by the Canadian Centre for Occupational Health and Safety that all employers must follow to ensure the safety of workers against bloodborne pathogens (8)

Cell: the basic unit of life (23)

Cell membrane: a membrane that surrounds the cytoplasm and gives the cell its shape (23)

Central nervous system (CNS): the brain and spinal cord; responsible for receiving information, processing it, and issuing instructions (compare with *peripheral nervous system*) (28)

Cerebral palsy: a developmental disability caused by damage to the cerebrum, the part of the brain involved with motor control (34)

Cerebrospinal fluid (CSF): a clear fluid that circulates around the brain and spinal cord and acts as a "shock absorber" to protect these structures (28)

Cerumen: a waxy substance that helps to protect the external auditory canal by trapping dirt and other particles; commonly referred to as "ear wax" (29)

Cesarean section: delivery of a baby through a surgical incision made in the mother's abdomen (40)

Chain of infection: the six key conditions that must be met for a person to get a communicable infection (pathogen, reservoir, portal of exit, method of transmission, portal of entry, and susceptible host) (7)

Chain of survival: the series of events that must take place in an emergency situation to increase the person's ability to survive the emergency without any permanent damage (12)

Charge nurse: a registered nurse (RN/RPN registered psychiatric nurse) or licensed practical nurse (LPN) who supervises the other nurses for a particular shift (2)

Chemical digestion: the process of breaking down food through the use of chemical substances such as enzymes (compare with *mechanical digestion*) (31)

Chemical restraint: any medication that alters a person's mood or behaviour, such as a sedative or tranquilizer (compare with *physical restraint*) (10)

Chemotherapy: the use of medications to destroy malignant cancer cells (37)

Cheyne-Stokes respiration: very irregular, shallow breaths, in an alternating fast–slow pattern; often seen in people who are dying (22)

Chronic bronchitis: a disorder caused by long-term irritation of the bronchi and bronchioles, such as that caused by inhaling tobacco smoke; one of two forms of chronic obstructive pulmonary disease (COPD) (26)

Chronic illness: an illness that is ongoing and often needs to be controlled through continuous medication or treatment (6)

Chronic obstructive pulmonary disease (COPD): a general term used to describe two related lung disorders, emphysema and chronic bronchitis; the leading cause of COPD is smoking (26)

Chronic pain: slow, diffuse, constant pain (29)

Chyme: the liquid substance produced by the digestion of food in the stomach (20)

Circulation: the continuous movement of the blood through the blood vessels; powered by the pumping action of the heart (27)

Circumcision: a procedure involving the removal of the foreskin, the fold of loose skin that covers the head of the penis; often performed on male infants for religious or cultural reasons (17)

Civil laws: laws concerned with relationships between individuals (4)

Client: a person who is receiving the services of a home health care agency (1)

Clinical death: the state of not having a pulse or breathing; can sometimes be reversed with prompt emergency treatment that restarts the heart and breathing (compare with *biological death*) (12)

Closed bed: an empty, made bed (15)

CNS: see *central nervous system*

Coagulation: clotting of the blood (27)

Coitus: sexual intercourse (6)

Collagen: a protein that supports connective tissue, such as that found in the dermis; loss of collagen contributes to the formation of wrinkles (24)

Colonies: groups of bacteria (7)

Colostomy: an alternate way of eliminating feces from the body; done when only part of the large intestine must be removed due to disease; after removing the diseased part of a person's large intestine, an artificial opening, called a stoma, is made in the abdominal wall and the remaining portion of the large intestine is connected to it (compare with *ileostomy*) (31)

Colostrum: a thin yellowish fluid that contains extra calories and proteins as well as antibodies and is produced by the mother's breasts immediately following delivery of the baby; after 2 to 3 days, colostrum is replaced by breast milk (40)

Comatose: the state of being in a coma, a state of unconsciousness from which a person cannot be aroused (10)

Communicable disease: a disease that can be spread from one person to another (7)

Communication: the exchange of information (5)

Competency evaluation: an examination consisting of a written portion and a skills portion that must be passed at the end of the personal support worker training course to obtain certification (2)

Conception (fertilization): occurs when the male and female sex cells join, forming a cell that contains the complete number of chromosomes (33)

Condom catheter: a device used to manage urinary incontinence in men; it consists of a soft plastic or rubber sheath, tubing, and a collection bag for the urine (20)

Conduction disorders: conditions that affect the pathway that the heart uses to transmit the electrical impulses that cause contraction (27)

Conductive hearing loss: hearing loss that results when something prevents sound waves from reaching the receptors in the cochlea of the ear (compare with *sensorineural hearing loss*) (29)

Confidentiality: keeping personal information that someone shares with you to yourself (4)

Conflict: discord resulting from differences between people; can occur when one person is unable to understand or accept another's ideas or beliefs (5)

Congenital: adjective used to describe a disorder that a person is born with (34)

Conjunctivitis ("pink eye"): infection and inflammation of the conjunctiva, a clear membrane that lines the inside of the eyelids and covers most of the surface of the eye; characterized by redness, swelling, itching, burning, and excessive tearing (29)

Constipation: a condition that occurs when the feces remain in the intestines for too long, resulting in hard, dry feces that are difficult to pass (20)

Contact precautions: used when caring for people infected with pathogens that can be transmitted directly (by touching the person), or indirectly (by touching fomites); include using barrier methods whenever contact with the infected person or items contaminated with wound drainage or body substances is necessary (7)

Contaminated: adjective used to describe an object that is soiled by pathogens (7)

Contractures: a condition that occurs when a joint is held in the same position for too long a time; the tendons shorten and become stiff, possibly causing permanent loss of motion in the joint (11)

Coordinated body movement: using the weight of the body to help with movement; the "C" in the ABCs of good body mechanics (9)

COPD: see *chronic obstructive pulmonary disease*

Coping mechanisms: conscious and deliberate ways of dealing with stress (compare with *defense mechanisms*) (35)

Coronary artery disease: a disorder that occurs when the arteries that supply the heart (the coronary arteries) narrow as a result of atherosclerosis, preventing adequate blood flow to the heart muscle (27)

CPR: see *cardiopulmonary resuscitation*

Cradle cap: see *seborrheic dermatitis*

Criminal laws: laws concerned with the relationship between the individual and society (4)

CSF: see *cerebrospinal fluid*

Culture: the beliefs (including religious or spiritual beliefs), values, and traditions that are customary to a group of people; a view of the world that is handed down from generation to generation (6)

Cuticle: the skin along the edges of the nail (18)

Cyanosis: blue or grey discolouration of the skin, lips, and nail beds; develops when the skin does not receive enough oxygen and is a sign of a respiratory or circulatory disorder (24)

Cyanotic: adjective used to describe skin, lips, or nail beds that have a blue or grey tinge (22)

Cystitis: infection of the bladder (32)

Cytoplasm: the jelly-like substance within a cell within which the organelles float (23)

D

Dandruff: excessive itching and flaking of the scalp (18)

Defamation: the act of making untrue statements that hurt another person's reputation (4)

Defecate: to have a bowel movement (20)

Defense mechanisms: unconscious ways of dealing with stress (compare with *coping mechanisms*) (35)

Definitive surgery: surgery that is done when the person's medical problem is known and the best way to address it is through surgery (39)

Dehydration: too little fluid in the tissues of the body (compare with *edema*) (19)

Delegate: to authorize another person to perform a task on your behalf (2)

Delirium: a temporary state of confusion (36)

Delusions: false ideas or beliefs, especially about oneself (35)

Dementia: the permanent and progressive loss of the ability to think and remember (36)

Dendrites: short extensions from the body of a neuron that *receive* information from other neurons (compare with *axon*) (28)

Denial: one of the stages of grief; the person refuses to accept the diagnosis or feels that a mistake has been made (21)

Dental caries: dental cavities or tooth decay, caused by poor oral hygiene (17)

Deodorant: a grooming product that covers or masks odour (17)

Depression: *(1)* an alteration in a person's mood that causes him or her to lose pleasure or interest in all usually pleasurable activities such as eating, working, or socializing; a feeling of hopelessness (35); *(2)* one of the stages of grief; the person fully realizes that death will be the end result of the illness and experiences sadness and regret (21)

Dermatitis: a general term for inflammation of the skin (24)

Dermis: the deepest layer of skin, where sensory receptors, blood vessels, nerves, glands, and hair follicles are found (24)

Depth of respiration: the quality of each breath (16)

Development: changes that occur psychologically or socially as a person passes through life (6)

Developmental disability: a permanent disability that affects a person before he or she reaches adulthood (that is, before 18 to 22 years of age) and interferes with the person's ability to achieve developmental milestones (34)

Diabetes mellitus: an endocrine disorder that results when the pancreas is unable to produce enough insulin (30)

Diabetic retinopathy: a complication of diabetes that can lead to blindness (29)

Dialysis: a procedure that is done to remove waste products and fluids from the body when a person's kidneys fail and can no longer perform this task (32)

Diaphoretic: adjective used to describe a person who has a medical condition that causes him to sweat a great deal (17)

Diaphragm: *(1)* the large flat surface of the stethoscope that is used to hear loud, harsh sounds (16); *(2)* the strong, dome-shaped muscle that separates the chest cavity from the abdominal cavity and assists in breathing (26)

Diarrhea: the passage of liquid, unformed stool (20)

Diastole: the resting phase of the cardiac cycle; during which the myocardium relaxes, allowing the chambers to fill with blood (compare with *systole*) (27)

Diastolic pressure: the pressure that the blood exerts against the arterial walls when the heart muscle relaxes; the second blood pressure measurement that is recorded (compare with *systolic pressure*) (16)

Dietitian: a person who has a degree in nutrition (19)

Digestion: the process of breaking food down into simple elements (nutrients) (19)

Digital examination: examination that is done when a person is thought to have a fecal impaction; a finger is inserted into the person's rectum to feel for the impacted mass (20)

Director of nursing (DON): the registered nurse who directs all of the nursing care within a facility (2)

Disability: impaired physical or emotional function (23)

Disaster: a sudden, unexpected event that causes injury to many people, major damage to property, or both (9)

Discharge: the official release of a patient or a resident from a health care facility to his or her home (14)

Discharge planning: the process used by the members of the health care team to help prepare a patient or resident to leave the facility; helps to make sure that the person continues to receive quality care, either from a home health care agency or from family members, after the discharge (14)

Disease: a condition that occurs when the structure or function of an organ or an organ system is abnormal (23)

Disinfection: the use of strong chemicals to kill pathogens on non-living objects that come in contact with body fluids or substances, such as bedpans, urinals, and over-bed tables; one of the techniques of medical asepsis (compare with *antisepsis, sanitization,* and *sterilization*) (7)

Disoriented: the state of being unable to answer basic questions about person, place, or time; a state of confusion (compare with *oriented to person, place, and time*) (12)

Diuresis: excessive urine output of urine; also called *polyuria* (20)

DNR: see *do not resuscitate order*

Do not resuscitate (DNR) order: an order written on a person's chart specifying the person's wishes that the usual efforts to save his life will not be made; also called a *no code order* (21)

Down syndrome: a developmental disability that is the result of having 47 chromosomes instead of 46; people with this disorder have mental retardation and certain key physical features, such as almond-shaped eyes and square hands with short, stubby fingers (34)

Draw sheet: a small, flat sheet that is placed over the middle of the bottom sheet, covering the area of the bed from above the person's shoulders to below his or her buttocks; see also *lift sheet* (15)

Droplet precautions: used when caring for people infected with pathogens that can be transmitted by direct exposure to droplets released from the mouth or nose (for example, when the person coughs, sneezes, or talks) (7)

Durable power of attorney for health care: a type of advance directive that transfers the responsibility for handling a person's affairs and making medical decisions to a family member, friend, or other trusted individual, in the event that the person is no longer able to make these decisions on his or her own behalf (21)

Dysmenorrhea: painful menstruation (33)

Dyspnea: laboured or difficult breathing (16)

Dysrhythmia: an irregular pulse rhythm (16)

Dysuria: painful or difficult urination (20)

E

Early morning care: care provided after a person wakes up to prepare him or her for breakfast or early testing or treatment (17)

Eczema: a type of chronic dermatitis that is usually accompanied by severe itching, scaling, and crusting of the surface of the skin (24)

Edema: too much fluid in the tissues of the body (compare with *dehydration*) (19)

Edentulous: without teeth (17)

Egg (ovum, ova): female sex cell (33)

Egocentric: an adjective used to describe someone who places himself at the center of the world and often overestimates his importance to others; a common character trait during adolescence (41)

Ejaculation: the forceful release of semen from the body; method by which sperm cells leave the man's body through the penis (33)

Elder abuse: physical, emotional, or sexual abuse of an older person (4)

Elective: adjective used to describe a surgical procedure that is planned for and scheduled ahead of time (39)

Embolus: a blood clot in a vessel that breaks off and moves from one place to another (27)

Emergency: a condition that requires immediate medical or surgical evaluation or treatment to prevent the person from dying or having a permanent disability (12)

Emergency medical services (EMS) system: a network of resources (including people, equipment, and facilities) that is organized to respond to an emergency (12)

Emergent: adjective used to describe surgery that must be performed immediately to prevent the person from dying or becoming disabled (39)

Empathy: the ability to imagine what it would feel like to be in another person's situation (3)

Emphysema: a disorder caused by long-term exposure of the alveoli to toxins, such as tobacco smoke; one of two forms of chronic obstructive pulmonary disease (COPD) (26)

EMS system: see *emergency medical services system*

Endocardium: the smooth inner lining of the heart wall (27)

Endotracheal tube: a device that is inserted into a person's nose or mouth and extends to the trachea; used when a person must receive mechanical ventilation for a short time (26)

Enema: the introduction of fluid into the large intestine by way of the anus for the purpose of removing stool from the rectum (20)

Enteral nutrition: placing food directly into a person's stomach or intestines, using a nasogastric tube, nasointestinal tube, gastrostomy tube, jejunostomy tube, or percutaneous endoscopic gastrostomy (PEG) tube (19)

Enzymes: substances that have the ability to break chemical bonds (31)

Epicardium: the smooth outermost layer of the heart wall (27)

Epidermis: the outer layer of the skin (24)

Epidural block: anesthesia given through a catheter that is placed in the spinal canal (40)

Epilepsy: a disorder characterized by chronic seizure activity (28)

Episiotomy: an incision made in the perineum to enlarge the vaginal opening, making delivery of the baby's head easier (40)

Erythema: redness of the skin (24)

Erythrocytes: red blood cells; responsible for carrying oxygen to all of the tissues of the body (27)

Esophageal (cardiac) sphincter: a circle of muscular tissue that surrounds the place where the esophagus enters the stomach and keeps food from going back up the esophagus after it has entered the stomach (31)

Esophagus: a long narrow tube that serves mainly as a passageway for food to get from the pharynx to the stomach (31)

Ethics: moral principles or standards that govern conduct (4)

Eupnea: a normal respiratory rate (16)

Evening (hour of sleep, hs) care: care provided in preparation for sleep (17)

Excoriation: an abrasion, or a scraping away of the surface of the skin; can be caused by trauma, chemicals, or burns (24)

Exhalation (expiration): the phase of respiration during which carbon dioxide is transported out of the lungs [compare with *inhalation (inspiration)*] (16)

Exploratory surgery: surgery that is performed when a person has a significant medical problem but the doctors do not know exactly how bad the problem is or exactly what is causing it (39)

Exposure control plan: a plan that states what actions must be taken if an employee is exposed to blood or other body fluids while on the job (8)

F

Facemask: a device used for delivering oxygen that is made of soft, moulded plastic material that fits over the nose and mouth (26)

Failure to thrive: failure of an infant to grow and develop both physically and emotionally, as a result of not being held and talked to (41)

False imprisonment: confining another person against his or her will (4)

Fanfolded: adjective used to describe the top sheet, blanket, and bedspread of a closed bed when they have been turned back (toward the foot of the bed) (15)

Fat-soluble: adjective used to describe a substance that dissolves in fat (for example, certain vitamins) (19)

Febrile: adjective used to describe the state of having a fever, or increased body temperature (16)

Fecal impaction: a condition that occurs when constipation is not relieved (20)

Fecal (bowel) incontinence: the inability to hold one's feces, or the involuntary loss of feces from the bowel (20)

Feces: the semi-solid waste product of digestion; stool (20)

Fetal alcohol syndrome: a combination of physical and mental problems that affect children whose mothers consumed alcohol during pregnancy (34)

Fibre supplement: a tablet or drink additive that is used to add bulk to the feces, causing them to hold fluid, and preventing constipation (20)

Fidelity: an ethical principle that requires health care workers to act with integrity to earn others' trust (4)

Filtrate: the liquid that forms the basis for urine (32)

First aid: the care given to an injured or sick person while waiting for more advanced help to arrive (12)

Fissure: a crack in the skin (24)

Five rights of delegation: a set of guidelines that help nurses to make good decisions about which tasks to delegate and to whom (2)

Fixation: the process of holding a broken bone in one position until the fracture heals; may be *external* (accomplished through the use of a cast) or *internal* (accomplished through the use of metal plates, screws, rods, pins, or wires attached to the bone) (25)

Flatulence: the presence of excessive amounts of flatus (gas) in the intestines, causing abdominal distension (swelling) and discomfort (20)

Flatus: gas that is formed as part of the digestion process (20)

Flow metre: a device used to set the rate at which oxygen is delivered to a patient or resident who is receiving oxygen therapy (26)

Fluid balance: a state where the amount of fluid taken into the body equals the amount of fluid that leaves the body (19)

Flushing: redness of the skin (24)

Fomite: a non-living object that has been contaminated (soiled) by pathogens (7)

Footboard: a padded board that is placed upright at the foot of the bed; used to keep the person's feet in proper alignment (15)

Foreskin: the fold of loose skin that covers the head of the penis (17)

Fowler's position: one of the basic positions in which the head of the bed is elevated to between 45 and 60 degrees; variations include *semi-Fowler's (low Fowler's) position* and *high Fowler's position* (11)

Fracture: a broken bone (25)

Fracture pan: a wedge-shaped bedpan that is used when a person has an injury or disability that makes it too uncomfortable or dangerous to use a regular bedpan (20)

Fragile X syndrome: an inherited type of mental retardation caused by a defect in the X chromosome (34)

Fraud: deception that could cause harm to another person (4)

Frequency: the term used to describe voiding that occurs more often than usual (20)

Friction: a term used to describe the force created when two surfaces (such as a sheet and a person's skin) rub against each other; can lead to skin breakdown (11)

Functional (modular) nursing: a model for organizing the health care team's efforts in which each member of the health care team carries out the same assigned task for all patients or residents (compare with *primary nursing* and *team nursing*) (2)

G

Gallbladder: a small pouch-like organ that is attached to the liver; it stores bile produced by the liver that is not secreted directly into the duodenum (31)

Gas exchange: the transfer of oxygen into the blood, and carbon dioxide out of it (26)

Gastrostomy tube: a tube used for enteral nutrition that is inserted into the stomach through a surgical incision in the abdomen (19)

Gatches: the joints at the hips and knees of the mattresses of most adjustable beds that allow the mattress to "break" so that the person's head can be elevated or his knees bent (13)

General anesthesia: a loss of consciousness brought on by the administration of a combination of inhaled and injected drugs (compare with *local anesthesia* and *regional anesthesia*) (39)

General lighting: lighting that supplies overall illumination (light), allowing a person to see and move about safely (compare with *task lighting*) (13)

Gingivitis: inflammation of the gums (17)

Glaucoma: a disorder of the eye that occurs when the pressure within the eye is increased to dangerous levels (29)

Glomerulus: part of the nephron, the functional unit of the kidney where blood is filtered to form urine (32)

Glucose: the body's most basic type of fuel; supplied by carbohydrates and sometimes referred to as "blood sugar" (19)

Goals: descriptions of what interventions (care actions that are taken to help a patient or resident) are meant to achieve (5)

Goitre: enlargement of the thyroid gland (30)

Graduate: a measuring device used to measure fluids (19)

Grand mal seizure: a seizure characterized by generalized and violent contraction and relaxation of the body's muscles [compare with *petit mal (absence) seizure*] (12)

Grief: mental anguish, specifically associated with loss (21)

Grooming: activities related to maintaining a neat and attractive appearance, such as shampooing and styling the hair, shaving, and applying makeup (18)

Grounded: an adjective used to describe electrical equipment that has a way of returning stray electrical current to the outlet so that the risk of electrical shock is reduced (9)

Growth: changes that occur physically as a person passes through life (6)

H

Halitosis: bad breath that does not go away (17)

Hallucinations: episodes when a person sees, feels, hears, or tastes something that does not really exist (35)

Hangnails: broken pieces of cuticle (18)

HAV: see *hepatitis A virus*

HBV: see *hepatitis B virus*

HCV: see *hepatitis C virus*

HDV: see *hepatitis D virus*

Head nurse: a registered nurse (RN), or a registered psychiatric nurse (RPN), who is in charge of a department or section (2)

Health Canada: the federal department responsible for the development of policies and programs to ensure the health and wellness of the Canadian population (1)

Health care–associated infections (HAIs): infections that patients or residents get while receiving treatment in a hospital or other health care facility, or that health care workers get while performing their duties within a health care setting (7)

Health care team: group of people with different types of knowledge and skill levels who work together to provide holistic care to the patient or resident (1)

Heart failure: a condition that occurs when the heart is unable to pump enough blood to meet the body's needs (27)

Heimlich manoeuver: abdominal thrusts; used to clear an obstructed airway in an adult or a child older than 1 year who is choking (12)

Hematuria: blood in the urine (20)

Hemiplegia: paralysis on one side of the body (compare with *paraplegia* and *quadriplegia*) (10)

Hemoglobin: a protein found in red blood cells that combines with oxygen to carry it to the tissues of the body (27)

Hemoptysis: the coughing up of blood or blood-stained sputum (26)

Hemorrhage: severe bleeding (12)

Hemorrhagic shock: shock that results from massive blood loss (12)

Hemostasis: the process of stopping blood loss from the circulatory system (27)

Hemothorax: a condition that occurs when blood builds up in the space between the lungs and the chest wall (26)

Hepatitis: inflammation of the liver (8)

Hepatitis A virus (HAV): a virus that is transmitted through the oral–fecal route and causes a form of acute hepatitis (8)

Hepatitis B virus (HBV): a bloodborne virus that causes a form of hepatitis that is acute in most people but may become chronic; a serious health threat for the health care worker (8)

Hepatitis C virus (HCV): a bloodborne virus that causes a form of chronic hepatitis that can eventually lead to end-stage cirrhosis (a fatal liver disease), liver failure, or liver cancer (8)

Hepatitis D virus (HDV): a bloodborne virus that is found only in people who are already infected with hepatitis B virus (HBV)

Hepatitis E virus (HEV): a virus that is transmitted through the oral–fecal route and causes a form of hepatitis (8)

Hernia: a disorder that occurs when an internal organ bulges through a weakness in the muscular wall of the abdominal cavity (31)

Heterosexual: a person who is sexually attracted to members of the opposite sex (6)

HEV: see *hepatitis E virus*

High Fowler's position: one of the basic positions in which the head of the bed is elevated to between 60 and 90 degrees (11)

HIV: see *human immunodeficiency virus*

HIV-positive: the state of being infected with human immunodeficiency virus (HIV) (38)

Holistic care: an adjective used to describe care of the whole person, physically and emotionally (1)

Homebound: adjective used to describe a person who cannot leave the house without a lot of help from another person (42)

Home health care agency: an agency that provides skilled care in a person's home (1)

Homeostasis: a state of balance (23)

Home support worker: personal support worker who provides skilled care in the home (42)

Homosexual: a person who is attracted to members of the same sex (6)

Hormones: chemicals that act on cells to produce a response (30)

Hospice organization: a health care organization that provides care for people who are dying, and their families (1)

Hospital: a health care facility that provides treatment for people with acute medical or surgical conditions (1)

Human immunodeficiency virus (HIV): a virus transmitted in blood and other body fluids (such as semen) that targets the T cells of the immune system; most people infected with HIV go on to develop acquired immunodeficiency syndrome (AIDS), a fatal illness (8)

Human resources (HR) department (personnel): the department within an organization that is concerned with matters related to employees; often responsible for hiring new employees (3)

Hydrocephalus: a condition that results from the build up of cerebrospinal fluid (CSF); sometimes called "water on the brain" (34)

Hygiene: personal cleanliness (3)

Hyperalimentation: see *total parenteral nutrition*

Hyperglycemia: a state of having too much glucose in the bloodstream (30)

Hyperopia: farsightedness; trouble seeing objects that are close (compare with *myopia*) (29)

Hypertension: high blood pressure; a blood pressure that is consistently greater than 140 mm Hg (systolic) and/or 90 mm Hg (diastolic) (16)

Hyperthyroidism (Graves disease): a condition caused by the excessive secretion of thyroxine, one of the thyroid hormones; characterized by increased hunger accompanied by weight loss, an irregular heartbeat, an inability to sleep, irritability, confusion, increased perspiration, and intolerance to heat (30)

Hyperventilation: increased rate and depth of breathing (16)

Hypoglycemia: a dangerous drop in blood glucose levels (30)

Hypotension: low blood pressure; a blood pressure that is consistently lower than 90 mm Hg (systolic) and/or 60 mm Hg (diastolic) (16)

Hypothyroidism: a condition caused by the low secretion of thyroxine, one of the thyroid hormones; characterized by fatigue, weakness, depression, anorexia, weight gain, constipation, and intolerance to cold (30)

Hypoventilation: decreased rate and depth of breathing (16)

Hypoxic: the state of being deficient of oxygen (26)

Hysterectomy: surgical removal of the uterus (33)

I

Ileostomy: an alternative way of eliminating feces from the body; done when the entire large intestine must be removed due to disease; after removing the person's diseased large intestine, an artificial opening, called a stoma, is made in the abdominal wall and the end of the small intestine is connected to it (compare with *colostomy*) (31)

Impotence (erectile dysfunction): the inability to achieve or maintain an erection long enough to engage in sexual activity (33)

Incident (occurrence) report: a preprinted document that is completed following an accident involving a patient or resident (10)

Indwelling catheter: a urinary catheter that is left inside the bladder to provide continuous urine drainage; also known as a retention catheter or a Foley catheter (20)

Infection: disease caused by pathogenic microbes (7)

Infection control: basic practices designed to decrease the chance that an infection will spread from one person to another in a health care facility (7)

Infertility: the inability to become pregnant or to carry a pregnancy to full term (33)

Influenza: an acute respiratory infection caused by the influenza virus; characterized by a sore throat, dry cough, stuffy nose, headache, body aches, weakness, and fever; commonly known as "the flu" (26)

Informed consent: permission granted by a patient or resident to begin treatment or perform a procedure after receiving a full explanation of the treatment or procedure from the health care provider (4)

Ingestion: the intake of food or fluids (19)

Inhalation (inspiration): the phase of respiration during which oxygen is taken into the lungs [compare with *exhalation (expiration)*] (16)

Intake and output (I&O) flow sheet: a document used for recording measurements of all of the fluids that enter and leave the body (19)

Intentional tort: a violation of civil law committed by a person with the intent to do harm (4)

Intentional wound: a wound that is the result of a planned surgical or medical intervention (compare with *unintentional wound*) (24)

Interventions: actions that are taken by the care team to help the patient or resident (5)

Interview: a meeting between an employer and a potential employee, during which information is exchanged regarding the organization, the job, and the potential employee's qualifications for the job (3)

Intimacy: a feeling of emotional closeness to another human being (6)

Intra-operative phase: one of three phases of care for a person who is having surgery; the phase during which the surgery is actually performed (compare with *pre-operative phase* and *post-operative phase*) (39)

Intravenous (IV) therapy: an alternative method of providing fluids and nutrition; fluids are given through a small catheter (tube) that is inserted into a vein (usually in the back of the hand) (19)

Invasion of privacy: the act of violating another person's right to keep certain information and aspects of himself away from the examination of others (4)

Ischemia: the state that occurs when the flow of oxygen-rich blood to the tissues is interrupted, leading to an oxygen deficiency in the tissues (27)

Isolation precautions: guidelines, based on a pathogen's method of transmission, that health care workers follow to contain the pathogen and limit others' exposure to it as much as possible (7)

J

Jaundice: a yellow discolouration of the skin and the whites of the eyes; usually associated with liver disorders (24)

Jejunostomy tube: a tube used for enteral nutrition that is inserted into the jejunum (part of the small intestine) through a surgical incision in the abdomen (19)

Joint: the area where two bones join together (25)

Justice: an ethical principle that requires health care workers to be fair and treat people equally regardless of race, religion, culture, disability, or ability to pay (4)

K

Kardex: a card file that contains condensed versions of each patient's or resident's medical record (5)

Keratin: a substance that causes mature skin cells to thicken and become resistant to water (24)

Kidney stones (renal calculi): a painful disorder characterized by the formation of clumps of minerals ("stones") in the kidney and bladder (32)

Korotkoff sounds: sounds that are heard while taking a person's blood pressure (16)

L

Labour: the process of giving birth to a baby, during which the mother's uterus contracts to push the baby out (40)

Lactation: the process by which the glandular tissue of the female breast produces milk (33)

Larceny: the act of stealing another person's property (4)

Laryngitis: inflammation of the larynx (the "voice box") (26)

Larynx: part of the respiratory airway; also known as the "voice box" (26)

Lateral position: one of the basic positions in which the person lies on his or her side (11)

Laws: rules that are made by a controlling authority, such as the province/territory or federal government, with the intent of preserving basic human rights (4)

Laxative: a medication that chemically stimulates the bowels to move; a treatment for constipation (20)

Lesion: a general term used to describe any break in the skin (24)

Leukemia: a general term for a group of disorders characterized by the excessive production of white blood cells that are abnormal in structure (27)

Leukocyte: white blood cell (27)

Liability: the responsibility of an individual to act within the confines of the law (4)

Libel: written statements that injure someone's reputation; a form of defamation (4)

Licensed practical nurse (LPN): a specially trained person who is licensed by the province or territory to provide routine care for the sick under the supervision of a registered nurse (RN) or a registered psychiatric nurse (RPN); completes a 1- to 2-year program in a vocational school, community college, or hospital (2)

Life-sustaining treatment: treatments that will prolong life, such as mechanical ventilation, cardiopulmonary resuscitation (CPR), and the placement of a feeding tube or intravenous (IV) line for the provision of nutrition (21)

Lift sheet: a draw sheet that is used to help lift or reposition a person who needs assistance with moving in bed (15)

Ligaments: very strong bands of fibrous tissue that cross over the joint capsule, attaching one bone to another and stabilizing the joint (25)

Litigation: the lawsuit, or legal action, taken against a person who is accused of breaking a law (4)

Liver: an organ that performs several important functions in the body, including the secretion of bile (a substance needed for digestion of fats), the production of clotting factors (chemicals that help our blood to clot), and the clearance of toxins (such as alcohol and drugs) from the body (31)

Living will: a type of advance directive that states a person's wish that death not be artificially postponed (21)

Local anesthesia: a loss of sensation in only a very small part of the body brought on by the injection of drugs (compare with *general anesthesia* and *regional anesthesia*) (39)

Lochia: vaginal discharge following the birth of a baby (40)

Logrolling: a technique for turning a person in which the person's body is moved in one fluid motion to keep the spine in alignment (11)

Long-term care facility: a health care facility that provides care for people who are unable to care for themselves at home, yet do not need to be hospitalized; sometimes referred to as a "nursing home" (1)

LPN: see *licensed practical nurse*

Lungs: the primary organs for respiration, the process the body uses to obtain oxygen from the environment and remove carbon dioxide (a waste gas) from the body (26)

Lymph: fluid in the lymph vessels (vessels that return the fluid that leaks into the tissues to the bloodstream) (27)

Lymph nodes: masses of lymphatic tissue that "clean" the lymph by removing bacteria and other large particles before returning the fluid to the bloodstream (27)

M

Macular degeneration: a vision disorder that results from the build-up of deposits in the macula (part of the retina) and eventually leads to blindness (29)

Macule: a small, flat, reddened skin lesion (24)

Magical thinking: a thought process that is common among preschoolers; the child believes that if he wishes for something hard enough, it will happen (41)

Malignant: adjective used to describe a cancerous tumour (that is, a tumour that has the ability to progress or invade other tissues) (compare with *benign*) (37)

Malpractice: negligence committed by people who hold licenses to practice their profession, such as doctors, nurses, lawyers, dentists, and pharmacists (4)

Mastectomy: surgical removal of a breast (33)

Mastication: chewing (31)

Masturbation: stimulation of the genitals for sexual pleasure or release, by a means other than sexual intercourse (6)

Materials Safety Data Sheet (MSDS): a document that summarizes key information about a chemical, such as its composition, which exposures may be dangerous, what to do if an exposure should occur, and how to clean up spills (9)

Mechanical digestion: the process of breaking down food through the use of physical means, such as chewing (compare with *chemical digestion*) (31)

Mechanical ventilation: a life-sustaining treatment in which a machine breathes for a person who cannot breathe on his or her own (26)

Medical asepsis: techniques that are used to physically remove or kill pathogens (see also *sanitization, antisepsis, disinfection,* and *sterilization*) (7)

Medical record: a legal document where information about a patient's or resident's current condition, the measures that have been taken by the medical and nursing staff to diagnose and treat the condition, and the patient's or resident's response to the treatment and care provided are recorded; also called a "medical chart" (5)

Medicare: the unofficial term used to describe Canada's official national health insurance program legislated by the Canada Health Act (1)

Melanin: a dark pigment that gives our skin, hair, and eyes colour (24)

Menarche: the onset of the first menstrual period (6)

Meninges: the three layers of connective tissue that cover and protect the brain and spinal cord (28)

Menopause: the cessation of menstruation and fertility that women typically experience in their early 50s (6)

Menorrhagia: excessive bleeding during a menstrual period, either in terms of the amount of blood lost or the number of days that bleeding lasts (33)

Menstrual period: the monthly loss of blood through the vagina that occurs in the absence of pregnancy (33)

Mental illness: a disorder that affects a person's mind, causing the person to act in unusual ways, experience emotional difficulties, or both (35)

Mental retardation: the state of having below-average intellectual functioning (that is, a decreased ability to reason, think, and understand) and problems with adaptive skills (that is, skills needed to live and work, such as communication skills, social skills, and self-care skills) (34)

Metabolism: the word used to describe the physical and chemical changes that occur when the cells of the body change the food that we eat into energy (16)

Metastasis: the process by which cancer cells spread from their original location in the body to a new location, which may be quite distant from the first (37)

Methicillin-resistant *Staphylococcus aureus* (MRSA): a type of bacteria that has become resistant to methicillin, a powerful antibiotic (7)

Microbe (microorganism): a living thing that cannot be seen with the naked eye; examples include bacteria and viruses (7)

Micturition: the process of passing urine from the body; also known as *urination* and *voiding* (20)

Midstream ("clean catch") urine specimen: a method of collecting urine that prevents contamination of the urine by the bacteria that normally exist in and around the urethra (20)

Mission: the officially stated purpose of a health care facility or organization (1)

Mitered corner: a corner that is made by folding and tucking the sheet so that it lies flat and neat against the mattress (15)

Morning (a.m.) care: care provided in the morning, to ready the person for the day, such as completion of personal hygiene and grooming activities, and bedmaking (17)

Motor nerves: nerves that carry commands from the brain down the spinal cord and out to the muscles and organs of the body (28)

MRSA: see *methicillin-resistant* Staphylococcus aureus

MS: see *multiple sclerosis*

Mucous membrane: a special type of epithelial tissue that lines many of the organ systems in the body and is coated with mucus (26)

Mucus: a slippery, sticky substance that is secreted by special cells and serves to keep the surfaces of mucous membranes moist (26)

Multiple sclerosis (MS): a disorder of the nervous system in which the myelin sheaths that cover the nerves are damaged, resulting in faulty transmission of nerve impulses (28)

Munchausen syndrome by proxy: a form of physical abuse seen in children; the child's caregiver (usually the mother) deliberately does things to make the child appear ill (41)

Muscle tone: the steady contraction of the skeletal muscles that helps us to maintain an upright posture, such as sitting or standing (25)

Muscular dystrophy: a general term for a group of disorders that cause the skeletal muscles to become more and more weak over time (25)

Myelin: a fatty, white substance that protects the axon and helps to speed the conduction of nerve impulses along the axon (28)

Myocardial infarction: a "heart attack"; occurs when one or more of the coronary arteries become completely blocked, preventing blood from reaching the parts of the heart that are fed by the affected arteries (27)

Myocardium: the thick, muscular middle layer of the heart wall; responsible for the pumping action of the heart (27)

Myopia: nearsightedness; trouble seeing objects that are far away (compare with *hyperopia*) (29)

N

Nasal cannula: a device used to deliver oxygen to a patient or resident; consists of two prongs of soft plastic tubing that are inserted into the nostrils (26)

Nasal cavity: the inside of the nose (26)

Nasogastric tube: a tube used for enteral nutrition that is inserted through the nose, down the throat, and into the stomach (19)

Nasointestinal tube: a tube used for enteral nutrition that is inserted through the nose, down the throat, and into the small intestine (19)

Nasopharyngeal airway: a soft rubber tube that is inserted into a person's nose and extends back toward the throat to create an opening that air can flow through (26)

Necrosis: tissue death as a result of a lack of oxygen (24)

Need: something that is essential for a person's physical and mental health (6)

Negligent: adjective used to describe a person who fails to do what a "careful and reasonable" person would do in any given situation (4)

Neonate: a newborn infant, 28 days or younger (6)

Nephron: the basic functional unit of the kidney; consists of a glomerulus and a series of tubules (32)

Neuron: a cell that can send and receive information (28)

Nits: the eggs of head lice, seen on the hair, near the scalp, in people with *pediculosis capitis* (head lice infestation) (18)

No code order: an order written on a person's chart specifying the person's wishes that the usual efforts to save his life will not be made; see also *do not resuscitate (DNR) order* (21)

Nocturia: the need to get up more than once or twice during the night to urinate, to the point where sleep is disrupted (20)

Nocturnal emission: the harmless involuntary discharge of semen during sleep; commonly called a "wet dream" (6)

Nonmaleficence: an ethical principle that requires health care workers to avoid harming those in their care (4)

Non-regulated health care profession: does not have a professional self-governing college (2)

Nonverbal communication: a way of communicating that uses facial expressions, gestures, and body language, instead of written or spoken language (5)

Normal (resident) flora: the harmless microbes that live in and on the body and help it to function properly (compare with *transient flora*) (7)

Nosocomial infections: infections that patients or residents get while receiving treatment in a hospital or other health care facility; a type of health care–associated infection (HAI) (7)

NPO status: a doctor's order specifying that a patient or resident is to have "*nils per os*" (nothing by mouth) (19)

Nucleus: the cell's "brain"; it contains all of the information the cell needs in order to do its job, grow, and reproduce (23)

Nurse's bag: a bag used by the home health worker to transport necessary supplies and equipment to each client's home (42)

Nursing diagnosis: a statement that describes a problem the person is having that can be identified and treated by the nursing staff independently (5)

Nursing history: a report that is completed by the nurse when a patient or resident is admitted to a health care facility that gathers information about the person's preferences, abilities, disabilities, and habits (14)

Nursing process: a process that allows members of the care team to communicate with one another regarding the patient's or resident's specific needs (in regard to care), what steps will be taken to meet those needs, and whether the steps were effective in meeting the person's needs; consists of five parts: assessment, diagnosis, planning, implementation, and evaluation (5)

Nutrients: substances in foods and fluids that the body uses to grow, to repair itself, and to carry out processes essential for living (19)

Nutrition: the process of taking in and using food (19)

Nutritional supplement: a flavored shake or drink that is used to supply extra calories or protein; often served with meals or as a snack in between meals (19)

O

Obese: the state of being extremely overweight (19)

Objective data: information that is obtained directly, through measurements or by using one of the five senses (sight, smell, taste, hearing, touch) (5)

Observation: something that you notice about the patient or resident, typically related to a change in the person's physical or mental condition (5)

Obsessive-compulsive disorder: an anxiety disorder that causes a person to suffer intensely from recurrent unwanted thoughts (obsessions) that are usually associated with rituals the person feels obligated to complete constantly (compulsions) (35)

Occult: adjective used to describe something that is hidden or cannot be seen with the naked eye; often used in reference to blood in a urine or stool sample (20)

Occupied bed: a bed with a person in it (15)

OCD: see *obsessive-compulsive disorder*

Oliguria: the state of voiding a very small amount of urine over a given period of time (20)

Open bed: a bed ready to receive a patient or resident (15)

Opportunistic microbes: microbes that are considered normal (resident) flora when they are in or on one part of the body, but can cause infection if they move out of that area and into or onto another part of the body (7)

Oral–fecal route: a method of transmitting an infection; occurs when feces containing a pathogen contaminate food or water, which is then consumed by another person (8)

Organ: a group of tissues functioning together for a similar purpose (23)

Organelles: structures inside of the cell that help the cell to make the energy it needs to stay alive and to rid itself of waste products (23)

Organism: a living thing, such as an animal or a plant (23)

Organ system: a group of organs that work together to perform a specific function for the body (23)

Oriented to person, place, and time: the state of being able to answer basic questions about person, place, or time; alert (compare with *disoriented*) (12)

Oropharyngeal airway: a hard plastic device that is inserted into a person's mouth to stop the tongue from falling back into the throat; used to keep the airway open (26)

Orthostatic hypotension: a sudden decrease in blood pressure that occurs when a person stands up from a sitting or lying position (16)

Osteoporosis: a disorder characterized by the excessive loss of bone tissue (25)

Ostomy: a surgically created opening between an internal structure and the skin, usually located on the abdomen (see also *ileostomy* and *colostomy*) (31)

Otitis externa: an infection of the lining of the external auditory canal; commonly referred to as "swimmer's ear" (29)

Otitis media: an infection of the middle ear that is common in young children (29)

Otosclerosis: an inherited form of hearing loss (29)

Over-bed table: a table that fits over a bed or a chair and can be raised or lowered as needed (13)

Ovulation: the release of a ripe, mature egg from the female ovaries each month (33)

P

PACU: see *post-anesthesia care unit*

Palliative care: care that focuses on relieving uncomfortable symptoms, not on curing the problem that is causing the symptoms (21)

Pallor: paleness of the skin (24)

Pancreas: an organ that produces substances that aid in digestion, as well as the hormones insulin and glucagon (31)

Panic disorder: a mental health disorder in which a person experiences episodes of sudden, overpowering fright (panic) and anxiety, usually accompanied by chest or abdominal pain, a rapid heart rate, shortness of breath, and/or dizziness (35)

Papule: a small, raised, firm skin lesion that can be easily felt by passing your fingers lightly over the affected area (24)

Paraplegia: paralysis from the waist down (compare with *quadriplegia* and *hemiplegia*) (10)

Parkinson's disease: a progressive neurologic disorder that is characterized by tremor and weakness in the muscles and a shuffling gait (28)

Pathogen: a microbe that can cause illness (7)

Patient: a person who is receiving health care in a hospital, clinic, or extended-care facility (1)

Pediculosis capitis: head lice (18)

Pelvic inflammatory disease (PID): infection of the fallopian tubes and abdominal cavity that can lead to infertility (33)

Percutaneous endoscopic gastrostomy (PEG) tube: a special type of gastrostomy tube that is inserted into the stomach with the aid of an endoscope (19)

Pericardium: a double-layered protective sac that surrounds the heart (27)

Perineal care (peri-care): cleaning the perineum and anus, as well as the vulva (in women) and the penis (in men) (17)

Perineum: the area from the bottom of the vagina to the anus (in women) or the area from the root of the penis to the anus (in men) (17)

Periodontitis: infection and inflammation of the soft tissue and bones that support the teeth; can lead to tooth loss (17)

Peri-operative period: the term used to describe all three phases of the surgical process as a whole—the pre-operative, intra-operative, and post-operative phases (39)

Peripheral nervous system (PNS): the nerves outside of the brain and spinal cord; receives information from the environment, and carries commands from the brain and spinal cord to the other organs of the body, such as the muscles (compare with *central nervous system*) (28)

Peripheral vascular disease: a disorder characterized by pain and cramping in the legs, caused by atherosclerosis of the arteries that supply blood to the legs (27)

Peristalsis: involuntary wave-like muscular movements, such as those that occur in the digestive system to move chyme (partially digested food) through the intestines (20)

Perseveration: the inappropriate and constant repetition of a phrase or act; often seen in people with dementia (36)

Personal protective equipment (PPE): barriers that are worn to physically prevent microbes from reaching a health care provider's skin or mucous membranes, such as gloves, gowns, masks, and protective eyewear (7)

Petit mal (absence) seizure: a seizure characterized by a sudden, brief break in consciousness or activity (compare with *grand mal seizure*) (12)

Phantom pain: the feeling that a body part is still present, after it has been surgically removed (amputated) (25)

Pharyngitis: inflammation of the throat (pharynx) (26)

Pharynx: throat region (26)

Phobia: an excessive, abnormal fear of an object or situation (35)

Physical abuse: the repetitive and deliberate infliction of physical injury on another person, such as that caused by striking, biting, slapping, shaking, or failing to meet a dependent person's physical needs (for example, for food, water, and cleanliness) (compare with *psychological [emotional] abuse* and *sexual abuse*) (4)

Physical restraint: a device that is attached to or near a person's body to limit a person's freedom of movement or access to his or her body (compare with *chemical restraint*) (10)

Physiology: the study of how the body parts work (23)

Placenta: the structure that develops from the inside lining of the uterus during pregnancy and participates in the exchange of gases and nutrients between the mother and the fetus (40)

Plaque: a fatty deposit that builds up on the inside of the artery wall, blocking blood flow to the tissues and making the artery wall brittle and prone to breaking (27)

Plasma: the liquid part of the blood (27)

Pleura: the membrane that lines the chest cavity and covers the outside of the lungs (26)

Pleurisy: inflammation of the pleura, the membrane that lines the chest cavity and covers the lungs (26)

Pneumonia: inflammation of the lung tissue, caused by infection with a virus or a bacterium, and resulting in impaired gas exchange (26)

Pneumothorax: the build-up of air in the space between the lungs and the chest wall (26)

PNS: see *peripheral nervous system*

Podiatrist: a doctor who specializes in the care of the feet (18)

Polyuria: excessive urine output; see also *diuresis* (20)

Post-anesthesia care unit (PACU): the recovery room where patients are taken following surgery so that they can be closely monitored by the health care team to make sure that they are recovering without complications from the surgery or the anesthesia (39)

Postmenopausal bleeding: uterine bleeding after menopause (33)

Postmortem care: the care of a person's body after the person's death (22)

Post-operative phase: one of three phases of care for a person who is having surgery; the phase after the surgery is actually performed (compare with *pre-operative phase* and *intra-operative phase*) (39)

Postpartum period: the 6-week period of time following the birth of a baby (40)

Post-procedure actions: steps that are routinely performed at the end of each patient or resident care procedure, called "Finishing Up" actions in this book (compare with *pre-procedure actions*) (9)

PPE: see *personal protective equipment*

Pre-eclampsia/eclampsia: dangerously high blood pressure in a pregnant woman (40)

Prenatal care: the health care given to a woman in the months leading up to the birth of her baby (40)

Pre-operative phase: one of three phases of care for a person who is having surgery; the phase before the surgery is actually performed (compare with *intra-operative phase* and *post-operative phase*) (39)

Pre-operative teaching: teaching done by members of the health care team to prepare a person and his or her family members for surgery; during pre-operative teaching, the person learns about the surgical procedure, its benefits and possible risks, and what can be expected during the post-operative recovery period (39)

Pre-procedure actions: steps that are routinely performed before each patient or resident care procedure; called "Getting Ready" actions in this book (compare with *post-procedure actions*) (9)

Presbycusis: age-related hearing loss (29)

Presbyopia: age-related loss of the eye's ability to focus on objects that are close (29)

Pressure points: bony areas where pressure ulcers are most likely to form; include the heels, ankles, knees, hips, toes, elbows, shoulder blades, ears, the back of the head, and along the spine (24)

Pressure-relieving mattress: a mattress that is placed on top of the regular mattress to help prevent skin breakdown in patients and residents who must stay in bed for long periods of time (15)

Pressure ulcer: a difficult-to-heal (and possibly even fatal) sore that forms when part of the body presses against a surface (such as a mattress or chair) for a long period of time; also known as pressure sores and decubitus ulcers (11)

Pre-term labour: labour that begins too early, before the fetus can survive on its own (40)

Primary nursing: a model for organizing the nursing team's efforts in which one nurse is assigned several patients or residents, and is responsible for planning and carrying out all aspects of care for those people [compare with *functional (modular) nursing* and *team nursing*] (2)

Procedure: a series of steps followed in a particular order when providing care to a patient or resident that helps to ensure that the care provided is safe and correct (9)

PRN (as-needed) care: personal hygiene care that is provided whenever a patient or resident needs it, throughout the day or night (17)

Professional: a person who has credentials, obtained through education and training, that enable him or her to become licensed or certified to practice a certain profession; also, a person who demonstrates a professional attitude (3)

Professionalism: the attitude of being a professional, characterized by a positive outlook and a commitment to doing one's best at all times (3)

Prognosis: a doctor's prediction of the course of a person's disease, and his or her estimation of the person's chances for recovery (37)

Prone position: one of the basic positions in which the person lies on his abdomen with his head turned to one side (11)

Prosthetic devices: artificial replacements for legs, feet, arms, or other body parts (23)

Psychiatrist: a doctor who specializes in the diagnosis and treatment of mental illness (35)

Psychological (emotional) abuse: the repetitive and deliberate infliction of emotional injury on another person, such as that caused by threatening a person with physical harm or abandonment, teasing a person in a cruel way, or preventing a person from interacting with others (compare with *physical abuse* and *sexual abuse*) (4)

Psychologist: a health care professional who is trained to provide counselling services for people with mental illness (35)

Puberty: the period during which the secondary sex characteristics appear and the reproductive organs begin to function (6)

Pulmonary circulation: the pattern of circulation that takes blood from the heart to the lungs to pick up oxygen and release carbon dioxide (compare with *systemic circulation*) (27)

Pulmonary embolism: a potentially fatal condition caused by blocking of the pulmonary artery by an embolus (a blood clot in a vessel that breaks off and moves from one place to another) (39)

Pulse: the wave of blood sent through the arteries each time the heart beats (16)

Pulse amplitude: the force or quality of the pulse (16)

Pulse deficit: the difference between the apical pulse rate (the pulse that is measured by listening over the apex of the heart with a stethoscope) and the radial pulse rate (the pulse that is measured by placing the middle two or three fingers over the radial artery, located on the inside of the wrist) (16)

Pulse points: the points where the large arteries run close enough to the surface of the skin to be felt as a pulse (12)

Pulse pressure: the difference between the systolic and diastolic pressures (16)

Pulse rate: the number of pulsations that can be felt over an artery in 1 minute; an indication of the heart rate (one of the vital signs) (16)

Pulse rhythm: the pattern of the pulsations and the pauses between them (16)

Pustule: a small, blister-like skin lesion that contains pus, a thick, yellowish fluid that is a sign of infection (24)

Pyelonephritis: a kidney infection (32)

Pyloric sphincter: a circle of muscular tissue that surrounds the place where the stomach empties into the small intestine and helps to prevent food from returning to the stomach once it enters the small intestine (31)

Q

Quadriplegia: paralysis from the neck down; compare with *paraplegia* and *hemiplegia* (10)

R

Race: a general characterization that describes skin colour, body stature, facial features, and hair texture (6)

RACE fire response plan: the general actions that are taken in the event of a fire emergency (remove to safety, activate the alarm, contain the fire, extinguish or evacuate) (9)

Radiation therapy: a type of therapy that uses energy transmitted by waves to destroy cancer cells (37)

Range of motion: the complete extent of movement that a joint is normally capable of without causing pain (25)

Rash: a group of skin lesions (24)

Reciprocity: the principle by which one province or territory recognizes the validity of a license or certification granted by another province or territory (2)

Recording: communicating information about a patient or resident to other health care team members in written form; sometimes called *charting* (5)

Rectal suppository: a small, wax-like cone or oval that is inserted into the anus, which dissolves at body temperature, stimulating peristalsis or lubricating and softening the stool (20)

Reduction: the word used to describe the process of bringing the ends of a broken bone into alignment (25)

Reference list: a list of three or four people who would be willing to talk to a potential employer about a job candidate's abilities (3)

Referred (radiating) pain: pain that is felt somewhere other than where it originated (29)

Regional anesthesia: a loss of sensation in part, but not all, of the body brought on by the injection of drugs (compare with *general anesthesia* and *local anesthesia*) (39)

Registered nurse (RN): a specially trained person who is licensed by the province or territory to develop care plans and coordinate all aspects of patient or resident care, as well as to provide that care; holds a baccalaureate degree from a liberal arts college or university (4 years) or an associate degree from a junior or community college (2 years) (2)

Registered nurse's assistant (RNA): another term used in some parts of Canada [see also *licensed practical nurse (LPN)* (2)

Registered psychiatric nurse (RPN): a specially trained person who is licensed by the province or territory to develop care plans and coordinate all aspects of patient or resident care, with a focus on mental health issues; holds a baccalaureate degree from a liberal arts college or university (4 years) or an associate degree from a junior or community college (2 years) (2)

Regress: to return to an earlier stage of development, as when an older child who is experiencing stress as a result of being hospitalized begins demonstrating behaviours from when she was younger, such as thumb-sucking or bedwetting (41)

Regulated health care profession: self-governed and associated with a professional organization called a college (2)

Rehabilitation: the process of helping a person with a disability to return to his or her highest level of physical, emotional, or economic function (23)

Reincarnation: the idea that a person's spirit or soul will live again on Earth in the form of an animal or human being yet to be born (22)

Religion: a person's spiritual beliefs (6)

Reminiscence therapy: a technique used for interacting with people who have dementia, in which the person with dementia is encouraged to remember and share experiences from his or her past with others (36)

Renal: related to, involving, or located in the region of the kidneys (32)

Renal calculi: see *kidney stones*

Reporting: the spoken exchange of information between health care team members (5)

Reproduction: the process by which a living thing makes more living things like itself (33)

Rescue breathing: a basic life support (BLS) technique in which the rescuer blows air into the victim's mouth to perform the function of breathing for the victim until the victim begins breathing again on her own (12)

Resident: a person who is living in a long-term care facility or assisted-living facility (1)

Resident inventory sheet: a document that lists and briefly describes all of the resident's personal belongings; completed when a resident is admitted to a long-term care facility (14)

Respiration: the process the body uses to obtain oxygen from the environment and remove carbon dioxide (a waste gas) from the body (26)

Respiratory arrest: the condition where breathing has stopped (12)

Respiratory rate: the number of times a person breathes in 1 minute (one breath is both an inhalation and an exhalation); one of the vital signs (16)

Respiratory rhythm: the regularity with which a person breathes (16)

Respiratory therapy: any treatment that is used to help a person achieve satisfactory respiration (26)

Respite care: home care that gives the primary caregiver an opportunity to rest or leave the home for a short period of time (42)

Restorative care: measures that health care workers take to help a person regain health, strength, and function; the means by which rehabilitation is achieved (23)

Restraint alternatives: measures taken to avoid the use of chemical or physical restraints (10)

Résumé: a brief document that gives a possible employer general information about a job candidate's education and work experience (3)

Reverse Trendelenburg's position: one of the basic positions in which the head of the mattress is raised so the person's head is higher than her feet (compare with *Trendelenburg's position*) (13)

Right: something a person is entitled to receive (4)

Rigor mortis: the stiffening of the muscles that usually develops within 2 to 4 hours of death (22)

Rugae: folds in the lining of the stomach (31)

S

Salivary glands: glands located near the mouth that produce and secrete saliva, a substance that helps with chewing and swallowing by moistening the food (31)

Sanitization: practices associated with basic cleanliness, such as handwashing, cleansing of eating utensils and other surfaces with soap and water, and providing clean linens and clothing; one of the techniques of medical asepsis (compare with *antisepsis, disinfection,* and *sterilization*) (7)

SCD: see *sequential compression device*

Schizophrenia: a mental health disorder that affects how a person thinks, feels, and acts; the person has difficulty determining what is real from what is imaginary (35)

Scope of practice: the range of tasks that a nursing assistant is legally permitted to do (2)

Seborrheic dermatitis (cradle cap): severe scaling of the scalp with thick, yellow, crusty patches (18)

Sebum: an oily substance secreted by glands in the skin that lubricates the skin and helps to prevent it from drying out (24)

Semi-Fowler's (low Fowler's) position: one of the basic positions in which the head of the bed is elevated approximately 30 to 45 degrees (11)

Sense organs: a general term used to describe the eyes, the ears, the nose, and the taste buds (29)

Sensorineural hearing loss: hearing loss that occurs when the receptors in the ear are unable to receive stimuli or transmit nerve impulses (compare with *conductive hearing loss*) (29)

Sensory nerves: nerves that carry information from the internal organs and the outside world to the spinal cord and up into the brain so that the brain can analyze the information (28)

Sensory receptors: specialized cells or groups of cells associated with a sensory nerve (29)

Septic shock: shock caused by a severe bacterial infection that involves the entire body (12)

Sequential compression device (SCD): a device that is applied to the calves to help prevent pooling of blood in the lower legs; often used following surgery to prevent cardiovascular complications (39)

Sex: the physical activity one engages in to obtain sexual pleasure and reproduce (6)

Sex cell (gamete): special cells contributed by each parent that contain half of the normal number of chromosomes (33)

Sexual abuse: forcing another person to engage in sexual activity [compare with *psychological (emotional) abuse* and *physical abuse*] (4)

Sexuality: how a person perceives his or her maleness or femaleness (6)

Sexually transmitted infection (STI): an infection that is most commonly transmitted by sexual contact; also known as venereal disease (33)

Shaken baby syndrome: severe brain damage or death in an infant or toddler resulting from violent shaking that causes the child's brain to hit the inside of his skull repeatedly (41)

Shearing: a term used to describe the force created when something or someone is pulled across a surface that offers resistance; can lead to skin breakdown (11)

Shock: the condition that results when the organs and tissues of the body do not receive enough oxygen-rich blood; see also *cardiogenic shock, hemorrhagic shock, anaphylactic shock,* and *septic shock* (12)

Shroud: a covering used to wrap the body of a person who has died (22)

Signs: objective observations (that is, observations based on information that is obtained directly, through measurements or by using one of the five senses) (compare with *symptoms*) (5)

Sims' position: one of the basic positions in which the person lies on his side with his head turned to one side and his knee sharply bent and supported by a pillow; the corresponding arm is bent at the elbow with the hand in front of the face, palm down, resting on a pillow; the lower leg is straight and the lower arm extends out from the side with the hand down near the hips and the palm turned upward (11)

Sitz bath: a hot water soak for the perineal area (40)

Skeleton: the framework for the body formed by the bones (25)

Slander: spoken statements that injure someone's reputation; a form of defamation (4)

Sperm cell: male sex cell (33)

Sphygmomanometer: a device used to measure blood pressure (16)

Spina bifida: a congenital defect of the spinal column that occurs when the vertebrae do not close properly during development, leaving the spinal cord exposed (34)

Sputum: mucus and other respiratory secretions that are coughed up from the lungs, bronchi, and trachea; also known as phlegm (26)

Standard precautions: precautions that a health care worker takes with each patient or resident to prevent contact with bloodborne pathogens; include the use of barrier methods (such as gloves) as well as certain environmental control methods (7)

STI: see *sexually transmitted infection*

Sterilization: the process of completely eliminating microbes from the surface of an object using an autoclave or chemicals; one of the techniques of medical asepsis (compare with *antisepsis, disinfection*, and *sanitization*) (7)

Stethoscope: a device that amplifies sound and transfers it to the listener's ears (16)

Stomach: a hollow, muscular pouch for holding food (31)

Stomatitis: inflammation of the mouth, often seen in people who are receiving chemotherapy (37)

Stool: a term used to refer to fecal material after it has left the body (20)

Stool softener: a medication that helps to prevent constipation by keeping fluid in the feces (20)

Straight catheter: a urinary catheter that is inserted and then removed immediately, after the urine in the bladder has drained out (20)

Stress: a physical or emotional factor that changes the body's normal balance or equilibrium (35)

Stroke: a disorder that occurs when blood flow to a part of the brain is completely blocked, causing the tissue to die; also known as a "brain attack" or cerebrovascular accident (CVA) (28)

Stump: the end of an amputated limb that is left after surgery (25)

Sub-acute care unit (skilled nursing unit, skilled nursing facility): a unit within a hospital or a long-term care facility, or a separate facility, that provides care focused on rehabilitation and helping the patient to move from hospital care to home care (1)

Subcutaneous tissue: the layer of fat that supports the dermis (the deepest layer of the skin) (24)

Subjective data: information that cannot be objectively measured or assessed (5)

Suctioning: the process of removing fluid and mucus from a person's airway (26)

Suicide: the act of taking one's own life intentionally and voluntarily (35)

Sundowning: the worsening of behavioural symptoms in the late afternoon and evening (as the sun goes down) of a person with dementia (36)

Supine (dorsal recumbent) position: one of the basic positions in which the person lies on his back, with the bed flat and the head supported by a pillow (11)

Supportive care: treatments that will not prolong life, but will make a person more comfortable, such as oxygen therapy, nutritional supplementation, pain medication, range-of-motion exercises, grooming and hygiene, and positioning assistance (21)

Supportive devices: *(1)* devices used when positioning a person to help the person maintain proper body alignment, such as pillows or rolled sheets, towels, or blankets (11); *(2)* devices that help to stabilize a weak joint or limb; used in physical therapy to help a person with a disability regain function (23)

Suprapubic catheter: a urinary catheter that is inserted into the bladder through a surgical incision made in the abdominal wall, right above the pubic bone (20)

Surgical bed: a closed bed that has been opened to receive a patient or resident who will be arriving by stretcher; the top sheet, blanket, and bedspread are folded toward the side of the bed, leaving one side open and ready to receive the person (15)

Symptoms: subjective observations (that is, observations that are based on information that cannot be measured or observed firsthand, such as a patient's or resident's complaint of pain) (compare with *signs*) (5)

Synapse: the gap between the axon of one neuron and the dendrites of the next (28)

Syncope: fainting (12)

Systemic circulation: the pattern of circulation that takes blood from the lungs to the rest of the body to release oxygen and pick up carbon dioxide (compare with *pulmonary circulation*) (27)

Systole: the active phase of the cardiac cycle, during which the myocardium contracts, sending blood out of the heart (compare with *diastole*) (27)

Systolic pressure: the pressure that the blood exerts against the arterial walls when the heart muscle contracts; the first blood pressure measurement that is recorded (compare with *diastolic pressure*) (16)

T

Tachycardia: a heart rate that is faster than normal (more than 100 beats/min in an adult) (16)

Tachypnea: a respiratory rate that is higher than normal (more than 24 breaths/min in an adult) (16)

Tactile receptors: receptors found in the skin that are stimulated when something comes in contact with the surface of the body and presses on them, causing them to change shape (29)

Task lighting: bright light directed toward a specific area, used for activities that require good lighting to prevent eyestrain (compare with *general lighting*) (13)

Tasks: growth and development milestones that must be completed before a person can move on to the next stage of growth and development (6)

TB: see *tuberculosis*

T cells: special white blood cells (leukocytes) that play a role in the immune response to invading pathogens; the main target of the human immunodeficiency virus (HIV) (8)

Team nursing: a model for organizing the care team's efforts in which a team leader (a registered nurse) determines all of the nursing needs for the patients or residents assigned to the team, and assigns tasks according to each team member's skills and level of responsibility [compare with *functional (modular) nursing* and *primary nursing*] (2)

Tendons: bands of connective tissue that attach the skeletal muscles to the bones (25)

Terminal illness: an illness or condition from which recovery is not expected (6)

Tetany: a condition that occurs when the body's calcium level drops too low; characterized by cramping of the skeletal muscles and an irregular heartbeat (30)

Thrombi (singular, *thrombus*): blood clots that form in the small blood vessels, blocking the flow of blood and depriving the tissues of oxygen and nutrients (27)

Thrombocytes: pinched-off pieces of larger cells that are found in the red bone marrow and are responsible for clotting of the blood; also called platelets (27)

Thrombophlebitis: a condition characterized by inflammation and pain in the legs, caused by a thrombus in one of the veins of the legs (39)

TIA: see *transient ischemic attack*

Tinea capitis: a fungal infection of the scalp (18)

Tinea pedis: a fungal infection of the skin and nails, commonly known as "athlete's foot" (18)

Tinnitus: ringing in the ear (29)

Tissue: a group of cells similar in structure and specialized to perform a specific function (23)

Toe pleat: loosening of the top linens over a person's feet to relieve pressure and promote comfort (15)

Tort: a violation of civil law (4)

Total parenteral nutrition (TPN, hyperalimentation): an alternative method of providing fluid and nutrition; nourishment is delivered directly into the bloodstream through a large catheter (tube) inserted into a large vein near the heart (19)

TPN: see *total parenteral nutrition*

Trachea: the passage that carries air from the larynx down into the chest toward the lungs; commonly known as the "windpipe" (26)

Tracheostomy: a surgically created opening in the neck that opens into the trachea; often used with a tracheostomy tube (instead of an endotracheal tube) when a person must be on a mechanical ventilator for more than a week or so (26)

Traction: a treatment for fracture in which the ends of the broken bone are placed in the proper alignment and then weight is applied to exert a constant pull and keep the bone in alignment (25)

Transfer: *(1)* to move a person from one place to another, for example, from the bed to a wheelchair (11); *(2)* to move a patient or resident within or between health care settings (14)

Transfer belt (gait belt): a webbed or woven belt with a buckle that is used to assist a weak or unsteady person with standing, walking, or transferring; called a *gait belt* when used to help a person walk (11)

Transient flora: microbes that are picked up by touching contaminated objects or people who have an infectious disease [compare with *normal (resident) flora*] (7)

Transient ischemic attack (TIA): a temporary (transient) episode of dysfunction caused by decreased blood flow to the brain (28)

Transmission-based precautions: precautions that a health care worker takes when a person is known to have a disease that is transmitted in a certain way; include airborne precautions, droplet precautions, and contact precautions (7)

Transsexual: a person who believes that he or she should be a member of the opposite sex (6)

Transvestite: a person who becomes sexually excited by dressing as a member of the opposite sex (6)

Trapeze bar: a device that is attached to the overhead frame of a person's bed; used to assist with movement (25)

Trendelenburg's position: one of the basic positions in which the foot of the mattress is raised so that the person's head is lower than her feet (compare with *reverse Trendelenburg's position*) (13)

Tuberculosis (TB): an airborne infection caused by a bacterium that usually infects the lungs (8)

Tumour: an abnormal growth of tissue; the cells that form the tumour may be benign or malignant (37)

Type 1 diabetes mellitus: a type of diabetes caused by destruction of the insulin-producing cells of the pancreas (30)

Type 2 diabetes mellitus: a type of diabetes caused by the inability of the cells of the body to respond to insulin; the pancreas still produces some insulin (30)

U

Ulcer: a shallow crater on the surface of the skin that is formed when the tissue dies and is shed (24)

Umbilical cord: a cord that supplies the growing fetus with nutrients and oxygen, and removes waste (40)

Unintentional tort: a violation of civil law that occurs when someone causes harm or injury to another person or that person's property without the intent to cause harm (4)

Unintentional wound: an unexpected injury that usually results from some type of trauma (compare with *intentional wound*) (24)

Unit: a patient's or resident's room (13)

Unresponsive: adjective used to describe a person who is unconscious and cannot be aroused, or conscious but not responsive when spoken to or touched (12)

Urethritis: infection of the urethra, the passageway that carries urine from the bladder to the outside of the body (32)

Ureterostomy: an alternative way of eliminating urine from the body; a surgical procedure in which the ureters are brought through the abdominal wall by way of small incisions and sutured in place (32)

Urgency: a need to urinate immediately (20)

Urgent: adjective used to describe surgery that is planned and scheduled ahead of time, but must be done as soon as possible to prevent the person's condition from getting worse (39)

Urinal: a device used for urination when a man is unable to get out of bed (20)

Urinalysis: examination of the urine under a microscope and by chemical means (20)

Urinary incontinence: the inability to hold one's urine, or the involuntary loss of urine from the bladder (20)

Urinary retention: the inability of the bladder to empty either completely during urination, or at all (20)

Urination: the process of passing urine from the body; also known as *micturition* and *voiding* (20)

Urine: formed by the kidneys; consists of waste products that have been filtered from the bloodstream, along with excess fluid (32)

Urostomy: an alternative way of eliminating urine from the body; a surgical procedure in which the ureters are attached to a small portion of the small intestine, one end of the segment of intestine is sealed off, and the other end is brought through the abdominal wall and sutured into place to create a stoma (32)

V

Validation therapy: a technique used for interacting with people who have dementia, in which the caregiver acknowledges the person's reality; rather than correcting the person, the caregiver attempts to distract the person and redirect the conversation whenever possible (36)

Value: a cherished belief or principle (4)

Vancomycin-resistant enterococcus (VRE): a type of bacteria that has become resistant to vancomycin, a powerful antibiotic (7)

Varicose veins: a condition that results from pooling of blood in the veins just underneath the skin, causing them to become swollen and "knotty" in appearance (27)

Vascular (multi-infarct) dementia: a type of dementia caused by the loss of function in multiple areas of the brain due to tissue death caused by a lack of adequate oxygen and nutrients (36)

Vector: a living creature, such as an insect, that can transmit disease (7)

Veins: vessels that return blood to the heart (27)

Ventilation system: a system that provides fresh air and keeps air circulating throughout a building (13)

Ventricles: the lower chambers of the heart (27)

Venules: the smallest veins (27)

Verbal communication: a way of communicating that uses written or spoken language (5)

Vernix: a protective, cheese-like substance that is present on the skin of newborns (40)

Vertigo: dizziness (29)

Vesicle: a small, blister-like skin lesion that contains fluid (24)

Villi (singular, *villus*): tiny, finger-like structures on the lining of the small intestine that increase the small intestine's ability to absorb nutrients (31)

Virulence: the strength or disease-producing potential of a pathogen (7)

Vital signs: certain key measurements that provide essential information about a person's health (16)

Voiding: the process of passing urine from the body; also known as *urination* and *micturition* (20)

VRE: see *vancomycin-resistant enterococcus*

W

Water-soluble: adjective used to describe a substance that dissolves in water (for example, certain vitamins) (19)

Weight bearing: a term used to refer to a person's ability to stand on one or both legs (11)

Will: a legal statement that expresses a person's wishes for the management of his or her affairs after death (21)

Work ethic: a person's attitude toward his or her work (3)

Wound: an injury that results in a break in the skin (and usually the underlying tissues as well) (24)

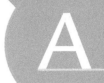
Answers to the
What Did You Learn? Exercises

Chapter 1: The Canadian Health Care System
Multiple choice: 1-c, 2-d, 3-b, 4-c, 5-a
Matching: 1-a, 2-c, 3-d, 4-b, 5-e

Chapter 2: The Personal Support Worker
Multiple choice: 1-b, 2-b, 3-c, 4-b, 5-b, 6-c

**Chapter 3: Professionalism and
Job-Seeking Skills**
Multiple choice: 1-b, 2-c, 3-b, 4-d, 5-a, 6-d, 7-b,
8-c, 9-c, 10-d, 11-a, 12-b, 13-c

Chapter 4: Legal and Ethical Issues
Multiple choice: 1-b, 2-a, 3-d, 4-b, 5-d, 6-d, 7-c,
8-a, 9-b, 10-a
Matching: 1-e, 2-a, 3-d, 4-b, 5-c

Chapter 5: Communication Skills
Multiple choice: 1-b, 2-a, 3-d, 4-b, 5-c, 6-a, 7-b,
8-c, 9-b, 10-b
Matching: 1-e, 2-a, 3-d, 4-c, 5-b

Chapter 6: Those We Care For
Multiple choice: 1-d, 2-a, 3-a, 4-b, 5-c, 6-a,
7-d, 8-b
Matching: 1-d, 2-c, 3-f, 4-g, 5-a, 6-b, 7-e

**Chapter 7: Communicable Disease and
Infection Control**
Multiple choice: 1-d, 2-b, 3-b, 4-a, 5-d, 6-c, 7-d,
8-d, 9-a, 10-c, 11-b, 12-b, 13-c
Matching: 1-c, 2-d, 3-f, 4-g, 5-e, 6-a, 7-h, 8-i,
9-j, 10-b

Chapter 8: Bloodborne and Airborne Pathogens
Multiple choice: 1-d, 2-d, 3-d, 4-b

Chapter 9: Workplace Safety
Multiple choice: 1-a, 2-b, 3-d, 4-a, 5-c, 6-c, 7-c,
8-a, 9-a, 10-c, 11-b, 12-b, 13-b, 14-d

**Chapter 10: Patient and Resident
Safety and Restraints**
Multiple choice: 1-d, 2-b, 3-c, 4-b, 5-b, 6-c,
7-c, 8-b

**Chapter 11: Postioning, Lifting, and
Transferring Patients and Residents**
Multiple choice: 1-a, 2-a, 3-d, 4-c, 5-d, 6-d,
7-d, 8-c, 9-b, 10-c, 11-d, 12-b, 13-d, 14-c,
15-d, 16-a

**Chapter 12: Basic First Aid and
Emergency Care**
Multiple choice: 1-d, 2-b, 3-c, 4-c, 5-b, 6-d,
7-d, 8-d
Matching: 1-g, 2-f, 3-i, 4-b, 5-c, 6-e, 7-j,
8-h, 9-d, 10-a

**Chapter 13: The Patient or
Resident Environment**
Multiple choice: 1-c, 2-d, 3-c, 4-b, 5-a, 6-c, 7-d
Matching: 1-c, 2-b, 3-a

**Chapter 14: Admissions, Transfers,
and Discharges**
Multiple choice: 1-c, 2-b, 3-a, 4-d, 5-b, 6-c,
7-c, 8-c, 9-c

Chapter 15: Bedmaking
Multiple choice: 1-b, 2-d, 3-c, 4-b, 5-c, 6-c,
7-a, 8-d

Chapter 16: Vital Signs, Height, and Weight
Multiple choice: 1-c, 2-a, 3-b, 4-c, 5-d, 6-d, 7-a,
8-c, 9-d, 10-d, 11-b, 12-c

Chapter 17: Cleanliness and Hygiene
Multiple choice: 1-a, 2-c, 3-d, 4-d, 5-c, 6-d, 7-b,
8-a, 9-d, 10-d, 11-d, 12-c
Matching: 1-g, 2-b, 3-f, 4-d, 5-c, 6-e, 7-a

Chapter 18: Grooming
Multiple choice: 1-c, 2-a, 3-a, 4-c, 5-b, 6-d, 7-d,
8-c, 9-d, 10-c, 11-a, 12-d
Matching: 1-d, 2-b, 3-e, 4-c, 5-a

Chapter 19: Basic Nutrition
Multiple choice: 1-c, 2-b, 3-c, 4-b, 5-b, 6-a, 7-c,
8-c, 9-b, 10-c, 11-b, 12-d
Matching: 1-c, 2-f, 3-a, 4-e, 5-d, 6-b

Chapter 20: Assisting With Urinary and Bowel Elimination
Multiple choice: 1-b, 2-a, 3-a, 4-a, 5-c, 6-d, 7-b, 8-d, 9-a, 10-c
Matching: 1-i, 2-j, 3-e, 4-f, 5-b, 6-c, 7-g, 8-d, 9-h, 10-a

Chapter 21: Caring for People Who Are Terminally Ill
Multiple choice: 1-d, 2-d, 3-d, 4-a, 5-c, 6-d
Matching: 1-b, 2-c, 3-a

Chapter 22: Caring for People Who Are Dying
Multiple choice: 1-c, 2-c, 3-b, 4-b, 5-a, 6-d, 7-b, 8-a
Matching: 1-d, 2-e, 3-b, 4-c, 5-a

Chapter 23: Basic Body Structure and Function
Multiple choice: 1-d, 2-d, 3-c, 4-d
Matching: 1-f, 2-j, 3-a, 4-d, 5-e, 6-c, 7-k, 8-b, 9-h, 10-g, 11-i

Chapter 24: The Integumentary System
Multiple choice: 1-d, 2-c, 3-a, 4-d, 5-b, 6-d, 7-b, 8-a
Matching: 1-g, 2-j, 3-i, 4-f, 5-a, 6-h, 7-e, 8-d, 9-c, 10-b

Chapter 25: The Musculoskeletal System
Multiple choice: 1-b, 2-b, 3-d, 4-b, 5-d, 6-b, 7-d, 8-c, 9-d, 10-c, 11-b, 12-b
Matching: 1-f, 2-c, 3-d, 4-e, 5-b, 6-a

Chapter 26: The Respiratory System
Multiple choice: 1-c, 2-c, 3-d, 4-a, 5-c, 6-a, 7-b, 8-d
Matching: 1-f, 2-g, 3-e, 4-a, 5-d, 6-b, 7-i, 8-c, 9-j, 10-h

Chapter 27: The Cardiovascular System
Multiple choice: 1-a, 2-d, 3-c, 4-d
Matching: 1-g, 2-d, 3-h, 4-j, 5-a, 6-b, 7-c, 8-i, 9-e, 10-f

Chapter 28: The Nervous System
Multiple choice: 1-b, 2-a, 3-b, 4-c, 5-d, 6-c, 7-b, 8-c, 9-c
Matching: 1-g, 2-i, 3-b, 4-h, 5-a, 6-c, 7-e, 8-d, 9-f

Chapter 29: The Sensory System
Multiple choice: 1-b, 2-b, 3-d, 4-c, 5-d, 6-d, 7-a, 8-b, 9-a
Matching: 1-c, 2-b, 3-g, 4-a, 5-e, 6-h, 7-d, 8-f, 9-i, 10-j

Chapter 30: The Endocrine System
Multiple choice: 1-d, 2-a, 3-b, 4-b, 5-d, 6-a
Matching: 1-h, 2-b, 3-c, 4-i, 5-e, 6-f, 7-g, 8-j, 9-a, 10-d

Chapter 31: The Digestive System
Multiple choice: 1-c, 2-d, 3-c, 4-a, 5-a, 6-d, 7-a, 8-a, 9-c

Chapter 32: The Urinary System
Multiple choice: 1-b, 2-d, 3-c, 4-a, 5-a, 6-a, 7-d, 8-b, 9-b
Matching: 1-e, 2-d, 3-a, 4-b, 5-c

Chapter 33: The Reproductive System
Multiple choice: 1-d, 2-b, 3-a, 4-c
Matching: 1-c, 2-e, 3-f, 4-h, 5-a, 6-g, 7-b, 8-d, 9-j, 10-i

Chapter 34: Caring for People With Developmental Disabilities
Multiple choice: 1-b, 2-b, 3-a, 4-b, 5-c, 6-a, 7-c, 8-b, 9-b, 10-a

Chapter 35: Caring for People With Mental Illness
Multiple choice: 1-c, 2-b, 3-c, 4-a, 5-b, 6-b, 7-a
Matching: 1-e, 2-b, 3-d, 4-c, 5-g, 6-f, 7-a

Chapter 36: Caring for People With Dementia
Multiple choice: 1-d, 2-a, 3-b, 4-c, 5-d, 6-d, 7-a, 8-b, 9-a, 10-d

Chapter 37: Caring for People With Cancer
Multiple choice: 1-a, 2-d, 3-b
Matching: 1-c, 2-e, 3-a, 4-f, 5-b, 6-g, 7-d

Chapter 38: Caring for People With HIV/AIDS
Multiple choice: 1-d, 2-a, 3-d, 4-b, 5-b

Chapter 39: Caring for Surgical Patients
Multiple choice: 1-b, 2-d, 3-d, 4-c, 5-a, 6-c, 7-b, 8-a

Chapter 40: Caring for Mothers and Newborns
Multiple choice: 1-c, 2-c, 3-d, 4-c, 5-d, 6-d, 7-b, 8-a
Matching: 1-b, 2-c, 3-a

Chapter 41: Caring for Pediatric Patients
Multiple choice: 1-b, 2-d, 3-a, 4-c
Matching: 1-c, 2-e, 3-d, 4-a, 5-b

Chapter 42: Introduction to Home Health Care
Multiple choice: 1-a, 2-c, 3-c, 4-d, 5-c, 6-a
Matching: 1-b, 2-e, 3-f, 4-a, 5-c, 6-d

Chapter 43: Safety and Infection Control in the Home Health Care Setting
Multiple choice: 1-b, 2-a, 3-c, 4-b, 5-b, 6-b

Introduction to the Language of Health Care

All professions have their own sets of words and abbreviations that are used to describe objects and situations that are specific to that particular profession. The health care profession is no different. In fact, the health care profession has so many unique words and abbreviations, you might think that health care professionals are speaking a different language from everyone else!

Understanding the words and abbreviations that are unique to the health care profession is essential if you expect to be able to communicate effectively with the other members of the health care team. Not knowing these words and abbreviations will make it difficult for you to read and follow orders for patient or resident care. In addition, you will need to know these words and abbreviations to accurately record and report.

In this appendix, you will learn some tricks that will allow you to figure out the meaning of many unfamiliar words you may hear or read. We will also introduce you to some commonly used medical words and abbreviations. Finally, you should always make it a point to look up new words or abbreviations in a medical dictionary as soon as you hear or read them. Or, you can ask the nurse to explain the meaning of the word or abbreviation to you. Before long, you will become very comfortable using and understanding the language of the health care profession!

MEDICAL TERMINOLOGY

Although the strange-sounding language of the health care profession may seem overwhelming at first, it is really quite easy to pick up. Some medical words come from the names of people (for example, Down syndrome, Alzheimer's disease, Parkinson's disease, Papanicolaou smear). Other words come from Greek or Latin words, just as many everyday English, Spanish, French, and Italian words do. For example, you know what a rhinoceros looks like, right? A rhinoceros is a large animal with a huge horn growing out of its nose (Fig. B-1). *Rhin-* comes from the Greek word for "nose," and *-ceros* comes from the Greek word *keras*, or "horn." Now where else might you find the Greek word *rhin-*? Well, if the mucous membranes on the inside of your nose are inflamed because you have a cold or allergies, the doctor might say that you have *rhinitis* (*rhin-*, nose + *itis*, inflammation). If a movie star has had a "nose job," then her publicist may tell the press that the celebrity has had *rhinoplasty*, the medical term for a nose job (*rhin-*, nose + *-plasty*, surgical repair).

Perhaps you have noticed a pattern here. Big words can be broken down into smaller parts, and if you know the meaning of the individual parts, you can figure out the meaning of the entire word. There are four types of word parts (Fig. B-2):

- **Roots** contain the essential, basic meaning of the word. For example, *cardi-* means "heart." Common roots are listed in Table B-1, at the end of this appendix.
- **Suffixes** are attached to the end of a root to make the root more specific. For example, *carditis* is "inflammation of the heart" (*cardi-*, heart + *-itis*, inflammation). Common suffixes are listed in Table B-2, at the end of this appendix.
- **Prefixes** are attached to the beginning of a root to make the root more specific. For example, *pericarditis* is "inflammation of the sac that surrounds the heart" (*peri-*, around + *cardi-*, heart + *-itis*, inflammation). Common prefixes are listed in Table B-3, at the end of this appendix.
- **Combining vowels** are often added in between the root and the suffix to make the new word easier to pronounce. When a word has more than one root, combining vowels may also be used between the roots. For example, *cardiomyopathy* is "disease of the heart muscle" (*cardi-*, heart + *o* + *my-*,

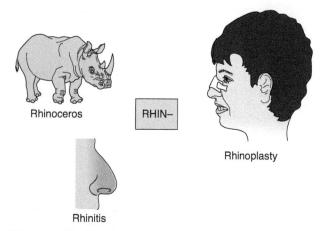

Figure B-1

Many of the words you use in everyday conversation have the same Greek or Latin origins as medical words that you may be less familiar with. For example, the Greek word *rhin-* means "nose." You see *rhin-* in words such as *rhinoceros, rhinitis,* and *rhinoplasty.* When you are trying to figure out the meaning of a new medical word, think about similar-sounding words that you may already know!

muscle + *o* + *-pathy,* disease). The combining vowel is usually "o," but "a" or "i" may also be used sometimes. The combining vowel that is used most often with each root is listed in Table B-1.

You will come across many medical words as you study each chapter in this textbook. When you come across a term in your reading that is new to you, try using what you have learned about the different word parts to guess the

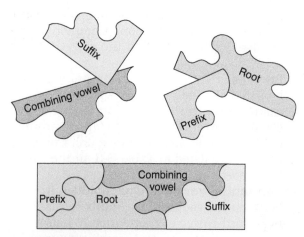

Figure B-2

Big words can be broken down into smaller parts, and if you know the meaning of the individual parts, then you can figure out the meaning of the entire word.

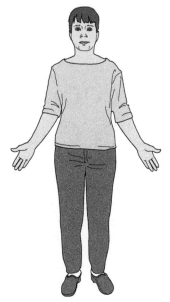

Figure B-3

When describing the location of one part of the body in relation to another, we imagine the body to be in normal anatomical position. In normal anatomical position, the person is standing upright, facing forward, with the legs slightly apart and the arms at the sides, with the palms facing forward.

word's meaning. Then look up the word in the glossary and see how well you did!

ANATOMICAL TERMS

Anatomy is the study of the structure of the body. To describe the location of one body part in relation to another, health care professionals use specific terms. To ensure that these terms always have the same meaning to everyone, we always imagine the body to be in *normal anatomical position* when we describe it. A person who is in normal anatomical position is standing upright and facing forward, with his feet slightly spread apart, and with his arms to the sides and the palms facing forward (Fig. B-3). *Anatomical planes* are used as standard points of reference when describing the body. A *plane* is a flat surface, like a pane of glass. Health care professionals use three main imaginary planes to divide the body (Fig. B-4):

- The **sagittal plane** is a vertical plane that divides the body into right and left sides. A sagittal plane that divides the body into exact right and left halves is sometimes called the *mid-sagittal plane.*

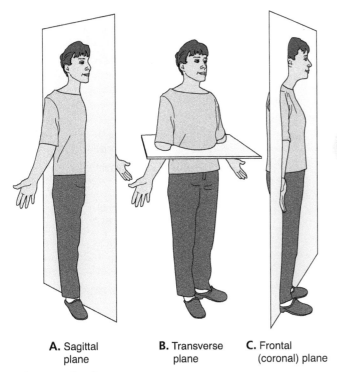

A. Sagittal plane   **B.** Transverse plane   **C.** Frontal (coronal) plane

Figure B-4

The body is divided into imaginary planes, which are used as points of reference when describing the location of one body part with relation to another. **(A)** The sagittal plane is a vertical plane that divides the body into right and left segments. Shown here is the mid-sagittal plane, which divides the body into equal right and left halves. **(B)** The transverse plane is a horizontal plane that divides the body into upper and lower segments. **(C)** The frontal (coronal) plane is a vertical plane that divides the body into front and back segments.

- The **transverse plane** is a horizontal plane that divides the body into upper and lower segments.
- The **frontal (coronal)** plane is a vertical plane that divides the body into front and back segments.

DIRECTIONAL TERMS

When describing the body, health care professionals often need to describe something that is above, under, to the side of, or farther away from something else. To do this, they use standard directional terms. Directional terms are used to describe the location of one body part in relation to another. When we use directional terms, we need a point of reference that stays the same. If not, just changing a person's body position would change a directional reference. This is where normal anatomical position and the anatomical planes come in.

Using the anatomical planes as reference points gives us the following directional terms (Fig. B-5):

- **Medial:** closer to the mid-sagittal plane of the body (toward the inner side). For example, the nose is medial to the eyes.
- **Lateral:** farther away from the mid-sagittal plane of the body (toward the outer side). For example, the ears are lateral to the nose.

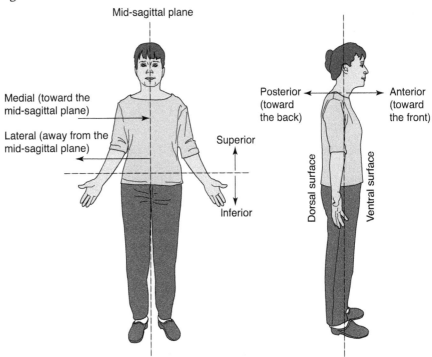

Figure B-5

Directional terms are used to describe the location of one body part in relation to another.

- **Superior:** closer to the top of the body (closer to the head). For example, the chin is superior to the breast.
- **Inferior:** farther away from the top of the body (closer to the feet). For example, the belly button is inferior to the breast.
- **Anterior:** toward the front, or *ventral surface,* of the body. For example, the abdomen is anterior to the buttocks.
- **Posterior:** toward the back, or *dorsal surface,* of the body. For example, the buttocks are posterior to the abdomen.

Two other directional terms are used to describe the location of one body part in relation to another. These terms describe the relationship between parts of the extremities (the arms and legs) and their points of attachment to the body (the shoulders and hips):

- **Proximal:** closer to the point of origin in relation to something else (for example, the elbow is proximal to the wrist)
- **Distal:** farther away from the point of origin in relation to something else (for example, the wrist is distal to the elbow)

Like other words used in the health care profession, many of these directional terms have similar meanings to words you use every day. For example, *distal* sounds like *distant,* or "farther away." Similarly, *proximal* sounds like *proximity,* which means "close by." If you find the terms *ventral* and *dorsal* hard to remember, just think of a shark swimming close to the surface of the water. The shark's dorsal fin, the fin located on the shark's back, is usually visible above the water.

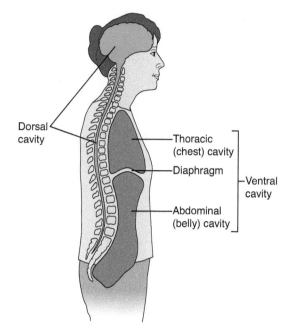

Figure B-6
The body has two major cavities, the dorsal cavity (*blue*) and the ventral cavity (*pink*). The diaphragm divides the ventral cavity into the thoracic (chest) cavity and the abdominal (belly) cavity.

TERMS USED TO DESCRIBE BODY CAVITIES

A *cavity* is a hollow space. In the body, cavities contain organs. There are two major cavities inside the body. The *dorsal cavity,* which contains the brain and spinal cord, is toward the back of the body. The *ventral cavity* is toward the front of the body (Fig. B-6). The ventral cavity is divided by the diaphragm into the *thoracic (chest) cavity* and the *abdominal (belly) cavity.*

- The thoracic cavity contains the lungs, the heart, and the large blood vessels that enter and leave the heart. Most of the esophagus is also contained in the thoracic cavity.
- The upper abdominal cavity contains the stomach, liver, pancreas, spleen, large intes-

tine, and small intestine. The lower abdominal cavity contains the urinary bladder, the rectum, and the female reproductive organs. The kidneys lie behind the abdominal cavity. Sometimes the upper and lower abdominal cavity are referred to together as the *abdominopelvic cavity.*

TERMS USED TO DESCRIBE THE ABDOMINAL AREA

Many patients or residents will experience pain or discomfort in the abdominal area. Often, knowing exactly where the pain or discomfort is occurring can provide clues to the source of the person's symptoms. Therefore, health care professionals use a number of different words to describe the abdominal area. The abdominal area can be described in terms of quadrants (fourths) or regions (Fig. B-7). Quadrants are typically used to describe general information, such as where a person is experiencing pain. Regions are used when it is necessary to be very specific (for example, when describing where an incision is located).

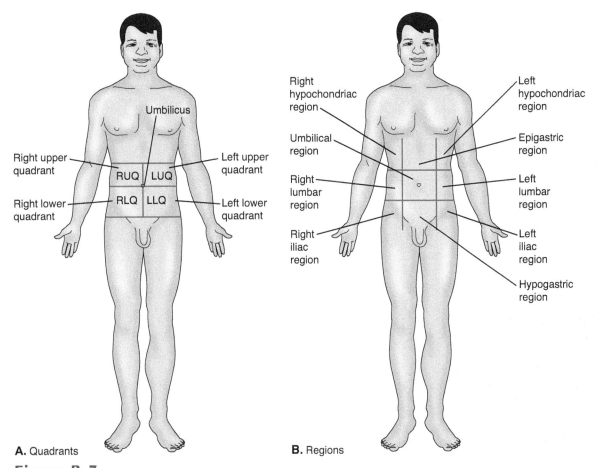

A. Quadrants   **B.** Regions

Figure B-7

The abdominal area can be described in terms of **(A)** quadrants or **(B)** regions. (Remember that when you are using the terms *right* and *left*, these terms are used in relation to the patient's or resident's right or left, not your right or left.)

QUADRANTS

Quad means "four." The simplest way to describe the abdominal area is to divide it into fourths, or quadrants. The quadrants are named according to their location: right upper quadrant (RUQ), left upper quadrant (LUQ), right lower quadrant (RLQ), and left lower quadrant (LLQ). By using these quadrants as reference, you can describe where your patient or resident is experiencing pain by saying, "Mrs. Jones is complaining of a sharp pain in her RUQ."

REGIONS

The abdomen can also be divided into smaller sections, called *regions*, for the purpose of description. There are nine regions (three rows of three):

- The upper row consists of the right and left hypochondriac regions and the epigastric

region. The hypochondriac regions are named for their relationship to the ribs: *hypo-* means "below" and *chondr/o-* means "cartilage" (of the ribs). The epigastric region is named for its relation to the stomach: *epi-* means "above" and *gastric* means "stomach."

- The middle row consists of the right and left lumbar regions and the umbilical region. The right and left lumbar regions are named for the region of the spinal column in that area. The umbilical region is named for the umbilicus, or belly button.

- The lower row consists of the right and left iliac regions and the hypogastric region. The iliac regions are named after the iliac crest, the bone that forms the hip bones. The iliac regions are also sometimes called the inguinal (groin) regions. The hypogastric region is named for its relation to the stomach: *hypo-* means "below" and *gastric* means "stomach."

ABBREVIATIONS

Abbreviations are shortened versions of words or phrases. Health care professionals use abbreviations to make recording more efficient. Some abbreviations come from English words. For example, you just learned that *RUQ* means "right upper quadrant." Other abbreviations come from Latin or Greek words, and therefore may seem foreign at first. For example, *bid* is the abbreviation for "twice daily," from the Latin words **b**is (twice) **i**n (a) **d**ie (day). And *NPO*, which means "nothing by mouth," comes from the Latin words **n**ils (nothing) **p**er (by) **o**s (mouth). As with other terms used in health care, you can often remember the meaning of a new abbreviation by relating it to an everyday word that you already know. For example, *bid, tid,* and *qid* are abbreviations that describe how many times a day an action is to be carried out. The abbreviation *bid* means "twice daily." Now think of how many wheels a *bi*cycle has: two, right? Similarly, the abbreviation *tid* means "three times daily." How many wheels does a *tri*cycle have? *Qid* would mean "four times daily."

Abbreviations that are commonly used in health care settings are listed in Table B-4, at the end of this appendix. Although abbreviations can help us save time and space when recording, it is very important to use only abbreviations that are approved for use in your facility. Otherwise, other members of the health care team may be confused by your meaning. In addition, if you are unsure of the meaning of an abbreviation that you read in a patient's or resident's care plan, please either look the abbreviation up or ask the nurse to explain it to you. It is important not to just guess at the meaning, because guessing could cause harm to the patient or resident.

Some abbreviations are easy to confuse, especially when they are handwritten. For example, *qd* (daily), *qid* (four times a day), and *qod* (every other day) might be easily mistaken for one another. Imagine what could happen if a patient or resident is supposed to receive a medication daily (*qd*) but someone misreads the abbreviation and gives the medication four times a day (*qid*)! To help prevent errors like this from occurring, the Joint Commission on Accreditation of Healthcare Organizations (JCAHO) has published a list of abbreviations that should not be used (Table B-5A; also see Table B-5B). Health care organizations that are accredited by JCAHO or are seeking accreditation will not use these abbreviations.

Table B-1 Common Roots and Their Combining Vowels

ROOT / COMBINING VOWEL	MEANING	ROOT / COMBINING VOWEL	MEANING
abdomin / o	abdomen	choledoch / o	bile duct
aden / o	gland	chondr / o	cartilage
adip / o	fat	col / o	colon
adren / o	adrenal glands	cost / o	ribs
angi / o	vessel (usually blood or lymph)	crani / o	cranium (skull)
arteri / o	artery	cutane / o	skin
arthr / o	joint	cyan / o	blue
blephar / o	eyelid	cyst / o	bladder
bronchi / o	bronchus	dent / o	teeth
calc / o	calcium	dermat / o	skin
carcin / o	cancer	dipl / o	double
cardi / o	heart	electr / o	electric
cephal / o	head	encephal / o	brain
cerebr / o	cerebrum (brain)	enter / o	intestine (usually the small intestine)
chol / e	bile, gall	erythr / o	red
cholecyst / o	gallbladder		

Table B-1 Common Roots and Their Combining Vowels (*Continued*)

ROOT / COMBINING VOWEL	MEANING	ROOT / COMBINING VOWEL	MEANING
esophag / o	esophagus	oste / o	bone
femor / o	femur (thigh bone)	ot / o	ear
gastr / o	stomach	pancreat / o	pancreas
gingiv / o	gum	pelv / i / o	pelvis
gluc / o	sugar, glucose	pharyng / o	pharynx (throat)
glyc / o	sugar, glucose	phleb / o	vein
gynec / o	woman, female	pleur / o	pleura
hemangi / o	blood vessel	pneum / o	lung, air
hemat / o	blood	proct / o	anus, rectum
hepat / o	liver	pyel / o	renal pelvis
hydr / o	water	radi / o	x-rays, radiation
hyster / o	uterus	ren / o	kidney
irid / o	iris	retin / o	retina
lapar / o	abdomen	rhin / o	nose
laryng / o	larynx (voice box)	salping / o	fallopian tube
leuk / o	white	scler / o	hardening, sclera (white of the eye)
lingu / o	tongue	sigmoid / o	sigmoid colon
lip / o	fat	spermat / o	sperm
lith / o	stone, calculus	spin / o	spine
lumb / o	lower back	spondyl / o	vertebra (backbone)
lymphangi / o	lymph vessel	stern / o	sternum (breastbone)
lymph / o	lymph	stomat / o	mouth
mamm / o	breast	tend / o	tendon
mast / o	breast	therm / o	heat
megal / o	enlargement	thorac / o	chest
melan / o	black	thromb / o	blood clot
mening / o	meninges	thyr / o	thyroid gland
men / o	menses, menstruation	toxic, tox / o	poison
muc / o	mucus	trache / o	trachea (windpipe)
myel / o	spinal cord, bone marrow	tympan / o	tympanic membrane (eardrum)
my / o	muscle	ureter / o	ureter
myring / o	tympanic membrane (eardrum)	urethr / o	urethra
nas / o	nose	ur / o	urine
necr / o	death	uter / o	uterus
nephr / o	kidney	vagin / o	vagina
neur / o	nerve	vascul / o	blood vessel
noct / o	night	vas / o	vas deferens, vessel
odont / o	teeth	ven / o	vein
oophor / o	ovary	ventricul / o	ventricle (of brain or heart)
ophthalm / o	eye	vesic / o	bladder
orchi / o	testis	vertebr / o	vertebra (backbone)
os / o	mouth		

Table B-2   Common Suffixes

SUFFIX	MEANING	SUFFIX	MEANING
-al	pertaining to	-oid	resembling
-algia	pain	-oma	tumour
-ar, -ary	pertaining to	-opia	vision
-cele	hernia, swelling	-osis	abnormal condition
-centesis	surgical puncture	-pathy	disease
-cyte	cell	-pause	cessation
-derma	skin	-penia	decrease
-dipsia	thirst	-pepsia	digestion
-ectomy	excision, removal of	-pexy	fixation
-edema	swelling	-phagia	swallow, eat
-emesis	vomiting	-phasia	speech
-emia	blood	-phobia	fear
-gram	record	-plasty	surgical repair
-graphy	process of recording	-plegia	paralysis
-ia	condition	-pnea	breathing
-ic	pertaining to	-rrhaphy	suture
-ism	condition	-rrhea	flow, discharge
-ist	specialist	-scope	instrument to view
-it is	inflammation	-scopy	visual examination
-lith	stone, calculus	-stenosis	structure, narrowing
-logist	specialist in the study of	-stomy	forming a new opening
-logy	study of	-therapy	treatment
-lysis	separation, destruction, loosening	-tome	instrument to cut
-malacia	softening	-tomy	incision, cut into
-megaly	enlargement	-tripsy	crushing
-meter	measure, instrument for measuring	-uria	urine, urination

Table B-3   Common Prefixes

PREFIX	MEANING	PREFIX	MEANING
a-, an-	without, not, absent	macro-	large
ab	away from	micro-	small
amb-, ambi-	both, on two sides	neo-	new
auto-	self	para-	near, beside, around
bi-	two, double	peri-	around
brady-	slow	poly-	many, much
dys-	bad, painful, difficult	post-	after, behind
epi-	above, upon	pre-	before
hemi-	half, partly	quadri-	four
hyper-	excessive	sub-	under, below
hypo-	under, below	supra-	above
inter-	between	tachy-	rapid
intra-	within	tri-	three

Table B-4 Common Medical Abbreviations

ABBREVIATION	MEANING	ABBREVIATION	MEANING
ab	antibody	disch	discharge
abd	abdomen	DJD	degenerative joint disease
ac	before a meal	DNR	do not resuscitate
ADLs	activities of daily living	DOA	dead on arrival
ad lib	as desired	DOB	date of birth
Adm (adm)	admitted or admission	DON	director of nursing
AFB	acid-fast bacillus (usually tuberculosis)	drsg	dressing
AIDS	acquired immunodeficiency syndrome	Dx	diagnosis
AKA	above-the-knee amputation	ECG (EKG)	electrocardiogram
AM (am)	morning	EEG	electroencephalogram
amb	ambulate, ambulatory	ER	emergency room
AMI	acute myocardial infarction (heart attack)	F	Fahrenheit
		FBS	fasting blood sugar
amt	amount	FF	force fluids
ap	apical	fl (fld)	fluid
approx	approximately	ft	foot or feet
ASAP	as soon as possible	Fx	fracture
as tol	as tolerated	gal	gallon
ax	axillary	GB	gallbladder
bid	twice a day	GI	gastrointestinal
BKA	below-the-knee amputation	GSW	gunshot wound
BM (bm)	bowel movement	GU	genitourinary
BP, B/P	blood pressure	h (hr)	hour
B.R.	bed rest	H_2O	water
BRP	bathroom privileges	HBV	hepatitis B virus
BSC	bedside commode	HIV	human immunodeficiency virus
C	centigrade, Celsius	HOB	head of bed
c̄	with	HS (hs)	hour of sleep (bedtime)
CA	cancer	ht	height
cath	catheter, catheterize	ICU	intensive care unit
CBC	complete blood count	IDDM	insulin-dependent diabetes mellitus
CBR	complete bed rest	in	inch
cc	cubic centimetre	I&O	intake and output
CCU	coronary care unit	IV	intravenous
CHD	coronary heart disease	L	left, litre
CHF	congestive heart failure	lab	laboratory
cl liq	clear liquids	lb	pound
c/o	complains of	lg	large
COPD	chronic obstructive pulmonary disease	liq	liquid
CPR	cardiopulmonary resuscitation	LLQ	left lower quadrant
CVA	cerebral vascular accident (stroke)	LMP	last menstrual period
dc (d/c)	discontinue		

(continued)

Table B-4   Common Medical Abbreviations (*Continued*)

ABBREVIATION	MEANING	ABBREVIATION	MEANING
lt	left	qt	quiet
LUQ	left upper quadrant	R	rectal
meds	medications	RBC	red blood cell, red blood cell count
MI	myocardial infarction (heart attack)	rehab	rehabilitation
mid noc	midnight	resp	respiration
min	minute	RLQ	right lower quadrant
mL	millilitre	ROM	range of motion
NB	newborn	RR	recovery room
neg	negative	rt (R)	right
nil	none	RT	respiratory therapy
no	number	RUQ	right upper quadrant
noc, noct	night	Rx	treatment
NPO (npo)	nothing per mouth (nils per os)	$\bar{s}$	without
N&V	nausea and vomiting	$\bar{ss}$	half
O_2	oxygen	SOB	shortness of breath
OB	obstetrics	Spec (spec)	specimen
OJ	orange juice	SSE	soapsuds enema
OOB	out of bed	ST	speech therapy
O	oral	STAT, stat	at once, immediately
OR	operating room	STI	sexually transmitted infection
OT	occupational therapy	Surg	surgery
oz (Oz)	ounce	Sx	symptoms
PAR	post-anesthesia recovery	tbsp	tablespoon
pc	after a meal	tid	three times a day
Peds	pediatrics	TIA	transient ischemic attack
per	by, through	TLC	tender loving care
PM (pm)	afternoon or evening	TPN	total parenteral nutrition
po (per os)	by mouth	TPR	temperature, pulse, and respirations
post op	postoperative	tsp	teaspoon
pre op	preoperative	Tx	treatment
prep	preparation	ty	tympanic
prn	as necessary	UA (u/a)	urinalysis
Pt (pt)	patient	UK	unknown
PT	physical therapy	URI	upper respiratory infection
q	every	UTI	urinary tract infection
qd	every day	VS (vs)	vital signs
qh	every hour	WA	while awake
q2h, q3h, q4h, etc.	every 2 hours, every 3 hours, every 4 hours, etc.	WBC	white blood cell, white blood cell count
qhs	every night at bedtime	w/c	wheelchair
qid	four times a day	WNL	within normal limits
qod	every other day	wt	weight
qs	sufficient quantity		

Table B-5A The Joint Commission's Official "Do Not Use" List

DO NOT USE	POTENTIAL PROBLEM	USE INSTEAD
U (unit)	Mistaken for "0" (zero), the number "4" (four), or "cc"	Write "unit"
IU (International Unit)	Mistaken for IV (intravenous) or the number 10 (ten)	Write "International Unit"
Q.D., QD, q.d., qd (daily)	Mistaken for each other	Write "daily"
Q.O.D., QOD, q.o.d, qod (every other day)	Period after the Q mistaken for "I" and the "O" mistaken for "I"	Write "every other day"
Trailing zero (X.0 mg)	Decimal point is missed	Write X mg
*Lack of leading zero (.X mg)		Write 0.X mg
MS	Can mean morphine sulfate or magnesium sulfate	Write "morphine sulfate"
MSO_4 and $MgSO_4$	Confused for one another	Write "magnesium sulfate"

This list applies to all orders and all medication-related documentation that is handwritten (including free-text computer entry) or on preprinted forms.
*Exception: A "trailing zero" may be used only where required to demonstrate the level of precision of the value being reported, such as for laboratory results, imaging studies of lesions, or catheter/tube sizes. It may not be used in medication orders or other mdication-related documentation.
Source: The Joint Commission on Accreditation of Healthcare Organizations (2006).

Table B-5B Additional Abbreviations, Acronyms, and Symbols for Possible Future Inclusion in the Official "Do Not Use" List

DO NOT USE	POTENTIAL PROBLEM	USE INSTEAD
> (greater than)	Misinterpreted as the number "7"(seven) or the letter "L"	Write "greater than"
< (less than)	Confused for one another	Write "less than"
Abbreviations for drug names	Misinterpreted due to similar abbreviations for multiple drugs	Write drug names in full
Apothecary units	Unfamiliar to many practitioners Confused with metric units	Use metric units
@	Mistaken for the number "2" (two)	Write "at"
cc	Mistaken for U (units) when poorly written	Write "mL" or "millilitres"
μg	Mistaken for mg (milligrams), resulting in one thousand-fold overdose	Write "mcg" or "micrograms"

Source: The Joint Commission on Accreditation of Healthcare Organizations (2006).

Index

Note: A t following a page number indicates tabular material, an f indicates a figure, a p indicates procedure material, and a b indicates a boxed feature.

A

Abandonment, 799, 799f
Abbreviations, medical, 842
  common, 845t–846t
  "Do Not Use" List of, 842, 847t
  "Do Not Use" List of, additional, 842, 847t
ABC fire extinguisher, 155, 155f
ABCs of emergency care, 216, 217b
Abdominal area terminology, 840–842, 841f
  quadrants in, 841, 841f
  regions in, 841–842, 841f
Abdominal cavity, 840, 840f
Abdominal thrusts
  in conscious adults, children >1 year, 224p
  general points on, 221–222
Abdominopelvic cavity, 840, 840f
Abduction, 510t
Abduction pillow, 516, 517f
Absence seizure, 219
Absorption, 372
  by digestive system, 636–637, 637f
  by skin, 485
Abuse, 51–52
  elder, 52
  home health care and, 806
  perpetrators of, 52
  physical, 51
  psychological (emotional), 51
  reporting of, 52
  risk factors for, 51–52
  sexual, 51
  signs of, 52b
Accessory structures, 482–484, 483f
Accidents, 161–166. See also specific accidents
  in home health care, 804–806
  preventing, 163–165
    burns, 165
    falls, 163, 163f, 164b–165b
    poisonings, 165
  reporting of, 166, 167f
  risk factors in, 161–163, 161f
    limited awareness of surroundings, 162
    medication, 162
    mobility, poor, 162
    paralysis, 162
    sensory impairment, 162
Accountability, 28
Acquired immunodeficiency syndrome (AIDS), 134, 135f
Acromegaly, 625–626, 626f
Active-assistive range-of-motion exercises, 523–524
Active range-of-motion (AROM) exercises, 523

Activities of daily living (ADLs). See also specific disorders
  with AIDS, 734, 734f
  with dementia, 711–713, 711f
  with developmental disability, 687
  with mental illness, 700
Activity therapy, for dementia, 716–717, 716f
Acute illness, 81
Acute pain, 599
Addison's disease, 626
Adduction, 510t
Adjustable beds, 241–243, 242f, 243f
Admissions, 251–257
  admissions process in, 252–253, 253f
  definition of, 251
  making patient/resident feel welcome in, 253
  nursing history in, 253, 254f–255f
  room preparation for, 253, 256, 256f
  sensitivity in, 251–252, 252f
  welcoming new resident in, 251–252, 252f
    communication skills in, 257
    decorating room in, 257
    greeting and introduction in, 256, 256f
    room preparation in, 253, 256, 256f
    settling into new home in, 256, 257f
Admission sheet, 69, 252, 253f
Adolescents, 87–88, 88f
  emotional needs in, 783, 783f
  physical needs in, 782–783
  safety needs in, 783
Adrenal cortex, 624
Adrenal gland disorders, 626–627, 626f
Adrenal gland function, 624, 624f
Adrenal glands, 620, 621f
Adrenaline, for shock, 220, 221f
Adrenocorticotropic hormone (ACTH), 622, 622f
Adrenocorticotropic hormone (ACTH) excess, in Cushing's syndrome, 626–627, 626f
Adulthood
  later, 89, 89f
  middle, 88, 88f
  older, 89, 89f
  young, 88, 88f
Advance directives, 440–442, 442f
Aerobic bacteria, 105
Afferent, 648, 650f
Afterlife, 451
Afternoon care, 315
Against medical advice (AMA), 258
Age
  on accident risk, 161–162
  on disease risk, 471

"Age spots," 486, 486f
Aging. *See specific topics*
Agitation, 709, 709f
Agoraphobia, 696
AIDS. *See HIV/AIDS*
AIDS awareness, 732–733, 732f
AIDS dementia, 706t
Airborne diseases, 136–138
Airborne pathogens, 136–138
    definition of, 136
    in sneeze, 136–137, 137f
    tuberculosis as, 137–138, 138f
Airborne precautions, 118–119, 120b
Airflow beds, 492–493, 493f
Airway
    definition of, 541
    in emergency care, 217b
    larynx, 542, 542f
    nasal cavity, 541, 542f
    pharynx, 541–542, 542f
    purpose of, 541
    trachea and bronchi, 542, 542f, 543f
Airway obstruction, 220–222, 222f
Airway obstruction clearing, 222f, 224p–229p
    in adults and children >1 year, 221–222, 222f
    in conscious
        adults and children >1 year, chest thrusts,
            226p
        infants, 227p–228p
    in infants, 222
    in unconscious
        adults and children >1 year, foreign body, 225p
        infants, 228p–229p
Alcohol abuse, 692, 694f
    fetal alcohol syndrome from, 684
    in residents, 694f
Alcohol-based hand rubs, 116, 809, 810f
Alcohol intake, in personal support worker, 30, 30f
Aldosterone, 624, 624f
Alignment, body, 141–142, 142f, 182, 182f
Alopecia, 355, 725–726, 726f
Alternating pressure beds, 493, 493f
Alveoli (alveolus), 542–543
    definition of, 181, 216
    in emphysema, 548
    gas exchange in, 544, 544f
    structure of, 543f
Alzheimer's disease, 705–707
    brain scan of, 705f
    causes of, 705–706, 706t
    plaques and tangles in, 705, 706f
    stages of, 707b
Ambulate, 189
Ambulation assistance, 189–191
    devices for, 190t, 191
    guidelines for, 191b
    post-operative, 753
    procedure for, 209p–210p
AM care, 315
Amebic dysentery, 106t, 107
Amenorrhea, 665
Amino acids, 374
Amplitude, pulse, 286
Amputation, 521–522, 522f
    from diabetes, 522f
    prosthetic devices after, 522, 522f
Amyotrophic lateral sclerosis (ALS), 591

Anaerobic bacteria, 105
Anaesthesia, surgical, 742–743
    general, 742–743
    local, 743
    regional, 743
Anaphylactic shock, 220
Anatomical planes, 838–839, 839f
Anatomical position, 838
Anatomical position, normal, 838, 838f
Anatomical terms, 838–840. *See also specific terms*
Anatomy, 465, 838
Androgens, 624, 624f
Anemia, 574–575, 575f
Anger, 437, 438t
Angina pectoris, 577
Angioplasty, balloon, 577, 579f
Ankle restraint, 173–174, 176p
Anorexia, 379
Anorexia nervosa, 697, 698f
Answers, to *What Did You Learn?* exercises,
    835–836
Antepartum (prenatal) period, 760–763
    complications in, 762
    definition of, 760
    emotional needs in, 762–763, 763f
    humanist health care in, 761
    phases (trimesters) of, 760, 761f
    physical needs in, 762
    routine care in, 760–761
Anterior, 839f, 840
Anterior chamber, 601, 602f
Antibiotics, 109
Antibodies, 109
Antidiuretic hormone (ADH), 621,
    622f
Anti-embolism stockings, 752, 755p–756p
Antimicrobial agents, 109
Antiperspirant, 323
Antisepsis, 112, 113f
Anuria, 405
Anus, 635f, 636
Anxiety disorders, 695–696
    definition and scope of, 695, 697
    obsessive-compulsive disorder, 695–696
    panic disorder, 695, 695f, 697
    phobias, 696
Aortic valve, 570, 570f
Aphasia, from stroke, 589
Apical pulse, 285f, 286–287
    measurement procedure for, 304p
    in newborn, 767
Aponeurosis, 509
Appearance, personal, 31–32, 32f, 33b
Appendages, 482, 483–484, 483f
Appendicitis, 636
Appendix, 635f, 636
Appetite
    definition of, 378–379
    loss of, 379
    taste and smell on, 601
Aqueous humor, 602, 602f
Arachnoid mater, 584
Areola, 766
Arteries, 285, 567, 568f
    aging on, 574
    pulse in, 285, 285f
    structure of, 567, 567f

Arterioles, 567, 568f
Arteriosclerosis, 576
Arthritis, 515–517
    gout, 517
    joint replacement with, 516–517, 516f, 517f
    osteoarthritis, 515–517
    overview and definition of, 515
    rheumatoid, 517, 517f
Ascending colon, 635, 635f
Ascorbic acid, 373t
Asepsis
    medical, 112–116
        antisepsis in, 112, 113f
        definition of, 112
        disinfection in, 112–113, 113f
        handwashing in, 115–116, 115f, 119b,
            122p–123p
        sanitization in, 112–113, 113f, 114b
        sterilization in, 112–113, 113f
    surgical, 116
As-needed care, 315
Aspiration, 221
Aspiration pneumonia, 546
Assault, 50, 50f
Assessment, in nursing process, 76
Assisted-living facilities. *See also specific topics*
    definition and function of, 9, 9f
    resident's unit in, 238, 238f
Assistive devices. *See also specific devices*
    in rehabilitation, 475, 476f
    for walking, 189–191, 190t, 191b
Asthma, 547–548, 548f
Astigmatism, 602, 602f, 603, 603f
Atelectasis, 750, 751f
Atherosclerosis, 575–576, 575f
Athlete's foot, 106t, 107
Atria, 569, 570f, 571f
Atrophy, 513, 513f
Attitude, 26–27
Auricle, 609, 610f
Autism, 683
Automated sphygmomanometers, 293
Autonomy, 53
Autopsy, 455
Axillary temperature, 284, 301p–302p
Axon, 583, 583f

B

Bacilli, 105, 105f
Back
    lifting safety for, 142–144, 144f, 145b–146b
    nursing injuries to, 142–143
Back supports, 144, 144f
Bacteria, 105, 105f, 106t
    aerobic, 105
    anaerobic, 105
Bag bath, 327, 328f
Bag technique, 807–808, 807f
Balance
    in body mechanics, 142, 143f
    ear in, 610
    emotional, 692, 692f
    fluid, 388–389, 484
Balanced diet, 375
Baldness, 355
Balloon angioplasty, 577
Balloons, as suffocation risk

in preschoolers, 781
in toddlers, 778
Barium, 639
Barium enema, 639, 640f
Barrel chest, 548
Barrier, 116
Barrier methods, 116–118
    gloves, 117, 117f, 119b, 123p
    gowns, 117, 119b, 124p–125p
    masks, 117–118, 118f, 119b, 126p
    personal protective equipment, 116
    personal protective equipment, removing multiple
        articles of, 118, 127p
    protective eyewear, 118, 118f, 119b
Basic human needs, 89–94. *See also* Needs, basic
    human
Basic life support (BLS) measures, 216–217, 217b
Bath blanket, 24, 265
Bathing, 322–328
    bag bath in, 327, 328f
    bed bath technique in, 326–327, 328f
        complete, 340p–342p
        partial, 342p–343p
    frequency and method of, 323
    guidelines for, 324, 325b–326b
    humanistic care in, 327–328
    of newborns, 770–771, 771f
    purposes of, 322
    shower chair in, 326, 327f, 795, 795f
    standard techniques for, 324
    supplies for, 323–324
    tub bath or shower technique for, 326, 327f,
        338p–339p
    whirlpool tubs for, 326, 327f
Bath mitt, 324, 324f
Bath oils, 323
Bathrooms, in health care facilities, 236, 237f
Battery, 50
Bed, 241–244, 243f
    adjustable, 241–243, 243f
    adjustment of, 243, 243f
    airflow, 492–493, 493f
    alternating pressure, 493, 493f
    casters of, 243
    Circ-O-Lectric, 493–494, 493f
    closed (unoccupied), 269–270, 270f,
        272p–274p
    gatches in, 242, 242f
    linens for, 263–265 (*See also* Linens, bed)
    mattress positions in, 242–243, 242f
    occupied, 270f, 271, 274p–276p
    open, 270, 270f
    regular (nonadjustable), 243–244
    side rails of, 242f, 243
    sitting on edge of, 191, 208p–209p
    surgical, 270, 270f
    wheels and wheel locks on, 243, 244f
Bed bath, 326–327, 328f
    complete, 340p–342p
    partial, 342p–343p
Bed cradle, 265, 265f
Bed linens, 263–265
    bath blanket, 265
    bed protectors, 264
    bedspreads, 264
    blankets, 264
    bottom and top sheets, 263

Bed linens (continued)
   draw sheets, 264, 264f
   for evacuating bedridden, 154, 155b
   handling of, 265–266, 266f, 267b–268b
   lift sheet, 264
   mattress pads, 263
   pillows and pillowcases, 264
Bedmaking, 263–276
   bed cradle in, 265, 265f
   footboard in, 265, 265f
   linen handling in, 265–266, 266f, 267b–268b
   linens in, 263–265 (See also Bed linens)
   pressure-relieving mattress in, 265
   techniques for
      for closed (unoccupied beds), 269–270,
         272p–274p
      guidelines for, 269b
      humanistic health care for, 271
      mitered corner in, 258f, 268–269
      for occupied beds, 271, 274p–276p
      for open beds, 270
Bed monitoring system, pressure-sensitive, 172f, 173
Bedpans, 398, 399f, 420p–421p
Bed protectors, 264
Bedside commode, 398, 398f
Bedside table, 244, 245f
Bed sores, 180, 181f, 487–494. See also Pressure
      ulcers
Bedspreads, 264
Bed transfers
   from bed to wheelchair
      one worker, 200p–202p
      two workers, 202p
   to stretcher, 204p–205p
   to/from stretcher, 188
   to/from wheelchair, 188
      one worker, 188
      two workers, 188
   from wheelchair, 203p–204p
Beliefs
   culture on, 94
   spiritual, 95
Bell, stethoscope, 286f, 287
Belly cavity, 840, 840f
Belt restraint, 174
Beneficence, 53
Benign tumour, 721–722
Biceps muscle, 509–511, 511f, 512f
Bicuspid valve, 570, 570f
bid, 842, 845t
Bile, 636
Binging, 697
Biological death, 216
Biopsy
   for cancer, 724f, 725
   of reproductive system, 667
Bipolar disorder, 697
Birthing suite, 237f
Bisexual, 92
Bladder, 649, 650f
Bladder infection, 652
Bladder muscle tone, 651
Bladder outlet, 649
Bladder training, 413–414
Bladder tumours, 654–655, 656f
Blankets, 264
Bleeding, uncontrolled severe, 220

Bleeding disorders, 574–575
Blindness, 605–606, 606f, 607b–608b
Blood, 565–567, 566f, 575f
Bloodborne diseases, 131–136. See also specific
      diseases
   in body fluids, 131
   CCOHS Bloodborne Pathogens Standard for, 136,
      136b
   hepatitis, 131–134, 132f, 133f (See also Hepatitis)
   HIV/AIDS, 134, 135t, 673, 731–736 (See also
      HIV/AIDS)
   protecting yourself from, 134–136, 136b
   transmission of, 131
Bloodborne pathogens
   definition of, 131 (See also specific pathogens)
   transmission via, 131
Bloodborne transmission, 131
Blood cells, 565–567, 566f
   aging on number of, 574
   muscle production of, 512
   red, 565–566, 566f
      impaired production of, 574
      increased destruction of, 574
   white, 108, 108f, 566, 566f
Blood disorders, 574–576, 575f
Blood flow, resistance to, 289
Blood glucose
   high, 627 (See also Diabetes mellitus)
   low, 627
   monitoring of, 627, 628f
Blood loss, chronic, 574
Blood pH, 651
Blood pressure, 289–294
   abnormal and normal findings in, 293–294
   in children, 296t
   definition of, 289
   diastolic, 289
   factors in, 289
   measurement of, 290–293
      automated sphygmomanometers in, 293
      bulb in, 290, 290f
      cuff in, 290f, 290t
      guidelines for, 292b
      Korotkoff sounds in, 291, 291b
      manometer in, 290, 290f
      manual sphygmomanometers in, 290–292, 290f
      procedure for, 290–293, 305p–306p
      stethoscope in, 291
   in newborn, 767, 767f
   systolic, 289
Blood spills, 119b
Blood sugar, 374
Blood vessel disorders, 575–576
   atherosclerosis, 575–576, 575f
   venous, 576
Blood vessels, 567, 567f
Blood volume, on blood pressure, 289
Body
   of stomach, 634–635, 635f
   of uterus, 663
Body alignment, 141–142, 142f, 182, 182f
Body cavity terms, 840, 840f
Body fluids
   bloodborne diseases in, 131
   definition of, 131
   spills of, 119b
Body language, 62, 62f

Body mechanics, 141–142
    alignment in, 141–142, 142f, 182, 182f
    balance in, 142, 143f
    coordinated body movement in, 142, 143f
    guidelines for injury protection in,
        145b–146b
Body movement, coordinated, 142, 143f
Body powder, 323
Body structure and function, 465–472
    cells in, 466–467, 467f
    health and disease in, 469–471
    organization of, 466–469, 466f
    organs in, 468–469
    organ systems in, 469, 470f
    tissues in, 467–468, 467f, 468t
Body temperature. See Temperature, body
Bonding period, 764, 764f
Bones
    flat, 506, 508f
    irregular, 506, 508f
    layers of, 506–507, 508f
    long, 506, 508f
Bony prominences, 487, 488f
Booster seat, 781
Booties, heel, 492, 492f
Bottom sheets, 263
Bowel elimination, 414–419
    bowel habits in, 414
    enema administration for, 417–418, 418f,
        428p–429p
    enema for, 416–418, 417f, 418f
    feces in, 414
    normal, 414, 414f
    problems with
        constipation, 415
        diarrhea, 414–415
        fecal impaction, 415, 416f
        fecal incontinence, 416–417
        flatulence, 415–416, 416f
    rectal suppositories for, 418
Bowel habits, 414
Bowel incontinence, 416–417
Bowman's capsule, 648, 650f
Bradycardia, 287
Bradypnea, 288
Braille, 606, 606f
Brain, 584–585, 585f
Brainstem, 584–585
Breaking point, 692
Breast cancer, 666, 666f
Breastfeeding, 766, 766f
Breasts, 663, 663f
Breast self-exam (BSE), 666, 666f
Breathing, 287–288. See also Cardiopulmonary
        resuscitation (CPR); Respiration
    deep, postoperative therapeutic, 750, 751f
    in emergency care, 217b
    exhalation in, 287–288
    functions of, 287–288
    inhalation in, 287
    process of, 287–288
    rescue, 216, 217b, 225p
Briefs, incontinence, 412–413, 413f
Bronchiole, 542, 542f–544f
Bronchitis, 546
Bronchitis, chronic, 548–549
Bronchoscopy

for cancer, 725
for lung cancer, 549, 550f
Bronchus (bronchi), 542, 542f, 543f
Bruises, from restraints, 169
Brushing
    hair (See Hair care)
    teeth, 330p–331p
Buddhism, death and dying practices in, 452t
Bulb, sphygmomanometer, 290, 290f
Bulimia nervosa, 697
Burns, 497–498. See also Wound
    from electrical appliances, 150, 152f, 165
    first-degree, 497
    prevention of, 165 (See also Fire safety)
    second-degree, 497
    third-degree, 497–498, 498f

C
Calcitonin, 622, 623
Calcium
    dietary, 373t
    muscle storage of, 511–512
    parathyroid hormone on, 623
Calcium salts, 652
Calculi, renal, 652–653, 653f
Call light system, 245–246, 246f
Calories, 372
Canada Health Act, 5–6, 6b
Canada Privacy Act, 51
Canada's Food Guide, 375, 376f–377f
Canadian Centre for Occupational Health and Safety
        (CCOHS), on hepatitis B virus, 133–134, 133f
Canadian Charter of Rights and Freedoms, 46
Canadian Human Rights Law, 35
Cancer, 721–728. See also specific types
    benign tumours in, 721–722
    care for
        emotional needs in, 727–728
        physical needs in, 726–727
    causes of, 722–723
    of cervix, 666
    definition of, 721
    detection of, 723
    of digestive system, 639
    humanistic health care for, 726
    malignant tumours in, 722
    metastasis of, 722, 722f
    of ovary, 666
    prognosis in, 728
    routine exams and screening for, 724–725, 724f
    structure of, 721, 721f
    treatment of, 725–726
        chemotherapy in, 725–726, 725f, 726f
        radiation therapy in, 725f, 726
        side effects from, 726
        surgery in, 724
    types of, 722
    warning signs of, 723–724, 723f
Cane, 190t
Capillaries, 567
Capillary bed, 567, 568f
Carbohydrates, 374
Carbon dioxide, on breathing, 287
Carcinogens, 722
Cardiac arrest, 216
Cardiac contraction, aging on, 574
Cardiac cycle, 572–573

Cardiac muscle, 468, 468t
Cardiac output, on blood pressure, 289
Cardiac rehabilitation, 579
Cardiac risk factors, 576
Cardiac sphincter, 634–635, 634f
Cardiogenic shock, 220
Cardiopulmonary resuscitation (CPR), 216
Cardiovascular complication prevention,
        postoperative, 751–752
    anti-embolism stockings in, 752, 755p–756p
    leg exercises in, 752, 752f
    sequential compression device for, 751–752, 751f
    for thrombophlebitis and pulmonary embolism, 751
Cardiovascular system, 469, 470f, 565–574
    aging on, 573–574
    function of, 571–573
        protection, 573
        regulation, 573
        transport, 571–573
    immobility on, 181f, 182
    structure of, 565–571 (See also specific structures)
        blood, 565–567, 566f
        blood vessels, 567, 567f, 568f
        heart, 569–571
        lymphatic system, 567–569
Cardiovascular system disorders, 574–579
    blood, 574–575, 575f
    blood vessel, 575–576
        atherosclerosis, 575–576, 575f
        venous, 576
    cardiac rehabilitation for, 579
    diagnosis of, 578–579, 579f
    heart, 576–578
        angina pectoris, 577
        conduction disorders and pacemakers, 578, 578f
        coronary artery disease, 577
            development of, 577
            risk factors for, 576
        heart failure, 577–578
        myocardial infarction, 577, 577f
        risk factors for, 576
Care plan, 75. See also specific disorders
Caries, 316
Carrier
    HBV, 133
    for infants, 778
Car seat
    for infants, 772, 772f, 778
    for preschoolers, 781
    for toddlers, 780
Cartilage
    definition of, 507
    in joints, 509f
    tracheal, 542
Case manager, 793
Cast care, 520b
Casters, bed, 242f, 243, 243f
Castile soap, 417
Cataracts, 604–605, 605f
Catastrophic reactions, 709
Catheter care, urinary, 407–411
    catheter removal in, preparation for, 411
    guidelines for, 410b
    providing, 408, 411, 426p–427p
    urine drainage bag in, 407–408, 408f–409f
    urine drainage bag emptying in, 411,
        427p–428p

Catheterization, urinary, 405–411. See also Urinary
        catheterization
Catheters
    condom, 413, 413f
    definition of, 405
    indwelling, 406f, 407
        double-lumen, 407, 407f
        triple-lumen, 407, 407f
        urinary, 408f–409f
    straight, 406–407, 406f
    suprapubic, 406f, 407
Cavities, 316, 840, 840f
CCOHS Bloodborne Pathogens Standard, 136,
        136b
Cecum, 635, 635f
Cell membrane, 467, 467f
Cells, 466, 467f
Celsius thermometer, 282, 282f
Central nervous system (CNS), 583–585, 585f
Cerebellum, 585, 585f
Cerebral palsy, 683–684, 684f
Cerebrospinal fluid (CSF), 584
Cerebrovascular accident (CVA), 218
Cerebrum, 584, 585f
Cerumen, 609
Cerumen impaction, 609
Cervical cancer, 666
Cervix, 663
Cesarean section, 763, 763f
Chain of infection, 109–112, 110f
    breaking, 111–112, 111f
    method of transmission in, 110, 110f
    pathogen in, 110, 110f
    portal of entry in, 110–111
    portal of exit in, 110
    reservoir in, 110
    susceptible host in, 111
Chain of survival, 222–223
Chair
    in resident's room, 244
    shower, 326, 327f, 795, 795f
    with tray table, 168f
Chair scale, 294–295, 295f, 308p–309p
Charge nurse, 17
Chart, medical, 69
Charting. See Recording
Chemical digestion, 636
Chemical restraint, 166. See also Restraints
Chemoreceptors, 543, 601
Chemotherapy, 725–726, 725f, 726f
Chest cavity, 840, 840f
Chest compressions, 225p
Chest pain, 218
Chest thrusts, in conscious adults and children 1>
        year, 226p
Chest tube drainage system, 549, 550f
Chest tubes, 549, 550f
Chest x-ray, 579
Chewing
    aging on, 637
    problems with, 384
Cheyne-Stokes respiration, 446
Chicken pox, 498
Child abuse, 783–785, 785b
    physical, 784
    psychological (emotional), 784
    reporting of, 785b, 787

risk factors for, 784
sexual, 784
Child-proofing, 778
Children, accident risk in, 162
Chlamydia, 672
Choking, 220–222, 222f
Choroid, 602, 602f
Christianity, death and dying practices in, 452t
Chronic bronchitis, 548–549
Chronic disease, on disease risk, 472
Chronic illness, 81
Chronic obstructive pulmonary disease (COPD),
     548–549
Chronic pain, 599
Chyme, 414, 636
Cilia, tracheal, 542
Ciliary body, 602, 602f
Circ-O-Lectric bed, 493–494, 493f
Circulation, 571–572
  cardiac cycle in, 572–573
  coronary, 570–571, 571f
  in emergency care, 217b
  pulmonary, 571–572, 572f
  systemic, 571, 572, 572f
Circulatory system. *See* Cardiovascular system
Circumcision, 322, 322f
Circumcision care, 768, 768f
Civil laws
  definition of, 48
  violations of, 48–51, 49f–50f
    assault in, 50, 50f
    battery in, 50
    defamation in, 49–50, 49f
    false imprisonment in, 50
    fraud in, 50
    invasion of privacy in, 50–51, 50f
    larceny in, 51
    unintentional tort and negligence in,
      48–49, 49f
Claudication, 576
"Clean catch" urine specimen, 403, 423p–424p
Cleaning solutions, 797, 797f
Cleanliness, 31–32, 32f, 33b, 314–345. *See also*
    specific types of care
  humanistic health care in, 315–316
  oral care in, 316–318, 330p–334p
  perineal care in, 318–322, 334p–338p
  of resident unit, 239, 239f
  scheduling routine care in, 315
  skin care in, 322–328
    bathing in, 322–328, 338p–343p
    massage in, 328–329, 344p–345p
  value of, 314
Cleanser, soapless, 323
Cleansing enema, 417, 417f
Clear liquid diet, 379
Clients
  in facility, 9, 81
  in home health care, 792
Clinical death, 216
Clitoris, 662f, 663
Closed bed, 270f, 272p–274p
Closed captioning, 609
Closed fracture, 518, 518f
Closed reduction, 519
Closed wounds, 494–495
Closet, resident's, 244–245, 245f

Coagulation, 566–567
Cocci, 105, 105f
Cochlea, 610, 610f
Code of ethics, for personal support workers, 53b
Coitus, 93
Cold applications, 524–526, 524t, 526f
  procedures for
    dry, 536p
    moist, 535p
Collagen, 486
Collection device, 390, 390f
Colon, 634f, 635–636, 635f
Colonies, 105
Colonoscopy, for cancer, 724, 724f
Colostomy, 640–641, 640f
Colostrum, 766
Comatose, 162
Combing hair, 366p–367p
Combining vowels, 837–838, 838f, 842t–843t
Comfort, resident unit, 238–241
  cleanliness in, 239, 239f
  lighting in, 240–241, 240f
  noise control in, 241, 241f
  odour control in, 239–240
  room temperature in, 240
  ventilation in, 240, 240f
Comfort measures, for dying, 448–449
Commercial enema, 417
Comminuted fracture, 518f, 519
Commode, bedside, 398, 398f
Commode hat, 390, 390f, 405
Communicable, 109–110
Communicable disease, 104–112. *See also specific*
    diseases
  chain of infection in, 109–112, 110f
  chain of infection in, breaking, 111–112,
    111f
  defenses against, 107–109, 108f
    antibiotics, 109
    immune system, 107–109
    integumentary system, 107, 484
    nonspecific, 107–108
    specific, 109
  microbes in, 104–107 (*See also* Microbes)
Communication, 58–75
  among health care team members, 67–77
    objective data in, 67, 67f
    observation in, 67–68, 67f–68f
    recording in, 69–75 (*See also* Recording)
    reporting in, 68–69, 68f
    subjective data in, 67–68, 68f
  definition and types of, 58–59, 59f
  effective, 59–65, 60f
    blocks to, 64
    conflict and, 64–65, 65f
    conflict resolution in, 65, 66f
    with co-workers, 59
    with patients and residents, 59
    responsibilities for, 59–60, 60f
  enhancement of
    body language in, 62, 62f
    encouraging people to talk in, 61–62
    open-ended questions in, 61–62
    receiver as good listener in, 61, 61f
    in sender, clear messages as, 61,
      62f
    tone of voice in, 62–64

Communication *(continued)*
  in new resident admission, 257
  nonverbal, 58–59
  telephone, 66–67, 66f, 66t
  verbal, 58
Compensation, 693
Competency evaluation, 17
Complex carbohydrates, 374
Compound fracture, 518, 518f
Compulsions, 695
Computerized charting, 75, 75f
Conception, 661
Conditions. *See specific conditions*
Condom catheters, 413, 413f
Conduction, 583
Conduction disorders, 578, 578f
Conduction system
  cardiac, 570
  coronary circulation, 570–571, 571f
Conduction time, aging on, 586
Conductive hearing loss, 609
Confidentiality
  definition and scope of, 50–51, 50f, 53
  of medical record, 74
Conflict, 64–65, 65f
Conflict resolution, 64–65, 65f, 66f
Congestive heart failure, 577–578
Conjunctivitis, 604, 604f
Connective tissue, 467
Conscientiousness, 28
Consciousness, checking for, 215
Consent, informed, 50
Consistent-carbohydrate diabetes meal plan, 380
Constipation, 415, 637
Contact dermatitis, 498
Contact lenses, 603, 603f, 608, 609f
Contact precautions, 120, 127p
Contagious, 109–110
Contaminated, 110, 110f
Continuing care aide, 20t
Continuous infusion pump, enteral feeding via,
    387, 387f
Contraction, heart, aging on, 574
Contractures, from lack of exercise, 523, 523f
Control centres
  for respiration, 288
  for temperature, 281
  for vital signs, 280
Conversion, 693
Convulsions, 219, 219f
Cooperativeness, 29
Coordinated body movement, 142, 143f
Coping mechanisms, 692–693, 693f, 694f
Cornea, 602, 602f
Coronal plane, 839, 839f
Coronary artery disease
  angina pectoris, 577
  myocardial infarction, 577, 577f
Coronary circulation, 570–571, 571f
Corpus callosum, 584, 585f
Corpus luteum, 664, 664f
Corrective lenses, 603, 603f
Cortex, adrenal, 624, 624f
Cough, smoker's, 545
Coughing
  as defense mechanism, 107–108
  postoperative therapeutic, 750, 751f

Counseling, grief, 440, 440f
Courtesy, 28
Cover letter, 35, 37f
Cradle cap, 355
Cream, 323
Creutzfeldt-Jakob disease, 706t
Criminal laws, 48, 51–52
  definition of, 48
  violation of, 51–52, 52b
Critical care unit (CCU), 236, 237f
Cross-contamination, 114b
Cuff, blood pressure, 290, 290f, 290t
Culture, 94–96, 94b
  on diet, 378
  sensitivity and, 108
Curative, 726
Curtains, privacy, 246
Cushing's syndrome, 626–627, 626f
Cuticle, 350
Cuticle scissors, 351, 351f
Cyanosis, 446, 482
Cystitis, 652
Cystoscopy, 657
Cysts, ovarian, 665–666
Cytoplasm, 467, 467f

D
Dandruff, 355
Dangling, 191, 208p–209p
Data. *See also* Record; Recording
  objective, 67, 67f
  subjective, 67–68, 68f
Deafness, 611–612. *See also* Hearing loss
  communicating with resident with, 612–613, 612f
  definition and forms of, 611–612
  hearing aids for, 613, 613f, 614b, 616p
  sign language for, 612–613, 612f
Death
  approaching, signs of, 446–447
  clinical, 216
  culture, religion, and, 452t
"Death rattle," 446
Decubitus ulcers, 487–494. *See also* Pressure ulcers
Deep breathing, postoperative therapeutic, 750, 751f
Deep touch, 599
Deep venous thrombosis (DVT), 576
Defamation, 49–50, 49f
Defecate, 414
Defense mechanisms, 693–694
  antibiotics and, 109
  against communicable disease, 107–109, 108f
  nonspecific, 107–108, 108f
  specific, 109
Definitive surgery, 742
Degenerative diseases, 471
Dehydration, 388, 650
Delegation, 20–22
  accepting/declining a task in, 21–22, 22b
  definition of, 20
  five rights of, 20, 21t
  by nurse, 19–20
  refusal of, 21
  scope of practice and, 21, 22b
Delirium, 704
Delivery
  during, 763–764, 763f
  immediately following, 764, 764f

Delusions, 697, 708
Dementia, 587, 703–717
  behaviors in, 707–710
    agitation, 709, 709f
    catastrophic reactions, 709
    delusions and hallucinations, 708–709
    "normal," 707
    pacing, 708, 708f
    repetition, 708
    rummaging, 708
    sexual behaviors, inappropriate, 709
    situations causing, 710b
    sundowning, 709
    wandering, 708, 708f
  causes of, 705–706, 706t
  communication with, 709
  definition of, 704, 705f
  vs. delirium, 704
  managing difficult behaviors in, 710, 711t
  stages of, 704
  types of, 705–707, 706t
    Alzheimer's disease, 705–707 (See also
      Alzheimer's disease)
    vascular dementia, 706–707, 706t
Dementia care
  ADL assistance in, 711–713, 711f
  on caregiver, 717
  for emotional and social needs, 715–717
    activity therapy in, 716–717, 716f
    music therapy in, 717
    pet therapy in, 717, 717f
    reminiscence therapy in, 715–716, 715f
  guidelines for, 712b–713b
  for physical needs, 711–715
    bathing, 714, 714f
    dressing, 714
    eating, 714–715, 715f
    elimination, 715
    general points on, 711–713, 711f
Dendrites, 583, 583f
Denial, 437, 437f, 438t, 693
Dental caries, 316
Dentures, oral care with, 317, 317b, 332p–333p
Deodorant, 323
Depression, 696–697, 696f
Dermatitis, 498
Dermatitis, seborrheic, 355
Dermis, 483, 483f
Descending colon, 635, 635f
Development, 84. See also Growth and development
Developmental disabilities, 680–687
  autism, 683
  care with, 685–686
  causes of, 680b
  cerebral palsy, 683–684, 684f
  communication with, 686–687, 687f
  congenital vs. acquired, 680, 680t
  definition of, 680
  Down syndrome, 683, 683f
  fetal alcohol syndrome, 684
  fragile X syndrome, 684
  humanistic health care with, 686
  hydrocephalus, 684–685, 685f
  mental retardation, 682–683, 682f
  rehabilitation with, 687
  special needs with, 680–682, 681f
    education, 680–681, 681f

emotional and social needs, 681–682
    protection of rights, 681
  spina bifida, 684, 685f
Diabetes mellitus, 627–629
  amputations from, 521–522, 522f
  causes of, 627
  complications of, 629
  epidemiology of, 627
  management of, 627–629, 628f
    blood glucose monitoring in, 627, 628f
    diet in, 628–629
    exercise in, 629
    medication in, 627, 628f, 629
  type 1, 627–629
  type 2, 629
Diabetic diet, 380
Diabetic retinopathy, 605
Diagnosis, nursing, 76
Dialysis, 654, 654f
Diapering, of newborns, 770
Diaphoretic, 315
Diaphragm, 542f, 543
  quadrants and, 841, 841f
  of stethoscope, 286–287, 286f
Diarrhea, 414–415
Diastole, 572
Diastolic blood pressure, 289
Diencephalon, 584, 585f
Diet
  balanced, 375
  cancer and, 722
  for diabetes mellitus, 628–629, 628f
  for healthy heart, 573, 573f
  special, 379–380
Dietitian, 379
Digestion, 372
  aging on, 637
  mechanisms of, 636
Digestive system (tract), 414, 414f, 469, 470f,
      633–637
  aging on, 637
  function of
    absorption, 636–637, 637f
    digestion, 636
    excretion, 637
  layers of, 633, 634f
  structure of, 633–636
    bile, 636
    gallbladder, 634f, 636
    large intestine, 634f, 635–636, 635f
    layers, 633, 634f
    liver, 634f, 636
    mouth, pharynx, and esophagus, 633–634, 634f
    overview of, 633, 634f
    pancreas, 634f, 636
    salivary glands, 634f, 636
    small intestine, 634f, 635, 635f
    stomach, 634–635, 634f
Digestive system disorders, 637–639
  cancer, 639
  diagnosis of, 639, 640f
  gallbladder, 638–639, 638f
  hernias, 638, 638f
  ulcers, 638
Digital examination, 415, 416f
Dilation and curettage (D&C), 667
Dining experience, standards relating to, 381, 381b

Directional terms, 839–840, 839f, 840f
Director of nursing (DON), 17
Disability, 472, 472f. *See also* Rehabilitation;
    Restorative care
  developmental, 680–687 (*See also* Developmental
    disabilities)
  on grooming, 349
  rehabilitation and, 472
Disaster, 156
Disaster preparedness, 156–157
  evacuating the building in, 155–156
  plan for, 157
Discharge, 258–259, 259f
Discharge planning, 259, 259f
Disease
  acute *vs.* chronic, 471
  categories of, 471
  definition of, 471
  health *vs.*, 469, 471
  mild *vs.* severe, 471
  risk factors for, 471–472
Disease transmission, 131–138
  airborne, 136–138 (*See also* Airborne diseases)
  bloodborne, 131–136 (*See also* Bloodborne diseases)
  method of, 110, 110f
Disinfection, 112–113, 113f
Disoriented, 215
Displacement, 693–694
Distal, 840
Diuresis, 404–405
Diuretic, 405
Dividers, room, 246
Do not resuscitate (DNR) order, 441
Dopamine, in Parkinson's disease, 590
Doppler ultrasound, 579
Dorsal cavity, 840, 840f
Dorsal recumbent position, 182f, 183, 183f
Dorsal surface, 839f, 840
Dorsiflexion, 510t
Double-bagging, 127p
Double-lumen indwelling catheters, 407, 407f
Dowager's hump, 514, 515f
Down syndrome, 683, 683f
Draw sheets, 264, 264f
Dress
  for application submission, 37
  for work, 31–32, 32f, 33b
Dressing, 362p–364p
Dressing changes, 497, 501p–502p
Droplet precautions, 119–120
Drying hair, 356, 357f
Duchenne's muscular dystrophy, 517–518
Duodenal ulcer, 638
Duodenum, 635, 635f
Durable power of attorney for health care, 441, 441f
Dura mater, 584
Dwarfism, pituitary, 625
Dying, 446–458
  communication with, 449–450
  Dying Person's Bill of Rights in, 448b
  emotional needs in, 450–451
    culture and religion in, 451, 452t–453t
    humanistic care in, 450–451
    individual differences in, 450
    listening in, 450, 450f
    loneliness in, 450, 450f
    spirituality in, 451, 452t–453t

family assistance with, 449–450, 449f, 454
family care in, 451, 454, 454f
family member care in, 451, 454, 454f
humanistic health care in, 450–451
physical needs in, 448–450
postmortem care in, 454–458 (*See also* Postmortem
    care)
resident/patient care in, 447–448, 447f
sensory changes in, 449
signs of approaching death in, 446–447
Dying Person's Bill of Rights, 448b
Dysentery, amebic, 106t, 107
Dysmenorrhea, 665
Dyspnea, 288
Dysrhythmia, 286
Dysuria, 404

E
Ear
  aging on, 610–611
  function of, 610
  structure of, 609–610, 610f
Ear disorders, 609–612
  cerumen impaction, 609
  deafness, 611–612 (*See also* Deafness)
  Ménière's disease, 611
  otitis externa, 611
  otitis media, 611
Eardrum, 609, 610f
Early morning care, 315
Ear wax, 609
Eating
  assistance with, 382–383, 382f, 383f
  on musculoskeletal system, 512
  post-operative assistance with, 753
Eating disorders, 697–698, 698f
Eating habits, 375–379
Echocardiography, 579
Eczema, 498
Edema, 389
Edentulous, 316
Education
  of personal support worker, 16–17, 16f
  special, 680–681, 681f
Efferent, 648, 650f
Egg, 661, 662–663
Egocentric, 783
Ejaculation, 670
Elbow pads, 492, 492f
Elder abuse, 52
Elderly, accident risk in, 162
Elective surgery, 742
Electrical appliances, burn risk with, 150,
    152f, 165
Electrical fire, 156t
Electrical shock prevention, 150, 152f
Electrocardiography (ECG, EKG), 579, 579f
Electroencephalography (EEG), 592, 593f
Electronic thermometers, 283, 283f
Electron microscope, 105
Elimination, 397–429
  bowel, 414–419 (*See also* Bowel elimination)
  equipment for, 397–398, 398f, 399f
  guidelines for assisting with, 401b–402b
  humanistic health care for, 400
  post-operative care for, 753
  promoting normal

fundamentals of, 399–400
guidelines for, 401b–402b
skin, 485
stool specimens in, 403, 425p
urinary, 403–414 (*See also* Urinary elimination)
urine specimens in, 402–403, 422p–423p
Embolism, pulmonary, 576, 751
Embolus, 575, 751
Emergencies, medical, in home health care,
804–806
Emergency care
ABCs of, 216, 217b
basic life support in, 216–217, 217b
Emergency medical services (EMS) system activation,
215
Emergency situations, 217–222
airway obstruction (choking), 220–222
airway obstruction clearing, 221–222, 222f,
224p–229p
fainting (syncope), 218–219, 218f
heart attack (myocardial infarction), 217–218
hemorrhage, 220
responding to, 214–215, 215f
activating EMS system in, 215
humanistic health care in, 216
oriented to person, place, and time in, 215
reporting unusual signs and symptoms in,
214–215, 215f
steps of response in, 215
seizures, 219, 219f
shock, 220, 221f
stroke, 218
Emergent surgery, 742
Emery board, 351, 351f
Emotional abuse, 51
Emotional balance, 692, 692f
Emotional health, on disease risk, 472
Emotional needs. *See specific age groups and topics*
Emotional rehabilitation, 475–477, 477f
Empathy, 29
Emphysema, 548, 548f
Endocardium, 569
Endocrine disorders, 471
Endocrine glands, 620, 621f. *See also specific glands*
Endocrine system, 469, 470f, 620–625. *See also
specific glands*
aging on, 625
functions of, 621–625
adrenal glands, 624, 624f
pancreas, 624–625
parathyroid glands, 623
pineal gland, 622
pituitary gland, 621–622, 622f
sex glands, 625
thymus gland, 623–624
thyroid gland, 622–623, 623f
glands in, 620, 621f
structure of, 621f
Endocrine system disorders, 625–629
acromegaly, 625–626, 626f
adrenal gland, 626–627, 626f
diabetes mellitus, 627–629 (*See also* Diabetes
mellitus)
thyroid gland, 626
Endometrial cancer, 666
Endometrium, 663
Endoscope, 386

Endoscopy
for cancer, 724–725, 724f
of digestive system, 639
Endospore, 105
Endotracheal intubation, 557–558,
558f
Endotracheal tube, 557–558, 558f
Enema, 416–418
administration of, 417–418, 418f, 428p–429p
types of, 417, 417f
use of, 416–417
Enema bag, 417f
Enteral nutrition, 386–388, 386f, 388f
Enterococcus, 109
Enterococcus, vancomycin-resistant (VRE), 109
Environment, in cancer, 722
Environment, resident's, 236–247
comfort of, 238–241
cleanliness in, 239, 239f
lighting in, 240–241, 240f
noise control in, 241, 241f
odour control in, 239–240
room temperature in, 240
ventilation in, 240, 240f
furniture and equipment in, 241–246 (*See also*
Furniture and equipment)
humanistic health care for, 247
patient's unit in, hospital, 236, 237f
personal items in, 246–247
resident's unit in, 236–238
in assisted-living facilities, 238, 238f
in home health care, 238, 238f
in hospital, 236, 237f
in long-term care facilities, 237–238, 238f
risk factors in, 161–163, 161f
Enzymes, 636
Epicardium, 569
Epidermis, 483, 483f
Epididymis, 668, 669f
Epidural block, 764
Epigastric region, 841, 841f
Epiglottis, 542, 633
Epilepsy, 590–591
Epinephrine
actions of, 624
adrenal source of, 624, 624f
for shock, 220, 221f
EpiPen Auto-Injector, 220, 221f
Episiotomy, 765
Epithelial tissue, 467
Equipment. *See* Furniture and equipment; *specific
equipment*
Erectile dysfunction, 670
Erections, aging on, 670
Erythema, 498
Erythrocytes, 565–566, 566f
Escherichia (E.) coli, 104–105
Esophageal sphincter, 634–635, 634f
Esophagus, 633–634, 634f
Estradiol, 624
Ethical dilemma, 53, 54f
Ethical issues, 52–54
code of ethics in, 53b
issues in, 52–53
personal ethics in, 53, 54f
professional ethics in, 53, 53b
protecting yourself from, 53–54

Ethics, 53, 54f
Etiquette, telephone, 66t
Eupnea, 288
Eustachian tube, 609, 610f
Evacuation, fire-related, 155–156
Evaluation, in nursing process, 77
Evening care, 315
Eversion, 510t
Exchange, of information, 60
Excoriation, 498–499, 499t
Excretion, 637. *See also* Bowel elimination;
    Elimination; Urination
Exercise
    for diabetes mellitus, 629
    for healthy heart, 573, 573f
    on musculoskeletal system, 512, 513f
    for personal support worker, 30, 30f
    for respiratory health, 545, 545f
Exhalation, 287–288
Expiration, 287–288
Exploratory surgery, 742
Exposure control plan, 136b
Expressive aphasia, 589
Extended-care patients, 83
Extension, 510t
External auditory canal, 609, 610f
External fixation, 519, 519f
External urethral sphincter, 649
Eye, 601–604
    aging on, 602, 604f
    function of, 602–603, 602f
    structure of, 602–603, 602f
Eyebrows, 602, 602f
Eye disorders, 604–606
    blindness, 605–606, 606f, 607b–608b
    cataracts, 604–605, 605f
    conjunctivitis (pink eye), 604, 604f
    diabetic retinopathy, 605
    glaucoma, 605
    macular degeneration, 605
Eyeglass care, 606–608, 608f
Eyeglasses, 603, 603f
Eyelashes, 602, 602f
Eyelids, 602, 602f
Eyes, prosthetic, 608–609, 609f
Eye socket, 602
Eyewear, protective, 118, 118f, 119b

F
Facemasks, oxygen, 555, 555f
Face shields, 118, 118f, 119b
Fahrenheit thermometer, 282, 282f
Failure to thrive, 777
Fainting, 218–219, 218f
Fallopian tubes, 662–663, 662f
Falls, 163–165
    assisting with, 149, 149b
    care after, 149b
    prevention of, 148–149, 163, 163f
        assessment in, 163, 163f
        cleaning up spills in, 148, 148f
        guidelines for, 164b–165b
    risk evaluation for, 163, 163f
False imprisonment, 50
Families
    nontraditional, 776–777
    traditional, 776

Fanfolded, 270, 270f
Farsightedness, 603, 603f
Fatigue, infection and, 111
Fats, 374
Fat-soluble, 374
Febrile, 285
Fecal impaction, 415, 416f
Fecal incontinence, 416–417
Feces, 414, 637
Feedback, 58, 59f, 60
Feeding, of newborns, 768–770, 769f
Feeding syringe, 715, 715f
Femoral hernias, 638, 638f
Fertilization, 661, 664
Fetal alcohol syndrome, 684
Fever, 108, 285
Fibre, 373
Fibre supplements, 415
Fibrinogen, 575
Fibroids, uterine, 665–666
Fidelity, 53
Fight-or-flight response, 281
Filtrate, 648
Filtration, in elderly, 651
Fimbriae, 662, 662f
Finances, on diet, 378
Fire
    fuel for, 150, 152f
    oxygen in, 152, 152f, 153b, 154f
    types of, 156t
Fire extinguisher, 155, 155f
Fire safety, 151–157
    electrical appliances and, 150, 152f
    guidelines for, 152, 153b, 154
    preventing fires in, 151–154, 152f, 153b
    reacting to fire emergency in, 154–156
        evacuation in, 155–156
        evacuation in, bed linen, 154, 155b
        extinguishing fires in, 154f, 155, 156t
        RACE fire response plan in, 154–155,
            154f
    smoking and, 153b
First-degree burns, 497
Fissure, 499, 499t
Fistula, 654
Five rights of delegation, 20, 21t
Fixation, fracture, 519–520, 519f, 520b
Fixed joints, 507, 509f
Flat bones, 506, 508f
Flatulence, 415–416, 416f
Flatus, 414
Flexion, 510t
Flora
    normal (resident), 104
    transient, 115
Flossing teeth, assisting with, 330p–331p
Flow meter, oxygen, 551, 551f
Flu, 546–547, 546f
Fluid balance, 388–389, 484
Fluids, 388–391
    dehydration and, 388
    drinking, 651, 652f
    edema and, 389
    fluid balance in, 388–389, 484
    intake/output measurements and recording in,
        389–391, 390f, 404–405, 405f
    NPO status and, 389

offering, 389
skin in, 484
Flushing, 482
Foley catheters, 406f, 407
Folic acid, 373t
Follicle, 664
Follicle-stimulating hormone (FSH), 622, 664
Fomites, 110, 110f
Food
choices of, 375–379
culture and, 95
measuring and recording intake of, 384–385, 385f
Food handling, in home health care, 808, 809f
Food labels, 375, 378f
Food poisoning, preventing, 808, 809f
Footboard, 265, 265f
Foot care, 351–352, 352f, 361p–362p
Force fluids, 389
Foreskin, 322, 322f, 669
Fowler's position, 183, 184f, 242, 242f, 561
Fracture, 518–521
closed, 518, 518f
comminuted, 519
definition of, 518
greenstick, 518, 518f
impacted, 518, 518f
open (compound), 518, 518f
from restraints, 169, 171
spiral, 518f, 519
stress, 518
treatments for
reduction and fixation, 519–520, 519f, 520b
traction, 520–521, 521f
Fracture pan, 398, 399f, 420p–421p
Fragile X syndrome, 683–684, 684f
Fraud, 50
Freely movable joints, 508
Frequency, urinary, 404
Friction
cause of, 185
pressure ulcers and, 491f, 492
Frontal plane, 839, 839f
Full liquid diet, 379–380
Functional incontinence, 412
Functional nursing, 19
Fundus
stomach, 634, 635f
uterine, 663
Fungi, 106t, 107
Furniture and equipment, 241–246. *See also specific furniture and equipment; specific types*
beds, 241–244, 242f, 244f
call light and intercom systems, 245–246, 246f
chairs, 244
closet, 244–245, 245f
other equipment, 246
over-bed tables, 244, 244f
privacy curtains and room dividers, 246
storage units, 244–245, 245f

G
Gait belt
application of, 199p–200p
use of, 187
Gallbladder, 634f, 636
Gallbladder disorders, 638–639, 639f
Gallstones, 638–639, 639f

Gametes, 661
Gangrene, 522, 522f
Gas, 414
Gas exchange, 543–544
in alveoli, 544, 544f
in emphysema, 548
Gastric ulcer, 638
Gastroscopy, for cancer, 725
Gastrostomy tube, 386–387, 386f
Gatches, 242, 242f
Gauze dressings, 496, 496f
Gender, on disease risk, 471
General anaesthesia, 742–743
General lighting, 240, 240f
General sense, 598–601
definition of, 598
pain, 599–601, 600f
position, 599
touch, 598–599, 599f
Genetics
in cancer, 722
on disease risk, 471
Genital herpes, 672, 672f
Genital warts, 672
Geography, on diet, 378
Geriatric patients, 83
Gigantism, pituitary, 625, 625f
Gingivitis, 316
Glans penis, 669
Glasses, 603, 603f
Glass thermometers, 281–283, 281f, 282f
Glaucoma, 605
Glomerulus, 648, 650f
Glossary, 815–834
Gloves, 117, 117f, 119b, 123p
Glucocorticoids, 624, 624f
Glucometer, 627, 628f
Glucose, 374
Glucose, blood
high, 627 (*See also* Diabetes mellitus)
low, 627
monitoring of, 627, 628f
Glycerin rectal suppositories, 418
Goals
life, 91–92
in nursing process, 76–77
patient and resident, 92
Goggles, 118, 118f, 119b
Goitre, 623, 623f
Gonadotropins, 622, 622f
Gonads. *See also specific glands*
in endocrine system, 620, 621f
functions of, 625
Gonorrhea, 672
Gout, 517
Gowns, 117
changing of, 364p
putting on, 124p
removing, 125p
in standard precautions, 119b
Graduate, 390, 390f, 405, 405f
Graft, 654
Grand mal seizures, 219, 219f
Graphic sheet, 69–70, 71f–72f
Graves' disease, 626
Greenstick fracture, 518, 518f
Grey hair, 486, 486f

Grief, 437–440
  of caregiver, 440, 440f, 442, 442f
  counseling for, 440, 440f
  definition of, 437
  of family, 440
  of resident, 439–440
  stages of, 438–440
    acceptance, 438t, 439, 439f
    anger, 437–438, 438f, 438t
    bargaining, 438, 438t, 439f
    denial, 437, 437f, 438t
    depression, 438–439, 438t, 439f
Grief counseling, 440, 440f
Grooming, 349–368. *See also specific types*
  definition and scope of, 349
  dressing and undressing in
    changing hospital gown, 364p
    clothing choice, 352, 353f
    dressing, 352–353, 353f, 362p–364p
    dressing with IV line, 353, 354f
    shoehorns and graspers, 353, 353f
    undressing, 353
  foot care in, 351–352, 352f, 361p–362p
  hair care in, 354–357 (*See also* Hair care)
  hand care in, 350–351, 351f, 360p–361p
  humanistic health care in, 350
  illness and disability on, 349
  make-up in, 358–359
  personal routines and practices in, 349
  shaving
    in men, 357–358, 367p–368p
    in women, 358
Grounded, 150, 152f
Ground-fault breakers, 150, 152f
Grouping
  by age, 82, 82f
  by illness or medical condition, 81–82, 82f
  by special health care needs, 82, 82f
Growth, 84
Growth and development, 83–89
  in adolescence (13–20 years), 87–88, 88f
  definition of, 83–89
  in infancy, 85, 86f
  in later adulthood (60–75 years), 89, 89f
  in middle adulthood (40–60 years), 88, 88f
  in older adulthood (75+ years), 89, 89f
  in preschool (3–5 years), 86, 86f
  principles of, 85, 85b
  psychological stages of, 85, 86f
  in school-age years (6–12 years), 87, 87f
  stages of normal progression in, 84–85, 84f
  tasks in, 85
  in toddlerhood, 85–86, 86f
  in young adulthood (20–40 years), 88, 88f
Growth hormone, 621–622, 622f

H
Hair, 483f, 484
Hair, grey, 486, 486f
Hair care, 354–357
  abnormalities and, 355
  combing in, 366p–367p
  drying in, 356, 357f
  personal preferences in, 355
  preventing tangles in, 357, 357f
  salons and barbershops for, on-site, 354, 355f
  self-care in, 355, 355f

  shampooing in, 356, 356f, 365p–366p
  styling in, 355f, 356–357, 357f
  texture and length of hair in, 354–355
Hair loss, 355, 724f, 725–726, 726f
Halitosis, 316
Hallucinations, 697, 708–709
Hand care, 350–351
  cutting nails in, 350–351, 351f
  procedure for, 360p–361p
  tools for, 350–351, 351f
Handrails, toilet, 397, 398f
Hand rubs, alcohol-based, 809, 810f
Handwashing, 115–116, 115f
  in home health care, 809, 810f
  in standard precautions, 119b
  techniques of, 115, 122p–123p
Hangnails, 351
Head injuries, 591, 591f
Head lice, 355
Head nurse, 17
Head tilt/chin lift maneuver, 225p
Health, 469–470
Health, of personal support worker
  emotional, 31, 31f
  physical, 29–31, 30f
Health Canada, 6, 6b
Health care aide, 20t
Health care–associated infections (HAIs), 112
Health care language. *See* Language, health care;
    specific terms
Health care organizations, 7–10. *See also specific*
    organizations
  assisted-living facilities, 9, 9f
  home health care agencies, 9, 9f
  hospice organizations, 9–10
  hospitals, 7
  long-term care facilities, 8, 8f
  missions of, 7
  structure of, 10, 10f
  sub-acute care units, 7–8, 8f
Health care support worker, 20t
Health care system. *See also specific topics*
  Canada Health Act in, 5–6, 6b
  government role in, 6, 6b
  Health Canada in, 6, 6b
  health care organizations in, 7–10 (*See also* Health
      care organizations)
  health care team in, 10–11, 11f
  history of, 4–6, 5f
  Medicare in, 6–7
  paying for health care in, 6–7
Health care team, 10–11, 11f
Hearing, 609–611
  aging on ear in, 610–611
  in dying, 449
  ear disorders on, 609–612
  ear function in, 610
  ear structure in, 609–610, 610f
Hearing aids, 613, 613f, 614b, 616p
Hearing loss, 611–612. *See also* Deafness
  communicating with resident with, 612–613,
      612f
  conductive, 611
  definition and forms of, 611–612
  hearing aids for, 613, 613f, 614b, 616p
  sensorineural, 611
  sign language for, 612–613, 612f

Heart, 569–571
  atria of, 569, 570f, 571f
  conduction system of, 570
  diet and exercise for, 573, 573f
  immobility on, 181f, 182
  tissue layers of, 569
  valves of, 570, 570f, 571f
  ventricles of, 569–570, 570f, 571f
Heart attack, 217–218, 577, 577f
Heart block, 578, 578f
Heart disorders, 576–578
  angina pectoris, 577
  cardiac rehabilitation for, 579
  conduction disorders, 578, 578f
  coronary artery disease, 577
    development of, 577
    risk factors for, 576
  diagnosis of, 579, 579f
  heart block and pacemakers, 578f
  heart failure, 577–578
  myocardial infarction, 577, 577f
  risk factors for, 576
Heart failure, 577–578
Heart rate, newborn, 767
Heart valves, 570, 570f
Heat applications, 524–527, 524t, 527f, 537p
Heat loss, 281
Heel booties, 492, 492f
Height, 294
  definition of, 294
  measurement of
    in children, 296, 296t
    scales in, 294–296
    with tape measure and sling scale, 294–296, 296f, 309p–310p
    with upright scale, 294, 295f, 307p–308p
Heimlich maneuver, 221–222, 222f, 224p
Helicobacter pylori, 638
Helminths, 106t, 107
Hematuria, 404
Hemiplegia, 162, 588–589
Hemispheres, 584
Hemodialysis, 654, 654f
Hemoglobin, 565–566, 574–575
Hemoptysis, 546
Hemorrhage, 220
Hemorrhagic shock, 220
Hemostasis, 567
Hemothorax, 551
Hepatitis, 131–134
  definition and causes of, 131, 132f
  hepatitis A virus (HAV), 132, 132f
  hepatitis B virus (HBV), 133–134, 133f
    vs. HIV, 135t
  hepatitis C virus (HCV), 134
  hepatitis D virus (HDV), 134
  hepatitis E virus (HEV), 134
  seriousness of, 132
Heredity
  in cancer, 722
  on disease risk, 471
Hernias, 638, 638f
Herpes simplex, 672, 672f
Heterosexual, 92
Hiatal hernias, 638, 638f
Hiatus, 634
High-Fowler's position, 183, 184f

Hinduism, death and dying practices in, 453t
Hip replacement surgery, 516–517, 517f
History
  medical, 69
  nursing, 69
HIV/AIDS, 673, 731–736. See also HIV/AIDS
  AIDS from HIV in, 731
  caring for person with, 734–736
    activities of daily living in, 734, 734f
    emotional needs in, 735, 735f
    humanistic health care in, 736
    physical needs in, 734, 735f
    standard precautions in, 734, 735f
  definition of, 730
  as global health crisis, 732–733, 732f, 733f
  Kaposi's sarcoma in, 731, 732f
  protecting rights with, 733
  risk for, 732
HIV encephalopathy, 706t
HIV-positive, 731
Holistic care, 10
Homebound, 793
Home health care, 238, 238f, 791–799
  client in, 792
  financing of, 792–793
  health care team in, 793–794, 793f
  for homebound, 793
  home support worker in, 791, 792, 797–799 (See also Home support worker)
  infection control in, 806–810 (See also Infection control, in home health care)
  responsibilities in, 794–797
    home environment in, 794–795
    homemaking in, 796–797, 796f, 797f
    overview of, 794
    personal care in, 795, 795f
    record keeping in, 794
    types of care in, 794
  safe home guidelines in, 804, 805b–806b
  workplace safety in, 804–806, 805b–806b
Home health care agencies, 9, 9f
Homemaker flow sheet, 796
Homemaking, in home health care, 796–797, 796f, 797f
Homeostasis
  principle of, 469
  urinary system in, 650–651
Home support worker. See also Home health care
  abandonment and, 799, 799f
  definition of, 791, 792
  nurse's bag for, 798, 798f
  in nursing team, 20t
  qualities of, 797–799
    ability to set professional boundaries, 799
    ability to work independently, 797–798
    planning, 798
    reliability, 798–799, 799f
  supplies and equipment for, 798, 798f
Homosexual, 92
Honesty, 29
Hormone, 619, 621. See also specific hormones
Hormone replacement therapy (HRT), 665
Hospice care, 441–442, 442f
Hospice organizations, 9–10
Hospital gown. See Gowns
Hospitals, 7
Host, susceptible, 111

Hot foods, 165
Hot liquids, 165
Hour of sleep care, 315
House diet, 379
Housekeeping, in home health care, 796–797, 796f, 797f
hs care, 315
Human immunodeficiency virus (HIV). *See also* HIV/AIDS
   as bloodborne pathogen, 134, 135f
   vs. hepatitis B virus, 135t
Humanistic approach, 96–97
Humanistic health care, 96
   bathing in, 327–328
   for cancer, 726
   with chronic obstructive pulmonary disease, 549
   developmental disabilities in, 686
   for dying, 450–451
   elimination in, 400
   for emergencies, 216
   grooming in, 350
   with HIV/AIDS, 736
   hygiene and cleanliness in, 315–316
   infection control in, 120
   linen changes in, 271
   meal time in, 379
   for ostomy, 641
   for patient's/resident's environment, 247
   perineal care in, 320
   for pregnancy, 761
   in rehabilitation and restorative care, 475
   restraint use in, 171
   transfers in, 188
Human resources (HR) department (personnel), 37, 37f
Human rights, basic, 46–47
Human Rights Law, Canadian, 35
Humidity bottle, 552b, 553
Huntington's chorea, 706t
Hydration, 650, 651, 651f
   dehydration and, 388
   edema in, 389
   fluid balance in, 388–389, 484
   intake/output measurement and recording in, 389–391, 390f, 404–405, 405f
   NPO status and, 389
   offering fluids in, 389, 389f
   skin and, 484
Hydrocephalus, 684–685, 685f
Hydrochloric acid, stomach, 636
Hygiene, personal, 31–32, 32f, 33b, 314–345
   assisting with, 808–809
   humanistic health care in, 315–316
   oral care in, 316–318, 330p–334p
   perineal care in, 318–322, 334p–338p
   post-operative assistance with, 753
   professional, 31–32, 32f, 33b
   scheduling routine care in, 315
   skin care in, 322–328
      bathing in, 322–328, 338p–343p
      massage in, 328, 344p–345p
   value of, 314
Hyperalimentation, 388, 388f
Hyperglycemia, 627
Hyperopia, 603, 603f
Hypertension, 293
Hyperthyroidism, 626

Hyperventilation, 288
Hypochondriac regions, 841, 841f
Hypogastric region, 841–842, 841f
Hypoglycemia, 627
Hypotension, 293–294
Hypotension, orthostatic, 293–294
Hypothalamus, 584, 585f
Hypothyroidism, 626
Hypoventilation, 288
Hypoxic, 559
Hysterectomy, 668

I
Ideal job, 32–35, 34f
Ileal conduit, 656
Ileostomy, 640, 640f
Ileum, 635, 635f
Iliac regions, 841, 841f
Illnesses
   acute, 81
   chronic, 81
   terminal, 81
Imaging studies
   for cancer, 724–725, 724f
   of digestive system, 639
   of female reproductive system, 667, 667f, 668f
   of urinary system, 657, 657f
Immobility, complications of, 180–182, 181f
Immune disorders, 471
Immune system, 107–109
Impacted fracture, 518, 518f
Impaction, fecal, 415, 416f
Implantation, 664
Implementation, in nursing process, 77
Impotence, 670
Imprisonment, false, 50
Incentive spirometry, 750–751, 751f
Incident report, 166, 167f
Incontinence, fecal, 416–417
Incontinence, urinary, 411–414
   causes of, 411
   definition of, 411
   functional, 412
   managing, 412–414
      bladder training in, 413–414
      condom catheters in, 413, 413f
      pads and briefs in, 412–413, 413f
   overflow, 412
   reflex, 412
   on resident and caregiver, 411–412
   from restraints, 171
   stress, 412
   urge, 412
   urinary retention in, 412
Incus, 609–610, 610f
Individual taste, on diet, 378
Indwelling catheters, 407, 408f–409f
   catheter care in, 407–411
      catheter removal in, preparation for, 411
      guidelines for, 410b
      providing, 408, 411, 426p–427p
      urine drainage bag emptying in, 411, 427p–428p
      urine drainage bag in, 407–408, 408f–409f
   systems for, 408f–409f
   types of, 406f
Indwelling medical devices. *See also specific types*
   infection from, 111

Infancy, 85, 86f
Infant care
    emotional needs in, 777, 778f
    physical needs in, 777
    safety needs in, 777–778
Infarct (infarction), 577, 577f, 706
Infection, 109. *See also specific types*
    chain of, 109–112, 110f
    health care–associated, 112
    from indwelling medical devices, 111
    nosocomial, 112
    respiratory, 546f, 547b
    respiratory, aging on, 545–546
    secondary, 499
    urinary system, 652, 652f
Infection control, in health care setting, 112–120,
        122p–127p. *See also* Chain of infection
    barrier methods in, 116–118, 123p–127p
        gloves, 117, 117f, 119b, 123p
        gowns, 117, 119b, 124p–125p
        masks, 117–118, 118f, 119b, 126p
        personal protective equipment in, 116
        personal protective equipment in, multiple articles
            of, 118, 127p
        protective eyewear, 118, 118f, 119b
    definition of, 112
    handwashing in, 115–116, 115f, 119b, 122p–123p
    infections in, 112
    isolation precautions in, 118–120
    medical asepsis in, 112–116 (*See also* Asepsis,
        medical)
    microbes in, 104–107 (*See also* Microbes)
    standard precautions in, 118, 119b
    surgical asepsis in, 116
Infection control, in home health care, 806–810
    sanitary environment in, 807–809
        bag technique in, 807–808, 807f
        cleaning equipment and household surfaces in,
            807f, 808
        food handling in, 808, 809f
        personal hygiene assistance in, 808–809
    standard precautions in, 809–810, 810f
Infection site, 108, 108f
Infectious disease, 471. *See also specific types*
Inferior, 839f, 840
Infertility, female, 665
Influenza, 546–547, 546f
Informed consent, 50
Infusion pump, enteral feeding via, 387, 387f
Ingestion, 372
Inguinal hernias, 638, 638f
Inhalation, 287
Inheritance, in cancer, 722
Injury, physical. *See specific types*
Injury protection, 144, 145b–146b
Inner ear, 610, 610f
Inspiration, 287
Instability, in Parkinson's disease, 590, 590f
Insulin, 627, 628f, 629
Intake and output (I&O) flow sheet, 389–390, 405
Integumentary system, 469, 470f, 482–487
    aging on, 485–487
        fragile, dry skin, 486–487, 487f
        nail thickening, 487
        physical appearance, 486, 486f
        temperature regulation, 487
    as defense mechanism, 107

definition of, 482
    in fluid balance, 484
    function of, 484–485, 485f
    hair in, 483f, 484
    immobility on, 180, 181f
    nails in, 484
    in protection, 484
    sebaceous glands in, 483, 483f
    skin color in, 482
    skin in, 483, 483f
    sweat glands in, 483f, 484
Integumentary system disorders, 487–502
    burns, 497–498
    lesions, 498–499, 499t
    pressure ulcers, 487–494 (*See also* Pressure ulcers)
    wounds, 494–497 (*See also* Wound)
        definition of, 494
        healing of, 495–497 (*See also* Wound healing)
        intentional, 494, 494f
        unintentional, 494, 494f
Intensive care patients, 83
Intensive care unit (ICU), 236, 237f
Intentional tort, 49
Intentional wound, 494, 494f
Intercom system, 245–246, 246f
Intercostal muscles, 543
Internal fixation, 519f, 520
Internal urethral sphincter, 649
Interstitial cell-stimulating hormone (ICSH), 669
Interventions, in nursing process, 76–77
Interviews, job, 40–42
    dress for, 41, 41f
    posture in, 41
    preparation for, 40
    purpose of, 40
    questions from interviewer in, 41, 42b
    questions to interviewer in, 41–42
    thank-you note after, 42, 42f
    time for, 41
Intimacy, 92, 93f
Intra-operative phase, 743
Intravenous pyelography (IVP), 657, 657f
Intravenous (IV) therapy, 385–386, 385f
Intubation, endotracheal, 557–558, 558f
Invasion of privacy, 50–51, 50f
Inventory sheet, resident, 256–257, 257f
Inversion, 510t
Iodine
    dietary, 373t
    on thyroid gland, 622–623
Iron, dietary, 373t
Irregular bones, 506, 508f
Ischemia (ischemic), 571, 587
Islam, death and dying practices in, 452t
Islets of Langerhans, 624
Isolation precautions
    double-bagging in, 127p
    standard precautions in, 118, 119b
    transmission-based precautions in, 118–120,
        120b, 127p

J
Jacket restraint, 168f
Jaundice, 482
Jejunostomy tube, 386–387, 386f
Jejunum, 386, 635, 635f
Job applications, 36–40, 38f–39f

Job description, 17, 18f–19f
Job interviews, 40–42. *See also* Interviews, job
Job openings, finding, 35
Job-seeking skills, 32–42
    applications in, submitting, 36–40, 38f–39f
    cover letter in, 35, 37f
    ideal job in, defining, 32–35, 34f
    interviews in, 40–42 (*See also* Interviews)
    job openings in, finding, 35
    leaving a job in, 42
    reference list in, 35–36
    résumés in, 35, 36f
Joint Commission's Official "Do Not Use" List, 842, 847t
Joint Commission's Official "Do Not Use" List additions, 842, 847t
Joint replacement surgery, 516–517, 516f, 517f
Joints, 507, 509f
    cartilage in, 509f
    fixed, 507, 509f
    freely movable, 508
    slightly movable, 507, 509f
    wear and tear on, 514
Judaism, death and dying practices in, 453t
Judgmental attitude, 64
Justice, 53

K
Kaposi's sarcoma, 731, 732f
Kardex, 75, 76f
Keratin, 483, 483f
Kidney failure, 653–655
    care of person with, 654–655, 654f, 655b
    causes of, 653–654
    signs of, 654
Kidney infection, 652
Kidneys, 648–649
Kidney stones, 652–653, 653f
Kilocalories, 372
Kitchen skills, on diet, 378
Knee replacement surgery, 516–517, 516f
Knot, quick-release, 173, 174f
Korotkoff sounds, 291, 291b
Kübler-Ross, Elisabeth, 437–440

L
Labels, food, 375, 378f
Labia, 662f, 663
Labour, 763
Labour, pre-term, 762
Lacrimal glands, 602
Lactation, 663
Language, health care, 837–847
    anatomical terms in, 838–840
        abdominal area, 840–842, 841f
        body cavities, 840, 840f
        directional, 839–840, 839f, 840f
        planes, 838–839, 839f
    combining vowels in, 837–838, 838f, 842t–843t
    importance of, 837
    medical abbreviations in, 842
        common, 845t–846t
        Do Not Use list, 842, 847t
    medical terminology in, 837–838, 838f
    prefixes in, 837, 838f, 844t
    roots in, 837, 838f, 842t–843t
    suffixes in, 837, 838f, 844t

Lap buddy, 168f
Lap restraint, 168f, 174, 177p
Larceny, 51
Large intestine, 634f, 635–636, 635f
Laryngitis, 542
Larynx, 542, 542f
Later adulthood, 89, 89f
Lateral, 839, 839f
Lateral position, 182f, 183–184, 183f
Laws, 48–51
    civil
        definition of, 48
        violations of, 48–51, 49f–50f
    criminal, 48, 51–52
        definition of, 48
        violation of, 51–52, 52b
    definition of, 47
Laxative, 415
Learn, desire to, 29
Leaving job, 42
Left hypochondriac region, 841, 841f
Left iliac region, 841, 841f
Left lower quadrant (LLQ), 841, 841f
Left lumbar region, 841, 841f
Left-sided heart failure, 577–578
Left Sims' position, 418, 418f
Left upper quadrant (LUQ), 841, 841f
Legal issues, 46–52. *See also specific topics*
    abuse in (*See* Abuse)
    basic human rights in, 46–47
    laws in, 48–51 (*See also* Laws)
        civil, 48–51, 49f–50f
        criminal, 48, 51–52, 52b
    patients' rights in, 47
    protecting yourself from, 53–54, 54f
    residents' rights in, 47–48
Leg bag, 408
Leg exercises, postsurgical, 752, 752f
Lenses
    corrective, 603, 603f
    of eye, 602
Lesions, 498–499, 499t
Letter, cover, 35, 37f
Leukemia, 575
Leukocytes, 108, 108f, 566, 566f
Liability, 48
Libel, 49
Lice, 106t, 107
Lice, head, 355
Licensed practical nurse (LPN), 17, 20t
Lifestyle
    in cancer, 722
    on disease risk, 471–472
Life support, basic, 216–217
Life-sustaining treatments, 441
Lifting
    back safety in, 142–144, 144f, 145b–146b
    mechanical, transferring with, 188–189, 188f, 206p–207p
Lift sheet, 186b, 264
Ligaments, 508, 509f
Light, call, 245–246, 246f
Lighting
    general, 240, 240f
    task, 241
Linen handling, 265–266, 266f, 267b–268b
Linens, bed, 263–265

bath blanket, 265
bedmaking with, 268–276 (*See also* Bedmaking, techniques for)
bed protectors, 264
bedspreads, 264
blankets, 264
bottom and top sheets, 263
draw sheets, 264, 264f
for evacuating bedridden, 154, 155b
handling of, 266f, 267b–268p
humanistic health care for, 271
lift sheet, 264
mattress pads, 263
pillows and pillowcases, 264
Lipids, 374
Liquid diet
clear, 379
full, 379–380
Liquids, thickened, 384
Lithotripsy, 654
Litigation, 48
Liver, 634f, 636
"Liver spots," 486, 486f
Living will, 441, 441f
Lobes, lung, 543
Local anaesthesia, 743
Lochia, 765
Lochia alba, 765
Lochia serosa, 765
Logrolling, 185–187, 198p–199p
Long bones, 506, 508f
Long-term care facilities, 8, 8f
Lotions, 323
Lou Gehrig's disease, 591
Low-cholesterol diet, 380
Low-Fowler's position, 183, 184f
Lumbar regions, 841, 841f
Lumpectomy, 668
Lung cancer, 549
chest tube drainage system for, 549, 550f
diagnosis of, 549, 550f
Lungs, 542–543
immobility on, 181–182, 181f
structure of, 542–543, 543f
Luteinizing hormone (LH), 622, 664
Lymph, 567
Lymphatic system (lymphatics), 567–569, 569f
Lymph nodes, 568, 569f

M
Macular degeneration, 605
Macule, 498, 499t
Mad cow disease, 706t
Magical thinking, 781
Mainstreaming, 680, 681f
Make-up application, 358–359
Malaria, 106t, 107
Malignant melanoma, 723, 723f
Malignant tumour, 721
Malleus, 609–610, 610f
Malpractice, 49
Mammary glands, 663, 663f
Mammography, 667, 668f
Manic depression, 697
Manicure, 350, 351f
Manometer, 290, 290f
Manual sphygmomanometers, 290–292, 290f

Masks, 117–118, 118f, 119b, 126p
Massage, 328, 344p–345p
Mastectomy, 668
Mastication, 636
Masturbation, 93
Materials Safety Data Sheet (MSDS), 150, 151f
Mattress, pressure-relieving, 265
Mattress pads, 263
Meal preparation, in home health care, 796, 796f
Meal time, 380–385
eating assistance in, 382–383, 382f, 383f
feeding dependent residents in, 383–384, 384f, 392p–393p
food intake measurements and recording at, 384–385, 385f
humanistic health care for, 379
importance of, 380–381, 381f
preparing for, 381–382
standards relating to, 381, 381b
thickened liquids in, 384
Mechanical digestion, 636
Mechanical lift, transferring with, 188–189, 188f, 206p–207p
Mechanical ventilation, 556–559
endotracheal intubation in, 557–558, 558f
general care measures with, 559–560
need for, 556
observation in, 560
tracheostomy in, 558–559, 558f
ventilators in, 556–557, 557f
Medial, 839, 839f
Medical abbreviations, 842, 845t–847t
common, 845t–846t
"Do Not Use" List of, 842, 847t
"Do Not Use" List of, additional, 842, 847t
Medical asepsis, 112–116
antisepsis in, 112, 113f
definition of, 112
disinfection in, 112–113, 113f
handwashing in, 115–116, 115f, 119b, 122p–123p
sanitization in, 112–113, 113f, 114b
sterilization in, 112–113, 113f
Medical emergencies, in home health care, 804–806
Medical history, 69
Medical patients, 83
Medical record (chart), 69
Medical terminology, 837–838, 838f. *See also* Language, health care; *specific terms*
Medicare, 6–7
Medication, on accident risk, 162
Medication administration record (MAR), 69
Medulla, 584–585, 585f
adrenal, 624, 624f
breathing control by, 543
Melanin, 483, 483f, 486
Melatonin, 622
Memory
aging on, 587, 587f
changes in, 587
Menarche, 87
Ménière's disease, 611
Meninges, 584
Menopause, 88
Menorrhagia, 665
Menstrual period, 664, 664f
Mental disorders, 471

Mental health, 691–694. *See also specific topics*
  coping mechanisms in, 692–693, 693f, 694f
  defense mechanisms in, 693–694
  emotional balance in, 692, 692f
  stress in, 691–692, 692f
  stress management in, 692, 693f
Mental illness, 690–700
  activities of daily living with, 700
  anxiety disorders, 695–696
    definition and scope of, 695
    definition of, 697
    obsessive-compulsive disorder, 695–696
    panic disorder, 695, 695f, 697
    phobias, 696
  bipolar disorder (manic depression), 697
  care with, 698–699, 699f
  causes and treatment of, 693–694, 694–695
  definition of, 690
  depression, 696–697, 696f
  eating disorders, 697–698, 698f
  in elderly, 698, 699f
  listening and observing with, 698–699
  vs. mental health, 691–693 (*See also* Mental
    health)
  schizophrenia, 697
  substance abuse, 692, 694f
Mental retardation, 682–683, 682f
Message, 58, 59f. *See also* Communication
Metabolic disorders, 471
Metabolism, 281, 372
Metastasis, 722, 722f
Methicillin-resistant *Staphylococcus aureus* (MRSA),
  109
Method of transmission, 110, 110f
Microbes, 104–107
  bacteria, 105, 105f, 106t
  fungi, 106t, 107
  on hands, 115
  normal (resident) flora, 104
  opportunistic, 105
  parasites, 106t, 107
  pathogens, 104
  types of, 104–107, 106t
  viruses, 105–107, 106t
Microorganism, 104–107. *See also*
  Microbes
Microscope, electron, 105
Micturition, 403
Midbrain, 584, 585f
Middle adulthood, 88, 88f
Middle ear, 609–610, 610f
Mid-sagittal plane, 838, 839f
Midstream urine specimen, 403, 423p–424p
Mild mental retardation, 682, 682f
Military time, 73, 73f, 74b
Mineralocorticoids, 624, 624f
Minerals, 373, 373t, 374. *See also specific*
  minerals
Mission, 7
Mitered corner, 268–269, 268f
Mitral valve, 570, 570f
Mitt restraint, 168f
Mobility. *See also* Exercise
  lack/impairment of
    on accident risk, 162
    complications of, 180–182, 181f
  for pressure ulcer prevention, 491f, 492

Moderate mental retardation, 682
Modular nursing, 19
Molds, 106t, 107
Moles, cancerous, 723, 723f
Montgomery ties, 497, 497f
Morning care, 315
Motor nerves, 585
Mouth, 633, 634f
Movement
  coordinated body, 142, 143f
  terminology for, 510t
  voluntary, 509, 512f
Mucosa, 633, 634f
Mucous membranes
  in airways, 541
  in dying, caring for, 448
  skin, 107
Mucus, 541
Multi-infarct dementia, 706–707, 706t
Multiple sclerosis (MS), 591
Munchausen syndrome by proxy, 784
Muscle layer, digestive tract, 633, 634f
Muscles
  immobility on, 180–181, 181f
  loss of mass in, 513–514, 513f
Muscle tissue, 467–468, 468t
Muscle tone
  of bladder, 651
  definition and function of, 509
Muscular dystrophy, 517–518
Muscular system, 469, 470f, 508–514, 509f
Musculoskeletal system, 506–514
  aging on, 512–514
    bone tissue loss in, 513
    exercise and eating in, 512, 513f
    joint wear and tear in, 514
    muscle mass loss in, 513–514, 513f
  functions of, 509–512, 512f
  joints in, 507–508, 509f
  muscular system in, 508–514, 511f
  range-of-motion exercises for, 523–524 (*See also*
    Range-of-motion exercises)
    contractures and, 523, 523f
    guidelines for, 525b
    procedure for, 524, 530p–535p
    types of, 523–524
  skeletal system in, 506–508
Musculoskeletal system disorders, 513–523
  amputations, 521–522, 522f
  arthritis, 515–517
    gout, 517
    osteoarthritis, 515–517
    osteoarthritis and joint replacement, 516–517,
      516f, 517f
    overview and definition, 515
    rheumatoid, 517, 517f
  fractures, 518–521 (*See also* Fracture)
  muscular dystrophy, 517–518
  osteoporosis, 514, 515f
  rehabilitation for, 527–528
Music therapy, for dementia, 717
Myasthenia gravis, 517
Myelin, 583, 583f
Myocardial infarction, 217–218, 577, 577f
Myocardium, 569
Myomas, 664–665
Myopia, 603, 603f

N

Nail clippers, 350, 351f
Nail polish, 351
Nails, 484
Nail thickening, 487
Narrative nurse's notes, 69, 70f
Nasal cannula, 552b, 553f, 554–555, 555f
Nasal cavity, 541, 542f
Nasogastric tube, 386–387, 386f
Nasointestinal tube, 386–387, 386f
Nasopharyngeal airway, 555–556, 556f
Nearsightedness, 603, 603f
Necrosis, 487
Needlesticks, 131
Needs, 89
Needs, basic human, 89–94. *See also specific topics*
  definition of, 89
  Maslow's hierarchy of human needs in, 89–92
    definition and overview, 89, 90f
    love and belonging, 91, 91f
    physiologic, 90, 90f
    safety and securityu, 90, 91f
    self-actualization, 91–92, 92f
    self-esteem, 91, 91f
  sexuality and intimacy in, 92–94, 93f
Negligence, 48–49, 49f
Neoplastic disease, 471
Nephrons, 648, 650f
Nervous system, 469, 470f, 583–587
  aging on, 586–587, 587f
  function of, 586
  structure of
    brain, 584–585, 585f
    cells, 583
    central nervous system, 583–585, 584f, 585f
    peripheral nervous system, 584, 584f, 585–586
    spinal cord, 585
Nervous system disorders, 587–592
  amyotrophic lateral sclerosis, 591
  diagnosis of, 592, 592f, 593f
  epilepsy, 590–591
  head injuries, 591, 591f
  multiple sclerosis, 591
  Parkinson's disease, 589–590, 590f
  rehabilitation for, 592–593, 593f
  spinal cord injuries, 592
  stroke, 588–589, 589f
  transient ischemic attacks, 587–588
Nervous tissue, 468
Neurons, 583, 583f
Neurotransmitters, in mental illness, 693
Newborn care, 766–772
  bathing in, 770–771, 771f
  burping in, 770, 770f
  for circumcision, 768, 768f
  diapering in, 770
  feeding in, 768–770, 769f
  putting baby down to sleep in, 771–772, 771f, 772f
  security in, 767, 768f
  transporting in, 772, 772f
  for umbilical cord stump, 767–768, 768f
  vital signs in, 767
Niacin, 373t
Nightingale, Florence, 15, 16f
Nitroglycerin, 577
Nits, 355
No-code, 441

Nocturia, 404
Nocturnal emissions, 87
Noise control, in resident unit, 241, 241f
Nonmaleficence, 53
Non-regulated health care professions, 15–16
Nonspecific defense mechanisms, 107–108, 108f
Nonverbal communication, 58–59
Norepinephrine, 624, 624f
Normal anatomical position, 838, 838f
Normal flora, 104
Nosocomial infections, 112
NPO status, 389, 747, 747f
Nucleus, 467, 467f
Nurse's bag, 798, 798f
Nurse's notes, narrative, 69, 70f
Nursing
  functional (modular), 19
  history of, 15, 16f
  primary, 17–19
Nursing diagnosis, 76
Nursing history, 69, 253, 254f–255f
Nursing home attendant, 20t
Nursing homes, 8, 8f
Nursing process, 75–77
Nursing team, 17–20
  functional nursing model for, 19
  members of, 17, 20t
  personal support worker duties in, 20
  primary nursing model for, 17–19
  team nursing model for, 19–20
Nutrients, 372. *See also specific types*
Nutrition, 372–393
  balanced diet in, 375
  Canada's Food Guide on, 375, 376f–377f
  in elderly
    chewing problems in, 384
    loss of appetite in, 379
    swallowing problems in, 384
  enteral, 386–388, 386f, 387f
  fluids and hydration in, 388–391
    dehydration, 388
    edema, 389
    fluid balance, 388–389, 484
    intake/output measurements and recording in, 389–391, 390f, 404–405, 405f
    with NPO status, 389
    offering fluids, 389
  food choices and eating habits in, 375–379
  food labels in, 375, 378f
  IV therapy in, 385–386, 385f
  meal time in, 380–385
    eating assistance in, 382–383, 382f, 383f
    feeding dependent residents in, 383–384, 384f, 392p–393p
    food intake measuring and recording at, 384–385, 385f
    humanistic health care for, 379
    importance of, 380–381, 381f
    preparing for, 381–382
    standards relating to, 381, 381b
    thickened liquids in, 384
  nutrients in, 372, 374–375 (*See also specific nutrients*)
  personal support worker in, 30, 30f
  post-operative, 753
  special diets in, 379–380
  total parenteral, 388, 388f

Nutritional disorders, 471
Nutritional supplements, 380

O

Obese, 375
Object check, 225p
Objective data, 67, 67f
Observation, 67–68
Obsessions, 695
Obsessive-compulsive disorder, 695–696
Obstetrical patients, 83
Occult, 404
Occupation, on disease risk, 472
Occupied bed, 270f, 271, 274p–276p
Occurrence report, 166, 167f
Odour control, in resident unit, 239–240
Oil glands, 483, 483f
Oil retention enema, 417, 417f
Oils, bath, 323
Older adulthood, 89, 89f
Oliguria, 404
Open bed, 270, 270f
Open-ended questions, 61–62
Open fracture, 518, 518f
Open reduction, 520
Open Reduction, Internal Fixation (ORIF), 520
Opportunistic microbes, 105
Oral care, 316–318
    with dentures, 317, 317b, 332p–333p
    with natural teeth, 316, 330p–331p
    timing of, 316
    for unconscious person, 318
        guidelines for, 318b
        procedures for, 333p–334p
        tongue blade for, 318, 318f
Oral–fecal route, 132, 132f
Oral temperature, 283–284, 298p–299p
Orange stick, 350, 351, 351f
Orbit, 602
Order sheet, physician's, 69
Organelles, 467, 467f
Organism, 466, 466f
Organs, 468–469
Organ systems, 469, 470f
Oriented to person, place, and time, 215
Oropharyngeal airway, 555–556, 556f
Orthostatic hypotension, 293–294
Ossicles, 609–610, 610f
Osteoarthritis, 515–517
Osteoporosis, 514, 515f
Ostomy, 640, 640f
Ostomy appliance, 640–641, 641f
Ostomy care, 639–645
    humanistic care in, 641
    ostomy appliance in, 639, 641, 641f
    procedure for, 643p–645p
    types of ostomies in, 639–641
Otitis externa, 611
Otitis media, 611
Otosclerosis, 611
Outer ear, 609, 610f
Outlets, with ground-fault breakers, 150, 152f
Ovarian cancer, 666
Ovarian cysts, 664
Ovaries, 662, 662f
Over-bed tables, 244, 244f
Overflow incontinence, 412

Oviduct, 662, 662f
Ovulation, 662, 664, 664f
Ovum (ova), 661
Oxygen
    in basic life support, 216
    fires from, 152, 152f, 153b, 154f
Oxygen concentrators, 554, 554f
Oxygen therapy, 551–556
    doctor and nurse role in, 551
    facemasks in, 555, 555f
    fire safety with, 152, 154, 154f
    flow meter in, 551, 551f
    flow rate in, 551–552, 551f, 552b
    forms of, 551
    guidelines for, 552b
    humidity bottle in, 552b, 553
    mechanical ventilation in, 556–559
    nasal cannulas in, 552b, 553f, 554–555, 555f
    nasopharyngeal airway in, 555–556, 556f
    oropharyngeal airway in, 555–556, 556f
    oxygen concentrators for, 554, 554f
    pressurized tanks for, 54f, 553–554
    pulse oximetre in, 553, 553f
    value of, 551
    wall-mounted delivery systems for, 553, 554f
Oxytocin, 621, 622f

P

Pacemaker, 570, 578, 578f
Pacing, 708, 708f
Pads, incontinence, 412–413, 413f
Pain, 599–601, 599f. *See also specific disorders*
    acute, 599
    chronic, 599
    management of, with cancer, 727
    radiating, 599
    referred, 599, 600f
    treatments for
        with cancer, 727
        cold applications, 524–526, 524t, 526f,
            535p–536p (*See also* Cold applications)
        heat applications, 524–527, 524t, 527f, 537p (*See
            also* Heat applications)
Palliative, 726
Palliative care, 441, 442f
Pallor, 482
Pancreas, 636
    functions of, 624–625, 636
    location of, 620, 621f, 634f
Panic, 695
Panic disorder, 695, 695f
Pap test, 667
Papule, 498, 499t
Paralysis, on accident risk, 162
Paraplegia, 162, 592
Parasites, 106t, 107
Parathyroid glands, 620
    function of, 623
    location of, 621f
Parathyroid hormone (PTH), 623
Parkinson's disease, 589–590, 590f, 706t
PASS, 155
Passive range-of-motion (PROM) exercises, 523, 525b,
    530p–535p
Pathogens, 104, 110, 110f. *See also specific types*
    airborne, 136–138 (*See also* Airborne diseases)
    bloodborne, 131–136 (*See also* Bloodborne diseases)

Patients, 7
Patients' rights, 47
Patient's unit, hospital, 236, 237f
Pediatric patients, 83, 776–785
    adolescents
        emotional needs in, 783, 783f
        physical needs in, 782–783
        safety needs in, 783
    child abuse in, 783–785, 785b
        physical, 784
        psychological (emotional), 784
        reporting of, 785b, 787
        risk factors for, 784
        sexual, 784
    family stress and, 776, 777f
    growth and development in, 776
    infant care in
        emotional needs in, 777, 778f
        physical needs in, 777
        safety needs in, 777–778
    preschooler care in
        emotional needs in, 780–781
        entertainment in, 780, 780f
        physical needs in, 780
        safety needs in, 781
    school-age children
        emotional needs in, 782, 782f
        overview of, 781
        physical needs in, 781–782
        safety needs in, 782
    toddler care in
        emotional needs in, 779–780, 779f
        physical needs in, 779
        regression in, 778–779
        safety needs in, 780
    understanding of, 776
Pediculosis, 106t, 107
Pediculosis capitis, 355
Pelvic inflammatory disease (PID), 672
Pelvis, renal, 649
Penetrating ulcer, 638
Penile cancer, 670
Penis, 322, 322f, 669, 669f
Percutaneous endoscopic gastrostomy (PEG) tube,
        386–387, 387f
Pericardium, 569
Perineal (peri) care, 318–322
    bath blanket for, 320, 320f
    culture and, 320
    definition and scope of, 318–319, 319f
    for females, 322, 334p–336p
    gender of worker for, 320
    guidelines for, 321b–322b
    humanistic care in, 320
    for males, 322, 322f, 336p–338p
    postpartum, 765–766
    for pressure ulcer prevention, 491, 491f
    reasons for, 319
    telling patient about, 319
Perineum, 318, 319f, 662f, 663
Periodontitis, 316
Peri-operative period, 743, 744f. See also specific
        phases
Peripheral nervous system (PNS), 584, 584f,
        585–586
Peripheral vascular disease, 576
Peristalsis, 414

Peritoneal dialysis, 654, 654f
Perpetrators, of abuse, 52
Perseveration, 708
Personal effects
    admission inventory of, 256–257, 257f
    storage of, 244–245, 245f
Personal ethics, 53, 54f
Personal hygiene. See Hygiene, personal
Personal items, 246–247
Personal protective equipment (PPE), 116. See also
        specific types
    gloves, 117, 117f, 119b, 123p
    gowns, 117, 119b, 124p–125p
    in home health care, 809–810
    masks, 117–118, 118f, 119b, 126p
    protective eyewear, 118, 118f, 119b
    removing multiple articles of, 118, 127p
Personal safety, in home health care, 810–811
Personal stories, operating room nurse, 99
Personal support worker, 15–22
    delegation to, 20–22
    education of, 16–17, 16f
    history of nursing and, 15, 16f
    non-regulated health care professions and,
        15–16
    in nursing team, 17–20, 20t (See also
        Nursing team)
    regulated health care professions and, 15
    responsibilities of, 17, 18f–19f
Petit mal seizures, 219, 219f
Pet therapy, for dementia, 717, 717f
Phantom pain, 523
Pharyngitis, 541
Pharynx, 541–542, 542f, 633, 634f
Phlegm, 546
Phobias, 696
Phosphorus, dietary, 373t
pH scale, 650–651
Physical abuse, 51
Physical examination, for personal support worker,
        30–31, 30f
Physical health, 29–31, 30f
Physical injury. See specific types
Physical injury protection, 144, 145b–146b
Physical needs. See specific age groups and topics
Physical rehabilitation, 475, 476f
Physical restraint, 166, 168f. See also Restraints
Physical therapy. See also Rehabilitation
    supportive devices in, 475, 476f
Physician's order sheet, 69
Physician's progress notes, 69
Physiology, 466
Pia mater, 584
Pick's disease, 706t
Pillowcases, 264
Pillows, 264
Pineal gland
    function of, 622
    location of, 620, 621f
Pink eye, 604, 604f
Pinna, 609, 610f
Pinworms, 106t, 107
Pituitary dwarfism, 625
Pituitary gigantism, 625, 625f
Pituitary gland
    function of, 621–622, 622f
    location of, 620, 621f

Planes, 838–839, 839f
    anatomical, 838–839, 839f
    frontal (coronal), 839, 839f
    sagittal, 838, 839f
    transverse, 839, 839f
Planning, in nursing process, 76
Plantar flexion, 510t
Plaques
    in Alzheimer's disease, 705, 706f
    cardiovascular, 575, 575f
Plasma, 565, 566f
Plastic bags, as suffocation risk, 778
Platelet count, low, 574–575
Platelets, 566–567, 566f
Pleura, 543
Pleurisy, 546
Plugs
    grounded, 150, 152f
    three-prong, 150, 152f
Pneumonia, 546, 547b
Pneumothorax, 550–551
Podiatrist, 351, 352f
Poisoning
    prevention of, 165
    in toddlers, 780
Polyuria, 404–405
Pons, 584, 585f
Portal of entry, 110–111
Portal of exit, 110
Position, 599
Position, anatomical, 838
Positioning, 180–187
    basic positions in, 182–184, 183f (See also
        Positions, basic)
    of dying, 449
    immobility and, 180, 181f
    of newborn for sleeping, 771–772, 771f, 772f
    post-operative assistance with, 752–753
    repositioning in, 185–187 (See also Repositioning)
    supportive devices for, 182
Positions, basic, 182–184
    body alignment in, 141–142, 142f, 182,
        182f
    Fowler's, 183, 183f, 184f, 242, 242f
    high-Fowler's, 183, 184f
    lateral, 182f, 183–184, 183f
    prone, 182f, 183f, 184
    reverse Trendelenburg's, 242f, 243
    semi-Fowler's (low Fowler's), 183, 184f
    Sims', 183f, 184
    sitting, 183f, 184
    supine (dorsal recumbent), 183, 183f
    Trendelenburg's, 242–243, 242f
Post-anaesthesia care unit (PACU), 749, 749f
Posterior, 839f, 840
Postmenopausal bleeding, 666
Postmortem care, 454–458
    autopsy in, 455
    on care worker, 455–456
    definition of, 454
    holistic approach to, 447, 447f
    need for, 454–455
    postmortem kit for, 455, 455f
    preparation for viewing in, 455, 455f
    shroud preparation in, 455, 456f, 457p–458p
Postmortem kit, 455, 455f
Post-operative patient care, 749–753

    ambulation in, 753
    elimination in, 753
    hygiene in, 753
    immediately after surgery, 749–750, 749f
    nutrition in, 753
    positioning in, 752–753
    in post-anaesthesia care unit, 749, 749f
    preventing complications in
        cardiovascular, 751–752, 755p–756p (See also
            Cardiovascular complication prevention,
            postoperative)
        leg exercises for, 752, 752f
        respiratory, 750–751, 751f
    room preparation for, 749, 749f
    vital signs in, 749–750, 750f
Post-operative phase, 743
Postpartum period, 764–772
    care of mother in, 764–766
    definition of, 764
Post-procedure actions, 144, 147b–148b
Postural instability, in Parkinson's disease,
    590, 590f
Potassium, dietary, 373t
Powder, body, 323
Power strips, grounded, 150, 152f
Precautions
    airborne, 118–119, 120b
    for bloodborne diseases, 134–136, 136b
    contact, 120, 127p
    droplet, 119–120
    standard (See Standard precautions)
    transmission-based, 118–120, 120b, 127p
Pre-clampsia/eclampsia, 762
Prefixes, 837, 838f, 844t
Pregnancy, 760–772
    antepartum (prenatal) period in, 760–763 (See also
        Antepartum (prenatal) period)
        complications in, 762
        definition of, 760
        emotional needs in, 762–763, 763f
        humanist health care in, 761
        meeting emotional needs in, 762–763, 763f
        meeting physical needs in, 762
        phases (trimesters) of, 760, 761f
        physical needs in, 762
        routine care in, 760–761
    delivery in
        during, 763–764, 763f
        immediately following, 764, 764f
    labour in, 763
    postpartum period in, 764–772 (See also Newborn
        care)
        care of baby in, 766–772 (See also Newborn
            care)
        care of mother in, 764–766
Prenatal care, definition of, 760
Pre-operative patient care, 743–749
    emotional preparation in, 743–746
        fears, concerns, and worries in, 743–744
        informed decision and consent in, 744,
            745f
        pre-operative teaching in, 744, 744f
        support in, 746
    physical preparation in, 746–749
        days leading up to surgery, 746
        evening before surgery, 746, 746f
        immediately before surgery, inpatients, 748–749

immediately before surgery, outpatients, 747–748, 747f, 748f
morning of surgery, 747
Pre-operative phase, 743
Pre-operative teaching, 744, 744f
Pre-procedure actions, 144, 146b–147b
Presbycusis, 610–611
Presbyopia, 604, 604f
Preschool, 86, 86f
Preschooler care
emotional needs in, 780–781
entertainment in, 780, 780f
physical needs in, 780
safety needs in, 781
Pressure points, for pressure ulcers, 487, 488f
Pressure-reducing devices, 492, 492f
Pressure-relieving mattress, 265
Pressure-sensitive bed monitoring system, 172f, 173
Pressure ulcers, 487–494. See also Wound
beds for
airflow, 492–493, 493f
alternating pressure, 493, 493f
Circ-O-Lectric, 493–494, 493f
definition of, 487
development of, 487, 488f
from immobility, 180, 181f
locations of, 487, 489f
prevention of, 490–492, 491f
repositioning for prevention of, 186b–187b (See also Repositioning)
risk factors for, 488
stages of, 488–490, 490f
Pressurized tanks, oxygen, 553–554, 554f
Pre-term labour, 762
Primary nursing, 17–19
Privacy, invasion of, 50–51, 50f
Privacy curtains, 246
PRN care, 315
Probe, thermometer, 283, 283f
Procedure, 144. See also specific procedures
Professional, 26
Professional appearance, 31–32, 32f, 33b
Professional ethics, 53, 53b
Professionalism, 26–32
accountability in, 28
attitude in, 26–27
conscientiousness in, 28
cooperativeness in, 29
courtesy in, 28
definition of, 26
desire to learn in, 29
emotional health in, 31, 31f
empathy in, 29
honesty in, 29
personal hygiene and appearance in, 31–32, 32f, 33b
physical health in, 29–31, 30f
punctuality in, 27–28, 28f
reliability in, 28
respectfulness in, 28–29
work ethic in, 27–29, 27f
Profound mental retardation, 682
Progeny, 107
Prognosis, with cancer, 728
Progress notes, physician's, 69
Projection, 692–693, 694
Prolactin, 622, 622f

Pronation, 510t
Prone position, 182f, 183f, 184
Prostate cancer, 670
Prostate gland enlargement, 651, 670
Prosthetic devices
after amputation, 522, 522f
general information on, 475, 476f
Prosthetic eye, 608–609, 609f
Prosthetic eye care, 609, 609f
Protective eyewear, 118, 118f, 119b
Protectors, bed, 264
Protein, 374
Protozoa, 106t, 107
Proximal, 840
Psychiatric disorders, 471
Psychiatric patients, 83
Psychiatrist, 694
Psychological abuse, 51
Psychological stages, of childhood, 86f
Psychologists, 694
Puberty, 87
Pulmonary circulation, 571–572, 572f
Pulmonary embolism, 576, 751
Pulmonary valve, 570, 570f
Pulse, 285–287
definition and origin of, 285
factors in, 286
newborn, 767
normal and abnormal findings in, 287
qualities of, 285–286
Pulse amplitude, 286
Pulse deficit, 287
Pulse measurement
apical pulse, 285f, 286–287, 304p
points of, 220, 285, 285f
radial pulse, 285f, 286, 287, 303p
stethoscope in, 286–287
Pulse oximetre, 551f, 553
Pulse points, 220, 285, 285f
Pulse pressure, 289
Pulse rate
in adults, 285
in children, 296t
Pulse rhythm, 285–286
Punctuality, 27–28, 28f
Pupil, 602, 602f
Purging, 697
Pustule, 498, 499t
Pyelonephritis, 652
Pyloric sphincter, 634f, 635
Pylorus, 635, 635f

Q
qd, 842, 846t
qid, 842, 846t
qod, 842
Quadrants, 841, 841f
Quadriplegia, 162, 592
Quality of life, 96–97
Questions, open-ended, 61–62
Quick-release knot, 173, 174f

R
Race, 94
RACE fire response plan, 154–155, 154f
Radial pulse, 285f, 286, 287, 303p

Radiating pain, 599, 600f
Radiation therapy, for cancer, 724–725
Radiography, chest, 579
Range of motion, 507
Range-of-motion exercises, 523–524
　contractures and, 523, 523f
　guidelines for, 525b
　procedure for, 524, 530p–535p
　types of, 523–524
Rash, 498
Rationalization, 693, 694
Reality orientation, 710, 711t
Receiver
　in communication, 58, 59f, 60
　as good listener, 61, 61f
Receptive aphasia, 589
Receptors
　sensory, 598
　tactile, 599, 599f
Reciprocity, 17
Record. See also Data
　medical, 69, 74
　medication administration, 69
Recording, 69–75. See also Data
　admission sheet in, 69
　computerized charting in, 75, 75f
　facility or agency policies on, 73
　graphic sheet in, 69–70, 71f–72f
　guidelines on, 74b
　in home health care, 794
　Kardex in, 75, 76f
　medical history in, 69
　medical record (chart) in, 69
　medication administration record in, 69
　miscellaneous documents in, 70
　narrative nurse's notes in, 69, 70f
　nursing history in, 69
　physician's order sheet in, 69
　physician's progress notes in, 69
　sample of, 70–73
　of subject data, 68
　time in, 73, 73f, 74b
Recreational drugs, 30, 30f
Rectal suppositories, 418
Rectal temperature, 284, 299p–300p
Rectum, 635f, 636
Red blood cells, 565–566, 566f
　impaired production of, 575
　increased destruction of, 575
Reduction, fracture, 519–520
Reference list, 35–36
Referred pain, 599, 600f
Reflex incontinence, 412
Regional anaesthesia, 743
Regions, abdominal, 841–842, 841f
Registered nurse (RN), 17, 20t
Registered nurse assistant (RNA), 17
Registered nurse's assistant (RNA), 20t
Registered psychiatric nurse (RPN),
　17, 20t
Regression
　in mental illness, 694
　in toddlers, 778–779
Regular diet, 379
Regulated health care professions, 15
Rehabilitation
　cardiac, 579

　with developmental disabilities, 686, 687
　devices in, 475, 476f
　disability in, 472
　for musculoskeletal disorders, 527–528
　for nervous system disorders, 592–593, 593f
　stroke, 589
Rehabilitation and restorative care, 472–478
　definitions of, 472
　disability in, 472f
　emotional rehabilitation in, 475–477, 477f
　guidelines for, 474b
　humanistic care in, 475
　personal support worker role in, 473–474.473f
　physical rehabilitation in, 475, 476f
Rehabilitation patients, 83
Reincarnation, 451
Reliability, 28
Religion, 94f, 95–96, 95f, 378
Reminiscence therapy, 715–716, 715f
Renal, 648
Renal calculi, 652–653, 653f
Renal failure, 653–655, 656b
　care of person with, 654–655, 654f, 655b
　causes of, 653–654
　signs of, 654
Renal pelvis, 649
Repetition, 708
Rephrasing, 62
Report, incident (occurrence), 166, 167f
Reporting, 68–69, 68f
　of abuse, 52
　of accidents, 166, 167f
　of child abuse, 785b, 787
　in communication among health care team
　　members,
　　68–69, 68f
　of subject data, 67–68, 68f
　of unusual signs and symptoms, 214–215,
　　215f
Repositioning, 185–187
　friction in, 185
　guidelines for, 186b–187b
　logrolling in, 185–187, 198p–199p
　moving to side of bed in
　　one worker, 185, 193p
　　two workers, 185, 193p–194p
　moving up in bed in
　　one worker, 185, 195p
　　two workers, 185, 196p
　for pressure ulcer prevention, 490, 491f
　raising head and shoulders in, 185,
　　196p–197p
　shearing in, 185
　turning onto side in, 185, 197p–198p
Repression, 693, 694
Reproduction, 660
Reproductive system, 469, 470f
Reproductive system, female, 661–665
　aging on, 664–665
　function of, 664, 664f
　structure of, 662–663, 662f
Reproductive system, male
　aging on, 670
　function of, 669–670
　structure of, 668–669, 669f
Reproductive system disorders, female, 665–666
　amenorrhea, 665

cancer, 666, 666f
cysts and noncancerous growths, 665–666
diagnostic procedures for, 667, 667f, 668f
dysmenorrhea, 665
infertility, 665
menorrhagia, 665
sexually transmitted infections, 671–673, 672f
surgical procedures in, 668
Reproductive system disorders, male
cancer, 670, 671f
diagnostic procedures for, 671
impotence, 670
sexually transmitted infections, 671–673, 672f
Rescue breathing, 216, 217b, 225p
Reservoir, 110
Resident flora, 104
Resident inventory sheet, 256–257, 257f
Residents, 8. *See also specific topics*
admission of, 251–257 (*See also* Admissions)
definition of, 81
Resident safety. *See* Safety, resident
Resident's environment. *See* Environment, resident's
Residents' rights, 47–48
Resident's unit, 236–238
in assisted-living facilities, 238, 238f
decorating room in, 257
in long-term care facilities, 237–238, 238f
preparation of, for admission, 253, 256, 256f
Resistance, to blood flow, 289
Resistance training, 514
Respectfulness, 28–29
Respiration, 287–289, 542. *See also* Cardiopulmonary
resuscitation (CPR)
definition of, 287
depth of, 288
in emergency care, 217b
exhalation in, 287–288
factors in, 288
functions of, 287–288
inhalation in, 287
measurement of, 288, 305p
newborn, 767
normal and abnormal findings in, 288
process of, 287–288
Respiratory arrest, 216
Respiratory exercises, postoperative, 750–751,
751f
Respiratory rate
in adults, 288
in children, 296t
Respiratory rhythm, 288
Respiratory system, 469, 470f, 541–546
aging on, 544–546
exercise on, 545, 545f
function of
gas exchange, 543–544, 544f
ventilation, 543
immobility on, 181, 181f
structure of, 541–543 (*See also specific parts*)
airway, 541–542, 542f
lungs, 542–543, 543f
toxins on, 545
Respiratory system disorders, 546–551
asthma, 547–548, 548f
cancer, 549, 550f
chronic obstructive pulmonary disease,
548–549

comfort with, promoting, 560f, 561
general care measures for, 559–560
hemothorax, 551
infections, 546f
aging on, 545–546
sputum specimen collection in, 546, 547b
observation for, 560
pneumothorax, 550–551
Respiratory therapy, 551–559
advanced training in, 551
definition of, 551
general care measures in, 559–560
observation in, 560
oxygen in, 551–556, 552b (*See also* Oxygen therapy)
suctioning in, 559, 559f
Respite care, 792, 793f
Restorative care, 472–473. *See also* Rehabilitation
Restraints, 166–177
alternatives to, 171–173, 172f
ankle or wrist, 173–174, 176p
applying
lap or waist (belt), 174
vest, 173
wrist or ankle, 173–174
chemical, 166
complications with, 169–171
guidelines and standards for, 168, 169f,
170b–171b
humanistic health care for, 171
jacket, 168f
lap or waist (belt), 168f, 177p
mitt, 168f
nerve damage from, 169
physical, 168f
quick-release knot for, 173, 174f
use of, 166–169, 169f, 170b–171b
vest, 168f, 175p–176p
wrist, 168f
Résumés, 35, 36f
Retention, urinary, 412
Retina, 602, 602f
Reverse Trendelenburg's position, 242f,
243
Rheumatoid arthritis, 517, 517f
Riboflavin, 373t
Right hypochondriac region, 841, 841f
Right iliac region, 841, 841f
Right lower quadrant (RLQ), 841, 841f
Right lumbar region, 841, 841f
Rights
basic human, 46–47
Canadian Charter of Rights and Freedoms,
46
Canadian Human Rights Law, 35
definition of, 46
with developmental disabilities, 681
Dying Person's Bill of Rights, 448b
five rights of delegation, 20, 21t
with HIV/AIDS, 733
patients', 47
residents', 47–48
Right-sided heart failure, 577
Right upper quadrant (RUQ), 841, 841f
Rigidity, in Parkinson's disease, 590,
590f
Rigor mortis, 455
Ringworm, 106t, 107

Risk factors
  for abuse, 51–52
  for accidents, 161–163, 161f (*See also under*
    Accidents)
  age as
    on accident risk, 161–162
    on disease risk, 471
  cardiac, 576
  for child abuse, 784
  for coronary artery disease, 576
  for disease, 471–472
  for pressure ulcers, 488
  in resident's environment, 161–163, 161f
Rocky Mountain spotted fever, 105
Rods, bacterial, 105, 105f
Room dividers, 246
Room preparation, resident's, 253, 256, 256f
Room temperature, 240
Roots, 837, 838f, 842t–843t
Rotation, 510t
Roundworms, 106t, 107
Routine care scheduling, 315
Rubra lochia, 765
Rugae, 635
Rummaging, 708

S
Safe home guidelines, 804, 805b–806b
Safety, resident, 161–177
  accidents in, 161–166 (*See also* Accidents)
    reporting of, 166, 167f
    risk factors in, 161–163
  restraints for, 166–177 (*See also* Restraints)
Safety, workplace
  home health care, 804–806
    abusive situations in, 806
    accidents and medical emergencies in, 804–806
    personal safety in, 810–811
    safe home guidelines in, 804, 805b–806b
  institution, 141–158
    ABCs of good body mechanics in, 141–142, 142f,
      143f
    chemical injury prevention in, 149–150
    disaster preparedness in, 156–157 (*See also*
      Disaster preparedness)
    electrical shock prevention in, 150, 152f
    fall assistance in, 149, 149b
    fall prevention in, 145b–146b, 148–149
    fire safety in, 151–157 (*See also* Fire safety)
      extinguishing fires in, 154f, 155, 156t
      oxygen therapy and, 152, 154, 154f
      preventing fires in, 151–154, 152f, 153b
      reacting to fire emergency in, 154–156, 154f,
        155b, 156t
    lifting and back safety in, 142–144, 144f,
      145b–146b
    procedures for
      post-procedure actions in, 144, 147b–148b
      pre-procedure actions in, 144–148, 146b–147b
    protecting yourself from physical injury in, 144,
      145b–146b
Safety needs. *See specific age groups and topics*
Sagittal plane, 838, 839f
Saline enema, 417, 417f
Salivary glands, 634f, 635
Salt water enema, 417, 417f
Sanitary environment, in home health care, 807–809

  cleaning equipment and household surfaces in,
    807f, 808
  client personal hygiene assistance in, 808–809
  food handling in, 808, 809f
  proper bag technique in, 807–808, 807f
Sanitization, 112–113, 113f, 114b
Sanitoriums, 137
Scabies, 106t, 107
Scales, 294–296
  chair, 294–295, 295f, 308p–309p
  sling, 295–296, 296f, 309p–310p
  upright, 294, 295f, 307p–308p
Schizophrenia, 697
School-age children
  emotional needs in, 782, 782f
  overview of, 781
  physical needs in, 781–782
  safety needs in, 782
School-age years, 87, 87f
Sclera, 602, 602f
Scope of practice, 21, 22b
Scrotum, 668, 669f
Seat belt, 168f, 177p
Sebaceous glands, 483, 483f
Seborrheic dermatitis, 355
Sebum, 483
Secondary infection, 499
Second-degree burns, 497
Seizures, 219, 219f
Semicircular canals, 610, 610f
Semi-Fowler's position, 183, 184f, 561
Sender, in communication, 60, 61, 62f
Sensation, skin in, 485
Sense organs, 598
Senses, 598–617
  general sense, 598–601
    definition of, 598
    pain, 599–601, 600f
    position, 599
    touch, 598–599, 599f
  hearing, 609–611
    aging on ear in, 610–611
    in dying, 449
    ear disorders on, 609–612 (*See also* Ear disorders)
    ear function in, 610
    ear structure in, 609–610, 610f
  sight, 601–605
    aging on eye in, 602, 604f
    contact lens care in, 608, 609f
    eye disorders in, 604–606 (*See also* Eye disorders)
    eye function in, 602–603, 603f
    eyeglass care in, 606–608, 608f
    eye structure in, 602–603, 602f
    prosthetic eye care in, 609, 609f
  special, 598
  taste and smell, 601, 601f
Sensor device, newborn, 767, 768f
Sensorineural hearing loss, 611
Sensory impairment, on accident risk, 162
Sensory nerves, 585
Sensory receptors, 598
Sensory system, structure of, 598
Septic shock, 220
Sequential compression device (SCD), 751–752, 751f
Serosa, 633, 634f
Severe mental retardation, 682
Sex, 92

Sex cells, 661
Sex cells, male, 668, 669f
Sex glands. *See also specific glands*
    functions of, 625
    structures and locations of, 620, 621f
Sex hormones, 625. *See also specific hormones*
Sexual abuse, 51
Sexual behaviors, inappropriate, with dementia, 709
Sexual intercourse, 93
Sexuality, 92–94, 93f
Sexually transmitted diseases (STDs). *See* Sexually transmitted infections (STIs)
Sexually transmitted infections (STIs), 671–673, 672f
    in adolescents, 783
    definition of, 671–672
    prevention of, 673
    types of, 672–673, 672f
Shaken baby syndrome, 784
Shampooing hair, 356, 356f, 365p–366p
Sharps, 119b
Shaving
    in men, 357–358, 357f, 367p–368p
    in women, 358
Shearing
    causes of, 185
    pressure ulcers and, 491f, 492
Sheath, thermometer, 282, 283, 283f
Sheet
    bottom and top, 263
    draw, 264, 264f
    lift, 264
Shivering, 511
Shock, 220, 221f
Shoehorns, 353, 353f
Short bones, 506, 508f
Shower chair
    in home health care, 795, 795f
    in hospital or institution, 326, 327f
Shroud, 455, 456f
Shunt, 654
Sickle cell anemia, 575, 575f
Side rails, bed, 242f, 243, 243f
Sight, 601–605
    aging on eye in, 602, 604f
    contact lens care for, 608, 609f
    eye disorders on, 604–606 (*See also* Eye disorders)
    eye function in, 602–603, 603f
    eyeglasses for, 603, 603f, 606–608, 608f
    eye structure in, 602–603, 602f
    prosthetic eye care for, 609, 609f
Sigmoid colon, 635, 635f
Sign language, 60, 612–613, 612f
Signs, reporting unusual, 214–215, 215f
Sikhism, death and dying practices in, 453t
Simple phobias, 696
Sims' position, 183f, 184
Sims' position, left, 418, 418f
Sing, 67
Sinoatrial node, 570
Sitting on edge of bed, 191, 208p–209p
Sitting position, 183f, 184
Sitz bath, 765
Skeletal muscle, 467, 468t, 508–509, 511f
Skeletal system, 469, 470f, 506–508
Skeletal traction, 521, 521f
Skeleton, 506, 507f
Skilled nursing facility, 7–8, 8f

Skilled nursing unit, 7–8, 8f
Skin, 483, 483f. *See also* Integumentary system
    as defense mechanism, 107
    immobility on, 180, 181f
    protection by, 484
Skin care, 322–328
    bathing in, 322–328 (*See also* Bathing)
    of dying, 448
    massage in, 328, 344p–345p
    for pressure ulcer prevention, 490, 491f
Skin disorders, 487–502. *See also* Integumentary system disorders
    pressure ulcers, 487–494
    wounds, 494–497 (*See also* Wound)
Skin tears
    prevention of, 186b–187b
    from restraints, 169
Skin traction, 521, 521f
Slander, 49
Sleep
    personal support worker, 30, 30f
    putting baby down to, 771–772, 771f, 772f
Slightly movable joints, 507, 509f
Sling scale, 295–296, 296f, 309p–310p
Small intestine, 634f, 635, 635f
Smell, 601, 601f
Smoker's cough, 545
Smoking
    cancer from, 723
    fire safety and, 153b
    personal support worker and, 30, 30f
    on respiratory system, 545
Smooth muscle, 467–468, 468t
Sneeze, 136–137, 137f
Soap, 323
Soapsuds enema, 417, 417f, 428p–429p
Social phobias, 696
Sodium, dietary, 373t
Sodium-restricted diet, 380
Soft diet, 380
Speaking, by dying, 449
Special diets, 379–380
Special education, 680–681, 681f
Special Olympics, 681–682
Special senses, 598
Specific defense mechanisms, 109
Speech, of dying, 449
Sperm, 668, 669f
Sperm cell, 661
Spheres, 105, 105f
Sphygmomanometers, 290, 290f
    automated, 293
    manual, 290–292, 290f
Spills, blood or body fluid, 119b
Spina bifida, 684, 685f
Spinal cord, 584f, 585, 585f
Spinal cord injuries, 592
Spinal nerves, 585–586
Spiral fracture, 518f, 519
Spirilla (spirals), 105, 105f
Spirometry, incentive, 750–751, 751f
Spleen, 568–569
Sputum, 546
Sputum specimen collection, 546, 547b
Stages of normal progression, 84f

Standard precautions, 118, 119b
  for bloodborne diseases, 134–136, 136b
  general, 118, 119b
  handwashing in, 119b
  in health care setting, 118, 119b
  with HIV/AIDS, 734, 735f
  in home health care, 809–810, 810f
    handwashing in, 809, 810f
    personal protective equipment in, 809–810
    sharps disposal in, 810
  isolation in, 118, 119b
  personal protective equipment in (*See* Personal
      protective equipment (PPE))
Stapes, 609–610, 610f
Staphylococcus aureus, 105, 105f
Staphylococcus aureus, methicillin-resistant (MRSA),
      109
Starches, 374
Stasis ulcers, 576
Stasis ulcers, venous, 499
Stent, 577
Sterilization, 112–113, 113f
Stethoscope, 286–287, 291
Stimulus, 598
Stockings, anti-embolism, 752, 755p–756p
Stoma, 386, 640, 641f
Stomach, 634–635, 634f
Stomach acid, 107, 636
Stomatitis, 727
Stones
  gallstones, 638–639, 639f
  kidney, 652–653, 653f
Stool, 414
Stool softener, 415
Stool specimen collection, 403, 425p
Storage units, 244–245, 245f
Straight catheters, 406–407, 406f
Strangulated hernia, 638
Strangulation, from restraints, 169
Strength, loss of, 475
Streptococcus pyogenes, 105
Stress, 111, 691–692, 692f
Stress fracture, 518
Stress incontinence, 412
Stress management, 692, 693f
Striations, 509
Stroke, 218, 588–589, 589f
Stump, 522f, 523
Styling hair, 355f, 356–357, 357f
Sub-acute care patients, 83
Sub-acute care unit, 7–8, 8f, 237f
Subcutaneous tissue, 483, 483f
Subjective data, 67–68, 68f
Submucosa, 633, 634f
Substance abuse, resident, 694f
Suctioning, airway, 559, 559f
Suffixes, 837, 838f, 844t
Suicide, 694, 699
Sundowning, 709
Superior, 839f, 840
Supination, 510t
Supine position, 183, 183f
Supplements, nutritional, 380
Supportive care, 441
Supportive devices. *See also specific devices*
  for body alignment, 182, 182f
  for rehabilitation, 475, 476f

Suppositories, rectal, 418
Suppression, 693, 694
Suprapubic catheter, 406f, 407
Surgery, 741
  definitive, 742
  elective, 742
  emergent, 742
  exploratory, 742
  urgent, 742
Surgical asepsis, 116
Surgical bed, 270, 270f
Surgical patient care, 742–756
  anaesthesia in, 742–743
  peri-operative period in, 743, 744f
  phases of, 743
  post-operative, 749–753 (*See also* Post-operative
      patient care)
  pre-operative, 743–749 (*See also* Pre-operative
      patient care)
  types of surgeries in, 742
Surgical patients, 82–83
Survival, chain of, 222–223
Susceptible host, 111
Swallowing
  aging on, 637
  problems with, 384
Sweat glands, 483f, 484
Symptoms
  definition of, 67
  reporting unusual, 214–215, 215f
Synapse, 583, 583f
Syncope, 218–219, 218f
Synovial fluid, 508
Syphilis, 672–673
Syphilitic dementia, 706t
Systemic circulation, 571, 572, 572f
Systole, 572
Systolic blood pressure, 289

T
Table
  bedside, 244, 245f
  over-bed, 244, 244f
Tachycardia, 287
Tachypnea, 288
Tactile receptors, 599, 599f
Tagging, of defective items and equipment, 150, 152f
Talk. *See* Communication
Tangle prevention, hair, 357, 357f
Tangles, in Alzheimer's disease, 705, 706f
Tape measure, for height and weight measurement,
      295–296, 309p–310p
Tapeworms, 106t, 107
Tap water enema, 417
Task lighting, 241
Tasks, 85
Taste, 378, 601, 601f
Taste buds, 601
T cells, 134, 135f
Teaching, pre-operative, 744, 744f
Team nursing, 19–20
Tear prevention, skin, 186b–187b
Tears, 107
Telephone communication, 66–67, 66f, 66t
Telephone devices for the deaf (TDD), 612
Telephone etiquette, 66t
Temperature, bathing water, 165

Temperature, body, 281–285
  definition of, 281
  in elderly, skin regulation of, 487
  factors in, 281
  in infants, monitoring of, 777
  measurement of, 281–284
    armpit (axillary), 284, 301p–302p
    in children, 296
    ear (tympanic), 284, 302p–303p
    forehead (temporal), 284
    mouth (oral), 283–284, 298p–299p
    in newborn, 767, 767f
    rectum (rectal), 284, 299p–300p
    thermometers in, 281–283 (See also
        Thermometers)
  metabolism in, 281
  muscular contraction on, 511
  normal and abnormal findings in, 284–285, 285t
  regulation of, 281
  skin regulation of, 484–485, 485f
Temperature, room, 240
Temporal artery thermometer, 283, 283f
Temporal temperature, 284
Tendons, 509, 509f
Terminal illness, 81, 436
Terminally ill, 436–442
  Dying's Person's Bill of Rights for, 448b
  dying with dignity in, 440–441, 440–442
    advance directives in, 440–442, 441f
    hospice care in, 441–442, 442f
  grief in, 437–440
    acceptance in, 438t, 439, 439f
    anger in, 437–438, 438f, 438t
    bargaining in, 438, 438t, 439f
    for caregiver, 440f, 441, 442, 442f
    counseling for, 440, 440f
    denial in, 437, 437f, 438t
    depression in, 438–439, 438t, 439f
    for family, 440
    for resident, 439–440
  home care for, 436, 437f
  listening and touch, 436–437
  wills for, 440
Terminology, medical, 837–838, 838f. See also
        Language, health care; specific terms
Testes, 668, 669f
Testicles, 668, 669f
Testicular cancer, 670, 671f
Testicular self-examination (TSE), 670, 671f
Testosterone, 625
Tetany, 623
Thalamus, 584, 585f
Thank-you note, after job interview, 42, 42f
Thermometers, 281–283
  Celsius, 282, 282f
  electronic, 283, 283f
  Fahrenheit, 282, 282f
  glass, 281–283, 281f, 282f
  temporal artery, 283, 283f
  tympanic, 283, 283f
Thiamin, 373t
Thickened liquids, 384
Third-degree burns, 497–498, 498f
Thoracic cavity, 840, 840f
Three-prong plugs, 150, 152f
Thrombocyte count, low, 574–575
Thrombocytes, 566–567

Thrombophlebitis, 751, 751f
Thrombosis, venous, 576
Thrombus (thrombi), 575, 751
Thrusts, abdominal, 221–222
Thymus gland, 568
  function of, 623–624
  location and structure of, 620, 621f
Thyroid gland
  function of, 622–623
  location and structure of, 620, 621f
Thyroid gland disorders, 626
Thyroid-stimulating hormone (TSH), 622, 622f
Thyroxine, 622–623
tid, 842, 846t
Time, recording of, 73, 73f, 74b
Time and travel log, 794
Tinea capitis, 355
Tinea corporis, 106t, 107
Tinea pedis, 106t, 107, 351
Tinnitus, 611
Tissues, 467–468, 467f, 468t
Tobacco smoke. See Smoking
Toddler care
  emotional needs in, 779–780, 779f
  physical needs in, 779
  safety needs in, 780
Toddlerhood, 85–86, 86f
Toenails, 351–352, 352f
Toe pleat, 276f, 276p
Toilet
  handrails on, 397, 398f
  higher seats on, 397–398, 398f
Toileting, for pressure ulcer prevention, 491, 491f
Tone, muscle, 509
Tongue blade, padded, 318, 318f
Top sheets, 263
Tort, 48
  intentional, 49
  unintentional, 48, 49f
Total abdominal hysterectomy (TAH), 668
Total parenteral nutrition (TPN), 388, 388f
Total vaginal hysterectomy (TVH), 668
Touch
  deep, 599
  sense of, 598–599, 599f
Trachea, 542, 542f, 543f
Tracheostomy, 558–559, 558f
Tract, 633
Traction, 520–521, 521f
Tracts, 585
Traditions, culture on, 94
Transfer belt, 187, 199p–200p
Transfers, resident, 187–189, 257–258
  from bed
    to stretcher, 188, 204p–205p
    to wheelchair (one worker), 188, 200p–202
    to wheelchair (two workers), 188, 202p
  definition of, 257
  fall prevention in, 148–149, 149b
  guidelines for, 188, 189b
  humanistic health care in, 18
  means of, 258   ⌐, 206p–207p
  with mechanical lift, 18
  planning for, 188
  reason and types   ⌐, 18, 205p
  stress in, 257–   ed, 18, 205p
  from stretch⌐

Transfers, resident *(continued)*
  transfer belt in, 187, 199p–200p
  weight bearing in, 187
  from wheelchair to bed, 188, 203p–204p
Transient flora, 115
Transient ischemic attacks (TIAs), 587–588
Transmission, 131–138
  airborne, 136–138 (*See also* Airborne diseases)
  bloodborne, 131–136 (*See also* Bloodborne diseases)
  method of, 110, 110f
Transmission-based precautions, 118–120, 120b,
      127p
Transparent dressings, 496, 496f
Transport. *See also* Car seat
  cardiovascular, 571–573
  of newborn, 772, 772f
Transsexual, 92–93
Transverse colon, 635, 635f
Transverse plane, 839, 839f
Transvestite, 93
Trapeze bar, 521
Tremor, in Parkinson's disease, 590, 590f
Trendelenburg's position, 242–243, 242f
Tricuspid valve, 570, 570f
Trigone, 649
Trimesters, of pregnancy, 760, 761f
Triple-lumen indwelling catheters, 407, 407f
Tube feeding, 386–388, 386f
Tuberculosis (TB)
  airborne precautions for, 118–119, 120, 120b
  airborne transmission of, 137–138, 138f
Tubules, renal, 648–649, 650f
Tumours. *See also* Cancer; *specific cancers*
  benign, 721–722
  bladder, 654–655, 656f
  definition of, 721
  malignant, 722
  urinary system, 654–655, 656f
Tunica externa, 567, 567f
Tunica intima, 567, 567f
Tunica media, 567, 567f
Tympanic membrane, 609, 610f
Tympanic temperature, 284, 302p–303p
Tympanic thermometers, 283, 283f
Typhus, 105

U
Ulcers, 499, 499t, 638. *See also* Pressure ulcers
Ultrasound, of female reproductive system, 667, 667f
Umbilical cord stump care, 767–768, 768f
Umbilical hernias, 638, 638f
Umbilical region, 841, 841f
Unconscious person, oral care for, 318
  guidelines for, 318b
  procedures for, 333p–334p
  tongue blade for, 318, 318f
Unintentional tort, 48, 49f
Unit, 237   wound, 494–495, 494f
Unit, resident's,
  decorating room 238
  in long-term care fac
  preparation of, on adm 237–238
Unoccupied bed, 272p–274   253, 256, 256f
Unresponsive, 215
Upper respiratory tract. *See* Resp
Upper respiratory tract cancer, 549   system

Upright scale, 294, 295f, 307p–308p
Ureteroscopy, 657
Ureterostomy, 656f
Ureters, 649
Urethra, 649, 650f, 651f
Urethra infection, 652
Urethral orifice, 649
Urethritis, 652
Urge incontinence, 412
Urgency, urinary, 404
Urgent surgery, 742
Uric acid, 517, 652
Urinals, 398, 399f, 421p–422p
Urinalysis, 402, 403f, 657
Urinary catheterization, 405–411
  catheter care in, 407–411
    catheter removal in, preparation for, 411
    guidelines for, 410b
    providing, 408, 411, 426p–427p
    urine drainage bag emptying, 411, 427p–428p
    urine drainage bag in, 407–408, 408f–409f
  catheters in, 406–407, 406f, 407f
  uses of, 405
Urinary diversion, 656, 656f
Urinary elimination, 403–414
  bedpans for, 398, 399f, 420p–421p
  catheterization for, 405–411 (*See also* Catheters;
      Urinary catheterization)
  equipment for, 397–398, 398f, 399f
  guidelines for assisting with, 401b–402b
  humanistic health care for, 400
  incontinence in, 411–414 (*See also* Incontinence,
      urinary)
  normal, 403–404, 404f
  obtaining urine specimens in, 402–403, 422p–423p
  output measurements of, 390, 390f, 404–405, 405f
  problems with
    anuria, 405
    dysuria, 404
    frequency and urgency, 404
    hematuria, 404
    nocturia, 404
    oliguria, 404
    polyuria, 404–405
  promoting normal
    fundamentals of, 399–400
    guidelines for, 401b–402b
  urinals for, 398, 399f, 421p–422p
  urination habits in, 404
  urine characteristics in, 404
Urinary meatus, 649
Urinary retention, 412
Urinary system, 469, 470f, 648–651
  aging on, 651
  function of, 650–651
  overview of, 403, 404f
  structure of, 649f
    bladder, 649, 650f
    kidneys, 648–649
    ureters, 649
    urethra, 649, 650f, 651f
Urinary system disorders, 651–657
  diagnosis of, 657, 657f
  infections, 652, 652f
  kidney failure, 653–655, 654f, 655b, 656b
  kidney stones, 652–653, 653f
  tumours, 655–657, 656f

Urinary tract infections (UTIs), 652, 652f
Urination, 403
Urination habits, 405
Urine, 649
    characteristics of, 404
    output measurements of, 390f, 391, 404–405, 405f
    straining of, 653, 653f
    with urinary tract infection, 652, 652f
Urine drainage bag
    care and use of, 407–408, 408f–409f
    emptying of, 411, 427p–428p
Urine specimen collection, 402–403, 422p–424p
Urostomy, 656, 656f
Uterine fibroids, 665–666
Uterine prolapse, 665–666
Uterine tubes, 662–663, 662f
Uterus, 662f, 663
Uterus, prolapsed, 665–666

V
Vaccine, hepatitis B virus, 133, 133f
Vagina, 662f, 663
Vaginal discharge, postpartum, 765
Vaginal opening, 662f, 663
Vaginal orifice, 662f, 663
Validation therapy, 710, 711t
Values
    culture on, 94, 95
    definition of, 53
Valves, heart, 570, 570f
Vancomycin-resistant enterococcus (VRE), 109
Varicose veins, 574
Vascular dementia, 706–707, 706t
Vas deferens, 668–669, 669f
Vector, 110
Veins, 567, 568f
    aging on, 573
    structure of, 567, 567f
Venereal diseases, 671–673, 672f
Venereal warts, 672
Venous disorders, 576
Venous stasis ulcers, 499
Venous thrombosis, 576
Venous ulcers, 576
Ventilation, 543
    aging on, 545
    in resident unit, 240, 240f
Ventilation, mechanical, 556–559
    chest tubes in, 549, 550f
    endotracheal intubation in, 557–558, 558f
    general care measures with, 559–560
    need for, 556
    observation in, 560
    tracheostomy in, 558–559, 558f
    ventilators in, 556–557, 557f
Ventilation system, 240, 240f
Ventilator, 556–557, 557f
Ventral cavity, 840, 840f
Ventral surface, 839f, 840
Ventricles, 569–570, 570f, 571f
Venules, 567, 568f
Verbal communication, 58
Vernix, 764
Vertigo, 611
Vesicle, 498, 499t
Vessels, blood, 567, 567f
Vestibular apparatus, 610, 610f

Vestibule, 610, 610f
Vest restraint, 168f, 173, 175p–176p
Villi, 636, 637f
Virulence, 112
Viruses, 105–107, 106t
Vision. *See also* Eye; Eye disorders
    of dying, 449
    normal, 602, 603f
Vision impairment, on accident risk, 162
Vital signs, 280–294. *See also specific signs*
    in antepartum care, 762
    blood pressure, 289–294, 305p–306p
    body temperature, 281–285, 298p–303p
    changes in, 280
    in children, 296, 296t
    control centres for, 280, 281, 288
    indications of, 280
    measurement and recording of, 280–281
    in newborn care, 767
    normal ranges of, 280
    in post-operative patient care, 749–750, 750f
    pulse, 285–287, 303p–304p
    respiration, 287–289, 305p
Vitamin A, 373t
Vitamin B$_1$, 373t
Vitamin B$_2$, 373t
Vitamin B$_3$, 373t
Vitamin B$_{12}$, 373t
Vitamin C, 373t
Vitamin D, 373t, 485
Vitamin E, 373t
Vitamin K, 373t, 374
Vitamins, 373t, 374
    fat-soluble, 374
    water-soluble, 374
Vitreous humor, 602
Vocational training, of disabled, 681, 681f
Voiding, 403
Voluntary movement, 509, 512f
Vomit
    choking from, 221
    output measurements of, 391
Vowels, combining, 837–838, 838f, 842t–843t
Vulva, 662f, 663

W
Waist restraint, 168f, 174, 177p
Walker, 190t
Walking
    assisting with, 189–191, 209p–210p
        devices for, 190t, 191
        guidelines for, 191b
        procedure for, 209p–210p
    post-operative assistance with, 753
Wall-mounted delivery system, oxygen, 553, 554f
Wandering, 708, 708f
Wandering monitoring system, 172f, 173
Warning signs, of cancer, 723–724, 723f
Warts, genital (venereal), 672
Wastes. *See* Elimination
Water, dietary, 374–375
Water-soluble, 374
Water temperature, for bathing, 165
Weight, 294–296
    definition of, 294
    measurement of, 307p–320p
        with chair scale, 294–295, 296f, 308p–309p

Weight (continued)
    scales in, 294–296
        with tape measure and sling scale, 295–296, 296f, 309p–310p
        with upright scale, 294, 295f, 307p–308p
Weight bearing, 187
Weightlifting, 143–144, 144f
What Did You Learn? exercise answers, 835–836
Wheelchair
    transfers from bed to
        one worker, 200p–202p
        two workers, 202p
    transfers to bed from, 188, 203p–204p
    transfers to/from, 188
        one worker, 188
        two workers, 188
    with tray table, 168f
Wheel-locks, on bed, 243, 244f
Wheels, bed, 242f, 243, 244f
Whirlpool tubs, 326, 327f
White blood cells, 108, 108f, 566, 566f
Wills, 440
Windpipe, 542, 542f
Work ethic, 27–29, 27f

Workforce, entering. See Job-seeking skills
Workplace safety. See Safety, workplace
Worms, 106t
Wound. See also Burns; Pressure ulcers
    closed, 494–495
    definition of, 494
    intentional, 494, 494f
    unintentional, 494–495, 494f
Wound closure, 495
Wound drain, 495–496, 496f
Wound dressing, 496–497, 496f
Wound dressing changes, 497, 501p–502p
Wound healing, 495–497
    dressing changes in, 497, 501p–502p
    requirements for, 495
    wound closure in, 495
    wound drains in, 495–496, 496f
    wound dressings in, 496–497, 496f
Wrinkles, 486, 486f
Wrist restraint, 168f, 173–174, 176p

Y
Young adulthood, 88, 88f